T0329325

CHOU'S
ELECTROCARDIOGRAPHY
IN CLINICAL PRACTICE

CHOU'S ELECTROCARDIOGRAPHY IN CLINICAL PRACTICE

Adult and Pediatric

SIXTH EDITION

BORYS SURAWICZ, M.D., M.A.C.C.
Professor Emeritus
Indiana University School of Medicine
Indianapolis, Indiana

TIMOTHY K. KNILANS, M.D.
Associate Professor, Pediatrics
University of Cincinnati School of Medicine
Director, Clinical Cardiac Electrophysiology and Pacing
The Children's Hospital Medical Center
Cincinnati, Ohio

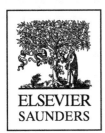

ELSEVIER
SAUNDERS

SAUNDERS
ELSEVIER

1600 John F. Kennedy Blvd.
Ste 1800
Philadelphia, PA 19103-2899

CHOU'S ELECTROCARDIOGRAPHY IN CLINICAL PRACTICE ISBN: 978-1-4160-3774-3
SIXTH EDITION

Notice

Knowledge and best practice in this field are constantly changing. As new research and experience broaden our knowledge, changes in practice, treatment, and drug therapy may become necessary or appropriate. Readers are advised to check the most current information provided (i) on procedures featured or (ii) by the manufacturer of each product to be administered, to verify the recommended dose or formula, the method and duration of administration, and contraindications. It is the responsibility of the practitioner, relying on their own experience and knowledge of the patient, to make diagnoses, to determine dosages and the best treatment for each individual patient, and to take all appropriate safety precautions. To the fullest extent of the law, neither the Publisher nor the Editors assume any liability for any injury and/or damage to persons or property arising out of or related to any use of the material contained in this book.

The Publisher

Library of Congress Cataloging-in-Publication Data

Surawicz, Borys, 1917-
    Chou's electrocardiography in clinical practice / Borys Surawicz, Timothy K. Knilans. — 6th ed.
        p. ; cm.
    Includes bibliographical references and index.
    ISBN 978-1-4160-3774-3
    1. Electrocardiography—Interpretation. 2. Heart—Diseases—Diagnosis. I. Knilans, Timothy K. II. Chou, Te—Chuan, 1922- Electrocardiography in clinical practice. III. Title. IV. Title: Electrocardiography in clinical practice.
        [DNLM: 1. Electrocardiography—methods. 2. Heart Diseases—diagnosis. WG 140 S961c 2008]
    RC683.5.E5C454 2008
    616.1'207547—dc22

                                                                2007048392

Executive Publisher: Natasha Andjelkovic
Editorial Assistant: Isabel Trudeau
Project Manager: Mary Stermel
Design Direction: Karen O'Keefe Owens
Marketing Manager: Todd Liebel

Working together to grow
libraries in developing countries

www.elsevier.com | www.bookaid.org | www.sabre.org

ELSEVIER   BOOK AID International   Sabre Foundation

Printed in the United States

Last digit is the print number: 9 8 7 6 5 4

This edition is dedicated to Dr. Te-Chuan Chou, the author of the first four editions, as a mark of respect for his scholarship and understanding of this subject.

CONTRIBUTING AUTHORS

Lawrence E. Gering, M.D., F.A.C.C.
Owensboro Mercy Health System
Owensboro, Kentucky; and
Riverview Hospital
Noblesville, Indiana

Timothy K. Knilans, M.D.
Associate Professor, Pediatrics
University of Cincinnati School of Medicine
Director, Clinical Cardiac Electrophysiology
and Pacing
The Children's Hospital Medical Center
Cincinnati, Ohio

Borys Surawicz, M.D., M.A.C.C.
Professor Emeritus
Indiana University School of Medicine
Indianapolis, Indiana

Morton E. Tavel, M.D., F.C.C.P.
The Indiana Heart Institute
Care Group, Inc.
Indianapolis, Indiana

CONTENTS

PREFACE

After the publication of his textbook *Clinical Electrocardiograpy* in 1956, Dr. Louis Katz was said to declare that electrocardiography was fully explored, implying no need for further investigations in this field. Similar verdicts have been pronounced in subsequent years, proving them to be consistently wrong in the face of the continuing flow of new information about the electrocardiogram (ECG) in synchrony with the continuing progress in other areas of cardiology.

As envisioned by the author of the first four editions, Dr. Chou, this text is primarily clinical, with sufficient basic science foundation and bibliography to understand the genesis of diverse ECG patterns. In the 7 years since the publication of the fifth edition, valuable new information emerged that necessitated complete revision of the sections dealing with ST-elevation myocardial infarction (STEMI) and non-STEMI, stress test, QT interval, and pacemakers. Dr. Timothy Knilans updated the section on pediatric electrocardiography, most extensively the chapter on cardiac arrhythmias. Given that the backbone of an ECG textbook are the illustrations, many figures in this edition were added and replaced.

I am indebted to Drs. HJJ Wellens, APM Gorgels, and PA Doevedans, authors of the monograph *The ECG in Acute Myocardial Infarction and Unstable Angina*, for their permission to reproduce several figures, and to Dr. Serge S. Barold for allowing us to include new information and figures in the chapter on cardiac pacemakers. I am grateful to Mrs. Terri Scott for her invaluable secretarial assistance.

BORYS SURAWICZ, M.D., M.A.C.C.

1 Normal Electrocardiogram: Origin and Description

Origin of the Electrocardiogram
Depolarization and Repolarization
Dipoles
Potential Decline with Increasing
Distance from the Heart
Solid Angle Theorem
Volume Conductor

Methods of Recording
ECG Leads
Vectorcardiography
Magnetocardiography
Body Surface Mapping
Signal-Averaged ECG

Normal ECG
P Wave
PR Interval
Ventricular Activation (QRS Complex)

Common Normal Variants
$S_1S_2S_3$ Pattern
RSR^1 Pattern in Lead V_1
"Early Repolarization" Variant
Poor R Wave Progression in Precordial
Leads
Athlete's Heart
Obesity and Edema

Origin of the Electrocardiogram

The waveform of the electrocardiogram (ECG) recorded from the body surface depends on the properties of the generator (i.e., cardiac action potential), the spread of excitation, and the characteristics of the volume conductor. The electrocardiographic theory attempts to integrate these three elements.[1]

Figure 1–1 shows the temporal relation between the atrial and ventricular action potentials and the surface ECG. The P wave is derived from atrial depolarization, the QRS complex from ventricular depolarization, the ST segment from phase 2 (plateau), and the T wave from phase 3 of the ventricular action potential. The activity of the conducting system is not represented on the surface ECG. Intracardiac electrodes can be used to record His bundle potential and signals from other parts of the conducting system.

DEPOLARIZATION AND REPOLARIZATION

Potential differences generated during cardiac activity set up currents in the conductors surrounding the heart. A simplified electrocardiographic

theory is based on an elementary model of a single fiber surrounded by a homogeneous medium. In such fibers, during resting the positive and negative boundaries are equal and opposite in sign for the extent of the conductor. This means that the polarized surface is closed, and no potential is recorded (Figure 1–2, top tracing). When the excitation wave invades the fiber and reverses the charges across the membrane, currents flow outside the fiber, inside the fiber, and across the membrane, as indicated by the arrows in Figure 1–1 (second tracing from top). This creates potential differences of depolarization, which disappear when the double layer again becomes homogeneous in the fully activated state, as shown in the middle tracing of Figure 1–2. Subsequently a transition from an activated to a resting state occurs, a process of repolarization shown in Figure 1–2 (fourth and fifth tracings from top).

DIPOLES

The heart contains about 10^{10} cells. Each instant of depolarization or repolarization represents different stages of activity for a large number of cells, and an electromotive force generated at each

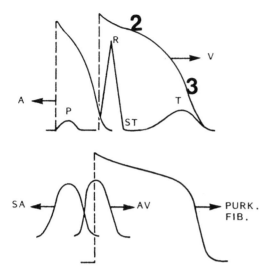

ECG AND ACTION POTENTIALS

MANIFEST: ATRIUM(A), VENTRICLE(V)
CONCEALED: SA NODE, AV NODE, PURK. FIB.

Figure 1–1   Timing of cardiac action potentials recorded during inscription of an ECG complex. The action potentials responsible for the atrial and ventricular activation are designated *manifest* and those responsible for impulse initiation and propagation as *concealed*. See text.

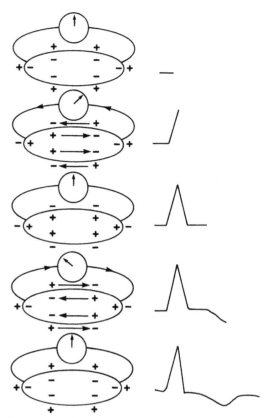

Figure 1–2   Resting state, depolarization, and repolarization in a single cell, the two ends of which are connected to a galvanometer. On the right are ECG deflections resulting from the polarization changes in the diagram on the left. (From Surawicz B: Electrocardiogram. *In:* Chatterjee K, Parmley WW [eds]: Cardiology. Philadelphia, JB Lippincott, 1991, by permission.)

instant represents a sum of uncanceled potential differences. A potential difference between two surfaces or between two poles carrying opposite charges forms a dipole, the magnitude (moment), polarity, and direction of which can be represented by a vector.* The ECG records the sequence of such instantaneous vectors attributed to an imaginary dipole that changes its magnitude and direction during impulse propagation. During activity the recording electrode is influenced by the potential difference across the boundary; the record of activity, represented by an instantaneous vector, depends on the position of the electrode within the electrical field created by the dipole.

Figure 1–3 represents an electrical field with a central location of a dipole in an ideal homogeneous medium. The solid lines represent positive and negative isopotential lines. The maximum potentials are given values of +20 and –20. They are in close proximity to the poles of the dipole (i.e., the source and the sink). The potentials decrease with increasing distance from the dipole. The vertical interrupted line that transects the dipole is a zero potential line. The leads to the right of this line record positive potentials,

---

*A dipole is a source-sink pair separated by a short distance.

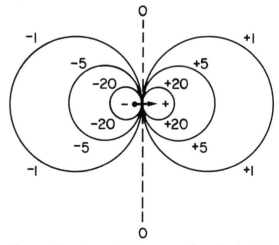

Figure 1–3   Electrical field generated by a dipole (-/+). (From Surawicz B: Electrocardiogram. *In:* Chatterjee K, Parmley WW [eds]: Cardiology. Philadelphia, JB Lippincott, 1991, by permission.)

and those to the left of the line record negative potentials. An electrode connecting two points on the isopotential line records no potential differences.

In the prototype model of Einthoven et al.,[2] the postulated generator of cardiac activity was a single dipole at the center of the triangle, and the postulated volume conductor was both homogeneous and unbounded. This oversimplified model remains useful for teaching electrocardiography at the elementary level. It does not explain, however, the three-dimensional (3D) distribution of cardiac electrical activity in the heart at each point in time during the cardiac cycle. It has been suggested that the electromotive forces generated by ventricular excitation can be expressed more properly by the electrical field of several dipoles rather than by that of a single dipole.[3]

POTENTIAL DECLINE WITH INCREASING DISTANCE FROM THE HEART

It has been established that in the volume conductor with the properties of the human thorax, the potential declines approximately in proportion to the square of the distance. This means that, for practical purposes, all points on the torso situated at a distance of more than two diameters of the heart are approximately "electrically" equidistant from the generator. Thus the remoteness of the electrodes placed on the extremities is sufficient to minimize the nondipolar components of the ECG caused by the proximity effect. At the

same time it can be understood that the anterior precordial leads, owing to their proximity to the heart, are influenced by the local potentials generated in the structures lying directly underneath the corresponding electrodes.

SOLID ANGLE THEOREM

The basic concept applicable to the analysis of the body surface potentials states that at any given point, the recorded potential is determined by the product of a solid angle subtended at this point by the boundary between the opposing charges and the charge density per unit area across the boundary (Figure 1–4). This means that for any given charge density, the deflection recorded by the electrode facing the boundary increases with increasing surface of the boundary and, conversely, that for any given dimension of the boundary surface, the magnitude of the recorded deflection increases with increasing charge density across the boundary. The solid angle theorem has been found useful for analysis of potential differences caused by injury currents[4] (see Chapter 7).

VOLUME CONDUCTOR

The conductivity of tissues surrounding the heart influences the amplitude of the ECG deflections. Tissues with low conductivity decrease the amplitude of the ECG deflections. Low voltage is present when the lungs are hyperinflated or when the heart is insulated by a large amount of fat. Low voltage can also be caused by pericardial

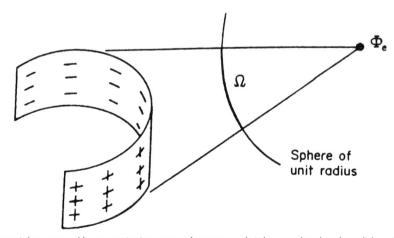

Figure 1–4 Potentials generated by an excitation wave of sources and sinks are related to the solid angle of the excitation wave as seen from the field point. The solid angle is the fraction of a unit sphere subtended by a three-dimensional object. The symbol is the potential generated by the illustrated source-sink boundary. This potential is determined by the charge density across the boundary, the solid angle, and the reciprocal of the square of the distance from the boundary to the field point. (From Barr RC: Genesis of the electrocardiogram. *In:* Macfarlane PW, Lawrie TD [eds]: Comprehensive Electrocardiology. New York, Pergamon, 1989. Copyright 1989 Elsevier Science, by permission.)

and pleural effusions or edema owing to the short-circuiting action of these well-conducting fluids.

Methods of Recording

ECG LEADS

To study the electromotive forces generated during the propagation of cardiac impulses, it is necessary to attach the leading electrodes to the heart or to the body surface. When one or both electrodes are in contact with the heart, the ECG leads are called *direct*. When the electrodes are placed at a distance of more than two cardiac diameters from the heart, the leads are called *indirect*. *Semidirect* leads designate an arrangement in which one or both electrodes are in close proximity but not in direct contact with the heart. The leads are considered *bipolar* when both electrodes face sites with similar potential variations and *unipolar* when potential variations of one electrode are negligible in comparison with those of the other. Of the 12 standard ECG leads, I, II, and III are indirect and bipolar; aV_R, aV_L, and aV_F are indirect and unipolar; and V_1 through V_6 are semidirect and unipolar.*

The three standard limb leads were designed by Einthoven to represent three sides of an equilateral triangle in which the heart is positioned at the center (Figure 1–5). As stated previously, this concept arose from an assumption that the electromotive forces of the heart could be represented by a single vector centered in this triangle. According to Einthoven's law, the magnitude of the deflection in lead II equals the sum of deflections in leads I and III. Figure 1–6 illustrates this point.

Although a more accurate system of electrode placement at points equidistant from the heart has been proposed by other investigators, the use of Einthoven's leads has become universally entrenched. The unipolar chest leads were introduced by Wilson for the purpose of diminishing the influence of the distant reference electrode. He constructed a zero potential electrode (V) by connecting the three limb electrodes through equal resistances of 5000 ohms to a central terminal. Wilson and coworkers[5] developed the system of unipolar chest leads and unipolar limb leads taken from the central

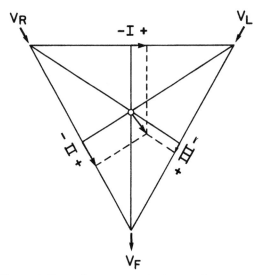

Figure 1–5   Einthoven's triangle showing the projection of a vector on the axes of three standard limb leads. (From Surawicz B: Electrocardiogram. *In:* Chatterjee K, Parmley WW [eds]: Cardiology. Philadelphia, JB Lippincott, 1991, by permission.)

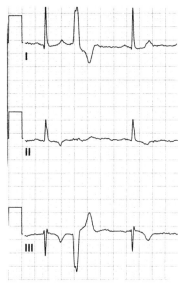

Figure 1–6   Einthoven's law. Note an isoelectric QRS complex in lead II as a result of equal amplitudes of opposite polarity in leads I and III.

terminal to the individual limb electrodes (V_R, V_L, V_F). Subsequently, Goldberger[6] disconnected the resistors placed between the limb and the central terminal and thus augmented (a) the voltage of these leads about 1.5 times (aV_R, aV_L, aV_F). The relation between the standard and unipolar augmented leads is as follows:

---

*The use of the term *unipolar* in reference to ECG leads is controversial because the potential at the central terminal pole is not negligible.

$$aV_R + aV_L + aV_F = 0$$

The direction of lead I is 0 degrees; lead II, 60 degrees; lead III, 120 degrees; lead aV_F, 90 degrees; lead aV_L, −30 degrees; and lead aV_R, −150 degrees.

Lead Display

The traditional sequence of lead display in a standard 12-lead ECG is: I, II, III, aV_R, aV_L, aV_F, and V_1–V_6. This sequence displays logically the precordial leads, but not necessarily the limb leads, where the displayed panoramic clockwise sequence would be: aV_L, I, −aV_R, II, aV_F, and III. The latter display was endorsed by a large number of leading electrocardiographers[7] but has not yet prevailed to alter the established tradition.

Vectors and Electrical Axis

The electromotive force generated by the heart at any instant can be represented by the vector force of a single equivalent dipole situated at this point. This vector points from the negative to the positive potential (coincident with the direction of the impulse propagation), and its magnitude is proportional to the magnitude of the electromotive force. The voltage registered in a given lead corresponds to the projection of the cardiac vector on the axis of the lead (see Figure 1–5). The maximum deflection is registered when the vector is parallel, and the minimum deflection is seen when the vector is perpendicular to the lead axis.

The maximum QRS vector is used to define the main axis. This vector usually corresponds to the R axis. The mean QRS axis is the average of all instantaneous vectors during the QRS complex. The general phrase "electrical heart axis in the frontal plane" is sometimes used in reference to the main axis and sometimes to the mean axis. This designation is meaningful only when one dominant deflection is present in at least one of the limb leads. When the QRS complex is biphasic in all leads, the meaning of the average QRS axis changes because the vectorcardiographic QRS loop (see later discussion) is nearly circular. Such a biphasic pattern with an indeterminate axis is described preferably as a sequence of two main axes corresponding to the initial and terminal deflections.

The semidirect precordial leads introduced by Wilson record the potential differences between the chest electrodes and the central terminal (V) electrode at locations shown in Figure 1–7.

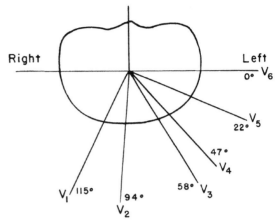

Figure 1–7 Directions of the lead axes of leads V_1 through V_6.

Intrinsic and Intrinsicoid Deflections

When the electrical activity on the cardiac surface is recorded by means of a unipolar lead, the activation front approaching the electrode registers an upright deflection, but as soon as the activation front reaches the electrode, the direction changes and the electrogram records a rapid negative deflection, which is referred to as *intrinsic*. The validity of this concept, proposed by Lewis et al. in 1914, was supported by the experiments of Dower.[8]

Dower showed that an electrode placed on the surface of the guinea pig heart inscribes a negative deflection that coincides with the upstroke of the ventricular action potential in the immediately subjacent cell. In Dower's study, the intrinsic deflection was marked more sharply on the left than on the right surface of the heart.[8]

The transition from positive to negative is less abrupt in semidirect unipolar precordial leads than in direct leads, which makes the intrinsic deflection less rapid and less distinct. For this reason, this deflection was designated by McLeod et al. in 1930 as *intrinsicoid*. The onset of an intrinsicoid deflection in the precordial leads corresponds to the peak of the tall R wave or the nadir of the deep S wave. The onset of an intrinsicoid deflection may be delayed if the duration of the excitation wave spreading toward the recording electrode is prolonged owing to increased ventricular wall thickness. In the right precordial leads the upper limit of normal is 0.035 second, and in the left precordial leads it is 0.045 second. This interval is used mostly to diagnose ventricular hypertrophy and bundle branch block when the onset of the intrinsicoid deflection is delayed.

Esophageal Leads

The esophageal leads can be viewed as an approximation of nearly direct left atrial leads because only a thin wall of the esophagus separates the electrode from the posterior wall of the left atrium. The left atrial origin of the esophageal electrograms has been documented by comparing the esophageal leads with the simultaneously recorded direct left atrial leads inserted transseptally during cardiac catheterization.[9]

Left atrial depolarization can be represented by a single vector directed inferiorly and anteriorly. Consequently, as the unipolar esophageal electrode is moved caudad, the points above the atrium record a negative deflection and the points below the atrium record a positive deflection; the intermediate points overlying the left atrium record a diphasic deflection.

VECTORCARDIOGRAPHY

The vectorcardiographic display is based on the assumption that the electrical activity of the heart may be approximated by a fixed location, a variable amplitude, and a variable orientation of the current dipole within a finite homogeneous torso. If the vectors during one cardiac cycle are displayed with their origin on a common zero point, their ends form a vector loop beginning at and returning to this point. Because each of the principal ECG components—the P wave, QRS complex, T wave, and U wave—starts from and returns to the same baseline, four loops can be recorded, one for each of these four deflections. If the ST segment is displaced from the baseline, the QRS loop does not return to the point of origin of the T loop and the loop remains open. Because the P, T, and U loops are of much lower amplitude than the QRS loop, their analysis requires considerable amplification.

To obtain a vectorcardiogram (VCG), two leads must be recorded simultaneously. The modern VCG system employs a set of three orthogonal leads, one in the right to left direction (x lead), one in the head to foot direction (y lead), and one in the front to back direction (z lead). Sets of appropriate resistors are used to "correct" these leads for the varying distances of the electrodes from the heart. The leads can be combined to form three loops: one in the frontal plane using the x and y leads, one in the sagittal plane using the y and z leads, and one in the horizontal plane using the x and z leads. To follow the direction of instantaneous vectors, it is customary to interrupt the loop at 2.0- or 2.5-ms intervals.

In addition to the enhanced accuracy of the orthogonal lead system and the ability to measure accurately the direction of instantaneous vectors at frequent intervals, the VCG displays the rotation of the loop, which adds valuable information not available from inspection of the scalar ECG.

Although in principle the scalar ECG and the VCG have essentially the same content, under certain circumstances the VCG displays a diagnostic pattern more distinctly than does the scalar ECG.[10] Thus the VCG may help clarify the diagnosis by providing more accurately measured intervals and by displaying the rotations of the QRS loop and its components. These details pertain most often to analysis of the early portion of the QRS complex. The VCG has been most useful for clarifying the diagnosis of inferior, anteroseptal, and posterior myocardial infarction and infarction complicated by bundle branch or fascicular blocks. VCG is also more sensitive for detecting left atrial enlargement (the magnitude of the maximum posterior P vectors in the horizontal and sagittal planes) and right ventricular hypertrophy (demonstration of a clockwise QRS loop displaced anteriorly and to the right).[11]

Notwithstanding the occasional diagnostic superiority of the VCG compared with the scalar ECG, the net yield of such advantages in clinical practice is not sufficient to overcome the disadvantages of the more costly equipment, the longer time needed to apply the electrodes and produce the record, and the occasional need to supplement the loops made from orthogonal leads by semidirect precordial leads. Such minor inconveniences combined with the increasing availability of technology for the assessment of wall motion abnormality and myocardial perfusion have resulted in a declining use of VCG in clinical practice. The necessity of using the scalar ECG for analysis of cardiac rhythms is another factor contributing to this trend.

The VCG is a useful teaching tool for explaining the scalar ECG, but equally instructive is the vectorial display of the magnitude and direction of the scalar ECG components. Plotting the vectors of the individual components of the QRS complex sequentially from the same point of origin allows us to trace a vectorcardiographic loop. Conversely, scalar ECG components can be derived from the VCG.

MAGNETOCARDIOGRAPHY

Magnetic signals are generated during depolarization and repolarization. The magnetic signals have a common basis with the ECG and therefore are similar in form and distribution. Unlike a conventional ECG, however, the magnetocardiogram can differentiate between displacement of the baseline and displacement of the ST segment (see Chapter 7). Otherwise, magnetocardiographic and ECG signals correlate closely with one another.[12] This may explain the virtual absence of magnetocardiograms in clinical practice.

BODY SURFACE MAPPING

Body surface mapping, facilitated by the use of a computer, provides detailed information about the distribution of QRS, ST, and T potentials on the body surfaces. Modern mapping systems analyze data at 1-ms intervals and print isopotential maps at 5-ms intervals. It has been shown that an array of 32 leads is sufficient to obtain an accurate isopotential map.[13] Another method is a body surface Laplacian map that utilizes circular electrodes and measures a two-dimensional (2D) projection image of the 3D distribution of cardiac electrical sources onto the body surface in millivolts per square millimeters (mV/mm^2).[14] Perhaps the most promising application of mapping is to measure the dispersion of QT intervals to assess the dispersion of ventricular repolarization (see later discussion).

SIGNAL-AVERAGED ECG

The main purpose of the signal-averaged ECG (SAECG) is detection of signals of microvolt amplitude. This requires reduction of noise, the principal source of which is skeletal muscle. The amplitude of noise is typically 5 to 20 μV; that is, it has a magnitude similar to that of high-frequency (>25 Hz) cardiac potentials.[15] Details of the technique can be found in instruction manuals and review articles, including the work of Simson.[15] Averaging the highly amplified voltages isolates signals of repetitive forms and cancels the random nonrepetitive noise. The average signals are high-pass filtered to reduce the large amplitude, low-frequency signal content such as the ST segment. Filters of 25 to 100 Hz are used predominantly, most commonly the 40 Hz frequency (Figure 1–8). If the cutoff is lower (i.e., 25 Hz) the specificity increases but the sensitivity declines.

High-pass filtering is referred to as the *time domain analysis* because it provides information about the duration of such intervals as the filtered QRS complex. The frequency domain

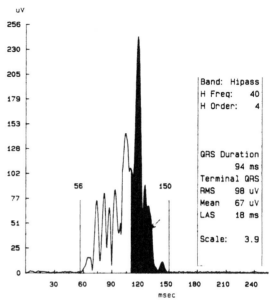

Figure 1–8 Signal-averaged ECG with normal values.

obtained by fast Fourier transform provides a display of amplitude versus frequency. The use of time domain is more prevalent, but the frequency domain is not without merit. The averaging is performed on several hundred complexes, usually in the orthogonal x, y, and z leads. The square root of the sum of $X^2 + Y^2 + Z^2$ is the vector magnitude commonly referred to as "filtered QRS complex." In the presence of ventricular late potentials at the microvolt level in the ST segment, the filtered QRS complex is prolonged. The duration of this interval represents the variable of most clinical interest aside from the amplitude of low potentials. It has been established empirically that abnormal potentials are less than 20 to 25 μV amplitude. A third variable usually included in routine analysis of the SAECG is the duration of the terminal portion of the filtered QRS complex of less than 40 μV amplitude. In the absence of intraventricular conduction disturbances, the frequently used criteria for abnormal durations are >114 to 120 ms for the duration of the filtered QRS complex and >38 ms duration of the low-amplitude signals. The criteria for abnormality are highly dependent on technique.[13] Figure 1–8 shows a normal SAECG recorded with the filter setting at 40 Hz frequency. The duration of the filtered QRS complex is 94 ms; the terminal QRS portion of less than 40 μV amplitude is 18 ms; and the amplitude of low potentials is 67 μV.

Normal ECG

P WAVE

Atrial activation begins in the sinoatrial (SA) node or the neighboring atrial pacemakers (see Chapter 2). It spreads in a radial fashion to depolarize the right atrium, the interatrial septum, and then the left atrium.[16,17] The last region of the left atrium to be activated is the tip of the left atrial appendage, or the posteroinferior left atrium beneath the left inferior pulmonary vein.[16] Three specialized pathways that contain Purkinje fibers have been identified as connecting the SA node to the atrioventricular (AV) node: the anterior, middle, and posterior internodal pathways. An interatrial pathway, the Bachmann bundle, connects the right and left atria. For practical purposes, the early part of the P wave may be considered to represent the electrical potential generated by the upper part of the right atrium, and the late part as that by the left atrium and the inferior right atrial wall.

The initial portion of the P wave, corresponding to depolarization of the right atrium, is directed anteriorly. The portion corresponding to depolarization of the left atrium and the inferior right atrial wall is directed posteriorly. Because both deflections are directed downward and to the left, they tend to fuse and form a single deflection in the frontal plane. However, careful inspection or amplification usually reveals a notch on the summit of the normal P wave (see Figure 1–15). The orientation of the two components is better visualized in the right precordial leads. In normal adults the duration of the P wave, which represents the duration of atrial activation, varies from 0.08 to 0.11 second.[18] In a study that involved a large population, a significant number of subjects had a duration of 0.12 to 0.13 second. For practical purposes, however, a value >0.11 second can usually be considered abnormal.[19]

The P axis in the frontal plane (determined from the limb leads) varies from 0 to +75 degrees,[20] with most falling between +45 and +60 degrees. Therefore the P wave is always upright in leads I and II and inverted in lead aV$_R$. In lead III it may be upright, diphasic, or inverted. When it is diphasic, the initial deflection is positive and the second component is negative. A diphasic P wave in lead III is present in 7 percent of the normal population.[21] The P wave in lead aV$_L$ is also variable in polarity. A negative P wave is relatively common in this lead. When it is diphasic, the deflection is negative-positive. In lead aV$_F$ the P wave is usually upright, but a diphasic or flat P wave is seen occasionally.

In the precordial leads, the P wave is often diphasic in leads V$_1$ and V$_2$. The early right atrial forces are directed anteriorly and the late left atrial forces posteriorly. Therefore the diphasic P wave has a positive-negative configuration. When the amplitude of one of the two components is low, the P wave appears entirely positive or entirely negative in lead V$_1$, but the P wave in lead V$_2$ is seldom entirely negative. In the remaining precordial leads, the P wave is always upright due to the essentially right-to-left spread of the atrial activation impulse.

The amplitude of the P wave in the limb leads seldom exceeds 0.25 mV or 25 percent of the normal R wave in normal individuals at rest, but the normal range is wide due to such factors as the position of the heart, proximity to the recording electrodes, degree of atrial filling, extent of atrial fibrosis, and other extracellular factors that influence the amplitude of ECG deflections on the body surface. In the precordial leads, the positive component of the P wave is less than 0.15 mV. In lead V$_1$ the negative deflection is usually less than 0.1 mV.

PR INTERVAL

The PR interval is measured from the beginning of the P wave to the beginning of the QRS complex. The term "PQ interval" is preferred by some electrocardiographers because it is the period actually measured unless the Q wave is absent. The PR interval spans the time required for the propagating impulse to advance from the atria through the AV node, bundle of His, bundle branches, and the system of Purkinje fibers until the ventricular myocardium begins to depolarize (Figure 1–9). It does not include the duration of conduction from the SA node to the right atrium (SA conduction).

In adults the normal PR interval is 0.12 to 0.20 second.[22] It is generally shorter in children and longer in older persons. The relation between heart rate and the duration of the PR interval is discussed in Chapter 19. The interval should be measured in the lead with the largest, widest P wave and the longest QRS duration. Such a selection avoids inaccuracies incurred by using the leads in which the early part of the P wave or QRS complex is isoelectric. Because most modern electrocardiographs record several leads simultaneously, the points of onset of the P wave and the QRS complex can be verified by examining the other simultaneously recorded leads.

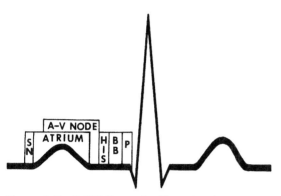

Figure 1–9 P-QRS-T complex illustrating the sequence of activation of the atria and the specialized conduction fibers. His = bundle of His; P = Purkinje fibers; SN = sinoatrial node. (From Damato AN, Lau SH: Clinical value of the electrocardiogram of the conduction system. Prog Cardiovasc Dis 13:119, 1970, by permission of the authors and Grune & Stratton.)

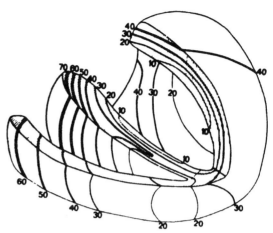

Figure 1–10 Total excitation in the adult normal human heart. The heart is depicted in the position it may occupy in the body. Portions of the right ventricle, septum, and left ventricle are removed, showing the opened left and right ventricular cavities. Movement of the isochrones can be clearly seen. Isochrones in the septal region near the atrioventricular sulcus are hypothetical, but some data are compatible with the location shown. (From Durrer D: Electrical aspects of human cardiac activity: a clinical-physiological approach to excitation and stimulation. Cardiovasc Res 2:1,1968. Copyright 1968 Elsevier Science, by permission.)

His bundle recordings have shown that most of the AV conduction time is consumed by impulse conduction through the AV node (i.e., proximal to the His bundle). The duration of the AH interval (i.e., the time between the intracavitary potential recorded from the lower part of the right atrium and the His bundle spike) is 50 to 130 ms.[23–25] The HV time, or the interval between the His spike and the onset of ventricular deflections, is 35 to 55 ms.

The PR interval includes atrial depolarization (P wave) and atrial repolarization (T_p), which is directed opposite to the P-wave axis. When the amplitude of atrial repolarization is low, the segment between the end of P and the onset of the QRS complex is, for practical purposes, horizontal. When atrial repolarization is more clearly expressed (e.g., during exercise-induced tachycardia) (see Chapter 10), the PR segment slopes downward in the conventional leads except in lead aV_R.[26] In normal subjects, at normal heart rates the magnitude of the PR segment depression is usually less than 0.08 mV, and the magnitude of elevation is less than 0.05 mV. Taller P waves are more likely to be associated with a greater degree of PR segment depression.

VENTRICULAR ACTIVATION (QRS COMPLEX)

Ventricular activation, excitation, and *depolarization* are synonyms for a process that determines the duration and configuration of the QRS complex on the ECG. Figure 1–10 shows the opened right and left ventricular cavities after a portion of the right ventricle, septum, and left ventricle has been removed.[27] The boundaries of activation are arranged concentrically. Purkinje fibers penetrate 3 to 4 mm into the apical and middle portions of the septum on both sides, but the basal and posterior septum are devoid of functioning Purkinje fibers. Activation can be divided into three phases: early, later, and latest.

Early Activation

The earliest sites of activation, represented by the 10-ms isochrones, are located in the middle-left side of the septum, high on the anterior paraseptal wall at about one third of the distance from the apex to the base. At 20 ms the excitation wavefront reaches the apex, anterior left ventricular wall, right ventricular septal surface near the attachment of the anterior papillary muscle, and part of the right ventricular free wall. Thus the two excitatory waves in the septum propagate in opposite directions: one from the low middle-left side to the right, and the other, which starts slightly later, from the lower right septal surface propagating to the left.

Later Activation

At 30 ms, invasion of the subendocardial layer of the apical half of the diaphragmatic wall is completed, and there is regular outward spread in a large part of the anterior wall and in a small part of the inferior wall. The opposing septal forces in the apical portion of the septum have met and have disappeared, and the basal portion of the septum is activated slowly toward both outflow tracts. The slowness of this activation is reflected in the close spacing of the isochrones.

At 40 ms, large portions of the surface of the anterior left ventricle and the right ventricle have undergone activation, and excitation begins in the subendocardial layers of the basal region of the left ventricular diaphragmatic wall. At this time the general direction of the excitation wave shifts inferiorly and laterally.

Latest Activation

From 50 ms on, the right ventricular and the septal forces are directed toward the base; the left ventricular forces have a more posterior direction. The last 30 ms (not shown) complete these movements with little change in direction. Figure 1–10 shows that most of the endocardial surface of the left ventricle is depolarized within 40 ms, which suggests that about half of the normal QRS complex is generated after completion of the endocardial activation.

Relation to the Morphology of the QRS Complex

Unlike the shape of the P wave, which can be explained by a single dipole reflecting a relatively simple pattern of activation sequence, genesis of the QRS complex is more complicated. This is because the electromotive forces forming the QRS complex are generated within a massive 3D structure by impulses propagating simultaneously in several directions. Most of the electrical forces during depolarization undergo cancellation, and the QRS complex is formed by residual noncanceled potentials, which in some idealized models have been represented by a single dipole but more often conform to models of two or more dipoles.

In the precordial leads the QRS complex is influenced by the proximity to the underlying portions of the heart that undergo excitation (customarily expressed in terms of a solid angle subtended by the excited area facing the electrode) and by the properties of the volume conductor (i.e., the geometry and the resistivity of the tissues between the heart and the electrode on the body surface). These variables must be considered when the morphology of the QRS complex is correlated with the spread of ventricular activation.

Therefore accurate reconstruction of the QRS complex from the maps depicting spread of excitation may not be feasible. In an oversimplified scheme the QRS is represented by three vectors (Figure 1–11). The interval corresponding to the earliest 20 to 30 ms of the QRS complex, directed rightward and anteriorly, represents more than septal depolarization, which means that this component of the QRS complex should not be referred to as "septal depolarization." The major ventricular forces are represented by a leftward-directed vector. The thickness of the left ventricular wall compared with that of the right ventricular wall and the relative positions of these two chambers explain why in the normal heart the R wave represents predominantly the uncanceled transmural excitation potentials of the left ventricle. The terminal portion of the normal QRS complex represents posterobasal depolarization of the septum and both ventricles and can be represented by a superiorly oriented QRS deflection that may be directed anteriorly or posteriorly. This means that the r^1 in the right precordial leads and the S in the left precordial leads are normal components of the QRS complex and can be variously expressed in different individuals.

QRS Duration

The duration of the QRS complex represents the duration of ventricular activation. It should be measured from the lead with the widest QRS complex because in certain leads the initial or terminal vectors may be perpendicular to the lead axis, creating an isoelectric segment and

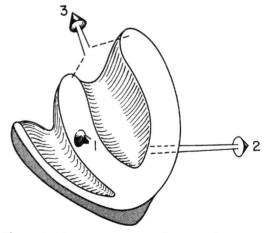

Figure 1–11 Representative resultant spatial vectors of ventricular activation. Vector 1 represents the resultant force of initial septal and paraseptal activation; vector 2, activation of the free wall of the ventricles; and vector 3, basal portion of the ventricles.

spuriously narrowing the QRS complex. The widest QRS complex is present usually in the precordial leads, especially leads V_2 and V_3. Another difficulty when obtaining an accurate value of QRS duration is caused by an overlap of ventricular depolarization and repolarization at the end of the QRS complex. This means that the transition from the QRS complex to the ST segment is gradual rather than sharp. Lepeschkin and Surawicz[28] proposed several methods of defining the J point, but these methods have not been compared with the currently employed computer measurements. If the measurement is made manually, it is recommended that the earliest and latest points be determined in simultaneously recorded leads. The interval determined in such manner is usually slightly longer than that obtained from the single-channel trace. With the single-channel recording, it is recommended that the widest complex in any of the

12 leads with the sharpest onset and termination be chosen.

In normal adults the QRS duration varies between 0.07 and 0.10 second and measures 0.08 second in about 50 percent of adults.[20] A duration of 0.11 second is sometimes observed in healthy subjects. The QRS duration is slightly longer in males than in females and in large, tall subjects than in small, short subjects.[28,29]

QRS Axis

By convention, the QRS axis represents the direction of the mean QRS vector in the frontal plane. It is determined using the hexaxial reference system derived from the Einthoven equilateral triangle (Figure 1–12). Two methods are generally used. One method is to find a lead with an isoelectric complex or a lead in which the algebraic sum of the deflections is zero. The

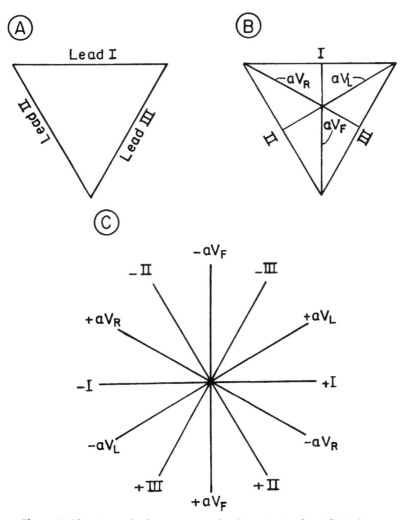

Figure 1–12 Hexaxial reference system. See Figure 1–5 and text discussion.

QRS axis is perpendicular to this lead, and its positive terminus points toward the limb lead with the largest net positive deflection. The other method is to use the algebraic sum of the deflections in two leads, usually leads I and III, to plot the axis (see Figure 1–5). The results obtained from these two methods are not necessarily the same. Furthermore, the direction of the axis may be different when a different pair of leads is used. A variance of up to ±35 degrees is occasionally obtained in the same individual.[30]

The normal QRS axis in the frontal plane is about +60 degrees (range −30 to +105 degrees).[19,31] A slight to moderate left axis is about +30 to 0 degrees; slight to moderate right axis, about +90 to +120 degrees; marked left axis, about −60 degrees; and marked right axis, about +150 degrees. An axis in the range of −60 to −90 degrees is best designated as left superior and an axis in the range of −180 to −90 degrees as right superior.

The mean QRS axis tends to shift leftward with increasing age. In an individual younger than 30 years, the axis is seldom superior to 0 degrees. After age 40 the axis is seldom to the right of +90 degrees. There is also an association between the QRS axis and body weight. A thin person is likely to have a more vertical axis, and overweight individuals tend to have a more leftward axis. The leftward shift of the QRS axis with aging is particularly prevalent in overweight subjects and is more pronounced in older obese men than in older obese women.

QRS Morphology and Amplitude

Analogous to the QRS axis, the morphology and amplitude of the QRS complex are significantly affected by some constitutional variables. With advancing age, the amplitude of the QRS complex decreases, but the changes are less apparent after age 40.[13,32] Men generally have a larger QRS amplitude than women.[33] African Americans tend to have higher voltage than Caucasians.[13,20,32] Table 1–1 shows the normal ranges* of the Q, R, S, and T wave amplitudes in men and women of different age groups, as compiled by Lepeschkin.[22]

Limb Leads

The morphology of the QRS complex in the limb leads depends on the orientation and amplitude

---

*Minor differences exist between some of the values listed in Table 1–1 and those discussed in the following paragraphs.

of the instantaneous QRS vectors in the frontal plane. The direction of the mean QRS vector or axis determines the polarity of the major deflection. Because the normal range of the QRS axis is between −30 and +105 degrees, lead I usually records a dominant R wave, except in young subjects with a rightward axis, in whom an R/S ratio of less than 1 may be seen (Figure 1–13). This is even more pronounced in lead aV_L, in which the entire QRS may be negative if the QRS axis is +90 degrees or more. Such a pattern is believed to characterize the vertical position of the heart. In lead II the R deflection is invariably prominent if the axis is normal, as the projection of the mean vector is always on the positive side of this lead. In contrast, the vector points toward the negative side of lead aV_R, which therefore always records a negative deflection. An essentially upright complex is more common in lead aV_F, especially in young individuals.

Because of the orientation of the lead III axis, the morphology of the QRS complex in this lead is variable. The normal QRS vector may project on the positive or negative side of the lead axis. When the QRS axis is between +30 and +75 degrees, the mean QRS vector is almost perpendicular to lead III. A slight shift of the direction of the QRS vector may change its projection on the lead from the positive to the negative side or vice versa, with a corresponding change in the polarity of the complex. The respiratory variation of the morphology also is most pronounced in this lead (Figure 1–14). For the same reason, notching and slurring of the QRS complex may be seen normally in this lead and, albeit less frequently, in the other inferior leads.

Q Wave

A Q wave is inscribed in a lead when the initial QRS vectors are directed away from the positive electrode. Q waves are more likely to be seen in the inferior leads when the QRS axis is vertical and in leads I and aV_L when the QRS axis is horizontal. The Q wave is present in one or more of the inferior leads (leads II, III, aV_F) in more than 50 percent of normal adults and in leads I and aV_L in fewer than 50 percent.[19,31] In lead aV_R the initial negativity usually is part of the QS deflection.

The duration of the Q wave is of considerable importance in the diagnosis of myocardial infarction. With the exception of leads III and aV_R, the Q waves in the limb leads normally do not exceed 0.03 second in duration. Indeed, in less than 5 percent of the normal population the Q wave duration exceeds 0.02 second in these

TABLE 1–1	Normal Amplitudes of Q, R, S, and T Waves			
Lead	Age (Years)	Q Wave	R Wave	S Wave	T Wave
---	---	---	---	---	---
I	12–16	1.0 (0–3.0)	5.9 (0–12.0)	1.3 (0–10.0)	2.4 (1.6–6.0)
	16–20	0.3 (0–1.3)	4.3 (1.8–9.5)	1.0 (0–3.5)	2.1 (0.2–3.7)
	20–30 ♂	0.3 (0–2.6)	5.7 (1.3–12.9)	1.3 (0–4.0)	2.1 (0.9–4.1)
	20–30 ♀	0.1 (0–1.0)	4.8 (1.3–9.5)	0.8 (0–3.2)	2.1 (0.5–4.0)
	30–40 ♂	0.2 (0–1.2)	5.4 (1.8–11.3)	1.2 (0–4.2)	2.0 (0.6–3.7)
	30–40 ♀	0.2 (0–1.1)	5.1 (1.4–15.0)	0.6 (0–2.9)	2.0 (0.9–3.8)
	40–60 ♂	0.2 (0–1.1)	6.0 (2.0–11.6)	0.7 (0–3.0)	1.9 (0.7–3.5)
	40–60 ♀	0.2 (0–1.2)	6.2 (2.0–12.5)	0.3 (0–2.1)	1.9 (0.7–3.2)
II	12–16	1.0 (0–2.5)	13.5 (3.5–24.5)	1.4 (0–7.0)	3.3 (–0.2 to +6.1)
	16–20	0.5 (0–2.8)	9.5 (2.9–15.8)	1.4 (0–6.3)	2.7 (0.2–5.7)
	20–30 ♂	0.5 (0–2.1)	11.7 (4.7–19.1)	1.4 (0–4.8)	2.9 (0.8–5.8)
	20–30 ♀	0.3 (0–2.2)	9.9 (3.9–15.9)	0.6 (0–2.9)	2.4 (0.7–4.4)
	30–40 ♂	0.3 (0–1.3)	9.3 (4.0–17.0)	1.3 (0–4.3)	2.7 (1.0–5.0)
	30–40 ♀	0.2 (0–1.3)	8.7 (2.1–15.5)	0.8 (0–3.2)	2.2 (0.6–4.9)
	40–60 ♂	0.3 (0–1.2)	7.5 (1.9–15.5)	0.8 (0–3.8)	2.3 (0.8–4.3)
	40–60 ♀	0.2 (0–1.5)	8.1 (2.6–15.3)	0.7 (0–3.1)	2.2 (0.8–4.1)
III	12–16	1.6 (0–5.0)	9.0 (1.0–26.0)	1.1 (0–9.0)	0.8 (–1.6 to +3.5)
	16–20	0.6 (0–4.6)	6.8 (1.2–15.0)	1.1 (0–4.9)	0.8 (–1.9 to +3.9)
	20–30 ♂	0.6 (0–2.6)	7.1 (0.8–15.8)	1.1 (0–6.0)	0.8 (–0.9 to +3.0)
	20–30 ♀	0.6 (0–2.2)	6.0 (0.5–14.2)	0.6 (0–4.3)	0.3 (–0.7 to +2.1)
	30–40 ♂	0.5 (0–2.0)	5.0 (0.3–12.4)	1.4 (0–8.5)	0.7 (–1.5 to +2.9)
	30–40 ♀	0.3 (0–1.0)	4.5(0.1–12.7)	0.8 (0–4.5)	0.4 (–1.8 to +2.0)
	40–60 ♂	0.4 (0–2.4)	3.2 (0.1–11.9)	1.6 (0–7.5)	0.4 (–1.2 to +2.2)
	40–60 ♀	0.4 (0–2.0)	3.6 (0.1–11.8)	1.4 (0–6.0)	0.3 (–1.1 to +1.7)
aV$_R$	12–16	7.9 (0–14.0)	1.2 (0–3.0)	2.5 (0–19.0)	–2.9 (–5.2 to –0.5)
	16–20	2.1 (0–9.0)	1.2 (0–4.7)	4.3 (0–11.1)	–2.0 (–4.8 to –0.1)
	20–30 ♂	2.5 (0–11.5)	0.6 (0–3.2)	9.0 (0–16.1)	–2.5 (–5.0 to –0.8)
	20–30 ♀	2.5 (0–11.5)	0.5 (0–1.8)	6.9 (0–11.6)	–2.2 (–5.0 to –0.7)
	30–40 ♂	2.1 (0–9.0)	0.6 (0–3.2)	7.6 (0–12.0)	–2.3 (–4.2 to –1.0)
	30–40 ♀	2.1 (0–9.0)	0.5 (0–2.2)	6.2 (0–14.6)	–2.1 (–3.5 to –0.9)
	40–60 ♂	2.0 (0–8.5)	0.5 (0–2.2)	6.8 (0–11.0)	–2.1 (–3.4 to –0.8)
	40–60 ♂	2.0 (0–8.5)	0.4 (0–1.6)	6.8 (0–12.5)	–2.0 (–3.6 to –0.7)
aV$_L$	12–16	1.0 (0–6.0)	2.4 (0–12.0)	3.0 (0–20.0)	1.1 (–1.0 to +3.6)
	16–20	0.5 (0–2.5)	1.9 (0.2–6.0)	2.0 (0–8.0)	0.6 (–1.8 to +3.6)
	20–30 ♂	0.3 (0–3.5)	2.0 (0.1–8.3)	2.7 (0–8.7)	1.7 (–0.8 to +2.1)
	20–30 ♀	0.3 (0–3.5)	1.9 (0.1–7.2)	2.0 (0–9.2)	1.0 (–0.4 to +2.2)
	30–40 ♂	0.3 (0–2.3)	2.4 (0.1–8.5)	1.8 (0–6.8)	1.8 (–1.0 to +2.1)
	30–40 ♀	0.1 (0–1.3)	2.3 (0.3–9.2)	1.0 (0–4.5)	1.0 (–0.4 to +3.0)
	40–60 ♂	0.2 (0–1.3)	3.4 (0.2–9.3)	1.1 (0–4.6)	1.1 (–0.5 to +2.2)
	40–60 ♀	0.2 (0–1.4)	3.3 (0.2–8.5)	0.7 (0–3.9)	0.7 (–0.1 to +2.6)
aV$_F$	12–16	1.3 (0–3.0)	10.2 (0.1–21.8)	1.0 (0–4.0)	2.3 (–0.7 to +5.4)
	16–20	0.8 (0–3.8)	7.7 (1.8–14.0)	1.0 (0–4.9)	1.8 (–0.6 to +5.2)
	20–30 ♂	0.5 (0–2.2)	8.8 (1.0–16.9)	0.7 (0–4.9)	1.1 (–0.2 to +3.5)
	20–30 ♀	0.3 (0–1.6)	7.6 (1.8–15.6)	1.0 (0–2.1)	0.5 (–0.1 to +3.1)
	30–40 ♂	0.3 (0–1.3)	6.7 (1.0–14.8)	0.8 (0–4.4)	1.0 (0.4–3.8)
	30–40 ♀	0.3 (0–1.2)	6.2 (1.0–13.9)	1.2 (0–2.6)	0.5 (0.1–3.2)
	40–60 ♂	0.2 (0–1.2)	4.7 (0.3–12.6)	0.9 (0–4.1)	0.9 (0–3.1)
	40–60 ♀	0.2 (0–11)	5.3 (0.3–13.4)	1.0 (0–3.9)	0.8 (–0.2 to +2.6)
V$_1$	12–16	0	5.6 (0–16.0)	13.8 (5.0–26.0)	–1.5 (–4.0 to +7.0)
	16–20	0	4.6 (0.4–16.7)	11.7 (1.8–25.1)	0.9 (–3.5 to +6.0)
	20–30 ♂	0	3.3 (0.3–8.9)	11.4 (5.0–18.0)	0.9 (–2.2 to +3.9)
	20–30 ♀	0	1.6 (0–5.3)	7.4 (1.6–14.2)	–0.7 (–2.1 to +2.0)
	30–40 ♂	0	2.2 (0.2–5.4)	9.1 (3.2–17.6)	0.7 (–1.4 to +3.3)
	30–40 ♀	0	1.6 (0–5.8)	7.6 (3.8–14.3)	–0.6 (–2.6 to +1.2)
	40–60 ♂	0	1.7 (0.1–4.9)	8.6 (2.9–16.7)	0.9 (–1.3 to +3.9)
	40–60 ♀	0	1.4 (0.1–4.0)	7.2 (2.3–15.1)	–0.2 (–1.9 to +1.5)

Table continued on following page

TABLE 1-1	Normal Amplitudes of Q, R, S, and T Waves (Continued)			
Lead	Age (Years)	Q Wave	R Wave	S Wave	T Wave
V_2	12–16	0	9.1 (2.0–21.0)	20.1 (4.0–51.0)	4.5 (−4.3 to +13.5)
	16–20	0	7.3 (0.5–20.5)	16.2 (2.6–45.5)	3.9 (−3.8 to +14.1)
	20–30 ♂	0	7.4 (1.7–13.9)	18.0 (6.7–29.1)	6.5 (1.1–12.3)
	20–30 ♀	0	4.6 (1.1–9.2)	12.4 (4.0–23.2)	3.1 (0–4.1)
	30–40 ♂	0	5.4 (0.6–12.1)	15.2 (6.1–27.8)	6.2 (2.0–11.1)
	30–40 ♀	0	3.7 (0.4–10.1)	11.3 (4.2–19.8)	2.9 (0–7.5)
	40–60 ♂	0	4.6 (0.6–12.0)	12.7 (5.2–23.3)	5.5 (1.7–10.1)
	40–60 ♀	0	3.6 (0.2–9.1)	9.4 (2.4–18.0)	3.0 (0.1–6.5)
V_3	12–16	0.1 (0–1)	11.8 (2.0–33.0)	14.1 (3.0–34.0)	4.1 (0–13.0)
	16–20	0.1 (0–1)	8.5 (1.6–23.3)	10.7 (0.9–28.9)	5.1 (−3.7 to +13.5)
	20–30 ♂	0 (0–0.4)	11.6 (2.2–26.6)	10.6 (6.7–22.0)	6.5 (1.9–11.7)
	20–30 ♀	0 (0–0.4)	8.2 (2.3–17.5)	6.1 (4.0–14.2)	3.5 (0–8.6)
	30–40 ♂	0 (0–0.5)	9.4 (2.2–22.5)	10.0 (6.1–22.0)	6.3 (3.1–11.5)
	30–40 ♀	0 (0–0.5)	7.1 (0.8–23.3)	5.1 (4.2–11.9)	3.1 (0.5–7.7)
	40–60 ♂	0 (0–0.4)	8.4 (1.4–11.6)	9.8 (5.2–19.0)	6.0 (2.1–10.7)
	40–60 ♀	0 (0–0.4)	7.1 (1.0–17.7)	6.0 (2.4–13.5)	3.4 (0.1–7.4)
V_4	12–16	0.5 (0–3.0)	23.5 (5.0–51.0)	7.0 (1.0–30.0)	7.2 (0–17.2)
	16–20	0.1 (0–1.0)	12.7 (3.1–30.1)	6.3 (0.2–15.0)	4.7 (−3.6 to +12.6)
	20–30 ♂	0.3 (0–2.9)	16.6 (6.1–27.7)	6.1 (0–15.0)	5.6 (1.5–11.8)
	20–30 ♀	0.1 (0–0.7)	11.5 (5.0–19.6)	2.9 (0–8.5)	3.6 (1.0–7.8)
	30–40 ♂	0.2 (0–1.7)	14.8 (5.2–29.2)	5.7 (1.1–12.1)	5.4 (2.0–9.9)
	30–40 ♀	0.2 (0–1.4)	11.8 (4.1–25.9)	2.4 (0–7.8)	3.3 (0.8–7.0)
	40–60 ♂	0.1 (0–1.0)	14.2 (5.2–25.6)	6.3 (0.8–14.1)	5.4 (1.6–10.4)
	40–60 ♀	0.2 (0–1.3)	12.4 (3.7–23.6)	2.8 (0–7.7)	3.5 (1.0–6.3)
V_5	12–16	1.3 (0–4.0)	18.2 (5.0–35.0)	2.5 (0–12.0)	5.7 (0.5–11.5)
	16–20	0.5 (0–2.8)	11.4 (4.1–26.5)	2.2 (0–8.1)	3.8 (0.2–10.6)
	20–30 ♂	0.7 (0–3.1)	15.3 (5.9–24.0)	2.2 (0–6.4)	3.8 (0.8–8.1)
	20–30 ♀	0.3 (0–1.2)	11.5 (5.2–18.7)	1.0 (0–4.0)	3.0 (1.0–5.5)
	30–40 ♂	0.4 (0–2.0)	14.3 (8.1–24.8)	2.3 (0–6.7)	3.7 (1.3–7.0)
	30–40 ♀	0.3 (0–1.8)	11.8 (5.0–27.2)	0.8 (0–3.2)	2.9 (0.8–5.9)
	40–60 ♂	0.3 (0–1.6)	14.1 (5.9–25.0)	2.4 (1.0–6.9)	3.9 (1.3–7.8)
	40–60 ♀	0.3 (0–1.2)	12.4 (5.0–20.9)	1.0 (0–5.0)	2.9 (0.9–5.1)
V_6	12–16	1.3 (0–2.5)	12.5 (4.0–27.0)	1.0 (0–6.0)	4.0 (0.8–7.2)
	16–20	0.6 (0–4.2)	13.5 (7.0–21.0)	1.2 (0–5.0)	3.8 (0.8–7.1)
	20–30 ♂	0.7 (0–2.6)	11.6 (3.7–19.3)	0.9 (0–3.7)	2.6 (0.5–5.9)
	20–30 ♀	0.4 (0–1.8)	9.6 (5.2–16.3)	0.3 (0–1.8)	2.4 (0.9–5.0)
	30–40 ♂	0.5 (0–1.6)	10.9 (5.9–18.3)	0.8 (0–2.8)	2.5 (0.8–4.5)
	30–40 ♀	0.3 (0–1.5)	9.2 (4.0–20.2)	0.3 (0–1.7)	3.3 (0.6–4.7)
	40–60 ♂	0.4 (0–1.5)	10.5 (4.9–17.8)	0.7 (0–2.9)	2.6 (0.8–4.9)
	40–60 ♀	0.3 (0–1.4)	9.6 (3.6–16.8)	0.3 (0–2.6)	2.3 (0.7–4.6)

Adapted from Lepeschkin E. *In*: Altman PE, Dittmer DS (eds): Respiration and Circulation. Bethesda, Md, Federation of American Societies for Experimental Biology, 1971, p 277.

♂ = male; ♀ = female.

Results are given as means, with the ranges in parentheses.

leads.[20] In lead III, Q wave duration is occasionally as long as 0.04 second but rarely is it 0.05 second. This lead accounts for most of the erroneous diagnoses of myocardial infarction.

The amplitude of the Q waves is less than 0.4 mV in all limb leads except lead III, in which it may reach 0.5 mV.[20,31,32] The depth of the Q wave is less than 25 percent of the R wave, but lead III is the exception. An example of a normal Q wave in several limb and precordial leads is shown in Figure 1–15.

R Wave

The maximum R wave amplitude is recorded in the lead in which the axis is most parallel and has the same polarity as the maximum vector. The upper limit for the R wave in lead I is 1.5 mV; in lead aV_L, 1.0 mV; and in leads II,

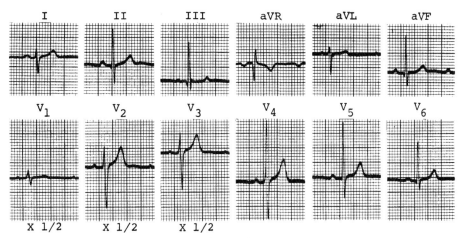

Figure 1–13 Normal ECG from a healthy 22-year-old man, illustrating rightward QRS axis in the frontal plane. The R/S ratio in V_1 is 1. Note ST-segment elevation in leads V_1–V_3.

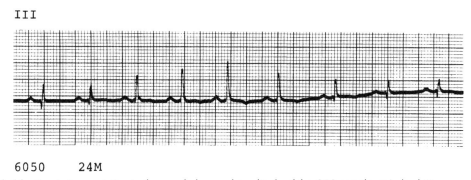

6050   24M

Figure 1–14 Respiratory variation in the morphology and amplitude of the QRS complexes in lead III.

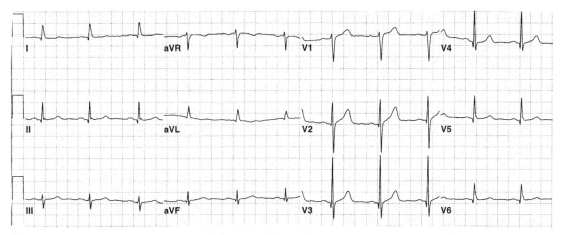

Figure 1–15 ECG of a 58-year-old man who has no evidence of structural heart disease and no abnormal findings on the echocardiogram. Note the Q waves in leads I, II, aV_L, aV_F, and V_2–V_6. Also note the slight notching of the P wave in leads II and III.

III, and aV_F, 1.9 mV. Larger amplitudes are occasionally seen in young subjects.[34]

S Wave

The S wave is most prominent in lead aV_R. An amplitude up to 1.6 mV may be seen in this lead in young subjects. A relatively large S wave sometimes is present also in leads III and aV_L, depending on the QRS axis. The magnitude usually does not exceed 0.9 mV. In leads I, II, and aV_F the S wave amplitudes are less than 0.5 mV.[31] If the amplitude of the entire QRS complex is less than 0.5 mV in all limb leads, the voltage is considered abnormally low.

Precordial Leads

The QRS complexes in the precordial leads represent projections of the QRS vectors in the horizontal plane. Figure 1–7 shows the directions of the lead axes of V_1 through V_6. As the dominant left ventricular forces are directed leftward, the right precordial leads (V_1 and V_2) record predominantly negative deflections (S waves), and the left precordial leads (V_5 and V_6) record upright deflections (R waves). Early activation of the anterior wall and late excitation of the posterior wall explain the initial positivity and terminal negativity of the complexes in the leads with an axis directed essentially anteriorly (e.g., V_1–V_4). The R wave progressively increases in amplitude from lead V_1 toward leads V_5 and V_6, and the S wave decreases from the right toward the left precordial leads.

Transitional Zone

The transitional zone is located at the site of the lead in which the amplitudes of the positive and negative deflections are of equal magnitude. It is related to the direction of the QRS axis in the horizontal plane, which during routine interpretation of the ECG is not expressed in degrees. As in the frontal plane, the QRS axis is perpendicular to the transitional lead. In normal adults the transitional zone usually is located between leads V_2 and V_4, with lead V_3 being the most common site. Slight notching of the complex is occasionally observed in the transitional lead. A transitional zone located to the right of lead V_2 is referred to as *counterclockwise rotation*. If the transitional zone is displaced leftward and beyond lead V_5, clockwise rotation is present. A leftward shift of the transition zone tends to occur in older subjects.

An R/S ratio of more than 1 in lead V_1 generally is considered abnormal in adults. According to Lamb's data, 6.4 percent of normal men and 1.5 percent of normal women have an R/S ratio of 1 in V_1. About 25 percent of men and 12 percent of women have a ratio of 1 in V_2. In leads V_5 and V_6, an R/S ratio less than 1 is usually abnormal, occurring in fewer than 2.5 percent of normal subjects.[20]

Q Wave

Small Q waves are present in the left precordial leads in more than 75 percent of normal subjects. They are seen most frequently in lead V_6, less frequently in leads V_5 and V_4, and rarely in V_3. Q waves in these leads are present more often in young subjects than in subjects older than 40 years. Q waves are likely to be present in more leads when the transitional zone is located on the right side of the precordium. The duration of the Q waves is 0.03 second or less. The amplitude usually is less than 0.2 mV, although it may reach 0.3 mV or even 0.4 mV. The deeper Q waves are seen more often in young adults.[22] An amplitude of 0.4 mV or more may be encountered in teenagers. In the posterior leads V7–V9, Q wave duration of ≥ 0.03 second was seen in 20 percent of normal male subjects.[35]

R Wave

The R wave increases in amplitude from the right toward the left precordium. The R wave may be absent in lead V_1, and a QS complex is recorded. A QS deflection, however, is rare in lead V_2. The upper limit of the R wave amplitude in V_1 is 0.6 mV, although in young adults the R wave may be taller.[36–38] The tallest R wave is most commonly seen in lead V_4, followed by lead V_5, whereas the voltage is generally lower in lead V_6 than in lead V_5. Echocardiographic studies suggest that the proximity of the left ventricle to the chest wall is a major determinant of the R wave amplitude in leads V_5 and V_6 in normal subjects.[39]

S Wave

The S wave is deepest in the right precordial leads, usually in lead V_2. The S wave amplitude decreases as the left precordium is approached. Although the upper limits of the S wave amplitude in leads V_1, V_2, and V_3 have been given as 1.8, 2.6, and 2.1 mV, respectively,[31] an amplitude of 3.0 mV is recorded occasionally in healthy individuals.[36] An S wave is often absent in leads V_5 and V_6. An S wave of less than 0.3 mV in lead V_1 is considered abnormally small. If the amplitude of the entire QRS complex is less than 1.0 mV in each of the precordial leads, the voltage is considered abnormally low.

ST Segment

The ST segment is the interval between the end of the QRS complex (J point, or ST junction) and the beginning of the T wave. In the limb leads, the ST segment is isoelectric in about 75 percent of normal adults.[19] ST segment elevation or depression up to 0.1 mV generally is considered within normal limits.[34] ST segment elevation is more common and is usually present in the inferior leads. ST segment depression seldom is seen in leads I, II, or aV_F because the ST vector in the frontal plane, if present, is directed inferiorly and usually leftward.

In the precordial leads, some ST segment elevation is seen in more than 90 percent of normal subjects.[19] The magnitude of the ST segment elevation is usually proportional to the QRS amplitude. Therefore it tends to be somewhat greater in men than in women,[13] particularly in young individuals. The elevation is most prominent (up to 0.3 mV or more) in leads V_2 and V_3. In the left precordial leads, the elevation rarely exceeds 0.1 mV. ST elevation exceeding 0.2 mV is uncommon in subjects older than 40 years. However, in body surface maps with 150 torso electrodes, maximum ST voltages at 40 ms into the ST segment averaged 0.2 mV, which was nearly twice as much as ST segment voltage sensed by the six standard precordial electrodes.[40]

Any ST segment depression in the precordial leads is considered abnormal, as the normal ST vector in the horizontal plane is directed anteriorly and leftward. In the posterior leads V7–V9, prevalence of ST segment elevation of 0.5 to 1.0 mm at 80 ms after J point in normal young men was 8.9 percent in lead V_7, 5.8 percent in lead V_8, and 3.1 percent in lead V_9.[35]

Definition of Baseline

The line connecting two consecutive points at the beginning of the QRS complex (i.e., the QQ interval) includes three segments that in the absence of tachycardia may be nearly isoelectric: (1) ST segment; (2) TP segment (from the end of the T wave to the onset of the P wave); and (3) PQ segment (from the end of the P wave to the onset of the QRS complex).

The ST segment corresponds to the plateau of the ventricular action potential and is isoelectric only in its central part because at the beginning of the ST segment the plateau potentials overlap with ventricular depolarization and at the end of the ST segment the plateau potentials overlap with rapid ventricular repolarization. The most common causes of ST segment deviation are (1) tachycardia because of the overlap with atrial repolarization; (2) delayed repolarization secondary to slow depolarization (e.g., ventricular hypertrophy, bundle branch block, preexcitation); and (3) myocardial ischemia, which can cause a shift of the ST segment (systolic injury current) or of the TQ segment (diastolic injury current). The cause of the shift can be recognized when the record is made with direct-current (DC) coupled amplifiers or a magnetocardiograph, but not on the ECG recorded with conventional equipment. Therefore the true baseline remains unknown, and the reference for measuring the ST segment shift is the line connecting the two consecutive points at the beginning of the QRS complex.

The TP interval can serve as a useful baseline when abnormal deviation of the PQ segment caused by a systolic or diastolic atrial injury current (e.g., during acute pericarditis or atrial infarction) is suspected (see Chapters 9 and 11).[26] In such cases there is no assurance that the diastolic ventricular potential has remained unchanged.

Use of the PQ interval as baseline offers no advantages over use of the TP segment; both represent the same level of ventricular diastolic potential. The accuracy of the PQ segment as baseline may be diminished by the presence of atrial repolarization.

T Wave

The T wave represents the uncanceled potential differences of ventricular repolarization.[33] The ventricular recovery process proceeds in the general direction of ventricular excitation. Hence one would expect the polarity of the T wave to be opposite that of the QRS complex with a zero net area of the ventricular complex (i.e., QRS and T). In the normal heart, however, the mean QRS vector and the mean T vector form a narrow angle, and the area of the ventricular complex has a positive value. This indicates that the duration of repolarization must be greater in some parts of the ventricles than in others. This difference was designated the *ventricular gradient*. For a discussion of the sources of the ventricular gradient, the reader is referred to other texts.[3,41] As a rule, the inhomogeneities of repolarization occur within small distances over the entire surface of the heart, and most are probably within the ventricular wall.[3,41] To explain the normal polarity of the T wave, it must be assumed that in the region(s) responsible for T wave shape, the fibers depolarized earlier repolarize later than the fibers that are depolarized later (i.e., a reversed sequence of repolarization versus the sequence of depolarization).

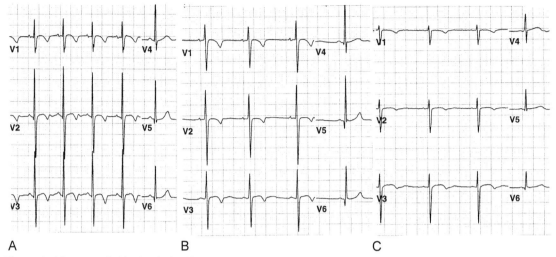

Figure 1–16 Precordial leads of a healthy 4-year-old child (**A**), a healthy 13-year-old Caucasian male (**B**), and a healthy 16-year-old African-American adolescent (**C**). Note the negative T waves in leads V_1–V_3.

In normal individuals the T vector is oriented leftward, inferiorly, and (in most adults) anteriorly. In children and young adults (especially females), the orientation may be slightly posterior but becomes increasingly anterior with advancing age. Because the T vector is directed leftward and inferiorly in the frontal plane, the T waves are always upright in leads I and II and inverted in lead aV_R. They may be upright or inverted in leads III and aV_L, depending on whether the T vector is more vertical or more horizontal. In lead aV_F, the T wave usually is upright but occasionally is flat or slightly inverted. In the horizontal plane the T vector is directed leftward and usually anteriorly. Therefore the T waves are always upright in left precordial leads V_5 and V_6. In about 5 percent of women the T wave is inverted in lead V_1.[19] An inverted, diphasic, or flat T wave is much less common in lead V_2 (less than 10 percent), is seen only occasionally in V_3, and is exceptional in lead V_4 (seen mostly in young patients). In adult men, T wave inversion in the right precordial leads is relatively uncommon. In Lamb's series,[20] fewer than 1 percent of adult men had inverted T waves in lead V_1.[20] When T wave inversion is present in two or more of the right precordial leads in the normal adult, the ECG resembles that of normal children and adolescents (Figure 1–16), and the phenomenon is called *persistent juvenile pattern* (Figure 1–17).

In the limb leads, the tallest T wave is seen most often in lead II. The T wave amplitude is normally less than 0.6 mV in all limb leads.[22]

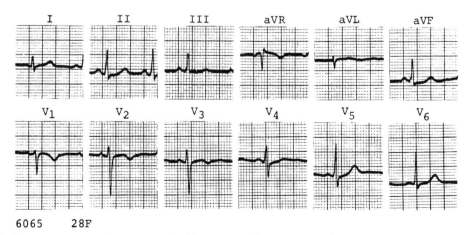

6065   28F

Figure 1–17 Persistent juvenile pattern in a healthy 28-year-old woman. Note the negative T waves in leads V_1–V_3.

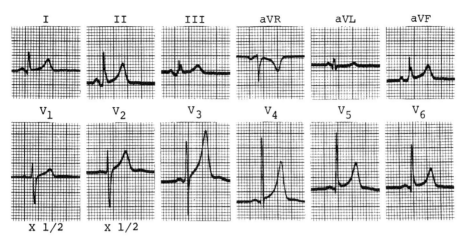

Figure 1–18 Tall T waves, especially in leads V_1–V_6, in a healthy 22-year-old man. Also note the elevated J point in leads V_2–V_4.

In leads I and II the amplitude should be not less than 0.05 mV. In women, the ascent of the T wave is slightly slower than in young and middle-aged men and the T wave amplitude is slightly lower than in men. The T waves in the precordial leads are tallest in leads V_2 and V_3. In men, the amplitude in these leads has an average value of about 0.6 mV but may reach 1.0 mV or more (Figure 1–18). It is significantly lower in men older than 40 years. In women the amplitude is generally lower, with an average of 0.3 to 0.4 mV; it is seldom above 0.8 mV. Although Lepeschkin's data (see Table 1–1) show that the T wave amplitude does not change appreciably with advancing age, others found a significant decrease.[13,31,42] For both genders the T waves tend to be lower in the left precordial leads than in the mid-precordial leads. They seldom, however, are considered normal when the T wave amplitude is less than 10 percent of the R wave amplitude. In the posterior leads (V_7–V_9), the T wave is upright.[35]

The normal upright or inverted T wave is asymmetric. The slope of the initial portion is more gradual than that of the terminal portion (Figure 1–19). The ascent of an upright T wave and the descent of the inverted T wave are slightly concave. A normal T wave in the right precordial leads may be diphasic, with an upright first portion and an inverted second portion. A negative-positive diphasic T wave is abnormal, but a positive-negative T wave does not always indicate normality.

QT Interval

The QT interval represents the duration of ventricular electrical systole. It is measured from the beginning of the QRS complex to the end of

the T wave.[43,44] The lead with a large T wave and a distinct termination is used. In practice, it is often difficult to obtain an accurate measurement. A multichannel recorder is helpful because it allows more accurate determinination of the onset of the QRS complex and the end of the T wave.[43–45] Recent scientific statement from the American Heart Association Electrocardiography and Arrhythmias Committee recommends "global" measurements of intervals, including QT, from simultaneously acquired 12 leads.[45a] Theoretically the QT value in all standard limb leads should be the same, but differences occur because of different projections of the ventricular complex on the limb axis in different leads. For

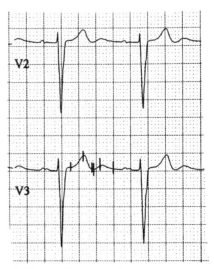

Figure 1–19 Configuration of a normal T wave and normal U wave. Note that the T wave has a steeper descent than ascent, whereas the U wave has a steeper ascent than descent.

instance, when the vectors are perpendicular to the QRST axis, an isoelectric segment may be recorded at the onset of the QRS complex, at the end of the T wave, or both, thereby causing artificial shortening of the QT interval. In the precordial leads, differences in the QT interval may be due to differences in the proximity to the heart and differences in local repolarization duration at the sites facing the recording electrode. The latter factors probably account for most of the so-called QT dispersion, which is a computed value of the difference between the longest and shortest QT intervals among 12 standard leads.[46]

Because the adjustment of the QT interval to changes in the RR interval occurs gradually rather than instantaneously,[3,47] the QT measurement represents a steady-state value only when the rhythm remains regular for several cycles. The QT interval includes the QRS duration, and although a prolonged QRS complex does not detract from the accuracy of the QT measurement, it may change the interpretation of the measured value. Subtraction of the QRS duration from the QT interval (JT interval) may be necessary when estimating the duration of repolarization independent of the duration of depolarization. This procedure introduces potential inaccuracy, however, because of the difficulties inherent in determining the end of the QRS complex.[28]

The QT interval decreases with increasing heart rate. Of the many formulas proposed to describe this relation, the most widely used formula for correcting the rate is that of Bazett, in which

$$QT_c = k\sqrt{RR}$$

the k value,[48] as modified by Shipley and Hallaran,[49] is 0.397 for men and 0.415 for women. It has been suggested that the QTc interval should be expressed in seconds, similar to the QT interval.[50] Many investigators consider the upper limit of normal for QTc for both genders to be 0.44 second. This value, however, is lower than the upper limit of the normal QTc values of approximately 0.46 second for men and 0.47 second for women as suggested by Lepeschkin.[21] The Bazett formula can be used to study the effect of interventions modifying the k value. When studying the effect of drugs and interventions, this type of evaluation may be more informative than the QT measurements alone determined at only one RR interval. The appropriate k value can be found by regression analysis of the measured intervals using the function defined by Bazett's formula with a k value serving as a reference.[51] Several investigators

found that the Bazett formula tends to overcorrect at rapid heart rates and undercorrect at slow heart rates.[52] More accurate values have been obtained with other formulas, such as the cubic root, quadratic, exponential, or linear formulas. It has been shown, however, that all of the 20 tested formulas were not as accurate as the formulas individualized for each person,[53] but the reported inaccuracies were in the range of 4 to 5 ms, which is usually of negligible practical importance.

In more than 5000 adults aged 28 to 62 years who formed the original cohort of the Framingham Heart Study,[54] a linear equation was more accurate than the Bazett formula. Table 1–2 (from the Framingham study) shows the average values and ranges in men and women. It can be used without any correction if one wishes to compare the measured QT interval with the values in this large cohort of presumably normal subjects.

The time of day can influence the measurement, as QT is longer in the evening and at night.[52,55,56] Morganroth et al.[57] found that for individual subjects the QTc varied over 24 hours of ambulatory monitoring by an average of 76 ms (range 35 to 108 ms).[57] Molnar et al.[58] reported that during ambulatory monitoring the upper limit for the mean QTc interval was 439 ms in normal men and 452 ms in normal women. The average maximum QTc interval was 495 ms, and the average QTc range, 95 ms. The QTc interval and the QTc variability reached a peak shortly after awakening.

Sleep prolonged the QT interval by 18 ms at a heart rate of 60 beats/min and by 21 ms at a heart rate of 50 beats/min compared with the waking state.[59] This diurnal variation is thought to be related to autonomic tone.

Considerable variability may be due to measurement differences among observers.[60] Because of the difficulty of obtaining exact measurements of the QT interval on many ECGs and because of varying normal limits given by various investigators, rigid adherence to a precise value for normality is not warranted. In addition, appreciable differences in QT interval measurements have been found in evolving automated algorithms from different manufacturers of electrocardiographs.[60a] For these reasons, minor deviation from the usual normal limits may not be clinically significant.

Differences between Ventricular Repolarization in Men and Women.

Bidoggia et al.[61] described differences between male and female ventricular repolarization patterns in adults, identifying several variables.

TABLE 1–2	Mean Predicted QT Values at Various RR Cycle Lengths					
		QT for Men (Seconds)			QT for Women (Seconds)		
RR (Seconds)	Heart rate (Beats/min)	Mean Value	Lower Limit*	Upper Limit*	Mean Value	Lower Limit	Upper limit
0.50	120	0.299	0.255	0.343	0.311	0.267	0.354
0.55	109	0.307	0.263	0.351	0.318	0.274	0.362
0.60	100	0.314	0.270	0.358	0.326	0.282	0.370
0.65	92	0.322	0.278	0.366	0.334	0.290	0.378
0.70	86	0.330	0.286	0.374	0.341	0.297	0.385
0.75	80	0.337	0.293	0.381	0.349	0.305	0.393
0.80	75	0.345	0.301	0.389	0.357	0.313	0.401
0.85	71	0.353	0.309	0.397	0.364	0.321	0.408
0.90	67	0.361	0.317	0.404	0.372	0.328	0.416
0.95	63	0.368	0.324	0.412	0.380	0.336	0.424
1.00	60	0.376	0.332	0.420	0.388	0.344	0.432
1.05	57	0.384	0.340	0.428	0.395	0.351	0.439
1.10	55	0.391	0.347	0.435	0.403	0.359	0.447
1.15	52	0.399	0.355	0.443	0.411	0.367	0.455
1.20	50	0.407	0.363	0.451	0.418	0.374	0.462
1.25	48	0.414	0.370	0.458	0.426	0.382	0.470
1.30	46	0.422	0.378	0.466	0.434	0.390	0.478
1.35	44	0.430	0.386	0.474	0.441	0.397	0.486
1.40	43	0.438	0.394	0.482	0.449	0.405	0.493
1.45	41	0.445	0.401	0.489	0.457	0.413	0.501
1.50	40	0.453	0.409	0.497	0.465	0.421	0.509

From Dajie A, Larson MG, Goldberg RJ, et al: An improved method for adjusting the QT interval for heart rate (the Framingham Heart Study). Am J Cardiol 70:797, 1992, by permission.

*Upper and lower 95% limits.

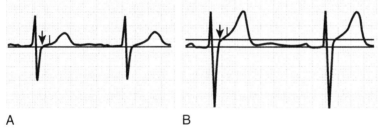

A   B

Figure 1–20   Female and male patterns in lead V_2. The arrow marks the J point, the short vertical line marks the point 60 ms after the J point, and the oblique line connects these two points for measurement of the ST angle. **A,** Female pattern: The J point is at the level of the Q-Q line, and the ST angle is 19 degrees. **B,** Male pattern: The J point is > 0.1 mV above the Q-Q line, and the ST angle is 36 degrees. (From Surawicz B, Parikh SR: Prevalence of male and female patterns of early ventricular repolarization in the normal ECG of males and females from childhood to old age. J Am Coll Cardiol 40:1870, 2002. With permission.)

Surawicz and Parikh[62,63] examined normal ECGs of 529 males and 544 females, aged 5 to 96 years, and applied two variables to analyze the early repolarization pattern (i.e., the J point amplitude and the angle of the ST takeoff in the precordial lead with the tallest T wave). They identified the following three patterns: the male pattern characterized by J point elevation >0.1 mV and ST angle >20 degrees (Figure 1–20), the female pattern with the J point < 0.1 mV above the baseline and ST takeoff <20 degrees, and an "indeterminate" pattern with J point elevation <0.1 mV and ST angle >20 degrees (not shown). The distribution of these patterns in females, as shown in Figure 1–23, reveals a large predominance of female pattern in all age groups. The distribution in males shows an age-dependent predominance of male pattern in males (see Figure 1–21) with a rise at puberty and subsequent gradual decline at middle age concomitant with rise of female pattern

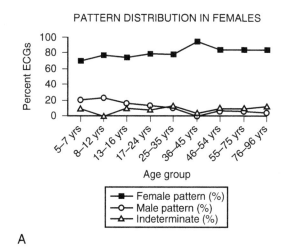

A

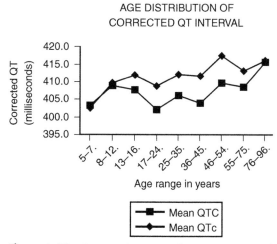

Figure 1–22 Average QTc intervals in nine groups of males and females. See text discussion. (From Surawicz B, Parikh SR: Differences between ventricular repolarization in men and women: description, mechanism and implications. Ann Noninvas Electrocardiol 8:333, 2003. With permission.)

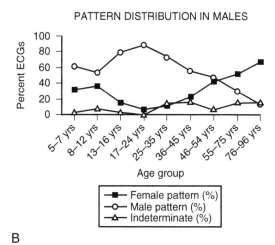

B

Figure 1–21 Pattern distribution in different age groups of females and males. See text discussion. (From Surawicz B, Parikh SR: Prevalence of male and female patterns of early ventricular repolarization in the normal ECG of males and females from childhood to old age. J Am Coll Cardiol 40:1870, 2002. With permission.)

and a reversal of distribution at an old age (i.e., distribution similar to that in women). These age-dependent gender differences were attributed to the effect of rise and fall of testosterone levels in males, in whom the hormone appeared to be responsible for the shortening of the QTc interval by shortening the duration of ventricular action potential.[64] Figure 1–22 shows that gender differences of QTc appear during puberty, diminish during age 56 to 75 years, and disappear in the oldest age group.

U Wave

The U wave is a small, low-frequency diastolic deflection that begins usually with the second heart sound at the onset of ventricular relaxation and after the end of the T wave.[65] The T-U junction is situated at or close to the isoelectric baseline, but it may be slightly depressed or slightly elevated. The duration of the QU end interval increases with increasing RR interval.[66] The U wave is usually a monophasic positive or negative deflection, although it may be diphasic (i.e., positive-negative or negative-positive).

Within the normal range of heart rates (i.e., from 50 to 100 beats/min), the interval from the end of the T wave to the apex of the U wave (aU) measures 90 to 110 ms. The timing of aU does not change after a sudden increase in cycle length (e.g., during atrial fibrillation or after a premature complex, which may result in encroachment of the T wave on the U wave). Within the range of heart rates from 50 to 100 beats/min, the interval from the end of the T wave to the end of the U wave ranges from 160 to 230 ms.

Unlike the normal T wave, the ascent of the U wave is either shorter than or equal to the duration of the descent (Figure 1–19). The U wave vector is directed similarly to the T wave vector; that is, the normal U wave is occasionally negative in leads III and aV_F; in leads I, aV_R, and aV_L, the U wave is usually isoelectric.

In 98 percent of cases, the amplitude of the largest U wave (usually in lead V_2 or V_3) ranges from 3 to 24 percent (average 11 percent) of T wave amplitude. Generally, the U wave amplitude varies directly with the T wave amplitude and, to a lesser degree, with the QRS amplitude.[65]

The U wave is usually better visualized in the semidirect leads (e.g., precordial, esophageal, intracoronary) than in the indirect leads, but the timing of the U wave is the same in all leads, and the increased U wave amplitude tends to reflect the overall increase in ECG amplitude. The U wave amplitude seldom exceeds 0.2 mV and is strongly rate dependent. In 500 randomly selected ECGs with a normal QT interval, the U wave was discernible in more than 90 percent of cases when the heart rate was less than 65 beats/min, in about two thirds of cases when the heart rate was 80 to 95 beats/min, and in about 25 percent of cases when the heart rate was within 80 to 95 beats/min. The U wave was seldom detectable when the heart rate exceeded 95 beats/min.[65] Detection of a low-amplitude U wave during rapid heart rate can be facilitated by enlarging the tracing.

In some cases it is difficult to differentiate the U wave from the second peak of a notched T wave. Lepeschkin prepared a nomogram that shows the predicted intervals between the onset of the Q wave to the apex of the T wave (aT) and U wave (aU) at various heart rates.[66] By measuring the intervals from the Q wave to the two peaks and comparing them with the predicted intervals on the nomogram, a notched T wave usually can be distinguished from a T-U complex. Furthermore, the apices of a notched T wave usually are less than 0.15 second apart, whereas the interval between the apices of the T and U waves is more than 0.15 second.[66]

The origin of the U wave has been disputed. Its characteristics are not compatible with the Purkinje or ventricular muscle repolarization hypothesis. The timing of the U wave during ventricular relaxation and the links between the U wave and mechanical events favor the mechanoelectrical hypothesis of U wave genesis. Unfortunately, little research has been done to test this hypothesis.[65]

Common Normal Variants

$S_1S_2S_3$ PATTERN

In a large number of normal adults the S wave is present in all standard limb leads. The S waves are recorded when the terminal QRS vectors, originating from the outflow tract of the right ventricle or the posterobasal septum, are directed superiorly and rightward. Hiss et al.[19] found an $S_1S_2S_3$ pattern in more than 20 percent of normal subjects. The incidence of a true $S_1S_2S_3$ pattern, in which the S wave amplitude equals or

exceeds the R wave amplitude in each of the three standard limbs, is much lower. More commonly, the amplitude of the S waves in leads II and III is greater than that of the R waves in these leads, but the S_1 is smaller than R_1.

When the R/S ratio equals 1 in all three standard limb leads, the frontal plane mean QRS axis cannot be determined. Such QRS axis is usually referred to as an *indeterminate axis*. The $S_1S_2S_3$ pattern should be distinguished from abnormal left axis deviation. In the latter case, the S_3 is larger than the S_2, whereas the reverse is true in the $S_1S_2S_3$ pattern.

An $S_1S_2S_3$ pattern also is seen in patients with right ventricular hypertrophy or pulmonary emphysema. In some healthy persons the $S_1S_2S_3$ pattern is associated with an RSR^1 complex in lead V_1. This combination of findings resembles a pattern seen in patients with right ventricular hypertrophy.

RSR^1 PATTERN IN LEAD V_1

An RSR^1 (or rSr^1 pattern) in lead V1 with a QRS duration of less than 0.12 second is found in 2.4 percent of healthy individuals[67] (see Figure 5–13). The incidence of this pattern is higher in leads V_{3R} and V_{4R}. The secondary R wave has been attributed to physiologic late activation of the crista supraventricularis of the right ventricular outflow tract, the base of the interventricular septum, or both. The RSR^1 pattern in lead V_1 also is seen in patients with organic heart disease, including those with right ventricular hypertrophy and other pathologic states. The differential diagnosis of the RSR^1 pattern in lead V_1 is discussed in Chapter 5.

"EARLY REPOLARIZATION" VARIANT

A small degree of ST segment elevation, especially in the precordial leads, is present in most healthy individuals. Occasionally, however, the elevation is more pronounced in some of the leads and mimics the changes associated with myocardial injury or pericarditis (see Figure 1–23). This is usually a variant of a normal male pattern, discussed previously, and is under consideration in the differential diagnosis of acute myocardial ischemia (see Chapter 7) and pericarditis (see Chapter 11). The term "early repolarization" lacks precise definition because there are no defined criteria for the upper limits of ST elevation in normal young males with male pattern. It has been suggested that the pattern of early repolarization is an electrocardiographic predictor of enhanced aerobic fitness.[68]

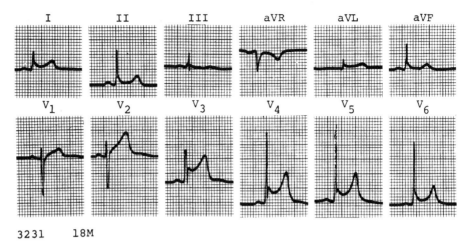

3231   18M

Figure 1–23   ST segment elevation is observed in most leads as a normal variant in an 18-year-old man. Note the notching and slurring of the terminal portion of the QRS complex.

POOR R WAVE PROGRESSION IN PRECORDIAL LEADS

The widely used term "poor R wave progression" is not helpful. In many cases the abnormally low R amplitude extending from the right into the middle or left precordial leads indicates myocardial infarction of the anterior wall. Such a pattern occurs also in the presence of left ventricular hypertrophy and in normal subjects (see Figure 1–24) without cardiac or pulmonary disease. It may be caused by a shift of the transitional zone to the left or by an atypical (abnormally high) placement of the mid-precordial chest electrodes. For this reason it is advisable to report the most likely cause of "poor R wave progression" in each case. This pattern is discussed also in Chapter 8 in the context of pseudoinfarction patterns.

ATHLETE'S HEART

The ECGs of trained athletes often presents findings considered abnormal by usual standards. One of the best-known and most common physiologic changes in athletes is slowing of the heart rate, attributed to an increase in vagal tone. Sinus bradycardia with a heart rate of 30 to 40 beats/min at rest is not uncommon, especially in highly trained endurance athletes.[69,70] Sinus pauses longer than 2 seconds are observed on the ambulatory ECG of more than one third of athletes.[69,70] First-degree atrioventricular (AV)

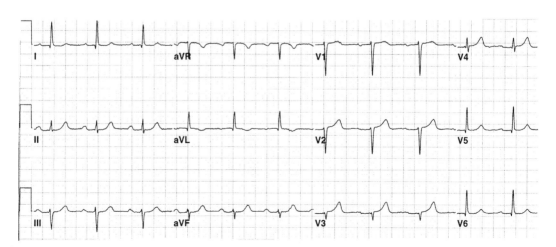

Figure 1–24   ECG of a 78-year-old woman who has no evidence of structural heart disease and no echocardiographic abnormalities. Note the low R wave in lead V_3 in a low-amplitude QRS complex inscribed near the transition zone.

block is seen in a similar percentage of these athletes.[69] Second-degree AV block with Wenckebach phenomenon may also occur.[69-71] Junctional escape complexes or junctional escape rhythm may be present. The bradyarrhythmias and AV conduction delays generally become less pronounced or disappear upon cessation of training.[42,71]

Echocardiographic studies in athletes often show an increase in the left and right ventricular mass and cavity dimensions, increased left ventricular wall thickness, and left atrial enlargement.[72-74] Ventricular dilatation is seen more frequently when the training is primarily isotonic rather than isometric.

Increased P wave amplitude and notching are noted occasionally on the ECG. The QRS voltage is increased to suggest left or right ventricular hypertrophy. The reported incidence of left or right ventricular hypertrophy varies considerably depending on the criteria used for the diagnosis.[42,74] An increase in QRS voltage may occur after only a few months of training, and the voltage decreases after deconditioning, although slowly.[42]

The normal variant of ST segment elevation is believed to be more prevalent among trained athletes. The T waves are often tall, especially in the precordial leads. These ST segment and T wave changes may regress after cessation of training.[42] Inverted or biphasic T waves in the precordial or limb leads may be present in athletes who lack objective evidence of coronary artery disease[75,76] (Figure 1-25). These T wave changes often are labile and may be normalized by physiologic and pharmacologic maneuvers.[77]

In an Italian study of 1005 consecutive athletes who were participating in 38 sporting disciplines, ECGs were distinctly abnormal in 14 percent and mildly abnormal in 26 percent of subjects. Diffuse T wave abnormalities without evidence of structural heart disease were present in 27 athletes.[78] In a Spanish study,[79] 26 athletes with negative T waves ≥2 mm in three or more leads had no evidence of heart disease and no adverse effects in the follow-up. In a study of 1282 professional football players,[80] frequent and complex ventricular tachyarrhythmias unassociated with structural heart disease and no adverse clinical effects were recorded in 355 trained athletes.[81]

OBESITY AND EDEMA

Most obese patients without clinical heart disease have normal ECGs, with the mean QRS vector shifting to the left with increasing obesity.[82] Both an increase and a decrease of voltage have been reported.[82,83] In morbidly obese subjects, the axes of P, QRS, and T waves are more leftward and low. QRS voltage, criteria for left ventricular hypertrophy, left atrial abnormalities, and T wave flattening were found to be significantly more common than in lean controls.[84] Figure 1-26 shows an ECG of a 45-year-old woman who weighs more than 400 lb. Of note is the left axis deviation and normal QRS voltage in the limb leads but attenuated QRS voltage in the precordial leads. QRS voltage is also decreased in the presence of anasarca.[85,86]

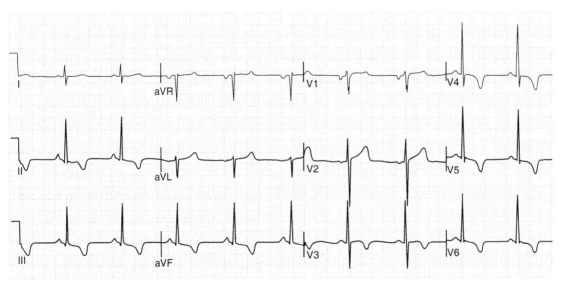

Figure 1–25 Abnormal ECG of a 49-year old male marathon runner without cardiac complaints. Cardiac examination, including blood pressure echocardiogram and nuclear stress test, was normal.

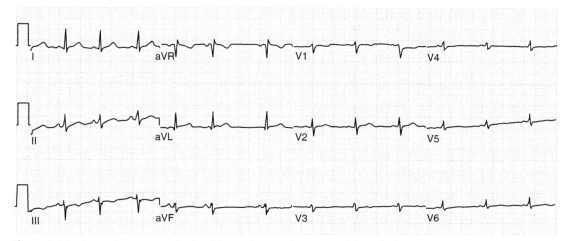

Figure 1–26   Low voltage due to obesity of the trunk. ECG of a 45-year-old, morbidly obese woman referred for bariatric surgery. ECG is normal. The voltage is within normal limits in the limb leads but below normal limits in leads V_1–V_6.

REFERENCES

1. Surawicz B: Electrocardiogram. *In:* Chatterjee K, Parmley WW (eds): Cardiology. Philadelphia, JB Lippincott, 1991.
2. Einthoven W, Fahr G, De Waart A: Ueber die Richtung und die manifeste Groesse der Potentialschwankungen im menschlichen Herzen und ueber den Einfluss der Herzlage auf die Form des Elektrokardiograms. Pfluegers Arch 150:275, 1913.
3. Surawicz B: Electrophysiologic Basis of ECG and Cardiac Arrhythmias. Baltimore, Williams & Wilkins, 1995.
4. Holland RP, Brooks H: TQ-ST segment mapping: critical review and analysis of current concepts. Am J Cardiol 40:110, 1977.
5. Wilson FN, Johnston FD, Macleod AG, et al: Electrocardiograms that represent the potential variations of a single electrode. Am Heart J 9:447, 1934.
6. Goldberger E: A simple, indifferent, electrocardiographic electrode of zero potential and a technique of obtaining augmented unipolar extremity leads. Am Heart J 23:483, 1942.
7. Anderson ST, Pahlm O, Selvester RH, et al: Panoramic display of the orderly sequenced 12-lead ECG. J Electrocardiol 27:347, 1994.
8. Dower GE: In defence of the intrinsic deflection. Br Heart J 24:55, 1962.
9. Binkley PF, Bush CA, Fleishman BL, et al: In vivo validation of the origin of the esophageal electrocardiogram. J Am Coll Cardiol 7:813, 1986.
10. Chou TC, Helm RA: Clinical Vectorcardiogram. Orlando, Grune & Stratton, 1967.
11. Chou TC: When is the vectorcardiogram superior to the scalar electrocardiogram? J Am Coll Cardiol 8:791, 1986.
12. Van Oosterom A, Oostendorp TF, Huiskamp GJ, et al: The magnetocardiogram as derived from electrocardiographic data. Circ Res 67:1503, 1990.
13. Green LS, Lux RL, Haws CW, et al: Effect of age, sex, and body habitus on QRS and ST-T potential maps of 1100 normal subjects. Circulation 71:244, 1985.
14. Li G, Lian J, Salla P, et al: Body surface Laplacian electrocardiogram of ventricular depolarization in normal subjects. J Cardiovasc Electrophys 14:16, 2002.
15. Simson MB: Signal-averaged electrocardiography. *In:* Zipes DP, Jalife J (eds): Cardiac Electrophysiology. From Cell to Bedside. Philadelphia, Saunders, 1990.
16. Boineau JP, Canavan TE, Schuessler RB, et al: Demonstration of a widely distributed atrial pacemaker complex in the human heart. Circulation 77:1221, 1988.
17. Durrer D, Van Dam RT, Freud GE, et al: Total excitation of the isolated human heart. Circulation 41:899, 1970.
18. Caceres CA, Kelser GA: Duration of the normal P wave. Am J Cardiol 3:449, 1959.
19. Hiss RG, Lamb LE, Allen MF: Electrocardiographic findings in 67,375 asymptomatic patients. Am J Cardiol 6:200, 1960.
20. Lamb LE: Electrocardiography and Vectorcardiography. Philadelphia, Saunders, 1965.
21. Lepeschkin E: Modern Eletrocardiography. The P-Q-R-S-T-U Complex. Baltimore, Williams & Wilkins, 1951.
22. Lepeschkin E: Duration of electrocardiographic deflections and intervals: man. *In:* Altman PE, Dittmer DS (eds): Respiration and Circulation. Bethesda, Md, Federation of American Societies for Experimental Biology, 1971, p 277.
23. Castellanos A Jr, Castillo C, Agha A: Contribution of His bundle recording to the understanding of clinical arrhythmias. Am J Cardiol 28:499, 1971.
24. Dhingra RC, Rosen KM, Rahimtoola SH: Normal conduction intervals and responses in 61 patients using His bundle recording and atrial pacing. Chest 64:55, 1973.
25. Narula OS, Scherlag RJ, Samet P, et al: Atrioventricular block: localization and classification by His bundle recordings. Am J Med 50:146, 1971.
26. Charles MA, Benziner TA, Glasser SP: Atrial injury current in pericarditis. Arch Intern Med 131:657, 1973.
27. Durrer D: Electrical aspects of human cardiac activity: a clinical-physiological approach to excitation and stimulation. Cardiovasc Res 2:1, 1968.
28. Lepeschkin E, Surawicz B: The measurement of the duration of the QRS interval. Am Heart J 44:80, 1952.
29. Surawicz B: Stretching the limits of the electrocardiogram's diagnostic utility. J Am Coll Cardiol 32:483, 1998.
30. Okomoto N, Kaneko K, Simonson E, et al: Reliability of individual frontal plane axis determination. Circulation 44:213, 1971.
31. Simonson E: The effect of age on the electrocardiogram. Am J Cardiol 29:64, 1972.
32. Pipberger HV, Goldman MJ, Littman D, et al: Correlations of the orthogonal electrocardiogram and vectorcardiogram with constitutional variables in 518 normal men. Circulation 35:536, 1967.

33. Franz MR, Bargheer K, Rafflebeul W, et al: Monophasic action potential mapping in human subjects with normal electrocardiograms: direct evidence for the genesis of the T wave. Circulation 75:381, 1987.
34. Kossman CE: The normal electrocardiogram. Circulation 8:920, 1953.
35. Chia B-L, Tan H-C, Yip JWL: Electrocardiographic patterns in posterior chest leads (V7, V8, V9) in normal subjects. Am J Cardiol 85:911, 2000.
36. Leatham A: The chest lead electrocardiogram in health. Br Heart J 12:213, 1950.
37. Manning GW, Smiley JR: QRS-voltage criteria for left ventricular hypertrophy in a normal male population. Circulation 19:224, 1964.
38. Langner PH: An octaxial reference system derived from a nonequilateral triangle for frontal plane vectorcardiography. Am Heart J 49:696, 1955.
39. Feldman T, Childers RW, Borow KM, et al: Change in ventricular cavity size: differential effects on QRS and T wave amplitude. Circulation 72:495, 1985.
40. Mirvis DM: Evaluation of normal variations in S-T segment patterns by body surface isopotential mapping: S-T segment elevation in the absence of heart disease. Am J Cardiol 50:122, 1982.
41. Surawicz B: The pathogenesis and clinical significance of primary T-wave abnormalities. In: Schlant RC, Hurst JW (eds): Advances in Electrocardiography. Orlando, Grune & Stratton, 1972.
42. Huston TP, Puffer JC, Rodney WM: The athletic heart syndrome. N Engl J Med 313:24, 1985.
43. Lepeschkin E, Surawicz B: The measurement of the QT interval of the electrocardiogram. Circulation 6:378, 1952.
44. Lepeschkin E, Surawicz B: The duration of Q-U interval and its components in electrocardiograms of normal persons. Am Heart J 46:49, 1953.
45. Cowan JC, Yosoff K, Moore M, et al: Importance of lead selection in QT interval measurement. Am J Cardiol 61:83, 1988.
45a. Kligfield P, Gettes LS, Bailey JJ, et al: Recommendations for the standardization and interpretation of the electrocardiogram. A scientific statement from the American Heart Association Electrocardiography and Arrhythmias Committee, Council on Clinical Cardiology, the American College of Cardiology Foundation and the Heart Rhythm Society. Rhythm 4:394, 2007.
46. Surawicz B: Will QT dispersion play a role in clinical decision-making? J Cardiovasc Electrophysiol 7:777, 1996.
47. Moleiro F, Castellanos A, Diaz JO, et al: Dynamics of QT intervals encompassing secondary repolarization abnormalities during sudden but transient lengthening of the RR intervals. Am J Cardiol 91:883, 2003.
48. Bazett HC: An analysis of the time-relations of electrocardiograms. Heart 7:353, 1920.
49. Shipley RA, Hallaran WR: The four-lead electrocardiogram in two hundred normal men and women. Am Heart J 11:325, 1936.
50. Molnar J, Weiss JS, Rosenthal JE: The missing second: what is the correct unit for the Bazett corrected QT interval? Am J Cardiol 75:537, 1995.
51. Ahnve S, Erhardt L, Lundman T, et al: Effect of metoprolol on QT intervals after acute myocardial infarction. Acta Med Scand 208:223, 1980.
52. Browne KF, Zipes DP, Heger JJ, et al: Influence of the autonomic nervous system on the QT interval in man. Am J Cardiol 50:1099, 1982.
53. Malik M: Problems of heart rate correction in assessment of drug-induced QT prolongation interval. J Cardiovasc Electrophysiol 12:411, 2001
54. Sagie A, Larson MG, Goldberg RJ, et al: An improved method for adjusting the QT interval for heart rate (the Framingham Heart Study). Am J Cardiol 70:797, 1992.
55. Bexton RS, Vallin HO, Camm AJ: Diurnal variation of the QR interval: influence of the autonomic nervous system. Br Heart J 55:253, 1986.
56. Rasmussen V, Jensen G, Jansen KF: QT interval in 24-hour ambulatory ECG recordings from 60 healthy adult subjects. J Electrocardiol 24:91, 1991.
57. Morganroth J, Brozovich FV, McDonald JF, et al: Variability of the QT measurement in healthy men, with implications for selection of an abnormal QT value to predict drug toxicity and proarrhythmia. Am J Cardiol 67:774, 1991.
58. Molnar J, Zhang F, Weiss JS, et al: Diurnal pattern of QTc interval: how long is prolonged? J Am Coll Cardiol 27:76, 1996.
59. Viitasalo M, Karlajinen J: QT intervals at heart rates from 50 to 120 beats/min during 24-hour electrocardiographic recordings in 100 healthy men: effects of atenolol. Circulation 86:1439, 1992.
60. Ahnve S: Errors in the visual determination of corrected QT(QTc) interval during acute myocardial infarction. J Am Coll Cardiol 5:699, 1985.
60a. Kligfield P, Hancock W, Helfenbein ED, et al: Relation of QT interval measurements in evolving automated algorithms from different manufacturers of electrocardiographs. Am J Cardiol 98:88, 2006.
61. Bidoggia H, Maciel JP, Cappaloza N, et al: Sex differences in the electrocardiographic pattern of cardiac repolarization. Possible role of testosterone. Am Heart J 140:678, 2000.
62. Surawicz B, Parikh SR: Prevalence of male and female patterns of early ventricular repolarization in the normal ECG of males and females from childhood to old age. Am Coll Cardiol 40:1870, 2001.
63. Surawicz B, Parikh SR: Differences between ventricular repolarization in men and women: description, mechanism and implications. Ann Noninvasive Electrocardiol 8:333, 2003.
64. Bai C-X, Kurokawa J, Tamagawa M, et al: Nontranscriptional regulation of cardiac repolarization currents by testosterone. Circulation 112:1701, 2005.
65. Surawicz B: U wave: facts, hypotheses, misconceptions, and misnomers. J Cardiovasc Electrophysiol 9:117, 1998.
66. Lepeschkin E: The U wave of the electrocardiogram. Mod Concepts Cardiovasc Dis 38:39, 1969.
67. Hiss RG, Lamb LE: Electrocardiographic findings in 122,043 individuals. Circulation 25:947, 1962.
68. Haydar ZR, Brantley DA, Gittings NS, et al: Early repolarization: an electrocardiographic predictor of enhanced aerobic fitness. Am J Cardiol 85:204, 2000.
69. Talan DA, Bauernfeind RA, Ashley WW, et al: Twenty-four hour continuous ECG recordings in long-distance runners. Chest 82:19, 1982.
70. Vittasalo MD, Kala R, Eisala A: Ambulatory electrocardiographic recordings in endurance athletes. Br Heart J 47:213, 1982.
71. Meytes I, Kaplinsky E, Yahini JH, et al: Wenckebach A-V block. A frequent feature following heavy physical training. Am Heart J 90:42, 1975.
72. Zeppilli P, Fenici R, Sassara M, et al: Wenckebach second-degree A-V block in top-ranking athletes: an old problem revisited. Am Heart J 100:281, 1980.
73. Maron BJ: Structural features of the athlete heart as defined by echocardiography. J Am Coll Cardiol 7:190, 1986.
74. Roeske WR, O'Rourke RA, Klein A, et al: Noninvasive evaluation of ventricular hypertrophy in professional athletes. Circulation 53:286, 1976.

75. Nishimura T, Kambara H, Chen CH, et al: Noninvasive assessment of T-wave abnormalities in precordial electrocardiograms in middle-aged professional bicyclists. J Electrocardiol 14:357, 1981.

76. Oakley DG, Oakley CM: Significance of abnormal electrocardiogram in highly trained athletes. Am J Cardiol 50:985, 1982.

77. Zeppilli P, Pirrami MM, Sassara MM, et al: T-wave abnormalities in top-ranking athletes: effects of isoproterenol, atropine and physical exercise. Am Heart J 100:213, 1980.

78. Pelliccia A, Maron BJ, Culasso F, et al: Clinical significance of abnormal electrocardiographic patterns in trained athletes. Circulation 102:278, 2000.

79. Grima-Serra R, Estorch M, Carrio I, et al: Marked ventricular repolarization abnormalities in highly trained athletes' electrocardiograms: clinical and prognostic implications. J Am Coll Cardiol 36:1310, 2000.

80. Choo JK, Abernethy WB II, Hutter AM: Electrocardiographic observations in professional football players. Am J Cardiol 90:198, 2002.

81. Biffi A, Pelliccia A, Verdile L, et al: Long-term clinical significance of frequent and complex ventricular arrhythmias in trained athletes. J Am Coll Cardiol 40:446, 2002.

82. Frank S, Colliver JA, Frank A: The electrocardiogram in obesity: statistical analysis of 1029 patients. J Am Coll Cardiol 7:295, 1986.

83. Alpert MA, Terry BE, Cohen MV, et al: The electrocardiogram in morbid obesity. Am J Cardiol 85:908, 2000.

84. Madias JE, Agarwal H, Win M, et al: Effect of weight loss in congestive heart failure from idiopathic dilated cardiomyopathy on electrocardiographic QRS voltage. Am J Cardiol 89:86, 2002.

85. Madias JE, Bazaz R, Agarwal H, et al: Anasarca-mediated attenuation of the amplitude of electrocardiographic complexes: a description of a heretofore unrecognized phenomenon. J Am Coll Cardiol 38:756, 2001.

86. Kudo Y, Yamasaki F, Kataoka H, et al: Effect of serum albumin on QRS wave amplitude in patients free of heart disease. Am J Cardiol 95:789, 2005.

2 Atrial Abnormalities

Atrial Depolarization

Atrial depolarization is represented by the P wave, which is a deflection of low amplitude and therefore difficult to scrutinize for morphologic details without amplification. The range of normal variations in shape, duration, and amplitude is fairly wide, which limits the specificity of P wave abnormalities. In addition, the wide availability of echocardiography, which is capable of precisely measuring atrial dimensions, has decreased the role of electrocardiography in diagnosing atrial abnormalities. Despite these problems, proper assessment of the P wave may be of great value for augmenting the utility of the electrocardiogram (ECG) as a diagnostic tool in clinical practice. The analysis of atrial abnormalities may be facilitated by a brief review of factors fundamental to the origin of the P wave.

UNICENTRIC AND MULTICENTRIC PACEMAKER

The prevailing notion until the early 1990s was that the normal impulse always originates in the core of the sinoatrial (SA) node and then spreads via the transitional cells and the crista terminalis to the rest of the atrial cells. The unicentric

hypothesis has been seriously challenged by Boineau and co-workers,[1] who studied atrial activation in patients undergoing open heart operations for Wolff-Parkinson-White (WPW) syndrome using a template containing 156 pairs of bipolar electrode pairs attached to the anterior and posterior surfaces of both atria. The maps obtained in these studies revealed an extensively distributed system of atrial pacemakers, mostly along the crista terminalis. The predominant clustering of sites was confined to a corridor 1.5 cm wide and 7.5 cm long, located along the junction between the superior vena cava and the right atrium, that extends posteriorly to the inferior limbus of the inferior vena cava. In 50 percent of subjects the impulse originated at more than one site (i.e., it was multicentric).

The important discovery of the multicentric origin of the P wave within a widely distributed area of the right atrium does not change the explanation of normal P wave morphology. This is because the unicentric and multicentric impulses originate predominantly on the posterior wall of the right atrium, and thus the differences in the propagation to the more distal sites are relatively small. This suggests that unless the impulse is formed on the anterior wall of the right atrium or in the left atrium, the relatively minor differences resulting from the change of the pacemaker site on the posterior wall of the right atrium are likely to escape recognition without detailed mapping of atrial activity.

ATRIAL ACTIVATION

A typical propagation from the region of the SA node proceeds along two pathways. One moves inferiorly along the crista terminalis of the posterior right atrium through the intercaval region to the posterior left atrium, and the other moves superiorly and anteriorly over Bachmann's bundle to the left atrium.

In the studies of Boineau et al.,[1] the total right atrial activation time was 57 ms, and the left atrial activation ended at 110 ms, resulting in an activation phase difference of 53 ms between the two atria. Normal P wave duration on the surface ECG in adults ranges from 70 to 140 ms.

Knowledge of the atrial activation sequence is of importance to diagnostic and ablation studies using intracardiac catheter electrodes. Josephson et al.[2] found the following average activation times in patients with normal P waves: high right atrium, 15 ms; mid-right atrium, 12 ms (in about half of individuals, activation at this site preceded the high right atrial site); low right atrium, 41 ms; atrioventricular (AV) junction (i.e., site of His bundle potential recording), 43 ms; and coronary sinus, 77 ms. In the retrograde direction the earliest excitation site was at the AV junction. The low right atrium was excited within 15 to 27 ms; the coronary sinus, within 21 to 55 ms; and the high right atrium, within 31 to 65 ms after the AV junction. Activation recorded by the electrode in the coronary sinus has been used to time left atrial activation. Similar information can be obtained by recording from the esophagus or pulmonary artery.[3]

Electroanatomic analysis of the sinus impulse propagation in the normal human atria confirmed the important role of Bachmann's bundle in interatrial propagation.[4]

CORRELATION WITH PRECORDIAL P WAVE MAPPING

Detailed precordial mapping using 150 disk electrodes by Mirvis[5] showed that P waves are negative on the upper anterior chest and positive on the lower part of the chest. The biphasic positive-negative configuration is seen in leads V_1 and V_2.

During the initial half of the P wave, the maximum is on the left mid-precordium and negative potentials are over the upper back.

Subsequently, the maximum migrates to the left and the negative potentials into the precordial area. Near the end of the P wave, the maximum shifts to the left back, and the minimum evolves in the left precordium. This pattern can be explained simply by the initial anteriorly directed right atrial activation front followed by the posteriorly directed left atrial activation front. Because each distribution had only a single maximum and a single minimum, the findings were consistent with a single dipole equivalent cardiac generator, as reported earlier by Taccardi.[6] The diphasic positive-negative P wave in leads V_1 and V_2 can be attributed to the electrode positions on the null line.

GENERAL APPROACH TO RECOGNIZING P WAVE ABNORMALITIES

It appears that the surface ECG reflects major trends in the direction of atrial excitation but cannot be relied upon to detect minor changes in the sequence of excitation. The normal P wave axis in the frontal plane is usually about 60 degrees. In leads I and II and the left precordial leads, the P wave is upright (Figure 2–1). In lead III, a biphasic P wave occurs in 7 percent of the normal population (Figure 2–2). The initial portion of the P wave corresponds to depolarization of the right atrial wall and is directed anteriorly. The terminal portion corresponds to depolarization of the left atrium and the inferior right atrial wall, and it is directed posteriorly. Because both deflections are directed downward and to the left, they tend to fuse and form a single deflection in the frontal plane. Careful inspection or amplification usually reveals a notch on the summit of the normal P wave. Visualization of these two components in normal persons is facilitated by inspecting the right precordial leads in which the P wave is usually biphasic (positive-negative) (see Figures 2–1 and 2–2) and by a vectorcardiographic display.[7] In the horizontal plane of the vectorcardiogram, the P wave loop is formed by an initially anteriorly directed right atrial portion and a terminal posteriorly directed left atrial portion.

The amplitude of the normal P wave usually does not exceed 0.25 mV, or 25 percent of the R wave, but the normal range is wide because of such variables as the position of the heart, proximity to the recording sites, degree of atrial filling, degree of atrial fibrosis, and other extracellular factors that influence the amplitude of ECG deflections on the body surface.

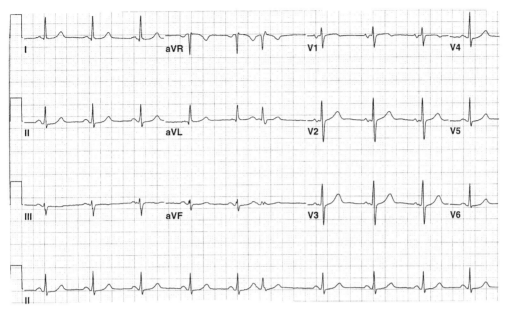

Figure 2–1 Normal P wave in a healthy 74-year-old woman. P wave duration is 120 ms. The P wave is positive in leads I, II, III, and V_3–V_6. It is positive-negative in leads V_1 and V_2. A premature atrial complex is conducted with aberration.

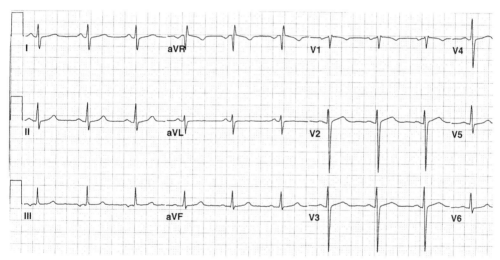

Figure 2–2 Normal P wave in a healthy 51-year-old man. P wave duration is 130 ms. The P wave is positive in leads I, II, and V_2–V_6. It is positive-negative in leads III and V_1.

P WAVE ABNORMALITIES ORIGINATING IN OR NEAR THE SINUS NODE

The normal thickness of the atrium is 1 to 2 mm. Each atrium weighs about 20 g, and the inter-atrial septum weighs 10 to 20 g. In response to increases in volume and pressure, atria primarily dilate and hypertrophy.

Many terms are used to interpret P wave abnormalities. The term *atrial enlargement* generally is used to imply the presence of atrial hypertrophy, dilatation, or both. As discussed later in the chapter, similar P wave changes may occur in the absence of such structural abnormalities. Hemodynamic alterations, heart rate, autonomic tone, position of the heart in the chest, conduction defects, and other factors may also be responsible for the changes. It has therefore been suggested that a less specific term, such as *atrial abnormality*, be used during the ECG diagnosis of P wave abnormalities. Atrial abnormalities can be grouped into three categories: (1) right atrial abnormalities; (2) left atrial abnormalities; and (3) interatrial conduction disturbances.

Right Atrial Abnormalities

Two ECG patterns are characteristic of a right atrial abnormality: right atrial hypertrophy and P pulmonale.

RIGHT ATRIAL HYPERTROPHY

ECG changes attributed to right atrial hypertrophy consist of tall P waves in both limb and right precordial leads, signifying a dominant anteriorly and inferiorly directed major P wave component. Because the right atrial forces are responsible for only the early part of the P wave, any increase in the duration of right atrial activation usually does not prolong the total duration of the P wave.

The ECG changes considered to be suggestive of right atrial hypertrophy correlate poorly with the clinical and anatomic findings. The two most common P wave changes in patients with congenital heart disease, tricuspid valve disease, or chronic cor pulmonale are (1) a P wave axis in the frontal plane of +75 degrees or more and (2) a positive deflection of the P wave in lead V_1 or V_2 > 0.15 mV (Figure 2–3). The characteristic pattern of P pulmonale (see later discussion) is less specific for right atrial hypertrophy.

RIGHTWARD DEVIATION OF THE P WAVE AXIS

Rightward or medial displacement of the P wave axis in the frontal plane is found in a significant number of patients with right atrial enlargement. The reported incidence is variable, as different values (+60 to +80 degrees) have been used to define the rightward displacement. The upper limit of +75 degrees is chosen here, based on the large series of normal subjects studied by Hiss and associates.[8] When the P axis is beyond +75 degrees, the P wave becomes small in lead I and negative in lead aV_L. It may become isoelectric in lead I if the axis is +90 degrees. An axis of more than +90 degrees is uncommon. It is significant that right atrial enlargement secondary to chronic obstructive pulmonary disease (COPD) is associated with a much higher incidence of rightward shift of the P wave axis than that due to other causes.[9] In fact, in patients with congenital heart disease, the P wave in lead I may be taller than that in lead III.[10] The term "P congenitale" has been used to describe this type of P wave. The right-axis deviation of the P wave is not specific for right atrial enlargement; it is frequently present in patients with pulmonary emphysema without cor pulmonale and with other conditions (discussed later).

TALL P WAVE IN LEAD V_1 OR V_2

The initial positive deflection of the P wave in the right precordial leads is normally less than 1.5 mm in amplitude.[11] An abnormally tall

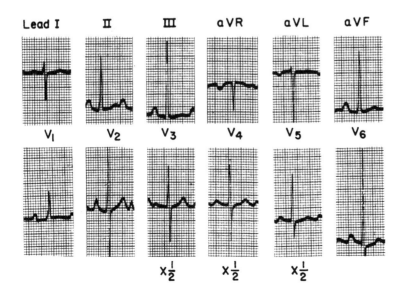

Figure 2–3 ECG of a 19-year-old woman with tetralogy of Fallot, showing right axis deviation, biventricular hypertrophy, and right atrial enlargement. Note the tall positive P waves in leads II, III, aV_F, and V_2.

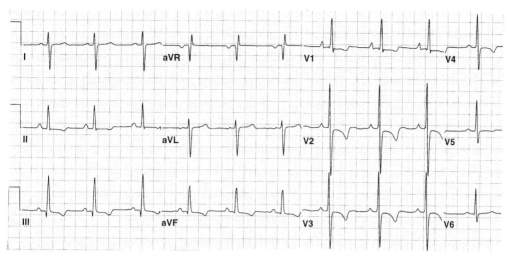

Figure 2–4   Pattern of right atrial enlargement. Note the tall positive P wave in lead V_1 in a 23-year-old man with pulmonary hypertension secondary to multiple pulmonary emboli in the setting of coagulopathy. ECG also shows right ventricular hypertrophy. Right atrial and right ventricular enlargements were confirmed by echocardiography.

P wave in leads V_1 or V_2 is seen in slightly more than 10 percent of patients with chronic cor pulmonale (Figure 2–4). In these patients a large negative component of the P wave simulating left atrial enlargement may be present (see later discussion). In such cases a negative or biphasic P wave in V_1 may be accompanied by a tall, peaked P wave in lead V_2. This sudden transition often leads one to suspect that the P wave changes in lead V_1 result from right, rather than left, atrial involvement. Biatrial enlargement should also be considered. This phenomenon also occurs occasionally in patients with isolated right atrial enlargement due to congenital heart disease, but monophasic, abnormally tall P waves in leads V_1 and V_2 are encountered more frequently in the latter condition than in patients with chronic cor pulmonale (Figure 2–3).[12] As a rule, an abnormally tall P wave in the right precordial leads is a more specific finding for right atrial enlargement than the diagnostic criteria based on the limb leads.[13] An initial positive component of the P wave in lead V_1 of >0.04 second has been also suggested as an indication of right atrial enlargement.[14]

P PULMONALE

The term *P pulmonale* is used to describe the tall, peaked ("gothic") P wave in leads II, III, and aV_F resulting in a P axis of more than 70 degrees (Figure 2–5). In patients with clinical evidence of chronic cor pulmonale, the P pulmonale pattern is present in about 20 percent of cases.[9,15]

A similar incidence exists in autopsy series.[9,17] The P pulmonale pattern is seen more frequently in patients with congenital heart disease, such as pulmonic stenosis, tetralogy of Fallot, Eisenmenger physiology, or tricuspid atresia, and in patients with pulmonary hypertension not caused by COPD. It has been reported that the tallest P waves are present in patients with an increase in both right atrial pressure and arterial desaturation.[12] On the other hand, volume overload of the right atrium without an increase in pressure is often associated with a near-normal P wave amplitude in the inferior leads, as in the case of atrial septal defect without pulmonary hypertension.[18]

P pulmonale is a widely recognized hallmark of diffuse lung disease.[19] Correlation with abnormal lung function was consistently better for the P wave axis than for the P wave amplitude, and the rightward axis shift was the most discriminating P wave change when evaluating the severity of COPD.[20] In patients with severe lung disease caused by interstitial pulmonary fibrosis, the P waves are usually normal,[21] suggesting that the axis shift is due to hyperinflation of the lungs.[17]

The P pulmonale pattern is most likely caused by the combination of a low diaphragm position and increased sympathetic stimulation. The former contributes to the vertical P axis, and the latter to increased amplitude. Because the influence of these two factors varies, the pattern of P pulmonale also tends to wax and wane in the same person depending on the heart rate or severity of bronchospasm.[22] Moreover,

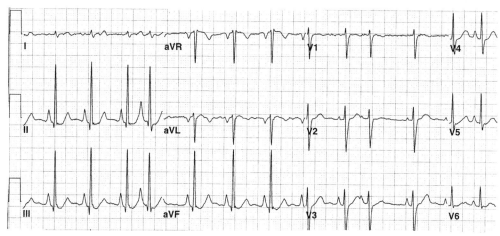

Figure 2–5 Typical P pulmonale pattern in a 71-year-old man with severe chronic obstructive airway disease. Atrial premature complexes are present.

arterial desaturation tends to increase the amplitude and peaking of the P wave.[10] The transient appearance of the P pulmonale has been observed in patients with acute pulmonary embolism.[23] The effect of emphysema on the position of the atria and the P wave amplitude and direction may be attributed to closer contact of the right atrium with the diaphragm and perhaps a change in the direction of the depolarization wavefront caused by stretching of atrial fibers. Sympathetic stimulation results in a more synchronous atrial depolarization, which causes increased amplitude and shorter duration of the P wave[24] (Figure 2–6).

There is no good overall correlation between P pulmonale and right atrial enlargement. P pulmonale may be present in the absence of heart or lung disease. A tall, peaked P wave may be seen in healthy subjects with asthenic body build and is probably related to the vertical position of the heart. The P wave amplitude often increases with

the standing position.[25] It may occur during expiratory efforts against pressure[26] or in patients with left pericardial defects who lack the restraining influence of the pericardium.[27] It also occurs during tachycardia and exercise (see Figure 2–6). Increased cardiac output and sympathetic stimulation may be responsible for the changes under these circumstances.[10]

For the reasons mentioned previously, there is no relation between the weight of the right atrium and the amplitude, duration, or axis of the P wave.[28] Chou and Helm[29] showed that in about half of the studied cases, P pulmonale was associated with conditions in which right atrial enlargement was not expected, and that in 36 percent of cases the P pulmonale pattern appeared to represent left atrial rather than right atrial enlargement. Figure 2–7 illustrates the pseudo P pulmonale pattern in patients with hypertensive disease with or without congestive heart failure. Figure 2–8 depicts a proposed mechanism for the appearance

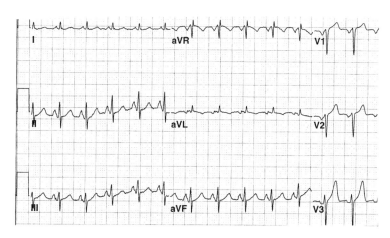

Figure 2–6 Tall, peaked narrow P waves resembling P pulmonale during tachycardia in a healthy 77-year-old woman. In the absence of tachycardia, the P wave amplitude and configuration were normal (not shown).

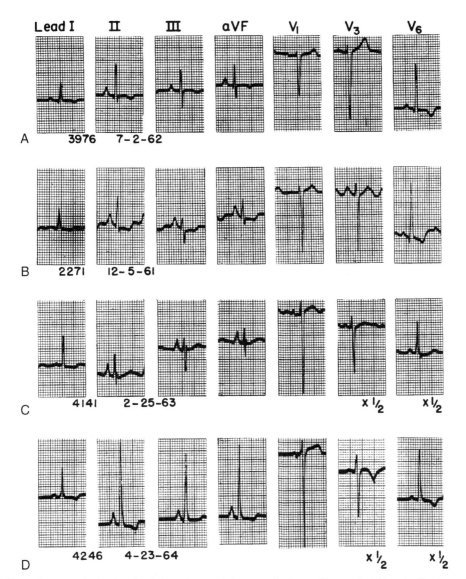

Figure 2–7   Tall P waves in the limb leads in patients with hypertensive heart disease mimicking the P pulmonale pattern. **A, B,** Records from patients with hypertensive heart disease without heart failure. **C, D,** Records from patients with hypertensive heart disease and early or questionable left ventricular failure. (From Chou T-C, Helm RA: The pseudo P pulmonale. Circulation 32:96, 1965.)

of the P pulmonale pattern in patients with left atrial enlargement.

The P pulmonale pattern has been described also in patients with coronary artery disease and angina pectoris.[30] Ischemia of the left atrial musculature was considered to be the cause of the increased voltage of the P wave and the rightward shift of the P wave axis.[26]

A prominent atrial T (Ta) wave often accompanies a tall P wave.[31] The amplitude of the negative deflection in the inferior leads may exceed 0.1 mV. Because the atrial T wave may last as

long as 0.45 second, the negative deflection in these leads may cause apparent depression of the ST segment (Figure 2–9).

ECHOCARDIOGRAPHIC CORRELATIONS

Kaplan et al.[32] correlated changes in right atrial volume in 100 patients with right atrial enlargement (average volume 147.6 mL) and 25 control subjects (average volume 35.0 mL) with various ECG criteria for right atrial enlargement. The best

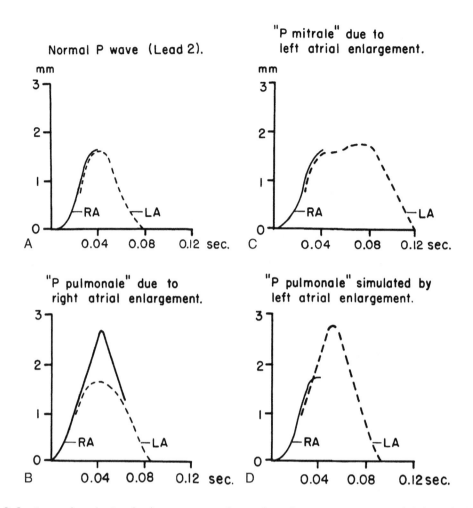

Figure 2–8   Proposed mechanism for the appearance of a P pulmonale pattern in patients with left atrial enlargement. **A,** Right and left atrial components of a normal P wave. **B,** P pulmonale pattern resulting from right atrial enlargement with an increase in the amplitude of the right atrial component of the P wave. **C,** P mitrale pattern associated with left atrial enlargement due to an increase in the left atrial component in amplitude and duration. Some associated intraatrial conduction defect may be responsible for prolongation of the P wave duration. **D,** Pseudo P pulmonale pattern in left atrial enlargement. The amplitude of the left atrial component is increased without marked prolongation of the duration of left atrial depolarization. (From Chou T-C, Helm RA: The pseudo P pulmonale. Circulation 32:96, 1965.)

predictors of right atrial enlargement were a P wave amplitude of >1.5 mm in lead V_1, a QRS axis of more than 90 degrees, and an R/S ratio of more than 1 in lead V_1 in the absence of complete right bundle branch block. The combined sensitivity of these criteria was 48 percent with 100 percent specificity.

Left Atrial Abnormality

The term *left atrial abnormality* describes an interatrial conduction disturbance in which the duration of the middle and terminal P wave components is prolonged owing to delayed left

atrial activation. Because of the direction of spread of the depolarization process and the anatomic orientation of the left atrium, the left atrial forces are directed leftward and posteriorly. An increase in the left atrial forces may therefore exaggerate these normal characteristics of the late portion of the P wave. The various criteria for diagnosis of left atrial enlargement (often called *abnormality*) are based essentially on these changes.

The wide separation between the anteriorly and posteriorly directed P wave components is reflected in a notched P wave in the limb leads and a prolonged interval between the peak and the nadir of the biphasic P wave in the right precordial leads. Intracardiac leads show that

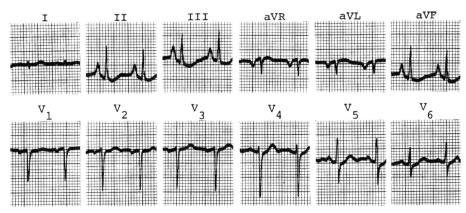

Figure 2–9 P pulmonale pattern in a 44-year-old woman with chronic obstructive lung disease. Frontal plane P axis is displaced toward the right (+85 degrees). ST segment depression in leads II, III, and aV_F is probably due to prominent atrial T waves. Negative P waves are visible in the right precordial leads.

activation of left atrial tissue recorded by the electrode in the coronary sinus is delayed by an average of 35 ms compared with a normal P wave (i.e., activation time 112 ms vs. 77 ms).[2] The delay probably takes place in Bachman's bundle because clamping of this bundle prolongs the interatrial conduction time to a similar degree.

The diagnostic criteria are as follows:

1. The P terminal force in lead V_1 is equal to or more negative than -0.04 mVsec (Figures 2–10 and 2–11). This measurement

(mVsec) is the product of the depth of the terminal negative deflection (in millivolts or millimeters) and its duration (in seconds).[33]

2. The P wave is notched with a duration of 0.12 second or more (P mitrale)[34] (see Figure 2–11).

3. Leftward shift of the P wave axis in the frontal plane to +15 degrees or beyond or a leftward shift of the terminal P forces in the frontal plane is present.

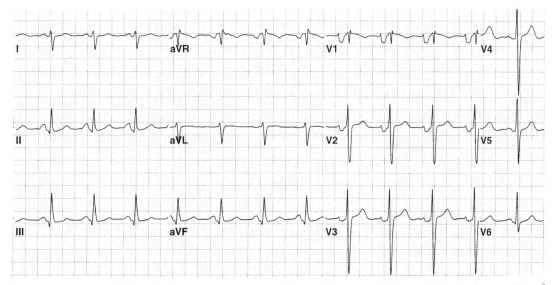

Figure 2–10 Pattern of left atrial enlargement in a 45-year-old man with severe mitral stenosis (mitral valve area 1.0 cm²), pulmonary artery pressure 60/30 mmHg, and right ventricular hypertrophy. P wave widening and notching is seen in leads I and II. In lead V_1 a small positive deflection is followed by a deep, wide negative deflection. Lead V_2 shows a relatively slow slope of the line connecting the positive peak with the negative nadir, reflecting the slow interatrial conduction characteristic of left atrial enlargement. See text discussion.

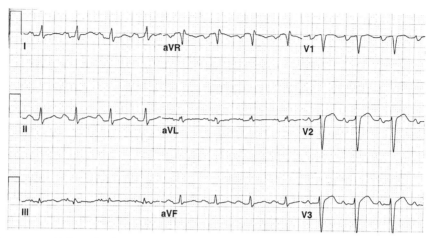

Figure 2–11   Pattern of left atrial enlargement in a 33-year-old man with severe dilated cardiomyopathy (left ventricular ejection fraction 15 percent). Enlargement of all four chambers was evident in the echocardiogram, but the ECG shows only left atrial enlargement, probably because the QRS voltage is diminished by massive obesity. P wave characteristics in the limb and right precordial leads are as in Figure 2–10.

CLINICAL AND ANATOMIC CORRELATION

P Terminal Force in Lead V1

Morris and associates[33] studied 100 normal subjects and 87 patients with aortic and mitral valve diseases. They found that the product of the amplitude and duration of the negative component of the P wave in lead V_1, which they termed the P terminal force at V_1 (TFP-V_1), is more negative than -0.03 mVsec in 2.5 percent of the normal population and in 92 percent of patients with left-sided valvular disease. In actual practice, the P terminal force may be determined by a visual estimate of the interval (i.e., the slope between the peak of the positive deflection and the nadir of the P wave). A terminal portion of the P wave in lead V_1 that occupies one small box on the recording paper in depth (-1.0 mm or 0.1 mV) and duration (0.04 second) yields a P terminal force of -0.04. Any terminal negative component of the P wave in lead V_1 of this magnitude or more suggests an increase in the delayed posterior left atrial depolarization.

In an evaluation of 62 patients with significant isolated mitral stenosis and left atrial enlargement proved at surgery,[35] the ECG met the Morris criterion in 68 percent of cases. Similar results have been obtained from other studies.[12,36] It has also been shown that the P terminal force correlates more closely with the left atrial volume than with left atrial pressure. This may explain the results of an anatomic correlation study[37] showing that an abnormal P terminal force in lead V_1 was present in only about half of the patients with increased left atrial weight.

A transient increase in the size of the negative component of the P wave in the right precordial leads is often seen in patients with left ventricular failure.[38] Romhilt and Scott[39] reported that signs of a left atrial abnormality satisfying the Morris criterion were present in 76 percent of patients during an acute episode of pulmonary edema.[27] It may be caused by an increase in left atrial pressure, as half of the patients no longer exhibited these P wave changes after 4 days of treatment.

Kasser and Kennedy[36] found that the Morris criteria[33] had limited specificity for predicting left atrial volume and pressure. In the experience of Chou,[13] a false-positive pattern of left atrial enlargement, suggested by a prominent negative P wave component in the right precordial leads, appeared most commonly in patients with COPD with or without cor pulmonale and no evidence of left-sided heart disease. A similar change occurs in patients with pectus excavatum[40] and in those with the straight-back syndrome.

Occasionally a prominent negative component of the P wave is seen in patients with a giant right atrium due to congenital heart disease. The markedly enlarged right atrium may be positioned on both the anterior and posterior views of the heart and more or less envelop the left atrium. The posterior atrial forces are now generated from the right atrium rather than the left atrium (Figure 2–12).

WIDE AND NOTCHED P WAVES

Prolongation of the P wave duration to 0.12 second or more in the limb leads reflects the same changes as the Morris criterion in the precordial

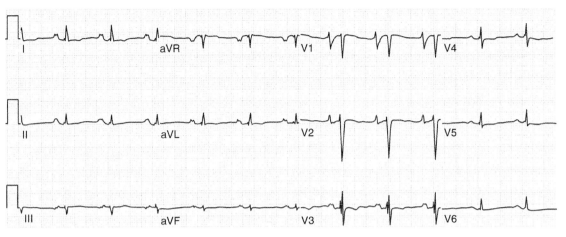

Figure 2–12   Pattern of right atrial enlargement with abnormal terminal P wave force in lead V₁ in a 25-year old woman who underwent corrective Fontan operation for tricuspid atresia in childhood. See text discussion.

leads (i.e., asynchrony of right and left atrial activation).[41] Prolonged P wave duration was present in about two thirds of patients with documented left atrial enlargement.[35,36] A significant positive relation appears to exist between the duration of the P wave and the degree of left atrial dilatation.[12,41] The correlation between P wave duration and left atrial volume is better than that with the left atrial pressure.[36] In autopsy studies, P wave duration also correlated better with the left atrial volume than with its weight.[9,42]

Minor notching or slurring of the P wave is found in one or more leads in most normal ECGs, particularly in the precordial leads. Definite bifid P waves with a peak-to-peak interval of more than 0.04 second, however, are not usually found in normal subjects.[43] Thomas and DeJong[43] observed prolongation of the interpeak interval in most patients with severe mitral stenosis. Other investigators found abnormal notching in slightly fewer than half of the

patients with left-sided heart disease.[33] Abnormal bifid P waves are also encountered in a significant number of patients with constrictive pericarditis,[43,44] probably due to atrial involvement by the compressing scar (Figure 2–13). In these patients the P wave duration may also be prolonged to mimic closely the P waves of patients with mitral disease.

The term *P mitrale* has been used to describe a P wave that is abnormally notched and wide because this P wave is commonly seen in patients with mitral valve disease, particularly mitral stenosis. The changes are most often present in leads I and II and the left precordial leads. The P mitrale pattern was observed in a third of patients with isolated mitral stenosis proved at surgery.[35] As indicated previously, these changes are not always due to dilatation or hypertrophy of the left atrium but rather may be caused by an intraatrial conduction defect secondary to atrial myocardial damage.[45]

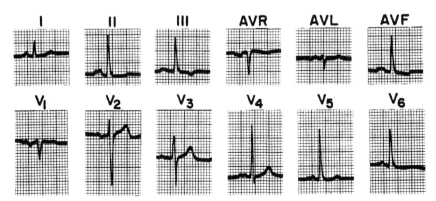

Figure 2–13   Abnormal notching and increased width of the P wave resembling P mitrale in a 58-year-old man with calcific constrictive pericarditis. The abnormal P wave is seen best in lead II.

Increased P wave duration in the limb leads is sometimes associated with increased P wave amplitude. An amplitude of more than 2.5 mm is seen in about 5 to 10 percent of patients with left atrial enlargement due to left-sided valvular heart disease, especially mitral valve disease or hypertensive heart disease.

When the duration of the P waves is not prolonged and the tall P waves are seen in inferior leads II, III, and aV_F, the changes closely mimic those of P pulmonale[29] (see Figure 2–6). In such cases an abnormal terminal force in lead V_1 and the presence of a left ventricular hypertrophy pattern aid in the differential diagnosis.

LEFTWARD SHIFT OF THE P WAVE AXIS

A leftward shift of the frontal plane P wave axis to less than +30 degrees or +15 degrees[31,35] is usually manifested by a late positive P deflection in lead aV_L and a negative terminal portion of the P wave in leads III and aV_F. These findings lack specificity and sensitivity. They occur in only about 10 percent of patients with left atrial enlargement caused by left-sided valvular disease and are present in about 5 percent of normal subjects. Conduction abnormalities in the atria or an ectopic atrial pacemaker may be responsible for some cases of abnormal leftward shift of the P vector.

ECHOCARDIOGRAPHIC CORRELATIONS

Chirife et al.[46] found that a P wave duration of >105 ms identified all patients with a left atrial dimension of >3.8 cm and had a specificity of 89 percent. In 307 patients studied by Waggoner et al.,[47] the combination of several ECG criteria had a predictive index of 63 percent for the presence and 78 percent for the absence of left atrial enlargement (left atrial dimension >4 cm). In 361 patients studied by Miller et al.,[48] the product of the amplitude and duration of the terminal component in lead V_1(PTF-V_1) of >0.06 mVsec correctly predicted left atrial enlargement in 80 percent of cases, with a positive predictive accuracy of 58 percent and a negative predictive accuracy of 83 percent. Velury and Spodick[49] found that among 51 patients with echocardiographic left atrial enlargement, the combined sensitivity of PTF-V_1 of >0.04 mVsec and P wave duration >100 ms was 82 percent. The criterion of increased PTF-V_1 alone had only 58 percent sensitivity, which suggested to the authors that in patients with left atrial enlargement, spatial vector forces other than those attributable to left atrial enlargement per se affect the ECG

configuration of the P wave in lead V_1. In the study of Lee et al[49a] biphasic P wave was specific for left atrial enlargement (92%), but sensitivity was low (12%).

Biatrial Enlargement: Diagnostic Criteria

The presence of biatrial enlargement may be suspected when signs of left and right atrial enlargement coexist. Because the two atria affect essentially different portions of the P wave, recognition of biatrial enlargement is not as difficult as in the case of biventricular hypertrophy. The diagnostic criteria are as follows:

1. The presence of a large diphasic P wave in lead V_1 with the initial positive component >1.5 mm and the terminal negative component reaching 1 mm in amplitude, >0.04 second in duration ("abnormal P terminal force"), or both (Figure 2–14)
2. The presence of a tall, peaked P wave (>1.5 mm) in the right precordial lead and a wide, notched P wave in the limb leads or left precordial leads (V_5 and V_6) (see Figure 2–14)
3. An increase in both the amplitude (≥2.5 mm) and duration (≥0.12 second) of the P wave in the limb leads

Atrial Enlargement in the Presence of Atrial Fibrillation

Thurmann and Janney[50] defined coarse f waves as those fibrillatory waves measuring >0.5 mm in amplitude and fine f waves as measuring ≤0.5 mm. They showed that coarse f waves in lead V_1 (≥1 mm) were associated with roentgenologic and anatomic evidence of left atrial enlargement or elevated left atrial pressure when available. However, in their study of 194 patients, 87 percent of those with coarse f waves in lead V_1 had rheumatic heart disease, and 88 percent of patients with fine f waves in lead V_1 had arteriosclerotic heart disease.

Skoulas and Horlick[51] noted that patients with untreated congestive heart failure often had coarse fibrillation, and the f waves became smaller with treatment. Atrial distension during failure was probably responsible for the increase in the size of the f waves. This phenomenon occurred more commonly in patients with coronary artery disease.

A significant correlation has been shown also between the coarse fibrillatory waves and an

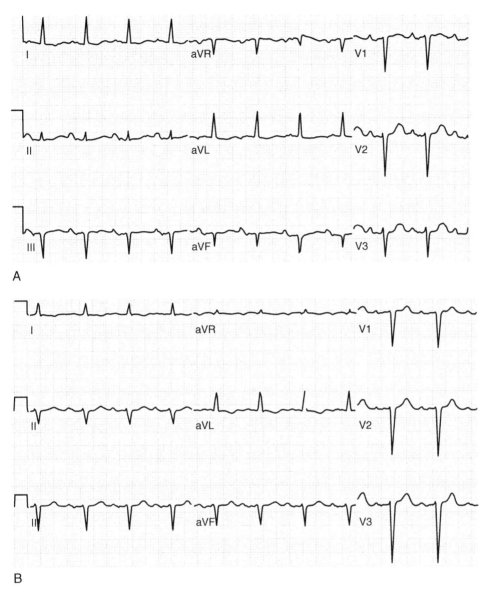

Figure 2–14   Two cases of echocardiographically documented biatrial enlargement. **A,** A 75-year-old woman with intermittent atrial flutter. **B,** A 62-year-old man with chronic rheumatic mitral and aortic valve disease. In both cases the P wave is wide and notched with a tall positive component and a wide shallow negative component in lead V_1.

abnormal P terminal force in lead V_1 during the sinus rhythm as defined by Morris and colleagues.[16,33] Fine f waves were usually associated with a normal P terminal force. Peter and associates suggested that the coarse fibrillatory waves (defined as ≥ 1 mm) should be considered signs of left atrial hypertrophy or "strain."[16] A few cases of coarse atrial fibrillation have been reported in patients with congenital heart disease and right atrial or biatrial enlargement.[52] Transient atrial fibrillation in patients with chronic cor pulmonale is often accompanied by large f waves in lead V_1.

NONSPECIFIC INTERATRIAL AND INTRAATRIAL CONDUCTION DISTURBANCES

In most cases the presence of a wide P wave is attributed to left atrial enlargement. In some cases, however, when a P wave of low or normal amplitude is considerably wider than normal and contains one or more notches (Figure 2–15), when the ECG criteria for left atrial enlargement are absent, and when no clinical suspicion or evidence of left atrial enlargement exists, the most proper ECG diagnosis is interatrial or intraatrial

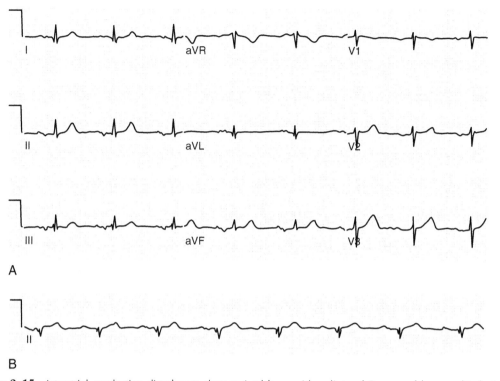

Figure 2–15   Intraatrial conduction disturbance characterized by a wide splintered P wave of low amplitude in two patients (ages 83 and 81 years). These patients had normal atrial dimensions on the echocardiogram and, except for age, no evidence of the heart diseases commonly associated with left atrial enlargement.

conduction disturbance (i.e., inter- or intraatrial block). This abnormality is not uncommon in patients with sick sinus syndrome and may be a precursor of atrial fibrillation.[53–55a] Abnormal notching of the P wave may also occur when there is an intraatrial conduction defect due to myocarditis, atrial ischemia, infarction, or fibrosis, which may also cause prolongation of the P wave. In one study interatrial block, defined as P wave duration ≥120 ms, was found in 40.6 percent of consecutive ECGs in hospitalized patients.[56]

In some cases the P wave duration can be wide. For instance, in a case reported by Soejima et al.,[57] the two components of a split P wave were separated by 400 ms; the first P wave represented activation of the lateral wall of the right atrium, and the second P wave represented activation of the medial right atrium and the left atrium.

In the early literature the term "interatrial conduction disturbance" referred to dissociated atrial rhythms[58] (see Chapter 14).

Atrial Repolarization

The atrial T wave (Ta) is usually directed opposite to the main P wave axis (i.e., Ta is negative in leads with an upright P wave) (Figure 2–16) and positive in leads with an inverted P wave. The atrial gradient (area under P + Ta) is normally close to zero. The Ta wave is frequently recognized in the presence of atrioventricular (AV) block. Hayashi et al.[59] found that in human subjects with AV block, the Ta/P wave amplitude ratio averaged 0.38. The duration of the Ta wave ranged from 230 to 384 ms and tended to be longer in a small subset of patients with "severe cardiovascular disease." In general, there is a direct correlation between the (P + Ta) and PP intervals,[59,60] suggesting that the (P + Ta) interval has the same meaning for the atria as the QT interval has for the ventricles.

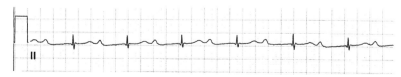

Figure 2–16   Atrial repolarization can be recognized as a shallow negative deflection after the P wave in a 90-year-old man with a long PR interval.

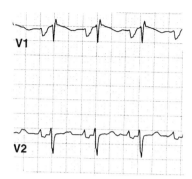

Figure 2–17 Slight ST segment elevation in lead V_1 and V_2 appears to be caused by the upsloping course of atrial repolarization following a negative P wave in a 55-year-old male heart transplant recipient.

The diagnostic importance of the relation between the P and Ta deflections (atrial gradient) is difficult to establish because the measurements require large amplification and can be carried out only in the presence of an AV block or a long PR interval.

As mentioned previously, atrial repolarization extending into the ST segment can cause a so-called false-positive ST segment depression,[61,62] particularly in the presence of a short PR interval.[63] Conversely, when the P wave is negative, atrial repolarization can simulate ST segment elevation. A possible example of such ST segment elevation is shown in Figure 2–17.

Summary

1. The increased amplitude of the positive P wave in the three standard limb leads and increased amplitude of the positive component of the biphasic or monophasic P wave in the right precordial leads suggests right atrial enlargement (or hypertrophy).

2. Vertical orientation of the P wave in limb leads with an increased amplitude but normal or subnormal duration (P pulmonale) attributed to low diaphragm position, hyperinflation of the lungs, and increased sympathetic stimulation are frequent findings in patients with COPD, bronchospasm, or acute cor pulmonale but may occur with or without right atrial enlargement.

3. Increased duration of the P wave with normal or increased P wave amplitude manifested by a notched P wave in limb leads or increased duration of the interval connecting the apex of the positive P wave component and the nadir of the negative P wave component in the right precordial leads signifies an interatrial conduction disturbance and suggests left atrial enlargement.

4. Increased duration (area) of the terminal negative P wave component in the right precordial leads suggests left atrial enlargement.

5. Increased amplitude of the negative terminal P wave component without an increased duration of this component and without an interatrial conduction disturbance is not a sign of left atrial enlargement.

6. Wide, notched, or polyphasic P waves of normal or low amplitude suggest an interatrial conduction disturbance with or without atrial enlargement.

REFERENCES

1. Boineau JP, Canavan TE, Schuessler RB, et al: Demonstration of a widely distributed atrial pacemaker complex in the human heart. Circulation 77:1221, 1988.
2. Josephson ME, Scharf DL, Kastor JA, et al: Atrial endocardial activation in man. Am J Cardiol 39:972, 1977.
3. Leier CV, Meacham JA, Schaal SF, et al: Interatrial conduction (activation) times. Am J Cardiol 44:442, 1979.
4. De Ponti R, Ho SY, Salerno-Uriarte JA: Electroanatomic analysis of sinus impulse propagation in normal human atria. J Cardiovasc Electrophysiol 13:1, 2002.
5. Mirvis DM: Body surface distribution of electrical potential during atrial depolarization and repolarization. Circulation 62:167, 1980.
6. Taccardi B: Body surface distribution of equipotential lines during atrial depolarization and ventricular repolarization. Circ Res 19:865, 1966.
7. Haywood LJ, Selvester RH: Analysis of right and left atrial vectorcardiograms. Circulation 33:577, 1966.
8. Hiss RG, Lamb LE, Allen MF: Electrocardiographic findings in 67:375 asymptomatic subjects. X. Normal values. Am J Cardiol 6:200, 1960.
9. Fowler NO, Daniels C, Scott RC, et al: The electrocardiogram in cor pulmonale with and without emphysema. Am J Cardiol 16:500, 1965.
10. Zimmerman HA, Bersano E, Dicosky C: The Auricular Electrocardiogram, Springfield IL, Charles C Thomas, 1968.
11. Leatham A: The chest lead electrocardiogram in health. Br Heart J 12:213, 1950.
12. DeOliveira JM, Zimmerman HA: Auricular overloadings: electrocardiographic analysis of 193 cases. Am J Cardiol 3:453, 1959.
13. Chou T-C: Electrocardiography. In: Clinical Practice. Adult and Pediatric, 4th ed. Philadelphia, Saunders, 1996, pp 23–36.
14. Dines DE, Parkin TW: Some observations on the value of the electrocardiogram in patients with chronic cor pulmonale. Mayo Clin Proc 40:745, 1965.
15. Kilcoyne MM, Davis AL, Ferrer MI: A dynamic electrocardiographic concept useful in the diagnosis of cor pulmonale: result of a survey of 200 patients with chronic obstructive pulmonary disease. Circulation 42:903, 1970.
16. Peter RH, Morris JJ Jr, McIntosh HD: Relationship of fibrillatory waves and P waves in the electrocardiogram. Circulation 33:599, 1966.
17. Surawicz B: Electrocardiographic diagnosis of chamber enlargement. J Am Coll Cardiol 8:711, 1986.
18. Sanchez-Cascos A, Deucher D: The P wave in atrial septal defect. Br Heart J 25:202, 1963.

19. Spodick DH: Electrocardiographic studies in pulmonary disease: establishment of criteria for the electrocardiographic inference of diffuse lung disease. Circulation 20:1073, 1959.

20. Calatayud JB, Abad JM, Khol NB, et al: P wave changes in chronic obstructive pulmonary disease. Am Heart J 79:444, 1970.

21. Ikeda K, Kubota K, Takahashi K, et al: P-wave changes in obstructive and restrictive lung disease. J Electrocardiol 18:233, 1985.

22. Harkavy J, Romanoff A: Electrocardiographic changes in bronchial asthma and their significance. Am Heart J 23:692, 1942.

23. Cutforth RH, Oram S: The electrocardiogram in pulmonary embolism. Br Heart J 20:41, 1958.

24. Irisawa H, Seyama I: The configuration of the P wave during mild exercise. Am Heart J 71:467, 1966.

25. Shleser IH, Langendorf R: The significance of the so-called P-pulmonale pattern in the electrocardiogram. Am J Med Sci 204:725, 1942.

26. Gross D: Contributions to the functional morphology of the P wave. Am Heart J 61:436, 1961.

27. Inoue H, Fujii J, Mashima S, et al: Pseudo right atrial overloading pattern in complete defect of the left pericardium. J Electrocardiol 14:413, 1981.

28. Mazzoleni A, Wolff L, Reiner L: Correlation between component cardiac weights and electrocardiographic patterns in 185 cases. Circulation 30:808, 1964.

29. Chou TC, Helm RA: The pseudo P pulmonale. Circulation 32:96, 1965.

30. Gross D: Electrocardiographic characteristics of P pulmonale waves of coronary origin. Am Heart J 73:453, 1967.

31. Wasserburger RH, Kelly JR, Rasmussen HK, et al: The electrocardiographic pentalogy of pulmonary emphysema: a correlation of roentgenographic findings and pulmonary function studies. Circulation 20:831, 1959.

32. Kaplan JD, Evans GT, Foster E, et al: Evaluation of electrocardiographic criteria for right atrial enlargement by quantitative two-dimensional echocardiography. J Am Coll Cardiol 23:747, 1994.

33. Morris JJ Jr, Estes EH Jr, Whalen RE, et al: P-wave analysis in valvular heart disease. Circulation 29:242, 1964.

34. Sodi-Pollares D, Calder RM: New Bases of Electrocardiography, St. Louis, Mosby, 1956.

35. Saunders JL, Calatayud JB, Schulz KJ, et al: Evaluation of ECG criteria for P-wave abnormalities. Am Heart J 74:757, 1967.

36. Kasser I, Kennedy JW: The relationship of increased left atrial volume and pressure to abnormal P wave on the electrocardiogram. Circulation 39:339, 1969.

37. Romhilt DW, Bove KE, Conradi S, et al: Morphologic significance of left atrial involvement. Am Heart J 83:322, 1972.

38. Sutnick AI, Soloff LA: Posterior rotation of the atrial vector: an electrocardiographic sign of left ventricular failure. Circulation 26:913, 1962.

39. Romhilt DW, Scott RC: Left atrial involvement in acute pulmonary edema. Am Heart J 83:328, 1972.

40. DeOliveira JM, Sambhi MP, Zimmerman HA: The electrocardiogram in pectus excavatum. Br Heart J 20:495, 1958.

41. Reynolds G: The atrial electrogram in mitral stenosis. Br Heart J 15:250, 1953.

42. Gordon R, Neilson G, Silverstone H: Electrocardiographic P wave and atrial weights and volumes. Br Heart J 27:748, 1965.

43. Thomas P, DeJong D: The P wave in the electrocardiogram in the diagnosis of heart disease. Br Heart J 16:241, 1954.

44. Dalton JC, Pearson RJ Jr, White PD: Constrictive pericarditis: a review and long-term follow-up of 78 cases. Ann Intern Med 45:445, 1956.

45. Wenger R, Hofmann-Credner D: Observations on the atria of the human heart by direct and semidirect electrocardiography. Circulation 5:870, 1952.

46. Chirife R, Feitosa GS, Frankl WS: Electrocardiographic detection of left atrial enlargement: correlation of P wave with left atrial dimension by echocardiography. Br Heart J 37:1281, 1975.

47. Waggoner AD, Adyanthaya AV, Quinones MA, et al: Left atrial enlargement: echocardiographic assessment of electrocardiographic criteria. Circulation 54:553, 1976.

48. Miller DH, Eisenberg RR, Kligfield PD, et al: Electrocardiographic recognition of left atrial enlargement. J Electrocardiol 16:15, 1983.

49. Velury V, Spodick DH: Axial correlates of PV1 in left atrial enlargement and relation to intraatrial block. Am J Cardiol 73:998, 1994.

49a. Lee KS, Appleton CP, Lester SJ, Adam TJ, Hurst RT, Morene CA, Altemose GT. Relation of electrocardiographic criteria for left atrial enlargement to two-dimensional echocardiographic left atrial volume measurements. Am J Cardiol. 99(1):113–8, 2007.

50. Thurmann M, Janney JG Jr: The diagnostic importance of fibrillatory wave size. Circulation 25:991, 1962.

51. Skoulas A, Horlick L: The atrial F wave in various types of heart disease and its response to treatment. Am J Cardiol 14:174, 1964.

52. Thurmann M: Coarse atrial fibrillation in congenital heart disease. Circulation 32:290, 1965.

53. Centurion OA, Isomoto S, Fukatani M, et al: Relationship between atrial conduction defects and fractionated atrial endocardial electrograms in patients with sick sinus syndrome. PACE 16:2022, 1993.

54. Liu Z, Hayano M, Hirata T, et al: Abnormalities of electrocardiographic P wave morphology and their relation to electrophysiological parameters of the atrium in patients with sick sinus syndrome. PACE 21(pt 1):9, 1998.

55. Agarwal YK, Aronow WS, Levy JA, et al: Association of interatrial block with development of atrial fibrillation. Am J Cardiol 91:882, 2003.

55a. Ariyarajah V, Apiyasawat S, Fernandes J, Kranis M, Spodick DH. Association of atrial fibrillation in patients with interatrial block over prospectively followed controls with comparable echocardiographic parameters. Am J Cardiol 99(3):390–2, 2007.

56. Frisella ME, Spodick DH: Confirmation of the prevalence and importance of a 12-lead investigation for diagnosis. Am J Cardiol 96:696, 2005.

57. Soejima K, Mitamura H, Miyazaki T, et al: A case of widely split double P waves with marked intra-atrial conduction delay. J Cardiovasc Electrophysiol 8:1296, 1997.

58. Cohen J, Scherf D: Complete interatrial and intratrial block (atrial dissociation). Am Heart J 70:23, 1965.

59. Hayashi H, Okajima M, Yamada K: Atrial T (Ta) wave and atrial gradient in patients with AV block. Am Heart J 91:689, 1976.

60. Debbas NMG, Jackson HSD, de Joghe D, et al: Human atrial repolarization: effects of sinus rate, pacing and drugs on the surface electrocardiogram. J Am Coll Cardiol 33:358, 1999.

61. Childers R: New and neglected aspects of atrial depolarization and repolarization. J Electrocardiol 30(Suppl):44, 1998.

62. Sapin PM, Koch G, Blauwet MB, et al: Identification of false positive exercise tests with use of electrocardiographic criteria: a possible role for atrial repolarization waves. J Am Coll Cardiol 18:127, 1991.

63. Myrianthefs MM, Nicolaides EP, Pitiris D, et al: False positive ST-segment depression during exercise in subjects with short PR segment and angiographically normal coronaries. J Electrocardiol 31:203, 1998.

3 Ventricular Enlargement

Before the advent of noninvasive methods capable of accurately estimating the dimensions, mass, and wall motion of cardiac chambers, electrocardiography in association with chest radiography and physical examination played a prominent role in assessing the size of the cardiac chambers. The electrocardiographic theory underlying the recognition of hypertrophy or dilation rests on a number of sound physical principles that may lead to meaningful correlations with the tissue mass, chamber diameter, and intracardiac blood volume.[1] There are, however, unavoidable limiting factors related to the variable orientation of the heart in the chest, variable properties of the volume conductor surrounding the heart, and nonspecificity of each depolarization and repolarization abnormality used for diagnosing hypertrophy or dilation.

As early as the 1950s and 1960s a wealth of autopsy and angiographic correlations firmly established the limits of the diagnostic accuracy of the electrocardiogram (ECG). With regard to left ventricular hypertrophy (LVH), it has been established that the ECG diagnosis is most accurate in patients with hypertensive and pure left-sided valvular heart disease in the absence of concomitant right ventricular hypertrophy (RVH), myocardial infarction, intraventricular conduction disturbances, and treatment with drugs altering depolarization and repolarization. Similar limiting factors play a role in the ECG diagnosis of RVH.

Left Ventricular Enlargement (Hypertrophy and Dilation)

In general, ECG criteria for the diagnosis of left ventricular enlargement are increased QRS amplitude (voltage), intraventricular conduction delay manifested by delayed intrinsicoid deflection in the precordial leads facing the left ventricle, widened QRS/T angle, and a tendency to left axis deviation (Figure 3–1).

VOLTAGE

The increased voltage is attributed to one or more of the following factors: increased left ventricular mass, increased left ventricular surface, increased intracavitary blood volume, and close proximity of the enlarged ventricle to the chest wall.

Left Ventricular Mass

The increase in the left ventricular mass exaggerates the leftward and posterior QRS forces. An increase in voltage may be due to the increase in the number[2] or size[3] of the fibers in the hypertrophied ventricle. The importance of fiber size was shown in the computer-generated ECG model where the amplitude of the R wave increased by 36 percent when the cell radius was increased by 15 percent without increasing the number of cells.[3] The enlarged cells and increased number of intercalated disks in the hypertrophied myocardium are believed to facilitate the intercellular current flow, which may be expected to increase the strength of the equivalent dipole generated by excitation of muscle layers. Consistent with this hypothesis was the finding of increased voltage recorded in the intramural electrograms from a hypertrophied human heart.[4]

In the presence of "pure" LVH (e.g., in children and young adults with isolated congenital

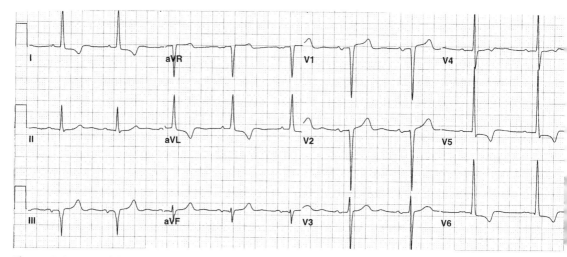

Figure 3–1 Typical left ventricular hypertrophy (LVH) pattern with secondary ST segment and T wave changes in a 67-year-old man with long-standing hypertension, bilateral carotid artery disease, bilateral renal artery disease, nonobstructive three-vessel coronary artery disease, and severe LVH but no history of myocardial infarction and no wall motion abnormalities. Q wave in lead III exemplifies a pseudoinfarction pattern. Note also the left atrial enlargement. PR interval, 220 ms; QRS, duration 102 ms; QTc, 415 ms.

aortic stenosis), the maximum spatial QRS vector significantly correlated with the peak left ventricular systolic pressure.[5] Because the QRS duration in this patient group was not increased, the increased voltage was believed to reflect an increased number of fibers in the hypertrophied myocardium.[2] In middle-aged and elderly patients, a significant correlation was observed between the QRS voltage and the left ventricular mass estimated from angiograms[6] and echocardiograms.[7–9]

Myocardial Surface

Hypertrophy increases the area of ventricular muscle in relation to the short-circuiting fluid surrounding the heart.[10] Increased surface area and wall thickness may be expected to increase the solid angle subtended by the precordial electrodes (see Chapter 1).

In a study of left ventricular angiograms in 93 patients with LVH, wall thickening sufficient to result in an increased left ventricular mass did not result in increased QRS voltage indicative of LVH unless sufficient concurrent chamber dilation was present.[11] This implied that there is a critical role for the geometric relation between wall thickness and chamber dilation, as would be expected from application of the solid angle theorem. However, a strict correlation between the left ventricular dimension and QRS voltage is not a universal finding. Thus Devereux et al.[12] found that the QRS voltage correlated only weakly with the size of the left ventricular chamber; for a given left ventricular mass, it

depended less on chamber dilation than on left ventricular weight, the depth of the left ventricle in the chest, and the patient's age.

Intracavitary Blood Volume

The QRS amplitude may be expected to increase in the presence of an increased end-diastolic blood volume owing to a mechanism postulated by Brody.[13] The Brody effect predicts that an increase in the intracardiac blood volume augments the initial (i.e., radial) QRS vectors and attenuates the late (i.e., tangential) QRS vectors. The validity of this principle was documented by correlating the R wave amplitude with the left ventricular volume, which was altered by pacing the heart at various rates.[14] Numerous studies using ventricular angiography,[6] nuclear imaging,[15,16] and echocardiography[8] have shown that the correlation of the QRS voltage with the left ventricular volume was either poor or not as good as the correlation with the left ventricular mass.

Proximity of the Heart to the Chest Wall

Feldman et al.[17] have shown that the R wave amplitude increased as the left ventricular lateral wall moved closer to the V_5 and V_6 electrodes and that the proximity of the left ventricle to the anterior chest wall was a major determinant of the R wave amplitude. Moreover, echocardiographic studies showed that the correlation between the ECG criteria for LVH and left ventricular mass calculated from the echocardiogram could be improved by correcting for the distance of the center of the left ventricular mass from the chest wall.[18]

INTRINSICOID DEFLECTION

In about 35 to 90 percent of LVH cases, the delayed onset of intrinsicoid deflections occurs $\geq$45 ms after the onset of the QRS complex,[10] which may be due to late activation of the hypertrophied left ventricle. The finding is not specific, however, because late ventricular activation in subjects with LVH also correlated with right ventricular thickness.[19]

REPOLARIZATION ABNORMALITIES

Deviation of the ST segment and the T wave in the direction opposite to the main QRS vector in the horizontal and frontal planes causes widening of the QRS/T angle. The combination of increased QRS amplitude and a wide QRS/T angle results in a pattern known as *left ventricular strain*. Even though the term "strain" is not appropriate to characterize an electrical event, use of this term has become entrenched in clinical practice. The ST and T changes in the left ventricular strain pattern are secondary to delayed propagation of the impulse in the conducting system, the hypertrophied myocardium, or both (see Chapter 23).

Diagnostic Criteria for Patients Aged 40 Years or Older

In most studies, high voltage in the precordial leads was the most sensitive criterion for the diagnosis of LVH. A recognition rate of up to 56 percent may be achieved, although it also was most frequently responsible for false-positive diagnoses.

If the duration of the QRS complex is <0.12 second, the following criteria are used for the diagnosis of LVH. They are based mainly on the studies of Sokolow and Lyon.[20]

The limb lead criteria are as follows:
1. R wave in lead I + S wave in lead III >2.5 mV
2. R wave in aV_L >1.1 mV
3. R wave in aV_F >2.0 mV
4. S wave in aV_R >1.4 mV

Precordial lead criteria are as follows:
5. R wave in V_5 or V_6 >2.6 mV
6. R wave in V_6 + S wave in V_1 >3.5 mV
7. Largest R wave + largest S wave in the precordial leads >4.5 mV

The most commonly used *voltage* criteria in the more recent literature are as follows:

S in V_1 + R in V_6 >3.5 mV
S in V_2 + R in V_6 >4.3 mV
S in V_1 >2.4 mV
S in V_6 >2.8 mV
R in aV_L >1.3 mV
    in addition to the Cornell criteria of:
R in aVL + S in V_3 >2.0 mV for females
    and >2.8 mV for males

Supporting criteria include the following:
8. Onset of the intrinsicoid deflection in V_5 or V_6 $\geq$0.05 second
9. ST segment depression and T wave inversion in the left precordial leads and in the limb leads in which major QRS deflection is upright in the presence of one or more of the above findings

Romhilt and Estes[21] proposed a point-score system that uses a combination of the various findings listed in Table 3–1. LVH is considered

TABLE 3–1	Point-Score System	
Measurement		**Points**
Amplitude: any of the following		3
Largest R or S wave in the limb leads $\geq$20 mm		
S wave in V_1 or V_2 $\geq$30 mm		
R wave in V_5 or V_6 $\geq$30 mm		
ST segment and T wave changes (typical pattern of left		
ventricular strain with the ST segment and T wave vector shifted		
in a direction opposite to the mean QRS vector)		
Without digitalis		3
With digitalis		1
Left atrial involvement: terminal negativity of the P wave		3
in V_1 is $\geq$1 mm in depth with a duration of $\geq$0.04 second		
Left axis deviation of −30 degrees or more		2
QRS duration $\geq$0.09 second		1
Intrinsicoid deflection in V_5 and V_6 $\geq$0.05 second		1

present if the points total 5 or more and is probably present if the points total 4.

Echocardiographic Criteria

Casale et al.[22] used the echocardiographically determined left ventricular mass measurements in 414 subjects as a standard to develop new ECG criteria for LVH and tested various correlations prospectively in an additional 129 subjects. The best criteria consisted of a combination of the sum of R amplitude in aV_L and S amplitude in V_3 to be >2.8 mV in men and >2.0 mV in women, associated with increased T wave amplitude in lead V_1. This combination had a sensitivity of 49 percent and a specificity of 93 percent, which was better than the respective values of 33 percent and 94 percent for the Sokolow-Lyon voltage criteria and 30 percent and 93 percent for the Romhilt-Estes score of 4 points or more. In the same study, ECG criteria based on a multiple logistic regression equation developed in the learning series and tested prospectively achieved 51 percent sensitivity, 90 percent specificity, and 76 percent overall accuracy for diagnosis of LVH. The innovative feature of these criteria is the separation by gender. A more accurate correlation was found subsequently using the product of either the Cornell voltage or 12-lead voltage system and the QRS duration.[23]

Framingham Heart Study investigators evaluated 10 ECG criteria for detecting LVH using ECG and echocardiographic measurements from 3351 adults.[24] The best performer for evaluating men was the Cornell voltage criterion multiplied by the QRS duration; for women, it was the voltage criteria in the limb leads. The sensitivity of the best criteria was about 95 percent, and the specificity varied from 32 to 51 percent. The authors found also that incorporation of obesity and age in gender-specific ECG algorithms consistently enhanced their performance for detecting hypertrophy.

Sensititivity and Specificity of Combined Criteria

To evaluate the sensitivity of the combined criteria, Scott and associates[25] studied 100 cases of isolated LVH with increased heart weight and left ventricular wall thickness at autopsy. Using one or more of the criteria listed previously (except criterion 7), 85 percent of the cases were correctly diagnosed. In this study, however, ST segment and T wave changes alone were also considered as indicative of LVH. In two later investigations[26,27] the sensitivities were 60 percent and 85 percent, respectively.

To test the specificity of listed criteria (except criterion 7), Chou et al.[28] reviewed the autopsy findings of 100 cases diagnosed as LVH by ECG less than 3 months before death. Cases with ST segment and T wave changes alone were not included. Taken together, 44 cases had isolated LVH, and 45 had combined ventricular hypertrophy. A false-positive diagnosis of LVH was made in 11 cases (11 percent). Selzer and associates[27] reported a slightly higher incidence (15 percent) of false-positive diagnoses. The point-score system,[21] tested in 360 autopsied hearts by the chamber dissection technique, gave a sensitivity of 54 percent, with only 3 percent false-positive diagnoses.

Sensitivity and Specificity of Individual Criteria

Mazzoleni and co-workers[29] examined the reliability of several of the individual criteria in the autopsied hearts with the chamber dissection technique. In 185 unselected adult patients, anatomic LVH was recognized in 22 percent by the criterion RV_5 or $V_6 + SV_1$ >3.5 mV and in 17 percent by the criterion RaV_L >1.0 mV.

A group of Cornell investigators[30] correlated antemortem ECGs with a left ventricular mass at autopsy in 220 patients. LVH was defined as an LV mass index >118 g/m^2 in men and >104 g/m^2 in women. They found that the product of the QRS duration and a 12-lead voltage (voltage-duration product) identified LVH more accurately than the voltage criteria alone, QRS duration criteria alone, or the Romhilt-Estes point score.

One of the most extensive anatomic correlation studies using the chamber dissection technique was conducted by Romhilt and associates.[32] A total of 33 ECG criteria for LVH were evaluated. The most sensitive (45 percent) was the R + S amplitude >4.5 mV. In other studies, increased QRS voltage correlated to variable degrees with the sum of the thickness of the septum and the posterior wall,[33–35] the posterior wall thickness alone,[36] or the calculated left ventricular mass.[37]

ST Segment and T Wave Changes

The two most commonly used repolarization criteria for the diagnosis of LVH are a QRS/T angle >100 degrees and a T wave that is upright in V_2 and more negative than −0.1 mV in V_6. The classic ST and T wave changes in LVH consist of ST segment depression with upward convexity and T wave inversion in the left precordial leads (Figures 3–1 to 3–4). Reciprocal changes are present in the right precordial leads with ST

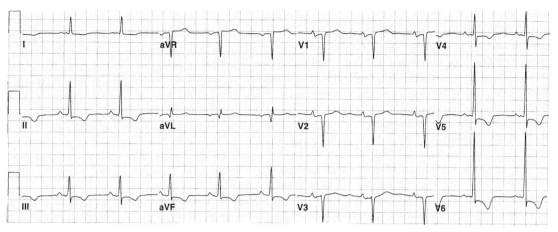

Figure 3–2 Typical left ventricular hypertrophy pattern with sharply inverted T waves suggestive of myocardial ischemia in a 78-year-old woman with hypertensive heart disease, intermittent atrial fibrillation, nonobstructive coronary artery disease, and no history of myocardial infarction suggested by the Q wave in aV_L. There is poor R wave progression and left atrial enlargement. PR interval, 183 ms; QRS duration, 74 ms; QTc, 403 ms.

segment elevation and a tall T wave. In the limb leads, the direction of the ST and T vectors is also directed opposite to the main QRS forces. Therefore ST segment depression and T wave inversion are seen in leads I and aV_L when the QRS axis is horizontal and in leads II, III, and aV_F when the QRS axis is vertical. These classic ST and T wave changes are usually found in patients with fully developed LVH.

If high QRS voltage and the secondary repolarization changes are both present, a false-positive diagnosis of LVH is seldom made.[27] Less pronounced repolarization changes, such as

slight ST segment depression or flat T waves in the left precordial leads, which usually precede frank ST segment deviation and T wave inversion during development of LVH, are also helpful, particularly when the voltage is increased.

A common diagnostic difficulty encountered in practice is recognition of the ST segment and T wave abnormalities caused by myocardial ischemia in the presence of the left ventricular strain pattern in patients with high-voltage QRS complexes suggestive of LVH. In theory, if the QRS area is strictly proportional to the ventricular mass and if the hypertrophy does not alter the

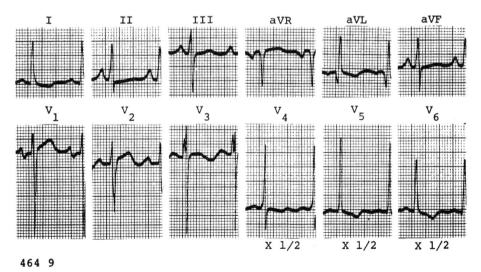

464 9

Figure 3–3 Left ventricular hypertrophy (LVH) with inverted U waves in a 33-year-old man with severe hypertension, cardiomegaly, and congestive heart failure. ECG shows high QRS voltage and notching of the R wave in lead V_3. With the addition of ST segment and T wave changes, the tracing is highly suggestive of LVH. U waves are inverted in leads V_4–V_6 and perhaps in leads V_2 and V_3. The P waves suggest left atrial enlargement.

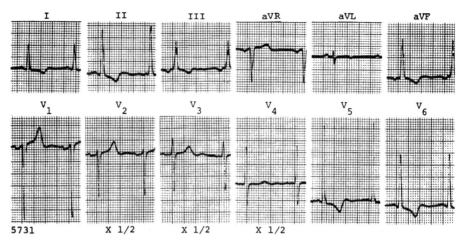

Figure 3–4 Aortic valve disease with left ventricular hypertrophy in a 61-year-old man with aortic stenosis and insufficiency. A peak systolic pressure gradient of 88 mmHg across the aortic valve was demonstrated during cardiac catheterization. Aortography revealed 3+ to 4+ aortic insufficiency. The coronary arteries were normal. The ECG shows high QRS voltage and the classic "strain pattern" of the ST segment and T waves. The P waves are suggestive of left atrial enlargement.

relation between the sequence of repolarization and the sequence of activation, the ventricular gradient should remain unchanged. This pattern occurs with uncomplicated hypertrophy, but the gradient does change when the ST and T wave changes are due to associated myocardial ischemia, which may be present even in the absence of coronary artery disease because of the following: (1) the increase in coronary artery diameter does not match the increased heart weight; (2) the unchanged capillary/fiber ratio increases the mean diffusion distance; and (3) the coronary vascular reserve is reduced owing to increased coronary vascular resistance.[38]

The morphology of the secondary T wave changes is distinctly different from that of the primary T wave changes and is suggestive of ischemia in about two thirds of the cases. In the remaining third of patients with documented LVH and normal coronary arteries, the negative T waves do not have the characteristic asymmetric configuration of secondary T waves (see Chapter 23) but instead resemble the primary terminally inverted T waves with an isoelectric or horizontally depressed ST segment, such as in the presence of subacute or chronic myocardial ischemia[39] (see Figures 3–2 and 3–4). In such cases one cannot use repolarization criteria to support the diagnosis of LVH. Repolarization changes attributed to myocardial ischemia can be distinguished from the secondary repolarization abnormalities caused by LVH if, instead of the expected secondary ST segment elevation and upright T wave, one encounters ST segment depression and T wave inversion in leads V_1 and V_2 (see Chapters 7 and 8). Favoring a

diagnosis of myocardial ischemia is the rapid appearance and disappearance of repolarization abnormalities in patients with coexisting coronary artery disease. It should be mentioned that transient or permanent T wave inversion in the right precordial leads in patients with LVH are occasionally caused by "right heart strain."

OTHER ECG CHANGES IN LVH

Incomplete Left Bundle Branch Block

In patients with LVH, Q waves often decrease in size or are absent (Figures 3–5 and 3–6). The Q wave was absent in about 50 percent of autopsied hearts with LVH resulting from various causes (T.C. Chou, 1960, unpublished data). The absence of the Q wave in the left precordial leads is related to leftward displacement of the initial QRS forces, which is also partly responsible for the decrease in the R wave in the right precordial leads.

When high QRS voltage and ST and T wave changes in LVH are accompanied by an increased QRS duration up to 0.11 second, an absence of Q waves with a delay in the onset of the intrinsicoid deflection in the left precordial leads, and (occasionally) notching of the QRS in the mid-precordial lead, the often-raised question is whether incomplete left bundle branch block (LBBB) coexists with hypertrophy. The problem is seldom of practical importance because incomplete LBBB is nearly always associated with marked LVH and therefore has the same significance as the LVH pattern with secondary ST and T wave changes.

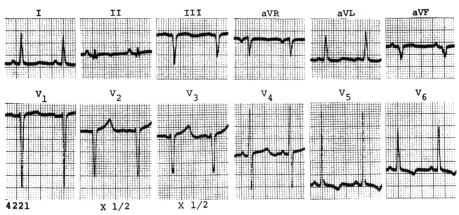

Figure 3–5 Coarctation of the aorta in a 36-year-old man who died shortly after unsuccessful correction of this congenital lesion. At autopsy there was also evidence of a healed dissecting aneurysm of the ascending aorta. The heart weighed 545 g and had marked left ventricular hypertrophy (LVH) and a moderate degree of dilatation. Left ventricular wall thickness was 25 mm. Coronary arteries revealed mild focal atherosclerosis with no significant narrowing of the lumen. Myocardium showed no evidence of fibrosis or infarction. Aortic valve was monocuspid with a centrally located orifice approximately 7 mm in diameter. This ECG was recorded 1 day before surgery. It shows rather typical changes of LVH. The QS deflections in leads III and aV$_F$ suggest inferior wall myocardial damage and, in view of the autopsy findings, represent a pseudoinfarction pattern. The poor progression of the R waves in the precordial leads also suggests the possibility of anterior myocardial damage, which was absent.

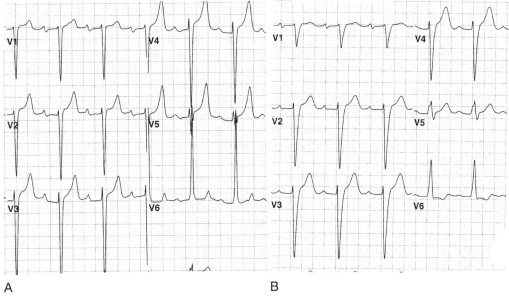

A   B

Figure 3–6 **A,** Left ventricular hypertrophy pattern with incomplete left bundle branch block (LBBB) (QRS, 110 ms; absent Q wave in lead V$_6$) in a 35-year-old man with alcoholic dilated cardiomyopathy (left ventricular ejection fraction 10 percent). **B,** Six months later the LBBB is complete. Standardization is half-normal. QRS duration is 156 ms. Pattern of left atrial enlargement and first-degree atrioventricular block are present in both **A** and **B**.

Abnormal Left Axis Deviation

When used alone, an abnormal left axis deviation of −30 degrees or more is a relatively insensitive, nonspecific sign of LVH. Grant[40] found no correlation between heart weight and left axis deviation.

Poor R Wave Progression in Precordial Leads

Poor progression of the R wave in the right and mid-precordial leads occurs commonly with LVH[41] and is associated with a leftward shift of the transitional zone in the precordial leads (i.e., R/S ratio <1 in V$_5$). Occasionally, R waves are absent in leads V_1, V_2, and even V_3, resulting in a QS deflection in these leads that mimics anteroseptal myocardial infarction (see Figures 3–2 and 3–5; also see Chapter 9).

Abnormal Q Wave in Inferior Leads

Occasionally, an abnormal Q wave is recorded in leads III and aV_F and less often in lead II, mimicking inferior myocardial infarction. Examples are shown in Figures 3–1 and 3–5. The mechanism of this pseudoinfarction pattern is not clear.

Notching and Prolongation of QRS Complex

In some patients the normal QRS complex is slightly prolonged and notched, especially in the mid-precordial leads, probably as a result of an intraventricular conduction defect (see Figure 3–3).

U Wave

The amplitude of a normal positive U wave may be increased in the right precordial leads, but the increase appears to be proportional to the overall increase in the amplitude of the ventricular complex. The U wave is often negative in the left precordial leads in patients with LVH, particularly when the latter is caused by systemic hypertension or regurgitation of the mitral or aortic valve (see Figure 3–3).[42]

Anatomic Correlations

Reichek and Devereux[43] found that the left ventricular mass estimated from M-mode echocardiography correlated well with the postmortem left ventricular weight in 34 subjects, and the respective sensitivities of the Romhilt-Estes point score and the Sokolow-Lyon voltage criteria were 50 percent and 21 percent, with a specificity of 95 percent for both criteria.

Several echocardiographic studies confirmed that the sensitivity and the specificity of the left ventricular strain pattern or of the Romhilt-Estes point score (particularly when the score was >5) was superior to the voltage criteria alone. The point score of Romhilt and Estes correlated with an increased left ventricular mass and was associated with a sensitivity of 57 percent and a specificity of 81 percent.[44] In two other studies[45,46] the left ventricular strain pattern had a sensitivity of 52 percent and a specificity of 95 percent.

Crow et al.[47] tested the performance of eight ECG criteria with the echocardiographic left ventricular mass index in a biracial population of men and women enrolled in the Treatment of Mild Hypertension Study. The ECG LVH sensitivity at 95 percent specificity was <34 percent. The Cornell voltage criteria showed the highest average sensitivity (17 percent). The ECG correlations with the LV mass index were consistently improved by including non-ECG variables, such as blood pressure and body mass index. The authors[47] thought that further refinement of the ECG criteria alone in Caucasian men was unlikely to improve its relation to the left ventricular mass. More recently, Budhwani et al.[48] correlated several traditional ECG criteria with the increased left ventricular mass estimated by echocardiography in 608 patients. Increasing number of the ECG criteria was associated with a greater mean left ventricular mass, but increased wall thickness and ventricular diameter did not influence significantly the frequency of any of the ECG criteria.

Echocardiographic studies exposed the shortcomings of the ECG in its ability to differentiate among concentric hypertrophy, eccentric hypertrophy, and dilation without hypertrophy and demonstrated that the QRS voltage may be increased in the presence of an increased left ventricular diastolic diameter and normal thickness of the left ventricular wall.[34] It appears that none of the tested criteria, such as the magnitude of the maximal QRS vector in the horizontal plane,[35] the QRS amplitude in the scalar ECG, or T wave changes, can distinguish reliably between concentric LVH and isolated left ventricular dilation. Echocardiography also showed that for a diagnosis of asymmetric LVH, the presence of prominent abnormal Q waves attributed to septal hypertrophy was a poor predictor of increased septal thickness or the septal wall/free wall ratio[31,49] (see Chapter 12). The echocardiogram is also superior to the ECG for detecting LVH in the presence of a ventricular conduction defect.

Systolic and Diastolic Overload of the Left Ventricle

Cabrera and Monroy introduced the concept of systolic and diastolic overload of the left ventricle.[50] Later writers used the terms *pressure overload* and *volume overload*. The ECG pattern of left ventricular systolic overload includes high voltage of the R wave and the classic secondary ST segment and T wave changes in the left precordial leads (see Figures 3–3 and 3–5). It occurs with such conditions as aortic stenosis, systemic hypertension, and coarctation of the aorta when the left ventricle contracts against increased resistance. With diastolic overload of the left ventricle, which is seen in patients with aortic insufficiency,

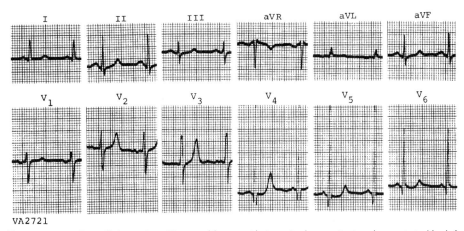

VA2721

Figure 3–7 Severe mitral insufficiency in a 52-year-old man with 4+ mitral regurgitation demonstrated by left ventricular angiography. The ECG reveals deep Q waves and tall R waves in the left precordial leads. ST segments and T waves are within normal limits. P wave changes are suggestive of left atrial enlargement. This tracing is a typical diastolic overload pattern of left ventricular hypertrophy.

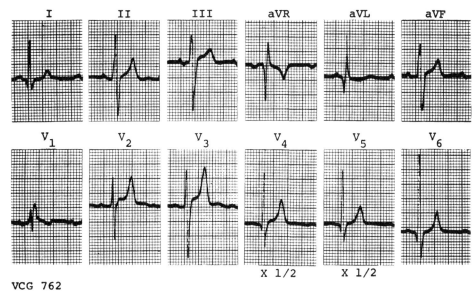

VCG 762

Figure 3–8 Ventricular septal defect in a 29-year-old man proved by cardiac catheterization. The ECG shows deep Q waves in leads I, aV$_L$, and V$_4$–V$_6$. There are tall R waves in the left precordial leads. The ST segment is slightly elevated, and the T waves are tall and peaked in most of the precordial leads. The findings are consistent with diastolic overloading of the left ventricle. An R^1 is present in lead V$_1$, suggesting possible right ventricular hypertrophy or incomplete right bundle branch block.

mitral insufficiency, and patent ductus arteriosus, the ECG usually exhibits high voltage of the R waves with prominent Q waves in the left precordial leads (Figure 3–7). The ST segment is usually elevated, with an upright, peaked T wave.

Although the concept of systolic and diastolic overload has enjoyed some popularity, its clinical application often has been disappointing, especially in patients with advanced acquired heart disease, severe dilatation, and hypertrophy. In young patients with congenital heart disease, correlation of the hemodynamic state and the

ECG pattern usually is better, particularly in patients with a ventricular septal defect without pulmonary hypertension whose ECG often shows a prominent Q wave followed by a tall R wave and an upright T wave (Figure 3–8).

PHYSIOLOGIC FACTORS AFFECTING THE RELIABILITY OF DIAGNOSTIC CRITERIA

Most of the present ECG criteria for LVH have been developed for populations with a high prevalence of heart disease. The Bayes theorem predicts that these criteria would result in a high incidence of false-positive ECG interpretations in a population with a low prevalence of heart disease. Indeed, in such populations none of the ECG signs of LVH are specific, and no QRS voltage criteria have more than 46 percent accuracy for the diagnosis of LVH.[51]

A common vexing problem stems from variations in precordial voltage. Such variations may be due to changes in electrode position but may also occur in the same individual at 24-hour intervals, even independent of electrode position, perhaps due to changes in respiration or heart rate.[52] The ST and T wave abnormalities are even less specific than the voltage. Moreover, the combination of increased voltage and a wide QRS/T angle can be present without hypertrophy due to delayed conduction in the left bundle branch system. This can be shown by applying early premature atrial stimuli, which causes a delay in the left bundle branch. The LVH pattern produced in this manner can be normalized by delaying conduction in the right bundle branch.[53]

Age

Age is one of the most important factors to be considered in the ECG diagnosis of LVH. Most of the voltage criteria were derived and tested against the older population. It is well known, however, that the QRS voltage is higher in adolescents and young adults than in older individuals (Figure 3–9). For example, from age 20 to 29 years, the normal 99th percentile for SV$_1$ + RV$_5$ or V$_6$ is 5.3 mV.[54] The voltage of SV$_2$ + RV$_5$ is more than 3.5 mV in 32 percent of normal men 20 to 39 years of age (T.C. Chou, 1960, unpublished data). It has been estimated that the amplitude of the maximum spatial QRS vector decreases by 6.5 percent for each decade of life from age 20 to 78.[55]

During routine interpretation of the ECG, LVH must be diagnosed with caution in patients under age 40 if only the voltage criteria are met, unless the amplitude is extremely high. Even the combination of high QRS voltage and ST and T wave changes, which is reliable in older subjects, cannot be applied with equal confidence in young subjects. The ST and T wave abnormalities may be due to other causes in the young patient, and the high amplitude of the QRS may be normal for the particular body build. It is therefore advisable to look for some other supporting evidence in the QRS complex such as abnormal left axis deviation, a delay in the onset of the intrinsicoid deflection in leads V$_5$ and V$_6$, an increase in QRS duration to 0.11 second, the presence of notching of the QRS complex in the mid-precordial leads, and especially poor progression of the R wave in the right and mid-precordial lead. Because most normal individuals have taller R waves in lead V$_5$ than in lead V$_6$, reversal of this order also is suggestive of an abnormality.

The correlation between the ECG and the left ventricular wall thickness in the elderly was determined in 671 autopsies of patients 65 to 116 years of age. The correlation was not affected by age in subjects younger than 85 years but was blunted in those older than 85.[56]

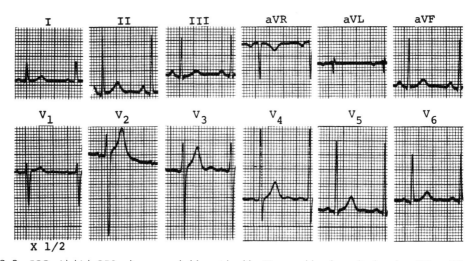

Figure 3–9 ECG with high QRS voltage recorded from a healthy 22-year-old male medical student. RV$_5$ + SV$_1$ = 46 mm; RV$_5$ + SV$_2$ = 49.5 mm.

Body Habitus

The voltage is reduced in persons with large breasts. A significant increase in R amplitude in leads V_1–V_5 occurred after left mastectomy and in leads V_3R and V_1 after right mastectomy.[57] On the basis of increased voltage, LVH would be erroneously diagnosed in nearly 50 percent of women after mastectomy.[57] Other factors that may alter voltage in the absence of hypertrophy are hematocrit, intraventricular conduction disturbance, and perhaps myocardial ischemia. A low hematocrit increases the QRS voltage and a high hematocrit decreases it because of changes in blood resistivity.[58]

Kilty and Lepeschkin[51] examined the effect of body build on the QRS voltage of the ECG. Using the ponderal index (height in inches divided by the cube root of weight in pounds) as a measure of body build, they found a highly significant correlation between body build and the voltage of $R_1 + S_3$, largest $R + S$ in the precordial leads, and largest $R + S$ in a single precordial lead. The precordial lead criterion $R + S$ >4.5 mV underdiagnoses LVH in obese people and overdiagnoses it in thin people. Others have also noted that most false-positive diagnoses of LVH occur in emaciated individuals.[51] The increased amount of adipose or muscle tissue in the chest wall affects the voltage as a result of an increased distance between the precordial electrode and the heart. An accumulation of adipose tissue around the heart of overweight persons may produce a similar effect[59] (see Figure 1–23).

The Cornell investigators[60] found that the ability of ECG criteria to detect LVH differs depending on the method used to index the left ventricular mass for body size and with the presence or absence of obesity. When the left ventricular mass was indexed to the body surface area or to height, the sensitivity of the Cornell product criteria increased from 39 to 52 percent with a matched specificity of 95 percent.

Gender and Race

Gender has a significant effect on the amplitude of the QRS complex. Men have higher amplitudes than women in both the limb leads and precordial leads, but especially in the latter.[59] In women it is sometimes important to know whether lead V_4 was recorded with the electrode on or underneath the breast. A significant reduction in voltage may occur if the electrode is placed on a large breast (Figure 3–10).

African-American subjects are reported to have higher QRS voltage than Caucasian subjects. In a study of 114 healthy adolescents[61] the upper limit for the S wave amplitude in lead V_1 was 3.4 mV in black males, 3.2 mV in white males, 2.6 mV in black females, and 1.6 mV in white females. The corresponding values for the R amplitude in lead V_6 were 3.0, 2.4, 2.2, and 2.4 mV.[62]

In another study of 15- to 19-year-old adolescents[61] the sum of S in V_1 and R in V_6 amplitudes averaged 3.69 mV in black males and 3.13 mV in white males. No significant differences were found between black and white females. The echocardiograms showed that the left ventricular posterior wall was thicker and the distance between the anterior chest wall and the mid-left ventricle was shorter in black males than in white males. No such racial differences were observed in females.

The Chicago Heart Association Detection Project in Industry collected data from 1391 black men and 19,216 white men.[63] The prevalence of an ECG LVH pattern was significantly higher in black men than in white men in each age group. The difference remained significant after adjustment for all possible risk factors. Examination of the data from National Health and Nutrition Surveys[64] also showed that black racial background was associated with a more than three-fold excess of LVH by the Cornell voltage criteria.

In a smaller study of 196 African-Americans, ages 54 to 100 years, Arnett et al.[65] found that the application of ECG algorithms was associated with misclassification of LVH and overestimation of the left ventricular mass by echocardiography. The diagnostic accuracy of the Cornell criteria in African-Americans was comparable to the accuracy reported in white subjects.

PATHOLOGIC STATES AFFECTING THE DIAGNOSIS OF LVH

The lung is a poor electrical conductor and attenuates the QRS voltage. In patients with chronic obstructive pulmonary disease (COPD), the voltage of the QRS complex may be markedly reduced. The presence of LVH often is not recognized in such patients. Pericardial effusion may also mask a ventricular hypertrophy pattern because of the short-circuiting effect of the pericardial fluid. Pulmonary edema may reduce the body surface potential by its short-circuiting effect.[66] A reduction of the amplitude of the complexes is also seen in patients with pleural effusion, generalized anasarca, or pneumothorax.

Myocardial damage in patients with coronary artery disease, secondary myocardial disease such as amyloidosis, or scleroderma-associated heart disease is often accompanied by low

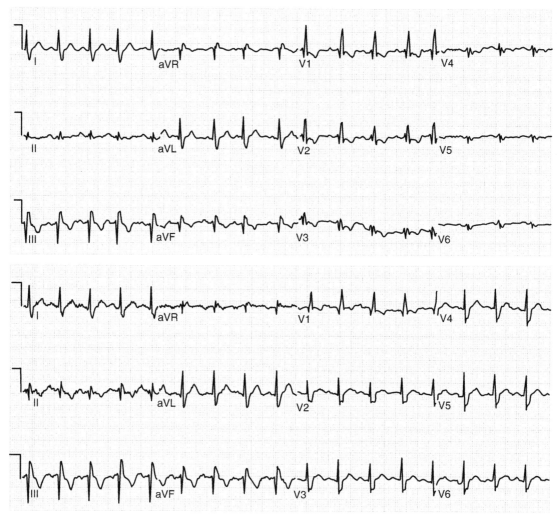

Figure 3–10 Difference in voltage in leads V_3–V_6 resulting from electrode placement under a large breast *(top)* and over the breast *(bottom)* in the ECG of a 60-year-old obese woman. The two ECGs were recorded 1 hour apart. Note the absence of an appreciable change in voltage in leads other than V_3–V_6.

voltage, which makes diagnosing LVH difficult. The presence of myocardial infarction did not affect ECG recognition of LVH by the voltage criteria in an autopsy series,[67] although changes in QRS amplitude during the acute stage are often present (see Chapter 7).

In most patients with RVH secondary to left ventricular disease, the effect is minimal and the diagnosis of LVH is not affected. When RVH is severe, however, the LVH pattern may not be apparent because of the canceling effect of the rightward forces.

ASSESSMENT OF THE SEVERITY OF VALVULAR LESIONS CAUSING LVH

Most attempts to correlate the ECG with the severity of a valvular lesion have been made in

patients with valvular aortic stenosis. Hugenholtz and associates[68] studied 95 patients (ages 6 weeks to 20 years) with congenital aortic stenosis. About three fourths of the patients with severe lesions and one fourth of those with mild lesions had evidence of LVH. Braunwald and associates[69] reported hemodynamic and ECG findings in 100 patients with congenital aortic stenosis. Their ages ranged from 2 to 51 years, with 36 patients younger than 10 years. No single ECG change was found to be reliable for determining the severity of the obstruction. The ECG was more helpful in patients younger than age 10 than in older individuals.

Roman and associates[70] correlated the ECG, echocardiographic, and radionuclide angiographic findings in 95 adults with severe, pure, chronic aortic insufficiency and no evidence of coronary artery disease. The correlation between the QRS voltage and the degree of left ventricular dilatation and dysfunction was weak.[70] In patients with chronic aortic regurgitation and massive cardiomegaly (heart weighing 1 kg or more), the usual QRS criteria for LVH were often absent.[43]

In patients with mitral insufficiency, the correlation between the severity of the mitral lesion and the ECG changes is generally poor. In a series of 65 cases of dynamically significant mitral insufficiency without significant mitral stenosis confirmed at surgery or autopsy, the ventricular complex was normal in 50 percent and suggestive of LVH in 30 percent, RVH in 15 percent, and combined ventricular hypertrophy in 5 percent of cases.[71]

LVH and Systemic Hypertension

In the early reports from the Framingham Study[72] the ECG was normal in almost half, borderline in one fifth, and definitely abnormal in one third of a group of 154 patients with a clinical diagnosis of hypertensive cardiovascular disease.[72] During the follow-up[73] the incidence of an LVH ECG pattern over a 14-year period of observation rose in proportion to the blood pressure elevation in all age groups. About half the patients with systolic pressures above 200 mmHg had or developed an LVH ECG pattern during the 14 years.

Ashizawa and associates[74] reported a 26-year follow-up study of 601 patients with hypertension and ECG changes of LVH with both high QRS voltage and ST segment and T wave changes. The patients were examined at 2-year intervals. In 60 subjects the ECG signs of LVH developed during the observation period. In 37 of the subjects, high QRS voltage appeared first, followed by ST and T wave changes. In 10 patients the ST and T wave changes occurred first; in the other 13 patients the QRS and ST segment and T wave changes appeared simultaneously. In 72 of the 601 subjects the LVH pattern regressed. The QRS voltage became normal in 36, ST segment and T wave changes disappeared in 25, and both high QRS voltage and ST segment and T wave changes disappeared in 11 patients. In about half of these 72 subjects, regression of the abnormal ECG findings, usually the QRS voltage, was associated with lowering the blood pressure. Regression of the ECG abnormalities during antihypertensive therapy was associated with lower morbidity and mortality.[75,75a]

Prognostic Value of ECG Changes

The ECG is of limited value for predicting the severity of the hypertension in individual patients. It is believed, however, that in the presence of both ST segment and T wave changes and high QRS voltage, patients usually have a higher blood pressure than those with high QRS voltage alone.[76]

In a study of 227 patients with untreated diastolic hypertension before the advent of echocardiography, the left ventricular mass was predicted by combining the surface area, gender, age, the S voltage in leads V_1 and V_4, and the duration of the terminal P wave component in lead V_1.[77] In the Framingham study[78] the mortality of hypertensive patients with a definitive LVH pattern (tall R wave, ST segment depression, flattened or inverted T wave, increased ventricular activation time in the left precordial leads) was much higher than in subjects without such findings, even though the blood pressure was the same. In an analysis of 4824 patients by Sullivan et al.,[79] the ECG pattern of LVH had an independent adverse effect on survival, even in patients without coronary artery disease.

In a study of 923 Caucasian untreated hypertensive patients[80] in whom the prevalence of echocardiographic LVH was 34 percent, the specificity of ECG for LVH was >90 percent and the sensitivity varied between 9 percent and 33 percent. The highest sensitivity was found when three highly specific criteria (Cornell voltage, Romhilt-Estes score, left ventricular strain pattern) were combined. Combination of these criteria was also most predictive of cardiovascular events in 1717 Caucasian hypertensive patients followed prospectively for up to 10 years.[81] In a long-term Losartan Intervention for Endpoint Reduction (LIFE) in Hypertension study of 8696 hypertensive subjects, ECG LV strain pattern identified patients at increased risk of developing congestive heart failure and dying, even in the setting of aggressive blood pressure lowering.[82]

PRESENCE OF LBBB

Klein et al.[83] used echocardiograms to develop criteria for diagnosing LVH in patients with LBBB. They found that the sum of the S amplitude in V_2 and the R amplitude in V_6 exceeding 4.5 mV had an 86 percent sensitivity and 100 percent specificity for LVH, and that the diagnosis of LVH was supported by the findings of left atrial enlargement and QRS duration >160 ms.

Right Ventricular Hypertrophy and Dilation

Right ventricular forces normally are directed anteriorly and rightward but are mostly masked by the dominant left ventricular potential. An increase in the right ventricular muscle mass modifies the resultant forces proportional to the severity of the hypertrophy. In mild cases, no apparent change may be detected in the ECG. If the RVH is severe, the normally dominant left posterior QRS forces may be replaced by prominent right anterior forces, and the QRS patterns in the left and right precordial leads are reversed. Intermediate degrees of abnormality may be observed when the hypertrophy is moderate. Because lead V_1 is more proximal to the right ventricular mass, it is the most sensitive lead for recording the changes. Tall R wave, small S wave, or a change in the R/S ratio may be observed. The onset of the intrinsicoid deflection in this lead may be delayed because of delayed activation of the right ventricular epicardium,[84,85] but the delay is seldom sufficiently pronounced to be of diagnostic usefulness.[85]

In some instances the increased rightward forces are directed posteriorly instead of anteriorly. In such cases no apparent abnormality is seen in lead V_1, but the left precordial leads may reveal deep S waves, and the increased rightward forces may be recognized in the limb leads as right axis deviation.

Secondary T wave change often occurs. The T waves are directed opposite to the main QRS vector (i.e., inverted in the right precordial leads and upright in the left precordial leads). These secondary T wave abnormalities may be accompanied by secondary deviations of the ST segment. In some instances, the ST and T changes may be seen without apparent QRS abnormalities and are attributed to myocardial ischemia of the right ventricle, or right ventricular strain.

THREE TYPES OF RVH

It is useful to subdivide the ECG manifestations of RVH and right ventricular dilation into three types: (1) typical RVH pattern with anterior and rightward displacement of the main QRS vector; (2) incomplete right bundle branch block (RBBB); and (3) posterior and rightward displacement of the main QRS axis, predominantly in patients with chronic lung disease.

Typical RVH Pattern

The typical RVH pattern is a mirror image of the LVH pattern, with right axis deviation in the frontal plane, tall R waves in the right precordial leads, deep S waves in the left precordial leads, and a slight increase in QRS duration (Figure 3–11). This pattern is characteristically present in patients with congenital pulmonary stenosis, tetralogy of Fallot, primary pulmonary hypertension, and other conditions in which the right ventricular mass tends to approach or exceed the left ventricular mass. The earliest portion of the QRS complex is usually unchanged because septal activation is normal. The anterior displacement of the main QRS vector manifested by tall R waves in the right precordial leads is attributed to a longer activation time of the hypertrophied right ventricular free wall.[86,87]

Intraoperative epicardial mapping of patients with RVH undergoing pulmonary thromboendarterectomy showed that right ventricular activation was delayed by an average of 36 ms.[84] In addition, the latest right ventricular epicardial activation occurred significantly later than the latest left ventricular activation (i.e., average of 75 ms vs. average of 64 ms). In some cases there was no discrete early right ventricular

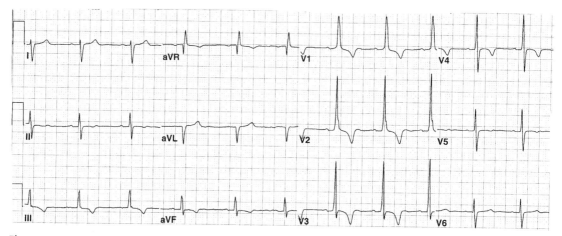

Figure 3–11 Typical right ventricular hypertrophy pattern with right axis deviation and negative T waves in leads V_1–V_4 in a 26-year-old man who had undergone corrective surgery for transposition of the great vessels during childhood.

breakthrough, but in these cases the latest right ventricular activation also occurred significantly later than the left ventricular activation.

Sensitivity and Specificity of Criteria for RVH

The sensitivity and the specificity of various criteria are generally inversely related.[88] The early criteria of Myers and associates[89] and Sokolow and Lyon[90] included the following:

1. R in V_1 >0.7 mV
2. S in V_1 <0.2 mV
3. S in V_5 or V_6 >0.7 mV
4. Sum of R in V_1 and S in V_5 or V_6 >1.05 mV
5. R in V_5 or V_6 <0.5 mV
6. R/S ratio in V_5 or V_6 <1
7. R in aV_R >0.5 mV
8. R/S ratio in V_5 divided by R/S ratio in V_1 <0.4
9. R/S ratio in V_1 (or V_3R) >1
10. qR pattern in V_1 (or V_3R)

Supporting criteria include the following:

11. Onset of intrinsicoid deflection in V_1 later than 0.04 second
12. Negative T wave in V_1 in the presence of R >0.5 mV
13. Right axis deviation >110 degrees

These criteria have high specificity but low sensitivity.[91,92] In the autopsy series in which the anatomic diagnosis was based mainly on right ventricular wall thickness, the ECG met one or more of the criteria in 23 to 100 percent.[93] Roman and colleagues[94] examined 118 hearts with an ECG diagnosis of RVH. There was a false-positive diagnosis in 60 percent of the cases. The criteria of R in V_1 + S in V_5 or V_6 >1.05 mV and S in V_5 or V_6 >0.7 mV were responsible for most of the erroneous diagnoses. Chou et al.[95] studied 97 patients in whom the presence of RVH was supported by hemodynamic data. The sensitivity of the ECG was 66 percent.

Burch and de Pasquale[96] found that none of the RVH criteria were satisfied in 40 percent of cases of autopsy-proven RVH due to cor pulmonale. Kilcoyne et al.[97] found that only 28 percent of 81 patients with cor pulmonale had an RVH pattern on the ECG.

Milnor[97a] modified the Sokolow and Lyon criteria and limited the variables to: QRS duration <0.12 second and a frontal axis of +110 to +180 degrees or −91 to ±180 degrees; or an R/S or R^1/S ratio in V_1 >1.0, with R or R^1 amplitude >0.5 mV. These criteria have the advantage of applicability in the presence of incomplete RBBB. They predicted RVH correctly in 24 of 32 autopsy-proven cases. A 79 percent sensitivity

and 73 percent specificity for diagnosing RVH was reported by Holt et al.[98] using the 12-dipole ECG derived from records made at 126 body sites.

Behar et al.[99] evaluated the usefulness of the Butler-Legget criteria for diagnosing RVH. These criteria are as follows: (1) P wave amplitude >0.25 mV in any of leads II, III, aV_F, V_1, or V_2; (2) R wave amplitude = 0.2 mV in lead I; (3) $A + R − PL = 0.7$ mV, where A (anteriorly directed deflection) is derived from lead V_1 or V_2, R (rightward deflection) is the S amplitude in lead I or V_6, and PL (posterolateral deflection) is the S amplitude in lead V_1. In patients with pulmonary hypertension, these criteria achieved 66 percent sensitivity for mitral stenosis, 97 percent sensitivity for pulmonary arterial obstructive disease, and 79 percent sensitivity for pulmonary disease. The specificity of these criteria was enhanced by ruling out posterior myocardial infarction using the Selvester QRS scoring system (see Chapter 8).

The explanation for the marked differences in the results probably lies in the patient population sampled. The lower sensitivity was obtained mostly from unselected adult patients in a general hospital.[92] In these patients, RVH most commonly develops as a result of left ventricular disease. The degree of hypertrophy usually is mild and likely to be masked by the dominant left ventricle. The higher sensitivity values mostly came from centers with large numbers of patients with congenital heart disease and a high incidence of severe RVH.[100]

Flowers and Horan[101] used the chamber dissection technique to examine 819 apparently unselected hearts, including 178 with RVH. The sensitivity and specificity of the individual criteria are summarized in Table 3–2, which indicates that the sensitivity of the individual criterion is low, generally less than 20 percent. The more sensitive signs, such as those based on changes in the left precordial leads, usually are associated with a larger number of false-positive diagnoses. By comparison, criteria based on abnormalities in lead V_1 are more specific but less sensitive.

Echocardiographic Correlations

Good correlations were found between the measurements of right ventricular wall thickness on the echocardiogram and autopsy findings.[102] The echocardiogram was reported to be more sensitive for detecting RVH than the ECG.[103] For increased right ventricular wall thickness, the sensitivity and the specificty of the echocardiogram were 93 percent and 95 percent, respectively. The corresponding values for the ECG

TABLE 3–2	Sensitivity, Specificity, and Correctness of ECG Criteria for Diagnosis of Right Ventricular Hypertrophy		
Criterion	Sensitivity (%)	Specificity (False-Positives) (%)	Correctness (%)
Right axis deviation ≥110 degrees	12	4	78
R/S V_1 (or V_{3R}) >1	6	2	78
RV_1 ≥7 mm	2	1	78
SV_1 ≤2 mm	6	2	78
qR in V_1	5	1	79
$RV_1 + SV_5$ or V_6 >10.5 mm	18	6	77
R/S V_5 or V_6 <1	16	7	77
OID in V_1 (or V_{3R}) = 0.035–0.055 second	8	6	76
RSR^1 in V_1 with R′ >10 mm	0	0	78
aVR ≥11.5 mm	0	0	78
RV_5 (or RV_6) <5 mm	13	13	71
SV_5 (or SV_6) ≥7 mm	26	10	76

Adapted from Flowers NC, Horan LG: IV. Hypertrophy and infarction: subtle signs of right ventricular enlargement and their relative importance. In: Schlant RC, Hurst JW (eds): Advances in Electrocardiography. Orlando, Grune & Stratton, 1972.
OID = onset of intrinsicoid deflection.

were 31 percent and 85 percent, respectively.[103] When the ECG and the echocardiogram were compared in 134 patients with RVH and in 78 patients without RVH, the ECG had 27 percent sensitivity and 88 percent specificity. In more than half the patients the diagnosis of RVH was difficult to establish on the ECG because of conduction disturbances or old myocardial infarction.[103]

Differential Diagnosis

Abnormal Right Axis Deviation. Other than RVH, the situations in which right axis deviation may be seen are as follows:
1. Normal young or slender adults
2. Chronic obstructive pulmonary disease (COPD) without cor pulmonale
3. Lateral myocardial infarction
4. Left posterior fascicular block

Right axis deviation occurs normally in infants and children. The mean QRS axis during the first 4 weeks of life is +110 degrees or more.[104] After 1 month the average axis is less than +90 degrees (although a significant number of children still have a QRS axis of up to +110 degrees). In the adult population, tall and slender subjects tend to have a rightward QRS axis. Hiss and colleagues[105] reported that 2 percent of normal subjects 20 to 30 years of age have an axis of +105 degrees. A frontal plane QRS axis of more than +110 degrees in older individuals is uncommon, however, and usually suggests abnormality. Even an axis

within the range from +90 to +110 degrees may indicate an abnormality in older patients, particularly if other ECG abnormalities coexist.

In patients with COPD the frontal plane axis may be within a range from +90 to +110 degrees in the absence of pulmonary hypertension. The recognition or exclusion of RVH in these patients is difficult. In patients with chronic lung disease without RVH, the amplitude of the entire QRS complex in lead I tends to be small.

In patients with lateral wall myocardial infarction, the loss of leftward forces may result in a rightward shift of the QRS vector. In these patients the initial R wave in lead I is usually absent, however, and abnormal Q waves are often observed also in the left precordial leads. Inverted T waves in leads I, aV_L, V_5, and V_6 are often present in patients with lateral myocardial infarction but are uncommon in patients with pure RVH.

Abnormal right axis deviation also is seen in patients with left posterior fascicular block. The differentiation of abnormal right axis deviation due to RVH from that secondary to left posterior fascicular block may not be possible without clinical information. If the P waves are suggestive of right atrial enlargement, however, the presence of RVH may be inferred. Left posterior fascicular block is favored if signs of inferior or posterior myocardial infarction are evident.

Tall R Wave, Small S Wave, Increased R/S Ratio in Lead V_1 in Conditions Other than RVH. One or more of the findings of a tall R wave, a small S wave, or an increased R/S ratio in lead V_1 may be seen in the following:

1. Normal young adults
2. True posterior infarction
3. Intraventricular conduction disturbances attributed to left septal fascicular block
4. Displacement of the heart due to pulmonary disease
5. Wolff-Parkinson-White pattern

A tall R wave with or without a small S wave in lead V_1 is a frequent finding in normal children. The average amplitude of the R wave in V_1 is more than 0.7 mV in children younger than 8 years.[106] The amplitude exceeds 0.7 mV in 20 percent of children between ages 8 and 12 and in 11 percent of those between ages 12 and 16. An amplitude of up to 1.6 mV may be seen in normal adolescents. The R/S ratio in V_1 is more than 1 in most children under 1 year of age,[106] but the ratio progressively decreases as age increases. In adults an R/S ratio of 1 or more was reported in fewer than 1 percent of the normal population.[107] Personal observations suggest that such a pattern is much more common, particularly among the younger and the obese populations. In lead V_2 an R/S ratio of >1 was observed in as many as 10 percent of adults.[108]

In patients with true posterior myocardial infarction, the polarity of the T wave in V_1 often is helpful in the differential diagnosis. Although exceptions do occur, an inverted T wave usually is seen in patients with RVH (see Figures 3–11 and 3–12; see also Figure 2–4), whereas an upright T wave in V_1 is likely to be associated with posterior myocardial infarction. The coexistence of abnormal right axis deviation in the frontal plane favors RVH. Occasionally, however, right axis deviation is observed in patients with posterior myocardial infarction when it is complicated by left posterior fascicular block. Because true posterior myocardial infarction is seldom encountered in the absence of inferior or lateral wall infarction, the differential diagnosis is usually not difficult.

An R wave of 0.7 mV or more occasionally is seen in lead V_1 in patients with autopsy-proven isolated LVH.[108] In such cases the S wave amplitude in lead V_1 is usually large. The cause of the tall R wave is unclear. In some cases it is associated with hypertrophic cardiomyopathy. These subjects often have a prominent R wave in the right precordial leads[107] and a small S wave in lead V_1, resulting in an R/S ratio of >1. Deep Q waves are usually present in the left precordial leads and in leads II, III, and aV_F. Hypertrophy of the interventricular septum is probably responsible for these abnormal forces.

Rightward displacement of the heart as a result of disease of the lung or pleura, such as massive pleural effusion or pneumothorax, may be accompanied by a tall R wave in lead V_1 (Figures 3–13 and 3–14) because lead V_1 is believed to record left, rather than right, ventricular potential. In the absence of structural heart disease, the T wave in V_1 is upright in the case of a displaced heart, whereas in patients with RVH the T wave in this lead is often inverted.

In patients with the Wolff-Parkinson-White pattern, the anterior direction of the delta wave resulting in an R or Rs pattern in lead V_1 is present in most subjects with posterior and leftward insertions of the atrioventricular bypass tract.

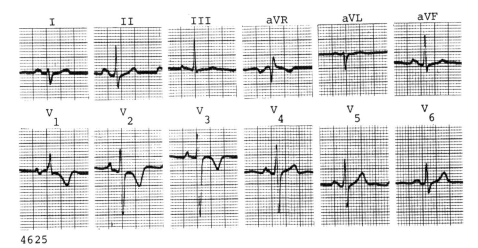

4625

Figure 3–12   Severe mitral stenosis in a 47-year-old man with severe mitral stenosis proved at surgery. On the ECG the P waves are consistent with biatrial enlargement. The abnormal right axis deviation with an R/S ratio of >1 in lead V_1 and the T wave inversion in the right precordial leads are consistent with right ventricular hypertrophy.

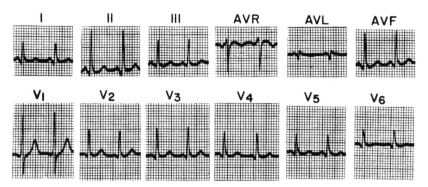

Figure 3–13   Tall R waves in the right precordial leads due to dextro displacement in a 28-year-old man with complete collapse of the right lung as a result of Hodgkin's disease. At autopsy the heart weight was normal, and there was no evidence of ventricular hypertrophy or myocardial damage.

qR Pattern in Lead V_1. The qR complex in V_1 is one of the most specific signs of severe RVH (see Figure 3–14). When the earliest part of the QRS complex is isoelectric, abnormal depolarization of the interventricular septum probably is responsible for the initial negativity of the complex.[109] It is possible that the right septal forces are now greater than those on the left, and the resultant vector is directed toward the left (opposite to the normal orientation). It has been also suggested that this complex is a manifestation of an enlarged right atrium that transmits to the right precordial leads the intracardiac potential from the right ventricle.[90] Indeed, in patients with this pattern the right atrium is frequently enlarged, and tricuspid regurgitation is commonly present. Others have ascribed this qR morphology to the extreme rotation of the heart such that the forces arising from the left ventricle are now recorded in the V_1 position.

Some normal adults have a QS rather than an rS deflection in lead V_1. If such an individual develops RBBB, a qR rather than an rSR^1 pattern will be recorded. If the QRS duration is 0.12 second or more, the conduction defect usually can be readily recognized. If the bundle branch block is incomplete with a QRS duration of 0.11 second or less, the differentiation becomes difficult. A similar problem exists in patients with anterior myocardial infarction and RBBB. The qR complex in these patients usually is accompanied by abnormal Q waves in the adjacent precordial leads.

Deep S Wave, Small R Wave, R/S Ratio <1 in Leads V_5 and V_6. In patients with COPD, the left precordial leads often display small R waves, deep S waves, and an R/S ratio of <1. These changes may be observed in the absence of pulmonary hypertension or cor pulmonale. When the lung disease is not associated with RVH,

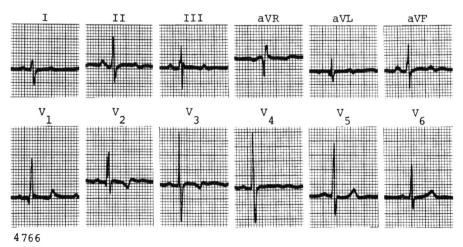

4766

Figure 3–14   Right ventricular hypertrophy caused by Eisenmenger syndrome. The patient is a 24-year-old man with a ventricular septal defect and severe pulmonary hypertension proved by cardiac catheterization. Abnormal right axis deviation with a qR pattern is apparent on the ECG in lead V_1, and T wave changes are visible in the right precordial leads.

however, the amplitude of the QRS complexes in the left precordial leads tends to be low.

A similar pattern in the left precordial leads may be seen in normal subjects and with various conditions associated with cardiomegaly and marked leftward shift of the transition zone. An rS pattern in leads V_5 and V_6 may be seen in patients with anterior myocardial infarction[110] (see Figure 4–7) and in those with left anterior fascicular block.[111]

ST Segment and T Wave Changes in RVH. With RVH, ST segment depression and T wave inversion are seen most commonly in the right precordial leads (see Figures 3–12 and 3–14). These changes also may be seen in leads II, III, and aV_F. If the T waves are biphasic in the right precordial leads, it is useful to note whether the configuration is of the positive-negative or negative-positive type. A negative-positive biphasic T wave is abnormal and often is seen in patients with RVH[112,113] (Figure 3–15), whereas the positive-negative configuration may be normal.

Systolic and Diastolic Overload Patterns. Cabrera and Monroy[50] called attention to the different ECG changes during systolic and diastolic overloading of the right ventricle. With systolic overloading, which was called *pressure overloading* by later investigators, lead V_1 exhibits a tall monophasic R wave or a diphasic RS, Rs, or qR complex. The T wave usually is inverted in this lead. This pattern typically is seen in patients with pulmonary stenosis, tetralogy of Fallot, or pulmonary hypertension (see Figures 3–14 and 3–15). With diastolic, or volume, overload of

the right ventricle, lead V_1 usually shows an rSR^1 pattern. This is the typical QRS complex in patients with an atrial septal defect, partial anomalous pulmonary venous return, or tricuspid insufficiency. The anatomic alteration consists mainly of a dilated right ventricle instead of hypertrophy as in the case of systolic overload.

The clinical application of this concept is of questionable value. As a rule, the hemodynamic correlation of these two ECG overload patterns is more satisfactory in congenital than acquired heart disease.[114]

$S_1S_2S_3$ Pattern as a Manifestation of RVH. The $S_1S_2S_3$ pattern is a frequently used descriptive term during ECG interpretation. It is seen in normal individuals and in patients with pulmonary emphysema or RVH. Chou et al.[112] proposed the criterion of an R/S ratio of <1 in leads I, II, and III or the S waves in these leads that exceed the upper limits of normal for the various age groups as defined by Simonson.[115*] S waves of low amplitude are more likely to be seen in normal subjects and deeper S waves in patients with RVH (Figure 3–16). Additionally, in patients with RVH and the $S_1S_2S_3$ pattern, the prominent late QRS forces are directed rightward and superiorly. The S wave amplitude is usually greater in lead II than in lead III.

---

*Upper limits of the normal amplitude of the S waves in leads I, II, and III:
  Age 20–29: S_1, 0.4 mV; S_2, 0.5 mV; S_3, 0.6 mV
  Age 30–39: S_1, 0.4 mV; S_2, 0.4 mV; S_3, 0.9 mV
  Age 40–49: S_1, 0.3 mV; S_2, 0.4 mV; S_3, 0.8 mV

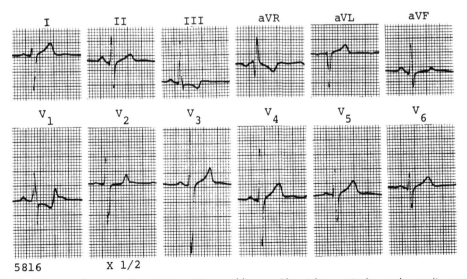

5816   X 1/2

Figure 3–15 Severe pulmonary stenosis in a 19-year-old man. The right ventricular peak systolic pressure was 132 mmHg. On the ECG, the findings suggestive of right ventricular hypertrophy are an abnormal right axis deviation and an R/S ratio >1 in V_1. The R wave in lead aV_R is >5 mm. Note the negative-positive biphasic T wave in lead V_1.

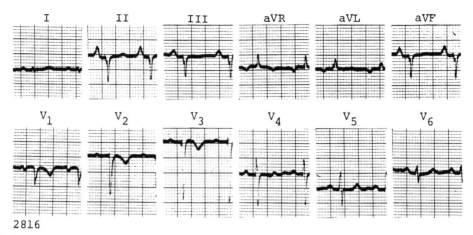

2816

Figure 3–16   RVH resulting from chronic cor pulmonale in a 67-year-old man with severe pulmonary emphysema and chronic cor pulmonale proved at autopsy. There was severe right ventricular hypertrophy and dilatation. Mild atherosclerosis of the coronary arteries was present without evidence of myocardial fibrosis or infarction. On the ECG the P wave is consistent with right atrial enlargement. There is an $S_1S_2S_3$ pattern, with the QRS axis in the frontal plane directed rightward and superiorly. The QS deflection in the right precordial leads with T wave inversion mimics anterior wall myocardial infarction. The R/S ratio in leads V_5 and V_6 is <1.

Incomplete RBBB

Incomplete RBBB, manifested by the rSR^1 pattern in the right precordial leads, is attributed to delayed activation of the hypertrophied right ventricular outflow tract (see Chapter 5). This pattern is most frequently due to factors other than RVH. It can signify hypertrophy, dilation, or overload of the right ventricle, perhaps most commonly in mitral valve disease with pulmonary hypertension (Figure 3–17) and atrial septal defect (see Chapter 12). In patients with pulmonic valvular stenosis, the R^1 voltage correlates with the severity of stenosis[116] (Figure 3–18). The prompt disappearance of this pattern observed in many cases within days after corrective surgery suggests that incomplete RBBB may result from slowing of intraventricular conduction due to stretching of the peripheral conducting system in the dilated ventricle (see Chapter 5).

In addition to RVH, an rSR^1 pattern in lead V_1 with the duration of the QRS complex <0.12 second is also seen in: (1) normal individuals; (2) acute right ventricular dilatation; (3) true posterior myocardial infarction; and (4) extracardiac abnormalities such as pectus excavatum. Further differential diagnoses of the incomplete RBBB pattern is discussed in Chapter 5.

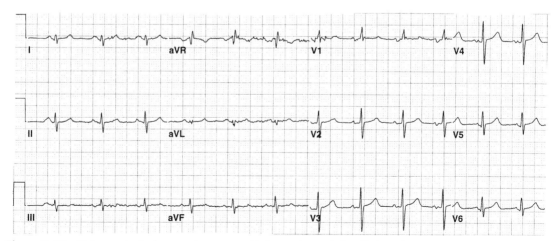

Figure 3–17   Right ventricular hypertrophy pattern with incomplete right bundle branch block in a 52-year-old man with mitral stenosis, mitral regurgitation, and pulmonary artery pressure of 100/42 mmHg. Left ventricular function and coronary arteriogram were normal. The QRS axis is intermediate. The P wave suggests left atrial enlargement.

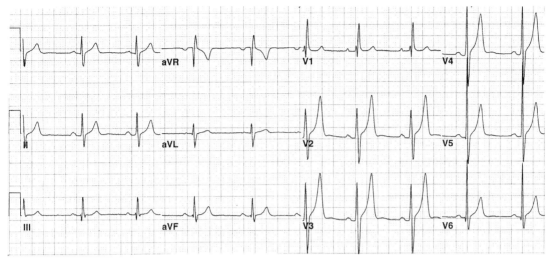

Figure 3–18 Incomplete right bundle branch block with increased R^1 amplitude in a 23-year-old man with moderately severe pulmonary valvular stenosis. Right ventricular pressure was 54/4 mmHg.

Patterns in the Presence of Chronic Lung Disease

The characteristic ECG pattern in patients with COPD is attributed to changes in the spatial orientation of the heart and the insulating effect of the overaerated lungs.[96] The changes induce peaked P waves in leads II, III, and aV_F; a low R wave amplitude in all leads; and a late QRS vector oriented superiorly and to the right resulting in a wide, slurred S wave in leads I, II, III, V_4, V_5, and V_6.[96,118,119] Pathognomonic of emphysema in the absence of myocardial infarction is low voltage with a posteriorly and superiorly oriented QRS vector and an axis of the P wave >60 degrees in the limb leads.[117] Atrial repolarization may become more prominent, as evidenced by depression of the Ta wave in lead II.[121] In the presence of an rSr^1 pattern in the right precordial leads, a slurred S wave in the left precordial leads and a prominent R wave in lead aV_R may indicate superimposed RVH.[117,120]

Severity of Chronic Lung Disease

The best criteria for judging the severity of COPD are (1) R in V_6 <0.5 mV; (2) R/S in V_6 <1.0; and (3) increased P wave amplitude in leads II and III[122] (Figure 3–19). In the orthogonal leads, low R wave amplitude and low R/S amplitude in the X lead, low voltage in the X and Y leads, and a rightward shift of the P axis identified COPD correctly in 75 percent of patients, with only 8 percent being

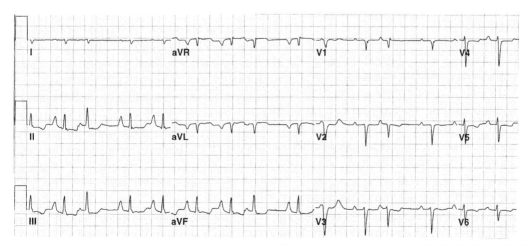

Figure 3–19 ECG pattern suggestive of severe respiratory insufficiency in a 63-year-old man with chronic obstructive lung disease, as described in the text. Premature atrial complexes are conducted with aberration.

false-positive diagnoses.[123] The best reported indicators of deteriorating pulmonary function in patients with COPD are (1) progressive reduction of the R wave and the R/S ratio in orthogonal lead X (may be applied to lead I), (2) progressive shift of the QRS axis in the superior direction, and (3) rightward shift of the P wave axis.

In a study of 263 cases of COPD followed for 13 years after an exacerbation of respiratory failure, Incalzi et al.[123] identified the strongest predictors of death to be an $S_1S_2S_3$ pattern, "right atrial overload" (defined as a P wave axis of +90 degrees or more), and an alveolar-arterial O_2 gradient >48 mmHg. The median survival of patients having either of these two ECG signs was 2.7 years; of those having both ECG signs, 1.33 years.

Chronic Cor Pulmonale

In an effort to detect early cor pulmonale, Kilcoyne and co-workers surveyed 200 patients with COPD.[97] One or more of the following ECG trends were suggested as indicators of right ventricular abnormality or dilation: (1) shift of the mean QRS axis to the right of +30 degrees; (2) T wave inversion in the right precordial leads; (3) ST segment depression in leads II, III, and aV_F; and (4) transient appearance of RBBB. These ECG manifestations usually were associated with an arterial oxygen saturation of less than 85 percent and a mean pulmonary arterial pressure of 25 mmHg or more.

The sensitivity of the ECG for diagnosing RVH in patients with chronic autopsy-proven cor pulmonale is about 60 to 70 percent,[94,124–128] whereas in clinical studies the rate of recognition may be only 28 percent. With moderate RVH the precordial leads display deep S waves in leads V_5 and V_6, but the R waves in the right precordial leads are not prominent. In the most severe cases of cor pulmonale, the QRS forces are oriented anteriorly and rightward, and tall R waves appear in the right precordial leads (Figure 3–20). Patients with cor pulmonale secondary to pulmonary thromboembolism, idiopathic pulmonary hypertension, or obesity hypoventilation syndrome are more likely to have a tall R wave in V_1 than are those with pulmonary emphysema[128,129] (Figures 3–21 and 3–22). The latter, however, more often have deep S waves in leads V_4, V_5, and V_6.

RVH IN OTHER CLINICAL CONDITIONS

Pulmonary Hypertension in Mitral Stenosis

In the absence of RVH secondary to pulmonary hypertension, the only ECG abnormality in patients with mitral stenosis is left atrial enlargement. In the experience of Chou,[130] the criteria for an RVH diagnosis, in descending order of frequency, are an R/S ratio in V_1 >1; a delay of onset of the intrinsicoid deflection in V_1; $RV_1 + SV_{5,6}$ >1.05 mV; S wave in V_1 <0.2 mV; R in V_1 > 0.7 mV; R/S ratio in V_5 or V_6 ≤1; right axis deviation ≥+110 degrees; rSR′ in V_1; RaVR ≥0.5 mV; and qR in V_1. Although exceptions often occur, there is correlation between the degree of pulmonary hypertension in mitral stenosis and the appearance of RVH on the ECG. Fowler and associates[131] found that when the mean pulmonary arterial pressure exceeded 42 mmHg, nearly all the patients exhibited a hypertrophy pattern, as indicated by an abnormal R/S ratio with delayed intrinsicoid deflection in lead V_1. Such evidence was not found in patients with a pulmonary artery pressure <28 mmHg. Others have shown

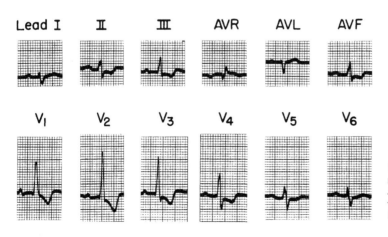

Figure 3–20   Severe chronic cor pulmonale with right heart failure secondary to pulmonary emphysema in a 54-year-old man. Note the qR pattern in lead V_1.

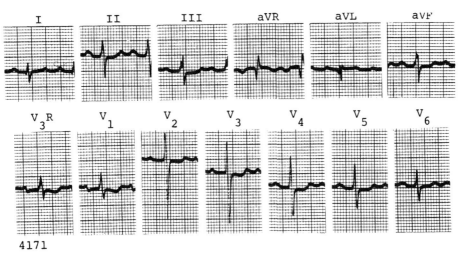

4171

Figure 3–21   Chronic cor pulmonale secondary to recurrent pulmonary embolism in a 56-year-old woman with a 6-year history of recurrent thrombophlebitis of the legs and pulmonary embolism. The diagnosis was verified at autopsy. The heart showed severe right ventricular hypertrophy and dilatation with marked right atrial hypertrophy. The ECG shows first-degree atrioventricular block. There is an $S_1S_2S_3$ pattern. The R/S ratio in lead V_1 is >1. Deep S waves are present in the left precordial leads. ST segment and T wave changes are present in the right and mid-precordial leads. The patient was not receiving digitalis at the time.

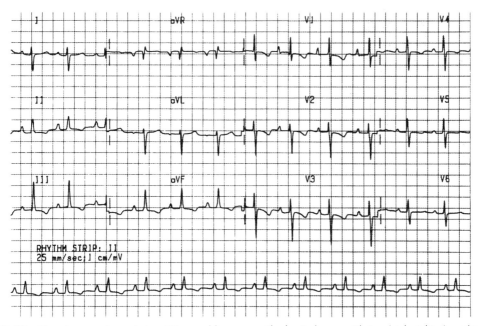

Figure 3–22   Chronic cor pulmonale in a 37-year-old woman with obesity-hypoventilation (pickwickian) syndrome. Her body weight ranged between 250 and 300 pounds, and she had a history of sleep apnea and syncope. There was clinical evidence of right ventricular failure. The pulmonary arterial pressure obtained during cardiac catheterization was at the systemic level. On the ECG the P waves are tall and peaked in leads II, aV_F, and V_1–V_3, suggestive of right atrial enlargement. The abnormal right axis deviation, R/S ratio in lead V_1 >1, and inverted T waves in leads V_1–V_4 are highly suggestive of right ventricular hypertrophy (RVH). T wave inversion in the inferior leads also is related to RVH.

that when the ECG displayed evidence of RVH, the mean pulmonary arterial pressure was uniformly 33 mmHg or higher, and the total pulmonary vascular resistance exceeded 800 or 1000 dynes·sec^{-1}·cm^{-5}.[132–134] The finding of a mean QRS axis that exceeded +90 degrees is thought by some to indicate moderate or severe pulmonary hypertension,[133] whereas incomplete RBBB or an rSR′ pattern is not a reliable indicator of the severity of the vascular obstruction. A monophasic R wave or qR complex in lead V_1 with T wave inversion is uncommon in patients with mitral stenosis, but its presence signifies advanced disease.

Congenital Heart Disease

The ECG diagnosis of RVH in congenital heart disease is generally accurate in more than 90 percent of cases.[93] The higher rate of RVH recognition in congenital heart disease than in acquired heart disease is due mainly to a higher right ventricular systolic pressure, greater right ventricular thickness, and the frequent absence of LVH in the congenital heart disease group.[135]

The relation between the ECG findings of RVH and the hemodynamic findings has been studied in patients with isolated pulmonary stenosis by several investigators.[136–139] According to Burch and DePasquale,[137] the ECG is normal in about 50 percent of patients with mild pulmonary stenosis and a peak right ventricular systolic pressure <60 mmHg. When the right ventricular pressure is elevated moderately or severely, most patients have an RVH pattern. A monophasic R wave or qR complex with T wave inversion in V_1 usually is seen in patients with severe lesions, whereas the less typical rSR^1 pattern is encountered more often in those with mild disease[136,138] (see Figure 3–18).

With an atrial septal defect, the basic pattern of rSR^1 in lead V_1 is common in patients who have mean pulmonary arterial pressures <20 mmHg, whereas most patients with a qR or rSR^1S^1 complex have higher pressures.[137,140] Additional discussion of the ECG findings with an atrial septal defect is included in Chapter 12.

▌ Combined Ventricular Hypertrophy

Partial cancellation of oppositely directed forces generated by LVH and RVH may result in a normal ECG pattern. For example, the development of RVH due to pulmonary hypertension sometimes obscures the previous LVH pattern. More often, however, recognition of the concurrent presence of LVH and RVH is possible because of the asynchrony of ventricular depolarization and because the semidirect precordial leads preferentially reflect the local potentials underlying the respective electrodes. A combined pattern of RVH and LVH is frequently present in patients with ventricular septal defect or patent ductus arteriosus in the presence of pulmonary hypertension (Eisenmenger

syndrome). In such cases, tall R waves may be present in both left and right precordial leads with a tall biphasic QRS in the mid-precordial leads (Katz-Wachtel pattern).[141]

Right axis deviation in the frontal plane in the presence of an LVH pattern suggests associated right ventricular enlargement. A less reliable indicator of possible right ventricular dilation in the presence of an LVH pattern is a shift of the transition zone in the precordial leads to the left. In adults with rheumatic heart disease, biventricular hypertrophy may be suspected in the presence of tall R waves in the left precordial leads and disproportionately small S waves (i.e., <1 mV in lead V_1) or inverted T waves in the right precordial leads. Such a pattern is characteristically present in patients with mitral stenosis and pulmonary hypertension who also have mitral regurgitation or aortic valve disease.

CLINICAL AND ANATOMIC CORRELATIONS

One of the following ECG criteria has been applied in a limited number of correlation studies:

1. ECG pattern meets one or more of the diagnostic criteria for isolated RVH or LVH.
2. Precordial leads show signs of LVH, but the QRS axis in the frontal plane is more than +90 degrees.[142]
3. The R wave is greater than the Q wave in lead aV_R, and the S wave is greater than the R wave in lead V_5, with T wave inversion in lead V_1 in conjunction with signs of LVH.[143]

In general, these criteria have low sensitivity for recognizing combined ventricular hypertrophy. In 172 cases of anatomic combined ventricular hypertrophy studied by four groups of investigators, the ECG was diagnostic in only 17 percent of cases.[143–146] It showed signs of isolated LVH or RVH in 28 percent of the cases. The secondary RVH in patients with left-sided heart disease is usually masked by the dominant LVH (Figure 3–23). Conversely, LVH, which is often seen in patients with chronic cor pulmonale, usually is not detectable on the ECG (Figure 3–24).

The specificity of the ECG diagnosis of combined ventricular hypertrophy is also limited. In a small autopsy series examined by Chou,[130] only 10 of 22 cases (45 percent) with an ECG diagnosis of combined hypertrophy had anatomic combined ventricular hypertrophy, with

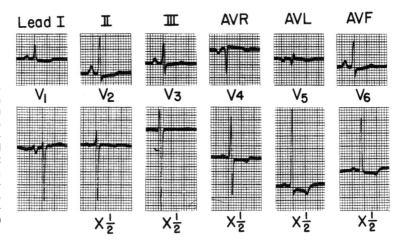

Figure 3–23 Anatomic combined ventricular hypertrophy with a left ventricular hypertrophy (LVH) pattern on the ECG in a 40-year-old man with advanced hypertensive cardiovascular disease and severe congestive heart failure. At autopsy the heart weighed 550 g, with marked hypertrophy and dilatation of all the heart chambers. The ECG shows left atrial enlargement and LVH. No evidence is seen of right ventricular hypertrophy.

the remainder showing isolated LVH. Jain et al.[147] studied 69 patients with biventricular hypertrophy identified by echocardiography. Among them, 17 (25 percent) had ECG findings compatible with biventricular hypertrophy, 25 (36 percent) had an LVH pattern, and 14 (20 percent) had an RVH pattern. An S wave in leads V_5 and V_6 >0.7 mV was the most frequent finding in the 17 patients with the ECG criteria for biventricular hypertrophy. The sensitivity of the ECG criteria for biventricular hypertrophy was 24.6 percent and the specificity was 86.4 percent. Figures 3–23 to 3–26 illustrate the spectrum of ECG changes seen in patients with anatomic combined ventricular hypertrophy.

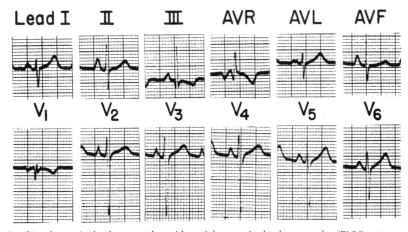

Figure 3–24 Combined ventricular hypertrophy with a right ventricular hypertrophy (RVH) pattern on the ECG in a 25-year-old extremely obese woman (400 lb). She was believed to have the pickwickian syndrome with chronic cor pulmonale and recurrent pulmonary embolism. At autopsy the heart weighed 615 g, with marked RVH and moderate left ventricular hypertrophy (LVH). The right ventricular wall was 9 mm thick, and the left ventricular wall was 19 mm thick. There also was marked right atrial hypertrophy and dilatation. On the ECG the P waves are consistent with right atrial enlargement. An abnormal right axis deviation with deep S waves in the left precordial leads suggests RVH. There is no evidence to suggest coexisting LVH.

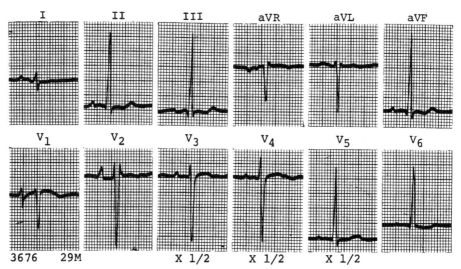

Figure 3–25   Rheumatic heart disease with combined ventricular hypertrophy in a 29-year-old man with severe aortic and mitral valve disease proved at cardiac catheterization and surgery. On the ECG the P waves are consistent with biatrial enlargement. The frontal plane QRS axis is +90 degrees. This finding, in the presence of signs of left ventricular hypertrophy, suggests coexisting right ventricular hypertrophy.

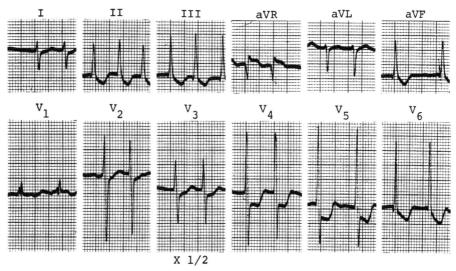

Figure 3–26   Combined ventricular hypertrophy demonstrated on the ECG in a 63-year-old man with severe mitral and aortic stenosis and mild aortic insufficiency. At autopsy the heart weighed 850 g, with hypertrophy and dilatation of all chambers. The left ventricular wall was 20 mm thick, and the right ventricular wall was 9 mm thick. Coronary arteries were patent, and there was no evidence of myocardial infarction. The ECG shows atrial fibrillation. The abnormal right axis deviation and the RSR[1] pattern in lead V_1 suggest right ventricular hypertrophy. The voltage of the R waves and the ST segment and T wave changes in the left precordial leads suggest left ventricular hypertrophy. Some of the ST and T changes are the result of a digitalis effect.

REFERENCES

1. Surawicz B: Electrocardiographic diagnosis of chamber enlargement. J Am Coll Cardiol 8:711, 1986.
2. Linzbach AJ: Heart failure from the point of view of quantitative anatomy. Am J Cardiol 5:370, 1960.
3. Thiry PS, Rosenberg RM, Abbott JA: A mechanism for the electrocardiogram response to left ventricular hypertrophy and acute ischemia. Circ Res 36:92, 1975.
4. Durrer D: The human heart: some aspects of its excitation. Transact Stud Coll Physicians Phila 33:159, 1966.
5. Hugenholtz PG, Gamboa R: Effect of chronically increased ventricular pressure on electrical forces of the heart. Circulation 30:511, 1964.
6. Baxley WA, Dodge HT, Sandler H: A quantitative angiocardiographic study of left ventricular hypertrophy and the electrocardiogram. Circulation 37:509, 1968.

7. McFarland TM, Alam M, Goldstein S, et al: Echocardiographic diagnosis of left ventricular hypertrophy. Circulation 57:1140, 1978.
8. Inoue H, Takenaka K, Murayama M, et al: Effects of acute changes in left ventricular size on surface potential in man. Jpn Heart J 23:279, 1982.
9. Wollam GL, Hull WD, Porter VD, et al: Time course of regression of left ventricular hypertrophy in treated hypertensive patients. Am J Med 75:100, 1983.
10. Lepeschkin E: Modern Electrocardiography. The P-Q-R-S-T-U Complex, Baltimore, Williams & Williams, 1951.
11. Antman EM, Green LH, Grossman W: Physiologic determinants of the electrocardiographic diagnosis of left ventricular hypertrophy. Circulation 60:386, 1979.
12. Devereux RB, Phillips MC, Casale PN, et al: Geometric determinants of electrocardiographic left ventricular hypertrophy. Circulation 67:907, 1983.
13. Brody DA: A theoretical analysis of intracavitary blood mass influence on the heart-lead relationship. Circ Res 4:731, 1956.
14. Daniels S, Iskandrian AS, Hakki AH, et al: Correlation between changes in R wave amplitude and left ventricular volume induced by rapid atrial pacing. Am Heart J 107:711, 1984.
15. Battler A, Froelicher V, Slutsky R, et al: Relationship of QRS amplitude changes during exercise to left ventricular function and volumes and the diagnosis of coronary artery disease. Circulation 60:1004, 1079.
16. Deanfield JE, Davies G, Mongiardi F, et al: Factors influencing R wave amplitude in patient with ischaemic heart disease. Br Heart J 49:8, 1983.
17. Feldman T, Childers RW, Borow KM, et al: Change in ventricular cavity size: differential effects on QRS and T wave amplitude. Circulation 72:495, 1985.
18. Horton JD, Sherber HS, Lakatta EG: Distance correction for precordial electrocardiographic voltage in estimating left ventricular mass. Circulation 55:509, 1977.
19. Carter WA, Estes EH Jr: Electrocardiographic manifestations of ventricular hypertrophy, a computer study of ECG-anatomic correlations in 319 cases. Am Heart J 68:173, 1964.
20. Sokolow M, Lyon TP: The ventricular complex in ventricular hypertrophy as obtained by unipolar precordial and limb leads. Am Heart J 37:161, 1949.
21. Romhilt DW, Estes EH: Point-score system for the ECG diagnosis of left ventricular hypertrophy. Am Heart J 75:752, 1968.
22. Casale PN, Devereux RB, Kligfield P, et al: Electrocardiographic detection of left ventricular hypertrophy: development and prospective validation of improved criteria. J Am Coll Cardiol 6:572, 1985.
23. Okin PM, Roman MJ, Devereux RB, et al: Electrocardiographic identification of increased left ventricular mass by simple voltage-duration products. J Am Coll Cardiol 23:417, 1995.
24. Norman JE, Levy D: Improved electrocardiographic detection of echocardiographic left ventricular hypertrophy: results of a correlated data base approach. J Am Coll Cardiol 26:1022, 1995.
25. Scott RC, Seiwert VJ, Simon DL, et al: Left ventricular hypertrophy: study of accuracy of current electrocardiographic criteria when compared with autopsy findings in one hundred cases. Circulation 11:89, 1955.
26. Rosenfeld I, Goodrich C, Kassebaum G, et al: The electrocardiographic recognition of left ventricular hypertrophy. Am Heart J 63:731, 1962.
27. Selzer A, Ebnother CL, Packard P, et al: Reliability of electrocardiographic diagnosis of left ventricular hypertrophy. Circulation 17:255, 1958.
28. Chou TC, Scott RC, Booth RW, et al: Specificity of the current electrocardiographic criteria in the diagnosis of left ventricular hypertrophy. Am Heart J 60:371, 1960.
29. Mazzoleni A, Wolff R, Wolff L, et al: Correlation between component cardiac weights and electrocardiographic patterns in 185 cases. Circulation 30:808, 1964.
30. Molloy TJ, Okin P, Devereux RB, et al: Electrocardiographic detection of left ventricular hypertrophy by the simple QRS voltage-duration product. J Am Coll Cardiol 20:1180, 1992.
31. Savage DD, Drayer HM, Henry WL, et al: Electrocardiographic findings in patients with obstructive and nonobstructive hypertrophic cardiomyopathy. Circulation 58:402, 1978.
32. Romhilt DW, Bove KE, Norris RJ, et al: A critical appraisal of the electrocardiographic criteria for the diagnosis of left ventricular hypertrophy. Circulation 40:185, 1969.
33. Cohen A, Hagan AD, Watkins J, et al: Clinical correlates in hypertensive patients with left ventricular hypertrophy diagnosed with echocardiography. Am J Cardiol 47:335, 1981.
34. Toshima H, Koga Y, Kimura N: Correlations between electrocardiographic, vectorcardiographic, and echocardiographic findings in patients with left ventricular overload. Am Heart J 94:547, 1977.
35. Browne PJ, Sridhar S, Dresser KB, et al: Hypertrophy or dilatation? A vectorial analysis of echocardiographically determined left ventricular enlargement. J Electrocardiol 11:117, 1978.
36. Geva B, Elkayam U, Fisman W, et al: Determination of left ventricular wall thickening in patients with chronic systemic hypertension: correlation of electrocardiography and echocardiography. Chest 76:557, 1979.
37. Bennet DH, Evans DD: Correlation of left ventricular mass determined by echocardiography with vectorcardiographic and electrocardiographic measurements. Br Heart J 36:981, 1974.
38. O'Keefe DD, Hoffman DT, Cheitlin R, et al: Coronary blood flow in experimental canine left ventricular hypertrophy. Circ Res 43:43, 1978.
39. Huwez FU, Pringle SD, Macfarlane PW: Variable patterns of ST-T abnormalities in patients with left ventricular hypertrophy and normal coronary arteries. Br Heart J 67:304, 1992.
40. Grant RP: Left axis deviation. Circulation 14:233, 1956.
41. Barker JM: The Unipolar Electrocardiogram: A Clinical Interpretation. Norwalk, CT, Appleton-Century-Crofts, 1952, p. 375.
42. Kishida H, Cole JS, Surawicz B: Negative U wave: a highly specific but poorly understood sign of heart disease. Am J Cardiol 49:2030, 1982.
43. Reichek N, Devereux RB: Left ventricular hypertrophy: relationship of anatomic, echocardiographic and electrocardiographic findings. Circulation 63:1391, 1981.
44. Kansal S, Roitman DI, Sheffield LT: A quantitative relationship of electrocardiographic criteria of left ventricular hypertrophy with echocardiographic left ventricular mass. Clin Cardiol 6:456, 1983.
45. Devereux RB, Reichek N: Repolarization abnormalities of left ventricular hypertrophy: clinical, echocardiographic and hemodynamic correlates. J Electrocardiol 15:47, 1982.
46. Devereux RB, Casale PN, Eisenberg RR, et al: Electrocardiographic detection of left ventricular hypertrophy using echocardiographic determination of left ventricular mass as the reference standard: comparison of standard criteria, computer diagnosis and physician interpretation. J Am Coll Cardiol 3:82, 1984.

47. Crow RS, Prineas RJ, Rautaharju P, et al: Relation between electrocardiography and echocardiography for left ventricular mass in mild systemic hypertension (results from treatment of mild hypertension study). Am J Cardiol 75:1233, 1995.

48. Budhwani N, Patel S, Dwyer EM Jr: Electrocardiographic diagnosis of left ventricular hypertrophy: the effect of left ventricular wall thickness, size, and mass on the specific criteria for left ventricular hypertrophy. Am Heart J 149:709, 2005.

49. Moro C, Tascon J, Muela A: Correlation between electrical and echocardiographic data in hypertrophic cardiomyopathy. Int J Cardiol 3:381, 1983.

50. Cabrera CE, Monroy JR: Systolic and diastolic loading of the heart. II. Electrocardiographic data. Am Heart J 43:669, 1952.

51. Kilty SE, Lepeschkin E: Effect of body build on the QRS voltage of the electrocardiogram in normal men: its significance in the diagnosis of left ventricular hypertrophy. Circulation 31:77, 1965.

52. Larkin H, Hunyor SN: Precordial voltage variation in the normal electrocardiogram. J Electrocardiol 13:347, 1980.

53. Piccolo E, Raviele A, Delise P, et al: The role of left ventricular conduction in the electrogenesis of left ventricular hypertrophy: an electrophysiologic study in man. Circulation 59:1044, 1979.

54. Manning GW, Smiley JR: QRS-voltage criteria for left ventricular hypertrophy in a normal male population. Circulation 29:224, 1964.

55. Pipberger HV, Goldman MJ, Littman D, et al: Correlations of the orthogonal electrocardiogram and vectorcardiogram with constitutional variables in 518 normal men. Circulation 35:536, 1967.

56. Yamashita S, Dohi Y, Miyagawa K, et al: Reliability of the electrocardiogram for detecting left ventricular hypertrophy in elderly. Am J Cardiol 81:650, 1998.

57. LaMonte CS, Friedman AH: The electrocardiogram after mastectomy. Circulation 32:746, 1965.

58. Rosenthal A, Restiaux NJ, Feig SA: Influence of acute variations in hematocrit on QRS complex of the Frank electrocardiogram. Circulation 44:456, 1971.

59. Levy D, Labib SB, Anderson KM, et al: Determination of sensitivity and specificity of electrocardiographic criteria for left ventricular hypertrophy. Circulation 81:815, 1990.

60. Okin PM, Roman MJ, Devereux RB, et al: Electrocardiographic identification of left ventricular hypertrophy: test performance in relation to definition of hypertrophy and presence of obesity. J Am Coll Cardiol 27:124, 1996.

61. Rao S: Racial differences in electrocardiograms and vectorcardiograms between black and white adolescents. J Electrocardiol 18:309, 1985.

62. Bailey MA, Su JJ, Guller B: Racial and sexual differences in the standard electrocardiogram of black vs white adolescents. Chest 75:474, 1979.

63. Xie X, Liu K, Stamler J, et al: Ethnic differences in electrocardiographic left ventricular hypertrophy in young and middle-aged employed American men. Am J Cardiol 73:564, 1994.

64. Rautaharju PM, Zhou SH, Calhoun HP: Ethnic differences in ECG amplitudes in North American white, black and Hispanic men and women: effect of obesity and age. J Electrocardiol 27(Suppl):20, 1994.

65. Arnett DK, Rautaharju P, Sutherland S, et al: Validity of electrocardiographic estimates of left ventricular hypertrophy and mass in African Americans (The Charleston Heart Study). Am J Cardiol 79:1289, 1997.

66. Rudy Y, Wood R, Plonsey R, et al: The effect of high lung capacity on electrocardiographic potentials. Circulation 65:440, 1982.

67. Scott RC: Ventricular hypertrophy. Cardiovasc Clin 5:220, 1973.

68. Hugenholtz PG, Lees MM, Nadas AS: The scalar electrocardiogram, vectorcardiogram, and exercise electrocardiogram in the assessment of congenital aortic stenosis. Circulation 26:79, 1962.

69. Braunwald E, Goldblatt A, Aygen MM, et al: Congenital aortic stenosis. I. Clinical and hemodynamic findings in 100 patients. Circulation 27:426, 1963.

70. Roman MJ, Kligfield P, Devereux RB, et al: Geometric and functional correlates of electrocardiographic repolarization and voltage abnormalities in aortic regurgitation. J Am Coll Cardiol 9:500, 1987.

71. Bentivoglio LG, Urricchio JF, Waldow A, et al: An electrocardiographic analysis of sixty-five cases of mitral regurgitation. Circulation 18:572, 1958.

72. Dawber TR, Kannel WB, Love DE, et al: The electrocardiogram in heart disease detection: a comparison of the multiple and single lead procedures. Circulation 5:559, 1952.

73. Kannel WB, Margolis JR: Electrocardiographic left ventricular hypertrophy and risk of coronary heart disease: the Framingham study. Ann Intern Med 72:813, 1970.

74. Ashizawa N, Seto S, Kitano K, et al: Effects of blood pressure changes on development and regression of electrocardiographic left ventricular hypertrophy: a 26-year longitudinal study. J Am Coll Cardiol 13:165, 1989.

75. Okin PM, Devereux RB, Jern S, et al: Regression of electrocardiographic left ventricular hypertrophy during antihypertensive treatment and the prediction of major cardiovascular events. JAMA 292:2343, 2004.

75a. Wachtell K, Okin PM, Olsen MH, Dahlof B, Devereux RB, Ibsen H, Kjeldsen SE, Lindholm LH, Nieminen MS, Thygesen K. Regression of electrocardiographic left ventricular hypertrophy during antihypertensive therapy and reduction in sudden cardiac death: the LIFE Study. Circulation 116(7):700–5, 2007.

76. Pringle SD, MacFarlane PW, McKillop JH, et al: Pathophysiologic assessment of left ventricular hypertrophy and strain in asymptomatic patients with essential hypertension. J Am Coll Cardiol 13:1377, 1979.

77. De Vries SO, Heesen WF, Beltman FW, et al: Prediction of left ventricular mass from the electrocardiogram in systemic hypertension. Am J Cardiol 77:974, 1966.

78. Kannel WB, Gordon T, Offutt D: Left ventricular hypertrophy by electrocardiogram: prevalence, incidence, and mortality in the Framingham study. Ann Intern Med 71:89, 1969.

79. Sullivan JM, Zwaag RV, El-Zeky F, et al: Left ventricular hypertrophy: effect on survival. J Am Coll Cardiol 22:508, 1993.

80. Schillaci G, Verdecchia P, Borgioni C, et al: Improved electrocardiographic diagnosis of left ventricular hypertrophy. Am J Cardiol 74:714, 1994.

81. Verdecchia P, Schillaci G, Borgioni C, et al: Prognostic value of a new electrocardiographic method for diagnosis of left ventricular hypertrophy in essential hypertension. J Am Coll Cardiol 31:383, 1998.

82. Okin PM, Devereux RB, Nieminen MS, et al: Electrocardiographic strain pattern and prediction of new-onset congestive heart failure in hypertensive patients. The Losartan intervention for endpoint reduction in hypertension (LIFE) study. Circulation 113:67, 2006.

83. Klein RC, Vera Z, De Maria AN, et al: Electrocardiographic diagnosis of left ventricular hypertrophy in the presence of left bundle branch block. Am Heart J 108:502, 1984.
84. Chen PS, Moser KM, Dembitsky WP, et al: Epicardial activation and repolarization patterns in patients with right ventricular hypertrophy. Circulation 83:104, 1991.
85. Wallace AG, Spach MS, Estes EH, et al: Activation of the normal and hypertrophied human right ventricle. Am Heart J 75:728, 1968.
86. Durrer D: The human heart: some aspects of its excitation. Transact Stud Coll Physicians Phila 33:159, 1966.
87. Kyriacopoulos JD, Conrad LL, Cuddy TE, et al: Activation of the free wall of the right ventricle in experimental right ventricular hypertrophy with and without right bundle branch block. Am Heart J 67:81, 1964.
88. Selzer A: Limitations of the electrocardiographic diagnosis of ventricular hypertrophy. JAMA 195:1051, 1966.
89. Myers GB, Klein HA, Stofer BE: The electrocardiographic diagnosis of right ventricular hypertrophy. Am Heart J 35:1, 1948.
90. Sokolow M, Lyon TP: The ventricular complex in right ventricular hypertrophy as obtained by unipolar precordial and limb leads. Am Heart J 38:273, 1949.
91. Murphy ML, Thenebudu PN, Blue LR, et al: Descriptive characteristics of the electrocardiogram from autopsied men free of cardiopulmonary disease: a basis for evaluating criteria for ventricular hypertrophy. Am J Cardiol 52:1275, 1983.
92. Walker JC Jr, Helm RA, Scott RC: Right ventricular hypertrophy. I. Correlation of isolated right ventricular hypertrophy at autopsy with the electrocardiographic findings. Circulation 11:215, 1955.
93. Scott RC: The electrocardiographic diagnosis of right ventricular hypertrophy: correlation with the anatomic findings. Am Heart J 60:659, 1960.
94. Roman GT Jr, Walsh TJ, Massie E: Right ventricular hypertrophy: correlation of electrocardiographic and anatomic findings. Am J Cardiol 7:481, 1961.
95. Chou TC, Masangkay MP, Young R, et al: Simple quantitative vectorcardiographic criteria for the diagnosis of right ventricular hypertrophy. Circulation 48:1262, 1973.
96. Burch GE, de Pasquale NP: The electrocardiographic diagnosis of pulmonary heart disease. Am J Cardiol 11:622, 1963.
97. Kilcoyne MM, Davis AL, Ferrer I: A dynamic electrocardiographic concept useful in the diagnosis of cor pulmonale. Circulation 42:903, 1970.
97a. Milnor WR: Electrocardiogram and vectorcardiogram in right ventricular hypertrophy and right bundle branch block. Circulation 16:348, 1957.
98. Holt JH, Barnard AC, Lynn MS, et al: A study of the human heart as a multiple dipole electrical source. III. Diagnosis and quantitation of right ventricular hypertrophy. Circulation 40:711, 1969.
99. Behar JV, Howe CM, Wagner NB, et al: Performance of new criteria for right ventricular hypertrophy and myocardial infarction in patients with pulmonary hypertension due to cor pulmonale and mitral stenosis. J Electrocardiol 24:231, 1991.
100. Woods A: The electrocardiogram in the tetralogy of Fallot. Br Heart J 14:193, 1952.
101. Flowers NC, Horan LG: IV. Hypertrophy and infarction: subtle signs of right ventricular enlargement and their relative importance. In Schlant RC, Hurst JW, editors: Advances in Electrocardiography, Orlando, Grune & Stratton, 1972.

102. Prakash R: Determination of right ventricular wall thickness in systole and diastole: echocardiographic and necropsy correlation in 32 patients. Br Heart J 40:1257, 1978.
103. Prakash R: Echocardiographic diagnosis of right ventricular hypertrophy: correlation with ECG and necropsy findings in 248 patients. Catheter Cardiovasc Diagn 7:179, 1981.
104. James FW, Kaplan S: The normal electrocardiogram in the infant and child. Cardiovasc Clin 5:295, 1973.
105. Hiss RG, Lamb LE, Allen MF: Electrocardiographic findings in 67,375 asymptomatic subjects. X. Normal values. Am J Cardiol 6:200, 1960.
106. Ziegler RF: Electrocardiographic Studies in Normal Infants and Children, Springfield, IL, Charles C Thomas, 1951.
107. Wigle ED, Baron RH: The electrocardiogram in muscular subaortic stenosis: effect of a left septal incision and right bundle-branch block. Circulation 34:585, 1966.
108. Chou TC, Scott RC, Booth RW, et al: Specificity of the current electrocardiographic criteria in the diagnosis of left ventricular hypertrophy. Am Heart J 60:371, 1960.
109. Fowler NO, Westcott RN, Scott RC: The Q wave in precordial electrocardiograms overlying the hypertrophied right ventricle: intracavity leads. Circulation 5:441, 1952.
110. Goodwin JF: The influence of ventricular hypertrophy upon the cardiogram of anterior cardiac infarction. Br Heart J 20:191, 1958.
111. Rosenbaum MB, Elizari MV, Lazzari JO: The Hemiblocks. Oldsmar, FL, Tampa Tracings, 1970, p. 94.
112. Chou TC, Co P, Helm RA: Vectorcardiographic analysis of T-wave inversion in the right precordial leads. Am Heart J 78:75, 1969.
113. McCaughan D, Primeau RE, Littmann D: The precordial T wave. Am J Cardiol 20:660, 1967.
114. Kamper D, Chou TC, Fowler NO, et al: The reliability of electrocardiographic criteria of chronic obstructive lung disease. Am Heart J 80:445, 1970.
115. Simonson E: Differentiation Between Normal and Abnormal in Electrocardiography, St. Louis, Mosby, 1961.
116. Ellison RC, Miettinen OS: Interpretation of RSR' in pulmonic stenosis. Am Heart J 88:7, 1974.
117. Selvester RH, Rubin HB: New criteria for the electrocardiographic diagnosis of emphysema and cor pulmonale. Am Heart J 69:437, 1965.
118. Schmock CL, Pomerantz B, Mitchell RS, et al: The electrocardiogram in emphysema with and without chronic airway obstruction. Chest 60:328, 1971.
119. Silver HM, Calatayud JB: Evaluation of QRS criteria in patients with chronic obstructive pulmonary disease. Chest 59:153, 1971.
120. Padmavati S, Raizada V: Electrocardiogram in chronic cor pulmonale. Br Heart J 34:658, 1972.
121. Wasserburger RH, Ward VG, Cullen RE, et al: The Ta wave of the adult electrocardiogram. An expression of pulmonary emphysema. Am Heart J 54:875, 1975.
122. Kerr A, Adicoff A, Klingeman JD, et al: Computer analysis of the orthogonal electrocardiogram in pulmonary emphysema. Am J Cardiol 25:34, 1970.
123. Incalzi RA, Fuso L, De Rosa N, et al: Electrocardiographic signs of chronic cor pulmonale: a negative prognostic finding in chronic obstructive pulmonary disease. Circulation 99:1600, 1999.

124. Armen RN, Kantor M, Weiser NJ: Pulmonary heart disease: with emphasis on electrocardiographic diagnosis. Circulation 17:164, 1958.
125. Caird FI, Wilcken DEL: The electrocardiogram in chronic bronchitis with generalized obstructive lung disease: its relation to ventilatory function. Am J Cardiol 10:5, 1962.
126. Millard FJC: The electrocardiogram in chronic lung disease. Br Heart J 29:43, 1967.
127. Phillips RW: The electrocardiogram in cor pulmonale secondary to pulmonary emphysema: a study of 18 cases proved by autopsy. Am Heart J 56:352, 1958.
128. Burwell CS, Robin ED, Whaley RD, et al: Extreme obesity associated with alveolar hypoventilation: a pickwickian syndrome. Am J Med 21:811, 1956.
129. Fowler NO, Daniels C, Scott RC, et al: The electrocardiogram in cor pulmonale with and without emphysema. Am J Cardiol 16:500, 1965.
130. Chou TC: Electrocardiography in Clinical Practice. Adult and Pediatric. 4th ed. Philadelphia, Saunders, 1996, p 63.
131. Fowler NO, Noble WJ, Giarratano SJ, et al: The clinical estimation of pulmonary hypertension accompanying mitral stenosis. Am Heart J 49:237, 1955.
132. Booth RW, Chou TC, Scott RC: Electrocardiographic diagnosis of ventricular hypertrophy in the presence of right bundle branch block. Circulation 18:169, 1958.
133. Scott RC, Kaplan S, Fowler NO, et al: The electrocardiographic pattern of right ventricular hypertrophy in chronic cor pulmonale. Circulation 11:927, 1955.
134. Semler HJ, Pruitt RD: An electrocardiographic estimation of the pulmonary vascular obstruction in 80 patients with mitral stenosis. Am Heart J 59:541, 1960.
135. Goodwin JF, Abdin ZH: The cardiogram of congenital and acquired right ventricular hypertrophy. Br Heart J 21:523, 1959.
136. Bassingthwaighte JB, Parkin TW, DuShane JW, et al: The electrocardiographic and hemodynamic findings in pulmonary stenosis with intact ventricular septum. Circulation 28:893, 1963.
137. Burch GE, DePasquale NP: Electrocardiography in the Diagnosis of Congenital Heart Disease. Philadelphia, Lea & Febiger, 1967, p 322.
138. Cayler GG, Ongley P, Nadas AS: Relation of systolic pressure in the right ventricle to the electrocardiogram: a study of patients with pulmonary stenosis and intact ventricular septum. N Engl J Med 258:979, 1958.
139. Gamboa R, Hugenholtz PG, Nadas AS: Corrected (Frank), uncorrected (cube), and standard electrocardiographic lead systems in recording augmented right ventricular forces in right ventricular hypertension. Br Heart J 28:62, 1966.
140. Barboza ET, Brandenburg RO, Swan HJC: Atrial septal defect: the electrocardiogram and its hemodynamic correlations in 100 proved cases. Am J Cardiol 2:698, 1958.
141. Katz LN, Wachtel H: The diphasic QRS type of electrocardiogram in congenital heart disease. Am Heart J 13:202, 1937.
142. Soulie P, Laham J, Papanicolis I, et al: Les principaux types electrocardiographiques de surcharge ventriculaire combinee. Arch Mal Coeur 42:791, 1949.
143. Pagnoni A, Goodwin JF: The cardiographic diagnosis of combined ventricular hypertrophy. Br Heart J 14:451, 1952.
144. Fraser HRL, Turner R: Electrocardiography in mitral valvular disease. Br Heart J 17:459, 1955.
145. Levine HD, Phillips E: An appraisal of the newer electrocardiography: correlations in one hundred and fifty consecutive autopsied cases. N Engl J Med 245:833, 1951.
146. Lipsett MB, Zinn WJ: Anatomic and electrocardiographic correlation in combined ventricular hypertrophy. Am Heart J 45:86, 1953.
147. Jain A, Chandna H, Silber EN, et al: Electrocardiographic patterns of patients with echocardiographically determined biventricular hypertrophy. J Electrocardiol 32:269, 1999.

4 Left Bundle Branch Block

PATHOGENESIS

After division of the left main bundle branch in dogs,[1-3] points adjacent to the interventricular groove anteriorly and posteriorly were activated from the right side without delay. Activation of the left septal surface was delayed by an average of 35 ms (range 15 to 68 ms). The delay at points located farther from the interventricular groove was approximately equal to that in the septum.[2] This finding suggests that activation occurred through the Purkinje system below the level of the block. Further studies showed that the time required for complete activation of the left septal surface was considerably shorter than the control value.[3] This is consistent with the concept that after block of the left bundle branch the homolateral subendocardial Purkinje system is activated simultaneously at multiple points, permitting rapid spread of activation to the adjoining muscle fibers of the left septal surface. These studies established the evidence of transseptal impulse propagation.

In humans, left bundle branch block (LBBB) caused the following changes in epicardial activation[4,5]: (1) right ventricular activation began earlier than normal with a breakthrough at 5 to 26 ms after the onset of the QRS complex; (2) consistent with the animal studies, part of the right septal surface activation was dependent on the left bundle branch; (3) a discrete left ventricular epicardial breakthrough was absent; (4) there was slow transseptal activation with anteroseptal crossing preceding the inferoseptal crossing by an average of 42 ms; (5) the distal left ventricular Purkinje system appeared to be engaged during the latter part of the QRS complex, as suggested by widely spread isochrones[5]; (6) the latest left ventricular activation occurred at 113 to 140 ms (average 124 ms), which was on average 20 ms before the end of the QRS complex.

Endocardial activation in LBBB was studied intraoperatively in patients with LBBB[6] and in the absence of LBBB when the LBBB pattern was simulated by right ventricular pacing.[7] The effects of preexisting LBBB and right ventricular pacing on the spread of excitation resembled each other, but the endocardial activation time was significantly longer during pacing from the right ventricular apex than from the right ventricular septum. These studies showed that: (1) right ventricular activation occurred before the onset of left ventricular activation; (2) the duration of total right ventricular activation was 36 ms, and right ventricular activation was completed 44 ms after the onset of the QRS complex; (3) left ventricular breakthrough occurred 44 to 58 ms after the onset of the QRS complex, most likely as a result of right-to-left transseptal activation (the transseptal time, defined as the interval from the right ventricular pacing stimulus to the earliest left ventricular activation, was 55 ± 17 ms in the absence of myocardial infarction); and (4) total left ventricular endocardial activation time averaged 61 ms in patients without organic heart disease, 81 ms in those with cardiomyopathy, and 119 ms in patients with previous anterior myocardial infarction. This suggests that the duration of left ventricular endocardial activation depends on the functional integrity of the distal specialized conduction system.[6] Rodriguez et al.[8] used a three-dimensional (3D) mapping system in patients with heart failure and found two types of left septal activation: endocardial activation via slowly conducting left bundle branch or high septal activation, probably via transseptal conduction from the right side. In some patients, right ventricular activation times were longer than left ventricular activation times.

HIS BUNDLE RECORDING

In the early study of Rosen et al.,[9] the HQ interval in patients with right bundle branch block (RBBB) and LBBB was prolonged by less than 3 ms, which means that the bundle branch blocks caused little delay of the onset of ventricular activation. Cannom et al.[10] compared the conduction times in the same subjects in the presence and absence of rate-dependent complete and rate-dependent incomplete LBBB. In both situations the presence of bundle branch block reversed the direction of septal depolarization. The complete LBBB increased the QRS duration by 40 to 70 ms and the incomplete LBBB by 30 ms. Change to a complete LBBB pattern was associated with a 10- to 30-ms increase in the HV interval, but change to incomplete LBBB caused no change in the HV interval.[10]

ECG CRITERIA

The World Health Organization (WHO) and the International Society and Federation for Cardiology (ISFC) Task Force[11] recommended the following criteria for diagnosis of uncomplicated LBBB:
1. The QRS duration is 120 ms.
2. Leads V_5, V_6, and aV_L show broad and notched or slurred R waves.
3. With the possible exception of lead aV_L, the Q wave is absent in left-sided leads.
4. The R peak time is prolonged by more than 60 ms in leads V_5 and V_6 but is normal in leads V_1 and V_2 when it can be determined.

The Q wave is absent because the initial QRS vector is directed to the left and most often anteriorly and superiorly. The slowing and notching of the mid-QRS portion is caused by slow transseptal conduction. The mass of the left ventricle

is activated in the left, posterior, and inferior direction. The polarity of the ST segment and the T wave is directed opposite to the main QRS axis, and the ventricular gradient is normal in persons with minimal heart disease but abnormal in those with severe heart disease.[12] Changes produced by the appearance of LBBB are shown in Figure 4–1 (see also Figure 3–6). Body surface maps[13] showed: (1) the location of the initial minimum to be on the right lateral or posterior chest, whereas normally the minima are located on the left lateral chest; (2) early appearance of the QRS minimum on the presternal areas (i.e., 16 ms vs. about 30 ms in normal subjects); (3) longer persistence of the QRS maximum in the left axillary region during the last two thirds of the QRS complex (i.e., 70 to 100 ms vs. 40 to 60 ms in normal subjects); (4) location of the earliest repolarization (presumably arising in the right ventricle) in the presternal region, whereas in normal subjects the early repolarization maximum occupies the left mammary or axillary regions; (5) location of the repolarization minimum during most of the ST-T interval in the left lateral region (i.e., the last areas to repolarize).

PATHOLOGY

Mauricio Rosenbaum divided LBBB into predivisional and divisional types. Studies of Lev et al.[14] showed that pathologic changes in the left bundle branch were caused by ischemic or mechanical (i.e., fibrosis of the cardiac skeleton) factors. In all studied cases the bundle was interrupted at the junction of the His bundle and left bundle branch. This suggests that LBBB is usually predivisional, a finding that is in agreement with the studies of Lenegre[15] and others.[14] The site at the junction with the His bundle is probably the most vulnerable portion of the left bundle branch because it is sandwiched between the connective tissue of the membranous septum and the summit of the ventricular septum.[14]

CLINICAL SIGNIFICANCE AND PROGNOSIS

The LBBB is encountered usually in patients with structural heart disease associated with hypertrophy, dilation, or fibrosis of the left ventricular myocardium, ischemic heart disease, and various cardiomyopathies[16–20] as well as advanced valvular heart disease. The incidence of LBBB was 14 percent among 250 patients with aortic stenosis.[19] LBBB can be caused by

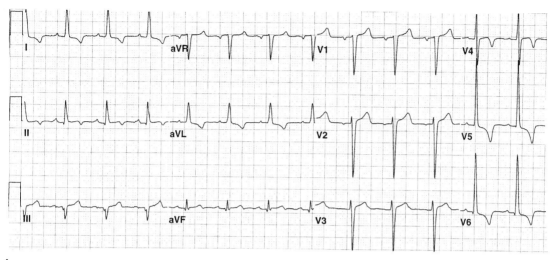

A

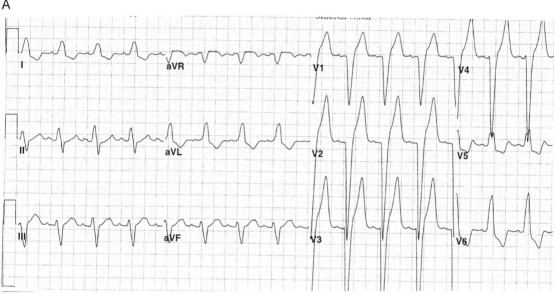

B

Figure 4–1   ECG of a 63-year-old man with critical aortic stenosis, aortic regurgitation, and normal coronary arteries without **(A)** and with **(B)** left bundle branch block (LBBB). **A,** Note the pattern of left ventricular hypertrophy and pseudoinfarction (QS in lead III). **B,** LBBB obliterates q in leads V_5 and V_6, obliterates the initial r in V_1 and V_2 (pseudoinfarction pattern), decreases the initial R amplitude in V_3 and V_4, shifts the QRS axis in the frontal plane to the left, and produces secondary ST segment and T wave changes.

toxic, inflammatory changes,[20] hyperkalemia,[21] or digitalis toxicity.[22]

LBBB can be also caused by primary degenerative disease of the conducting system (Lenegre disease) or sclerosis and calcification of the cardiac skeleton (Lev disease).[15,23,24] These conduction system diseases usually occur in elderly patients. In a general male population the prevalence of LBBB at age 50 was 0.4 percent, and at age 80 it was 6.7 percent.[25] In most subjects with LBBB, regional wall motion abnormalities (i.e., akinetic or dyskinetic segments in the septum, anterior wall, or at the apex) are present even in the absence of coronary artery disease, previous myocardial infarction, or cardiomyopathy, probably as a result of an abnormal sequence of activation.[26] LBBB is frequently produced by septal myectomy in patients with obstructive hypertrophic cardiomyopathy.[27]

The presence of LBBB has no adverse prognostic significance in subjects without evidence of structural heart disease.[28–31] Such patients fall primarily into a category of young subjects with idiopathic LBBB or older subjects with primary disease of the conducting system.

In a study of 67,375 asymptomatic U.S. Air Force cadets, Lamb et al.[32] found LBBB in 13 subjects who had no evidence of heart disease. Rotman and Triebwasser[29] followed a group of 121 Air Force flying personnel and applicants with LBBB; their age at the time of diagnosis ranged from 20 to 56 years, and 89 percent had no evidence of heart disease. After a mean follow-up of 8.8±4.8 years, most subjects remained free of cardiovascular disease. Coronary artery disease was found in 5 percent and hypertension in 9 percent; nine subjects (8 percent) died during the follow-up period.

In the Framingham study,[33] 55 subjects developed new LBBB at an average age of 62 years. Cardiovascular disease was manifest in 89 percent of these individuals at the time of the appearance of LBBB, and 50 percent died within 10 years of the onset of LBBB. Only 11 percent of subjects with LBBB remained free of cardiovascular abnormalities during the follow-up period (versus 48 percent in the control population). In another study of 550 patients with LBBB, only 12 percent had no demonstrable heart disease.[34] The markers of favorable prognosis were an absence of left atrial enlargement, QRS axis in the frontal plane of 0 degrees or more, and a normal electrocardiogram (ECG) before the development of LBBB.[33]

In patients with cardiomyopathy, coronary artery disease, and hypertension, the prognosis depends on the severity of the heart disease. McAnulty et al.[35] found in the prospective study that 21 percent of 104 patients with LBBB died within 2 years, and half of the deaths were sudden. Freedman et al.[36] reported that in patients undergoing coronary artery bypass surgery (CASS study) the presence of LBBB contributed independently to increased mortality. In patients with acute myocardial infarction (MI), the presence of LBBB is associated with increased mortality both in the hospital and during follow-up.[37–39] Additionally, in patients with acute MI undergoing emergency cardiac catheterization, LBBB was associated with greater morbidity and mortality despite treatment with primary angioplasty.[40]

QRS AXIS IN THE FRONTAL PLANE

The appearance of LBBB may cause no QRS axis shift in the frontal plane or variable degrees of left and superior axis shift (Figure 4–2).

The superior axis shift occurs more often in patients with preexisting left anterior fascicular block,[41] and there is an increased incidence of HV prolongation.[42] More advanced heart disease and higher mortality rates have been reported for patients with this pattern.[41,43] Rosenbaum's group[43] suggested that in some cases the LBBB with a superior axis is caused by predivisional LBBB with an additional delay in the left anterior division. Rosenbaum et al.[43] found that a marked shift of the QRS axis to the left may occur because of LBBB alone (see Figure 4–2). This took place in about 70 percent of their cases, and the shift ranged from 2 degrees to 160 degrees (average 40 degrees). Similar findings were reported by Swiryn et al.[44] among 231 patients with intermittent LBBB.

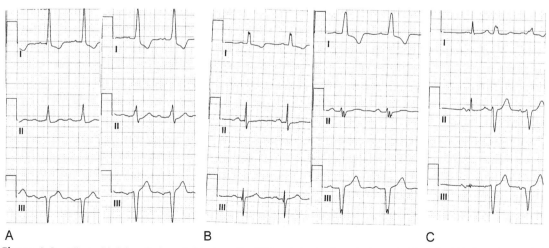

A　　　　　　　　　　　B　　　　　　　　　　　C

Figure 4–2　Effect of left bundle branch block on the QRS axis in the frontal plane. **A,** No axis shift. **B,** Left axis shift. **C,** Superior axis shift.

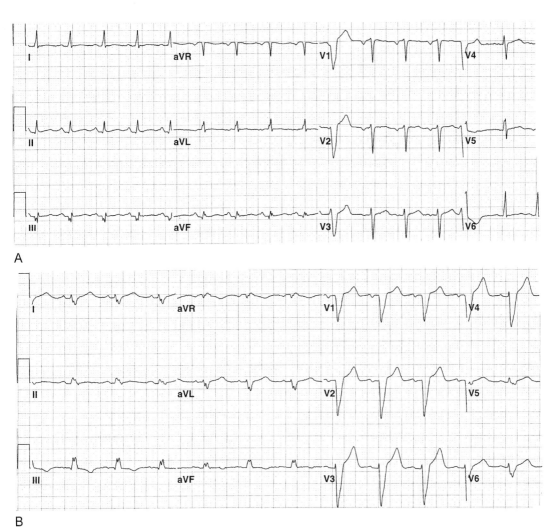

Figure 4–3   ECG of a 49-year-old man with inferior myocardial infarction before (**A**) and 2 days after (**B**) the appearance of left bundle branch block. There is a QRS axis shift to the right in the frontal plane and deep S waves in the left precordial leads.

According to Chou,[45] the axis shift in LBBB can be explained by the manner of the activation front arrival in the Purkinje network following the transseptal transmission. If the activation arrives first at the terminals of the posterior division of the LBB, the delayed excitation of the anterior and lateral wall of the left ventricle results in a leftward or superior shift of the QRS axis. If the activation front arrives first at the terminals of the anterior division or reaches both divisions simultaneously, the QRS axis is shifted rightward or remains normal.

Dhingra et al.[23] compared the clinical ECG findings in 49 patients with chronic LBBB and a normal frontal plane QRS axis (−29 to +90 degrees) and 53 patients with a superior axis (−30 to −90 degrees). The patients with the superior axis were older; had a higher incidence of coronary artery disease, cardiomegaly, and congestive heart failure; had higher mortality; and had longer average PR, AH, and HV intervals. No evidence of structural heart disease (i.e., "primary conduction system disease") was found in 8 of 49 patients with a normal axis and in none of 53 patients with a superior axis. There was no significant difference in the QRS duration or in the presence or absence of an atypical LBBB (Q in I, aV_L, or deep S in V_6) for the two groups.

A less common, atypical pattern is the LBBB with right axis deviation. This may be caused by right ventricular hypertrophy (RVH) or MI. The author has observed that the right axis shift often coincides with the appearance of deep S waves in the left precordial leads (see Figure 4–3).

ATYPICAL LBBB

The WHO criteria[10] apply predominantly to the typical LBBB pattern, but there are several atypical patterns. In a common atypical pattern, RS deflections are present in leads V_5 and V_6 (see Figure 4–3). In most cases of this type, a typical R pattern is present in leads I and aV_L and can also be recorded in leads V_7 and V_8.[45] It can be assumed therefore that the RS pattern in leads V_5 and V_6 corresponds to a transitional zone that is displaced to the left, which may be caused by cardiac dilatation or a ventricular aneurysm.

In a typical LBBB pattern, small R is present in the right precordial leads and in lead III. When the initial r wave amplitude is low or the initial r wave is absent, LBBB simulates MI of the anterior or inferior wall, respectively[46–48] (see Figure 4–1).

Another atypical manifestation is the presence of narrow q waves in lead aVL (Figures 4–4 and 4–5) and occasionally in lead I in the absence of MI. This suggests septal depolarization proceeding from left to right. Observations during right ventricular pacing, however, have shown that q waves in leads I and aV_L may be present in right ventricular paced complexes when the pacing site is located slightly above the apex.[49] It is therefore plausible that the initial front of transseptal activation is directed from right to left but is oriented superiorly and posteriorly, giving rise to a q wave in leads I and aV_L. There

is no experimental support for this hypothesis in patients with LBBB.

QRS DURATION

Because the normal QRS duration ranges in adults from 80 to 110 ms and the duration of transseptal transmission is about 40 ms, the QRS duration in the presence of LBBB may be expected to be within the range of 120 to 150 ms. It may be postulated therefore that subjects with LBBB and a QRS duration >150 ms have structural or functional abnormalities that delay transseptal transmission or cause additional slowing of conduction during later impulse propagation. Such conduction slowing may be caused by sodium channel–blocking drugs or by hyperkalemia. More often, however, patients with marked QRS prolongation (i.e., QRS duration >180 ms) have severe left ventricular structural abnormalities. There is no strict correlation between the QRS duration and the severity of left ventricular dysfunction. Figure 4–4 shows LBBB with a wide QRS complex. In an unpublished personal study, the QRS duration of patients with LBBB and ischemic cardiomyopathy was correlated with the left ventricular ejection fraction (LVEF) measured by angiography or echocardiography. In 11 patients with a QRS duration of 120 to 149 ms (average 135.2 ms), the LVEF ranged from 18 to 52 percent (average 31.4 percent), whereas in 12 patients with a QRS duration of 150 to 192 ms (average 162.2 ms), the LVEF ranged from 15 to 40 percent (average 26.4 percent). The difference failed to reach a level of statistical significance.

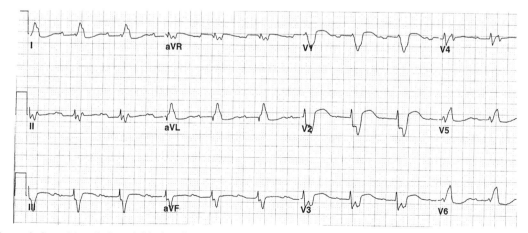

Figure 4–4   Left bundle branch block with a wide QRS complex (218 ms) in the absence of hyperkalemia or conduction-slowing drugs, recorded after cardioversion of atrial fibrillation. P waves suggest left atrial enlargement, and the PR interval is prolonged. There is a small q wave in the aV_L lead.

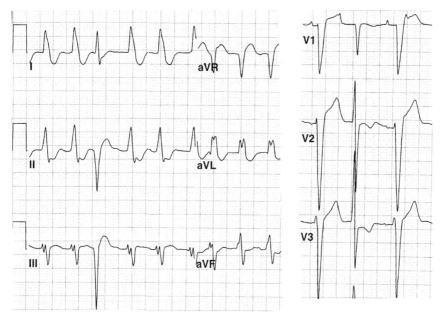

Figure 4–5   Two examples of premature ventricular complex with narrow QRS in the presence of left bundle branch block (LBBB). Note the small q wave in the aV$_L$ lead during LBBB on the tracing at the left.

QRS MORPHOLOGY IN PREMATURE VENTRICULAR COMPLEXES

Premature right ventricular complexes (PVCs) have LBBB morphology, and left ventricular PVCs have RBBB morphology. In the presence of LBBB, PVCs with a narrow or slightly widened QRS complex are common (see Figure 4–5). This may be due to fusion with a conducted impulse when PVCs arise late in the contralateral chamber during diastole or to an equal or a nearly equal delay in both bundle branches. The latter may occur when the PVC originates in the septum distal to the site of the LBBB or when the LBBB is caused not by an anatomic interruption but instead by a conduction delay.[12] A PVC with QR morphology in the left precordial leads suggests MI, even when the supraventricular complexes with LBBB morphology do not reveal the presence of infarction.[12]

Moulton et al.[50] showed that a PVC with a long QRS duration and a broad notch is a reliable marker of reduced left ventricular function. Similarly, a QRS duration of 180 ms or more in ventricular complexes elicited by pacing from the right ventricular apex correlates with increased severity of heart disease.[51] (See also Chapter 26.)

INCOMPLETE LBBB

Incomplete LBBB implies slowing of conduction in the left bundle branch. The presence of incomplete LBBB should be suspected when the ECG shows a pattern of left ventricular hypertrophy with slight QRS widening and absent Q waves in the left precordial leads and lead I. The WHO/ISFC Task Force[10] criteria for incomplete LBBB include (1) QRS duration >100 ms but <120 ms; (2) prolongation of the R peak time to 60 ms or more in the left precordial leads; and (3) absence of a Q wave in leads V$_5$, V$_6$, and I. According to Schamroth and Bradlow,[52] the diagnosis is justified when a transition can be observed during a short time interval from normal ventricular conduction to complete LBBB with an intermediate stage of various degrees of incomplete LBBB (Figure 4–6).

Cases of alternating or rate-dependent incomplete LBBB with reversal of the direction of the initial QRS portion have been reported.[53] Sodi-Pallares and co-workers[54] recorded intracavitary leads in humans with incomplete LBBB and showed reversal of the direction of the initial ("septal") activation similar to that seen in the presence of complete LBBB.

Reversal of the direction of the initial QRS force may not be a reliable indicator for a conduction delay in the left bundle branch. Leighton et al.[55] showed that in five patients with a pattern of incomplete LBBB on the surface ECG, intracavitary leads revealed a normal left-to-right and apex-to-base direction of the initial QRS vector and no evidence of electromechanical delay in the left ventricle.

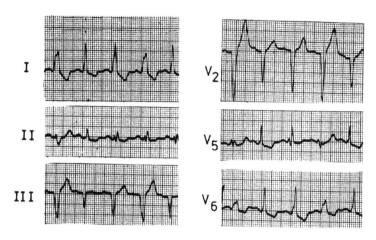

Figure 4–6 Wenckebach period of the left bundle branch.

In view of the controversy surrounding the existence and pathogenesis of the incomplete LBBB, it is appropriate to view the pattern of incomplete LBBB defined by the WHO[10] as a variant of left ventricular hypertrophy (LVH) pattern with additional conduction delay but with similar secondary ST segment and T wave changes.[52,56,57] Nevertheless, some pathologic studies show left bundle branch lesions in patients with incomplete LBBB.[45]

"CORRECTED TRANSPOSITION" OF GREAT VESSELS

In the presence of ventricular inversion and corrected transposition, the initial QRS force has the same direction as in LBBB because the ventricular conduction system is inverted. In the absence of other abnormalities of the conduction system, however, the duration of the QRS complex and other conduction intervals is normal.[58]

DIAGNOSIS OF LVH

The diagnosis of LVH in the presence of LBBB is difficult because LBBB can alter the amplitude of the QRS complex in either direction.[45] It has been suggested, however, that LVH can be suspected when the QRS amplitude is increased. Klein et al.[59] used echocardiograms to develop criteria for the diagnosis of LVH in patients with LBBB. They found that a sum of the S wave amplitude in lead V_2 and the R wave amplitude in V_6 exceeding 4.5 mV had 86 percent sensitivity and 100 percent specificity for LVH. These investigators also found that a diagnosis of LVH was supported by the findings of left atrial enlargement and a QRS duration >160 ms. Mehta et al.[60] also found left abnormality to be a useful predictor of LVH in patients with LBBB.[60]

Most patients with LBBB have anatomic LVH.[14,61–63] Scott and Norris[62] examined the hearts of 29 patients with LBBB. LVH was present anatomically in all patients, whereas the ECG criteria for LVH were present in only 17 of these cases (60 percent).

In some patients with asymmetric hypertrophic cardiomyopathy, Q wave amplitude and duration are increased, presumably due to septal hypertrophy (see Chapter 12). The appearance of LBBB results in obliteration of such Q waves (see Figure 4–16).

PRESENCE OF RVH

The presence of LBBB makes it difficult to recognize RVH. In some cases it can be suspected in the presence of right axis deviation but can be better recognized on the vectorcardiogram.[45]

Recognition of Myocardial Ischemia and Myocardial Infarction in the Presence of LBBB

It has been shown that an acute injury pattern can be recognized in patients with LBBB during percutaneous transluminal coronary angioplasty (PTCA) and spontaneous myocardial ischemia because the ST segment deviation becomes more pronounced under these conditions. Abnormal ST segment deviations can be concordant or discordant with the QRS polarity. The discordant ST segment deviation represents an exaggeration of normal ST segment deviation (i.e., higher than expected secondary ST elevation in the right precordial lead with a dominant S wave or higher than expected secondary ST depression in the leads with dominant R waves) (Figures 4–7 and 4–8).

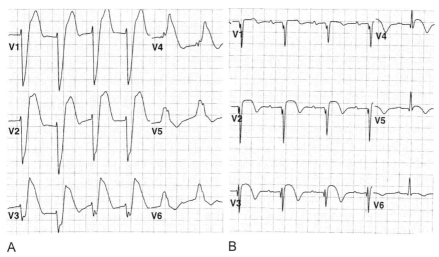

A   B

Figure 4–7 Precordial leads of an 84-year-old man with acute myocardial infarction of the anterior wall. **A,** Left bundle branch block (LBBB) with acute injury pattern causes discordant ST segment elevation, which in leads V_2 and V_3 exceeds 1 mV. **B,** One day later there is evolution of the infarction pattern without LBBB. Cardiac catheterization revealed severe three-vessel coronary artery disease with apical akinesis and a left ventricular ejection fraction of 30 percent.

The concordant ST segment deviation is the opposite of the expected secondary ST segment deviation (i.e., ST depression in the right precordial leads with dominant S wave or ST elevation in the leads with a dominant R wave) (Figures 4–9 and 4–10).

The concordant ST segment deviations are easily recognizable and create no diagnostic difficulties except in the transitional leads with an RS pattern in which ST segment depression or

elevation can be recorded in the presence of an uncomplicated LBBB. Sgarbossa et al.[64] studied the ECGs of 131 patients with acute MI and LBBB. They showed that the maximum sensitivity with a target specificity >90 percent was achieved when at least one lead showed >1 mm concordant ST segment elevation or >5 mm discordant ST segment deviation. In this study, concordant ST segment elevation >1 mm had a sensitivity of 73 percent, whereas discordant ST segment

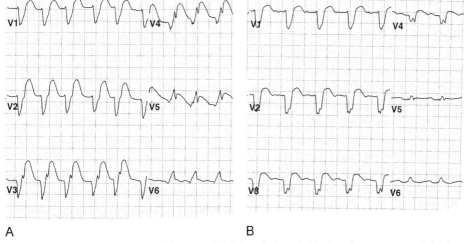

A   B

Figure 4–8 Precordial leads of a 45-year-old man with left bundle branch block and acute myocardial infarction of the anterior wall. **A,** Acute injury pattern manifested by discordant ST segment elevation, which is equal to or exceeds the QRS amplitude in leads V_2–V_4. **B,** One day later there is evolution of the infarction pattern with decreasing ST segment elevation and beginning terminal T wave inversion in leads V_2 through V_4. Note the Cabrera's sign (notch on the S ascent in leads V_2–V_4). Coronary angiography revealed a high-grade complex stenotic lesion in the proximal left anterior descending coronary artery. There was anterior apical akinesis with an estimated left ventricular ejection fraction of 40 percent.

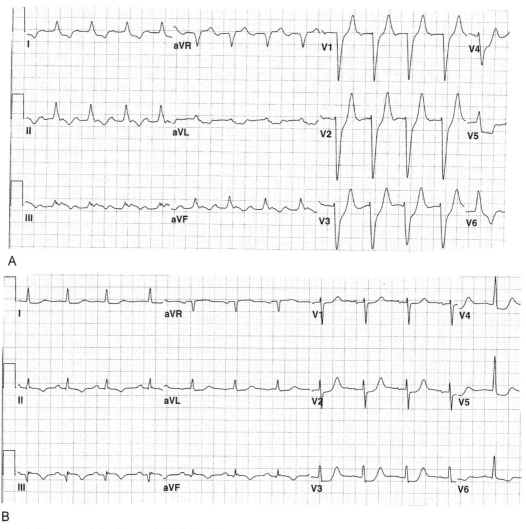

Figure 4–9 Myocardial infarction (MI) of the inferior wall documented by enzyme elevation in a 77-year-old woman. **A,** Left bundle branch block (LBBB) with ST segment elevation in lead III and concordant reciprocal ST segment depression in leads $V_1–V_4$. **B,** On the following day there is a typical pattern of inferior MI without LBBB, with ST segment elevation in leads III, aV_F, and reciprocal ST segment depression in leads I, aV_L, and $V_2–V_5$.

elevation >5 mm had a sensitivity of 31 percent, and concordant ST segment depression in leads V_1, V_2, or V_3 had a sensitivity of 25 percent.[64] The specificity of all patterns was 92 to 96 percent. The results of this study require a caveat because the amplitude of the ST segment deviation has been expressed in millimeters (assuming that 1 mm = 0.1 mV) rather than in percent of QRS amplitude, which influences the amplitude of the ST segment deviation. For example, in the presence of a deep S wave (e.g., 4 mV) in lead V_1 or V_2, an ST segment elevation of 5 mm (0.5 mV) may be normal for LBBB; but with a small S wave (e.g., 0.1 mV), an ST segment elevation of 3 mm (0.3 mV) may be abnormal. The same considerations apply to the magnitude of discordant ST segment depression in relation to the R amplitude in the leads with a dominant R wave.

Primary T Wave Abnormalities

Primary T wave abnormalities caused by myocardial ischemia or other factors are concordant (i.e., negative T wave in the leads with a dominant S wave or RS pattern) (see Figure 4–8). The significance of concordant T wave changes in the leads with a dominant R wave (i.e., upright T wave) is less certain. In the study by Sgarbossa et al.,[64] upright T waves in leads V_5 and V_6 had a sensitivity of 26 percent for the diagnosis of acute MI, but it is not clear whether this

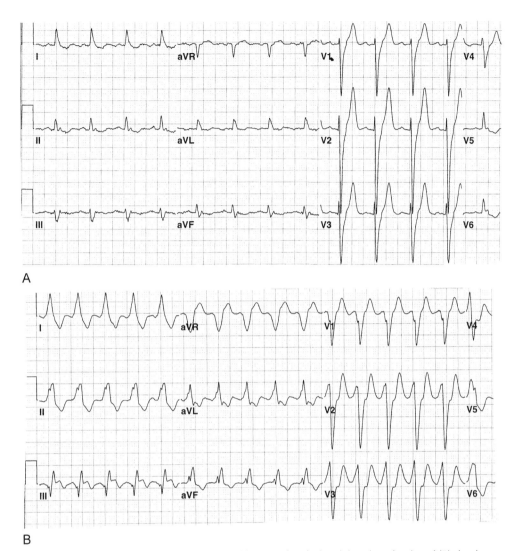

Figure 4–10 Left bundle branch block in a 68-year-old man 2 days before **(A)** and on the day of **(B)** development of an acute myocardial infarction of the inferior wall documented by enzyme elevation. In addition to Q wave and ST segment elevation in lead III, there is concordant reciprocal ST segment depression in leads V_2 and V_3.

T wave pattern resulted from MI. Upright T waves in the leads with a dominant R wave (i.e., leads I, aV_L, V_5, V_6) are frequently present in subjects with LBBB without MI or other structural myocardial disease. This may occur when the secondary repolarization change caused by LBBB fails to produce T wave inversion but lowers the amplitude of the upright T wave. It may also occur when the location of the transition zone of the QRS complex differs from that of the T wave. This situation can be recognized when the T wave remains upright in leads V_5 and V_6 but is negative in lead aV_L. In many cases, however, the mechanism of a persistent concordant T wave in the leads with an

R wave is unexplained by these mechanisms (Figure 4–11).

QRS Changes

The presence of LBBB makes it difficult to recognize MI because the QRS changes caused by LBBB can simulate a pattern of nonexistent MI (see Figure 4–1) or, alternatively, obscure a pattern of preexisting MI (Figure 4–12). Despite these difficulties, many investigators have reported certain atypical features of the QRS configuration attributed to MI, including the following:

1. Q waves in leads V_5 or V_6[65–70]
2. Wide Q waves in I or aV_L

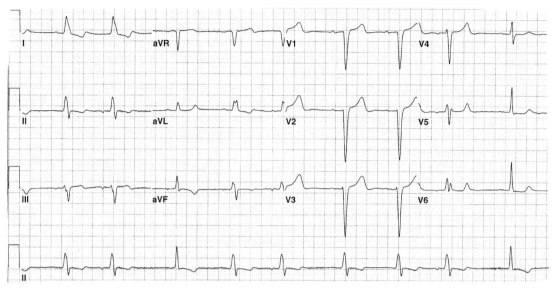

Figure 4–11   ECG of an 82-year-old woman with rate-dependent left bundle branch block (LBBB) that is present in the first two complexes and absent in the third complex following a longer RR interval. There is a late transition zone (between leads V_5 and V_6) and an upright T wave in lead V_6 with an upright QRS complex. The T wave amplitude is higher in the presence of LBBB than in its absence. The patient had severe three-vessel coronary artery disease and an aortic aneurysm.

3. Notching of the S wave in leads V_3 through V_5 (Cabrera's sign) (see Figure 4–8)
4. Small narrow R wave or series of "tiny notches" deforming the terminal portion of the QRS complex[69]
5. Notching of the R wave upstroke in leads I, aV_L, V_5, and V_6 (Chapman's sign)[66]
6. Q waves in leads III and aV_F[67,70] (Figure 4–13): Laham et al.[71] found that in patients with LBBB, a Q wave of 30 ms or longer duration in lead aV_F was present in 10 of 35 patients with inferior MI and in 4 of 131 patients without MI. Negative T waves were present in 30 of 35 patients with inferior MI and in 12 of 131 patients without inferior MI. The combination of abnormal Q waves and negative T waves in lead aV_F provided a sensitivity of 86 percent and a specificity of 91 percent for the diagnosis of inferior MI in the presence of LBBB (see Figure 4–10).

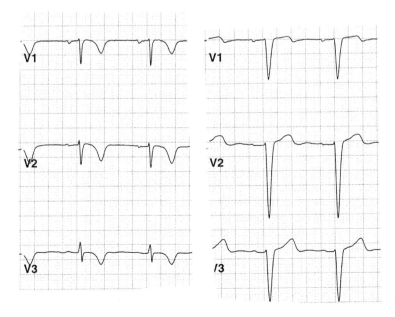

Figure 4–12   Left bundle branch block (LBBB) obscures evidence of myocardial infarction (MI). Leads V_1–V_3 of a 68-year-old woman with recent MI of the anterior wall before and 1 day later when the LBBB appeared.

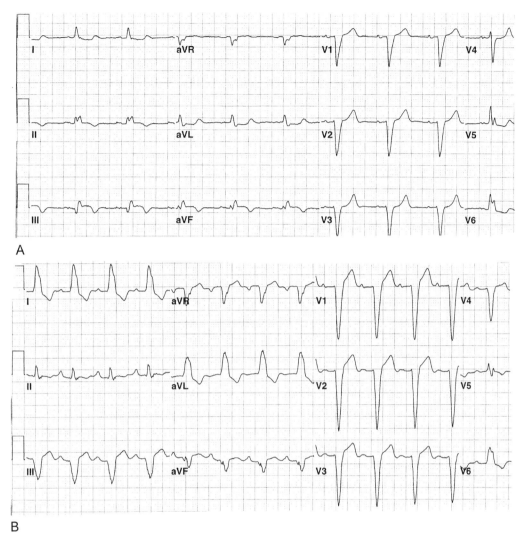

Figure 4–13 Myocardial infarction (MI) of the inferior wall in the presence of left bundle branch block (LBBB). **A,** ECG of a 78-year-old woman following a massive infarction of the inferior wall complicated by cardiogenic shock in the presence of three-vessel coronary artery disease and a left ventricular ejection fraction of 20 percent. There is a wide Q wave, ST segment elevation, and a negative T wave in lead III. **B,** ECG of a 67-year-old man with documented MI of the inferior wall, 100 percent occlusion of the proximal right coronary artery, 70 percent occlusion of the proximal left anterior descending coronary artery, hypokinesis of the anterior wall, akinesis of the inferior wall, and a left ventricular ejection fraction of 35 percent. Note the QS pattern in lead III.

7. Q wave in lead aV$_F$ exceeds 50 ms in duration[72-75]: Suspicion of MI is enhanced when generalized QRS widening exceeds 140 ms and in the presence of Q wave. Horan et al.[73] found that MI was present in 12 of 14 patients with complete or incomplete LBBB and a Q wave in the inferior leads, whereas Q waves in the anterior and lateral leads were not diagnostic of MI.

Kindwall et al.[74] evaluated the predictive value of various ECG criteria listed in the literature by pacing the right ventricle at two sites in patients with various types of MI. This procedure superimposed the LBBB pattern with a normal or superior axis on the MI pattern. The same procedure was carried out in persons without MI. The diagnostic usefulness of the following criteria has been examined: (1) notching of the S wave in leads V$_3$, V$_4$, and V$_5$ (Cabrera's sign); (2) notching of the R in leads I, aV$_L$, and V$_6$ (Chapman's sign); (3) notching of the S descent in leads II, III, and aV$_F$; and (4) abnormal R waves in lead I, aV$_L$, or V$_6$. The investigators concluded that Cabrera's sign is a fairly reliable predictor of previous MI and of an anterior site. Surprisingly, Q waves in leads I, aV$_L$, and aV$_F$ were useful only for localizing the site (anterior) but not for predicting the presence of MI. None of the remaining criteria provided useful information for recognizing a previous MI or locating its site. Because of the occasional q wave presence in leads I and aV_L in the absence of MI, the recognition of lateral or anterolateral MI may be particularly difficult. However, as shown in Figure 4–14, following the occurrence of anterolateral MI the Q wave in leads I and aV_L became wider, the R wave amplitude in leads V5 and V6 decreased, and a Q wave appeared in lead V_6, which is not known to be present in the absence of MI.

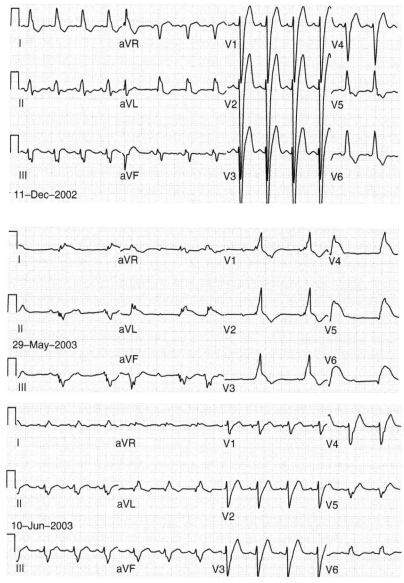

Figure 4–14 ECGs of a 65-year-old woman with left bundle branch block (LBBB) present before the occurrence of myocardial infarction (MI) *(top)*. The middle tracing was recorded on the day of MI caused by complete occlusion of LAD coronary artery at the site of the takeoff of the first diagonal branch showing complete A-V block with ventricular escape rhythm; there is an acute injury pattern with ST-elevation in leads I and aV_L, as well as a monophasic ("tombstone") pattern in leads V_4–V_6. Q waves are present in the leads I, aV_L, and V_5 and V_6. The patient underwent acute intervention with placement of stents in the proximal left anterior descending artery and in the ostium of the first diagonal branch. The bottom tracing, performed 6.5 months after MI, shows LBBB with Q wave in the leads I, and V_5 and V_6. Note that in comparison with the ECG before the MI *(top)*, the Q wave is now present in the lead V_6 and is wider in the leads I and aV_L. There is also a marked decrease of R amplitude in the leads V_5 and V_6.

ECG Diagnosis of Myocardial Ischemia and Myocardial Infarction in the Presence of Right Ventricular Paced Rhythm

It has been pointed out[49] that the diagnosis of remote MI during right ventricular pacing has major limitations. The problems of recognizing abnormal ST segment deviation, abnormal T wave polarity, and QRS abnormalities suggestive of a remote MI in the presence of right ventricular paced rhythm are similar to those encountered in the presence of LBBB.[76] Changes in the catheter position can alter the ECG pattern.[76] Barold et al.[69] suggested that in the presence of right ventricular pacing, MI should not be diagnosed if q waves are present only in leads I and aV$_L$. (See Chapter 26.)

Functional Bundle Branch Block

Cases of intermittent bundle branch block or an alternating LBBB and RBBB (Figure 4–15) prove that in some cases the blocked bundle branches can still conduct. Moreover, it is well known that bundle branch blocks can appear and disappear, depending on cycle length (e.g., acceleration- and deceleration-dependent blocks) (see Figures 4–11 and Figures 4–16 to 4–18), the presence of myocardial ischemia (e.g., exercise-induced block), changes in autonomic nervous tone, and other factors. Therefore in many cases a bundle branch block must be considered in terms of functional rather than anatomic integrity, meaning delayed conduction relative to conduction in other ramifications of the system. Halpern et al.[77] used isoproterenol to alter conditions for induction and termination of rate-dependent bundle branch block. Isoproterenol shortens the effective refractory period of the bundle branch and enhances the rate of diastolic depolarization. Therefore administration of isoproterenol shortens the cycle at which tachycardia-dependent bundle branch block appears and dissipates and the cycle at which the bradycardia-dependent bundle branch block manifests.

MECHANISM OF CYCLE LENGTH–DEPENDENT BUNDLE BRANCH BLOCK

The onset of tachycardia- or acceleration-dependent bundle branch block is best explained by voltage- or time-dependent refractoriness, whereas the perpetuation can be attributed to concealed transseptal conduction from the contralateral bundle branch.

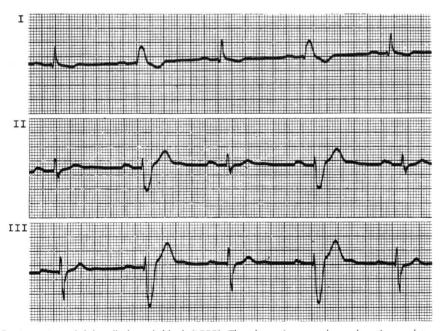

Figure 4–15   Intermittent left bundle branch block (LBBB). The alternating complexes show incomplete and complete LBBB. There is also a first-degree atrioventricular block.

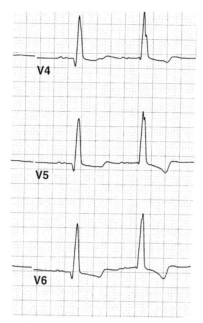

Figure 4–16 Rate-dependent left bundle branch block (LBBB) in a 65-year-old man with severe obstructive hypertrophic cardiomyopathy (intraventricular pressure gradient of 90 mmHg). The first complex preceded by a longer RR interval shows no LBBB and a wide Q wave attributed to septal hypertrophy. In the second complex, LBBB obliterates the Q wave.

The mechanism of bradycardia- or deceleration-dependent bundle branch block at critically long cycles is more controversial.[78] The phenomenon was first reported in 1915 by Wilson,[77] but the first rational hypothesis as to its cause emerged following the discovery of slow conduction and depressed excitability during diastolic depolarization of automatic pacemaker fibers.[79] Clinical observations are available that support this mechanism. For instance, Fisch and Miles[80]

reported cases in which a progressive increase in cycle length resulted in a progressive increase in QRS duration (i.e., change from an incomplete to a complete bundle branch block). In this particular study, definitive evidence of the mechanism (i.e., an automatic escape impulse arising at a critically long cycle) did not occur.

Diastolic depolarization cannot be the only factor responsible for the occurrence of bradycardia-dependent bundle branch block. Numerous laboratory and clinical observations are incompatible with such mechanisms, particularly when excitability decreases with time in the absence of any change of the diastolic membrane potential.[81] Gilmour et al.[82] studied this phenomenon in canine Purkinje fibers, atrial trabeculae, and cat papillary muscles depolarized to membrane potentials of -70 to -60 mV. The decline of action potential amplitude at long coupling intervals was attributed to slow recovery of the transient outward current (i_{to}) because it was prevented by 4-aminopyridine but not by isoproterenol, caffeine, or cesium.

WENCKEBACH PERIODICITY

In 1925 Scherf and Schookhoff demonstrated Wenckebach periodicity in bundle branches in dogs. Subsequently, Rosenbaum and Lepeschkin[83] postulated Wenckebach periodicity in humans with bilateral bundle branch block. Rosenbaum et al.[84] reported cases of manifest and concealed Wenckebach periods in bundle branches and recommended the following diagnostic criteria: (1) the "opening" impulse should be normally conducted in the affected bundle branch; (2) the second impulse should be conducted with a delay of no more than 40 to 60 ms; and (3) the last complex of the sequence should not be activated retrogradely. Figure 4–6 illustrates

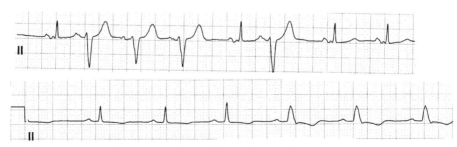

Figure 4–17 Examples of acceleration-dependent left bundle branch block (LBBB) *(top)* and deceleration-dependent LBBB *(bottom)*.

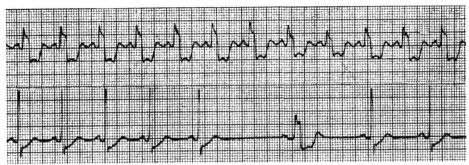

Figure 4–18   Example of tachycardia-dependent and bradycardia-dependent left bundle branch block in the same subject.

Wenckebach periodicity in the left bundle branch.

Lehmann et al.[85] showed that in subjects with normal function of the His-Purkinje system, incremental ventricular pacing permitted achievement of faster rates of input into the conducting system than did supraventricular pacing. Applying incremental ventricular pacing, these investigators established that a 2:1 and 3:2 retrograde Wenckebach block in the conduction system is a "physiologic" phenomenon.[85]

HOW COMPLETE IS "COMPLETE" BUNDLE BRANCH BLOCK?

Cannom et al.[86] tested refractory periods in patients in whom the effective refractory period (ERP) of the ventricular conduction system was longer than the functional refractory period (FRP) of the atrioventricular node. In patients with LBBB, they observed a shift of the mean QRS axis in the frontal plane to the left before the ERP of the ventricular conduction system was reached. This observation documented conduction through the left anterior fascicle during LBBB, but there was no similar evidence that left posterior division participates in conduction. However, conduction abnormalities in the right bundle branch during LBBB were demonstrated by long HV intervals and prolonged ERP of the ventricular conduction system. These examples of slow conduction through the left anterior division and through the right bundle branch, as well as similar observations reported by others, raise the question of the degree of completeness of the "complete" bundle branch block.

In 1974 Wu et al.[87] reported several cases in which premature stimuli changed the pattern of intraventricular conduction disturbance and restored conduction in a bundle branch or fascicle that had been blocked at a basic cycle length. They suggested that a "partial" bundle branch block depends on the discordance of conduction and refractory period. This means that the block occurs when a slowly conducting segment has a shorter refractory period.

In 1981 Barrett et al.[88] postulated that at least half of LBBBs are "incomplete" even though the duration of the QRS complex exceeds 120 ms.* Flowers[60] suggested that intraventricular conduction delays should be viewed in terms of asynchronous ventricular activation resulting from differences in delay in one bundle branch or one fascicle compared with the other. It should be recalled that in some cases bundle branch and fascicular blocks probably occur as a consequence of longitudinal dissociation in the His bundle.[81] Wu et al.[87] noted that variable degrees and sites of conduction delays combined with variable degrees and sites of abnormal refractoriness and excitability can result in "very complex sequences of ventricular activation." In practice, not infrequently widening of the QRS complex occurs in the presence of LBBB when the heart rate increases (Figure 4–19).

---

*This concept was postulated earlier by Scherf (personal communication by Dr. Charles Fisch).

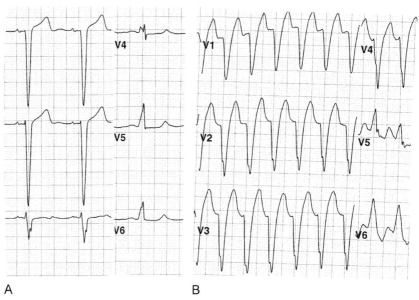

A   B

Figure 4–19   Effect of the heart rate on QRS duration in a 72-year-old man with left bundle branch block, severe obstructive two-vessel coronary artery disease, global hypokinesis, lateral wall akinesis, and a left ventricular fraction of 35 percent. In the tracings recorded 6 hours apart, the QRS duration at a heart rate of 65 beats/min is 128 ms **(A)**; at a heart rate of 151 beats/min, the QRS duration is 148 ms **(B)**.

REFERENCES

1. Amer NS, Stuckey JS, Hoffman BF, et al: Activation of the interventricular septal myocardium studied during cardiopulmonary bypass. Am Heart J 59:224, 1960.
2. Seidenstein M, Stuckey JS, Hoffman BF, et al: Activation of the epicardial surface of the left ventricle following left ventriculotomy and left bundle branch block. Am J Cardiol 10:101, 1962.
3. Venerose RS, Seidenstein M, Stuckey JH, et al: Activation of subendocardial Purkinje fibers and muscle fibers of the left septal surface before and after left bundle branch block. Am Heart J 63:346, 1962.
4. Sohi GS, Flowers NC, Horan LG, et al: Comparison of total body surface map depolarization patterns of left bundle branch block and normal axis with left bundle branch block and left-axis deviation. Circulation 67:660, 1983.
5. Wyndham CR, Smith T, Meeran MK, et al: Epicardial activation in patterns with left bundle branch block. Circulation 61:696, 1980.
6. Vassallo JA, Cassidy DM, Marchlinski F, et al: Endocardial activation of left bundle branch block. Circulation 69:914, 1984.
7. Vassallo JA, Cassidy DM, Miller JM, et al: Left ventricular endocardial activation during right ventricular pacing: effect of underlying heart disease. J Am Coll Cardiol 7:1228, 1986.
8. Rodriguez L-M, Timmermans C, Nabar A, et al: Variable patterns of septal activation in patients with left bundle branch block and heart failure. J Cardiovasc Electrophysiol 14:135, 2003.
9. Rosen KM, Rahimtoola SH, Sinno MZ, et al: Bundle branch and ventricular activation in man: a study using catheter recordings of left and right bundle branch potentials. Circulation 63:193, 1971.

10. Cannom DS, Wyman MG, Goldreyer BN: Initial ventricular activation in left-sided intraventricular conduction defects. Circulation 62:621, 1980.
11. Willems JL, Robles de Medina EO, Bernard R, et al: Criteria for intraventricular conduction disturbances and pre-excitation. J Am Coll Cardiol 5:1261, 1985.
12. Scott RC: Left bundle branch block: a clinical assessment. Part I. Am Heart J 70:535, 1965.
13. Musso E, Still D, Macchi G, et al: Body surface maps in left bundle branch block uncomplicated or complicated by myocardial infarction, left ventricular hypertrophy or myocardial ischemia. J Electrocardiol 20:1, 1987.
14. Lev M, Unger PN, Rosen KM, et al: The anatomic substrate of complete left bundle branch block. Circulation 50:479, 1974.
15. Lenegre J: Etiology and pathology of bilateral bundle branch block in relation to heart block. Prog Cardiovasc Dis 6:409, 1964.
16. Bauer GE: Bundle branch block: some usual and some unusual features. Australas Ann Med 13:62, 1964.
17. Marriott HJL: Electrocardiographic abnormalities, conduction disorders and arrhythmias in primary myocardial disease. Prog Cardiovasc Dis 7:99, 1964.
18. Chen C-H, Sakurai T, Fujita M, et al: Transient intraventricular conduction disturbances in hypertrophic obstructive cardiomyopathy. Am Heart J 101:672, 1981.
19. Wood P: Aortic stenosis. Am J Cardiol 1:553, 1958.
20. Brake CM: Complete left bundle branch block in asymptomatic airmen. Aerospace Med 40:781, 1969.
21. Cohen HC, Rosen KM, Pick A: Disorders of impulse conduction and impulse formation caused by hyperkalemia in man. Am Heart J 89:501, 1975.
22. Singh RB, Agraval BV, Somani PN: Left bundle branch block: a rare manifestation of digitalis intoxication. Acta Cardiol 31:175, 1976.

23. Dhingra RC, Amat-Y-Leon F, Wyndham C, et al: Significance of left axis deviation in patients with chronic left bundle branch block. Am J Cardiol 42:551, 1978.
24. Lev M: Anatomic basis for atrioventricular block. Am J Med 37:742, 1964.
25. Erikssen P, Hansson P-O, Eriksson H, et al: Bundle-branch block in a general male population: the study of men born in 1913. Circulation 98:2494, 1998.
26. Williams RS, Behar VS, Peter RH: Left bundle branch block: angiographic segmental wall motion abnormalities. Am J Cardiol 44:1046, 1979.
27. Quin JX, Shiota T, Lever HM, et al: Conduction system abnormalities in patients with obstructive hypertrophic cardiomyopathy following septal reduction interventions. Am J Cardiol 93:171, 2004.
28. Rodstein M, Gubner R, Mills JP, et al: A mortality study in bundle branch block. Arch Intern Med 87:663, 1951.
29. Rotman M, Triebwasser JH: A clinical and follow-up study of right and left bundle branch block. Circulation 51:477, 1975.
30. Wong B, Rinkenberger R, Dunn M, et al: Effect of intermittent left bundle branch block on left ventricular performance in the normal heart. Am J Cardiol 39:459, 1977.
31. Smith RF, Jackson DH, Harthorne JW, et al: Acquired bundle branch block in a healthy population. Am Heart J 80:746, 1970.
32. Lamb LE, Kable KD, Averill KH: Electrocardiographic findings in 67,375 asymptomatic subjects. V. Left bundle branch block. Am J Cardiol 6:130, 1960.
33. Schneider JP, Thomas HE, Kreger BE, et al: Newly acquired left bundle branch block: the Framingham study. Ann Intern Med 90:303, 1979.
34. Jain AC, Mehta MC: Etiologies of left bundle branch block and correlation with hemodynamic and angiographic findings. Am J Cardiol 91:137, 2003.
35. McAnulty JH, Rahimtoola SH, Murphy ES, et al: A prospective study of sudden death in "high risk" bundle-branch block. N Engl J Med 299:209, 1978.
36. Freedman RA, Alderman EL, Sheffield LT, et al: Bundle branch block in patients with chronic coronary artery disease: angiographic correlates and prognostic significance. J Am Coll Cardiol 10:73, 1987.
37. Abben R, Denes P, Rosen KM: Evaluation for criteria for diagnosis of myocardial infarction: study of 256 patients with intermittent left bundle branch block. Chest 75:575, 1979.
38. Hindman MC, Wagner GS, JaRo M, et al: The clinical significance of bundle branch block complicating acute myocardial infarction. I. Clinical characteristics, hospital mortality, and one year follow-up. Circulation 58:679, 1978.
39. Nimetz AA, Shubrooks SJ, Hutter AM, et al: The significance of bundle branch block during acute myocardial infarction. Am Heart J 90:439, 1975.
40. Guerrero M, Harjai K, Stone GW, et al: Comparison of the prognostic effect of left versus right versus no bundle branch block on presenting electrocardiogram in acute myocardial infarction patients treated with primary angioplasty in myocardial infarction trials. Am J Cardiol 96:482, 2005.
41. Lichstein E, Mahapatra R, Gupta PK, et al: Significance of complete left bundle branch block with left axis deviation. Am J Cardiol 44:239, 1979.
42. Spurrell RA, Krikler DM, Sowton E: Study of intraventricular conduction times in patients with left bundle branch block and left axis deviation and in patients with left bundle branch block and normal QRS axis using His bundle electrograms. Br Heart J 34:1244, 1972.
43. Rosenbaum MB, Elizari MV, Lazari JO: The Hemiblocks. Oldsmar, FL, Tampa Tracings, 1970.
44. Swiryn S, Abben R, Denes O, et al: Electrocardiographic determinants of axis during left bundle branch block: study in patients with intermittent left bundle branch block. Am J Cardiol 46:46, 1980.
45. Chou TC: Electrocardiography in Clinical Practice. Philadelphia, Saunders, 1991.
46. Pryor R: Recognition of myocardial infarction in the presence of bundle branch block. Cardiovasc Clin 6: 255, 1974.
47. Timmis GC, Gandagharan V, Ramos RG, et al: Reassessment of Q waves in left bundle branch block. J Electrocardiol 9:109, 1976.
48. Havelda CJ, Sohi GS, Flowers NC, et al: The pathologic correlates of the electrocardiogram: complete left bundle branch block. Circulation 65:445, 1982.
49. Sgarbossa EB: Recent advances in the electrocardiographic diagnosis of myocardial infarction: left bundle branch block and pacing. Pacing Clin Electrophysiol 19:1370, 1996.
50. Moulton KP, Medcalf T, Lazzara R: Premature ventricular complex morphology: a marker for left ventricular function and structure. Circulation 81:1245, 1990.
51. Sumiyoshi M, Nakata Y, Tikano T, et al: Clinical significance of QRS duration during ventricular pacing. PACE 15:1053, 1992.
52. Schamroth L, Bradlow WA: Incomplete left bundle branch block. Br Heart J 26:285, 1964.
53. Cannom DS, Wyman MG, Goldreyer BN: Initial ventricular activation in left-sided intraventricular conduction defects. Circulation 62:621, 1980.
54. Sodi-Pallares D, Estandia A, Soberson J, et al: Left intraventricular potential of the human heart. II. Criteria for diagnosis of incomplete bundle branch block. Am Heart J 40:655, 1950.
55. Leighton RF, Ryan JM, Goodwin RS, et al: Incomplete left bundle branch block: the view from transseptal intraventricular leads. Circulation 36:261, 1967.
56. Barold SS, Linhart JW, Hildner FJ, et al: Incomplete left bundle-branch block: a definite electrocardiographic entity. Circulation 38:702, 1968.
57. Teresawa F, Kuramochi M, Yazaki Y, et al: Clinical and pathological studies on incomplete left bundle branch block in the aged. Isr J Med Sci 5:732, 1969.
58. Gillette PC, Busch U, Mullins CE, et al: Electrophysiologic studies in patients with ventricular inversion and "corrected transposition." Circulation 60:939, 1979.
59. Klein RC, Vera Z, De Maria JE, et al: Electrocardiographic diagnosis of left ventricular hypertrophy in the presence of left bundle branch block. Am Heart J 108:502, 1984.
60. Mehta A, Jain AC, Mehta MC, et al: Usefulness of left atrial abnormality for predicting left ventricular hypertrophy in the presence of left bundle branch block. Am J Cardiol 85:354, 2000.
61. Flowers NC: Left bundle branch block: a continuously evolving concept. J Am Coll Cardiol 9:684, 1987.
62. Scott RC, Norris RJ: Electrocardiographic-pathologic correlation study of left ventricular hypertrophy in the presence of left bundle-branch block. Circulation 20:766, 1959.
63. Zmyslinski RW, Richeson JF, Akiyama T: Left ventricular hypertrophy in presence of complete left bundle-branch block. Br Heart J 43:170, 1980.
64. Sgarbossa EB, Pinski SL, Barbagelata A, et al, for the GUSTO-I Investigators: Electrocardiographic diagnosis of evolving acute myocardial infarction in the presence of left bundle branch block. N Engl J Med 334:481, 1996.

65. Hands ME, Cook EF, Stone PH, et al, and the MILIS Study Group: Electrocardiographic diagnosis of myocardial infarction in the presence of complete left bundle branch block. Am Heart J 116:23, 1988.

66. Chapman MG, Pearce ML: Electrocardiographic diagnosis of myocardial infarction in the presence of left bundle branch block. Circulation 16:558, 1957.

67. Dressler W, Roesler H, Schwager A: The electrocardiographic signs of myocardial infarction in the presence of bundle branch block. Am Heart J 39:217, 1950.

68. Rhoads DV, Edwards JE, Pruitt RD: The electrocardiogram in the presence of myocardial infarction and intraventricular block of the left bundle branch block type. Am Heart J 62:735, 1961.

69. Barold SS, Falkoff MD, Ong LS, et al: Electrocardiographic diagnosis of myocardial infarction during ventricular pacing. Cardiol Clin 5:403, 1987.

70. Fesmire FM: ECG diagnosis of acute myocardial infarction in the presence of left bundle branch block in patients undergoing continuous ECG monitoring. Ann Emerg Med 26:69, 1995.

71. Laham CL, Hammill SC, Gibbons RJ: New criteria for the diagnosis of healed inferior wall myocardial infarction in patients with left bundle branch block. Am J Cardiol 79:19, 1997.

72. Selvester RH, Wagner GS, Ideker RE: Myocardial infarction. In: MacFarlane PW, Lawrie TD (eds): Comprehensive Electrocardiology. New York, Pergamon, 1989.

73. Horan LG, Flowers NC, Tolleson WJ, et al: The significance of diagnostic Q waves in the presence of bundle branch block. Chest 58:214, 1970.

74. Kindwall KE, Brown JP, Josephson ME: Predictive accuracy of criteria for chronic myocardial infarction in pacing-induced left bundle branch block. Am J Cardiol 57:1255, 1986.

75. Havelda CJ, Sohi GS, Flowers NC, et al: The pathologic correlates of the electrocardiogram: complete left bundle branch block. Circulation 65:445, 1982.

76. Sgarbossa EB, Pinski SL, Gates KB, et al, for the GUSTO-I Investigators: Early electrocardiographic diagnosis of myocardial infarction in the presence of ventricular paced rhythm. Am J Cardiol 77:423, 1996.

77. Halpern MS, Chiale PA, Nan GY, et al: Effects of isoproterenol on abnormal intraventricular conduction. Circulation 62:1337, 1980.

78. El-Sherif N, Scherlag BJ, Lazzara R: Bradycardia-dependent conduction disorders. J Electrocardiol 19:1, 1976.

79. Singer DH, Lazzara R, Hoffman BF: Interrelationships between automaticity and conduction in Purkinje fibers. Circ Res 21:537, 1967.

80. Fisch C, Miles WM: Deceleration-dependent left bundle branch block; a spectrum of bundle branch conduction delay. Circulation 65:1029, 1982.

81. Surawicz B: Electrophysiologic Basis of ECG and Cardiac Arrhythmias. Baltimore, Williams & Wilkins, 1995.

82. Gilmour RF, Salata JJ, Davis JR: Effects of 4-amino-pyridine on rate-related depression of cardiac action potentials. Am J Physiol 251:H297, 1986.

83. Rosenbaum MB, Lepeschkin E: Bilateral bundle branch block. Am Heart J 50:38, 1955.

84. Rosenbaum MB, Elizari M, Lazzari E, et al: Wenckebach periods in the bundle branches. Circulation 60:79, 1969.

85. Lehmann MH, Denker S, Mahmud R, et al: Functional His-Purkinje system behavior during sudden ventricular rate acceleration in man. Circulation 68:767, 1983.

86. Cannom DS, Goldreyer BN, Damato AN: Atrioventricular conduction system in left bundle branch with normal QRS axis. Circulation 46:129, 1972.

87. Wu D, Denes P, Dhingra R, et al: Bundle branch block: demonstration of the incomplete nature of some "complete" bundle branch and fascicular blocks by the extrastimulus technique. Am J Cardiol 33:583, 1974.

88. Barrett PA, Yamaguchi I, Jordan JL, et al: Electrophysiological factors of left bundle branch block. Br Heart J 45:594, 1981.

5 Right Bundle Branch Block

Complete Right Bundle Branch Block

The delay or failure of impulse propagation in the right bundle branch causes delayed activation of the right ventricle, whereas the left ventricle is activated normally. The initial portion of the QRS complex remains unchanged despite absent right septal depolarization. The late QRS portion represents an unopposed slow conduction spread across the septum to the right ventricle in the anterior and either superior or inferior direction. The spatial QRS loop is divided into initial-rapid and late-slow (appendage-like) portions. The duration of the slow terminal QRS portion is 0.04 second or longer. It corresponds to the wide S wave seen in leads I, V_5, and V_6 and the R' in lead V_1. The terminal deflection may be upright or downward in the inferior leads but is always upright in lead aV_R and usually downward in lead aV_L.[1] A marked superior deviation of the terminal deflection, as shown in Figure 5–1, is relatively uncommon and is usually associated with the presence of structural heart disease.

The diagnostic criteria of the World Health Organization (WHO) and the International Society and Federation for Cardiology (ISFC) Task Force[2] are as follows: (1) QRS duration is 120 ms; (2) an rsr', rsR', or rSR' pattern in lead V_1 or V_2 and occasionally a wide and notched R wave; (3) S wave longer than 40 ms or longer than the duration of the R wave in leads V_6 and I; and (4) normal R peak time in leads V_5 and V_6 but $\geq$50 ms in lead V_1.

Body surface maps show an absence of right ventricular breakthrough. The right ventricle is activated by way of the septum. Activation occurs late, which suggests that utilization of the right ventricular Purkinje fibers is minimal and insufficient.[3]

The first normally inscribed QRS portion is sometimes called the "unblocked" part. It occupies the first 0.06 to 0.08 second of the QRS interval. Development of the right bundle branch block (RBBB) does not alter the initial component of the normally inscribed QRS complex, but the duration of the initial unblocked QRS portion varies. This can be best observed in lead V_1 when the electrocardiogram (ECG) is available before and after the onset of RBBB. Sometimes the initial rS deflection is fully preserved, but more often the S wave is shortened to a variable degree or it disappears entirely, with the initial r wave appearing as a notch on the ascent of the R' deflection (Figure 5–2). Sometimes the initial r deflection becomes invisible, and the QRS complex is transformed into a pure broad R wave or an Rs complex. Other variations include disappearance of the initial r wave, resulting in a qR pattern (Figure 5–3). The relation between the amplitude of R and R' also varies; that is, the R amplitude may be smaller than, equal to, or larger than the amplitude of R'.

In uncomplicated RBBBs there is usually little ST segment displacement. The T wave polarity is opposite to the terminal, slowly inscribed deflection of the QRS complex. It is upright in leads I, V_5, and V_6 and inverted in the right precordial leads. In the transitional precordial leads (e.g., V_3 or V_4) the T wave may be diphasic. This pattern may also occur in the right precordial leads. A negative T wave in the left precordial leads is always abnormal (Figure 5–4), but an upright T wave in the leads with an R' pattern (i.e., V_1 or V_2) is seen sometimes in the absence of factors that may explain its presence, such as an anterior myocardial infarction (Figure 5–5) or a posterior myocardial infarction (Figure 5–6A).

In the author's experience, an upright T wave in lead V_1 is sometimes seen in the presence of left ventricular hypertrophy or when the QRS

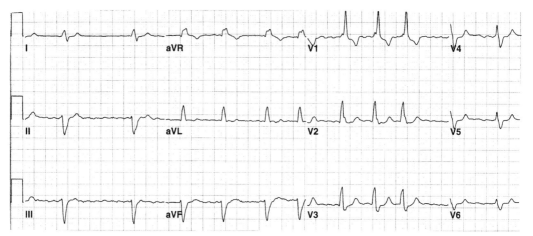

Figure 5–1   Right bundle branch block with superior axis deviation of the terminal QRS deflection in a 72-year-old man with moderately severe three-vessel coronary artery disease, diffuse hypokinesis of the left ventricle, and an estimated left ventricular ejection fraction of 40 percent. The rhythm is atrial fibrillation.

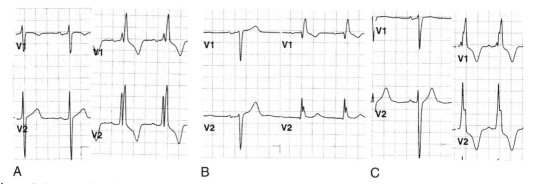

A   B   C

Figure 5–2   Examples of ECG changes in leads V_1 and V_2 produced by the appearance of right bundle branch block. **A,** Initial R wave remains unchanged in leads V_1 and V_2. **B,** Small portion of initial S wave is preserved in lead V_1. **C,** Initial small r wave appears as a notch on the ascent of the R wave.

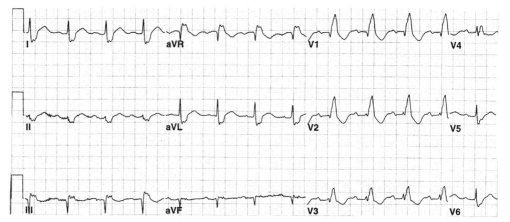

Figure 5–3   A qR pattern in lead V_1 in the absence of myocardial infarction in a 58-year-old man with normal left ventricular function and no cardiac catheterization evidence of obstructive coronary artery disease. The small r wave in lead V_2 suggests that the pattern in lead V_1 is caused by an isoelectric r. A similar explanation is plausible for the qR pattern in leads III and aV_F.

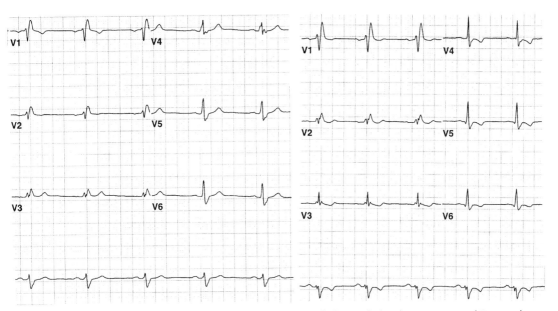

Figure 5–4   Right bundle branch block (RBBB) in a 68-year-old man before and after the appearance of T wave abnormalities caused by a non–Q wave myocardial infarction. At the bottom of each panel is lead II.

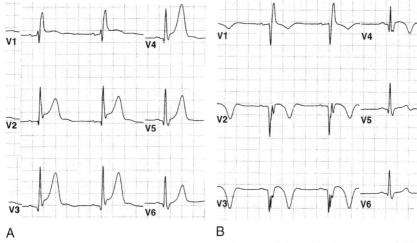

A   B

Figure 5–5   **A,** Transient appearance of an upright T wave in right precordial leads in the presence of right bundle branch block (RBBB) caused by an acute injury pattern of the anterior wall. **B,** ECG recorded 9 hours later shows evolution of a pattern of myocardial infarction of the anterior wall with persisting RBBB.

complex has an rsr's' morphology. In many subjects without demonstrable heart disease, an upright T wave in lead V_1 remains unexplained. One possibility is that the transition zone between the negative and the upright T wave is to the right of lead V_1 and a negative T wave can be found in lead V_3R or V_4R. This assumption is corroborated by the nearly ubiquitous T wave inversion associated with R' deflection in lead aV_R when the T wave is upright in lead V_1 (Figure 5–6B).

The presence of RBBB does not interfere with the recognition of Q wave anterior and inferior myocardial infarction (Figures 5–7 and 5–8) but may cause difficulty with the recognition of posterior myocardial infarction. A diagnosis of myocardial infarction of the inferior wall is sometimes suggested incorrectly when the initial r in leads III and aV_F is small or isoelectric (see Figure 5–3).

ANATOMIC CORRELATION

Good correlation has been shown between the ECG findings of RBBB and the histopathologic changes of the bundle branch.[4,5] Lev and

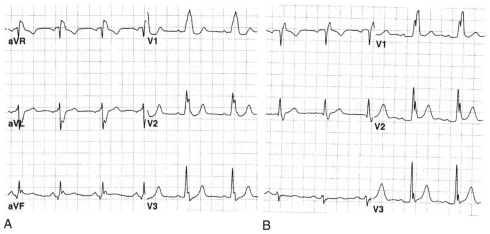

Figure 5–6 Two examples of an upright T wave in the right precordial leads in the presence of right bundle branch block. **A,** ECG of a 70-year-old man with a documented myocardial infarction of the posterior wall caused by obstruction of a large, obtuse marginal branch, marked hypokinesis of the posterobasal wall, and an estimated left ventricular ejection fraction of 30 percent. **B,** ECG of a 76-year-old man who had no evidence of structural heart disease except for a calcified aortic valve. The T wave is upright in the right precordial leads and inverted in the aV_R lead.

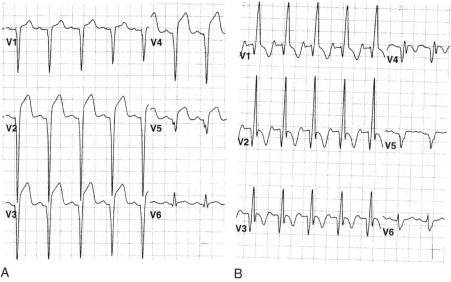

Figure 5–7 Precordial leads of a 41-year-old man with a large myocardial infarction of the anterior wall and a left ventricular ejection fraction of 25 percent before **(A)** and after **(B)** the appearance of right bundle branch block.

associates performed detailed pathologic examination of the conduction system in nine cases of RBBB, predominantly in patients with coronary artery disease; they found significant, albeit incomplete, lesions in all.[5] They emphasized that the ECG pattern of complete RBBB does not necessarily imply complete anatomic disruption of the continuity of the bundle branch. A unilateral delay of impulse propagation through a functionally altered portion of a bundle branch could produce a pattern of complete bundle branch block if this delay exceeds the time required for impulse propagation from the contralateral ventricle through the ventricular septum.[1] RBBB may occur after repair of the ventricular septal defect through the tricuspid valve and is attributed to injury of the proximal right bundle branch during the procedure.[6]

The RBBB pattern is not always caused by interruption of the main right bundle branch. For instance, after infundibular resection during surgical repair of tetralogy of Fallot, activation of

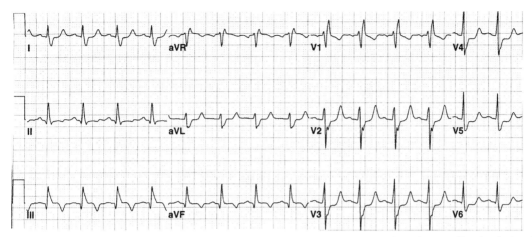

Figure 5–8 ECG of a 61-year-old man with a documented myocardial infarction of the inferior wall and right bundle branch block. Note the Q wave and ST segment elevation in leads II, III, and aV_F and reciprocal ST segment depression in leads V_2 through V_6. The patient had severe four-vessel coronary artery disease with total occlusion of the right coronary artery, inferior basal hypokinesis, and an estimated left ventricular ejection fraction of 45 percent.

the pulmonary outflow tract was delayed by more than 30 ms,[6] but there was no change in activation over the body of the right ventricle. This shows that the RBBB pattern was caused by interrupted conduction in the peripheral branches and not by damage to the proximal portion of the right bundle branch.

It is well known that RBBB is a common complication after right ventriculotomy. Krongrad and associates[7] noted that there was no relation between the length of the ventricular incision and the QRS duration, but the RBBB pattern appeared following an incision of 1 cm or less at a specific site. They suggested that disruption of the distal portion of the right bundle branch was responsible. It has been suggested also that damage to the more peripheral right ventricular Purkinje network may be a responsible mechanism.[6] The findings from electrophysiologic studies in postoperative patients provided additional support to the concept that ECG changes of RBBB may be caused by lesions at three levels: proximal branch, distal branch, and peripheral ramifications.[8]

Right ventricular hypertrophy alone can cause an RBBB pattern, and there is an increased incidence of RBBB among populations at high altitude.[9] There is ample evidence that the RBBB pattern can also be caused by distension of the right ventricle. RBBB is nearly always present in patients with Ebstein's anomaly (incidence, 80 to 95 percent) and in those with large atrial septal defect of the secundum type or an atrioventricular cushion defect (incidence, 90 to 100 percent).[9]

In patients with Ebstein's anomaly of the tricuspid valve, the ECG shows a bizarre form of

RBBB with a slurred terminal QRS portion of low amplitude resembling a second QRS complex attached to the preceding "normal" complex (see Chapter 12). Kastor et al.[10] found that in contrast to the usual RBBB, the activation of the right ventricular apex and right ventricular outflow tract was not delayed in patients with Ebstein's anomaly. The HV interval was prolonged in four of five patients, possibly as the result of a stretched conduction pathway. However, the slurred terminal QRS portion (i.e., the "second QRS complex") was caused by delayed depolarization in some portion of the large, stretched, thin-walled atrialized right ventricle.

Gatzoulis et al.[11] studied the effect of chronic right ventricular overload in patients who had RBBB after repair of tetralogy of Fallot. They found that in 21 of 41 patients with restrictive right ventricular Doppler physiology, the QRS duration averaged 129.3 ms, whereas in the remaining patients without restrictive physiology, the QRS duration averaged 157.5 ms. The increase in QRS duration developed with chronic right ventricular volume overload. This study suggests that the QRS duration in the presence of RBBB is affected by the degree of right ventricular distension.

RBBB IN THE GENERAL POPULATION

Many subjects with RBBB have no evidence of underlying heart disease. Such isolated RBBB occurs more commonly than does isolated left bundle branch block (LBBB). In a study of more than 122,000 apparently normal male Air Force personnel and applicants between the ages of

16 and 55 years, Hiss and Lamb found an incidence of RBBB of 1.8 per 1000.[12] The incidence increased with age. Below age 30 the incidence was 1.3 per 1000, and between ages 30 and 44 it ranged from 2.0 to 2.9 per 1000.[12]

In another report from the same institution, 394 subjects who had RBBB were 17 to 58 years old (mean, 36 years).[13] Fewer than 30 subjects in this group had evidence of coronary, hypertensive, or other organic heart disease. Of the 394 subjects, 372 were followed for an average of 10.8 years. During the follow-up, coronary heart disease or hypertension each developed in an additional 21 subjects (6 percent). Fourteen patients (4 percent) died, but in only three was the cause of death cardiac in origin.

The absence of an adverse prognosis has been confirmed in other groups of otherwise healthy young subjects with RBBB, some of whom were studied by cardiac catheterization and coronary angiography.[14,15] Moreover, many asymptomatic subjects with a change from a normal pattern to an RBBB pattern had no evidence of heart disease.[15] The cause of RBBB in these otherwise healthy individuals remains uncertain. The long, slender structure of the bundle makes it vulnerable to processes associated with aging. Eriksson and associates[16] prospectively studied 885 men who were 50 years old in 1963 and found that the prevalence of bundle branch block increased from 1 percent at age 50 to 17 percent at age 80. RBBB occurred nearly twice as often as LBBB (12.9 percent vs. 6.5 percent). These findings support the hypothesis that bundle branch block is a marker of slowly progressing degenerative myocardial disease.[16]

RBBB AND ACUTE MYOCARDIAL INFARCTION

The RBBB pattern occurs in 3 to 29 percent of patients with acute myocardial infarction[17] (Figures 5–9 to 5–11). It is often accompanied by left anterior fascicular block.[18] The important lesion is usually in the left anterior descending coronary artery.[19] A mortality rate of 36 to 61 percent has been reported in these patients. Hindman and associates reported an in-hospital mortality of 24 percent and a total 1-year mortality of 48 percent in patients with acute myocardial infarction and RBBB.[20] The time of onset of the RBBB in relation to infarction was uncertain in many cases. Several studies have shown that the mortality rate was higher in patients with new-onset RBBB than in those with an old RBBB. This is in contrast to the findings in patients with acute anterior myocardial infarction and LBBB, for whom the mortality rate with an old LBBB was higher than in those with recent-onset bundle branch block.[19]

During the thrombolytic era the overall meaning of RBBB in association with acute myocardial infarction has not changed, although a higher rate of new and transient RBBB and a lower rate of bifascicular block may reflect a beneficial effect of thrombolytic therapy.[21] Investigators analyzing the data of 297,832 patients from the National Registry of Myocardial Infarction[22] reported a 6.2 percent prevalence of RBBB in association with acute myocardial infarction. Compared with patients with myocardial infarction without RBBB and without ST segment elevation, RBBB was associated with a 69 percent increase in the risk of

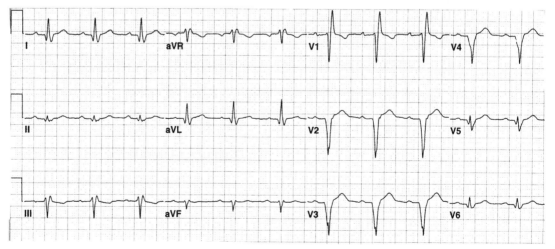

Figure 5–9   ECG of a 72-year-old man with a myocardial infarction of the anterior wall and right bundle branch block. Coronary angiography showed total occlusion of left anterior descending artery, 70 percent obstruction of the proximal left circumflex artery, and total occlusion of the proximal right coronary artery. Left ventricular ejection fraction was 25 percent.

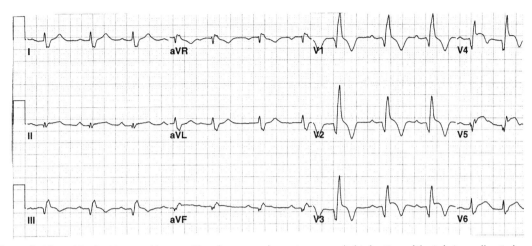

Figure 5–10   ECG of a 68-year-old man with a documented remote myocardial infarction of the inferior wall, a 1-day-old myocardial infarction of the anterior wall, and right bundle branch block.

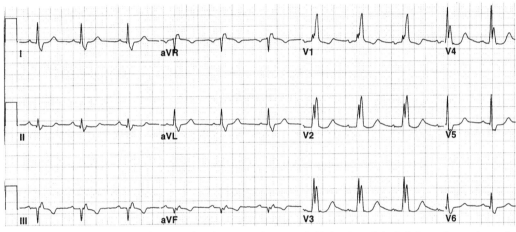

Figure 5–11   ECG of a 70-year-old man with a documented myocardial infarction of the inferior and posterior walls and right bundle branch block. Cardiac catheterization revealed severe obstructive three-vessel coronary artery disease, hypokinesis of the inferior wall, and an estimated left ventricular ejection fraction of 40 percent.

in-hospital death after adjustment for potential confounders.[22] In the study of Moreno et al.,[21] 74 of 681 consecutive patients with acute myocardial infarction undergoing thrombolytic therapy had RBBB. These patients tended to be older and to have a large myocardial infarction. In 46 percent of patients in whom the onset of RBBB was recent, 84 percent of the RBBBs resolved within 12 hours after admission. Patients with new-onset, irreversible RBBB had a poor prognosis with 73 percent mortality at the 1-year follow-up.

RBBB ASSOCIATED WITH OTHER HEART DISEASE

The RBBB may be caused by a variety of pathologic processes such as hypertension, coronary artery disease, rheumatic heart disease, acute and chronic cor pulmonale, myocarditis including Chagas disease, cardiomyopathies, sclerosis of the cardiac skeleton, and degenerative disease of the conducting system. Transient RBBB may result from trauma inflicted during right-sided cardiac catheterization. It has also been reported after nonpenetrating steering wheel injuries to the chest.[23,24] The frequent occurrence of RBBB after cardiac transplantation is discussed in Chapter 12.

The RBBB is reported to be the most common perioperative conduction defect after coronary artery bypass surgery.[25] Among 913 patients with perioperative ventricular conduction abnormalities reported by Chu and associates,[25] 156 (17 percent) had transient changes and 126 (14 percent) had persistent changes. Complete RBBB was found in 93 (60 percent) of the patients with transient changes and in 36 (29 percent) of those with persistent changes. Left anterior fascicular block was the next most common conduction defect, followed by incomplete RBBB. Chu et al.[25] found that development of new perioperative ventricular conduction abnormalities did not decrease the survival rate in patients followed for up to 3 years after operation. Not unexpectedly, RBBB developed in 62 percent of patients after transluminal septal myocardial ablation in patients with obstructive hypertrophic cardiomyopathy.[26]

The most common cause of RBBB in children is open heart surgery to correct tetralogy of Fallot or a ventricular septal defect. In survivors of tetralogy of Fallot repair, RBBB with a long QRS duration was a predictor of malignant ventricular arrhythmias and sudden cardiac death.[11]

The RBBB ECG pattern is prevalent in patients with atrial septal defect, coarctation of the aorta, and Ebstein's anomaly (see Chapter 12). RBBB occurs frequently in patients with arrhythmogenic right ventricular dysplasia and in some of their family members.[27] A characteristic distortion of the terminal portion of the QRS complex known as the *epsilon wave* may be seen in these patients.[28,29] The pattern of RBBB with ST elevation and occurrence of sudden cardiac death is known as *Brugada syndrome* (see Chapter 7). Hereditary bundle branch defect is an autosomal dominant trait with variable expression, and its prevalence is associated with a risk of progression to complete atrioventricular block.[30]

In patients with bundle branch reentrant tachycardia, ablation of the right bundle branch produces the RBBB pattern and prolongation of the HV interval. In 15 patients who had an LBBB pattern before ablation, the QRS duration increased after ablation from 138 ± 26 ms to 168 ± 13 ms, and the HV interval increased by 24 ± 16 ms. HV interval prolongation was not necessarily associated with QRS widening. The widened QRS complex seen with His-Purkinje damage was attributed to reduced synchronization of endocardial activation.[31]

An underappreciated cause of conduction delay in the right ventricle, resulting in an RBBB-like pattern, is right ventricular ischemia and infarction. Kataoka et al.[32] examined the ECGs of 31 patients with acute right ventricular or inferior infarction caused by severe proximal narrowing of the right coronary artery. Of six patients with acute right ventricular infarction and ST segment elevation in the right precordial lead, typical RBBB occurred in one; in three patients, terminal R' developed following return of the ST segment to baseline. In an accompanying

review of the literature, the authors found that among the 26 patients with ischemia or infarction of the right ventricle, 11 (42 percent) showed a pattern of right ventricular conduction delay in the right ventricle. Surawicz et al.[33] reported a case of transient RBBB with ST segment elevation during percutaneous transluminal angioplasty of the proximal right coronary artery.[33] In this case the pattern was attributed to a focal periischemic block; and the conduction delay represented by a wide R' deflection in the right precordial leads was not evident in the more distant left precordial leads. Two other examples of this phenomenon are shown in Figure 5–12.

PROGNOSIS

The prognosis of patients with RBBB depends on the presence or absence and the type of heart disease. In the absence of heart disease, the prognosis and the survival time are not much different from those of the general population.[34,35]

In the Framingham Study, Schneider and associates followed 70 persons who had RBBB during 18 years of observation.[36] Only 15 (21 percent) of these subjects had no clinically apparent cardiovascular abnormalities. The cardiovascular mortality among these 70 subjects was almost three times higher than that in an age-matched sample of the population at large.

Freedman et al.[35] evaluated 272 patients with chronic coronary artery disease and RBBB enrolled in the Coronary Artery Surgery Study (CASS). These patients had more extensive coronary artery disease and more impaired left ventricular function than those without a ventricular conduction defect, but the anatomic and functional abnormalities were less severe than those seen in patients with LBBB. In contrast to patients with LBBB and coronary artery disease, RBBB is not an independent predictor of the mortality rate.[1] Although the RBBB can develop during the course of acute anterior myocardial infarction, in most patients with coronary artery disease the RBBB is not caused by a left anterior descending coronary artery lesion.[1]

VENTRICULAR HYPERTROPHY IN THE PRESENCE OF RBBB

Unpublished studies of Chou[1] showed that the development of RBBB is associated with reduced amplitude of the R wave in the left precordial leads. Because the amplitude of the S wave in the right precordial leads also is frequently

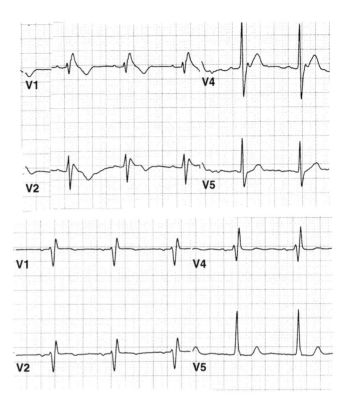

Figure 5-12 Two examples of "focal" right bundle branch block with a QRS duration that is longer in leads V_1 and V_2 than in lead V_5 (and other "remote" leads, which are not shown).

reduced, the presence of RBBB lowers the sensitivity and increases the specificity of the voltage criteria for the diagnosis of left ventricular hypertrophy. Booth et al. found that only 1 of 37 autopsied cases with a hypertrophied left ventricle and ECG pattern of complete or incomplete RBBB met the usual criteria for left ventricular hypertrophy.[37] Mehta et al.[38] found that the ECG pattern of a left atrial abnormality is an independent predictor of left ventricular mass and hypertrophy in the presence of RBBB.

The ability to diagnose right ventricular hypertrophy in the presence of RBBB also suffers from the lack of reliable criteria, even though in some clinical situations the mere presence of RBBB is suggestive of right ventricular hypertrophy (see Chapter 3). Barker and Valencia[39] considered right ventricular hypertrophy to be present if R' was > 1.5 mV in complete RBBB and > 1.0 mV in incomplete RBBB. Booth et al.[37] found that in seven patients with anatomic combined ventricular hypertrophy these criteria were not met, whereas two of three patients who met the criterion for complete RBBB had anatomic right ventricular hypertrophy.

In patients with transient RBBB, or when the ECGs before and after the development of the conduction defect are available, an R' > 1.5 mV may be observed during the block even though the control tracing shows no evidence of right ventricular hypertrophy.[40-42] Therefore it is generally agreed that the amplitude of R' in lead V_1 is not a reliable sign of right ventricular hypertrophy with complete RBBB. Studies of Chou and co-workers[43] in patients who developed RBBB after surgical correction of tetralogy of Fallot showed that abnormal right axis deviation of the initial unblocked QRS portion persisted after development of the conduction disturbance. This suggested that the pattern of abnormal right axis deviation (in the absence of left posterior fascicular block) may be considered a sign of right ventricular hypertrophy.

With incomplete RBBB, Milnor[44] suggested the following two criteria for diagnosis of right ventricular hypertrophy: (1) a rightward mean frontal plane QRS axis of +110 to +270 degrees or (2) an R/S or R'/S ratio in lead V_1 of > 1, provided the R or R' amplitude in V_1 is > 0.5 mV. In the study of Booth et al.,[37] the specificity of the Barker and Valencia[39] or the Milnor[44] criteria was about 60 percent. Carouso and associates[45] found that an R' > 1.0 mV was present in lead V_1 in only 3 of 24 cases of autopsy-confirmed right ventricular hypertrophy. Therefore the sensitivity of these criteria is low, and the incidence of false-positive diagnoses is fairly high.

Incomplete Right Bundle Branch Block

The WHO/ISFC Task Force[2] criteria for incomplete RBBB are the same as for complete RBBB, except that the QRS duration is <120 ms. When the QRS duration is ≤100 ms, the incomplete RBBB pattern is difficult to distinguish from that of a normal variant.

Liao and associates[46] followed 1960 Caucasian men with incomplete RBBB to evaluate their clinical course and prognosis. The men with incomplete RBBB were found to be at more risk of developing left axis deviation and complete RBBB. The likelihood of developing a complete RBBB in 11 years for men with incomplete RBBB was 5.1 percent compared with 0.7 percent of those without such a pattern. There was no demonstrable increase in cardiac deaths within 20 years among subjects with incomplete RBBB. The authors suggested that incomplete RBBB frequently represents a primary conduction system abnormality in middle-aged men.

INCOMPLETE RBBB AND rSr′ PATTERN IN RIGHT PRECORDIAL LEADS: CLINICAL SIGNIFICANCE

The presence of incomplete RBBB is usually suggested by the morphology of the ventricular complex in the right precordial leads, even though a wide terminal deflection in other leads is equally diagnostic. The characteristic pattern in lead V_1 is rSr′ with an inverted T wave and a QRS duration of <0.12 second. In most subjects exhibiting this pattern, the right bundle branch does not appear to be involved in any pathologic processes (Figure 5–13). When the QRS duration is normal, the rSr′ pattern in the right precordial leads is most often normal, where the r′ deflection represents normal terminal depolarization of the crista supraventricularis, proximal septum, and base of the heart. One of the reasons that some normal subjects exhibit this pattern and others do not may depend on the position of the heart relative to the sites of the exploring electrodes. Normal QRS duration is often seen in patients with chronic lung disease (Figure 5–14). The incidence of the rSr′ pattern increases as the precordial electrode is moved to the right. Andersen et al.[47] found this pattern in 4 percent of normal persons in lead V_3R and in 6 percent in lead V_4R. A higher incidence of the rSr′ pattern can be expected if one explores the regions superior to the routine location of the right precordial leads V_1 and V_2. Indeed, exploration of the upper chest and the subclavicular area may disclose a prevalence of the rSr′ pattern similar to that seen in lead aV_R, in which this pattern is considered normal. It follows that the differential diagnosis between an incomplete RBBB caused by a pathologic process and a normal variant rests more on clinical association and other ECG abnormalities (e.g., abnormal P waves, QRS amplitude, primary T wave abnormalities) than on the morphologic characteristics of the pattern. The likelihood of an abnormality increases with increased QRS duration. In addition, Tapia and Proudfit[48] suggested the following criteria for normality:

1. Amplitude of initial R <0.8 mV
2. Amplitude of r′ <0.6 mV
3. R/S ratio of <1.0

Nearly all the normal subjects in their study met these criteria. Approximately 80 percent of patients with congenital heart disease and 46 percent of patients with acquired heart disease had values exceeding these limits.

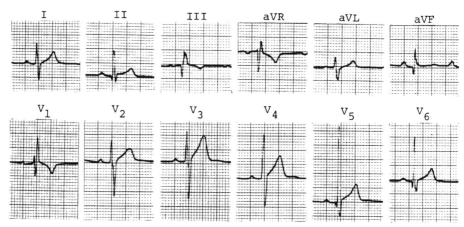

Figure 5–13 Note the rSR′ pattern in lead V_1 (incomplete right bundle branch block) in a healthy 23-year-old man.

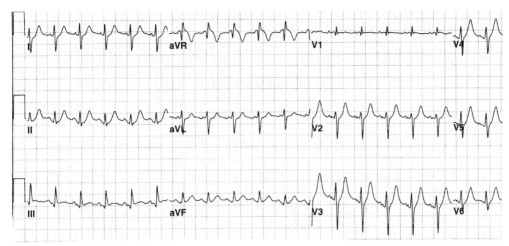

Figure 5–14 Incomplete right bundle branch block with a narrow QRS (72 ms) in a 47-year-old man with severe chronic obstructive lung disease and cor pulmonale.

The pathological incomplete RBBB is attributed to slowed conduction or delayed activation of the right ventricular conduction system or ventricular myocardium. The pattern appears transiently or permanently in some of the following clinical situations:

1. During atrial fibrillation, atrial flutter, supraventricular tachycardia, or in atrial premature complexes, incomplete (and complete) RBBB is the most common pattern of aberrant intraventricular conduction because the right bundle branch is the site of the longest action potential and the longest refractory period in the normal conducting system (see Chapter 17).

2. In the presence of massive pulmonary embolism or other forms of acute cor pulmonale, the transient appearance of incomplete RBBB is probably caused by acute distension of the right ventricle and a conduction delay in the stretched myocardium or the peripheral conducting system.

3. In patients with acute anteroseptal myocardial infarction, the appearance of RBBB (usually complete) is attributed to the ischemia caused by the coronary obstruction proximal to the septal branches supplying the conduction system.

4. In patients with acute inferior myocardial infarction involving the right ventricle, the appearance of incomplete RBBB (usually transient) is probably caused by slow conduction in the ischemic right ventricular myocardium (periischemic block).

5. In patients with right ventricular hypertrophy (e.g., in the presence of cor pulmonale, mitral stenosis, and various types of congenital heart disease), the pattern of complete or incomplete RBBB is likely caused by slow conduction in the hypertrophied or dilated right ventricle. Massing and James[49] cited the studies of Lenegre,[4] who found that the right bundle branch was histologically normal in 25 (76 percent) of 33 patients with the incomplete RBBB pattern and that 31 (94 percent) of the subjects had right ventricular hypertrophy. Moore et al.[50] reported that in dogs, incomplete RBBB was associated with increased focal thickness of the right ventricular free wall, whereas conduction in the right bundle branch and the activation time in the peripheral Purkinje system were normal.

6. The common occurrence of complete or incomplete RBBB in patients with a dilated right ventricle caused by an atrial septal defect, Ebstein's anomaly, or arrhythmogenic right ventricular dysplasia may be attributed to a conduction delay in the myocardium or the peripheral conducting system. A QRS morphology similar to that of incomplete RBBB also has been noted during right ventricular ventriculotomy, suggesting a more distal origin of the conduction abnormality.[7]

7. Lesions interrupting the continuity of the bundle branch may be expected to cause RBBB when the conducting system becomes damaged by myocarditis,

myocardial fibrosis, tumor, amyloid, and other degenerative processes.

8. The RBBB may be caused by congenital absence or atrophy of the bundle branch.

9. Various degrees of RBBB can be induced intermittently by applying pressure to the right septal surface during cardiac catheterization.[51]

10. An rSr' pattern is often recorded in subjects with skeletal abnormalities such as pectus excavatum and straight back syndrome. The r' is usually small.[1] The ECG changes are attributed to a change in the position of the heart as a result of the decrease in the anteroposterior diameter of the chest.[52-54]

11. Complete or incomplete RBBB appears frequently after coronary artery bypass surgery and in transplanted hearts. The former is usually transient, and the latter is often permanent. The mechanism of these conduction disturbances is inadequately understood.

REFERENCES

1. Chou TC: Electrocardiography in Clinical Practice, 4th ed. Philadelphia, Saunders, 1996.
2. Willems JL, Robles de Medina EO, Bernard R, et al: Criteria for intraventricular conduction disturbances and preexcitation. J Am Coll Cardiol 5:112, 1985.
3. Liebman J, Rudy Y, Diaz P, et al: The spectrum of right bundle branch block as manifested in electrocardiographic body surface potential maps. J Electrocardiol 17:329, 1984.
4. Lenegre J: Contribution a l'Etude des Blocs de Branche. Paris, JB Baillliere, 1958.
5. Lev M, Unger PN, Lesser ME, et al: Pathology of the conduction system in acquired heart disease: complete right bundle branch block. Am Heart J 61:593, 1961.
6. Okoromo EO, Guller B, Maloney JD, et al: Etiology of right bundle-branch block pattern after surgical closure of ventricular septal defects. Am Heart J 90:14, 1975.
7. Krongrad E, Heller SE, Bowman FO, et al: Further observations on the etiology of the right bundle branch block pattern following right ventriculotomy. Circulation 50:1105, 1974.
8. Horowitz LN, Alexander JA, Edmunds LH: Postoperative right bundle branch block: identification of three levels of block. Circulation 62:319, 1980.
9. Laham J: Les Blocs de Branche en Clinique. Paris, Malsone Editeur, 1985.
10. Kastor JA, Goldreyer BM, Josephson ME, et al: Electrophysiologic characteristics of Ebstein's anomaly of the tricuspid valve. Circulation 52:987, 1975.
11. Gatzoulis MA, Till JA, Somerville J, et al: Mechano-electrical interaction in tetralogy of Fallot: QRS prolongation relates to right ventricular size and predicts malignant ventricular arrhythmias and sudden death. Circulation 92:231, 1995.
12. Hiss RG, Lamb LE: Electrocardiographic findings in 122,043 individuals. Circulation 25:947, 1962.
13. Rotman M, Triebwasser JH: A clinical and follow-up study of right and left bundle branch block. Circulation 51:477, 1975.
14. Schaffer AB, Reiser I: Right bundle branch system block in healthy young people. Am Heart J 62:487, 1961.
15. Smith RF, Jackson DH, Harthorne JW, et al: Acquired bundle branch block in a healthy population. Am Heart J 89:746, 1970.
16. Eriksson P, Hansson PO, Eriksson H, et al: Bundle-branch block in a general male population: the study of men born 1913. Circulation 98:2494, 1998.
17. Moreno AM, Alberola AG, Tomas JG, et al: Incidence and prognostic significance of right bundle branch block in patients with acute myocardial infarction receiving thrombolytic therapy. Int J Cardiol 61:135, 1997.
18. Nimetz AA, Shubrooks SJ, Hutter AM, et al: The significance of bundle branch block during acute myocardial infarction. Am Heart J 90:439, 1975.
19. Simons GR, Sgarbossa W, Wagner G, et al: Atrioventricular and intraventricular conduction disorders in acute myocardial infarction: a reappraisal in the thrombolytic era. PACE 21:2651, 1998.
20. Hindman MC, Wagner GS, Jaro M, et al: The clinical significance of bundle branch block complicating acute myocardial infarction. I. Clinical characteristics, hospital mortality, and one-year follow-up. Circulation 58:679, 1978.
21. Moreno AM, Tomas JG, Alberola AG, et al: Incidence, clinical characteristics, and prognostic significance of right bundle-branch block in acute myocardial infarction: a study in the thrombolytic era. Circulation 96:1139, 1997.
22. Go AS, Barron HV, Rundle AC, et al: Bundle-branch block and in-hospital mortality in acute myocardial infarction. Ann Intern Med 129:690, 1998.
23. Jackson DH: Transient post-traumatic right bundle branch block. Am J Cardiol 23:877, 1969.
24. Kumpuris AG, Casale TB, Mokotoff DM, et al: Right bundle branch block: occurrence following nonpenetrating chest trauma without evidence of cardiac contusion. JAMA 242:172, 1979.
25. Chu A, Califf RM, Pryor DB, et al: Prognostic effect of bundle branch block related to coronary artery bypass grafting. Am J Cardiol 59:798, 1987.
26. Quin JX, Shiota T, Lever HM, et al: Conduction system abnormalities in patients with obstructive hypertrophic cardiomyopathy following septal reduction interventions. Am J Cardiol 93:171, 2004.
27. Hermida JS, Minassian A, Jarry G, et al: Familial incidence of late ventricular potentials and electrocardiographic abnormalities in arrhythmogenic right ventricular dysplasia. Am J Cardiol 79:1375, 1997.
28. Fontaine G, Guiraudon G, Frank R, et al: Arrhythmogenic right ventricular dysplasia: a previously unrecognized syndrome. Circulation 60(Suppl II):65, 1979.
29. Angelini P, Springer A, Sulbaran T, et al: Right ventricular myopathy with an unusual intraventricular conduction defect (epsilon potential). Am Heart J 101:680, 1981.
30. Stephan E, de Meeus A, Bouvagnet P, et al: Hereditary bundle branch defect: right bundle branch blocks of different causes have different morphologic characteristics. Am Heart J 133:249, 1997.
31. Mehdirad AA, Curtiss E, Tchou P: Interrelations between QRS morphology, duration, and HV interval changes following right bundle branch radiofrequency catheter ablation. PACE 21:1180, 1998.
32. Kataoka H, Tamura A, Yano S, et al: Intraventricular conduction delay in acute right ventriclar ischemia. Am J Cardiol 64:94, 1989.

33. Surawicz B, Orr CM, Hermiller JB, et al: QRS changes during percutaneous transluminal coronary angioplasty and their possible mechanisms. J Am Coll Cardiol 30:452, 1997.

34. Fleg JL, Das DN, Lakatta EG: Right bundle branch block: long-term prognosis in apparently healthy men. J Am Coll Cardiol 1:887, 1983.

35. Freedman RA, Alderman EL, Sheffield LT, et al: Bundle branch block in patients with chronic coronary artery disease: angiographic correlates and prognostic significance. J Am Coll Cardiol 10:73, 1987.

36. Schneider JF, Thomas HE, Kreger BE, et al: Newly acquired right bundle branch block: the Framingham study. Ann Intern Med 92:37, 1980.

37. Booth RW, Chou TC, Scott RC: Electrocardiographic diagnosis of ventricular hypertrophy in the presence of right bundle branch block. Circulation 18:169, 1958.

38. Mehta A, Jain AC, Morise AP, et al: Left atrial abnormality by electrocardiogram predicts left ventricular hypertrophy by echocardiography in the presence of right bundle-branch block. Clin Cardiol 21:109, 1998.

39. Barker JM, Valencia F: The precordial electrocardiogram in incomplete right bundle branch block. Am Heart J 38:376, 1949.

40. Dodge HT, Grant RP: Mechanisms of QRS prolongation in man: right ventricular conduction defects. Am J Med 21:534, 1956.

41. Scherlis L, Lee YC: Transient right bundle branch block: an electrocardiographic and vectorcardiographic study. Am J Cardiol 11:173, 1963.

42. Scott RC: The correlation between electrocardiographic patterns of ventricular hypertrophy and the anatomic findings. Circulation 21:256, 1960.

43. Chou TC, Schwartz D, Kaplan S: Vectorcardiographic diagnosis of right ventricular hypertrophy in the presence of right bundle branch block. In: Hoffman I, Hamby RI (eds): Vectorcardiography, 3rd ed. Amsterdam, North-Holland, 1976, p 21.

44. Milnor WR: The electrocardiogram and vectorcardiogram in right ventricular hypertrophy and right bundle branch block. Circulation 16:348, 1957.

45. Carouso G, Maurice P, Scebat L, et al: L'electrocardiogramme de l'hypertrophie ventriculaire droite. Arch Mal Coeur 44:769, 1951.

46. Liao Y, Emidy LA, Dyer A, et al: Characteristics and prognosis of incomplete right bundlle branch block. An epidemiologic study. J Am Coll Cardiol 7:492, 1986.

47. Andersen HR, Nielsen D, Hansen LG: The normal right chest electrocardiogram. J Electrocardiol 20:27, 1987.

48. Tapia FA, Proudfit WL: Secondary R waves in right precordial leads in normal persons and in patients with cardiac disease. Circulation 21:28, 1960.

49. Massing GK, James TN: Conduction and block in the right bundle branch: real and imagined. Circulation 45:1, 1972.

50. Moore EN, Boineau JP, Patterson DF: Incomplete right bundle branch block: an electrocardiographic enigma and possible misnomer. Circulation 44:678, 1971.

51. Penaloza D, Gamboa R, Sime F: Experimental right bundle branch block in the normal human heart: electrocardiographic, vectorcardiographic, and hemodynamic observations. Am J Cardiol 8:767, 1961.

52. De Leon AC, Perloff JK, Twigg H, et al: The straight back syndrome: clinical cardiovascular manifestations. Circulation 32:193, 1965.

53. De Oliveira JM, Sambhi MO, Zimmerman HA: The electrocardiogram in pectus excavatum. Br Heart J 20:495, 1958.

54. Ellsberg EI: Electrocardiographic changes associated with pectus excavatum. Ann Intern Med 49:130, 1958.

6 Other Intraventricular Conduction Disturbances

Fascicular Blocks
Left Anterior Fascicular Block
Left Posterior Fascicular Block
Uncertain Role of Midseptal Fascicles

Bilateral, Bifascicular, and Trifascicular Bundle Branch Block
Bilateral Bundle Branch Block
RBBB and Left Anterior Fascicular Block
RBBB and Left Posterior Fascicular Block

Trifascicular Block

Intraventricular Conduction Disturbances Associated with Myocardial Infarction and Periinfarction Block

Nonspecific Intraventricular Conduction Disturbances

Fascicular Blocks

The left bundle branch divides into two fascicles; one is superior and anterior, and the other is inferior and posterior. The fascicles branch into networks of Purkinje fibers. The anterior division activates the anterior and lateral walls of the left ventricle, and the posterior division activates the inferior and posterior walls.

Normally the left ventricle is activated simultaneously through the two divisions of the left bundle branch. A delay or interruption of the conduction in one of the divisions results in asynchronous activation of the left ventricle.

When the conduction is blocked or delayed in the anterior fascicle, the impulse spreads inferiorly through the posterior division.[1] When the conduction is blocked or delayed in the posterior fascicle, activation of the inferior and posterior wall is delayed and dependent on the impulse arriving from the anterolateral wall of the left ventricle. The late QRS vectors are directed inferiorly and rightward.

Rosenbaum et al.[2] introduced the term *hemiblocks* for electrocardiographic (ECG) patterns resulting from slowed or interrupted conduction at the level of these two fascicles. The distinct ECG morphologies of the two patterns that Rosenbaum et al. designated as hemiblocks explain the wide appeal of the fascicular block concept. The term *hemiblock* has not been universally adopted, however, mainly because the prefix "hemi-" excludes the possibility that more than two fascicles of the left bundle branch play a distinct role in impulse propagation (see later discussion). The World Health Organization (WHO)

and the International Society and Federation for Cardiology (ISFC) Task Force[3] accepted the more flexible term *fascicular block*.

LEFT ANTERIOR FASCICULAR BLOCK

Watt et al. established that interruption of the anterior division of the left bundle branch in the baboon resulted in a leftward axis shift in the frontal plane "to a degree sufficient to satisfy criteria for clinically significant left axis deviation in the human being."[1] The studies of Rosenbaum et al.[2] led to similar conclusions.

A block in the anterior fascicle prolongs the intraventricular conduction time by an average of about 20 ms (Figure 6–1). This means that the QRS duration may be normal or slightly prolonged in uncomplicated cases of left anterior fascicular block. In patients with intermittent left anterior fascicular block, the reported widening of the QRS was usually less than 20 ms when the left anterior fascicular block appeared[4] (Figure 6–2). Das[5] reported an average increase of 25 ms in 63 subjects who had an abnormal left axis deviation of −30 degrees or more. The degree of prolongation appeared to be in proportion to the degree of axis shift.

Because the initial septal and inferior wall activation is directed rightward and inferiorly, an initial q wave is recorded in lead I and an r wave in the inferior leads. The principal QRS force is directed to the left, posteriorly and superiorly, and is slightly delayed. Being relatively unopposed, this force assumes greater prominence. As a result of these changes in excitation there is: (1) Q in leads I, aV$_L$, or the left precordial leads (or some combination of these leads)

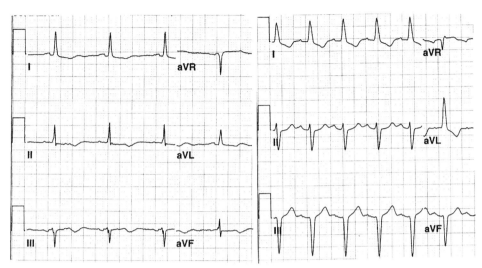

igure 6–1   ECG of a 78-year-old woman with a non-Q wave myocardial infarction. The two ECGs are recorded 1 day part: before and after development of a left anterior fascicular block, which causes an increase of QRS duration from 88 o 112 ms. The increased R wave amplitude in lead aV$_L$ simulates left ventricular hypertrophy.

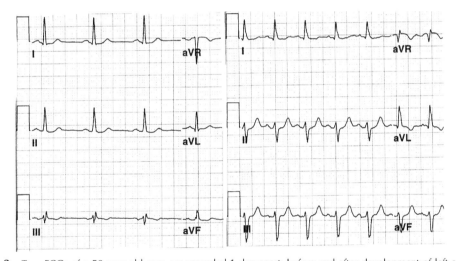

Figure 6–2   Two ECGs of a 50-year-old man are recorded 1 day apart, before and after development of left anterior fas- cicular block, which causes an increase in the QRS duration from 84 to 98 ms.

and R in leads III and aV$_F$; (2) prominent R in leads I and aV$_L$ and a deep S in leads III and aV$_F$. The main QRS axis in the frontal plane is between −30 and −90 degrees, although Rosenbaum et al's original criteria required the QRS axis to be between −45 and −85 degrees. Two other criteria of Rosenbaum et al are a QRS duration of ≤110 ms and a Q wave of ≤20 ms in leads I and aV$_L$.[2] When left anterior fascicular block developed transiently during coronary arteriography, the average QRS duration increased by 13 ms.[6] In practice, the Q wave amplitude is variable and the Q wave may become temporarily absent without other ECG

changes. In one study the Q wave was absent in leads I and aV$_L$ in 12 of 44 (27 percent) patients, with the average QRS axis in the frontal plane within −45 to −80 degrees.[7] In some of the remaining patients the Q wave was present only in lead I or only in lead aV$_L$.

In 222 newly developed cases of marked left axis deviation without apparent heart disease, Rabkin and associates[8] found that Q waves remained absent or unchanged from the previous tracings in leads I and aV$_L$ in most subjects (81 percent). It appears therefore that the direction of the initial QRS force may vary sufficiently to account for variable Q wave expression in different leads.

The leftward shift of the QRS axis results in a tall R wave in leads I and aV_L, as the major forces are directed toward the left arm. The large amplitude of the R wave in lead aV_L may cause a false-positive diagnosis of left ventricular hypertrophy (LVH) (see Figure 6–1). For the same reason, $R_1 + S_3$ may exceed 2.5 mV in the absence of LVH. In the precordial leads, the transitional zone may be displaced to the left, with decreased amplitude of the R waves and increased amplitude of the S wave in the left precordial leads (Figure 6–3). These changes are related to the superior displacement of the QRS forces. The lead axes of V_5 and V_6 are directed not only leftward but also slightly downward.[9] The low R amplitude may contribute to an erroneous diagnosis of an anteroseptal myocardial infarction (see Figure 6–3). Indeed, in practice the left anterior fascicular block ranks high among common causes of a "pseudoinfarction pattern." A less common but clinically important finding with a left anterior fascicular block is the appearance of a small q wave in the right precordial leads, suggesting an anterior myocardial infarction. This is attributed to the change in the orientation of the initial QRS forces. They are directed inferiorly and may project on the negative side of the lead axes of these leads. This explanation is supported by the fact that q waves are absent when these precordial leads are recorded one intercostal space below their routine locations.[1,10]

The proper limits of axis deviation have been debated in the literature, contributing to a multitude of recommendations. The WHO/ISCF Task Force[3] accepted an axis of −45 to −90 degrees, adding that some more liberal definitions of the left axis deviation (e.g., beginning at −30 degrees) have been accepted. Flowers[11] stated aptly that "there is no discrete point at which left axis deviation magically becomes left anterior fascicular block." The requirement to meet strict ECG criteria in terms of axis deviation can put the interpreter of the ECG in an uncomfortable situation. When one follows serial changes of the ECG, it is not unusual to observe almost daily shifts of the average left and superior axis deviation by as much as 30 degrees in either direction. Thus when adhering to a strict definition of left anterior fascicular block, one is frequently forced to change the ECG interpretation from left anterior fascicular block to left axis and vice versa without obvious changes in the subject's cardiac status.

With uncomplicated cases of left anterior fascicular block, an rS complex is recorded in the inferior leads. The S wave in lead III is larger than that in lead II, as the mean QRS axis is more parallel to the negative side of the lead III axis.[9] If S_2 is greater than S_3, the mean QRS axis is in the right superior quadrant of the frontal plane, and right axis deviation is present.

The pattern of left anterior fascicular block with an absent or low-amplitude initial R in leads II, III, and aV_F may be similar to that of inferior myocardial infarction. Patients with inferior myocardial infarction may show a QS or Qr deflection in the inferior leads. If the Q wave is deep, the calculated mean QRS axis may be superior to −30 degrees. Such a finding, however, does not represent left anterior fascicular block, even though the QRS axis is shifted leftward, because the initial forces rather than the terminal forces are displaced superiorly. When

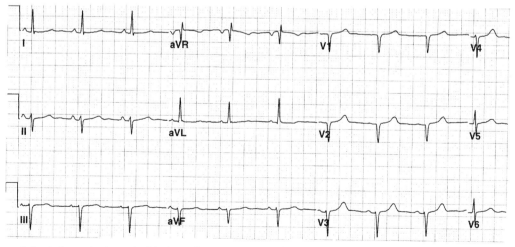

Figure 6–3 Left anterior fascicular block simulates an anteroseptal myocardial infarction in a 64-year-old woman who has no evidence of structural heart disease.

QS complexes are present in the inferior leads, left anterior fascicular block may coexist with the infarction. The most important distinction between the patterns is counterclockwise rotation in the frontal plane with left anterior fascicular block and clockwise rotation with inferior myocardial infarction. These patterns may be difficult to differentiate on the scalar ECG.

Warner et al.[12] proposed the following criteria for left anterior fascicular block when three leads are recorded simultaneously: (1) the QRS complex in leads aV_R and aV_L each end in an R wave; and (2) the peak of the terminal R in V_R occurs later than the peak of the terminal R in aV_L. This means that the terminal QRS forces are directed superiorly and are inscribed in a counterclockwise direction.

In the absence of coexisting repolarization abnormalities, the ST segment and T waves are not significantly different from those of normal individuals.

Superior (Left) Axis Deviation in the Frontal Plane

Figure 6–4 shows that the superior axis in the frontal plane is associated with several intraventricular conduction disturbances, not all of which are attributed to the block in the anterior fascicle of the left bundle branch. For instance, in most patients with ostium primum–type atrial septal defects or with complete forms of the common atrioventricular (AV) canal, the QRS

axis in the frontal plane is directed superiorly, as with left anterior fascicular block (Figure 6–4B). Burchell and associates[13] considered the possibility that the pattern was caused by an advancing excitation front in the posterolateral wall of the left ventricle occurring at a normal time without being counterbalanced by the excitation front in the anterior wall. Durrer et al.[14] proved the validity of this concept during operative mapping. They found that in patients with partial and complete forms of AV canal, the posterobasal region of the left ventricle was excited much earlier (i.e., 28 to 35 ms after the beginning of QRS) than the 70 ms or more in normal persons. The abrupt shift to the left and in an upward direction, which takes place approximately during the 30- to 40-ms interval, occurs after disappearance of the outward spreading excitatory forces in the posterobasal wall and is attributed to unopposed forces in the lateral and anterior parts of the ventricle. Thus the pattern simulating left anterior fascicular block in these patients is caused by preexcitation of the posterobasal region of the left ventricle resulting from an abnormal anatomic structure of the conducting system. Subsequently, Boineau et al.[15] confirmed these findings in a dog with ostium primum interatrial septal defect. Other congenital heart lesions associated frequently with superior axis deviation, possibly as a result of altered anatomy of the conducting system, are tricuspid atresia, common ventricle with transposition of the great vessels, corrected transposition of the

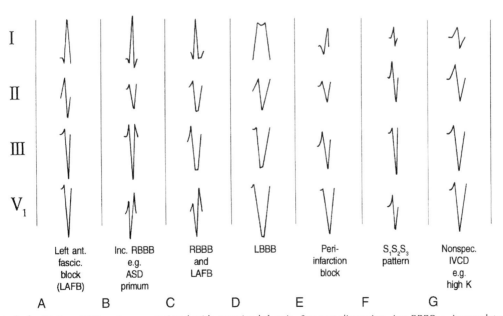

Figure 6–4 Various ECG patterns associated with superior left axis. See text discussion. Inc RBBB = incomplete right bundle branch block; IVCD = intraventricular conduction disturbance; LBBB = left bundle branch block.

great vessels with left-sided apex, and a Wolff-Parkinson-White (WPW) pattern.[16]

The $S_1S_2S_3$ pattern (Figure 6–4F), which causes a superior axis in the frontal plane, is usually associated with adults with chronic lung disease. The mean axis in these patients is often more than −90 degrees, which means that it is right superior rather than left superior. Although right ventricular hypertrophy may be present in adults and right or left ventricular hypertrophy in children with this pattern, changes in cardiac position or excitation sequence are more likely to explain this pattern than the presence of hypertrophy. The other causes of superior axis shown in Figure 6–4 (i.e., periinfarction block, bifascicular block, hyperkalemia) are discussed elsewhere.

Left Anterior Fascicular Block in the Absence of Heart Disease

The abnormal left axis deviation is one of the most common abnormal ECG findings. Among 67,375 Air Force men without symptoms, Hiss and associates found a frontal plane QRS axis of −30 to −90 degrees in 128 (1.9 percent).[17] In the Tecumseh study of 4678 persons older than 20 years, abnormal left axis deviation was found in 248 (5 percent).[18] It was more prevalent in men than in women, and the frequency increased with age for both genders. Figure 6–5 shows left anterior fascicular block in a 102-year-old woman who also had two other common age-related abnormalities (i.e., right bundle branch block and atrial fibrillation). Approximately 59 percent of the individuals with left

axis deviation had other findings suggestive of heart disease. The remainder had no other evidence of cardiac abnormalities.[18]

Eliot and associates[19] examined 195 apparently healthy men with a mean age of 41 years who had marked left axis deviation but no other ECG abnormality. During the initial investigation and the follow-up period of up to 22 months, 113 (58 percent) subjects were found to have cardiovascular disease or subclinical diabetes mellitus.

Among the 363 male insurance applicants age 30 and older with left anterior fascicular block examined by Corne et al.,[20] 194 (53 percent) had no cardiovascular abnormalities. There was no significant difference in the occurrence of heart disease between the group of subjects with a QRS axis of −31 to −59 degrees and the group with an axis of −60 to −90 degrees.

Left Anterior Fascicular Block in Patients with Coronary Artery Disease and Hypertension

Coronary and hypertensive heart diseases are the most common causes of abnormal left axis deviation. With acute myocardial infarction, isolated left anterior fascicular block occurs in about 4 percent of patients.[21–23] Another 5 percent of patients have left anterior fascicular block associated with right bundle branch block (RBBB).[21,23] The infarction, usually anteroseptal or anterolateral, is caused by left anterior descending coronary artery occlusion. Left anterior fascicular block can also occur in patients with inferior myocardial infarction.[24]

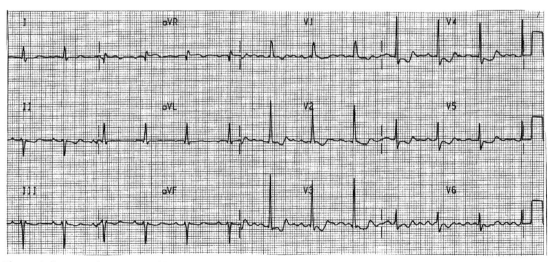

Figure 6–5 ECG of a 102-year-old woman shows three common manifestations of the aging heart: left anterior fascicular block, right bundle branch block, and atrial fibrillation.

ne explanation is that the His bundle receives dual blood supply from the septal branch of ne left anterior descending coronary artery and trioventral (AV) nodal artery. If there is longitu-inal dissociation of conduction in the His bun-le, ischemia of the His bundle caused by the bsent AV nodal artery supply may affect only ne part of the His bundle containing the fibers f the left anterior fascicle.[24] In patients with uspected coronary artery disease who were eferred for stress testing, isolated left anterior ascicular block was associated with myocardial schemia and an increased cardiac death during ollow-up.[25]

Other Causes of Left Anterior Fascicular Block

Left anterior fascicular block can be caused by all types of left-sided heart disease, but there is no direct relationship between left axis deviation and LVH.[26] In the absence of manifest heart dis-ase and in association with aging, left anterior ascicular block is attributed to degenerative dis-ase of the conducting system,[27] sclerosis of the eft side of the cardiac skeleton,[28] or myocardial fibrosis.[26,29] Demoulin et al.[30] found that subjects with left anterior fascicular block had more fibro-is in the ramifications of the left bundle branch divisions, but the lesions were not confined to he anterior division and in half the cases were not predominant in the regions of anterior rami-ications. This is consistent with earlier fin-dings showing that the ECG pattern occurred in patients with various lesions and no consistent nvolvement of specific regions in the ventricular myocardium or the conducting system.[31]

Castellanos et al.[32] observed cases in which catheter insertion into the right ventricle pro-duced a transient mechanical RBBB that was associated in two cases with left anterior fascicu-lar block and in two cases with left posterior fas-cicular block. Because the left ventricle was not mechanically disturbed, these observations sug-gest that left fascicular blocks can be caused by lesions involving the His bundle. This probably implies the existence of longitudinal dissociation in the His bundle.[32]

In patients with congenital heart disease, abnormal left axis deviation is most commonly seen in patients with endocardial cushion defects, which include atrial septal defect of the primum type, AV canal, and a common atrium (Figure 6–6). Left axis deviation occurs in about 4 percent of those with an isolated ventricular septal defect.[9] In patients with cyanotic heart disease, left axis deviation is seen typically in those with tricuspid atresia and often in patients with a single ventricle.[16] Isolated congenital left axis deviation without evidence of heart disease also has been reported.[33]

LVH in the Presence of Left Anterior Fascicular Block

As mentioned earlier, left anterior fascicular block can cause a false-positive diagnosis of LVH based on voltage criteria without associated secondary ST segment and T wave changes. Based on an echocardiographic study, Gertsch et al.[34] pro-posed that LVH is present if the amplitude of the S wave in lead III plus that of the largest QRS complex in the precordial leads is ≥3.0 mV. In their study of 50 patients with left anterior

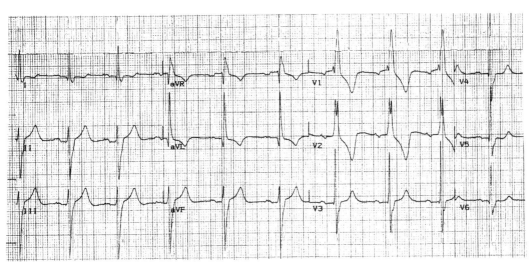

Figure 6–6   ECG of a 24-year-old woman with an endocardial cushion defect.

fascicular block (26 with and 24 without LVH), the specificity of the proposed criterion was 87 percent and the sensitivity was 96 percent.

LEFT POSTERIOR FASCICULAR BLOCK

Division of the left posterior fascicle in dogs and baboons produced a modest axis shift, a slight increase in QRS duration, and slight changes in QRS morphology. The axis shift was greater in primates than in dogs, but the ECG, although suggestive of inferior myocardial infarction (Q wave in lead III), was not clearly abnormal.[35]

In humans, a block in the posterior fascicle causes the excitation wave to first travel through the region of the anterior fascicle and then spread out inferiorly. The QRS prolongation is usually 20 ms or less.[1] The QRS interval therefore may remain within normal limits, although an uncomplicated left posterior fascicular block with a duration of 120 ms has been reported.[6]

In the ECG, depolarization forces are directed opposite to those in the left anterior fascicular block. The initial 10- to 20-ms deflection is directed superiorly and to the left, and the subsequent main QRS force is directed inferiorly, to the right and posteriorly. This causes an rS pattern in leads I and aV_L and a qR pattern in leads III and aV_F. The relatively deep S wave in lead I is a consistent finding, as the terminal QRS forces are invariably directed rightward.

The WHO/ISFC Task Force[3] criteria include a QRS axis in the frontal plane from +90 to ±180 degrees and a QRS duration of less than 120 ms. A Q wave should always be present in lead III; it may be small or absent in leads II and aV_F. In the precordial leads the transition zone is often displaced to the left, resulting in an RS complex in the left precordial leads.[36] The smaller R wave and deeper S wave in the left precordial leads resemble those seen with right ventricular hypertrophy (RVH). If Q waves are present in the left precordial leads before the block develops, they may disappear when the fascicular block causes a leftward shift of the initial QRS forces.[9]

Abnormal Right Axis Deviation

Rosenbaum and co-workers[2] suggested a QRS axis > +120 degrees as a criterion for the diagnosis of left posterior fascicular block, but they stated that the diagnosis may be considered with an axis of +90 or even +70 degrees. They indicated that the latter probably represents an incomplete form of left posterior fascicular block.

It is important to exclude other causes of abnormal right axis deviation before diagnosing left posterior fascicular block. RVH, pulmonary emphysema, a vertical heart, and extensive lateral wall myocardial infarction also may be accompanied by abnormal right axis deviation.

With RVH, a tall R wave or an rSR' pattern may be present with a negative T wave in the right precordial leads. Such a finding is uncommon with left posterior fascicular block unless posterior wall infarction or RBBB coexists.

The ECG pattern of chronic lung disease can usually be recognized by the presence of typical P waves, low QRS amplitude in the limb leads, and deep S waves in the left precordial leads.

With lateral wall myocardial infarction, a QS pattern rather than rS is recorded in leads I and aV_L. Moreover, the T waves in these leads are usually inverted, which is uncommon with uncomplicated left posterior fascicular block. The coexistence of lateral wall myocardial infarction and left posterior fascicular block has been reported.[9] In many instances, differentiation of left posterior fascicular block from the other entities cannot be accomplished by the ECG alone; supplementary clinical data are needed. The probability of left posterior fascicular block as the cause of an abnormal right axis deviation increases in a patient with left ventricular disease and no evidence of right-sided heart involvement.

The pattern of left posterior fascicular block is seldom recognized as an isolated finding in the absence of RBBB. Rosenbaum and co-workers[2] attributed the low incidence of the isolated left posterior fascicular block to the following characteristics of the left posterior division of the left bundle branch: (1) it is short and thick; (2) it has a dual blood supply from the anterior and posterior descending coronary arteries; (3) it is situated within the less turbulent left ventricular inflow tract; and (4) it is the first group of fibers to branch off the bundle of His.

The specificity of the left posterior fascicular block pattern as a marker of localized conduction disturbance increases when it appears during acute myocardial ischemia[37] or acute myocardial infarction.[38] The incidence of left posterior fascicular block in acute myocardial infarction is the lowest of all intraventricular conduction defects, varying from 0.2 to 0.4 percent.[38–40] Transient left posterior fascicular block has been observed during coronary arteriography when the contrast material was injected into the right coronary artery.[6]

Histopathologic studies of Demoulin and Kulbertus[41] in 13 cases (9 in association with RBBB) showed major alterations of the left-sided conduction system that consistently were maximal at the level of the posterior portion of the ft bundle branch. The changes were less widely spread but more pronounced and more proximately located than in subjects with left anterior fascicular block. Rizzon et al.[38] described the histologic changes affecting the myocardium and the conducting system in eight cases of left posterior fascicular block. The myocardial infarction was both anterior and posterior, and involved the septum in all cases. The relative rarity of the pattern and the location and extent of the infarction, associated with a left posterior divisional block pattern, suggested that the damage involved not only the posterior but also the midseptal division of the left bundle branch (see later discussion).

UNCERTAIN ROLE OF MIDSEPTAL FASCICLES

That the left bundle branch is anatomically subdivided into two fascicles has not been universally accepted. Several investigators, beginning with Tawara[42] and including Demoulin and Kulbertus,[41] Massey and James,[43] and more recently Nakaya and Hiraga,[44] described the branching portion of the left bundle branch as a diffuse, fanlike network broadly distributed over the septal surface. Consequently, it has been suspected that the network of midseptal fibers emanating from the left bundle branch participates jointly with the anterior and posterior fascicles in the genesis of the QRS complex.[45]

Figure 6–7[44] shows that by blocking the septal fibers, activation from the anterior and posterior fascicles arrives at the site previously activated by the midseptal division. This is expected to shift the QRS forces anteriorly, resulting in increased R amplitudes in leads V_1, V_2, and V_3.

Hoffman et al.[46] suggested that the anterior conduction delay is responsible for the pattern simulating posterior myocardial infarction (see Chapter 8) in patients in whom the presence of posterior infarction is difficult to explain because the coronary artery disease is limited to the left anterior descending coronary artery. The presence of a median septal (centroseptal) fascicular block is an attractive explanation for such an ECG pattern.[44] Possible examples are in Figures 5–6B, 6–5, and 6–12 after Q waves and little change in frontal plane QRS axis.[48]

Similarly, a delay in the middle fascicle may explain a certain type of ventricular aberration pattern with atrial premature complexes. This pattern consists of a prominent anterior precordial force without QRS prolongation and without incomplete RBBB.[47] It is also marked by absence of Q waves and left axis deviation.[48]

It can be concluded that even if the ECG pattern of the midseptal divisional block remains unproven, the concept of an anterior conduction delay presents an attractive explanation for the tall R waves in the right precordial leads in the absence of RVH, RBBB, preexcitation, and posterior myocardial infarction.

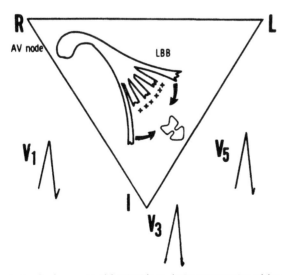

Figure 6–7   Mechanism of anterior displacement of the QRS loop during interruption of the midseptal fibers. Cardiac vector of activation of the apical area is directed anteriorly, to the left, and inferiorly. After block of the septal fibers, activation comes from the anterior and posterior divisions to the area activated by the midseptal fibers before interruption. Accordingly, the QRS vector is displaced to the left and anteriorly. V_1 and V_6 show a relatively tall R wave, but a deep S wave is not seen in the left precordial leads. I = inferior; L = left; LBB = left bundle branch; R = right. (From Nakaya Y, Hiraga T: Reassessment of the subdivision block, of the left bundle branch block. Jpn Circ J 45:503, 1981, by permission of the authors and publisher.)

Bilateral, Bifascicular, and Trifascicular Bundle Branch Block

BILATERAL BUNDLE BRANCH BLOCK

Strauss and Langendorf[49] analyzed the ECGs of a patient with Adam-Stokes disease, a variable degree of AV block, and varying combinations of right and left bundle branch blocks. They assumed that alternation was caused by a "partial block in the two main bundle branch systems with a shorter relative refractory phase of the bundle branch which has the longer absolute refractory period."

In 1954, Richman and Wolff[50] described a pattern of left bundle branch block (LBBB) in the limb leads and RBBB in the precordial leads and called it "left bundle branch block masquerading as right bundle branch block" (Figure 6–8). It is possible that the midseptal pathway block plays a role in such cases (see previous discussion).

Lepeschkin[51] categorized various combinations of first-, second-, and third-degree bilateral bundle branch block. In addition to the complete right and left bundle branch block varieties, he discussed other patterns, such as: (1) first-degree block in one branch and second-degree block in the other, causing alternation of right and left bundle branch block, one of which was constantly associated with a short PR interval; (2) first-degree block in one branch with a third-degree block in the other branch, resulting in a complete right bundle branch block with a prolonged PR, similar to the effect of an unequal bilateral first-degree block; and (3) several varieties of bilateral second-degree

block, exemplified by: (a) equal and asynchronous bilateral second-degree block manifested by alternation of right and left bundle branch block without alternation of PR intervals; (b) unequal synchronous bilateral second-degree block resulting in 2:1 AV block with bundle branch block in the conducted impulse; and (c) unequal and asynchronous bilateral second-degree block, a complicated pattern resulting in regularly recurring changes in the PR interval, changes in QRS morphology, occasional blocked QRS complexes, and QRS complexes of nearly normal configuration. Figure 6–9 illustrates a bilateral bundle branch block of similar complexity. Lepeschkin also discussed the possibility that all such patterns may be complicated by variable delays in "part of the left branch."

Intracardiac electrocardiography confirmed the existence of latent bilateral bundle branch blocks. Dhingra et al.[52] studied patients with chronic bifascicular block and found that in 21 patients (4 percent), atrial pacing induced additional block distal to the His bundle. In about 25 percent of these patients, the response was "functional"; in the others, conduction failed intermittently through the functioning fascicle (i.e., a bifascicular block "unmasked" by pacing). More recently, Dhala et al.[53] studied 14 patients after inadvertent or deliberate ablation of the right bundle branch (treatment for bundle branch reentrant tachycardia). They found that this procedure unmasked some delay in the left bundle branch as manifested by an axis shift to the right or to the left that was attributed to latent anterior or posterior fascicular block, respectively.

The study of Ohkawa et al.[54] showed that in 7 of 10 patients with complete AV block, severe

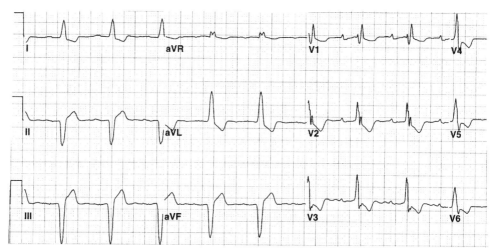

Figure 6–8 ECG of an 83-year-old man with first-degree atrioventricular block, right bundle branch block, and a pattern simulating left bundle branch block in the limb leads because of an absent S wave in lead I (masquerading pattern).

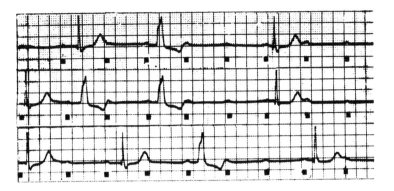

Figure 6-9 Continuous strip of lead II in a patient with high-degree atrioventricular (AV) block. Note the normal conduction (last QRS complex in the lower strip), right bundle branch block (first QRS complex in the upper strip and first and second QRS complex in the lower strip), left bundle branch block (second QRS complex in the upper strip, second and third in the middle strip, and third in the lower strip), and AV junctional escape (third QRS complex in the middle). Dots mark the P waves.

fibrosis affected both bundle branches. When the conduction in both bundle branches is interrupted, the resulting complete AV block is indistinguishable from a trifascicular block (see later discussion).

RBBB AND LEFT ANTERIOR FASCICULAR BLOCK

The RBBB with a left anterior fascicular block is the most common type of bilateral (and bifascicular) bundle branch block. The pattern fulfills the criteria for both entities. When impulse propagation is interrupted or delayed in the right bundle branch and the anterior division of the left bundle branch, ventricular activation begins in the region supplied by the left posterior division. The right

ventricle is depolarized late by the impulse propagating across the septum. The first portion of the QRS complex has the characteristics of an isolated left anterior fascicular block, and the last portion has the characteristics of an RBBB (Figure 6-10). Diagnostic criteria include the following:

1. Prolongation of the QRS duration to 0.12 second or longer
2. RSR′ pattern in lead V₁, with the R′ being broad and slurred
3. Wide, slurred S waves in leads I, V₅, and V₆
4. Frontal plane axis of the first 0.06 to 0.08 second of the QRS complex (representing the forces preceding delayed right ventricular activation) being −30 to −90 degrees
5. Initial r wave in the inferior leads

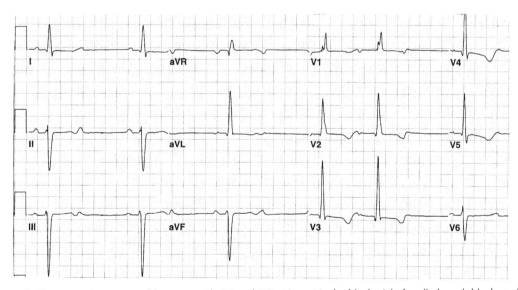

Figure 6-10 ECG of a 76-year-old woman with 2:1 and 3:2 atrioventricular block, right bundle branch block, and left anterior fascicular block. The patient had moderately severe calcific aortic stenosis, left ventricular hypertrophy, left ventricular ejection fraction of 55 percent, no wall motion abnormalities, and no evidence of myocardial ischemia (nuclear imaging). This patient meets the criteria of so-called Lev's disease.

The axis is determined using the early unblocked portion of the QRS complex, which is rapidly inscribed. The onset of the slurred portion of the QRS, which marks the inscription of the forces bypassing the blocked right bundle branch, can usually be recognized within 0.06 to 0.08 second after the onset of the QRS complex. It must be recalled that the concept of the "mean axis" is valid only when there is a single dominant deflection, which is usually the case in the presence of fascicular blocks.

The most frequent cause of RBBB with left anterior fascicular block is coronary artery disease, which in large series is responsible for 41 to 61 percent of cases.[55,56] In patients with acute myocardial infarction, it occurs in about 4.8 to 7.0 percent of cases.[21,23,24,39,57] The location of the infarction usually is anterior. This can be explained by the close proximity of the anterior division of the left bundle and the right bundle branch in the anterior part of the interventricular septum and by the common blood supply of the two structures via the septal branches of the left anterior descending coronary artery. Lenegre[27] correlated the ECG with the pathologic fascicular block. Myocardial infarction with either complete or partial destruction of the right and left bundle branch was found in all.

Another common cause of this bifascicular block is primary degenerative disease of the conducting system. Such patients have no symptoms and have normal-sized hearts. Histologic examination reveals a sclerodegenerative process limited to the conduction tissue. Rosenbaum and co-workers[2] named this entity *Lenègre's disease* in recognition of the French pathologist who first described the lesions in detail.[27]

Another pathologic process affecting the conduction system was called *Lev's disease* by Rosenbaum and co-workers.[2] Lev explained an intraventricular conduction defect by the presence of sclerosis of the left side of the cardiac skeleton, a condition usually seen in elderly subjects who tend to have no other evidence of heart disease.[28] With advancing age there is normally progressive fibrosis and calcification of the mitral annulus, central fibrous body, pars membranacea, base of the aorta, and summit of the muscular septum. Because the conduction system is adjacent to some of these structures, a fibrotic process at the summit of the muscular septum may injure the right bundle branch and the anterior division of the left bundle branch. Lenègre's disease and Lev's disease are often grouped together as primary conduction disease (see Figure 6–10). In the study of Dhingra and associates,[52] 86 (19 percent) of 452 patients with chronic bifascicular block had primary conduction disease. This diagnosis was assigned to 23 percent of 331 patients with RBBB and left anterior fascicular block and to 7 percent of 113 patients with complete LBBB.

Aortic valve disease, especially aortic stenosis, may be associated with bifascicular block.[58] Both fascicles may be involved by an extension of the fibrocalcific process of the aortic valve at the level of the pseudobifurcation (i.e., the point at which the right bundle branch separates from the most anterior fibers of the left bundle branch).[9] Myocardial fibrosis or an infiltrative process involving the conduction system may cause bifascicular block in patients with cardiomyopathy (idiopathic or secondary to a systemic disease). Hypertensive disease with or without coronary artery disease accounts for about 20 to 25 percent of patients with bifascicular block.[55,56] Among the congenital heart diseases, RBBB with a left anterior fascicular block occurs mainly with endocardial cushion defects (see Figure 6–6). It was also found in about 6 percent of patients with a ventricular septal defect and in 11 percent of patients with tetralogy of Fallot following corrective surgery.[59] The conduction defect has been observed also after tricuspid valve replacement,[60] after cardiac transplantation,[9] and during hyperkalemia.[61]

RBBB and Left Anterior Fascicular Block: Relation to Complete AV Block

The data from five prospective studies involving 950 patients[62] with chronic bifascicular block (predominantly RBBB and left anterior fascicular block) showed that sudden death occurred in 82 patients during an average follow-up of 1 to 3 years. The presence of complete AV block immediately before death was documented in only 6 patients but was suspected in 31. Among the 452 patients with chronic bifascicular block (277 of them included in one of the previously mentioned prospective studies) reported by Dhingra and coworkers,[52] the cumulative incidence of AV block at 5 years was 11 percent; in 7 percent the AV block developed spontaneously without an apparent precipitating cause. The site of the AV block varied, being trifascicular in fewer than half of the patients. A prolonged HV interval turned out to be an inconsistent precursor of trifascicular block.[63] Patients with primary conduction system disease had a lower incidence of complete AV block and a lower incidence of cardiac death and sudden death than those with organic heart disease.[36]

In patients with acute myocardial infarction, the incidence of complete AV block in patients with bifascicular block varied from 24 to 43 percent.[21,28] The mortality in these patients is high, even in the absence of complete AV block, and varies from 36 to 59 percent.[22,23,64,65]

RBBB AND LEFT POSTERIOR FASCICULAR BLOCK

The RBBB with left posterior fascicular block is a less common type of bilateral bundle branch block. The ECG pattern fulfills the criteria of both entities (Figure 6–11). Ventricular activation begins in the anterior and lateral wall of the left ventricle via anterior division of the left bundle branch. It is followed by excitation of the inferoposterior wall by retrograde conduction of the impulse from the anterior to the posterior division. The delayed excitation of the right ventricle depends on the impulse advancing transseptally from the left to the right side. The diagnostic criteria include the following:

1. Prolongation of the QRS to 0.12 second or longer
2. RSR' pattern in lead V_1, with the R' being broad and slurred
3. Wide, slurred S waves in leads I, V_5, and V_6
4. Frontal plane axis of the first half or 0.06 to 0.08 second of the QRS complex of +90 degrees or farther to the right, with an rS deflection in lead I and a qR deflection in leads III and aV_F

The bifascicular block involving the right bundle branch and the left posterior division of the left bundle branch is much less common than RBBB with left anterior fascicular block, but it is seen more frequently than an isolated left posterior fascicular block. The causes of RBBB with left posterior fascicular block are the same as those of RBBB with left anterior fascicular block, coronary artery disease being the most common.[1,65] The incidence of this conduction disturbance in patients with acute myocardial infarction is less than 0.8 percent.[21,23,24,38] In some of these cases, autopsy showed involvement of a large part of the entire intraventricular septum.[38]

The incidence of progression to complete AV block varies among studies, probably reflecting differences in the clinical condition of the patients. Among Rosenbaum's 30 patients (often with Chagas disease), complete or high-grade AV block developed in 16 and Stokes-Adams attacks in 18.[66] Scanlon et al.[56] reported that complete AV block developed in 8 of 49 cases followed for an average of 2 years, and Dhingra and co-workers[67] reported AV block in 2 of 21 patients during a similar follow-up period.

TRIFASCICULAR BLOCK

Trifascicular block may be suspected if there is a permanent block in one fascicle and an intermittent block in the other two fascicles. For example, if a patient with a chronic RBBB has a pattern of left anterior fascicular block and left posterior fascicular block on different occasions, the presence of disease in all three fascicles is implied (Figure 6–12). If the block in one of the three fascicles is incomplete, the ECG shows a bifascicular block with first- or second-degree AV block. However, such a pattern does not

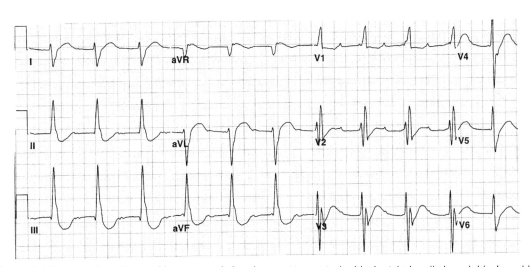

Figure 6–11   ECG of an 87-year-old woman with first-degree atrioventricular block, right bundle branch block, and left posterior fascicular block.

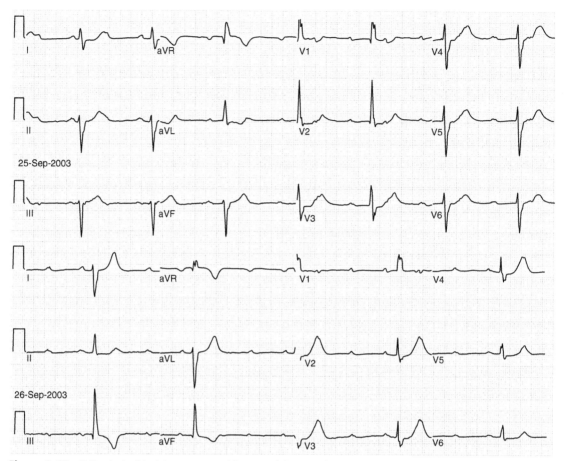

Figure 6–12 Trifascicular block in a 56-year-old man with history of syncope. *Top:* Sinus rhythm with a complete atrioventricular block (or dissociation). The escape pacemaker at the rate of 44 bpm is presumed to be located in the left posterior fascicle, resulting in the pattern of right bundle branch block (RBBB) and left anterior fascicular block. *Bottom:* Sinus rhythm with 3:1 AV block and P-R interval of 252 ms in the conducted complexes with the morphology of RBBB and left posterior fascicular block indicating that the conduction in the left anterior fascicle is not permanently blocked. The tall R in the lead V₂ at the top may be caused by left septal fascicular block because R is not as tall in the lower ECG even though RBBB appears unchanged.

always indicate that the first- or second-degree AV block is caused by involvement of the third fascicle because the conduction delay may be at the level of the AV node or the His bundle.

A complete trifascicular block results in a complete AV block (see Figure 6–12). The escape pacemaker often originates in the region of the left or right posterior fascicle, resulting in an escape rhythm with a pattern of RBBB plus left posterior fascicular block or RBBB plus left anterior fascicular block, respectively.

A definitive diagnosis of trifascicular block requires His bundle recording. Levitas and Haft[68] compared the results of His bundle recording in 89 patients with PR prolongation and bifascicular block with those of 172 patients with a normal PR interval and bifascicular block. Variable degrees of HV interval prolongation were recorded in the two groups. The authors concluded that it is difficult to determine whether trifascicular block is present in the individual patient from the body surface ECG.

Intraventricular Conduction Disturbances Associated with Myocardial Infarction and Periinfarction Block

See Chapter 8 for a discussion of intraventricular conduction disturbances associated with myocardial infarction and periinfarction block.

Nonspecific Intraventricular Conduction Disturbances

he WHO/ISFC Task Force[3] suggested "nonspecific intraventricular conduction delay" for a QRS duration that is longer than 0.11 second ut does not satisfy the criteria of either LBBB r RBBB. In a number of cases, such delays can e explained by the action of drugs or substances that cause slower depolarization (e.g., yperkalemia) or induce block of sodium channels. For example, it has been reported that tricyclic antidepressant drugs produce a fairly specific intraventricular conduction disturbance with a terminal QRS vector between 130 and 270 degrees.[69]

If the conduction delay is uniform, the QRS complex is uniformly widened and the QRS/T angle remains normal. However, not all nonspecific intraventricular conduction delays can be explained by factors known to slow conduction uniformly in the ventricular muscle. Atypical QRS widening that does not fit the criteria of either LBBB or RBBB may be caused by complex delays in the conduction system, regional conduction slowing in the myocardium, or a combination of the two (Figures 6–13 and 6–14). No systematic exploration or classification of such patterns has been attempted. Prolongation of the QRS duration up to 0.11 or even 0.12 second may be seen in healthy individuals (see Chapter 1).

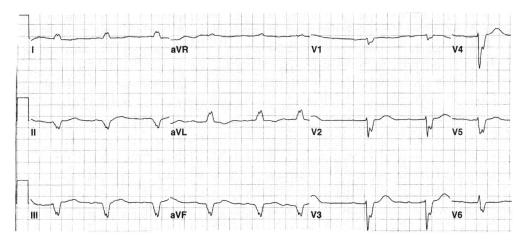

Figure 6–13 Undetermined intraventricular conduction disturbance. ECG of a 71-year-old man with end-stage cardiomyopathy and atrial fibrillation. QRS duration is 168 ms. The pattern resembles left bundle branch block, but the slowest portion of the QRS complex is at its end, as with right bundle branch block.

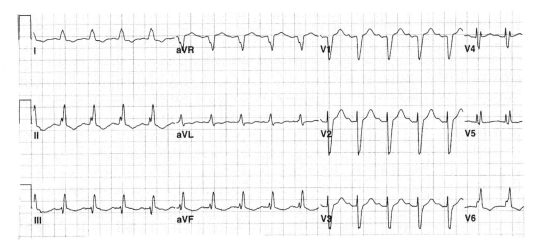

Figure 6–14 Undetermined intraventricular conduction disturbance. ECG of a 72-year-old woman with coronary artery disease and hypertension. QRS duration is 116 ms. The pattern resembles incomplete left bundle branch block (LBBB), but the initial slurred portion is wider than in a typical incomplete LBBB.

Notching of a QRS complex with a normal QRS duration should not be diagnosed as an intraventricular conduction disturbance. In most such cases, the notch can be explained by a nearly perpendicular projection of the depolarization vector inscribed at that time.

REFERENCES

1. Watt TB, Murao S, Pruitt RD: Left axis deviation induced experimentally in a primate heart. Am Heart J 70:381, 1965.
2. Rosenbaum MB, Elizari MV, Lazzari JO: The Hemiblocks: New Concepts of Intraventricular Conduction Based on Human Anatomical, Physiological and Clinical Studies. Oldsmar, FL, Tampa Tracings, 1971.
3. Willems JL, Robles de Medina EO, Bernard R, et al: Criteria for intraventricular conduction disturbances and preexcitation. J Am Coll Cardiol 5:1261, 1985.
4. Rosenbaum MB, Elizari MV, Levi RJ, et al: Five cases of intermittent left anterior hemiblock. Am J Cardiol 24:1, 1969.
5. Das G: Left axis deviation: a spectrum of intraventricular conduction block. Circulation 53:917, 1976.
6. Fernandez F, Scebat L, Lenègre J: Electrocardiographic study of left intraventricular hemiblock in man during selective coronary arteriography. Am J Cardiol 26:1, 1970.
7. Jacobson LB, LaFollette L, Cohn K: An appraisal of initial QRS forces in left anterior fascicular block. Am Heart J 94:407, 1977.
8. Rabkin SW, Mathewson FAL, Tate RB: Natural history of marked left axis deviation (left anterior hemiblock). Am J Cardiol 43:605, 1979.
9. Chou TE-C: Electrocardiography in Clinical Practice. Adult and Pediatric, 4th ed. Philadelphia, Saunders, 1996, pp 101–120.
10. McHenry PL, Phillips JF, Fisch C, et al: Right precordial qrS pattern due to left anterior hemiblock. Am Heart J 81:498, 1971.
11. Flowers NC: Left bundle branch block: a continuously evolving concept. J Am Coll Cardiol 9:684, 1987.
12. Warner RA, Hill NE, Mookherjee S, et al: Improved electrocardiographic criteria for the diagnosis of left anterior hemiblock. Am J Cardiol 51:723, 1983.
13. Burchell HB, Du Shane JW, Brandenburg RO: The electrocardiogram of patients with atrioventricular cushion defects (defects of the atrioventricular canal). Am J Cardiol 6:575, 1960.
14. Durrer D, Roos JP, Van Dam RT: The genesis of the electrocardiogram of patients with ostium primum defects (ventral atrial septal defects). Am Heart J 71:642, 1966.
15. Boineau JP, Moore EN, Patterson DF: Relationship between the ECG, ventricular activation, and the ventricular conduction system in ostium primum ASD. Circulation 68:556, 1973.
16. Pryor R, Blount SG: The clinical signficance of true left axis deviation: left intraventricular blocks. Am Heart J 72:391, 1966.
17. Hiss RG, Lamb LE, Allen MF: Electrocardiographic findings in 87,375 asymptomatic subjects. Am J Cardiol 6:619, 1965.
18. Ostrander LD: Left axis deviation: prevalence, associated conditions and prognosis. Ann Intern Med 75:23, 1971.
19. Eliot RS, Millhon WA, Millhon JJ: The clinical significance of uncomplicated marked left axis deviation in men without known disease. Am J Cardiol 12:767, 1963.
20. Corne RA, Beamish RA, Rollwagen RL: Significance of left anterior hemiblock. Br Heart J 40:552, 1978.
21. Atkins JM, Leshin SJ, Blomqvist G, et al: Ventricular conduction blocks and sudden death in acute myocardial infarction: potential indications for pacing. N Engl J Med 288:281, 1973.
22. Norris RM, Croxson MS: Bundle branch block in acute myocardial infarction. Am Heart J 79:728, 1970.
23. Scheinman M, Brenmann BA: Clinical and anatomic implications of intraventricular conduction blocks in acute myocardial infarction. Circulation 46:753, 1972.
24. Bosch X, Theroux P, Roy D, et al: Coronary angiographic significance of left anterior fascicular block during acute myocardial infarction. J Am Coll Cardiol 5:9, 1985.
25. Biagini E, Elhendy A, Schinkel AFL, et al: Prognostic significance of left anterior hemiblock in patients with suspected coronary artery disease. J Am Coll Cardiol 46:858, 2005.
26. Grant RP: Left axis deviation: an electrocardiographic-pathologic correlation study. Circulation 14:233, 1956.
27. Lenègre J: Etiology and pathology of bilateral bundle branch block in relation to complete heart block. Prog Cardiovasc Dis 6:409, 1964.
28. Lev M: Anatomic basis for atrioventricular block. Am J Med 37:742, 1964.
29. Corne RA, Parkin TW, Brandenburg RO, et al: Significance of marked left axis deviation: electrocardiographic-pathologic correlative study. Am J Cardiol 15:605, 1965.
30. Demoulin JC, Simar LJ, Kulbertus HE: Quantitative study of left bundle branch fibrosis in left anterior hemiblock: a stereologic approach. Am J Cardiol 36:751, 1975.
31. Entman ML, Estes EH, Hackel DB: The pathologic basis of the electrocardiographic pattern of parietal block. Am Heart J 74:202, 1967.
32. Castellanos A, Ramirez AV, Mayorga-Cortes A, et al: Left fascicular blocks during right heart catheterization using the Swan-Ganz catheter. Circulation 64:1271, 1981.
33. Gup AM, Granklin RB, Hill HE: The vectorcardiogram of children with left axis deviation and no apparent heart disease. Am Heart J 69:619, 1965.
34. Gertsch M, Theler A, Foglia E: Electrocardiographic detection of left ventricular hypertrophy in the presence of left anterior fascicular block. Am J Cardiol 61:1098, 1988.
35. Watt TB, Pruitt RD: Left posterior fascicular block in canine and primate hearts: an electrocardiographic study. Circulation 60:677, 1969.
36. Dhingra RC, Wyndham C, Bauernfeind R, et al: Significance of chronic bifascicular block without apparent organic heart disease. Circulation 60:33, 1979.
37. Bobba P, Salerno JA, Casari A: Transient left posterior hemiblock: report of four cases induced by exercise test. Circulation 66:931, 1972.
38. Rizzon P, Rossi L, Baissus C, et al: Left posterior hemiblock in acute myocardial infarction. Br Heart J 37:711, 1975.
39. Col JJ, Weinberg SL: The incidence and mortality of intraventricular conduction defects in acute myocardial infarction. Am J Cardiol 29:344, 1972.
40. Romhilt DW, Estes EH: Point-score system for the ECG diagnosis of left ventricular hypertrophy. Am Heart J 75:752, 1968.

1. Demoulin JC, Kulbertus HE: Histopathologic correlates of left posterior fascicular block. Am J Cardiol 44:1083, 1979.

2. Tawara S: Das Reizleitungssystem des Saeugetierherzens: eine anatomhistologische Studie ueber die Atrioventricular Buendel und die Purkinjeschen Faden. Jena, G Fischer, 1906.

3. Massing GK, James TN: Anatomical configuration of the His bundle and bundle branches in the human heart. Circulation 53:609, 1976.

4. Nakaya Y, Hiraga T: Reassessment of the subdivision block of the left bundle branch. Jpn Circ J 45:503, 1981.

5. Uhley HN, Rivkin LM: Electrocardiographic patterns following interruption of the main and peripheral branches of the canine left bundle of His. Am J Cardiol 13:41, 1964.

6. Hoffman I, Mehta J, Helsenrath J, et al: Anterior conduction delay: a possible cause for prominent anterior QRS forces. J Electrocardiol 9:15, 1976.

7. Reiffel JA, Bigger JT: Pure anterior conduction delay: a variant "fascicular" defect. J Electrocardiol 11:315, 1978.

8. Mac Alpin RN: In search of left septal fascicular block. Am Heart J 144:948,2002.

9. Strauss S, Langendorf R: Bilateral partial bundle branch block. Am J Med Sci 205:233, 1943.

10. Richman JL, Wolff L: Left bundle branch block masquerading as right bundle branch block. Am Heart J 47:383, 1954.

11. Lepeschkin E: The electrocardiographic diagnosis of bilateral bundle branch block in relation to heart block. Prog Cardiovasc Dis 6:445, 1964.

12. Dhingra RC, Wyndham C, Bauernfeind R, et al: Significance of block distal to the His bundle induced by atrial pacing in patients with chronic bifascicular block. Circulation 60:1455, 1979.

13. Dhala A, Gonzalez-Zuelgaray J, Deshpande S, et al: Unmasking the trifascicular left intraventricular conduction system by ablation of the right bundle branch. Am J Cardiol 77:706, 1996.

14. Ohkawa SI, Hackel DB, Ideker RE: Correlation of the width of the QRS complex with the pathologic anatomy of the cardiac conduction system in patients with chronic complete atrioventricular block. Circulation 63:938, 1981.

15. Lasser RP, Haft JL, Friedberg CK: Relationship of right bundle-branch block and marked left axis deviation (with left parietal or peri-infarction block) to complete heart block and syncope. Circulation 37:429, 1968.

56. Scanlon PJ, Pryor R, Blount SG: Right bundle-branch block associated with left superior or inferior intraventricular block: clinical setting, prognosis and relation to complete heart block. Circulation 42:1123, 1970.

57. Nimetz AA, Shubrooks SJ, Hutter AM, et al: The significance of bundle branch block during acute myocardial infarction. Am Heart J 90:439, 1975.

58. Thompson R, Mitchell A, Ahmed M, et al: Conduction defects in aortic valve disease. Am Heart J 98:3, 1979.

59. Downing JW, Kaplan S, Bove KE: Postsurgical left anterior hemiblock and right bundle-branch block. Br Heart J 34:263, 1972.

60. Aravindakshan V, Elizari MV, Rosenbaum MB: Right bundle branch block and left anterior fascicular block (left anterior hemiblock) following tricuspid valve replacement. Circulation 62:895, 1970.

61. Bashour T, Hsu I, Gorfinkel JH, et al: Atrioventricular and intraventricular conduction in hyperkalemia. Am J Cardiol 35:199, 1975.

62. Surawicz B: Prognosis of patients with chronic bifascicular block. Circulation 60:40, 1979.

63. Dhingra RC, Paliteo E, Strasberg B: Significance of the HV interval in 517 patients with chronic bifascicular block. Circulation 64:1265, 1981.

64. Godman MJ, Lassers BW, Julian DG: Complete bundle-branch block complicating acute myocardial infarction. N Engl J Med 282:237, 1970.

65. Scanlon PJ, Pryor R, Blount SG: Right bundle branch block associated with left superior or inferior intraventricular block: associated with acute myocardial infarction. Circulation 42:1135, 1970.

66. Rosenbaum MB: The hemiblocks: diagnostic criteria and clinical significance. Mod Concepts Cardiovasc Dis 39:141, 1970.

67. Dhingra RC, Denes P, Wu D, et al: Chronic right bundle branch block and left posterior hemiblock: clinical, electrophysiologic and prognostic observations. Am J Cardiol 36:867, 1975.

68. Levitas R, Haft JL: Significance of first degree heart block (prolonged PR interval) in bifascicular block. Am J Cardiol 34:259, 1974.

69. Niemann JT, Bessen HA, Rothstein RJ, et al: Electrocardiographic criteria for tricyclic antidepressant cardiotoxicity. Am J Cardiol 57:1154, 1986.

7 Acute Ischemia: Electrocardiographic Patterns

"Acute injury pattern" is an electrocardiographic (ECG) term that defines an abnormal ST segment elevation in two or more adjacent leads among the standard 12 leads (except lead aV_R). The term is derived from an injury current flowing between an injured (i.e., depolarized) tissue and a normally polarized tissue (see later discussion). The most common cause of injury current and the corresponding injury pattern is acute myocardial ischemia (e.g., during thrombotic, embolic, or spastic coronary occlusion). Transient injury current producing a similar ECG injury pattern may result from pressure exerted by pericardial fluid during acute pericarditis. The ECG injury pattern may be longlasting or permanent under various circumstances. Examples include (1) myocardial dyskinesis or ventricular aneurysm; (2) pressure exerted by fibrin or calcification during chronic pericarditis; (3) pressure exerted by a cardiac tumor; and (4) a variant pattern in a normal heart with the excessive asynchrony of early repolarization.

Systolic and Diastolic Currents of Injury

The diagram in Figure 7–1A is discussed in detail in Chapter 9. For purposes of this discussion it must be noted that under normal circumstances, small potential differences exist after the end of depolarization; that is, after the end of the QRS complex (a possible cause of junctional ST deviation) but not during the plateau (distal ST segment) and not during diastole (TP segment).[1] In contrast, the diagram in Figure 7–1B shows that there are two causes of ST segment deviation during myocardial ischemia: (1) shortening and decreased amplitude of the action potential and (2) depolarization (i.e., a less negative resting membrane potential). The shortening and decreased amplitude of the ventricular action potential create potential differences, resulting in a systolic current of injury. The depolarization creates potential differences resulting in a diastolic current of injury. The arrow on the left in Figure 7–1B shows that the potential

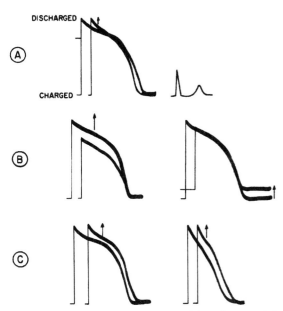

Figure 7–1 **A,** Normal ECG is derived from the potential differences between two ventricular action potentials (see Chapter 1). **B,** Potential differences responsible for systolic *(left)* and diastolic *(right)* currents of injury. **C,** Potential differences responsible for secondary repolarization are to the left and changes in the repolarization slope (e.g., digitalis effect) to the right. These changes are discussed in Chapter 9. (From Surawicz B, Saito S: Exercise testing for detection of myocardial ischemia in patients with abnormal electrocardiograms at rest. Am J Cardiol 41:943, 1978. Copyright 1978 Excerpta Medica, Inc., by permission.)

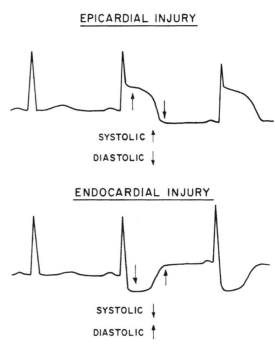

Figure 7–2 Effects of subepicardial and subendocardial injury on the ST segment and the baseline of the ECG. The direction of the arrows indicates the flow of current, not the ST segment vector. (From Surawicz B, Saito S: Exercise testing for detection of myocardial ischemia in patients with abnormal electrocardiograms at rest. Am J Cardiol 41:943, 1978. Copyright 1978 Excerpta Medica, Inc., by permission.)

difference produced by the systolic current of injury displaces the ST segment, and the arrow on the right shows that the potential difference produced by the diastolic current of injury displaces the baseline.

Figure 7–2 shows the effects of epicardial and endocardial injury on the ST segment, such as one would record in a standard limb or an anterior precordial ECG lead. Epicardial injury may cause elevation of the ST segment and depression of the baseline, whereas endocardial injury may cause depression of the ST segment and elevation of the baseline.

The conventional ECG recorded with alternating current (AC)-coupled amplifiers does not reveal displacement of the baseline and therefore does not detect differences between the ST segment displacement caused by the systolic and diastolic currents of injury.[4–7] Such differences can be discerned, however, using direct current (DC)-coupled amplifiers.

The magnetocardiogram has also been helpful for distinguishing the systolic from the diastolic "current of injury."[8] The magnetocardiogram showed that the ST depression during exercise-

induced ischemia results from a baseline shift, produced by a steady injury current that flows during the entire cardiac cycle but is interrupted during the ST interval. It appears, therefore, that the major change after coronary occlusion is "diastolic injury current" owing to depolarization in the ischemic areas, whereas shortening of the action potential during acute ischemia makes a smaller contribution to the ST segment displacement. The injury current arises at the ischemic border[9] and has been shown to create 12- to 20-mV potential gradients at the "electrical border" between the ischemic and normal myocardium in dogs with left anterior descending (LAD) coronary artery occlusion.[10]

In humans, isopotential body surface mapping has shown an early appearance of repolarization potentials at an average of 21.3 ms before the end of the QRS complex in patients with anterior infarction and 34.6 ms before the end of the QRS complex in patients with inferior infarction.[11] The topographic configuration of the isopotential maps was relatively simple, and in patients with both types of infarction the pattern was compatible with a single-dipole equivalent cardiac generator[11] (see Chapter 1).

Depression and Elevation of the ST Segment

Depression of the ST segment in the precordial leads reflects the posteriorly directed ST segment vector. The top diagrams on the left in Figure 7–3 show that this can be caused by subendocardial ischemia or subendocardial myocardial infarction (MI) of the anterior wall and by subepicardial ischemia or infarction of the posterior wall.

Boden and Spodick[12] listed the following causes of ST segment depression in the precordial leads: (1) reciprocal changes in the presence of inferoposterior or inferoseptal or basal (high lateral) acute MI; (2) anterior subendocardial myocardial ischemia or non-Q wave infarction; (3) posterior ("transmural") or posteroseptal acute MI; and (4) "benign" reciprocal changes (presumably a normal variant). Figure 7–4 shows diffuse ST segment depression attributed to subendocardial MI in a patient with a subtotal occlusion of the left main coronary artery.

Elevation of the ST segment in the precordial leads represents an anteriorly directed ST segment vector. Figure 7–5 shows that ST elevation may occur in the presence of subepicardial injury, infarction, pericarditis,[13] cardiac tumor, or transient ischemia during coronary spasm. The resulting systolic and diastolic currents injury cause elevation of the ST segment (sol arrow) and depression of the baseline (dashe arrow). The diagram on the right in Figure 7- shows that ST segment elevation also may caused by delayed repolarization in the subend cardial region or premature repolarization of t subepicardial region. Another rare cause of ST se ment elevation (not shown in Figure 7–5) is a upright Ta wave following a negative P wave (Figure 7–6).

Acute myocardial ischemia frequently produces an acute injury pattern. It must be emph sized that acute injury is not synonymous wit acute MI. Acute injury pattern can appear the absence of MI, as a precursor of MI, concom itant with the pattern of acute MI, or in the pre ence of a preexisting MI pattern.

The hallmark of acute injury is ST segmer elevation, which is usually accompanied reciprocal ST segment depression. An acu injury pattern can also produce a primary S segment depression (e.g., a subendocardial o posterior wall injury); the reciprocal ST segmer elevation in such cases may be detectable i

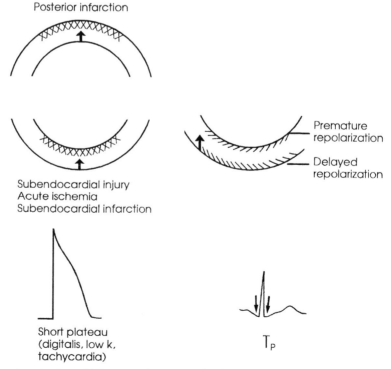

Posterior infarction

Subendocardial injury
Acute ischemia
Subendocardial infarction

Premature
repolarization

Delayed
repolarization

Short plateau
(digitalis, low k,
tachycardia)

T p

Figure 7–3 Several mechanisms of ST segment depression. The direction of the arrows indicates the flow of current, no the ST segment vector. (From Surawicz B, Saito S: Exercise testing for detection of myocardial ischemia in patients wit abnormal electrocardiograms at rest. Am J Cardiol 41:943, 1978. Copyright 1978 Excerpta Medica, Inc., by permission.)

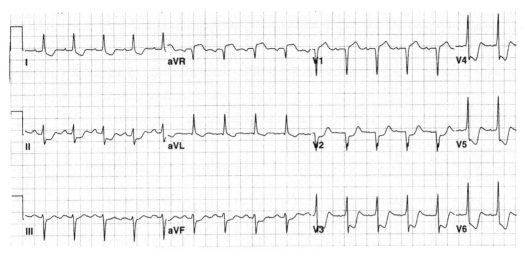

Figure 7–4 ECG of a 79-year-old woman with an apparent acute subendocardial myocardial infarction attributed to sub-total occlusion of the left main coronary artery, associated with global hypokinesis and an estimated left ventricular ejection fraction of 10 percent. ST segment is depressed in leads I, II, III, aV_L, aV_F, and V_2–V_6. Apparent "reciprocal" ST segment elevation is seen in leads aV_R and V_1.

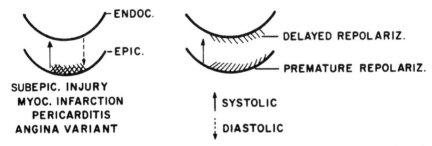

Figure 7–5 Several mechanisms of ST segment elevation. The direction of the arrows indicates the flow of current, not the ST segment vector. Endoc. = endocardium; epic. = epicardium; myoc. = myocardium; repolariz. = repolarization; subepic. = subepicardium. See text discussion. (From Surawicz B, Saito S: Exercise testing for detection of myocardial ischemia in patients with abnormal electrocardiograms at rest. Am J Cardiol 41:943, 1978. Copyright 1978 Excerpta Medica, Inc., by permission.)

leads aV_R and V_1 (see Figure 7–4). It has been suggested that ST segment elevation in leads V_{3R} through V_{5R} represents a reciprocal manifestation of acute posterolateral injury without right ventricular (RV) involvement.[16] In all other cases, however, the localization of ST segment elevation defines the primary site of the acute injury. The diagnosis of acute injury pattern is not made in the absence of ST segment elevation.

PQ Segment Elevation and Depression

Elevation of the PQ segment is usually attributed to atrial infarction (see Chapter 9). Depression of the PQ segment was found in 10 percent of patients with acute anterior wall MI[17] and in 8 percent of those with inferior wall MI.[18] In patients with both anterior and inferior MI, the presence of PQ segment depression was associated with a high incidence of pericarditis, large MI size, and more complications.

Localization of ST Segment Elevation and Reciprocal ST Segment Depression

The vector of the deviated ST segment is directed toward the site of ischemia. Thus ischemia or infarction of the anterior wall causes ST segment elevation in the anterior precordial leads (Figure 7–7), whereas ischemia or infarction of the inferior wall causes ST segment elevation in leads III, aV_F, and occasionally lead II (Figure 7–8). Right ventricular infarction causes segment elevation in the right precordial lead V_1[19] (Figure 7–9).

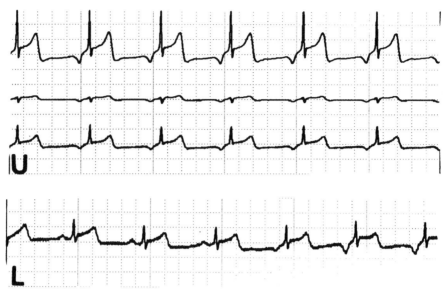

Figure 7–6   Two ECG strips recorded during ambulatory monitoring on two occasions. *Top,* P waves are negative in three leads. *Bottom,* Transition from the rhythm with an upright P wave to that of the inverted P wave in one of the monitor leads. ST segment elevation is simulated only in the presence of an inverted P wave, presumably because of atrial repolarization directed opposite to the inverted P wave.

ST segment elevation in the lead V_1 is also believed to be specific for anterior MI in which the first septal perforator is involved.[20]

ANTERIOR WALL MI AND OCCLUSION OF THE LAD CORONARY ARTERY

In patients with acute injury associated with an anterior MI, ST segment elevation is usually present in leads I, aV_L, a variable number (usually 3 to 6) of precordial leads (see Figures 7–7 and 7–10), and occasionally lead II. Reciprocal ST segment depression is nearly always present in leads III and aV_F.

In patients with an anterior MI, ST segment elevation in lead V_1 occurs less frequently than in leads V_2 and V_3. The presence of ST elevation in lead V_1 suggests that the conal branch of the right coronary artery is either absent or small and therefore does not reach the intraventricular septum.[21] Conversely, the absence of ST segment elevation in lead V_1 during acute anterior MI suggests the presence of a large conal branch of the right coronary artery protecting the septum from transseptal MI.[21]

Occlusion of the LAD artery "wrapped" around the apex could be recognized by the presence of ST segment elevation with positive T waves in lead III associated with ST segment elevation in aV_L during the early stage of infarction.[22] Figure 8–14 shows such a pattern in a patient in whom the infarction was believed to be related to the use of cocaine.

According to Wellens et al.,[23] the area perfused by LAD coronary artery can be divided into three main parts: (1) the basoseptal part, supplied by the first septal branch(es); (2) the lateral basal part, perfused by the first diagonal branch(es) or intermediate branch; and (3) the inferoapical part, receiving blood from the distal LAD, frequently "wrapped" around the apex. In the quoted study of Engelen et al.,[24] occlusions at different sites led to electrocardiographically four different patterns: (1) proximal to the septal and diagonal branches, which results in ischemia of all three areas, named above; (2) proximal before the first septal, but distal to the first diagonal branch, which leads to the ischemia of the septum and the inferoapical area, whereas the basolateral area remains free; (3) before the first diagonal but distal to the first septal branch, which leads to ischemia of the basolateral wall and the inferoapical wall but not the septum; and (4) distal to the first septal and diagonal branches, which leads to the ischemia of inferoapical area only. The incidence of these sites of occlusion in the study of Engelen et al. was as follows: 40%, 10%, 10%, and 40%, respectively.[2]

In an earlier study, Birnbaum et al.[25] attempted to predict the level of obstruction of the LAD artery in patients with acute anterior infarction. The culprit lesions were proximal to the first diagonal branch in 59 patients and distal to that artery in 38 patients. When the ST segment was elevated in the anterior precordial leads, the presence of ST elevation in leads I and aV_L was

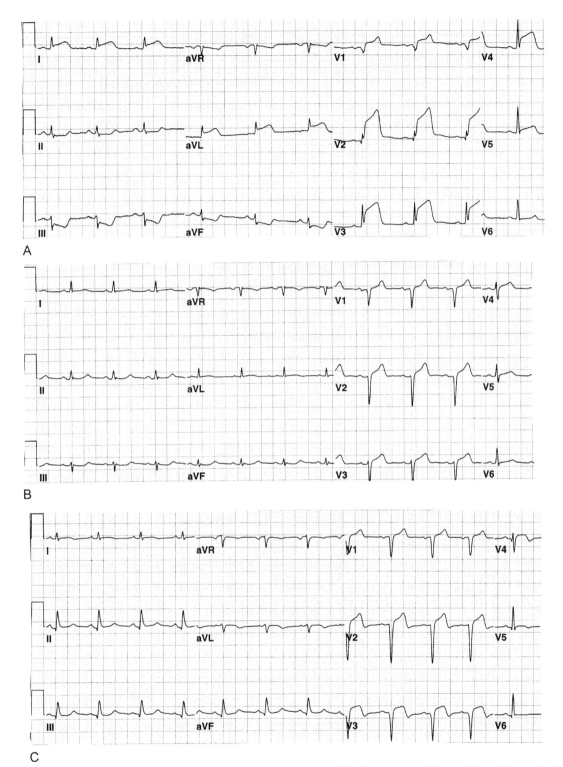

Figure 7–7   ECG of a 71-year-old man with an acute anterior myocardial infarction caused by occlusion of the proximal left anterior descending coronary artery. **A,** Day of infarction. Note the ST segment elevation in leads I, aV_L, and V_1–V_5 and the reciprocal ST segment depression in leads III and aV_F. **B,** Next day. Note the pseudonormalization. **C,** Following day. Note the typical evolution of a myocardial infarction in the anterior wall. Ventriculogram revealed an extensive infarction.

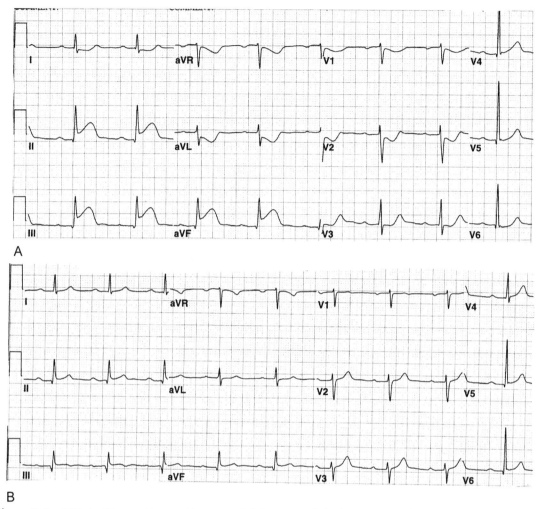

Figure 7–8   ECG of a 57-year-old man with an acute inferior myocardial infarction caused by occlusion of the right coronary artery. **A,** Day of infarction at 4:37 AM. Note the ST segment elevation in leads II, III, and aV_F and the reciprocal ST segment depression in leads I, aV_L, and V_1–V_3. PR interval was 280 ms. **B,** Same day at 12:08 PM, after percutaneous angioplasty of the right coronary artery. Note complete regression of the ST segment displacement.

predictive of a proximal lesion in 87 percent of cases; its absence was predictive of a distal obstruction in 73 percent of cases. The presence of reciprocal ST segment depression in the inferior leads was also suggestive of a proximal lesion.

The following is a synopsis of ECG findings described by Wellens et al.[23] in different types of LAD occlusion.

LAD Occlusion Proximal to the First Septal and First Diagonal Branch

This type of very proximal LAD occlusion often causes right bundle branch block (RBBB). ST vector is directed superiorly (Figure 7–11, *left*), causing ST elevation in leads aV_R, aV_L, V_1–V_3, or V_4,

and reciprocal ST depression in inferior leads as well as in leads V_5–V_6 (Figure 7–11, *right*).

LAD Occlusion Proximal to the First Septal but Distal to the First Diagonal or Intermediate Branch

This type of proximal LAD occlusion results in rightward direction of ST vector (Figure 7–12, *left*), and unlike in the occlusion distal to both the first septal and first diagonal, the ST segment is depressed in lead aV_L (Figure 7–12, *right*).

Distal LAD Occlusion

Figure 7–13 shows that the ST vector points inferiorly. To the left, the ST segment is elevated

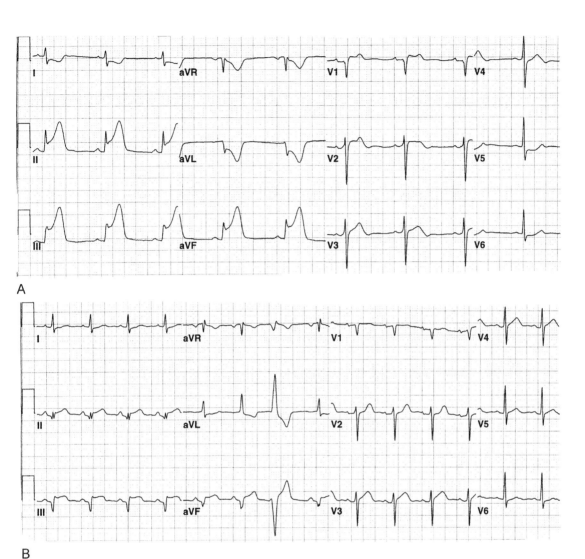

Figure 7–9   ECG of a 47-year-old man with an acute inferior and right ventricular myocardial infarction caused by isolated total proximal occlusion of the right coronary artery associated with closure of the right ventricular marginal branch. **A,** Day of infarction at 4:27 PM. Note the ST segment elevation in leads II, III, aV$_F$, V$_1$, and V$_2$ and reciprocal ST segment depression in leads I, aV$_L$, and V$_5$. **B,** Next day at 5:34 AM after successful angioplasty of the right coronary artery but an inability to open the right ventricular marginal branch. Right ventricular infarction was confirmed by echocardiography; residual ST segment elevation is present in leads II, III, aV$_F$, and V$_1$.

in the inferior and lateral precordial leads, but depressed in lead aV$_R$.

Occlusion of the First Diagonal Branch of the LAD Coronary Artery

Occlusion of the first diagonal branch causes ST elevation mainly in leads I and aV$_L$ and fewer changes in the precordial leads[26–28] (Figure 7–14).

Occlusion of the Main Septal Branch

Occlusion of the main septal branch causes ST segment elevation in leads V$_1$ and V$_2$ and

reciprocal ST segment depression in leads II, III, aV$_F$, V$_5$, and V$_6$.

LEFT MAIN CORONARY ARTERY OCCLUSION

Diagnosis of left main coronary artery occlusion is difficult. It can be suspected when ST elevation is present in all but inferior leads (Figure 7–15). Wellens et al.[23] suggested that left main coronary artery occlusion should be suspected when RBBB and other features of very proximal LAD occlusion are associated with signs of severe posterobasal ischemia. Yamaji et al.[29] and Gaitando

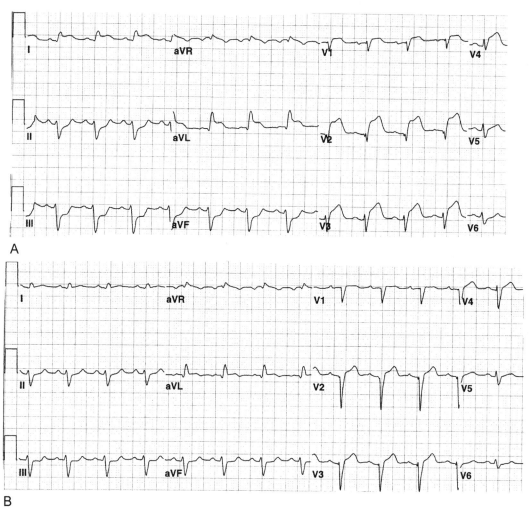

Figure 7–10 ECG of a 57-year-old man with an anterior myocardial infarction caused by total occlusion of the proxim left anterior descending (LAD) coronary artery. **A,** Day of infarction at 11:59 AM. Note the ST segment elevation in leads aV_L, and V_1–V_4 and the reciprocal ST segment depression in leads III and aV_F. **B,** Same day at 3:07 PM after angioplasty the LAD coronary artery. Note the lessened ST segment displacement. The QRS complex measures 118 ms in **A** (perii chemic block) and 90 ms in **B**.

et al.[29a] reported that left main occlusion should be suspected when ST elevation in lead aV_R is greater than in lead V_1. Other reported markers of left main coronary occluson were: diffuse ST segment depression[29b] (see Figure 7–4) and ST segment deviation in lead V_6 greater than or equal to ST segment deviation in lead V_1.[29c]

ST SEGMENT DEVIATION IN LEAD aV_R

Lead aV_R appears to be often overlooked, possibly because it has no adjacent neighboring lead among the limb leads to identify a discrete part of the LV. Lead aV_R faces predominantly superior-posterior wall of the left ventricle. Therefore ST segment in aV_R tends to be elevated

when it is depressed in anterior leads and tend to be depressed when the ST segment is elevate in anterior leads. These changes are note mostly when ST segment deviation is large an may be overlooked when the QRS amplitude i the lead aV_R is low, particularly when there i an rSR′ pattern with T wave directed opposit to the terminal QRS portion.

The literature has emphasized the ST eleva tion in lead aV_R in patients with left main CA! (see previous discussion) and an associatio with poorer outcome of MI in patients with pre dominant ST depression in anterior, lateral, o inferior leads who tended to have more exten sive CAD and wall motion abnormalities.[30,3] In my opinion, the vectorial analysis of the lea

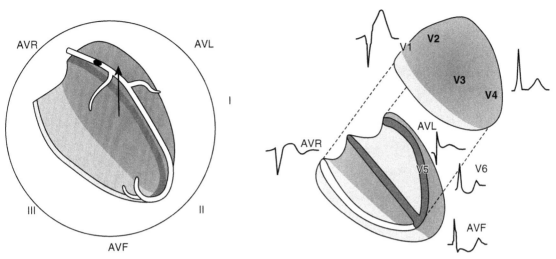

Figure 7–11   *Left panel:* Diagram of proximal left anterior descending coronary artery occlusion shows global ischemia of the whole anterior wall with ST vector pointing in a superior direction. *Right panel:* Related ECG changes with ST segment elevation in leads aV_R and V_1 and reciprocal ST segment depression in the inferior leads and V_5–V_6. (From Wellens HJJ, Gorgels APM, Doevedans PA [eds]: The ECG in Acute Myocardial Infarction and Unstable Angina. Norwell, MA, Kluwer Academic, 2003. With permission of authors and publisher.)

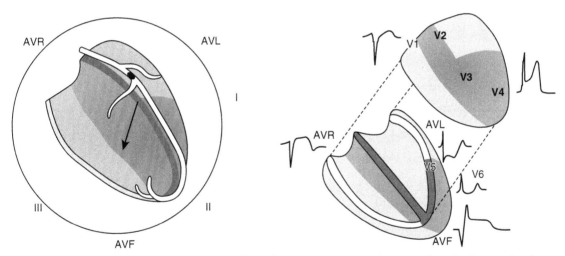

Figure 7–12   *Left panel:* Diagram of left anterior descending coronary artery occlusion involving the first septal perforator but not the first diagonal branch with ST vector pointing medially. *Right panel* shows related ECG change with ST elevation in the precordial and inferior leads and reciprocal ST segment depression in lead aV_L. (From Wellens HJJ, Gorgels APM, Doevedans PA [eds]: The ECG in Acute Myocardial Infarction and Unstable Angina. Norwell, MA, Kluwer Academic, 2003. With permission of authors and publisher.)

aV_R should be performed not in isolation, but rather in concert with changes in all available leads.

INFERIOR WALL MI AND OCCLUSION OF RCA OR LEFT CIRCUMFLEX CORONARY ARTERY

In the presence of acute injury associated with an inferior MI, the ST segment is elevated in leads II, III, and aV_F and occasionally in leads V_5 and V_6. Reciprocal ST segment depression is usually present in leads I and aV_L and often in one or more precordial leads, predominantly leads V_2–V_3. Changes in lead V_1 vary. ST segment elevation in lead V_1 may be caused by the presence of right ventricular MI, which can be suspected also when reciprocal ST segment depression in lead V_1 is absent[32–34] (Figures 7–16 and 7–17). The presence of ST segment depression

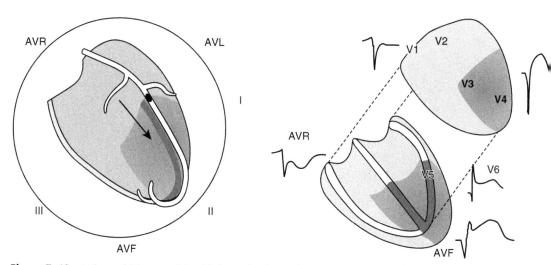

Figure 7–13 *Left panel:* Diagram of distal left anterior descending coronary artery occlusion with ST vector pointing inferiorly and to the left. Right panel shows related ECG changes with ST segment elevation in the lateral precordial and inferior leads and reciprocal ST segment depression in lead aV$_R$. (From Wellens HJJ, Gorgels APM, Doevedans PA [eds]: The ECG Acute Myocardial Infarction and Unstable Angina. Norwell, MA, Kluwer Academic, 2003. With permission of authors and publisher.)

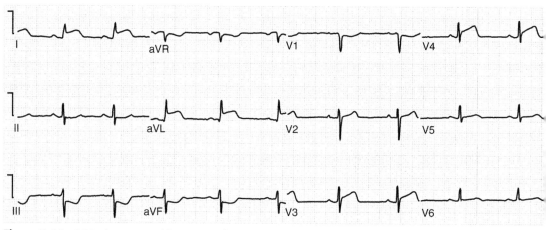

Figure 7–14 ECG of a 47-year-old woman with myocardial infarction anterior wall caused by ostial occlusion of large diagonal branch supplying a large territory of the ventricle. The dominant right coronary artery was normal. There was 40 percent narrowing of the left anterior descending coronary artery in the midportion with nonobstructive luminal lesions in the left circumflex artery. Left ventricular ejection fraction was 25 percent. The ECG shows pattern of anterosuperior infarction with ST segment elevation in leads I, aV$_L$, and V$_2$–V$_4$ with reciprocal ST segment depression in leads II, III, and aV$_F$.

in lead V$_1$ indicates either a reciprocal change alone or an association with posterior wall MI[26] (Figures 7–18 and 7–19).

In a study of 16,521 patients with an inferior MI, ST segment depression in the precordial leads was present in 61.1 percent of cases.[35] Reciprocal ST segment depression occurred more frequently in patients with a large MI and more wall motion abnormalities, and it was associated with high mortality.[35–37] The magnitude of the sum of ST depression voltage in leads V$_1$–V$_6$ added significant independent prognostic information, with the risk of 30-day mortality

increasing by 36 percent for every 0.5 mV of precordial ST segment depression.[32] In another study[38] the presence of ST segment elevation in lead V$_6$ in patients with acute inferior MI was associated with large infarct size and a high incidence of complications. Moreover, the mortality of patients with inferior MI was increased when maximal ST segment elevation occurred in leads V$_4$–V$_6$ but not in lead III.[37] In a study of 1153 patients with inferior MI who took part in the Global Utilization of Streptokinase and TPA for Occluded Arteries Study (GUSTO-I), subjects with maximum ST segment depression in leads

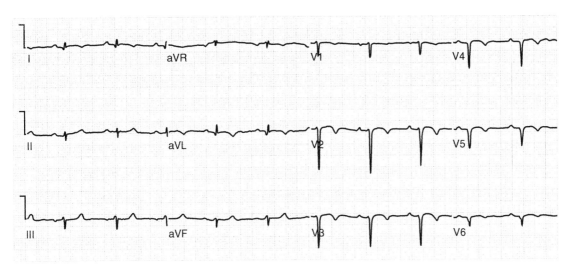

Figure 7–15   ECG of a 42-year-old woman admitted with acute chest pain. Coronary angiography revealed 90 percent ostial occlusion of the left main coronary artery with minor luminal irregularities in other large coronary branches. There was anterior hypokinesis with estimated left ventricular ejection fraction of 45 percent. There are Q waves in I, aV$_L$, and V$_3$–V$_6$ leads with small r in V$_1$–V$_3$ leads. The pattern in the inferior leads II, III, and aV$_F$ is normal.

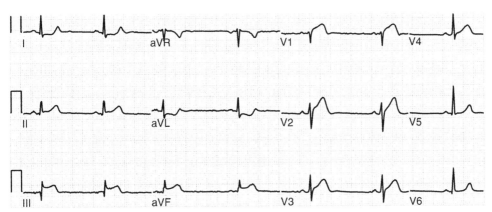

Figure 7–16   ECG of a 45-year-old man with inferior and right ventricular myocardial infarction caused by occlusion of the right coronary artery proximal to the right ventricular marginal branch and failure of thrombolytic treatment. No significant stenoses were present in the left coronary arteries. ST segment elevation is present in leads II, III, aV$_F$, and V$_1$–V$_3$; note also the reciprocal ST segment depression in leads I and aV$_L$.

V$_4$–V$_6$ had three-vessel disease more often than those without precordial ST segment depression or those with ST segment depression in leads V$_1$–V$_3$.[39]

RIGHT OR CIRCUMFLEX CORONARY OCCLUSION?

Inferior MI is caused by the occlusion of the dominant left circumflex artery in about 18% of cases.[40] Myocardial infarction caused by the dominant right coronary artery and the dominant left circumflex artery tends to produce similar Q wave changes (Figures 7–8, 7–9, and 7–16

to 7–21), but the pattern of ST segment elevation may be helpful for the differential diagnosis. This is shown in Figure 17–22, reproduced from the study of Wellens et al.[23] Although both vessels perfuse the inferior wall, the RCA territory covers the medial part including the inferior septum, whereas the circumflex territory covers the left posterobasal and lateral area. Thus in the case of RCA occlusion, the ST vector is directed inferiorly and rightward, whereas in the case of left circumflex occlusion, the ST vector points inferiorly and leftward. Accordingly, in RCA occlusion, the ST elevation is greater in lead III than in lead II with ST depression in lead I,

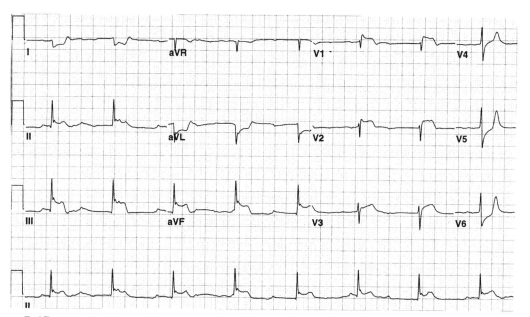

Figure 7–17 ECG of a 61-year-old woman resuscitated from cardiac arrest but who succumbed to cardiogenic shock on the same day. Acute injury pattern suggests inferior and right ventricular infarction. The latter was corroborated by the ST segment elevation in leads to the right of lead V₁. In the left precordial leads, ST segment elevation extends to lead V and reciprocal depression is present in leads I, aVL, and V5–V6. There is sinus tachycardia with complete atrioventricul (AV) dissociation and AV junctional rhythm at a rate of 56 beats/min.

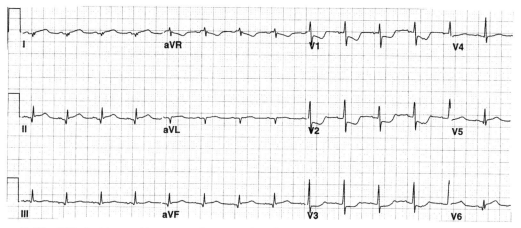

Figure 7–18 ECG of a 65-year-old woman with a posterolateral myocardial infarction attributed to complete occlusion the left circumflex coronary artery in its midportion and complete occlusion of the dominant right coronary artery. There w severe posterolateral hypokinesis with an estimated left ventricular ejection fraction of 10 percent. ST segment elevation present in leads I, aVL, and V6 and reciprocal ST segment depression in leads V1 through V3.

whereas in the case of circumflex occlusion, ST segment in lead I is either elevated or isoelectric. In the experience of these investigators,[23] ST depression in lead I was predictive of RCA occlusion in 86 percent of cases and an isoelectric or elevated ST segment in lead I was predictive of circumflex occlusion in 77 percent of cases.

Numerous earlier studies produced the same or similar results. Thus Huey et al.[41] compared the ECGs of 40 consecutive patients with acut MI caused by left circumflex artery occlusio with those of 107 patients with right coronar occlusion. In the patients with inferior MI, ST seg ment elevation in one or more of leads I, aVL, V and V6 was highly suggestive of occlusion of the le circumflex artery (see Figure 7–20). Bairey et al. also reported that ST segment elevation in the la eral leads identified circumflex artery occlusio as the cause of inferior MI.

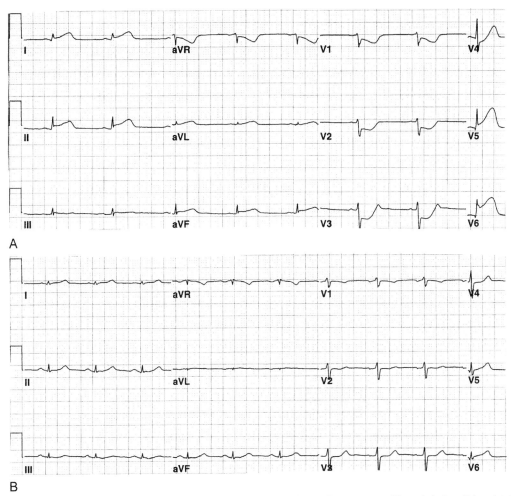

Figure 7–19 ECG of a 48-year-old man with acute occlusion of a large obtuse marginal branch before (**A**) and 3 hours after (**B**) emergency percutaneous coronary angioplasty. Note the ST segment elevation in leads I, aV$_L$, V$_5$, and V$_6$. Reciprocal ST segment depression in leads V$_1$–V$_3$ regress after angioplasty.

In patients with inferior MI, ST segment elevation in lead III exceeding that in lead II, particularly when combined with ST segment elevation in lead V$_1$, is a powerful predictor of occlusion of the right coronary artery proximal to the acute margin of the heart[42] (see Figure 7–9). Hertz et al.[43] reported the same results with an added finding that reciprocal ST depression in lead aV$_L$ was greater than in lead I.

Leads V$_5$ and V$_6$ are affected by posterolateral ischemia (Figures 7–23 and 7–24). ST segment elevation >0.2 mV in leads V$_5$ and V$_6$ in patients with inferior MI correlated with occlusion of an artery (right or circumflex) supplying a large territory of the myocardium with an expected high ischemic burden.[44] In patients with an inferior MI with ST segment elevation in leads II, III, and aV$_F$, the presence of additional ST segment elevation in leads V$_5$–V$_6$ or

leads I and aV$_L$ is a fairly sensitive and specific marker for left circumflex coronary artery occlusion.[42]

Depression of the ST segment in leads V$_1$–V$_3$ tends to indicate a large posterolateral perfusion defect,[32] probably owing to the involvement of posterior or posterobasal wall, and is more often associated with occlusion of the circumflex artery (71 percent) than of the RCA (40 percent).[45]

LATERAL, INFEROLATERAL, AND POSTEROLATERAL MI

Lateral wall involvement causes ST segment elevation in leads V$_5$ and V$_6$. It occurs more frequently in circumflex artery than right coronary artery occlusion, but independent of the vessel involved, ST elevation in these leads implies a larger ischemic area.[23]

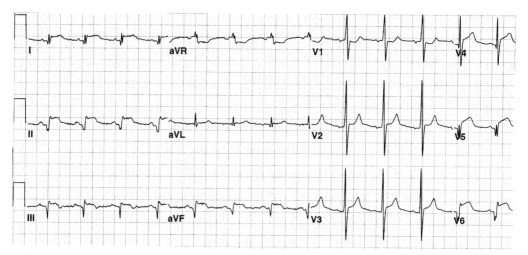

Figure 7–20   ECG of an 82-year-old man with an acute inferior and posterobasal myocardial infarction, apparently caus[e] by 95 percent occlusion of the dominant left circumflex artery and 95 percent occlusion of the mid-right coronary arter[y] Note the ST segment elevation in leads II, III, aV_F, and V_2–V_6 and the reciprocal ST segment depression in leads aV_R a[nd] V_1. Left ventricular ejection fraction is 20 percent.

Localizaton of ST segment elevation and reciprocal ST segment depression varies in patients with a lateral MI depending on the extent and location of the MI. Typically, ST segment elevation in patients with inferolateral MI is present in leads II, III, aV_F, V_5, and V_6 (see Figure 7–20). In many cases, however, ST segment elevation extends to the right of lead V_5 (i.e., leads V_2–V_4). The lead with maximal ST segment elevation, however, is usually V_6 or V_5. Reciprocal ST segment depression may be present in leads I, III, aV_L, and V_1–V_4, but it may also be absent.

In patients with high lateral MI caused by occlusion of the left circumflex coronary artery, the ST segment is usually elevated in leads I, aV_L, V_5, and V_6; it is depressed in leads III and aV_F and occasionally in lead V_1 (see Figure 7–23).

Posterior wall involvement causes reciprocal ST depression in right precordial leads. When present in patients with RCA occlusion, it indicates dominance of this vessel. In case of circumflex artery occlusion, the posterior wall is nearly always involved. Therefore absence of ST segment depression in the right precordial leads in inferior MI is strongly suggestive of RCA involvement.[23] In patients with posterolateral MI, ST segment elevation may be either absent or present in leads V_5 and V_6.

In patients with a so-called true posterior MI (i.e., without ECG evidence of inferior or lateral MI), ST segment elevation may be present in leads V_7–V_9 and reciprocal ST segment depression in leads V_1–V_3.[46] Routine recording of leads V_7–V_9 has been recommended in patients wit[h] suspected MI but with a nondiagnostic 12-lea[d] ECG.[47–49] ST elevation in posterior leads V_7–V_9 in patients with an inferior MI was associate[d] with a high incidence of posterolateral wa[ll] motion abnormalities, large infarct, and lo[w] ejection fraction.[49] In the study of Wung an[d] Drew,[50] posterior leads V_7–V_9 contributed signi[f]icant additional diagnostic information abov[e] and beyond the standard 12-lead ECG when [the] criterion of 0.05 mV instead of 0.1 mV ST eleva[-] tion was applied to the posterior leads.

ACUTE INJURY PATTERN IN BOTH ANTERIOR AND INFERIOR LEADS

In the GUSTO study, a pattern with combine[d] ST segment elevation in at least two of lead[s] V_1–V_4 and more than two leads of leads II, II[I] and aV_F was present in 179 of 2996 patients wit[h] acute MI. Of these patients, RCA occlusion wa[s] present in 59 percent and distal LAD occlusio[n] in 36 percent. Patients with combined anterio[r] and inferior ST segment elevation tended to hav[e] limited MI size and a more preserved L[V] function.[51]

ACUTE INJURY PATTERN IN RIGHT PRECORDIAL LEADS

Elevation of the ST segment in the right precor[-] dial leads V_{3R} and V_{4R} usually signifies the pres[-] ence of RV MI.[52,53] In patients with RV M[I] ST segment elevation may extend to additiona[l] right precordial leads V_{5R} and V_6R[52–55] and

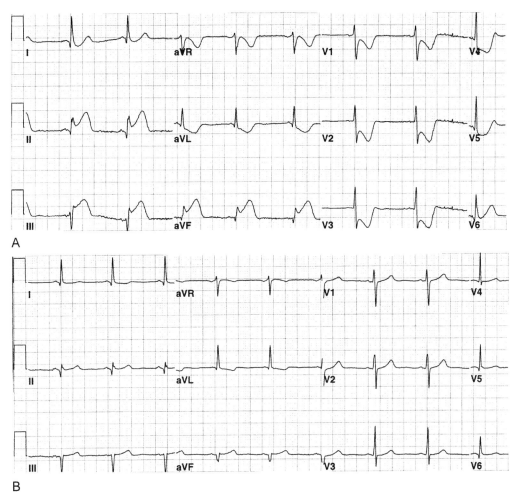

Figure 7–21   ECG of a 48-year-old man with an inferoposterior myocardial infarction caused by total occlusion of the large-caliber circumflex coronary artery. No significant stenoses were present in the left anterior descending and right coronary arteries, but there was a 90 percent stenosis of a small diagonal branch. **A,** Day of infarction. Note the ST segment elevation in leads II, III, and aV$_F$ and reciprocal ST segment depression in leads I, aV$_L$, and V$_1$–V$_6$. **B,** At 13 hours after angioplasty of the left circumflex artery. Note the regression of the ST segment deviation and the decrease in QRS duration from 104 ms to 86 ms.

sometimes to precordial leads V$_1$–V$_5$[45] (see Figure 7–24). In the presence of an inferior MI, a diagnosis of RV MI is supported by a discordant pattern of ST segment elevation in V$_1$ and ST segment depression in V$_2$.[56] ST segment elevation in leads V$_{3R}$ and V$_{4R}$ may be present in patients with acute anterior MI but seldom extends to lead V$_{5R}$.[57] Moreover, when the ST segment elevation caused by acute anterior MI is present in leads V$_{3R}$–V$_{5R}$, the magnitude of the ST segment elevation diminishes from V$_{3R}$ to V$_{5R}$, whereas in the presence of RV MI, the ST segment elevation is either the same or increases from V$_{3R}$ to V$_{5R}$.[58] Saw et al.[59] found that in patients with inferior MI, ST elevation in lead III greater than in lead II was more sensitive than lead V$_{4R}$ in diagnosing RV MI.

Isolated RV infarction is rare, but the diagnosis can be verified by echocardiography. In one reported case, ST segment elevation in the precordial leads was associated with minimal ST segment elevation in the inferior leads.[60] In another case, massive ST segment elevation in the precordial leads was associated with massive ST segment elevation in inferior leads.[44] Such cases are rare.

TOMBSTONING PATTERN

The term "tombstoning pattern of ST segment in acute MI" was apparently introduced by Wimalarathna.[61] It is used infrequently to label a purely monophasic pattern occurring most often in patients with proximal occlusion of

RIGHT CORONARY ARTERY MI   CIRCUMFLEX CORONARY ARTERY MI

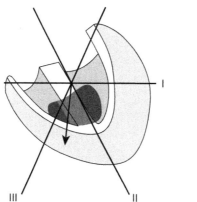
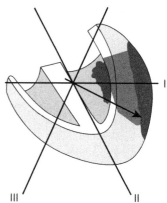

Figure 7–22 Schematic presentation of the ST segment vector in inferior wall myocardial infarction showing the differ-ence between the occlusion of right and left circumflex coronary artery and the corresponding ECG changes in the limb leads. See text discussion. (From Wellens HJJ, Gorgels APM, Doevedans PA [eds]: The ECG in Acute Myocardial Infarction and Unstable Angina. Norwell, MA, Kluwer Academic, 2003. With permission of authors and publisher.)

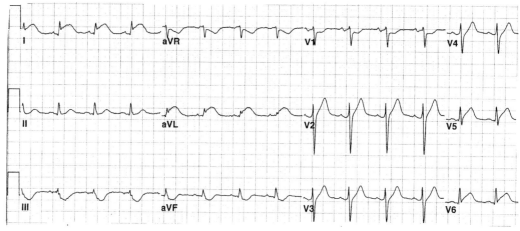

Figure 7–23 ECG of a 63-year-old man with a pattern of high lateral myocardial infarction probably caused by left circumflex artery disease. Coronary angiography showed 50 percent mid-left circumflex artery stenosis, 75 percent obtus marginal artery stenosis, 99 percent proximal left anterior descending artery stenosis, and aneurysmal dilatation of the righ coronary artery. ST segment elevation is present in leads I, aV_L, V_5, and V_6; reciprocal ST segment depression is present i leads III, aV_F, and V_1.

LAD coronary artery[62] and suggesting a large infarct and a low LV ejection fraction[63] (see Figures 7–29 and 7–30). It can be seen also in an agonal ECG (Figure 7–25).

BRUGADA AND OTHER RSR′ PATTERNS WITH ST ELEVATION IN THE RIGHT PRECORDIAL LEADS

In patients with an RSR′ pattern in the right precor-dial leads and absent anterior infarction, ST seg-ment elevation may be caused by septal ischemia (Figures 7–26 and 7–27) or by RV MI.[53–56,58] Other causes of such a pattern include the syn-drome associated with sudden cardiac death

described by Brugada and Brugada[64] an arrhythmogenic RV dysplasia (see Chapter 12 Brugada and Brugada[65] described a syndrom of RBBB, persistent ST segment elevation in lead V_1–V_3 (ocasionally in other leads), and sudde cardiac death that affects predominantly mal patients and is often familial. In some subject with this syndrome, the pattern appears inter mitently with transient normalization of th ECG. There are three types of the ECG patter in the most common, type 1, the ST segment i coved and the elevation is ≥0.2 mV; in typ 2 there is saddleback elevation of ≥0.1 mV and in type 3 the coved or saddleback elevatio is <0.1 mV.[66] The ST elevation is augmented b

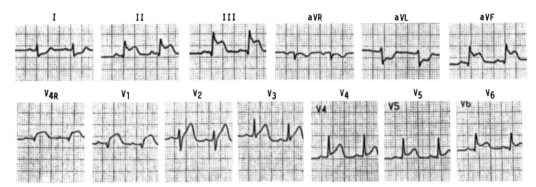

Figure 7-24 Acute inferoposterior myocardial infarction with right ventricular infarction in a 37-year-old man. ECG was recorded on the day of the onset of chest pain. A diagnosis of infarction was corroborated by serial cardiac enzyme changes. Radionuclide angiography revealed an akinetic inferoposterior wall of the left ventricle and severe hypokinesis of the right ventricle. The left ventricular ejection fraction was 48 percent and the right ventricular ejection fraction 11 percent. Physical examination revealed marked jugular venous distension. ST segment elevation is present in leads II, III, and aV$_F$ and reciprocal ST segment depression in leads I and aV$_L$. There is some ST segment elevation in the left precordial leads. Its cause is uncertain. Marked ST segment elevation in leads V$_1$ and V$_{4R}$ is suggestive of right ventricular infarction. ST segment elevation in all of the precordial leads subsided the next day.

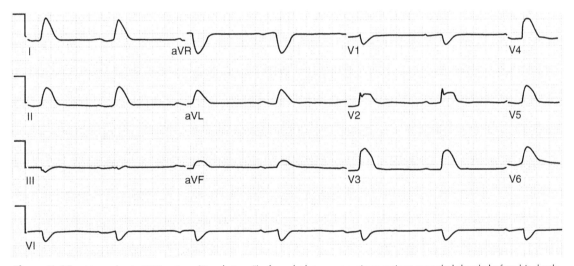

Figure 7-25 Monophasic ECG pattern ("tombstone") of a pulseless unconscious patient recorded shortly before his death.

selective stimulation of α-adrenergic or muscarinic receptors and by sodium channel–blocking antiarrhythmia drugs,[67] but reduced by β-adrenergic stimulation or α-adrenergic block.[68] Many of these patients have no evidence of structural heart disease. Mutations of the SCN5A gene, which encodes the cardiac sodium channel, have been identified in about 15 percent of patients with Brugada syndrome who have frequently bradyarrhythmic complications.[69,70] A similar ECG pattern was present in young male Southeast Asians who died unexpectedly during sleep[71] and in patients with familial cardiomyopathy (arrhythmogenic RV dysplasia) involving the right ventricle and the conducting system.[72–74]

Common to these conditions is QRS widening confined to selected leads with ST segment elevation (usually V$_1$–V$_3$) with normal QRS duration in remote leads such as I and V$_6$.[75] In patients with RV dysplasia, the shape of the terminal QRS portion in the right precordial leads has been likened to the Greek letter epsilon.

The pattern of RBBB with ST segment elevation in the right precordial leads is not entirely specific for RV ischemia or Brugada syndrome because it can occur with other conditions (Figures 7–28 and 7–30). Table 7–1 lists some of the conditions in which the Brugada type ECG pattern may be encountered. The largest number is probably in the unexplained category.[76]

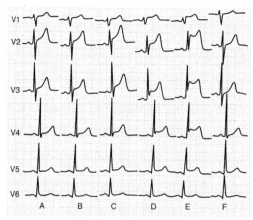

Figure 7–26 Selected electrocardiographic leads before **(A)**, during **(B–E)**, and after **(F)** balloon occlusion of the proximal left anterior descending coronary artery in a patient in whom ST segment elevation in leads V_1–V_3 during occlusion was associated with a QRS duration increase in these leads. (From Surawicz B, Orr CM, Hermiller JB, et al: QRS changes during percutaneous transluminal coronary angioplasty and their possible mechanism. J Am Coll Cardiol 30:452, 1997. American College of Cardiology, by permission.)

CORONARY SPASM, UNSTABLE ANGINA PECTORIS, NON-Q WAVE MI

Acute injury pattern is the diagnostic marker of coronary spasm, and the lead distribution of ST segment deviation during coronary spasm is the same as during myocardial ischemia caused by other types of coronary occlusion (Figure 7–29). ST segment elevation has been reported also in patients with syndrome X, normal coronary angiograms, and suspected spasm of coronary arterioles.[77] In the presence of unstable angina pectoris[78] and non-Q wave MI,[79] an acute injury pattern is present in a small number of patients. Other ECG changes accompanying these conditions are discussed in Chapters 8 and 9.

ST SEGMENT CHANGES AS A GUIDE TO THROMBOLYTIC THERAPY

The ECG plays a crucial role in identifying candidates for thrombolytic treatment.[80] The indication for emergent thrombolytic therapy of suspected acute MI is based on the presence of ST segment elevation of >0.1 mV in two limb leads or two or more anatomically contiguous precordial leads. In the cases of preexisting ST segment elevation, such as with left bundle branch block (LBBB), the same rule applies when the availability of the basic pattern allows recognition of the ST shift.[81] Regression of ST segment elevation parallels recanalization,[82–84] and incomplete resolution of ST segment elevation is a powerful independent predictor of early mortality.[85–88]

Reelevation of the ST segment is a sign of limited myocardial salvage and suggests extensive myocardial damage.[89–93] In some cases, in the presence of anterior ischemia, a transient increase in ST segment elevation (attributed to adenosine release) preceding and following the decrease during the first hour has no adverse consequences.[94,95] The magnitude of ST segment elevation, measured as a sum of the ST shift voltages, is related to the severity of myocardial ischemia and not to the size of the area at risk.[96]

Depression of the ST segment may be reciprocal or indicative of additional (presumably subendocardial) ischemia. Shah et al.[97] evaluate

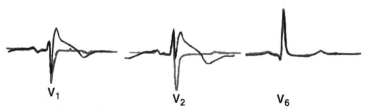

V_1 V_2 V_6

Figure 7–27 Superposition of the ECG before and during occlusion of the left anterior descending coronary artery in a patient whose ECG is shown in Figure 7–20. Note the increased QRS duration during occlusion in leads V_1 and V_2 but not in V_6. (From Surawicz B, Orr CM, Hermiller JB, et al: QRS changes during percutaneous transluminal coronary angioplasty and their possible mechanism. J Am Coll Cardiol 30:452, 1997. American College of Cardiology, by permission.)

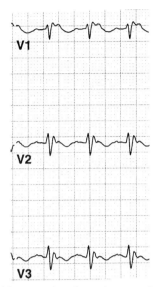

Figure 7–28 Example of an electrocardiogram (leads $V_1–V_3$) simulating the pattern of Brugada syndrome in a 61-year-old man after surgical replacement of the aortic valve and a coronary bypass for a 60 percent obstruction of the left main coronary artery.

the prognostic significance of the resolution of ST segment depression in patients with acute MI after thrombolytic treatment. They compared patients with ST segment depression resolving simultaneously with ST segment elevation (simultaneous group) and patients with ST segment depression persisting after ST segment elevation resolution (independent group). The in-hospital mortality was significantly higher in the independent group than in the simultaneous group or a control group without ST segment depression.

ST SEGMENT SHIFT DURING PERCUTANEOUS CORONARY ANGIOPLASTY

Balloon occlusion of the coronary artery during angioplasty lasts usually 1.5 to 3.0 minutes. The behavior of the ST segment during percutaneous transluminal coronary angioplasty (PTCA) is the same as during spontaneous myocardial ischemia, but the magnitude of the ST segment elevation expressed in percent of QRS amplitude tends to be smaller. Among patients with acute MI treated with direct angioplasty, there was a rapid decrease of ST segment elevation in those with myocardial reperfusion but not in those with a no-reflow phenomenon.[98]

Also, the average number of leads with ST segment elevation and those with reciprocal ST segment depression tends to be smaller during PTCA than during acute ischemia. The maximal ST segment elevation during balloon occlusion of the LAD coronary artery is located in lead V_2, V_3, or V_4 (see Figure 7–30) and, during occlusion of the RCA, in lead III. During occlusion of the diagonal branch of the LAD coronary artery, maximal ST segment elevation may be located in lead aV_L. The results of occlusion of the left circumflex coronary artery vary. In about one third of cases, an ST segment shift in the standard 12-lead ECG is absent; in another third, ST segment elevation is present in one or more standard leads; and in the remaining third of cases there is ST segment depression in leads V_2 and V_3, which is believed to represent a reciprocal change of ST segment elevation localized in the back.[99] The localization of the ST segment elevation predicts the site of the future loss of QRS voltage.[100]

In theory, an absence of ST segment displacement at the site of presumed acute injury may be due to cancellation by contralateral ST segment displacement in an opposite direction; but in practice such a mechanism is difficult to verify. The nonhomogeneous intensity of ischemia detracts from the accuracy of locating the site of ischemia. Thus it has been shown that balloon occlusion of the partially stenotic LAD coronary artery caused reversible ST segment elevation in the left precordial leads when the collateral circulation was poor or absent. The same procedure in similar patients with good collateral circulation produced ST segment depression in the same leads.[101,102] Studies during coronary artery angioplasty showed that the site of impaired perfusion could be identified with greater accuracy using a larger array of precordial leads.[102] For instance, ST segment elevation in the left axillary and back leads was specific for occlusions of the left circumflex and diagonal branches. ST segment elevation in lead V_{3R} was present in 82 percent of cases with an occluded right coronary artery.[103]

Kornreich et al.[102] used 120 leads to construct a body surface potential map in 131 patients with acute MI. They found that the most abnormal ST segment elevations and depressions at each MI location were localized in leads outside the standard precordial lead positions. This study supports the prevailing notion that a larger number of electrodes, such as are employed during mapping of the torso, can improve the diagnostic accuracy of the ECG.

It has been shown that ST segment behavior has a predictive value in patients with acute first anterior MIs caused by an LAD coronary artery lesion treated with rapid reperfusion by angioplasty. Kobayashi et al.[104] found that recovery of LV

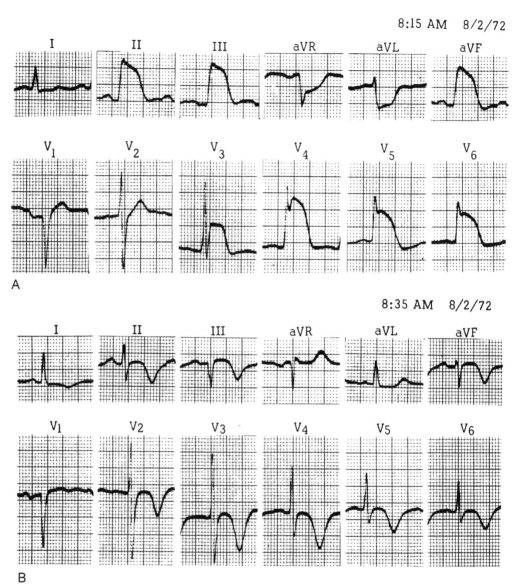

Figure 7–29   Variant angina. Patient had severe coronary artery disease involving all three major vessels, especially the anterior descending branch, as demonstrated by coronary arteriogram. **A,** Tracing recorded during angina at rest. **B,** Tracing recorded 20 minutes later, after the pain had subsided. The latter tracing is representative of the patient's baseline ECG. During angina (**A**), marked ST segment elevation is present in leads II, III, aV$_L$, and V$_1$–V$_6$ with reciprocal ST segment depression seen in leads aV$_R$ and aV$_L$. There is also an increase in the amplitude of the R wave in leads II, III, and aV$_F$, with disappearance of the S waves in leads showing marked ST segment elevation. The resulting complexes resemble the monophasic transmembrane potential. Many similar episodes were observed in this patient.

systolic function was better in patients in whom ST segment elevation resolved than in those in whom it did not. Santoro et al.[105] found that reduction in the ST segment elevation after direct coronary angioplasty was the only independent predictor of LV function recovery. Microvascular injury has been suspected to be the cause of persistent ST segment elevation after primary angioplasty for acute MI.[106,107] (Also see Chapter 8.)

PERSISTENT ST SEGMENT ELEVATION AFTER MI

After healing of the MI, ST segment elevation persists in about 60 percent of patients with an anterior infarction (Figure 7–31) and in about 5 percent of patients with an inferior MI.[108]

Persistent ST segment elevation correlates with the presence of asynergy.[21] It has been shown that ST segment elevation developed during balloon

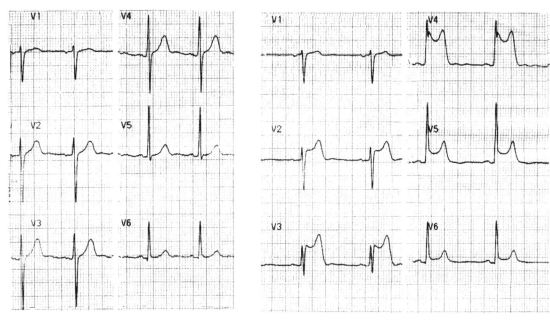

Figure 7–30   ECG leads V_1–V_6 before *(left)* and during *(right)* balloon occlusion of the left anterior descending coronary artery at midlevel. The maximal ST segment shift and maximal S amplitude decrease (percent of baseline value) are in lead V_4. (From Surawicz B, Orr CM, Hermiller JB, et al: QRS changes during percutaneous transluminal coronary angioplasty and their possible mechanisms. J Am Coll Cardiol 30:452, 1997. American College of Cardiology, by permission.)

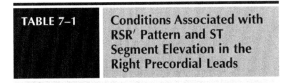

TABLE 7–1	Conditions Associated with RSR′ Pattern and ST Segment Elevation in the Right Precordial Leads

Brugada syndrome (types 1 to 3)
Arrhythmogenic right ventricular dysplasia
Southeast Asian males at risk of sudden cardiac death
Ischemia or infarction of the right ventricle
Anteroseptal ischemia or infarction
Pulmonary embolism
Hyperkalemia
Unexplained, not at risk of sudden cardiac death

inflation coincident with the new appearance of hypocontractility in a region of previously normal motion[109] and that there was a close association between the magnitude and extent of ST segment elevation and the extent of asynergy.[110] The most sensitive marker for anterior wall hypocontractility was ST segment elevation in lead V_2; for inferior wall hypocontractility, the most sensitive marker was ST segment elevation in lead III.

The widely held notion that persistent ST segment elevation is a marker of a ventricular aneurysm has not been supported by recent studies. Radionuclide imaging has shown similar global and regional wall motion abnormalities in patients with and without persistent ST segment elevation after MI.[111] If the aneurysm is defined as a "full-thickness scar that exhibits a localized convex protrusion during both phases of the cardiac cycle," two-dimensional echocardiography shows that the persistent ST segment elevation correlates with dyskinesia rather than with an aneurysm.[112]

The well-established relation between persistent ST segment elevation and the paradoxical motion of LV myocardium[112] suggests that stretch may play a role in the process, but the mechanism by which stretch might cause ST segment displacement has not been elucidated. The study of Toyofuku et al.[113] supports the hypothesis that stretch can cause ST segment elevation in the absence of ischemia. These investigators reported that in patients with arrhythmogenic right ventricular dysplasia (ARVD) who had no coronary artery disease, ST segment elevation was induced by exercise. In their study, significant ST segment elevation in the right precordial leads developed in 11 of 17 (65 percent) patients with severe RV asynergy; the finding proved to be helpful for diagnosing ARVD noninvasively.

The results of aneurysmectomy have not helped to locate the site of abnormal potential differences. In one study of 74 ECGs with ST segment elevation before aneurysmectomy, the pattern remained unchanged in 60.8 percent, improved in 25.7 percent, and became more

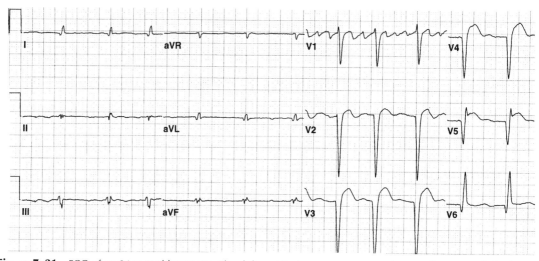

Figure 7–31   ECG of an 84-year-old woman with a left ventricular aneurysm, a massive anterior myocardial infarctio 5 years after onset. Present are atrial fibrillation, low voltage in the limb leads, intraventricular conduction disturbance su gestive of periinfarction block, and persistent ST segment elevation in leads V_2–V_6.

pronounced in 13.5 percent of the cases after aneurysmectomy. The average ST segment amplitude after aneurysmectomy in several studies was reduced by only one fourth[114] (Figure 7–32). Engel et al.[114] found that after an encircling endocardial ventriculotomy the ST segment elevation was unchanged, suggesting that the ST segment elevation did not originate in the injured tissue adjacent to the aneurysm. The authors admitted to the possibility, however, that the encircling procedure could have created new zones of injury.

RECOGNITION AND SIGNIFICANCE OF RECIPROCAL ST CHANGES WITH ACUTE MI

Depression of the ST segment in the presence of ST segment elevation can be a result of the process that caused the injury current responsible for ST segment elevation. Alternatively, it may be a marker of an independent additional area of injury in another location.

It has been shown that a subendocardial lesion associated with ST segment elevation in subendocardial electrograms causes a reciprocal ST segment depression in the epicardial electrograms, so long as a layer of nonischemic epicardial muscle is present. However, when ischemia becomes transmural, ST segment elevation occurs in the epicardial electrograms. During acute ischemia, reciprocal ST segment depression is present in all patients with an inferior MI (see Figure 7–9) and in 70 percent of patients

with an anterior MI (see Figures 7–7 and 7–10 When the magnitude of the ST segment elevatio is small because the overall amplitude of th complex is low, reciprocal ST segment depres sion may be more conspicuous than the culpr ST segment elevation (Figure 7–33).

Echocardiographic studies showed that recip rocal ST segment depression did not correla with remote wall changes, a finding compatibl with a truly reciprocal change; but this findin has not been universally confirmed. Thu nuclear imaging suggests that reciprocal ST seg ment change indicates an additional region c remote ischemia.[115] Moreover, angiographi studies performed within 2 weeks of an acut MI in 84 patients with inferior MI showed tha patients with anterolateral ST segment depres sion had larger infarcts and a higher incidenc of multivessel disease.[108] In the same study, th absence of reciprocal ST segment depressio "virtually precluded multivessel disease." Also among patients with anterior infarction, ST seg ment depression in inferior leads occurred i 45 percent and was associated with more exten sive infarction, increased morbidity, and a highe incidence of multivessel coronary disease.[116]

During the evolution of an inferior wal infarction associated with ST segment elevatio in lead III, an absent or a disproportionatel small reciprocal ST segment elevation in lead V_1 and V_2 was suggestive of an associated infarc tion of the right ventricle[117] (see Figures 7–ç and 7–16). The same principle was shown t be applicable when an anterior MI caused b

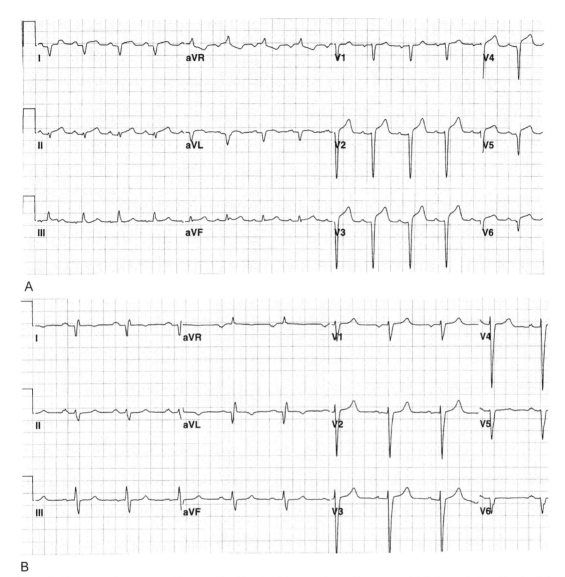

Figure 7–32 ECG of a 50-year-old man with akinesis of the anterior wall, apex, and inferior wall; hypokinesis of the lateral wall; and a left ventricular ejection fraction of 20 percent before (**A**) and after (**B**) aneurysmectomy. **A,** Note the absent r waves and elevated ST segment in leads I, aV$_L$, and V$_2$–V$_6$. **B,** Note regression of the ST segment elevation and reappearance of r waves in leads V$_2$–V$_4$.

occlusion of the LAD coronary artery was accompanied by ischemia of the inferior wall.[117] The latter was caused by continuation of the occluded LAD coronary artery beyond the apex of the heart onto the inferior wall of the left ventricle or by the LAD coronary artery supplying collaterals to the previously infarcted inferior wall. Under such circumstances, ST segment elevation in the anterior precordial leads was associated with attenuation or reversal of the reciprocal ST segment depression in the "inferior" leads.[118] In patients with acute MI, the sensitivity of MI detection increases significantly by co-existence of ST-segment elevation and reciprocal depression in the 12-lead ECG.[118a]

ABSENCE OF THE EXPECTED RECIPROCAL ST SEGMENT DEVIATION

In the presence of the three common types of Q wave MI (anterior, lateral, inferior), ST segment elevation is usually associated with reciprocal ST depression in one or more of the standard 12 leads. In the presence of posterior or anterior subendocardial MI, the acute injury pattern is manifested by ST segment depression

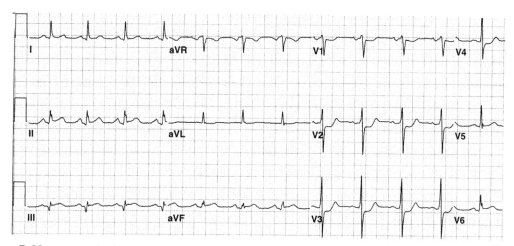

Figure 7–33 Low-amplitude ST segment elevation in low-amplitude complexes in leads III and aV$_F$ compared with mo[re] conspicuous reciprocal ST segment depression in leads V$_1$–V$_4$. ECG of a 45-year-old man with an inferior myocardial infar[c]tion attributed to occlusion of the proximal left circumflex coronary artery. Left ventricular ejection fraction was 45 perce[nt]

in one or more of the standard leads. The reciprocal ST segment elevation may be present only in the back in the case of subendocardial infarction and may be difficult to detect in the anterior leads in the case of posterior infarction because of the low amplitude of the ST segment deviation caused by the remote location of the infarction.

The apparent lack of expected reciprocal ST segment depression in the presence of ST segment elevation in one or more standard precordial leads may be attributed to one or more of the following factors:

1. Failure to examine leads aV$_R$ and V$_1$, which are probably relatively close to the posterobasal part of the left ventricle. These leads are often less carefully examined than the other 10 leads, and so the differences between normal and abnormal patterns in these leads may be less recognizable.
2. Difficulty of recognizing it owing to the low amplitude of the ventricular complex in the leads with expected ST segment deviation (Figure 7–34).
3. Obfuscation by secondary ST segment deviations caused by intraventricular conduction disturbance or ventricular hypertrophy. A common cause is wide terminal QRS deflection in the presence of incomplete or complete RBBB.
4. Coexistence of acute anterior and inferior injury patterns (Figure 7–35).
5. Diffuse ST segment elevation during the early stage of anterior infarction with transient extension of the ST segment elevation into the territory facing the inferior leads.
6. Associated pericarditis (Figures 7–36 and 7–37). It has been suggested[119] that the

disappearance of the reciprocal ST segme[nt] depression or appearance of the ST se[g]ment elevation in the leads with previou[s] ST segment depression in some cases faci[l]itates the diagnosis of infarction-relate[d] pericarditis.

ST SEGMENT ELEVATION: NORMAL VARIANT AND ACUTE PERICARDITIS

In some young men after onset of puberty a[n] excessive ST segment elevation occurs as a no[r]mal variant. Mehta et al.[120] described this pa[t]tern as an elevated concave ST segment, locate[d] commonly in the precordial leads (most conspi[c]uously in leads V$_1$–V$_3$) with reciprocal ST se[g]ment depression in lead aV$_R$. The pattern [is] often associated with tall peaked T waves, a slu[r] on the R wave, vertical electrical axis in the fron[]tal plane, and sinus bradycardia.[120] The inc[i]dence decreases with advancing age. A revie[w] of the literature suggests that, contrary to th[e] anecdotal reports, the pattern is equally commo[n] in all races.[120]

The term "early or premature repolarization," which is not clearly distinguishable from th[e] normal male pattern, is frequently applied t[o] this pattern.[121,122] The prematurity implies tha[t] the ST segment shift is attributed to shortenin[g] of ventricular action potentials in some epicar[]dial regions. Rapid early repolarization in thes[e] regions may be expected to produce potentia[l] differences, resulting in a current similar to th[e] injury current. Consequently, in partial suppor[t] of this theory are the observations that exer[]cise[123] and isoproterenol abolish the ST segmen[t] elevation, presumably as a result of diminishe[d]

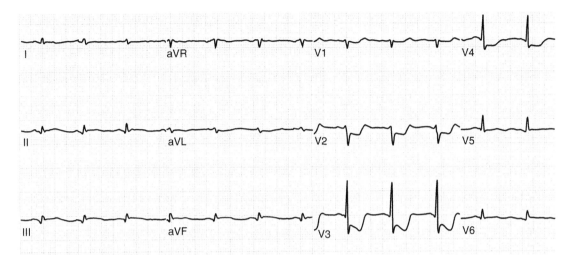

Figure 7–34 ECG of a 44-year-old woman with acute inferior myocardial infarction and low-voltage ECG. Note that both the ST segment elevation in leads II, III, and aV$_F$ and the reciprocal ST segment depression in leads V$_1$–V$_4$ are approximately of the same amplitude, in proportion to the QRS amplitude.

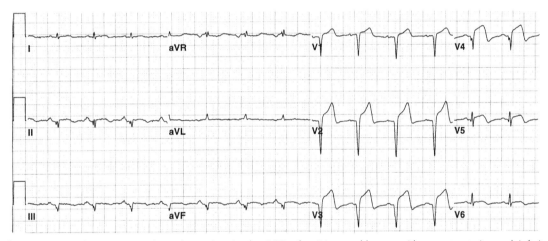

Figure 7–35 Absent reciprocal ST depression in the ECG of a 54-year-old man with recent anterior and inferior myocardial infarction and aneurysmal dilatation of the middle and apical portions of the septum and apical portions of the inferoanterior and lateral walls of the left ventricle. Estimated left ventricular ejection fraction was 15 percent.

difference between ventricular action potential durations. However, mapping studies have not substantiated the rationale for the term "early repolarization," because in normal young volunteers the overlap between the onset of ventricular repolarization and the end of QRS (which ranged from 4 to 16 ms) did not correlate significantly with the ST segment deviation in the precordial leads.[124]

The pattern of "early repolarization" (or normal "male" pattern) may simulate the changes of acute pericarditis, possibly because they may be caused by a similar mechanism. In both, inscription of the ST segment begins before QRS forces have returned to baseline,[122,125] but the ST segment elevation in pericarditis is usually present in both limb and precordial leads. In contrast, ST segment elevation in the "normal variant" is confined more frequently to the precordial lead[123,126] (see Figure 1–13). Moreover, the T wave amplitude in the left precordial leads tends to be greater in persons with "normal variant" than in those with acute pericarditis.[126] In practice, however, the distinction between these two patterns may be difficult.

Persistent multilead ST segment elevation is present in patients with spinal cord injury at the C5 to C6 levels (i.e., lesions that completely disrupt cardiac sympathetic influences).[127] These changes were reversed by low doses of infused isoproterenol. Although the mechanism

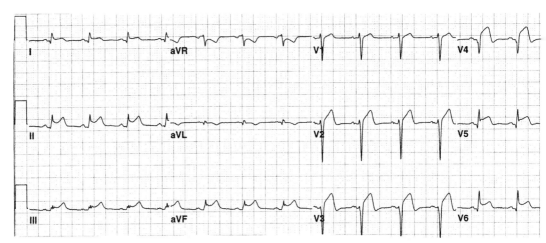

Figure 7–36 ECG of a 72-year-old man 2 days after acute anterior myocardial infarction caused by occlusion of the left anterior descending (LAD) artery at midlevel with associated pericarditis as evidenced by pericardial friction rub. Both proximal LAD and right coronary arteries were diseased but without critical stenoses. ST segment is elevated in all leads except V_1 and aV_R; in the latter the ST segment is depressed.

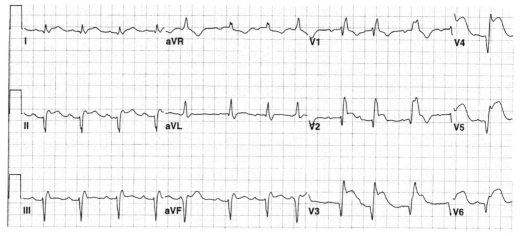

Figure 7–37 ECG of an 82-year-old woman recorded 2 days after the onset of anterolateral myocardial infarction documented by echocardiogram, which also showed a ventricular septal defect with a large left-to-right shunt and a small pericardial effusion. Patient died the next day. ST segment is elevated in leads I, II, III, aV_L, aV_F, and V_1–V_6; it was depressed in lead aV_R.

of ST segment elevation in these patients has not been clarified, the findings demonstrate that normal sympathetic tone modulates the course or sequence (or both) of ventricular repolarization.

ST SEGMENT ELEVATION: OTHER CAUSES

Table 7–2 lists additional causes of ST segment elevation encountered less frequently than the conditions discussed previously.

T WAVE CHANGES (HYPERACUTE T WAVE PATTERN)

Pointed tall or deeply negative "coronary" T waves associated with a prolonged QT interval may appear either before or after primary ST segment elevation has begun to subside (Figure 7–39A). These T wave abnormalities are attributed to prolongation of activity in the ischemic regions of the ventricle.[2,141] In some cases the increase in T wave amplitude may be modest and not easily recognized.[142] In the presence of posterior infarction

TABLE 7–2	Less Common Causes of ST Segment Elevation

Pulmonary embolism and acute cor pulmonale (usually lead III)
Cardiac tumor
Acute aortic dissection[128]
After mitral valvuloplasty[129]
Pancreatitis and gallbladder disease[130–132] and other catastrophic illnesses[133]
Myocarditis[133,134] (Figure 7–38)
Septic shock
Anaphylactic reaction[135]
J wave
Hyperkalemia ("dialyzable" current of injury)
With any marked QRS widening (e.g., antidepressant drug overdose[136] or class IC antiarrhythmia drugs[137,138])
After transthoracic cardioversion[139]
Following implantable cardioverter defibrillator shocks[140]

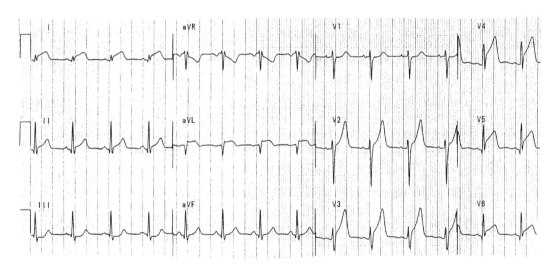

Figure 7–38   Acute injury pattern on the ECG of a 35-year-old man with presumed acute myocarditis presenting as the first manifestation of previously undetected human immunodeficiency virus (HIV) infection. Elevated levels of cardiac enzymes on admission suggested the diagnosis of myocardial infarction, but the patient had normal coronary arteries and no pericardial effusion. The ECG returned to normal within 5 days.

tall upright T waves in the precordial leads are similar to the "hyperacute" T waves seen during acute anterior ischemia (Figure 7–39B) but usually are less transient.

QT INTERVAL

During acute myocardial ischemia the QT interval may shorten, lengthen, or remain unchanged[25] (Figure 7–40). It has been reported that prolonged QT within the first few hours of symptoms predicts primary cardiac arrest in patients with acute MI.[143]

U WAVE

During acute myocardial ischemia the U wave may become inverted or increase in amplitude. The former occurs more often. Transient U wave inversion, however, may be caused not only by regional myocardial ischemia but also by an elevation of blood pressure.[144,145] It has been observed that during acute ischemia the inverted portion of the U wave appears late; that is, the U wave is positive-negative, whereas the U wave related to elevated blood pressure is negative-positive.[146]

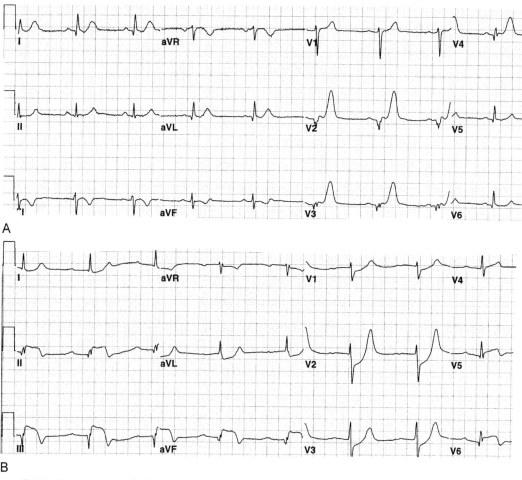

Figure 7–39   Two examples of tall T waves exceeding 1 mV in amplitude. **A,** Hyperacute stage of anterior myocardi infarction in a 63-year-old man with an occluded left anterior descending (LAD) coronary artery recorded durir the course of thrombolytic therapy. **B,** Acute inferior and posterolateral myocardial infarction in an 82-year-old ma with an occluded dominant right coronary artery, 90 percent stenosis of the mid-LAD artery, and absent collater circulation.

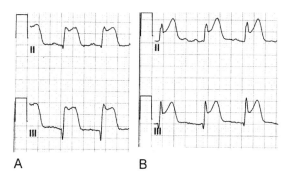

A   B

Figure 7–40   Variable QTc values during acute ischemia. **A,** Normal QT and QTc (344 and 418 ms, respectively) on a ECG of a 42-year-old man with acute inferior infarction caused by occlusion of the right coronary artery. **B,** Prolonge QT and QTc (394 and 451 ms, respectively) in a 49-year-old man with acute inferior infarction caused by occlusion of large right posterolateral branch of the right coronary artery.

The reports of U wave inversion during ischemia stem mostly from the observations during exercise or coronary spasm, whereas U wave inversion is seldom observed during PTCA or with spontaneous myocardial ischemia. Correlation with myocardial imaging showed that during exercise a negative U wave in the anterior precordial leads was both sensitive and specific for myocardial ischemia of the anterior wall, whereas a negative U wave in the inferior leads was specific but not sensitive for acute ischemia of the inferior wall.[147]

Increased U wave amplitude in the precordial leads is observed occasionally during spontaneous myocardial ischemia or during exercise-induced ischemia (see Chapter 10). It is believed to be a specific although not a sensitive marker of significant narrowing of the left circumflex or right coronary artery.[148] It is probably caused by increased compensatory wall motion of the nonischemic myocardium and increased sympathetic stimulation.

REVERSIBLE QRS CHANGES

The QRS changes during acute myocardial ischemia can be caused by: (1) ischemia of the conducting system; (2) impaired conduction in the ischemic myocardium; and (3) passive shift of the QRS deflections resulting from shift of the ST and TP segments. Bundle branch blocks and fascicular blocks may follow occlusion of the LAD coronary artery proximal to the first septal perforator, or after occlusion of an artery supplying collaterals to the myocardium supplied by the previously occluded proximal LAD coronary artery. These conduction disturbances are discussed in Chapters 4–6.

Elevation of the ST segment and decreased high-frequency components in the signal-averaged ECG[149] are frequently associated with decreased amplitude or disappearance of the S wave in the precordial leads (see Figures 7–8, 7–10, 7–11, and 7–41). Other changes may include the appearance or disappearance of the Q wave (Figure 7–42) and an increase in the R wave amplitude[150] (see Figure 7–41). In the leads with reciprocal ST segment depression, the S wave amplitude may increase and the R wave amplitude may decrease. These changes take place without changes in the QRS duration and are assumed to represent passive shifts of the QRS deflection. The term "periischemic block" applies to transient QRS changes associated with increased QRS duration.[28,151] Such changes occur less often than changes in QRS

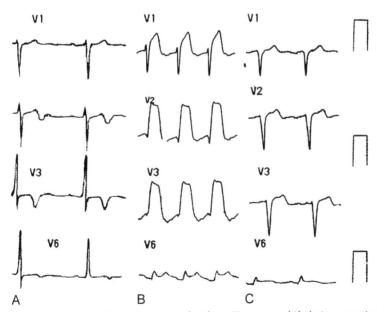

Figure 7–41 Transient appearance of a Q wave associated with an ST segment shift during acute ischemia. Four precordial ECG leads of an 80-year-old man with obstructive disease of the left anterior descending (LAD) coronary artery. The patient was admitted on day 1 (**A**) with a diagnosis of unstable angina pectoris and abnormal T waves. **B,** ECG recorded on day 2 after abrupt closure of an intracoronary stent inserted during coronary angioplasty at the midlevel of the LAD artery. **C,** ECG recorded on day 3 after an emergent coronary artery bypass graft. Note in **B** the transient appearance of a Q wave, an increase in R wave amplitude in lead V₂, and disappearance of the S wave in leads V₂ and V₃. Compared with the ECG in **A**, there is a marked decrease of R wave amplitude in all leads in **C**. (From Surawicz B: Reversible QRS changes during acute myocardial ischemia. J Electrocardiol 31:209, 1998, by permission.)

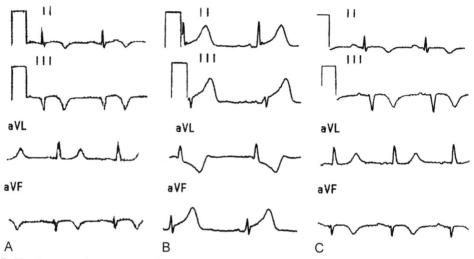

Figure 7–42 Transient disappearance of a QS wave associated with an ST segment shift during acute myocardial ischemia. Selected ECG leads from a 61-year-old woman with a remote inferior myocardial infarction, obstruction of the dominant right coronary artery at midlevel, and nonobstructive disease of the left anterior descending and left circumflex coronary arteries. She was admitted after a new onset of angina pectoris and treated with percutaneous transluminal coronary angioplasty (PTCA) of the right coronary artery. **A,** Before admission on 8/17/95. **B,** Before PTCA on 11/3/95 10:47 AM. **C,** After PTCA on 11/4/95 at 5:58 AM. Note the disappearance of the Q wave in lead III associated with the ST segment shift. The QRS patterns before **(A)** and after **(C)** development of an acute injury pattern are similar. (From Surawicz: Reversible QRS changes during acute myocardial ischemia. J Electrocardiol 31:209, 1998, by permission.)

configuration caused by a passive ST segment shift and sometimes are more pronounced in selected leads (e.g., V_1, V_2, III, aV_F) than in the remaining ECG leads (see Figure 7–23).

In a study by Surawicz,[150] reversible QRS changes encountered in 29 patients with acute MI included new Q waves in 3 cases, decreased Q wave amplitude in 2 cases, QS change to qRS or qR in 6, disappearance of QS or Q in 4, increased R amplitude in 9, decreased R amplitude in 6, decreased S amplitude by more than 75 percent in 18, and increased QRS duration in 4. Reversible changes of the initial QRS portion were present in 24 of 29 patients, and those of the terminal QRS portion occurred in a patients.

It has been reported that in patients with acute anterior infarction, distortion of the terminal QRS

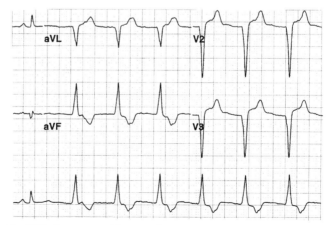

Figure 7–43 Portion of the ECG of a 58-year-old man with an acute anterior myocardial infarction attributed to occlusion of the left anterior descending artery after thrombolytic therapy. Rhythm strip in lead II shows an onset of accelerated ventricular rhythm with retrograde conduction to the atria.

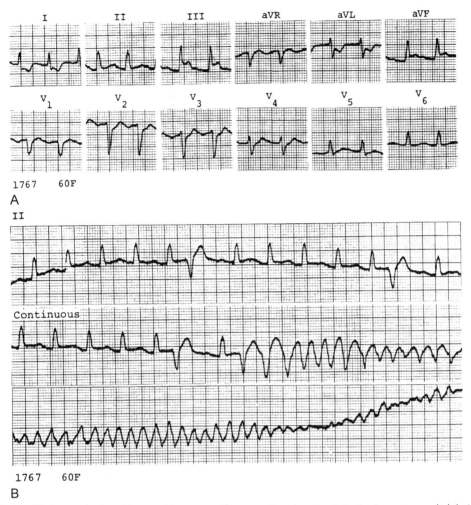

Figure 7–44   Variant angina in a 60-year-old woman with recurrent angina at rest. **A,** Tracing was recorded during one of the episodes, revealing ST segment elevation in leads II, III, and aV$_F$, with reciprocal ST segment depression in leads I, aV$_L$, V$_2$, and V$_3$. **B,** A few minutes later. Note the appearance of premature ventricular complexes and the development of ventricular tachycardia and fibrillation.

portion on admission predicts a high mortality rate[152] and a greater incidence of reflow impairment after emergency coronary angioplasty.[153] In another study, terminal QRS distortion on admission was a better predictor of final infarct size than ST segment measurements.[154]

VENTRICULAR ARRHYTHMIAS DURING ACUTE ISCHEMIA

Harris[155] showed that one-stage occlusion of the coronary artery in dogs caused ventricular fibrillation in 30 to 50 percent of the animals. Arrhythmias did not occur, however, when the occlusion was performed in two stages: first narrowing the vessel, and then closing it after 30 minutes. These observations may be pertinent to the current concept of ischemic preconditioning, which postulates that repetitive attacks of angina pectoris diminish the severity of myocardial ischemia following coronary occlusion.

Elevation of the ST segment is frequently associated with the appearance of premature ventricular contractions (PVCs), which may precipitate a sudden onset of ventricular fibrillation (VF) typically displaying the R-on-T phenomenon. These arrhythmias are sometimes called "occlusion arrhythmias." It is of interest that the "primary VF" during acute ischemia tends to be a unique, isolated event that rarely recurs after successful defibrillation and regression of the acute injury ECG pattern. In a large group of hospitalized patients with acute MI, the incidence of recurrent VF was 2.4 percent.

The increased heart rate exacerbates ventricular arrhythmias during acute ischemia, but the influence of the increased heart rate is difficult to dissociate from the effect of sympathetic stimulation, Bradycardia has no consistent effect on arrhythmia during acute ischemia, but long pauses may precipitate arrhythmias and initiate electrical alternans.

With experimental ischemia, reperfusion arrhythmias that occur after release of the occlusion are no less malignant than arrhythmias following sudden occlusion, and VF occurs frequently within a few seconds after the sudden release of coronary ligation. The reperfusion arrhythmias appear to be nonreentrant. In humans, however, life-threatening ventricular tachyarrhythmias occur seldom during reperfusion, and unlike after occlusion, the incidence of VF is low. The most common arrhythmias during reperfusion are PVCs and accelerated ventricular rhythms (Figure 7–43); these arrhythmias are seen more often after lysis of the occluding thrombus than after coronary angioplasty. In the study of Zehender et al.,[156] PVCs and couplets were seen in all 22 patients (100 percent) and ventricular tachycardia (VT) in 21 (95 percent) of 22 patients with acute infarction in whom reperfusion was achieved. Sustained VT or VF

was not observed in these patients, although V occurred in three of eight patients in whom cor nary occlusion persisted. Among 26 patients wi patent infarct-related arteries reported by Gress et al.,[157] all had PVCs and 21 (81 percent) had a accelerated ventricular rhythm or VT; but only patient required cardioversion for VF. Engel et al.[158] found that ventricular tachyarrhythmi associated with epicardial reperfusion strong correlated with worsening left ventricular fun tion after the acute phase of anterior wall N and hypothesized that they may represent a no invasive marker of cellular injury.

Airaksinen et al.[159] studied 152 patients du ing balloon occlusion of the coronary arte and recorded ventricular arrhythmia in only I patients (12 percent). There were no cases repetitive ectopic complexes. The group patients with ventricular arrhythmias had le severe coronary stenosis than the rest of th patients and no visible collaterals to th occluded vessel. Surawicz et al.[28] observed n ventricular arrhythmias while monitoring 2 patients with percutaneous coronary angioplast

Ventricular fibrillation has been reported aft relief of coronary spasm (Figure 7–44), but suc events are probably even more rare than durin coronary angioplasty.

REFERENCES

1. Cascio WE, Yan GX, Kleber AG: Passive electrical properties, mechanical activity, and extracellular potassium in arterially perfused rabbit ventricular muscle. Circ Res 66:1461, 1990.
2. Kleber AG, Janse MJ, Van Capelle FJ, et al: Mechanisms and time course of ST and TQ segment changes during acute regional myocardial ischemia in the pig heart determined by extracellular and intracellular recordings. Circ Res 42:603, 1978.
3. Surawicz B: Electrophysiologic Basis of ECG and Cardiac Arrhythmias. Baltimore, Williams & Wilkins, 1995.
4. Samson WE, Scher AM: Mechanism of ST segment alteration during acute myocardial injury. Circ Res 8:780, 1960.
5. Downar E, Janse MJ, Durrer D: The effect of acute coronary artery occlusion on subepicardial transmembrane potentials in the intact porcine heart. Circulation 56:217, 1977.
6. Kleber AG: Resting membrane potential, extracellular potassium activity and intracellular sodium activity during acute global ischemia in isolated perfused guinea pig hearts. Circ Res 52:442, 1983.
7. Taccardi B: Changes in cardiac electrogenesis following coronary occlusion. In: Marchetti G, Taccardi B (eds): Coronary Circulation and Energetics of the Myocardium. Basel, Karger, 1967.
8. Cohen D, Kaufman LA: Magnetic determination of the relationship between the ST segment shift and the injury current produced by coronary artery occlusion. Circ Res 36:414, 1975.
9. Smith GT, Geary G, Ruf W, et al: Epicardial mapping an electrocardiographic models of myocardial ischem injury. Circulation 60:930, 1979.
10. Cinca J, Figueras J, Senador E, et al: Transmural D electrograms after coronary artery occlusion and late embolization in pigs. Am J Physiol (Lond) 246:H47 1984.
11. Mirvis DM: Body surface distributions of repolarizatic forces during acute myocardial infarction. I. Isopotenti and isoarea mapping. Circulation 62:878, 1980.
12. Boden WE, Spodick DH: Diagnostic significance of pre cordial ST segment depression. Am J Cardiol 63:35! 1989.
13. Surawicz B, Lasseter KC: Electrocardiogram in pericard tis. Am J Cardiol 26:471, 1970.
14. Hams TR, Copeland GD, Brody DA: Progressive injur current with metastatic tumor of the heart. Am Heart 69:392, 1965.
15. Puletti M, Curione M, Pozzar F, et al: Atrial repolarizatio its role in ST elevation. J Electrocardiol 12:321, 1979.
16. Kataoka H, Tamura A, Mikurya Y: Central precordi ST-segment elevation in posterolateral myocardial infarc tion. Am Heart J 125:1202, 1993.
17. Nagahama Y, Sugiura T, Takehana K, et al: Clinical sig nificance of PQ segment depression in acute Q wav anterior wall myocardial infarction. J Am Coll Cardic 23:885, 1994.
18. Nagahama Y, Sugiura T, Takehana K, et al: PQ segmen depression in acute Q wave inferior wall myocardi infarction. Circulation 91:641, 1995.
19. Braat SH, Brugada P, den Dulk K, et al: Value of lead V₄ for recognition of the infarct coronary artery in acut

inferior myocardial infarction. Am J Cardiol 53:1538, 1984.

20. Kataoka H, Tamura A, Yano S, et al: ST elevation in the chest leads in anterior wall left ventricular acute myocardial infarction. Am J Cardiol 66:1146, 1990.

21. Ben Gal T, Sclarovsky S, Herz I, et al: Importance of the conal branch of the right coronary artery in patients with acute anterior wall myocardial infarction: electrocardiographic and angiographic correlation. J Am Coll Cardiol 29:506, 1997.

22. Porter A, Sclarovsky S, Ben-Gal T, et al: Value of T-wave direction with lead III ST segment depression in acute anterior wall myocardial infarction: electrocardiographic prediction of a "wrapped" left anterior descending artery. Clin Cardiol 21:562, 1998.

23. Wellens HJJ, Gorgels APM, Doevedans PA (eds): The ECG in Acute Myocardial Infarction and Unstable Angina. Boston, Kluwer Academic, 2003, pp 9–42.

24. Engelen DJM, Gorgels APM, Cheriex EC, et al: Value of the electrocardiogram in localizing the occlusion site in the left anterior descending coronary artery in acute anterior myocardial infarction. J Am Coll Cardiol 34:389, 1999.

25. Birnbaum Y, Sclarovsky S, Solodky A, et al: Prediction of the level of left anterior descending coronary artery obstruction during anterior wall myocardial infarction by the admission electrocardiogram. Am J Cardiol 72:823, 1993.

26. Lew AS, Hod H, Cercek B, et al: Inferior ST segment changes during acute anterior myocardial infarction: a marker of the presence or absence of concomitant inferior wall ischemia. J Am Coll Cardiol 10:519, 1987.

27. Iwasaki K, Kusachi S, Kita T, et al: Prediction of isolated first diagonal branch occlusion by 12-lead electrocardiography: ST segment shift in leads I and aVL. J Am Coll Cardiol 23:1557, 1994.

28. Surawicz B, Orr CM, Hermiller JB, et al: QRS changes during percutaneous transluminal coronary angioplasty and their possible mechanisms. J Am Coll Cardiol 30:797, 1997.

29. Yamaji H, Iwasachi S, Kusachi S, et al: Prediction of acute left main coronary occlusion by 12-lead electrocardiogram: aVR ST segment elevation with less V1 ST-segment elevation. J Am Coll Cardiol 38:1348, 2001.

29a. Gaitonde RS, Sharma N, Ali-Hasan S, et al: Prediction of significant left main coronary artery stenosis by the 12-lead electrocardiogram in patients with rest angina pectoris and the withholding of clopidogrel therapy. Am J Cardiol 92:846, 2003.

29b. Frierson JH, Dimas AP, Metzdorff M, et al: Critical left main stenosis presenting as diffuse ST segment depression. Am Heart J 125:1773, 1993.

29c. Mahajan N, Hollander G, Thekoott D, et al: Prediction of left main coronary artery obstruction by 12-lead electrocardiography: ST segment deviation in lead V6 greater than or equal to ST segment deviation in V1. Ann Nonivasive Electrocardiol 11:102, 2006.

30. Barrabes JA, Figueras J, Moure C, et al: Prognostic value of lead aVR in patients with a first non-ST-segment elevation acute myocardial infarction. Circulation 108:814, 2003.

31. Kosuge M, Kimura K, Ishikawa T, et al: Combined prognostic utility of ST segment in lead aVR and troponin T on admission in non-ST-segment elevation acute coronary syndromes. Am J Cardiol 97:334, 2006.

32. Wong CK, Freedman B, Bautovich G, et al: Mechanism and significance of precordial ST-segment depression during inferior wall acute myocardial infarction

33. Shah PK, Pichler M, Berman DS, et al: Non-invasive identification of a high risk subset of patients with acute inferior myocardial infarction. Am J Cardiol 46:915, 1980.

34. Goldberg HL, Borer JS, Jacobstein JS, et al: Anterior ST depression in inferior myocardial infarction: indicator of posterolateral infarction. Am J Cardiol 48:1009, 1981.

35. Peterson ED, Hathaway WR, Zabel KM, et al: Prognostic significance of precordial ST segment depression during inferior myocardial infarction in the thrombolytic era: results in 16,521 patients. J Am Coll Cardiol 28:305, 1996.

36. Bates ER, Clemmensen PM, Califf RM, et al: Precordial ST segment depression predicts a worse prognosis in inferior infarction despite reperfusion therapy. J Am Coll Cardiol 16:1538, 1990.

37. Birnbaum Y, Herz I, Sclarovsky S, et al: Prognostic significance of precordial ST segment depression on admission electrocardiogram in patients with inferior wall myocardial infarction. J Am Coll Cardiol 28:313, 1996.

38. Tsuka Y, Sugiura T, Yoshiteru A, et al: Clinical characteristics of ST-segment elevation in lead V_6 in patients with Q-wave acute inferior wall myocardial infarction. Coron Artery Dis 10:465, 1999.

39. Birnbaum Y, Wagner GS, Barbash GI, et al: Correlation of angiographic findings and right (V_1 to V_3) versus left (V_4 to V_6) precordial ST-segment depression in inferior wall acute myocardial infarction. Am J Cardiol 83:143, 1999.

40. Kontos MC, Desai PV, Jesse RL, et al: Usefulness of the admission electrocardiogram for identifying the infarct-related artery in inferior wall acute myocardial infarction. Am J Cardiol 79:182, 1997.

41. Huey BL, Beller GA, Kaiser DL, et al: A comprehensive analysis of myocardial infarction due to left circumflex artery occlusion; comparison with infarction due to right coronary artery and left anterior descending artery occlusion. J Am Coll Cardiol 12:1156, 1988.

42. Bairey CN, Shah PK, Lew AS, et al: Electrocardiographic differentiation of occlusion of the left circumflex versus the right coronary artery as a cause of inferior acute myocardial infarction. Am J Cardiol 60:456, 1987.

43. Herz I, Assali AR, Adler Y, et al: New electrocardiographic criteria for predicting either the right or left circumflex artery as the culprit coronary artery in inferior wall acute myocardial infarction. Am J Cardiol 81:1343, 1997.

44. Kataoka H, Kanzaki K, Mikutiya Y, et al: Massive ST-segment elevation in precordial and inferior leads in right ventricular myocardial infarction. J Electrocardiol 21:115, 1988.

45. Kosuge M, Kimura K, Ishikawa T, et al: New electrocardiographic criteria predicting the site of coronary artery occlusion in inferior wall acute myocardial infarction. Am J Cardiol 82:1318, 1998.

46. Casas RE, Marriott HJL, Glancy DL: Value of leads V_7–V_9 in diagnosing posterior wall acute myocardial infarction and other causes of tall R waves in V_{1-2}. Am J Cardiol 79:508, 1997.

47. Agarwal JB, Khaw K, Aurignac F, et al: Importance of posterior chest leads in patients with suspected myocardial infarction, but nondiagnostic, routine 12-lead electrocradiogram. Am J Cardiol 83:323, 1999.

48. Zalenski RJ, Rydman RJ, Sloan EP, et al: ST segment elevation and the prediction of hospital life-threatening

complications: the role of right ventricular and posterior leads. J Electrocardiol 31(Suppl):164, 1998.

49. Matetzky S, Freimark D, Feinberg MS, et al: Acute myocardial infarction with isolated ST-segment elevation in posterior chest leads V$_{7-9}$. J Am Coll Cardiol 34:748, 1999.

50. Wung S-F, Drew BJ: New electrocardiographic criteria for posterior wall acute myocardial ischemia validated by a percutaneous transluminal coronary angioplasty model of acute myocardial infarction. Am J Cardiol 87: 970, 2001.

51. Sadanandan S, Hochman JS, Kolodziej A, et al: Clinical and angiographic characteristics of patients with combined anterior and inferior ST-segment elevation on the initial electrocardiogram during acute myocardial infarction. Am Heart J 146:653, 2003.

52. Chou TC, Van der Bel-Kahn J, Allen J, et al: Electrocardiographic diagnosis of right ventricular infarction. Am J Med 70:1175, 1981.

53. Braat SH, Gorgels APM, Bar FW, et al: Value of the ST-T segment in lead V$_4$ in inferior wall acute myocardial infarction to predict the site of coronary artery occlusion. Am J Cardiol 60:140, 1988.

54. Kataoka H, Kanzaki K, Mikuriya Y: An ECG marker of underlying right ventricular conduction delay in the hyperacute phase of right ventricular infarction or ischemia. J Electrocardiol 23:369, 1990.

55. Forman MB, Goodin J, Phelan B, et al: Electrocardiographic changes associated with isolated right ventricular infarction. J Am Coll Cardiol 4:640, 1984.

56. Geft IL, Shah PK, Rodriguez L, et al: ST elevations in leads V$_1$ to V$_5$ may be caused by right coronary artery occlusion and acute right ventricular infarction. Am J Cardiol 53:991, 1984.

57. Mak KH, Chia BL, Tan ATH, et al: Simultaneous ST-segment elevation in lead V$_1$ and depression in lead V$_2$: a discordant ECG pattern indicating right ventricular infarction. J Electrocardiol 27:203, 1994.

58. Kataoka H, Tamura A, Yano S, et al: Intraventricular conduction delay in acute right ventricular ischemia. Am J Cardiol 64:94, 1989.

59. Saw J, Davies C, Fung A, et al: Value of ST elevation in lead III greater than lead II in inferior acute myocardial infarction for predicting in-hospital mortality and diagnosing right ventricular infarction. Am J Cardiol 87:448, 2001.

60. Porter A, Herz I, Strasberg B: Isolated right ventricular infarction presenting as anterior wall myocardial infarction on electrocardiography. Clin Cardiol 20:971, 1997.

61. Wimalaratna HSK: Tombstoning electrocardiographic pattern in acute myocardial infarction. Lancet 342:496, 1993.

62. Guo XH, Yap YG, Chen LJ, et al: Correlation of coronary angiography with "tombstoning" electrocardiographic pattern in patients with acute myocardial infarction. Clin Cardiol 23:347, 2000.

63. Balei B, Yesildag O: Correlation between clinical findings and the "tombstoning" electrocardiographic pattern in patients with anterior wall acute myocardial infarction. Am J Cardiol 92:1316, 2003.

64. Brugada J, Brugada P: Further characterization of the syndrome of right bundle branch block, ST segment elevation and sudden cardiac death. J Cardiovasc Electrophysiol 8:325, 1997.

65. Brugada P, Brugada J: Right bundle branch block, persistent ST segment elevation and sudden cardiac death: a distinct clinical and electrocardiographic syndrome. J Am Coll Cardiol 20:1391, 1992.

66. Eckardt L, Probst V, Smits JPP, et al: Long-term progno of individuals with right precordial ST-segment-elevati Brugada syndrome. Circulation 111:257, 2005.

67. Alings M, Wilde A: "Brugada" syndrome: clinical d and suggested pathophysiologicical mechanism. Circu tion 99:666, 1999.

68. Miayazaki T, Mitamura H, Miyoshi H, et al: Autonom and antiarrhythmic drug modulation of ST segment e vation on patients with Brugada syndrome. J Am C Cardiol 27:1061, 1996.

69. Frustaci A, Priori SG, Pieroni M, et al: Cardiac histolo cal substrate with clinical phenotype of Brugada sy drome. Circulation 112:3680, 2005.

70. Makiyama T, Akao M, Tsuji K, et al: Risk for brac arrhythmic complications in patients with Brugada sy drome caused by SCN5A gene mutations. J Am C Cardiol 46:2100, 2005.

71. Nademanee K, Veerakul G, Nimmannit S, et al: Arrhyt mogenic marker for the sudden unexplained death sy drome in Thai men. Circulation 96:2595, 1997.

72. Marcus FI, Fontaine GH, Guiradon G, et al: Right ve tricular dysplasia: a report of 24 adult cases. Circulati 65:384, 1982.

73. Corrado D, Nava A, Buja G, et al: Familial cardiomyop thy underlies syndrome of right bundle branch bloc ST segment elevation and sudden death. J Am Coll Ca diol 27:443, 1996.

74. Tada H, Aihara N, Ohe T, et al: Arrhythmogen right ventricular cardiomyopathy underlies syndrome right bundle branch block, ST-segment elevation, ar sudden death. Am J Cardiol 81:519, 1998.

75. Fontaine G, Andrade FR, Buraka M, et al: Right bund branch block in arrhythmogenic right ventricular dysp sia [abstract]. J Electroacardiol 28(Suppl):90, 1996.

76. Surawicz B: Brugada syndrome: manifest, conceale "asymptomatic," suspected, and simulated. J Am Cc Cardiol 38:775, 2001.

77. Murakami H, Urabe K, Nishimura M: Inappropria microvascular constriction produced transient ST-se ment elevation in patients with syndrome X. J Am Cc Cardiol 32:1287, 1998.

78. De Servi H, Arbustini E, Marsico F, et al: Correlatio between clinical and morphologic findings in unstab angina. Am J Cardiol 77:128, 1996.

79. Huey B, Gheorghiade M, Crampton RS, et al: Acute no Q wave myocardial infarction with early ST segment ele vation: evidence for spontaneous coronary reperfusio and implications for thrombolytic trials. J Am Coll Ca diol 9:18, 1987.

80. Curtis JP, Portnay EL, Wang Y, et al: The pre-hospit electrocardiogram and time to reperfusion in patien with acute myocardial infarction. J Am Coll Cardi 47:2544, 2006.

81. Stark K, Krucoff MW, Schryver B, et al: Quantification ST-segment changes during coronary angioplasty i patients with left bundle branch block. Am J Cardic 67:1219, 1991.

82. Blanke H, Scherff H, Karsch KR, et al: Electroca diographic changes after streptokinase-induced recanal zation in patients with acute left anterior descendin artery obstruction. Circulation 68:406, 1983.

83. Fernandez AR, Sequeira RF, Chakko S, et al: ST segmer tracking for rapid determination of patency of th infarct-related artery in acute myocardial infarctio J Am Coll Cardiol 26:675, 1995.

84. Andrews J, Straznicky I, French JK, et al: ST-segmer recovery adds to the assessment if TIMI 2 and 3 flow i predicting infarct wall motion after thrombolytic therap Circulation 101:2138, 2000.

85. Schroeder R, Wegscheider K, Schroeder K, et al: Extent of early ST segment elevation resolution: a strong predictor of outcome in patients with acute myocardial infarction and a sensitive measure to compare thrombolytic regimens. J Am Coll Cardiol 26:1657, 1995.
86. Pepine CJ: Prognostic markers in thrombolytic therapy: looking beyond mortality. Am J Cardiol 78:24, 1996.
87. Krucoff MW, Croll MA, Pope JE, et al: Continuous 12-lead ST-segment recovery analysis in the TAMI 7 study. Circulation 88:437, 1993.
88. Shah A, Wagner GS, Granger CB, et al: Prognostic implications of TIMI flow grade in the infarct related artery compared with continuous 12-lead ST-segment resolution analysis. J Am Coll Cardiol 35:666, 2000.
89. Krucoff MW, Parente AR, Bottner KR et al: Stability of multilead ST segment "fingerprints" over time after percutaneous transluminal coronary angioplasty and its usefulness in detecting reocclusion. Am J Cardiol 61:1232, 1988.
90. Kondo M, Tamura K, Tania H, et al: Is ST segment re-elevation associated with reperfusion an indicator of marked myocardial damage after thrombolysis? J Am Coll Cardiol 21:62, 1993.
91. Essen R, Merx W, Effert S: Spontaneous course of ST-segment elevation in acute anterior myocardial infarction. Circulation 59:105, 1979.
92. Ochiai M, Isshiki T, Hirose Y, et al: Myocardial damage after successful thrombolysis is associated with the duration of ST re-elevation at reperfusion. Clin Cardiol 18:321, 1995.
93. Kosuge M, Kimura K, Ishikawa T, et al: Relation of absence of ST reelevation immediately after reperfusion and success of reperfusion with myocardial salvage. Am J Cardiol 80:1080, 1997.
94. Schechter M, Rabinowitz B, Beker B, et al: Additional ST segment elevation during the first hour of thrombolytic therapy: an electrocardiographic sign predicting a favorable clinical outcome. J Am Coll Cardiol 20:1460, 1992.
95. Doevendans PA, Gorgels AP, van der Zee R, et al: Electrocardiographic diagnosis of reperfusion during thrombolytic therapy in acute myocardial infarction. Am J Cardiol 75:1026, 1995.
96. Steg PG, Faraggi M, Himbert D, et al: Comparison using dynamic vectorcardiography and MIBI SPECT of ST segment changes and myocardial MIBI uptake during percutaneous transluminal coronary angioplasty of the left anterior descending coronary artery. Am J Cardiol 75:998, 1995.
97. Shah A, Wagner GS, Califf RM, et al: Comparative prognostic significance of simultaneous versus independent resolution of ST segment resolution relative to ST segment elevation during acute myocardial infarction. J Am Coll Cardiol 30:1478, 1997.
98. Santoro GM, Valenti R, Buoanamici P, et al: Relation between ST-segment changes and myocardial perfusion evaluated by myocardial contrast echocardiography in patients with acute myocardial infarction treated with direct angioplasty. Am J Cardiol 82:932, 1988.
99. Shah A, Wagner GS, Green CL, et al: Electrocardiographic differentiation of the ST-segment depression of acute myocardial injury due to the left circumflex artery occlusion from that of myocardial ischemia of nonocclusive etiologies. Am J Cardiol 78:512, 1997.
100. Bell AJ, Briggs CM, Nichols P, et al: Relationship of ST-segment elevation to eventual QRS loss in acute anterior wall myocardial infarction. J Electrocardiol 20:177, 1993.
101. MacDonald RG, Hill JA, Feldman RL: ST segment response to acute coronary occlusion: coronary hemodynamic and angiographic determinants of direction of ST segment shift. Circulation 74:973, 1986.
102. Kornreich F, Montague TJ, Rautaharju PM: Body surface potential mapping of ST segment changes in acute myocardial infarction: implications for ECG enrollment criteria for thrombolytic therapy. Circulation 87:773, 1993.
103. Saetre HA, Startt-Selvester RH, Solomon JC, et al: 16-Lead ECG changes in coronary angioplasty. J Electrocardiol 24:153, 1991.
104. Kobayashi N, Ohmura N, Nakada I, et al: Further ST elevation at reperfusion by direct percutaneous transluminal coronary angioplasty predicts poor recovery of left ventricular systolic function in anterior wall AMI. Am J Cardiol 79:862, 1997.
105. Santoro GM, Antoniucci D, Valenti R, et al: Rapid reduction of ST-segment elevation after successful direct angioplasty in acute myocardial infarction. Am J Cardiol 80:685, 1997.
106. Claeys MJ, Bosmans J, Veenstra L, et al: Determinants and prognostic implications of persistent ST-segment elevation after primary angioplasty for acute myocardial infarction. Circulation 99:1972, 1999.
107. Matetzky S, Nnovikov M, Gruberg L, et al: The significance of persistent ST elevation versus early resolution of ST segment elevation after primary PTCA. J Am Coll Cardiol 34:1932, 1999.
108. Roubin GS, Shen WF, Nicholson M, et al: Anterolateral ST segment depression in acute inferior myocardial infarction. Am Heart J 107:1177, 1984.
109. Bar FW, Brugada P, Dassen WR, et al: Prognostic values of Q waves, R/S ratio, loss of R wave voltage, ST segment abnormalities, electrical axis, low voltage, and notching. J Am Coll Cardiol 4:17, 1984.
110. Cohen M, Scharpf SJ, Rentrop KP: Prospective analysis of electrocardiographic variables as markers for extent and location of acute wall motion abnormalities observed during coronary angioplasty in human subjects. J Am Coll Cardiol 10:17, 1987.
111. Lindsay J, Dewey RC, Talesnick BS, et al: Relation of ST segment elevation after healing of acute myocardial infarction to the presence of the ventricular aneurysm. Am J Cardiol 54:84, 1984.
112. Arvan S, Varat MA: Persistent ST segment elevation and left ventricular wall abnormalities: a 2-dimensional echocardiographic study. Am J Cardiol 53:1542, 1984.
113. Toyofuku M, Takaki H, Sunagawa K, et al: Exercise-induced ST elevation in patients with arrhythmogenic right ventricular dysplasia. J Electrocardiol 32:1, 1999.
114. Engel TR, Caine R, Kowey PR, et al: ST segment elevation with ventricular aneurysm. J Electrocardiol 17:75, 1984.
115. Pichler M, Shah PJ, Peter T, et al: Wall motion abnormalities and electrocardiographic changes in acute transmural myocardial infarction: implications of reciprocal ST segment depression. Am Heart J 106: 1003, 1983.
116. Haraphongse M, Tanomsup S, Jugdutt BI: Inferior ST segment depression during acute anterior myocardial infarction: clinical and angiographic correlations. J Am Coll Cardiol 4:467, 1984.
117. Lew AS, Laramee P, Shah PK, et al: Ratio of ST segment depression in lead V_2 to ST segment elevation in lead aVF in evolving inferior acute myocardial infarction: an aid to the early recognition of right ventricular ischemia. Am J Cardiol 57:1047, 1986.
118. Lew AS, Hod H, Cercek B, et al: Inferior ST segment changes during acute anterior myocardial infarction: a

marker of the presence or absence of concomitant inferior wall ischemia. J Am Coll Cardiol 10:519, 1987.

118a.Martin NM, Groenning BA, Murray HM, et al: ST-segment deviation analysis of the admission 12-lead electrocardiogram as an aid to early diagnosis of acute myocardial infarction with a cardiac magnetic resonance imaging gold standard. J Am Coll Cardiol 50:1021, 2007.

119. Oliva PB, Hammil SC, Edwards WD: Electrocardiographic diagnosis of postinfarction regional pericarditis. Circulation 88:896, 1993.

120. Mehta M, Jain AC, Mehta A: Early repolarization. Clin Cardiol 22:59, 1999.

121. Kambara H, Phillips J: Long term evaluation of early repolarization syndrome (normal variant RS-T segment elevation). Am J Cardiol 38:157, 1976.

122. Spodick DH: Differential characteristics of the electrocardiogram in early repolarization and acute pericarditis. N Engl J Med 295:523, 1976.

123. Spratt KA, Borans SM, Michelson EL: Early repolarization: normalization of the electrocardiogram with exercise as a clinically useful diagnostic feature. J Invasive Cardiol 7:238, 1995.

124. Mirvis DM: Evaluation of normal variations in ST segment patterns by body surface isopotential mapping: ST segment elevation in absence of heart disease. Am J Cardiol 50:122, 1982.

125. Shabetai R, Surawicz B, Hamill W: Monophasic action potentials in man. Circulation 38:341, 1970.

126. Ginzton LE, Laks MM: The differential diagnosis of acute pericarditis from normal variant: New electrocardiographic criteria. Circulation 65:1004, 1982.

127. Lehmann KG, Shandling AH, Yusi AU, et al: Altered ventricular repolarization in central sympathetic dysfunction associated with spinal cord injury. Am J Cardiol 63:1498, 1989.

128. Hirata K, Kyushima M, Asato H: Electrocardiographic abnormalities in patients with acute aortic dissection. Am J Cardiol 76:1212, 1995.

129. Ludman PF, Hildick-Smith D, Harcombe A, et al: Transient ST-segment changes associated with mitral valvuloplasty using the Inoue balloon. Am J Cardiol 79:1704, 1997.

130. Patel J, Movahed A, Reeves WC: Electrocardiographic and segmental wall motion abnormalities in pancreatitis mimicking myocardial infarction. Clin Cardiol 17:505, 1994.

131. Chandraratna PAN, Nimalasurya A, Reid CL, et al: Left ventricular asynergy in acute myocarditis: simulation of acute myocardial infarction. JAMA 250: 1428, 1983.

132. Dec GW, Waldman H, Southern J, et al: Viral myocarditis mimicking acute myocardial infarction. J Am Coll Cardiol 20:85, 1992.

133. Thomas I, Mathew J, Kumar VP, et al: Electrocardiographic changes in catastrophic abdominal illness mimicking acute myocardial infarction. Am J Cardiol 59:1224, 1987.

134. Chida K, Ohkawa S-I, Esaki Y: Clinicopathologic characteristics of elderly patients with persistent ST segment elevation and inverted T waves: evidence of insidious or healed myocarditis? J Am Coll Cardiol 25:1641, 1995.

135. Rich MW: Myocardial injury caused by an anaphylactic reaction to ampicillin/sulbactam in a patient with normal coronary arteries. Tex Heart Inst J 25:194, 1998.

136. Bolognesi R, Tsialtas D, Vasini P, et al: Abnormal ventricular repolarization mimicking myocardial infarction after heterocycling antidepressant overdose. Am J Cardiol 79:242, 1997.

137. Nakamura W, Segawa K, Ito H, et al: Class IC antiarrhythmic drugs, flecainide and pilsicainide, produce ST segment elevation simulating inferior myocard ischemia. J Cardiovasc Electrophysiol 9:855, 1998.

138. Krishanan S, Josephson ME: ST segment elevati induced by class IC antiarrhythmic agents: underlyi electrophysiologic mechanisms and insights into dr induced proarrhythmia. J Cardiovasc Electrophys 9:1167, 1998.

139. Kok L-C, Mitchell MA, Haines DE, et al: Transient elevation after transthoracic cardioversion in patie with hemodynamically unstable ventricular tachy rhythmias. Am J Cardiol 85:878, 2000.

140. Gurevitz O, Lipchenca I, Yaacoby E, et al: ST segme deviation following implantable cardioverter defibril tor shocks: incidence, timing and clinical significanc PACE 25:1429, 2002.

141. Wilson FN, MacLeod AG, Barker PS: The T deflecti in the electrocardiogram. Trans Assoc Am Physicia 46:29, 1931.

142. Goldberger AL: Hyperacute T waves revisited. Am Hea J 104:888, 1982.

143. Selker HP, Raitt MH, Schmid CH, et al: Time-depende predictors of primary cardiac arrest in patients wi acute myocardial infarction. Am J Cardiol 91:28 2003.

144. Kishida H, Cole JS, Surawicz B: Negative U wave highly specific but poorly understood sign of heart d ease. Am J Cardiol 49:2030, 1982.

145. Gerson MC, McHenry PL: Resting U wave inversion a marker of stenosis of the left anterior descending co onary artery. Am J Med 69:545, 1980.

146. Miwa K, Miyagi Y, Fujita M, et al: Transient termin U wave inversion as a more specific marker for myoca dial ischemia. Am Heart J 125:981, 1993.

147. Miyakoda H, Endo A, Kato M, et al: Exercise-induc U wave changes in patients with coronary artery di ease: correlation with tomographic thallium-201 my cardial imaging. Jpn Circ J 60:641, 1996.

148. Chikamori T, Takata J, Seo H, et al: Diagnostic signi cance of an exercise-induced prominent U wave acute myocardial infarction. Am J Cardiol 78:127 1996.

149. Petterson J, Pahlm O, Carro E, et al: Changes in high frequency QRS components are more sensitive tha ST-segment deviation for detecting acute corona occlusion. J Am Coll Cardiol 36:1827, 2000.

150. Surawicz B: Reversible QRS changes during acute my cardial ischemia. J Electrocardiol 31:209, 1998.

151. Wagner NS, Sevilla DC, Krucoff MW, et al: Transie alterations of the QRS complex and ST during percutan ous transluminal balloon angioplasty of the left anteri descending coronary artery. Am J Cardiol 62:1038, 198

152. Birnbaum Y, Kloner RA, Sclarovsky S, et al: Distortio of the terminal portion of the QRS on the admissic electrocardiogram in acute myocardial infarction an correlation with infarct size and long-term prognos (Thrombolysis In Myocardial Infarction 4 Trial). Am Cardiol 78:396, 1996.

153. Mager A, Sclarovsky S, Herz I, et al: QRS complex di tortion predicts no reflow after emergency angioplast in patients with anterior wall acute myocardial infarc tion. Coron Artery Dis 9:1999, 1998.

154. Birnbaum Y, Maynard C, Wolfe S, et al: Terminal QRS di tortion on admission is better than ST-segment measure ments in predicting final infarct size and assessing th potential effect of thrombolytic therapy in anterior wa acute myocardial infarction. Am J Cardiol 84:530, 1999.

155. Harris AS: Delayed development of ventricular ectopi rhythms following experimental coronary occlusion Circulation 1:1318, 1950.

156. Zehender M, Utzolino S, Furtwaengler A, et al: Time course and interrelation of reperfusion-induced ST changes and ventricular arrhythmias in acute myocardial infarction. Am J Cardiol 68:1138, 1991.

157. Gressin V, Gorgels A, Louvard Y, et al: ST-segment normalization time and ventricular arrhythmias as electrocardiographic markers of reperfusion during intravenous thrombolysis for acute myocardial infarction. Am J Cardiol 71:1436, 1993.

158. Engelen DJ, Gressin V, Krucoff MW, et al: Usefulness of frequent arrhythmias after epicardial recanalization in anterior wall acute myocardial infarction as a marker of cellular injury leading to poor recovery of left ventricular function. Am J Cardiol 92:1143, 2003.

159. Airaksinen KEJ, Ikaehaimo MJ, Huikuri HV: Stenosis severity and the occurrence of ventricular ectopic activity during acute coronary occlusion during balloon angioplasty. Am J Cardiol 76:346, 1995.

8 Myocardial Infarction and Electrocardiographic Patterns Simulating Myocardial Infarction

Myocardial Infarction

ORIGIN OF THE ABNORMAL INITIAL QRS DEFLECTION

The abnormal initial deflection in myocardial infarction (MI) is caused by loss of the voltage previously generated by the infarcted tissue. The loss of voltage is believed to cause transmission of the cavity potentials to the surface of the heart. Wilson et al.[1,2] suggested that epicardial Q waves were caused by passive transmission of intracavitary potentials through an electrically inactive myocardial tissue (Wilson's window theory). Another way of explaining this process is to state that the loss of voltage results in a new balance of electrical forces that become oriented away from the regions of complete or partial tissue loss toward the noninfarcted tissue. If this portion of the myocardium is depolarized early in the sequence of activation, an abnormal Q wave is recorded; the infarction is called *Q wave infarction*. Studies in experimental animals support both hypotheses of the abnormal Q wave (i.e., tissue loss and transmission of cavity potentials).

With anterior MI, abnormal Q waves appear in the anterior precordial leads; with inferior infarction, they appear in the "inferior" leads; with lateral infarction, they are in the "lateral" leads; and with posterior infarction they are in the leads on the posterior wall of the chest.

Because posterior chest leads are not recorded routinely, the presence of posterior infarction can be recognized in the form of reciprocal changes in the anterior precordial leads (abnormal R wave). However, because the posterobasal portion of the ventricles is depolarized not at the beginning of the QRS complex but later, the QRS abnormalities of the posterobasal infarction may become recognizable only during the late QRS portion.

MI WITH ABNORMAL Q WAVE

On the surface electrocardiogram (ECG), an abnormal Q wave is usually defined in adults as one that has a duration of 40 ms or more.[3–6] In the vectorcardiogram, where the duration of the Q wave can be measured more precisely, the Q wave is often considered abnormal when it measures 30 ms or more. In infants and children, the duration of an abnormal Q wave in leads I and aV_L caused by an anomalous left main coronary artery originating from the pulmonary artery was 30 ms or longer in all cases.[7]

Some electrocardiographers consider the amplitude of the Q wave a criterion of abnormality; for example, the Q wave is abnormal when its amplitude exceeds 25 percent of the following R wave.[3] Such a finding, however, has low specificity and cannot be used as a reliable marker of MI in practice. The definition of a wide Q wave does not apply to leads aV_R and V_1, which may normally lack the initial R wave. Additionally, in leads III, aV_F, and aV_L the initial R wave may be absent, and a QS or QR

deflection may represent a normal variant. The QS pattern in lead III is more prevalent in subjects with a horizontal heart position, many of whom are obese (Figure 8–1); the QS is more prevalent in lead aV_L in slender subjects with a vertical heart position (Figure 8–2). A Q wave is also considered abnormal, even if it is less than 30 ms in duration, when it is present in leads that normally display an initial R wave (e.g., leads V_2 and V_3), but this definition of abnormality does not apply when the transitional zone is shifted to the left or right[3] or when the electrodes are placed high with respect to the anatomic position of the heart (see later discussion).

The Q wave develops within 6 to 14 hours (mean 9 hours) after the onset of symptoms.[8] Bar et al.[9] found that the development of Q waves, loss of R waves, and QRS score were completed within the first 9 hours after onset of an acute MI. Most commonly the Q waves develop while the ST segment is still elevated and persist for a variable number of days, weeks, months, or years and often indefinitely. In one study of 251 men who survived 8 weeks after a Q wave MI, diagnostic Q waves persisted 3.5 years in 70 percent of patients.[10] The disappearance of Q waves in the remaining 30 percent of patients corroborates the reported 12 to 20 percent incidence of nondiagnostic ECGs in patients with previously documented Q wave MI.[3]

Kalbfleisch et al.[11] found that Q waves disappeared in 6.7 percent and became "equivocal" in 5.2 percent of 775 patients. Most of the reversion occurred within 2 years, and none occurred

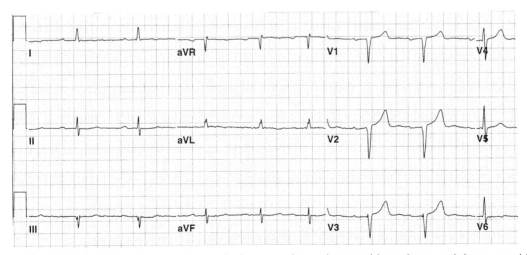

Figure 8–1 ECG of an obese 76-year-old man who has no evidence of structural heart disease and shows normal left ventricular function on the echocardiogram. Note the Q wave in lead III and QS pattern in leads V_1 and V_2 (i.e., poor R wave progression).

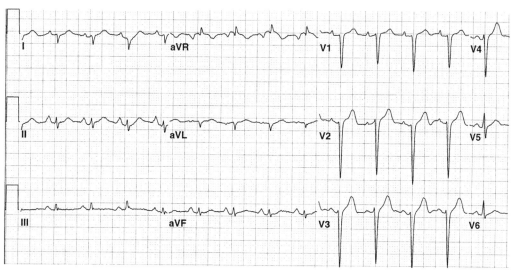

Figure 8–2   ECG of a slender 22-year-old man who has no evidence of structural heart disease and shows normal left ventricular function on the echocardiogram. Note the right axis deviation and QS pattern in lead aV_L.

after 6 years. In the study of Coll et al.,[12] 11 percent of patients lost their Q waves during a follow-up period averaging 65 months. In the present era of thrombolytic therapy and primary angioplasty for acute MI, the reversal of abnormal Q waves occurs more frequently (Figure 8–3). Iwasaki et al.[13] found that among 94 patients with acute anterior infarction treated with reperfusion, an abnormal Q wave (defined as >40 ms and >25 percent of the R wave amplitude) regressed within 6 to 60 months in one or more leads in 77 percent of the patients. The incidence of Q wave regression in patients with patent infarct-related artery (81 percent) was not significantly different from that in those with an occluded lesion (67 percent). Similarly, the incidence of QRS normalization was not affected by revascularization therapy.[14] Q wave regression did not correlate with hemodynamic improvement or the extent of regional wall motion changes and had no prognostic significance.[15]

Q WAVE VS. NON-Q WAVE INFARCTION

The terms *Q wave infarction* and *non-Q wave infarction* have replaced, in practice, the former designations "transmural" and "nontransmural" infarction.[15] The purely descriptive definitions (i.e., Q wave and non-Q wave MI) avoid any allusions to the area or thickness implied in the terms transmural and nontransmural MI.

When using the above terms it should be remembered that: (1) the mere presence of Q waves in any of the standard leads except

aV_R can occur normally, which means that the definition refers to a Q wave of abnormal duration; and (2) Q waves, even if absent in the surface leads, may be present in the epicardial leads without being transmitted to the body surface, because the lesion is not sufficiently large.[16] The terms imply that a Q wave MI is larger than a non–Q wave MI.

Indeed, Mirvis et al.[17] showed that the percentage of left ventricular (LV) infarcted myocardium and the average depth of infarction in dogs predicted the development of a Q wave significantly and independently. If these findings are applicable to humans, they suggest that Q waves may be present when there is an extensive nontransmural MI.

Magnetic resonance tomographic imaging showed that transmural scar was present in 87 percent of 30 patients with Q wave infarction and in 35 percent of 17 patients with non–Q wave infarction.[18] The tomographic transmural defect was significantly larger in patients with Q wave infarction than in those with non–Q wave infarction (34 vs. 18 percent of the LV circumference). This study shows that Q wave infarctions tend to be larger than non–Q wave infarctions, although a considerable overlap exists between the two groups, confirming that an absence of Q waves does not mean that the infarction is not transmural.[18] Moreover, epicardial maps constructed from 120 torso leads have shown that a non–Q wave MI is not a distinct entity but rather a small, less extensive MI.[19] Kornreich et al. found that 56 percent of patients with non–Q wave MIs had abnormalities of the

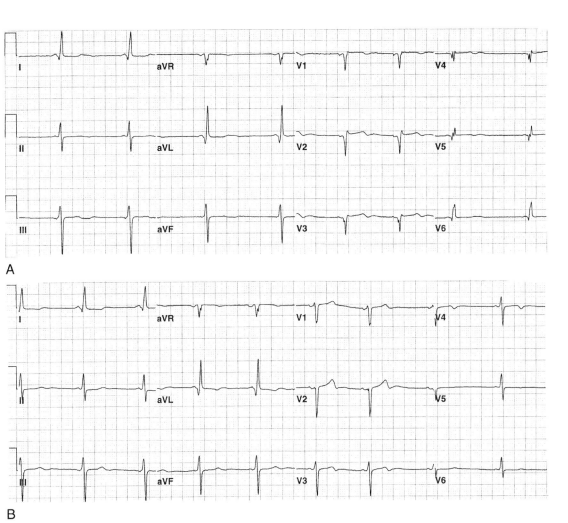

Figure 8–3 Rapid regression of Q waves after thrombolytic treatment. ECG of a 38-year-old woman with an anterior myocardial infarction caused by 90 percent ostial stenosis and 90 percent mid-level stenosis of the left anterior descending coronary artery. ECG in **B** was recorded 5 days after that in **A**. Q waves are no longer present in leads V_1–V_6.

initial QRS complex (i.e., abnormal Q waves, reduced R waves, or abnormally tall R waves in leads located outside the conventional electrode position).[19]

ECG LOCALIZATION OF MI

The Committee on Nomenclature of Myocardial Wall Segments of the International Society of Computerized Electrocardiography recommended adoption of a 12-segment LV subdivision based on the works of Selvester, Wagner, Ideker, and their colleagues. Figure 8–4 shows that each of the four walls of the left ventricle (anteroseptal, anterosuperior, posterolateral, inferior) is subdivided into three segments: the basal, middle, and apical.

Small infarcts, which represent about 20 percent of all infarcts, measure 2.0 to 2.5 cm across and are about 0.5 cm thick. They tend to produce small changes in the QRS wave forms (i.e., notches, slurs, and "bites" in the vector loop) but no diagnostic Q waves unless they are strategically located with respect to the recording electrode.[20] According to these investigators, the "classic" Q waves of MI appear when the infarct is (1) at least 3 to 4 cm in diameter and 5 to 7 mm thick and involving 50 percent of the transmural thickness and (2) located in the part of the heart that is activated during the initial 40 ms of the QRS complex. The infarcts limited to the base, representing 8 to 10 percent of all infarcts,[20] occur in the region depolarized 40 ms or later after the onset of the QRS and produce no abnormalities of the initial QRS complex.[21,22] In an additional 7 percent of infarcts, abnormalities of the initial QRS complex are absent because of the cancellation resulting from two infarcts localized at opposing sites.[20]

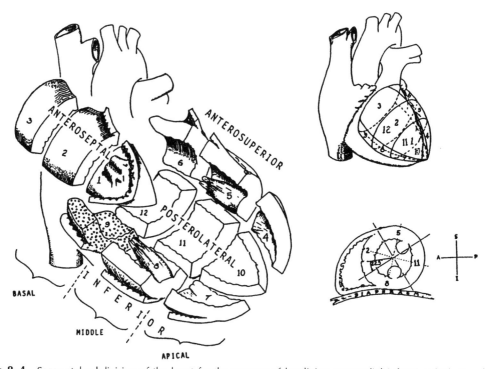

Figure 8–4 Segmental subdivision of the heart for the purpose of localizing myocardial infarction (MI). Based on the recommendations of the International Society of Computerized Electrocardiography, MIs can be localized as follows: basal anteroseptal = segment 3; middle anteroseptal = segment 2; apical anteroseptal = segment 1; apical posterolateral = segment 10; middle posterolateral = segment 11; basal posterolateral = segment 12; basal anterosuperior = segment 6; middle anterosuperior = segment 5; apical anterosuperior = segment 4; apical inferior = segment 7; middle inferior = segment 8; basal inferior = segment 9. (From Selvester RH, Wagner GS, Ideker RE: Myocardial infarction. *In:* MacFarlane PW, Lawrie TD [eds]: Comprehensive Electrocardiology. New York, Pergamon, 1989. Copyright 1989 Elsevier Science, by permission.)

DIAGNOSTIC CRITERIA FOR Q WAVE INFARCTION

Anterior MI Caused by Left Anterior Descending Coronary Artery Occlusion

The subdivision of anterior MI patterns based on the location of the ST segment elevation was described in Chapter 7. Because the distribution of Q waves tends to follow (albeit often in fewer leads), the subdivision based on the Q wave distribution is similar. Q waves in leads V_2–V_3 or V_2–V_4 are present in nearly all cases of anterior MI. The additional Q wave in lead aV_L (and occasionally in lead I) suggests an anterosuperior MI, whereas the additional Q wave in the lead V_5 or V_5–V_6 suggests an anterolateral MI. The term "anteroseptal MI" is not helpful because some portion of the septum is usually involved in the anterior MI caused by left anterior descending (LAD) occlusion.

Shalev et al.[23] failed to support the notion that a Q or a QS deflection >0.03 second in leads V_1–V_3 defines an anteroseptal infarction. These investigators compared ECG, echocardiographic, and cardiac catheterization findings in 80 patients whose disorder fit the traditional definition of acute anteroseptal MI. Their study showed that 92 percent of patients with ST segment elevation in leads V_1–V_3 had an anteroapical infarct, and the culprit narrowing was more frequently found in the mid to distal LAD coronary artery. They suggested that the ECG pattern traditionally termed "anteroseptal" should be called an *anteroapical infarction*, whereas the term *anteroseptal* should be defined as an extensive MI of the anterior wall associated with diffuse ST changes involving the anterior, lateral, and occasionally inferior leads.[2] In my opinion, the electrocardiographic terms *apical* and *anteroapical MI* are difficult to define (see later discussion). For instance, Warner et al.[24] found that abnormal Q waves (i.e., wider than 30 ms) in leads I, aV_L, V_5, and V_6 more often reflected an apical than a lateral MI. The term *anteroinferior* is applicable to anterior MI caused by LAD coronary artery "wrapped" around the apex (Figure 8–5; see also Figure 8–14).

A large anterior infarction combines the abnormalities of anterolateral and anterosuperior MIs (see Figures 7–7, 7–10, and 7–11).

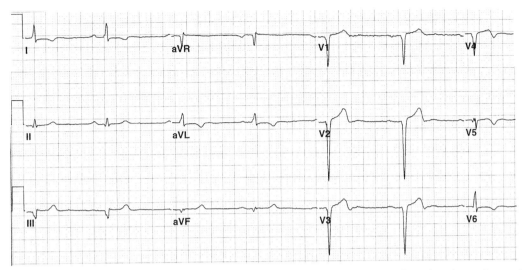

Figure 8–5   ECG of a 65-year-old man with an anterior infarction involving the inferior wall, attributed to occlusion of the left anterior descending artery "wrapping" around the apex. There was no critical obstructive disease in the dominant right and diminutive left circumflex arteries. Anterior wall and apex were akinetic with a left ventricular ejection fraction of 25 percent. Sinus bradycardia and first-degree atrioventricular block are present.

Posterior, Posterolateral Infarction, and Differential Diagnosis of Tall R Waves in Lead V₁

With the posterior or posterolateral MI, the initial QRS forces are directed anteriorly and to the right, causing an increased R wave in the right precordial leads and a Q wave in lead aV_L, V_5, or V_6. If the Q wave in these leads is absent, the diagnosis of posterior MI is uncertain because a tall R wave in the right precordial leads is a common normal variant.[25] If, however, right ventricular (RV) hypertrophy and right bundle branch block (RBBB) are excluded, the duration of the R wave in the right precordial leads is >40 ms, and the R/S amplitude is >1.0, the pattern is highly specific, although its sensitivity for basolateral MI is only 36 percent.[26] The sensitivity improves, however, when the T wave is upright in lead V_1[27,28] (Figure 8–6).

Casas et al.[29] summarized the characteristics of various ECG patterns associated with tall R waves as follows:

1. *True posterior infarction:* ST segment depression and upright T wave in leads V_1 and V_2, Q waves, and ST segment elevation in leads V_7–V_9
2. *Right ventricular hypertrophy:* Right axis deviation, right atrial enlargement, secondary ST segment and T wave changes, normal ECG in leads V_7–V_9
3. *Ventricular septal hypertrophy:* Associated Q waves, left ventricular hypertrophy (LVH), normal ECG or deep narrow Q waves in leads V_7–V_9

4. *Right bundle branch block:* Wide QRS, R peaks late in V_1, often broad S wave
5. *Wolff-Parkinson-White pattern:* Short PR, delta wave
6. *Normal variant:* No other abnormalities

Consideration of these guidelines is of some help but does not always resolve the diagnostic dilemma of tall R waves in the right precordial leads. For instance, a normal variant associated with right axis deviation simulates right ventricular hypertrophy. In another example of a difficult differential diagnosis, a smoothly ascending or notched wide R wave without an S wave may be caused by RBBB alone, RBBB with right ventricular hypertrophy, or RBBB with posterior infarction. Using cardiovascular magnetic resonance imaging (MRI), Bayes de Luna et al.[30] found that the RS morphology in lead V1 was caused by lateral MI and proposed to eliminate the term *posterior MI* in the presence of such pattern.

The term *high lateral infarction* has been applied to a pattern with Q waves confined to leads I, aV_L, and "high lateral" leads recorded two intercostal spaces above the standard lead positions (see Figure 7–23). Pearce et al.[31] showed that of 20 patients with such a pattern (the duration of the Q wave was not specified), only 2 had an MI at autopsy. Based on the correlations with cardiovascular MRI, Bayes de Luna et al.[30] proposed to substitute the term *limited anterolateral MI* for high lateral MI in the presence of Q wave confined to the lead aV_L.

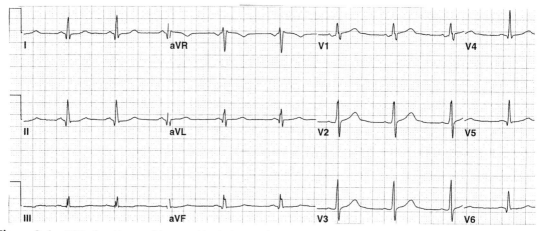

Figure 8–6 ECG of a 44-year-old man with single-vessel coronary artery disease and posterior myocardial infarction caused by occlusion of the posterior descending coronary artery. Estimated left ventricular ejection fraction was 50 percent. Note the tall R waves and upright T waves in leads V_1 and V_2 and the normal q waves in leads I, II, aV_L, aV_F, and V_4–V_6.

Inferior Infarction

With an inferior MI the initial QRS forces are directed superiorly, causing a Q wave in leads III, aV_F, and frequently in lead II (see Figures 7–8, 7–9, 7–16, and 7–21). The specificity of a Q wave ≥30 ms in leads aV_F and II is 96 percent, and the sensitivity is about 50 percent.[32] The abnormal superior force is much easier to demonstrate in the vectorcardiogram (VCG) than in the ECG for two reasons: (1) greater accuracy of the measurement of duration and (2) direct display of clockwise rotation. Of 100 patients with proven inferior MI that occurred several months or years earlier, the VCG detected the typical QRS abnormality in 90 and the ECG in only 42 patients.[33] Similar results have been reported by several other investigators.

The coexistence of inferior MI with left anterior fascicular block is easier to diagnose on the VCG than on the ECG. Both conditions produce superiorly directed QRS forces, but the initial forces of the inferior MI rotate in a clockwise direction, whereas with left anterior fascicular block the rotation is counterclockwise. When the two abnormalities coexist, the initial portion of the superiorly oriented QRS loop is rotated in a clockwise direction and is followed by a counterclockwise rotation of the terminal portion of the QRS loop. Warner et al.[34] empirically derived the following specific ECG criteria for the diagnosis of combined inferior MI and left anterior fascicular block in three simultaneously recorded limb leads: (1) leads aV_R and aV_L both end in an R wave with the peak of the terminal R wave in aV_R occurring later than the peak of the terminal R wave in aV_L; and (2) a Q wave of any magnitude is present in lead II.[34]

A large inferoposterior infarction combines abnormalities of the posterolateral and inferior MIs.

RIGHT VENTRICULAR INFARCTION

Isolated infarction of the RV free wall seldom occurs.[3,35,36] Symptomatic RV MI causing serious hemodynamic complications is usually associated with an acute MI of the inferior or inferoposterior wall.[3] Most pathologic studies showed that RV infarction is present in 14 to 36 percent of patients with LV inferior Q wave infarction, but no major RV MI is seen in hearts with an isolated anterior MI.[3,35,37–39] A small portion of the RV, however, was involved with equal frequency in anterior and inferior (posterior) LV infarction.

Cabin et al.[40] found RV infarction only in 13 percent of 97 hearts with anterior LV MI; the RV infarcts occupied 10 to 50 percent of the circumference of the RV free wall from base to apex. All LV infarcts involved the septum and were large.[3]

RV infarction usually causes loss of the R wave in leads V_{3R} and V_{4R} (see Figure 7–24). Lead V_{3R} appears to be more useful because the rS pattern is nearly always present normally in this lead, whereas in lead V_{4R} the initial r wave is absent in about 9 percent of normal persons.[41] An RBBB appearance has been described in some cases.[3] Chou pointed out that an old RV MI cannot be recognized on the ECG because of the lack of specific QRS changes and the transient nature of the ST segment elevation.[3]

Elevation of the ST segment in one or more of the right precordial leads is the most important diagnostic sign of RV MI. On the standard

12-lead ECG, ST segment elevation may be present in lead V_1 and in some instances also in leads V_2 and V_3[42,43] (see Figures 7–16, 7–17, and 7–24). The right-sided leads V_{3R}–V_{6R} are more sensitive for recognizing an acute RV infarction.[44,45] Lead V_{4R} appears to be the most useful among these leads.[3,45]

Zehender et al.[46] found ST segment elevation in lead V_{4R} in 107 (54 percent) of 200 consecutive patients with acute inferior infarction. Using autopsy findings, coronary angiography, hemodynamic measurements, and noninvasive imaging, they found that ST segment elevation in lead V_{4R} had a sensitivity of 88 percent, specificity of 78 percent, and diagnostic accuracy of 83 percent in the diagnosis of associated acute RV MI. Braat et al.[44] emphasized the transient nature of ST segment elevation in the supplementary right precordial leads because this finding was no longer present within 10 hours after the onset of chest pain in one half of their patients. It has been suggested that leads V_{3R}-V_{6R} be added routinely to the 12-lead ECG for the initial recordings in patients with acute inferior LV infarction.[3]

The pattern of acute RV infarction with ST segment elevation in leads V_1–V_3[42,43] closely resembles that of an acute anteroseptal infarction. Conversely, in some patients with anterior infarction the ST segment elevation extends into the V_{3R} and V_{4R} leads (see Chapter 7). Occasionally, ST segment elevation caused by RV MI extends from lead V_1 to lead V_5 or even to lead V_6.[42] A rare finding, reported by Chou,[3] was a QS pattern in leads V_1–V_3 observed by the author in four patients in whom the right coronary artery was completely occluded at its proximal portion, although no significant lesions were found in the left coronary arteries. This can be explained by the disappearance of the depolarization of the RV wall, which contributes to formation of the initial "septal" QRS deflection directed from left to right.

MI OF THE LEFT VENTRICLE INVOLVING VENTRICULAR PAPILLARY MUSCLES

Dabrowska et al.[47] correlated the ECG with autopsy findings in 53 patients with acute MI involving one or both LV papillary muscles and in 10 patients with acute MI without papillary muscle involvement. ST segment depression of >1 mm was found in 86.8 percent of patients with papillary muscle involvement and in only one patient without it. ST depression in the inferior leads was seen only in patients with anterolateral papillary muscle infarction, whereas ST segment depression in lead I or aV_L was seen

only in cases with posteromedial papillary muscle infarction.[47]

OTHER PATTERNS

Early terminology referred to the ECG pattern of *apical infarction* characterized by a Q wave in leads V_3 and V_4 together with Q waves in leads II, III, and aV_F. Rothfeld et al.[48] demonstrated low sensitivity of the above criteria: Among 62 patients in whom akinesia or dyskinesia was localized at the apex within 3 weeks after the onset of MI, 26 percent had no Q waves, 23 percent had Q waves in the "inferior" leads only, and 32 percent had Q waves in the "anterior" leads only. The pattern combining Q waves in both sets of leads was present in only 19 percent of patients with apical infarction.

Pure septal infarction was inadvertently produced by occlusion of the septal branch during percutaneous transluminal coronary angioplasty.[49] The resulting ECG changes consisted in the disappearance of the septal Q wave, ST segment elevation in leads V_1 and V_2, and reciprocal ST segment depression in leads II, III, aV_F, V_5, and V_6.[50] In one of the personally observed cases, alcohol injection into the first septal perforating artery for treatment of obstructive hypertrophic cardiomyopathy produced RBBB and changes in the initial QRS portion, mainly in leads I and aV_L, which suggests infarction of the basal septum (Figure 8–7). In a recent study, McCann et al. found that patients who developed RBBB after alcohol septal ablation had more extensive transmural septal infarctions.[50a]

It is important to emphasize that not all ECG patterns of MI encountered in practice fit the previously mentioned criteria for localizing the infarction. Various other abnormal patterns of the initial QRS complex may be present, causing difficulties of exact definition and precise localization of MI.

MULTIPLE INFARCTIONS

Myocardial infarction in more than one region of the ventricles is usually the result of an occlusion of more than one coronary artery, but progressive narrowing of the lumen, a distal embolus, or breakdown of the collateral circulation can cause extension of a previous infarction or a new infarction in the absence of involvement of an additional major artery.

The recognition of two independently occurring infarctions is not difficult when the infarctions differ in their age of onset or when the territories of the two infarctions are noncontiguous. Most

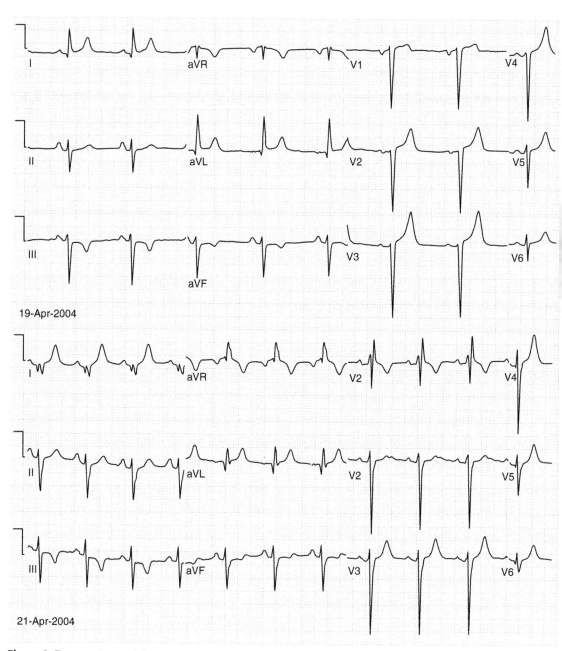

Figure 8–7　ECG changes following septal ablation with alcohol. *Top:* Before ablation, ECG is suggestive of left ventricular hypertrophy. *Bottom:* After ablation there is right bundle branch block and a pattern of basal septal myocardial infarction, suggested by increased duration and amplitude of Q wave in leads I and aV_L. In the remaining leads, the onset of QRS complex is essentially unchanged.

common difficulties arise in the presence of an atypical distribution of coronary blood flow. For instance, an LAD coronary artery extending inferiorly and supplying part of the inferior wall adjacent to the apex or a right coronary artery supplying the lower portion of the septum can give rise to a single inferoseptal MI simulating the presence of two independent infarctions.

The development of a new infarction may mask the signs of a previous infarction, particularly if the previous infarction is located on the opposite side of the ventricle (Figure 8–8). For example, loss of the posteriorly directed QRS forces caused by posterior infarction may produce an R wave in the anterior precordial leads, thereby obscuring the pattern of a preexisting

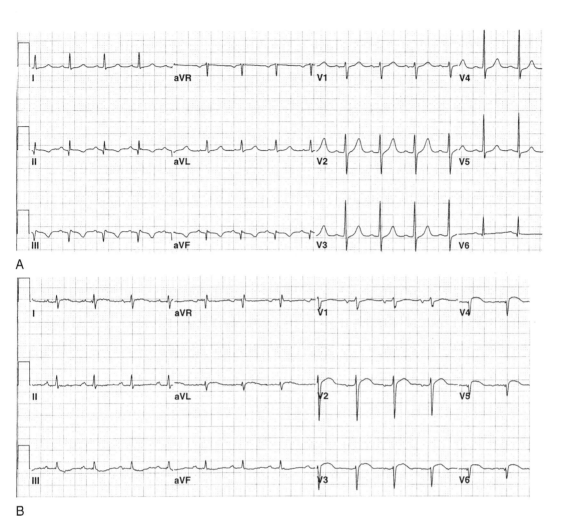

Figure 8–8   Effect of a new infarction on the pattern of a previous infarction. ECGs of a 72-year-old woman. **A,** One day after the onset of acute inferior infarction. Note the Q waves in leads II, III, and aV$_F$. **B,** Three weeks later on the day of acute lateral infarction, there is a right axis shift in the frontal plane, and the presence of the previous inferior infarction is no longer recognizable.

anterior infarction. In rare cases, two opposing initial vectors of two infarctions located at opposing sides cancel each other, making both infarctions unrecognizable.

OPTIMAL LEADS

Right-sided precordial leads, particularly leads V$_{3R}$ and V$_{4R}$, are helpful for establishing the diagnosis of an RV infarction. Zeymer et al.[50] assessed RV involvement by an ST segment elevation of >1 mV in lead V$_{4R}$ and the infarct size by the extent of ST segment deviation. RV involvement was present in 169 (32 percent) of 522 patients with inferior infarction. ST segment elevation of >1 mV in lead V$_{4R}$ was associated with large infarcts and high 30-day mortality rates. This study showed that the higher cardiac mortality rate with RV infarctions was related to

the large infarct size and more proximal right coronary artery lesion, and not to the presence of the RV infarction per se.[51]

Zalenski et al.[51] explored the contribution of ST segment elevation in the RV leads (V$_{4R}$–V$_{6R}$) and posterior (V$_7$–V$_9$) leads to the diagnosis of suspected acute MI in 533 patients. The study showed that addition of these leads modestly improved the recognition of acute MI. The authors calculated that an additional 14,000 patients with acute MI would be diagnosed on a national level (based on an annual hospitalized prevalence for acute MI of 700,000) if the RV and posterior leads were routinely recorded in all patients.[51]

Kornreich et al.[19] performed a discriminant analysis of torso maps derived from 120 leads in 308 patients with various types of MI. They concluded that six features from six torso sites accounted for a specificity of 96 percent and sensitivity of 94 percent. Unfortunately, each of these six positions were located outside the conventional electrode sites. Therefore it seems that the diagnostic accuracy for MI on the ECG would improve if the present lead system were altered. The firm entrenchment of the traditional recording system makes it unlikely that a "lead reform" can muster an influential constituency.

ABNORMALITIES DURING MIDDLE AND LATE PORTIONS OF THE QRS COMPLEX

Abnormalities during mid or late portions of the QRS complex can be caused by changes in the sequence of activation or slow activation within or outside the MI (or both). The QRS duration may remain unchanged if the infarction affects the normally late activated parts of the ventricle and alters the activation pattern but does not cause slowing of conduction. This appears to be uncommon. In most MIs with the abnormalities of the late QRS portion, the QRS duration is increased.

A ventricular conduction defect after MI was described in 1917 by Oppenheim and Rotschild (see Castle and Keane[52]). It was followed by debates in the literature on whether the conduction slowing resulted from interruption of the conduction in the terminal twigs of the Purkinje network, termed *arborization block*, or to slowing of conduction in the myocardium. In 1950 First et al.[53] introduced the term *periinfarction block* to explain the MI pattern in which the initial QRS abnormality (i.e., Q wave) is followed by a slow, slurred terminal deflection.

PERIINFARCTION BLOCK

Grant[54] proposed the following criteria for diagnosis of periinfarction block: (1) characteristic abnormality of the initial QRS portion (i.e., a Q wave); (2) abnormal terminal QRS force directed toward the infarct with an angle of 100 degrees or more between the initial and terminal QRS forces; and (3) little or no prolongation of the QRS complex. Grant suspected that the axis shift of the terminal QRS portion in patients with such a pattern was caused by left anterior or left posterior fascicular block. He coined the definitions *anterolateral periinfarction block* (Figure 8–9; see also Figure 7–31) and *diaphragmatic periinfarction block* (Figure 8–10). In the former, the Q waves diagnostic of MI in leads I and aV_L are followed by a terminal QRS force directed leftward and superiorly, producing an S wave in leads II, III, and aV_F. This pattern resembles the left anterior fascicular block. In the diaphragmatic periinfarction block, the Q waves diagnostic of MI in leads II, III, and aV_F are followed by terminal QRS forces directed rightward and inferiorly, producing an S wave in leads I and aV_L. This pattern resembles that of left posterior fascicular block.

The existence of an "arborization block" was questioned[55] because infarction in dogs did not alter the morphology of the Purkinje fiber spikes, even though the latter appeared sometimes 20 to 30 ms after the onset of the QRS complex. Also,

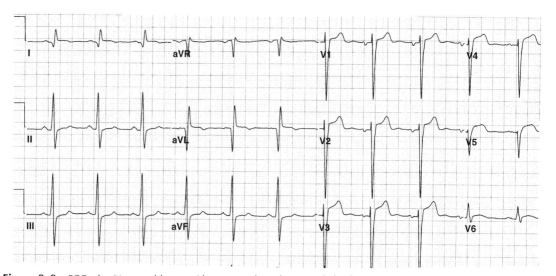

Figure 8–9 ECG of a 61-year-old man with a remote lateral myocardial infarction and QRS duration of 120 ms. Lateral periinfarction block is suggested by the wide R wave in leads I and aV_L. See text discussion.

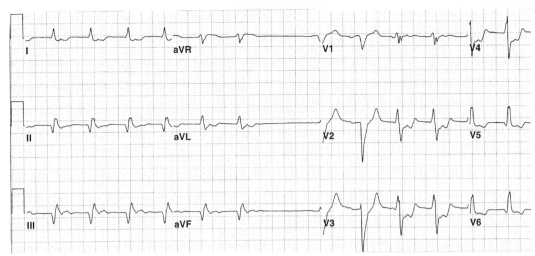

Figure 8–10   ECG of a 77-year-old woman with an inferior infarction resulting in extensive inferobasal akinesis attributed to total occlusion of the proximal right coronary artery. QRS duration is 136 ms. Inferior periinfarction block is suggested by wide R waves in leads II, III, and aV_F. There is an atrioventricular junctional rhythm with two sinus complexes recognizable by the different morphology of the ventricular complex.

in humans with transmural MI, the HV interval and the interval from the onset of the QRS complex to the onset of RV activation were unchanged.[56]

Subsequently, Vassallo et al.[57] found that the endocardial activation pattern was normal in patients with inferior MI and a QRS duration averaging 164 ms. In the same study, the activation pattern was either normal or delayed in the region of the infarction in patients with anterior MI and a QRS duration averaging 144 ms.[57] Thus studies in both experimental animals and humans led to the conclusion that the conduction delay in MI is localized not in the conducting system but in the myocardium.

The experimental studies of Kadish et al.[58] confirmed that conduction over the epicardial surface of the infarction was slow. These studies validate the concept of the periinfarction block. However, Durrer et al.[55] thought that the surface ECG would not be able to distinguish between the slow conduction around the infarction (periinfarction) and the slow conduction within the infarction (i.e., in the strands of viable myocardium within a mottled infarction). Therefore they proposed the ECG term *postinfarction block*. Despite its apparent merit, the term has not been used widely in the literature.

Slow conduction in the infarcted myocardium of humans has been amply documented. Vassallo et al.[57] found that in patients with a previously healed inferior MI and a history of ventricular tachycardia (VT), the area of delayed activation was in the inferoposterior basal region. Isochronal maps computed from 127 endocardial and

epicardial sites during sinus rhythm in 45 post-MI patients operated on for recurrent VT showed that the activation delay was present in 89 percent of patients, and terminal activation was topographically related to MI in 94 percent. Delayed activation beyond the QRS complex was observed on the endocardium and epicardium, respectively, in 11 and 31 percent of cases.[59]

Signal averaging has enabled us to establish the increased incidence of high-frequency components of low amplitude within the QRS complex in patients with acute and chronic MI.[60–62] The increased incidence of high-frequency components is attributed to fragmentation of the depolarization wave front by fibrous tissue, and the low amplitude is attributed to an overall decrease in electromotive force and slowing of ventricular conduction.[62]

In patients with a previously healed anterior MI and history of VT, late activation occurred throughout the inscription of the QRS complex and corresponded anatomically to the anterior free wall and the septum. Slow activation in the infarcted myocardium lasted longer than the activation at the sites of the latest normal activation, such as the posterior basal region.[57,58] The signal-averaged ECGs showed that the incidence of late potentials rises to a peak of 42 percent during the first week, followed by a decline to 13 percent by day 42.[63] Late potentials during the first week after infarction were associated with subsequent ventricular dilatation.[63]

The ECG pattern of periinfarction block, as defined by Grant,[54] is not specific for solid infarction because it is frequently associated with myocardial fibrosis.[52,64] Abnormalities in the middle and terminal portion of the QRS loop on the VCG can be helpful when diagnosing a previous inferior MI even in the absence of the diagnostic abnormalities of the initial QRS forces.[65,66] Abnormal slowing of conduction, manifested by increased duration of the QRS complex, can appear transiently during myocardial ischemia without infarction (e.g., during coronary angioplasty[67] or during coronary spasm[68] (see Chapter 7).

ANGIOGRAPHIC CORRELATIONS

Knowledge of the coronary anatomy can be helpful when interpretation of the ECG (Figure 8–11) shows myocardial perfusion patterns of the three major coronary artery systems in the three conventional echocardiographic views. The anatomy of the three principal coronary arteries supplying the heart varies among individuals, particularly with regard to the dominant artery, which by definition gives off the posterior descending coronary artery. The right coronary artery is dominant in about 90 percent of cases and the left circumflex artery in about 10

percent of cases. In a small percentage of hearts, the pattern of coronary supply is balanced because both right and left circumflex arteries give off parallel descending branches close to the interatrial groove. The dominant artery usually gives off the anterioventricular (AV) node artery. The sinus node artery arises in 55 percent of individuals from the right circumflex artery and in 45 percent from the left circumflex artery.

The dominant right coronary artery supplies the right side of the heart, the inferior wall, a variable amount of the lateral LV wall, and part of the posteromedial papillary muscle group of the mitral valve. Occlusion of the right coronary artery can cause inferior, posterior, inferoposterior, inferolateral, inferoposterior, and RV MI.

The left circumflex artery supplies most of the LV lateral wall and variable amounts of the inferior wall. Occlusion of this artery can cause posterior and lateral infarctions (posteroapical, posterolateral, posterobasal, posteroinferior, inferolateral, or high lateral). When the left circumflex artery is dominant, it crosses the crux of the heart, gives off the posterior descending artery, and perfuses about half of the ventricle. Its occlusion results in large inferoposterior and posterolateral infarctions.

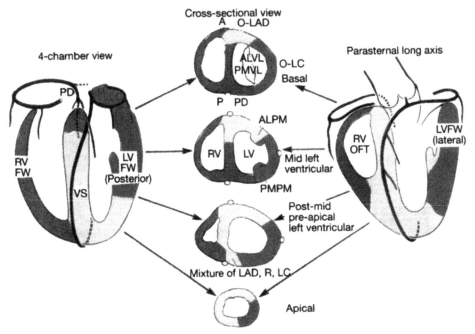

Figure 8–11 Myocardial perfusion patterns of the three major coronary artery systems in three conventional echocardiographic views: right coronary artery, left anterior descending artery, left circumflex artery. A = anterior; ALPM = anterolateral papillary muscle; LAD = left anterior descending; LC = left circumflex; LV = left ventricle; LVFW = left ventricular freewall; P = posterior; PMPM = posterior medial papillary muscle; PD = posterior descending; RV = right ventricle; RVOFT = right ventriclular outflow tract; VS = ventricular septum. Note that there is no designation of the inferior wall because the authors grouped the true posterior, inferior, and inferoapical infarctions under the more expansive term *posterior infarction*. (From Parker AB, Waller BF, Gering LE: Usefulness of the 12-lead electrocardiogram in detection of myocardial infarction: electrocardiographic-anatomic correlations. Part II. Clin Cardiol 19:141, 1996, by permission.)

A combination of an occlusion of dominant RCA and left circumflex artery causes an inferior and posterolateral MI as shown in Figure 8–12.

The LAD coronary artery supplies the anterior wall of the left ventricle, most of the septum, and the apex of the left ventricle. In approximately 30 percent of cases, there is an intermediate branch originating at the site of the division of the main stem entry. Figure 8–13 shows an ECG in a patient with occlusion of the intermediate branch.

Anteroseptal and anterior MIs are nearly always caused by occlusion of the LAD coronary artery, which is also often responsible for apical infarction and sometimes lateral infarction. Proximal occlusion can result in bundle branch block. Left anterior fascicular block occurs in about 8 percent of anterior MIs caused by LAD coronary artery occlusion.[20]

The AV node is supplied by the AV node artery, which subsequently ramifies to supply the His bundle, and, in many cases, the posterior

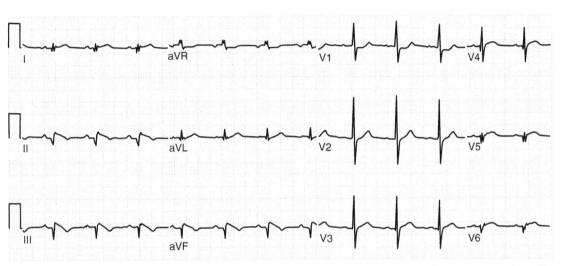

Figure 8–12   ECG of a 82-year old man with a pattern of inferior and posterolateral myocardial infarction, as evidenced by Q wave in leads I–III, aV$_F$, and V$_5$–V$_6$ with increased R wave amplitude in leads aV$_R$ and V$_1$–V$_3$. The dominant right coronary artery was occluded proximally, and there was a 95 percent narrowing of the left circumflex artery, whereas the left anterior descending coronary artery was widely patent. Estimated left ventricular ejection fraction of 20 percent.

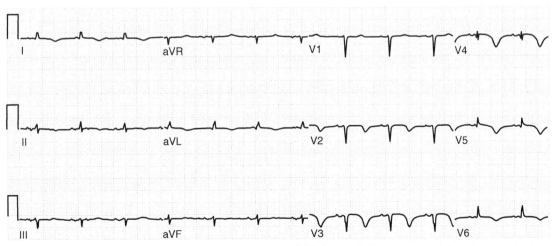

Figure 8–13   ECG of a 77-year old man with anterior myocardial infarction (MI) caused by ostial occlusion of the intermediate branch without major obstructions in other major coronary arteries. There was mid-anterolateral dyskinesis with contractile apex. Abnormal Q waves are present in the leads V$_2$ and V$_3$ with decreased R amplitude in leads V$_4$–V$_5$ and diffuse T wave abnormalities. The earlier ECG taken before MI was normal (not shown).

division of the left bundle branch. There are also marked individual variations. In the study of Frink and James[69] the His bundle was supplied in 9 of 10 human hearts by both the AV node artery and the first septal branch of the LAD artery and in one heart by the AV node artery alone. In the same series, the proximal right bundle branch was supplied by both AV node artery and the septal branch in five hearts, the septal branch alone in four, and the AV node artery alone in one. The anterior half of the left bundle branch was supplied dually in four hearts, entirely by septal branches in five, and by the AV node artery alone in one. The posterior half of the LBB was supplied by the AV node artery alone in five hearts, dually in four, and by the septal branch alone in one. In only one of the 10 studied hearts were both bundle branches supplied proximally by the anterior septal branches alone. This suggests that a bilateral bundle branch block may be caused by occlusion of the LAD artery proximal to the takeoff of the first septal branch alone or, more often, by distal occlusion of the LAD artery and an additional occlusion of the right coronary artery proximal to the takeoff of the AV node artery.

It should be noted that the conduction system appears to be more resistant to ischemia than the myocardium and that in patients with MI the appearance of a bundle branch block may be caused not only by ischemia but by edema, necrosis, and polymorphonuclear cell infiltration of the surrounding myocardium. The frequently observed transient nature of the intraventricular conduction disturbances in patients with acute MI can be attributed to both the resistance to ischemia and the frequent presence of a dual blood supply of the conduction system. In addition, collaterals exist within the septum between branches of the AV node artery and septal branches from the LAD artery and between the left anterior or descending artery and the branches of the posterior descending artery supplying the posterior parts of the septum. For all these reasons, it is difficult to predict the impact of any particular coronary occlusion on the extent and duration of the resulting intraventricular conduction disturbances. Perhaps the most remarkable phenomenon is that coronary occlusions proximal to the takeoff of the sinoatrial node artery or AV node artery create only exceptionally permanent sinoatrial or AV blocks.

The correlation between the site of coronary occlusion and the localization of the MI is generally good, but in the presence of chronic coronary artery disease, particularly in patients undergoing revascularization, the usefulness of the ECG at rest is limited. In fact, the ECG is frequently normal in the presence of significant coronary artery disease with obstruction of one or more coronary arteries. This can usually be explained by the presence of a collateral circulation.

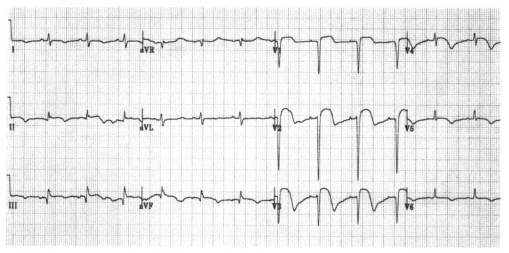

Figure 8–14 Acute anteroseptal and inferior myocardial infarction related to cocaine use. The patient is a 30-year-old woman known to be a cocaine user. She developed severe chest pain; the ECG recorded 90 minutes after the onset of pain reveals ST segment elevation in the anteroseptal and inferior leads (not shown). Coronary arteriogram reveals complete thrombotic occlusion of the proximal left anterior descending artery. Percutaneous transluminal angioplasty was performed with satisfactory results. The visualized artery was long and wrapped around the apex of the heart to supply a substantial part of the inferior wall. The ECG recorded on the next day shows signs of acute anteroseptal and inferior infarctions. There is a QS deflection in lead V_1. The R waves in leads V_2 and V_3 are small. The ST segment in leads V_1–V_3 is elevated, and the T waves are inverted in the entire precordial leads and lead I. In the inferior leads, Q waves are present with ST segment elevation and T wave inversion.

Fuchs et al.[70] correlated ECG and angiographic findings in patients with MI and single-vessel coronary artery disease. Sixty patients had abnormal Q waves. With two exceptions, the presence of an abnormal Q wave in leads I, aV_L, and V_1–V_4 was associated with disease of the LAD artery. The presence of Q waves in leads II, III, and aV_F was associated with left circumflex or right coronary artery disease.

In the study of Blanke and co-workers,[71] a typical ECG pattern of acute anteroseptal infarction was highly reliable for predicting that the LAD artery was the infarct-related vessel with a sensitivity of 90 percent and a specificity of 95 percent. Also, a typical pattern of acute inferior infarction correctly identified the right coronary or left circumflex artery as the infarct-related artery in 94 percent of cases. The presence of typical findings of infarction in inferior leads without evidence of posterior or lateral infarction was highly specific for right coronary artery disease. When the ECG showed a pattern of posterior or lateral infarction (or both) without a typical pattern of infarction in the inferior leads, the infarct-related artery was most likely the left circumflex. In 56 percent of patients with the left circumflex artery as the infarct-related vessel, ECG abnormalities were nondiagnostic. In all the patient subgroups, no apparent ECG differences were found between patients with total vs. subtotal occlusion of the infarct-related vessel.

In an unpublished study, Surawicz and Orr examined electrocardiographic-angiographic correlations in 71 consecutive patients with first MI caused by LAD coronary artery occlusion in the absence of ≥50 percent lesions in the remaining large coronary branches.

The culprit lesions were proximal to the first diagonal branch of the artery (and in about half of these, they were proximal to the first septal perforator) in 48 cases and distal to the takeoff of both the first diagonal and the first septal perforator in 23 cases. We subdivided the ECG patterns based on the new Q wave distribution into the following four types: type 1 with Q waves in leads V_2–V_3 or V_2–V_4 ($n = 28$) (Figure 8–15); type 2 with Q waves in V_2–V_3 or V_2–V_4 + Q in aV_L ($n = 16$) (Figure 8–16); type 3 with Q waves in V_2–V_5 or V_2–V_6 ($n = 11$) (Figure 8–17); and type 4 with Q waves in V_2–V_5 or V_2–V_6 + Q in aV_L ($n = 16$) (Figure 8–18). The occlusion was proximal in 50 percent of patients with types 1 and 3 patterns and in 83 percent of patients with types 2 and 4 patterns. The left ventricular ejection fraction (LVEF) was ≥35 percent in 60 percent of patients with type 1 pattern and in 16 to 20 percent of those with types 2, 3, and 4 patterns. These results show that types 2 and 4 patterns were the best predictors of proximal occlusion, and that types 2, 3, and 4 predicted a markedly depressed LV function. Added Q wave in the lead aV_L or in leads V_5–V_6 to the obligatory Q wave in the leads V_2–V_3 or V_2–V_4 was a marker of LVEF ≤35 percent. Acquired RBBB was present in 21 cases, of which all but 1 occurred in patients with occlusion before the first septal perforator (see Figure 8–18).

Not included into this material were subjects with isolated occlusion of the first diagonal branch (see Figure 7–14), of the intermediate branch (see Figure 8–13), and occlusion of artery "wrapped" around the apex (Figure 8–14).

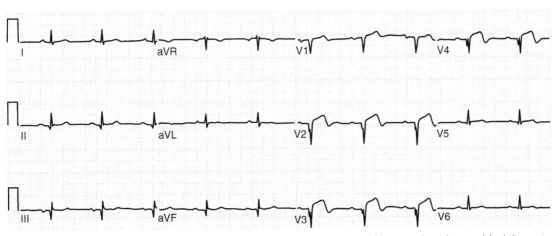

Figure 8–15   ECG type 1 pattern of anterior myocardial infarction in a 55-year-old man with occlusion of the left anterior descending coronary artery distal to the first septal perforator and diagonal branch and no major obstructions in other large coronary branches. Note the Q wave in leads V_2–V_4. The narrow q waves in the inferior leads are normal for this patient's body build. Estimated left ventricular ejection fraction of 40 percent.

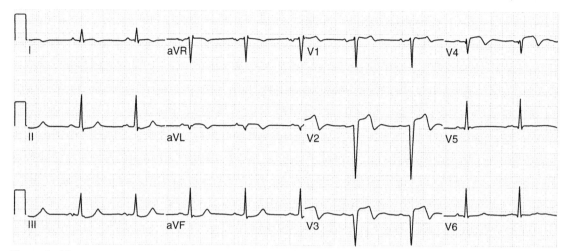

Figure 8–16   ECG type 2 pattern of anterior myocardial infarction in a 54-year-old man with proximal occlusion of the left anterior descending coronary artery and no major lesions in the remaining large coronary branches. Estimated left ventricular ejection fraction of 30 percent. Note the Q waves in leads V₂–V₄ and aV_L.

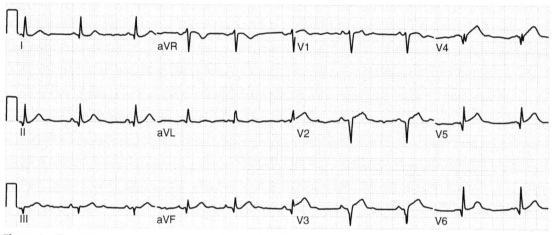

Figure 8–17   ECG type 3 pattern of anterior infarction in a 60-year-old man with complete occlusion of the left anterior descending coronary artery distal to the second diagonal branch and less than 50 percent obstruction in other coronary branches. Estimated left ventricular ejection fraction of 25 percent. Note the Q waves in leads V₂–V₆. ECG was normal shortly before myocardial infarction (not shown).

The most common new intraventricular conduction defect is left anterior fascicular block, which occurs predominantly in patients with LAD coronary artery occlusion. In patients with an inferior infarction and assumed newly developed left anterior fascicular block implied by a frontal axis shift from –30 to –90 degrees, there was also a high prevalence of LAD coronary artery stenosis, and the infarction was extensive.[72] Presumably the development of this conduction disturbance is caused by the loss of collateral circulation following occlusion of right coronary artery.[72]

Dunn et al.[73] examined ECGs of 84 patients with isolated circumflex artery occlusion. The ECG was abnormal in 82 of these patients; Q waves were present in 35 patients, a "true posterior infarction" pattern (initial R wave of 0.04 second or more in lead V₁ or V₂) in 43, ST-T wave abnormalities in 2, and LBBB in 2. Inferior abnormalities correlated with peripheral stenoses, and lateral abnormalities correlated with central stenoses. Figure 8–19 shows the ECG pattern of an inferior infarction in a 16-year-old girl with Kawasaki disease.

A true posterior infarction pattern was seen in patients with both central and peripheral stenoses. In patients with RV infarction, the right coronary artery is the infarct-related vessel (see Figures 7–16 and 7–24). In the experience of

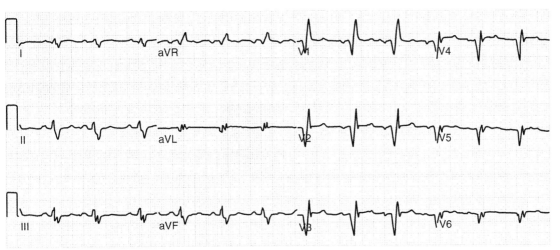

Figure 8–18 ECG type 4 pattern of anterior infarction in a 37-year-old man with 100 percent ostial occlusion of the left anterior descending coronary artery and no obstructing lesions in other major coronary branches. Note the right bundle branch block (not present before myocardial infarction) and Q waves in leads V_1–V_6 and aV_L. Estimated left ventricular ejection fraction of 10 percent.

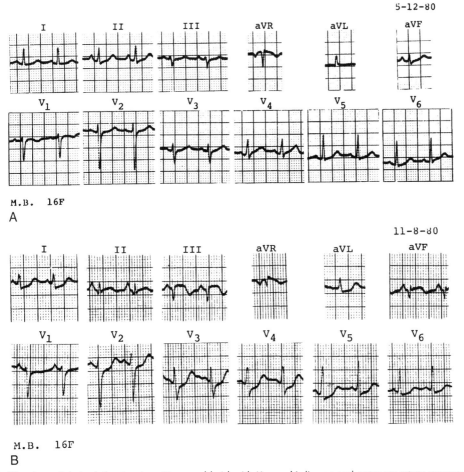

Figure 8–19 Acute inferior infarction in a 16-year-old girl with Kawasaki disease and coronary artery aneurysm demonstrated by coronary arteriography before the development of myocardial infarction. ECGs were obtained before (**A**) and after (**B**) the infarction occurred. Note the appearance of Q waves with ST segment elevation and T wave inversion in the inferior leads on the tracing of 11/8/80. (Courtesy of Dr. Samuel Kaplan.)

Chou,[3] the right coronary artery was occluded or nearly occluded at its proximal portion in nearly all patients with acute inferior and RV infarctions and impaired RV function. In cases of RV infarction associated with occlusion of the right coronary artery at its midportion, there was often no RV dysfunction even though the infarction was diagnosed by ECG.[3] In the study of Weinshel et al.,[74] RV infarction was present in patients with right coronary occlusion proximal to all of the free wall branches but not in patients in whom the obstruction occurred distal to all of the free wall branches.

Midgette et al.[75] used the database from a clinical trial to develop ECG predictors of the infarct-related artery in a group of patients considered candidates for thrombolytic therapy. They identified 12 sets of sums of ST segment deviation and T wave polarity. For example, the sum of the ST segment elevation in leads V_1 to V_4 was referred to as the *summary anterior ST segment elevation*, and the sum of the negative T wave amplitude in leads I, aV_L, and V_5 was referred to as the *summary lateral T wave negativity*. They found that in patients with a high summary anterior ST segment elevation and a low summary lateral T wave negativity, the LAD coronary artery was likely the infarct-related artery; in patients with a low summary anterior ST segment elevation and a high summary lateral T wave negativity, a right coronary artery lesion was likely; and in patients with both a low summary anterior ST segment elevation and a low summary lateral T wave negativity, the left circumflex artery was most likely the infarct-related vessel.

SUMMARY: ECG-ANGIOGRAPHIC CORRELATION FOR MI

The heart is shaped like a cone with walls of uneven thickness without identifiable landmarks separating different regions. In this chapter I suggested for orientations the following correlations:

Anteroseptal, anterior, extensive anterior infarction: Likely the LAD coronary artery. If leads I and aV_L are also involved in an anterior extensive infarct, the culprit lesion is likely to be proximal to the diagonal branch.

Inferior infarction: Right coronary artery (RCA) or, less likely, the left circumflex artery (LCX).

Inferoposterior infarction: RCA or LCX.

Inferior infarction plus right ventricular infarction: Proximal RCA.

Anterolateral, high lateral, inferolateral, posterolateral infarction: LCX.

Based on the recently performed correlations of the location and extent of MI with the cardiac magnetic resonance imaging (CMRI), it was recommended that increased R waves, representing the Q-wave equivalent in leads V_1 and V_2, indicate a lateral MI and that abnormal Q waves in leads aV_L and I without Q waves in lead V_6 indicate a mid-anterior MI. Therefore, the terms posterior and high-lateral MI are incorrect when applied to these patterns and should be changed to lateral wall MI and mid-anterior wall MI, respectively. The other 4 recommended locations are: septal (Q in V_1, V_2), apical-anterior (Q in V_1, V_2 to V_4–V_6), extensive anterior (Q in V_1, V_2 to V_{4-6}, aV_L, and sometimes I), and inferior (Q in II, III, and aV_F).[75a] The subdivisions of anterior MI in this classification, based on CMRI, is similar to what I proposed on the basis of correlations with ventriculograms (see page 177), but the propriety of terms—inferior, posterior, lateral and posterolateral—is expected to be further debated.

Evolution of ECG Patterns for Acute Q Wave MI

In a classic sequence of events, during MI the first ECG change is the "hyperacute" T wave (see Chapter 7) followed by ST segment elevation, Q waves (possibly abnormal R waves), decreased ST segment elevation with the beginning of T wave inversion, and return of the ST segment to baseline with symmetric T wave inversion and a prolonged QT interval. During the course of the transition from ST elevation to T wave inversion, a stage of pseudonormalization may occur when the ST segment deviation subsides and the T wave inversion has not yet occurred (see Figure 7–7). This classic sequence of events is often altered in various ways, particularly in patients undergoing thrombolytic therapy or primary coronary angioplasty (see Figures 7–8 to 7–10, 7–19, and 7–21).

The incidence of transient "hyperacute" T wave changes is low even when the ECG is monitored from the time of the onset of symptoms. The patterns of ST segment elevation are described in Chapter 7. As a rule, the ST segment elevation is recorded in a larger number of leads than in those with a developing abnormal Q wave. The extent, magnitude, and time course of ST elevation and the associated reciprocal ST segment depression are highly variable. In most cases the initial ST segment elevation decreases markedly during the first 7 to 12 hours after the onset of chest pain[76,77] and subsides within a few days. Mills et al.[78] found that

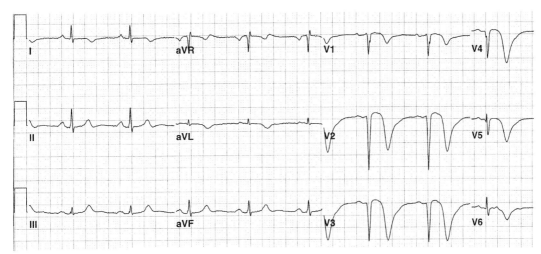

Figure 8–20   ECG of a 66-year-old woman recorded 2 days after myocardial infarction documented by the clinical course and elevation of cardiac enzymes, possibly caused by coronary spasm. Coronary arteries and left ventricular function were normal. Note the typical giant "coronary" T waves, with the QTc = 527 ms.

the ST segment elevation resolved within 2 weeks in 90 percent of patients with inferior infarction and in only 40 percent of those with anterior infarction. The modern treatment of acute MI has changed the course of ST segment evolution, but the significance of persistent ST segment elevation as a marker of suspected ventricular aneurysm has remained unchanged (see later discussion).

Abnormal T waves are usually more symmetric and more pointed than normal T waves. They are sometimes called "coronary" T waves and are usually associated with lengthening of the QT interval (Figure 8–20). Figure 8–21 shows that the characteristic morphology of a coronary T wave is not altered by ventricular pacing. In

patients with MI, pointed coronary T waves appear before or after the primary elevation of the ST segment has begun to subside. In the presence of an elevated ST segment, the site at which the T wave descent begins to form can be recognized by the presence of a notch at the summit of the repolarization wave (Figure 8–22). When the notch deepens, the negative deflection is formed. This negative deflection has a characteristic shape known as a "cove-plane" T wave.[3] With the increasing descent of the ST segment, the area of the negative T wave increases. When the ST segment becomes horizontal, a symmetric, sharply inverted T wave of varying amplitude is inscribed. Such T waves are distinctly different from the secondary T waves of ventricular

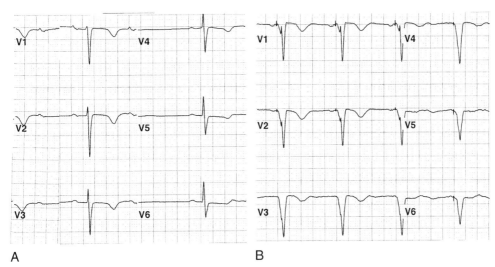

A   B

Figure 8–21   ECG leads V_1–V_6 of an 83-year-old woman with a remote anterior myocardial infarction before (**A**) and after (**B**) pacemaker implantation. Note the persistent T wave abnormality in the paced complexes.

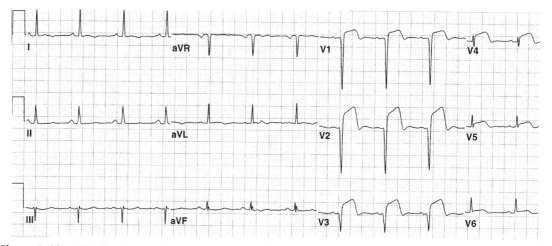

Figure 8–22 ECG of a 52-year-old woman recorded 3 days after onset of an acute anterior infarction caused by total occlusion of the left anterior descending coronary artery. Note the persistent ST segment elevation in the precordial leads with an incipient T wave inversion indicated by the terminal dip in leads V_1–V_3.

hypertrophy or intraventricular conduction disturbances but may be indistinguishable from primary T wave abnormalities caused by other processes (see Chapter 23).

Infarction T waves are attributed to prolongation of activity in the regions of the ventricle immediately adjoining the area of infarction (i.e., stunned myocardium).[79,80] The abnormal T wave after an MI is frequently called the "ischemic" T wave. However, the term *ischemia* has been used also to designate reversible ST segment depression with or without T wave abnormalities, such as those seen during an attack of angina pectoris. To distinguish between these two forms of abnormal repolarization, the term "postischemic T wave pattern" was proposed, but it has not gained popularity. Thus the term *ischemia* is applied in clinical practice to both the acute transient changes associated with ST segment deviations and the subacute or chronic stages of the process associated predominantly with T wave abnormalities.[80]

The T wave abnormalities that appear during stress-induced or spontaneous attacks of angina pectoris usually regress within minutes, but after MI they may persist for several days, weeks, months, or even years. The vector of abnormal T waves tends to be directed away from the area of abnormal (prolonged) repolarization, which means that the T wave becomes negative in leads I, aV_L, V_5, and V_6 in the presence of anterolateral infarction; in leads V_1–V_3 in the presence of "anteroseptal" infarction; in leads II, III, and aV_F in the presence of inferior infarction; and upright in the right precordial leads in the presence of posterior infarction. The correlation

between the distribution of T wave abnormalities and localization of myocardial lesions is not as reliable as the correlation between the distribution of Q waves and the region of the MI. U wave inversion, if present, occurs during the early stage of the MI. In the presence of an anterior MI, a negative U wave appears in the anterior precordial leads and in the presence of inferior infarction in leads III and aV_F. It has been reported that in patients with lateral MI caused by occlusion of the left circumflex coronary artery, the amplitude of a positive U wave is increased, a finding that is usually difficult to verify in practice.

INCREASED R AMPLITUDE

The frequently observed increase in R amplitude during myocardial ischemia and exercise-induced tachycardia has been attributed to altered conduction.[81,82] During the hyperacute phase of MI in dogs, R wave amplitude changes were associated with changes in the ventricular activation pattern.[83] A marked increase in R amplitude ("giant R waves") has been observed transiently during the hyperacute phase of MI in humans[84] (Figure 8–23).

The increase in R wave amplitude has also been attributed to ventricular dilation associated with myocardial ischemia. Studies in both experimental animals and humans, however, have shown that the increased R amplitude during acute ischemia is not caused by changes in the intracardiac blood volume.[80] For other explanations, see Chapter 7.

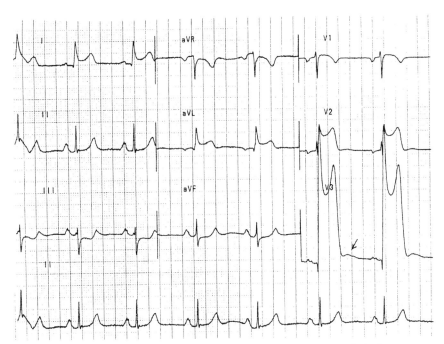

Figure 8–23   Increased R wave amplitude during the acute phase of an anterior myocardial infarction. Conventional ECG standardization is not shown. Arrow points to the U wave. (From Surawicz B: Electrophysiologic Basis of ECG and Cardiac Arrhythmias. Baltimore, Williams & Wilkins, 1995.)

Thrombolytic Treatment and Primary Angioplasty in Acute MI

Successful reperfusion results in myocardial salvage. Baer et al.[18] found, within 36 hours after admission, a 23.3 percent gain in the ECG-estimated infarct size in a successfully reperfused patient group compared with a 12.0 percent gain in the nonperfused patient group.

The most useful evidence of coronary reperfusion after thrombolytic therapy and successful primary angioplasty is reduction of the ST segment elevation.[85–99] Definition of ST segment recovery is facilitated by continuous analysis of the monitored ECG.[90] A decrease in the ST segment elevation of 0.2 mV or more may be observed within 30 minutes after the beginning of thrombolytic treatment and angioplasty[86,88,91] and may continue for 3 to 6 hours.[85,99] Additionally, resolution of an RBBB and AV block can be observed following successful reperfusion.

Persistent ST-segment elevation at 30 minutes after primary percutaneous transluminal coronary angioplasty (PTCA) was a marker of impaired reperfusion in patients with acute MI.[85,86] Also, incomplete ST segment resolution after stenting for acute MI was a marker of microcirculatory dysfunction and more extensive myocardial damage.[85]

Transient reelevation or fluctuation of ST segment elevation has been reported during the early phases of reperfusion before final resolution.[92,93] Maeda et al.[94] found that additional ST segment elevation immediately after reperfusion occurred in patients with severe ischemic myocardial damage before reperfusion and predicted a lesser degree of improvement in the LVEF. In other studies, ST segment reelevation after reperfusion predicted limited myocardial salvage.[95] In the GUSTO study, 243 of 734 patients had a new ST segment shift assessed as >0.1 mV deviation from the baseline within 6 to 24 hours after thrombolytic therapy.[96] Patients with a new shift 6 to 24 hours after treatment represented a high-risk group with increased 30-day and 1-year mortality.[96] In another large study, ST segment reelevation and slow resolution after direct PTCA was a negative predictor of the recovery of LV function.[97,98] It should be noted, however, that reperfusion may occur without a decrease in ST segment elevation, and a decrease in ST segment elevation may occur in the absence of reperfusion. Kircher et al.[99] studied 56 consecutive patients with acute MI 90 minutes after thrombolytic treatment. The rapid decrease in ST segment elevation alone as an indicator of successful reperfusion had a sensitivity of 52 percent, a specificity of 88 percent, and a predictive value of 88 percent. In the CADILLAC study, resolution of ST segment elevation after primary angioplasty correlated strongly with improved prognosis.[100]

During the early stages of reperfusion, a decrease in R wave amplitude or development of a Q wave is accelerated,[87,101,102] but after 12 hours or more the Q waves may be smaller or appear in fewer leads, and the reduced R wave amplitude is less pronounced in patients with reperfusion than in those without reperfusion. Raitt et al.[103] found that the appearance of abnormal Q waves early in the course of acute MI did not lessen the benefit of reduced infarct size after thrombolytic therapy. Conversely, Q wave regression in patients with an anterior infarction receiving thrombolytic treatment did not correlate with improvement of LV function and had no prognostic significance.[13] However, patients who did not develop Q waves after thrombolytic therapy in the GUSTO-1 trial had better prognosis and quality of life.[103] In patients treated with angioplasty, distortion of terminal QRS portion was associated with poor clinical outcome.[104]

Reperfusion is associated with the presence of ventricular premature complexes in nearly all cases. The most characteristic arrhythmia, however, is an accelerated ventricular rhythm[14] (see Figure 7–43).

In the study of Cercek et al.,[105] 90 percent of patients had accelerated ventricular rhythm, and 23 percent had ventricular tachycardia during the first 24 hours after reperfusion. Gorgels et al.[106] observed accelerated ventricular rhythm in 45 percent of 58 patients with successful reperfusion but in only 1 of 14 patients in whom the infarct-related artery remained occluded. Kircher et al.[99] found that the development of reperfusion arrhythmia had a sensitivity of 37 percent, a specificity of 84 percent, and a predictive value of 82 percent. Shah et al.[92] found that accelerated ventricular rhythm occurred in 49 percent of 69 patients who had a patent infarct-related artery with thrombolysis.

Gorgels et al.[106] suggested that the morphology of the QRS complex during ventricular arrhythmia may be useful for identifying the site of myocardial necrosis and the infarct-related artery. In their experience, reperfusion of the LAD coronary artery was associated with a variety of configurations, but the QRS duration was relatively short. During an accelerated ventricular rhythm after reperfusion of the right coronary artery, the QRS complex had a superior axis, and reperfusion of the left circumflex artery was never accompanied by LBBB QRS morphology.

Other arrhythmias during reperfusion include sinus bradycardia and both second- and third-degree AV block. The AV conduction disturbances are associated predominantly with restoration of flow in arteries supplying the inferoposterior left ventricle.[3]

Sensitivity and Specificity of the ECG

ECG criteria for various myocardial locations were established during the late 1940s by Myers and co-workers,[5,6,107–111] who reported extensive correlations between the ECG and autopsy findings. With few modifications these criteria are still in use today, although numerous factors limit the accuracy of the ECG for recognizing and localizing MI. Chou[3] listed factors that influence the accuracy of the ECG diagnosis and location of MI: (1) dimensions of the infarct; (2) age of the infarct; (3) thickness of the ventricular wall involved (i.e., whether it is transmural, intramural, or subendocardial); (4) location of the infarct; (5) presence or absence of multiple infarcts; (6) presence or absence of ventricular hypertrophy or dilation; and (7) presence or absence of ventricular conduction abnormality. Numerous other factors can be added to this list (e.g., presence or absence of pulmonary or pericardial effusion, pulmonary emphysema, drug effects, electrolyte disturbances, preexcitation, and ectopic rhythms). Diagnosis of MI in the presence of intraventricular conduction disturbances is discussed elsewhere (see Chapters 4 and 5).

In the studies reviewed by Chou.[3] the overall sensitivity of the ECG for recognizing autopsy-proven MI was 55 to 61 percent. These percentages probably represent average values because the incidence of the ECG missing the diagnosis of acute infarction is only 6 to 25 percent,[112–114] whereas the incidence of unrecognized old MI may be much higher. In a prospective, population-based cohort study from Iceland with a 4- to 20-year follow-up, at least a third of all MI was unrecognized.[115] In another series, definite ECG signs of MI were absent in 80 percent of patients with old infarcts.[112] In 9 studies reviewed by Sheifer et al.,[116] the incidence of clinically unrecognized MI ranged from 22 to 24 percent. Old anterior infarctions are usually more easily recognizable than inferior, posterior, or lateral infarcts.[3] Prediction of the exact location of infarction is often inaccurate.[117]

Intraventricular conduction disturbances and LVH account for the largest number of unrecognized infarctions, particularly when they modify the initial portion of the QRS complex. The term *poor R wave progression* is often applied to cases of possible previous anterior MI, implying that infarction could have diminished the amplitude of the R wave without producing a Q wave, or that a low-amplitude R wave did reappear in leads with previously recorded QS patterns (Figure 8–24).

More often, however, poor R wave progression is caused by an atypical electrode position in relation to the anatomic position of the heart (see Figure 8–1). The position of the heart also plays a role in the appearance of Q waves in the "inferior" leads, creating false patterns of an inferior MI. Conversely, in patients with an inferior infarction, a diminutive R wave may remain or reappear after the initial presence of a Q wave

in leads III and aV$_F$ and thus obscure the presence of a remote inferior infarction. In such cases, suspicion of the past inferior infarction is enhanced by the presence of a typical symmetric inverted T wave in leads II, III, and aV$_F$ or a first-degree AV block (or both).

The likelihood of correctly diagnosing an inferior infarction is enhanced when the Q wave is present not only in lead III but also in leads aV$_F$ and II. Because lead aV$_F$ represents half of the sum of leads II and III, the presence of a Q wave in both leads II and III always results in a Q wave in lead aV$_F$. When the Q wave is present in lead III but absent in lead II, the Q wave in aV$_F$ may be present or absent. Finally,

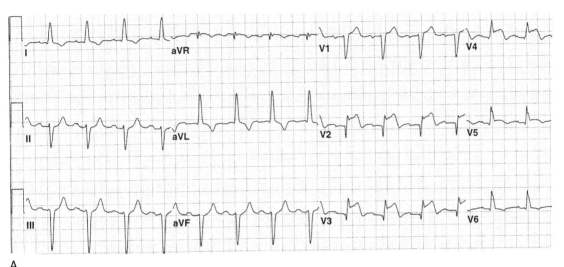

A

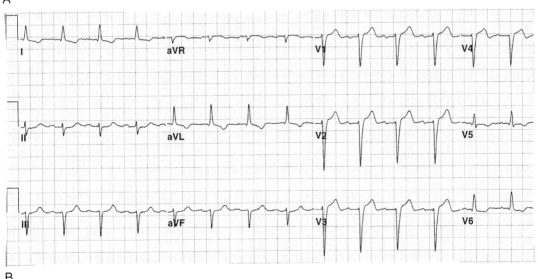

B

Figure 8–24   Poor R wave progression after anterior myocardial infarction on the ECG of an 83-year-old man. **A,** Recorded 2 hours after the onset of an acute infarction following thrombolytic therapy, it shows Q waves in leads V$_1$–V$_4$. **B,** Recorded 23 days later, the presence of previous anterior infarction is revealed by poor R wave progression (i.e., low r amplitude in leads V$_2$–V$_4$). Left anterior fascicular block was present on both occasions.

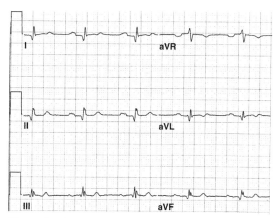

Figure 8–25 ECG limb leads of a 45-year-old man with anterolateral infarction attributed to diffuse disease of the left anterior descending artery with a 90 percent stenosis of the large diagonal branch; estimated left ventricular ejection fraction of 25 percent. Note the Q wave in leads I, II, aV$_L$, and aV$_F$ but not in lead III. See text discussion.

a Q wave in lead aV$_F$ may be present if there is a Q wave in lead II but not in lead III (Figure 8–25). In such cases, inferior infarction is unlikely. Disappearance of the Q wave in lead III or aV$_F$ (or both) during deep inspiration lessens the likelihood of inferior MI, but unfortunately this finding lacks specificity (Figure 8–26). Diagnosis of an old posterior wall MI is facilitated by the presence of an upright symmetric T wave in association with increased R amplitude in leads V$_1$ and V$_2$.

The incidence of false-positive diagnosis of MI varies among series. In the study of Gunnar et al.,[117] the overall incidence of false-positive diagnoses was 31 percent. Horan and co-workers[118] analyzed the ECGs of 768 patients without pathologic evidence of MI. Abnormal Q waves with duration >0.03 second were present in 11 percent of patients. MI was often falsely predicted when the abnormally wide Q waves or QS deflections were limited to leads V$_1$–V$_4$ alone (false prediction of anteroseptal infarction) or inferior leads alone (false prediction of an inferior infarction). If the abnormal Q waves were located in the anterolateral leads or at more than one location, the examiners seldom made a false prediction of MI. However, in a recent study of 479 consecutive patients with previous MI who were referred for nuclear stress testing, the presence of notched or fragmented QRS complexes of <120 ms duration was shown to have a higher sensitivity and a greater negative predictive value for diagnosis MI scar than the presence of Q waves in the 12-lead ECG.[118a]

ESTIMATION OF MI SIZE BY THE QRS SCORING SYSTEM

Selvester et al.[119] developed a QRS scoring system based on knowledge of the normal ventricular activation sequence. These investigators divided the ventricles into 20 segments (7 for the septum, 9 for the left ventricle, and 4 for the right ventricle). Each segment was represented in a computer model by a dipole (see Chapter 1 and Figure 8–4). Simulation of normal activation in the model produced tracings resembling normal VCGs. By increasing the strength of dipoles representing the left or right ventricular segments, Selvester et al. reproduced the patterns of LVH and RVH.[119]

Encouraged by these results, they simulated the loss of active myocardium by eliminating 1 or more of the 20 dipoles. The increasing amount of loss was reflected in increasing deviation from the normal pattern. They established that the VCG detected loss of as little as 0.1 percent of the LV muscle. Using a modification of this method, Wagner et al.[120] developed criteria for estimating the MI size from the standard 12-lead ECG and from the body surface map. Wagner et al.[120] found that a 29-point QRS scoring system, which included 37 criteria in 12 ECG leads, achieved 98 percent specificity in a population considered unlikely to have suffered MI when a score of 2 points or more was required to identify an MI. This means that the ECG criteria for MI are seldom met when MI is not likely to be present.

Subsequently, these investigators established that equally high specificity could be achieved for the diagnosis of a healed MI using only three

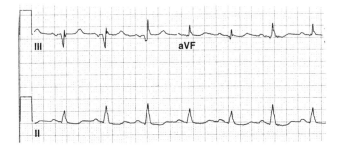

Figure 8–26 Respiratory variations of the QRS complex in leads III, aV$_F$, and II on the ECG of a 47-year-old man with a documented inferior infarction caused by complete occlusion of the right coronary artery. See text discussion.

criteria for the three common MI locations (anterior, inferior, posterolateral): (1) Q wave ≥ 30 ms in AV_F; (2) any Q or $R \leq 10$ ms and ≤ 0.1 mV in V_2; and (3) $R \geq 40$ ms in V_1.[121]

Wagner et al.[120] evaluated the predictive value of the scoring system for MIs verified anatomically during autopsy. In 19 of 21 patients with a single anterior MI and no conduction disturbances. the QRS score was predictive of the MI size, with a correlation coefficient (r) of 0.80. Each QRS score point represented about 3.5 percent of the infarcted left ventricle.[122] In 28 of 31 patients with a single inferior MI, the correlation coefficient was 0.74. The sensitivity of the Q wave ≥ 30 ms in lead III was 90 percent.[123] Moreover, in living subjects with pure anterior or inferior MI and absent LVH and intraventricular conduction disturbances, the QRS score correlated well with the extent of wall motion abnormalities determined by scintigraphy.[124] In 20 patients with a single posterolateral MI the correlation coefficient was 0.72, and each of the score points represented about 4 percent of the infarcted LV mass.[125]

These studies by Wagner's group[126] showed that the 29-point QRS scoring system for estimating MI size performed adequately in the presence of single infarcts with a previously normal ECG. The QRS score correlated less well with the anatomic findings in 32 patients with multiple infarcts $(r=0.44)$. In a later study, Pahlm et al.[127] established the reliability of the Selvester score for estimating the size of inferior and posterolateral infarcts, but for multiple infarcts all methods performed poorly. Another system for estimating MI size, developed by Cowan and co-workers,[128] provided a better correlation with anatomy $(r=0.94)$ even in patients with two or three infarcts. The discrepant results more likely reflect differences in patient selection rather than the superiority of one of the computerized scoring systems. Aldrich et al.[129] proposed formulas using quantitative ST segment deviation on the admission ECG to predict final infarct size in the absence of thrombolytic therapy. The correlations of these formulas with final infarct size were relatively weak.[130]

It has been shown that during thrombolytic therapy, the dynamics of Q wave formation and the QRS score were not reliable indicators for assessing reperfusion.[131,132] The QRS score was also unreliable for predicting the extent of LV asynergy in 315 patients with recent MI, particularly in those with an inferior MI.[133] In a follow-up study of 474 patients with MI without intraventricular conduction disturbances, ventricular hypertrophy, or atrial fibrillation, the QRS score and other ECG variables were not sufficiently

powerful to improve risk assessment when added to other clinical information routinely collated in the hospital.[134] In a study of 38 patients receiving thrombolytic therapy, the correlation of the 32-point QRS score with technetium pyrophosphate tomographic measurement revealed that the score was useful for immediate measurements of the ischemic area and subsequent infarct size.[135]

LIMITATIONS OF ECG FOR PREDICTING MI SIZE

The QRS score for estimating the extent, depth, and location of MI is based predominantly on assessment of the initial portion of the QRS complex. Some of the factors that may limit the predictive value of these abnormalities in patients with acute or chronic MI are as follows:

1. Intraventricular conduction disturbances may be present.
2. Hypertrophy of the myocardium surrounding the scar may cause relative "shrinkage" of the MI area.[136]
3. There may be cancellation of electrical forces by an infarction in another area.
4. Possible "revitalization" of electrically "depressed" areas of stunned or hibernating myocardium may interfere.[137] This may result in unmasking a previous cancellation (e.g., reappearance of Q waves of a previous inferior MI after revascularization of the anterior wall[138]) or reappearance of R waves after revascularization of the region with Q waves.[139] Similar effects may be caused by development of a collateral circulation.[140]
5. Infarct "expansion" may occur, in which the myocardial wall stretches and becomes thinner.[141]
6. An increase in intravascular volume may increase considerably the weight of an MI as a result of swelling.[142]
7. Q waves may appear transiently during acute MI,[143,144] including coronary spasm.[145]
8. Miscellaneous factors of uncertain etiology may affect the predictive value, such as the perioperative MI changes regressing more rapidly than those of nonoperative MI, even if the scores in both types are equal during the acute phase.[146]

PROGNOSTIC VALUE OF ECG FOR MI

Numerous studies have shown that the resting 12-lead ECG may have an independent predictive value in a patient with infarction. Some ECG characteristics of prognostic significance are as follows. First, Q wave infarctions are usually larger than non-Q wave infarcts.[147,148] Mortality is higher among patients with Q wave infarction than among those with a non-Q wave infarction during the early stage.[149] In nonrevascularized patients, the non-Q wave infarcts tend to recur and the recurrences are associated with increased mortality. As a result, the two types of infarction (not treated with revascularization) have similar long-term prognoses.[150]

Birnbaum et al.[150] compared the clinical findings and mortality of patients with acute MI with and without abnormal Q waves; 923 patients had abnormal Q waves in two leads or more, and 1447 patients had no Q waves. In patients with an anterior infarction, abnormal Q waves on the admission ECG were associated with high peak creatine kinase, high prevalence of heart failure, and increased mortality, whereas in patients with an inferior infarction, abnormal Q waves were not associated with an adverse prognosis.

Second, more leads with abnormal Q waves, wider and deeper Q waves, and a larger decrease in R wave amplitude are associated with a greater decrease in the LVEF. It has been shown that early and late mortality rates are higher for patients with an anterior infarction than for those with an inferior infarction even if the infarct size is comparable.[148,151]

Third, the absolute magnitude of the ST segment elevation at hospital admission was found to be of significant prognostic importance.[152] In patients with an inferior infarction, the amplitude of the ST segment elevation was predictive of in-hospital development of a high-degree AV block.[153] The degree of reciprocal ST segment depression also was related to infarct size and mortality independent of the ST elevation with both anterior and inferior infarctions.[3] In patients with an inferior infarction, the markers of a more serious prognosis include coexisting ST segment depression in leads V_1–V_4 and the presence of third degree AV block.[153]

Fourth, the presence of an extensive right ventricular infarction in patients with inferior infarction adversely affects the prognosis,[3] but this may be due to the large infarction size.[154] In a study of 200 consecutive patients with inferior infarction, Zehender et al.[44] found that the mortality rate for 107 patients with an associated RV infarction was 31 percent vs. 6 percent for 93 patients without an associated RV infarction. The incidence of cardiogenic shock, ventricular fibrillation, and complete AV block was also significantly higher among patients with an RV infarction than in those without it.

Other prognostic indicators include distortion of the terminal portion of the QRS complex,

found to be associated with a higher hospital mortality in patients with acute MI treated with thrombolytic agents and angioplasty,[155,156] and higher T wave amplitude on the presenting ECG. The latter finding was associated with lower 30-day mortality and a more benign hospital course, possibly because the presence of higher T waves in the presenting ECG may reflect earlier initiation of thrombolytic treatment.[156]

Other T wave abnormalities also have predictive value. In one study of patients with acute Q wave MI, those with ST segment elevation of >2 mm and positive T waves had large infarcts and a low incidence of recurrent ischemia, whereas patients with ST segment elevation of <2 mm and negative T waves had relatively smaller infarctions and a higher incidence of recurrent ischemia.[157] In another study,[158] persistent negative T waves in leads with Q waves in the chronic stage of MI indicated the presence of a transmural infarction with a thin fibrotic layer, whereas positive T waves indicated a nontransmural infarct containing viable myocardium within the layer. Tamura et al.[159] found that normalization of negative T waves in the infarct-related leads during healing of acute anterior infarction occurred in patients with small infarcts and was suggestive of functional recovery of viable myocardium.

Bundle branch block is associated with an adverse prognosis. In the multicenter registry of 1571 U.S. hospitals, the presence of LBBB ($n=$ 1997; 6.2 percent) was associated with a 34 percent increase in the risk of in-hospital death after adjustment for potential confounders.[160] In the Gusto-I trial the presence of bundle branch block also carried an independent 53 percent higher risk for 30-day mortality.[161] Complete in-hospital reversion of bundle branch block was seen in 12 percent and partial reversion in 12 percent of patients.[162] Complete reversion correlated with a recent onset of bundle branch block as evidenced by >2 mm ST segment depression in the inferior leads and a QRS duration <140 ms.[162] The frequency of advanced second- and third-degree AV block ranged in various studies from 5 to 16 percent and 8 to 16 percent, respectively.[164] In the TAMI trial, the mortality rate for patients with AV block was 20 percent, compared with 4 percent for patients without AV block.[163] Kosuge et al.[164] found that patients with complete AV block after inferior MI who had rapid atrial rate had a more extensive MI than those with a slow atrial rate.

LONG-TERM PROGNOSIS

In the GISSI-1 study, the survival rate at 10 years after hospital discharge was related to the extent of myocardial injury as determined by the number of leads with ST-segment elevation in 11,712 patients with MI who were randomized to streptokinase treatment or control.[165] The increased QRS duration (>108 ms) after MI has been identified as a risk factor for adverse effects. In the VALIANT trial, however, it appeared to be a marker rather than an independent predictor.[166] This conclusion is contradicted by the study from the Mayo Clinic, which showed that QRS duration >105 ms was associated with an increased risk of cardiac death after adjustment for other risk factors.[167] Also, the presence of RBBB and LBBB was associated with increased long-term mortality.[168] In patients with anterior MI and RBBB, increasing QRS duration was associated with increasing 30-day mortality.[168a]

VENTRICULAR ASYNERGY AND VENTRICULAR ANEURYSM

The ECG accurately predicts the site of ventricular asynergy in patients with coronary artery disease, but only in the absence of other types of heart disease, intraventricular conduction disturbances, or ventricular hypertrophy. Abnormal Q waves in the precordial leads are almost invariably accompanied by asynergy of the anterior segment of the left ventricle, whereas the incidence of asynergy is lower in patients with Q waves in the inferior leads. The presence of ST segment elevation with T wave inversion in a patient with an old MI indicates a greater degree of ventricular asynergy and more extensive myocardial scarring.[3,169,170] In the presence of abnormal Q waves and ST segment elevation with T wave inversion, dyskinesis was demonstrated in 68 percent of patients[170] (see Figure 7–31).

Pathologic Q waves are absent in about 25 to 50 percent of patients with ventricular asynergy.[171,172] Among patients with abnormal Q waves and associated ST segment elevation with T wave inversion, dyskinesis was demonstrated in 68 percent.[171] The incidence of dyskinesis in patients with an anterior wall MI is higher among those with a large number of precordial leads with abnormal Q waves. Mills et al.[78] found that persistent ST segment elevation was highly specific for asynergy, as only 1 of 30 patients with coronary disease and a normal ventriculogram had such pattern.

Anatomic correlations confirm the angiographic findings. In 64 cases of autopsy-proven ventricular aneurysm, the ECG location of the infarction correlated well with the anatomic site of the aneurysm.[172] Among the patients in whom the ECG was recorded more than 30 days after the onset of infarction, 79 percent of 50 patients with an anterior aneurysm, and 50 percent of 13 patients with a posterior (inferior) aneurysm had persistent ST segment elevation in the appropriate leads. Among 290 patients with an LV pseudoaneurysm, the incidence of ST segment elevation was 20 percent.[173]

Among patients undergoing surgical resection of a ventricular aneurysm,[175] the anatomic localization determined at the time of operation was correctly predicted by the ECG changes. Of 26 patients, 21 had abnormal Q waves and 22 had persistent ST segment elevation. Those with wide distribution of the abnormal Q waves had large aneurysms, but the size of the infarction could not be predicted by the magnitude of the ST segment elevation (see Figure 7–32). After aneurysmectomy there was usually a decrease in QRS duration and an increase in R wave amplitude. The number of leads with abnormal Q waves was reduced, and in some cases Q waves disappeared in all leads. The ST segment elevation also tended to decrease, and in about a third of cases it disappeared after aneurysmectomy. It can be concluded therefore that the ECG is a fairly sensitive tool for detecting of ventricular aneurysms, particularly at the more common anterior locations.[3]

The most helpful ECG sign is persistent ST segment elevation that lasts more than 1 month after the onset of acute MI.[172] The mechanism of such ST segment elevation is poorly understood. A prevailing hypothesis attributes ST displacement to an injury current generated during systole at the junction of the aneurysm with the surrounding myocardium. According to this theory, the outward (paradoxical) bulging of the aneurysm produces undue tension at the junction of the aneurysm and normal tissue, resulting in injury (depolarization?) of the surviving myocardium next to the border of the aneurysm.[3]

In some patients with dyskinesis, the ST segment becomes elevated after exercise.[3] The phenomenon of ST segment elevation reappearing during exercise-induced ischemia has been reproduced in pigs with a 1-month-old MI.[174] In this model, acute ischemia adjacent to chronic infarction induced ST segment elevation at the surface of the scar despite the virtual absence of viable tissue in the infarction. This suggests a passive ST segment potential transmission from the ischemic periinfarction area through the infarction.[175]

ECG FINDINGS PREDICTIVE OF CARDIAC RUPTURE

Oliva et al.[176] retrospectively and prospectively examined ECGs of 70 patients with cardiac rupture after MI. Patients with rupture had a significantly higher incidence of pericarditis, which was detectable on the ECG by progressive or recurrent ST segment elevation in the absence of recurrent ischemia. In patients with anterior infarction, free wall rupture did not occur when the ECG changes of infarction were confined to leads V_1 and V_2. When the anterior wall adjacent to the septum ruptured, the ECG showed changes in leads V_1–V_4. Of 30 patients with an inferior infarction, 27 had additional involvement of the adjacent lateral wall, or posterior wall, or both. Altogether, 55 patients (79 percent) had multisegment infarcts, with a mid-lateral or high lateral component in 88 percent. In the study of Yoshino et al., ST segment elevation in the lead aV_L was the only independent predictor of cardiac rupture.[177] In patients with anterior MI, ST elevation in inferior leads attributed to the LAD coronary artery extending beyond the apex ("wrapped LAD") correlated significantly with an increase in septal rupture.[178]

Figueras et al.[179] examined clinical and ECG features in patients who died of an acute MI with and without LV free wall rupture. Risk factors of an early rupture included advanced age and first transmural anterior infarction without conduction abnormalities or heart failure. ST segment elevation on admission was higher in patients with early rupture (1 day) than in those with later rupture. On day 2 the ST segment elevation decreased less in patients with the subsequent late rupture (>2 days) than in those without rupture. Among the entire group of 93 patients with rupture, the site of rupture was anterior in 38 percent, posterior in 33 percent, and lateral in 29 percent. Evidence of pericarditis was rarely seen except for extensive pericardial adhesions in 10 patients who died late (>4 days). Solodky et al.[180] characterized retrospectively the following six predictors of cardiac rupture: age, female gender, thrombolytic therapy, heart rate >100 bpm, and systolic blood pressure <100 mmHg. Patients with all these variables had a 26 percent incidence of cardiac rupture. The risks of this event included: female gender, age, and lack of previous angina. The occurrence of ventricular septal defect after thrombolytic therapy was reported by the same group of investigators.[181]

VENTRICULAR REMODELING AND REVERSE REMODELING

The term *remodeling* is used for a number of different processes at the molecular, cellular, and myocardial tissue levels, but at the gross pathologic level it implies post-MI processes that are responsible for ECG changes; namely, expansion of MI, ventricular dilatation, hypertrophy, and intraventricular conduction disturbance.[182] Figure 8–27 shows ECG remodeling in an example of increased QRS duration within a period of less than 2 years after MI.

Several studies have shown that prognosis and development of ischemic cardiomyopathy are affected by increasing QRS duration and distortion of the QRS complex.[183–185] Placement of left ventricular assist devices in patients with advanced heart failure was associated with a decrease in QRS duration and QT shortening (reverse remodeling).[186]

ECG Abnormalities Simulating MI

Abnormalities of the initial QRS portion simulating MI fall into four categories: (1) loss of viable myocardium caused by lesions other than MI; (2) altered distribution of the myocardial mass; (3) altered sequence of depolarization; and (4) altered position of the heart.

LOSS OF VIABLE MYOCARDIUM

A distinct ECG pattern similar to the posterolateral MI pattern is frequently present in Duchenne-type pseudohypertrophic muscular dystrophy (Figure 8–28). However, the tall R waves in the right precordial leads and the deep Q waves in the limb and left precordial leads are usually less wide than in patients with MI. This ECG pattern is sufficiently distinct to suggest the clinical diagnosis and is attributed to fibrous scarring of the posterolateral wall of the left ventricle.[187] Histologic abnormalities in cardiac muscle in such cases resemble those in the patient's skeletal muscle.

Sanyal et al.[188] found tall R waves with an abnormal R/S ratio in 64 percent and deep Q waves (>0.4 mV) in 44 percent of 75 patients with this condition. Similar ECG abnormalities are also frequently present in patients with Friedreich's ataxia[189] (Figure 8–29).

Other conditions associated with abnormalities of the initial QRS portion simulating MI include myocarditis,[190] myocardial contusion (Figure 8–30), scleroderma,[118] amyloidosis,[191] and primary and metastatic cardiac tumors.[192]

ALTERED DISTRIBUTION OF MYOCARDIAL MASS

Abnormal Q waves resembling Q waves in myocardial infarction are particularly common in patients with hypertrophic cardiomyopathy (see

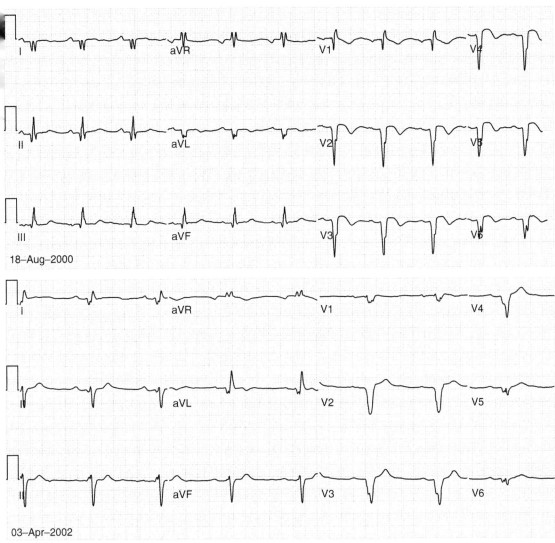

18–Aug–2000

03–Apr–2002

Figure 8–27   Example of ECG remodeling in a 53-year-old woman with an extensive anterior myocardial infarction and incomplete right bundle branch block caused by ostial occlusion of the left anterior descending coronary artery. *Top,* QRS duration = 118 ms; *bottom,* less than 2 years later, QRS duration = 168 ms. No intervening coronary events occurred during the period between the two records.

Chapter 12). Idiopathic hypertrophic subaortic stenosis, later renamed *obstructive cardiomyopathy,* became a subject of intense investigation during the early 1960s. During this period many investigators encountered the characteristic ECG pattern simulating MI with a deeper than normal Q wave in the "lateral" and "inferior" leads and a taller than normal R wave in the right precordial leads (Figure 8–31).

It has been assumed that these electrical forces represent an increased amplitude of depolarization in the hypertrophied septum. In support of this assumption are the observations

that the pattern regresses frequently after septotomy[193] or after development of hypertrophy of the free LV wall.[188] Braudo et al.[194] pointed out that strong forces representing activation of the LV free wall may cancel the oppositely directed large forces of septal depolarization. These investigators suggested that disappearance of the "pseudoinfarction" pattern parallels the natural course of the disease, which begins with isolated septal hypertrophy, followed by free wall hypertrophy in response to outflow obstruction.

Because depolarization of the RV free wall also occurs at about the same time as septal

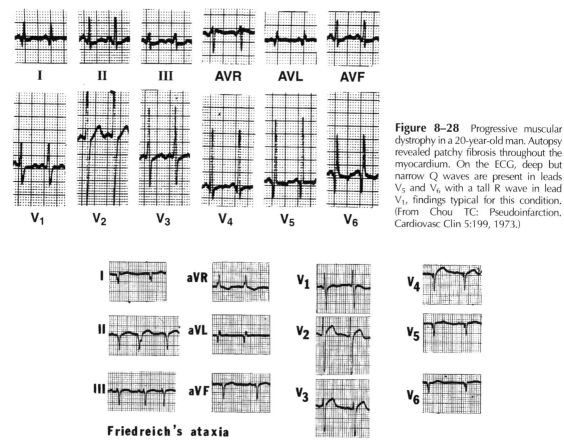

Figure 8–28 Progressive muscular dystrophy in a 20-year-old man. Autopsy revealed patchy fibrosis throughout the myocardium. On the ECG, deep but narrow Q waves are present in leads V_5 and V_6 with a tall R wave in lead V_1, findings typical for this condition. (From Chou TC: Pseudoinfarction. Cardiovasc Clin 5:199, 1973.)

Figure 8–29 ECG simulating myocardial infarction in a 39-year-old man with Friedreich's ataxia and no evidence of coronary artery disease. (From Surawicz B: Electrophysiologic Basis of ECG and Cardiac Arrhythmias. Baltimore, Williams & Wilkins, 1995.)

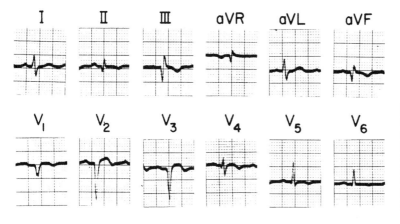

Figure 8–30 Myocardial contusion in a 34-year-old man who sustained nonpenetrating trauma to the chest. ECG is suggestive of anteroseptal and inferior myocardial infarction. Coronary arteriogram was normal. (From Chou TC: Pseudoinfarction. Cardiovasc Clin 5:199, 1973.)

depolarization, the thickness of the RV free wall also influences the amplitude of the initial QRS deflection.[195] Thus the variable interaction of septal, LV, and RV free wall forces creates variable patterns of initial depolarization and explains the lack of significant relation between the prominence of "septal" forces in the ECG and the thickness of the septum.[196,197] Goldberger[198] pointed out that with septal hypertrophy the T wave is directed opposite to the prominent septal depolarization force (i.e., is positive in the leads with a deep Q wave). This "septal hypertrophy and strain pattern" usually differs from the pattern of MI or LVH.[199]

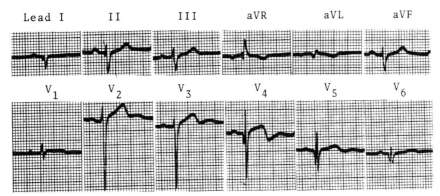

Figure 8–31 Idiopathic hypertrophic subaortic stenosis in a 23-year-old man. Intraventricular pressure gradient of 135 mmHg was demonstrated during isoproterenol infusion. ECG changes resemble those of anterolateral MI. (From Chou TC: Pseudoinfarction. Cardiovasc Clin 5:199, 1973.)

A qR pattern in the right precordial leads is often present in patients with severe RVH, usually in association with right atrial enlargement and tricuspid regurgitation (Figure 8–32). The genesis of this pattern is uncertain, but it may be related to abnormal septal depolarization.[3]

ALTERED SEQUENCE OF DEPOLARIZATION AND ABNORMAL POSITION OF THE HEART

The most common cause of abnormal Q waves without heart disease is an abnormal or atypical position of the heart in the chest. In stocky or obese persons with a high diaphragm position, this causes a deep Q wave or a QS deflection in lead III. Such "positional" Q waves can be recognized because they disappear during deep inspiration. However, it is not conclusive evidence against infarction because Q waves caused by remote inferior MI sometimes behave in the same manner.

Another variant simulating MI is an absent initial R wave in the right and mid-precordial leads. Such "poor R wave progression" can be caused by one of the following mechanisms: (1) right to left septal depolarization, such as incomplete or complete LBBB, LVH, dextrocardia, or "corrected" transposition of the great vessels; (2) inferior deviation of the initial QRS force; (3) downward displacement of the point of origin of the initial QRS force; (4) position of the recording electrodes; or (5) pseudo-Q wave caused by perpendicular orientation of the initial QRS deflection to the lead axis (i.e.,

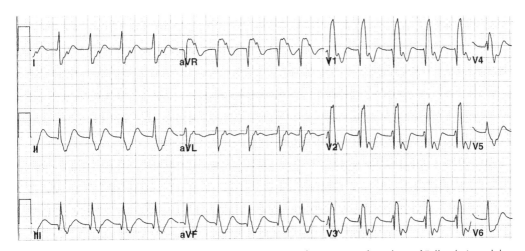

Figure 8–32 ECG of a 39-year-old man who had undergone surgical correction of tetralogy of Fallot during adolescence. There is right ventricular hypertrophy and right ventricular dilation with severe tricuspid regurgitation. The Q wave in lead V₁ simulates septal infarction. There is apparent atrioventricular junctional tachycardia with a single premature complex (sinus capture?) and right bundle branch block with a QRS duration of 202 ms.

an "isoelectric R wave"). Not infrequently, two or more of these factors occur together.

With LVH, QS deflections in the right precordial leads or poor R wave progression in the precordial leads not infrequently produce a pseudoinfarction pattern. In the presence of uncomplicated complete or incomplete LBBB, r waves in precordial leads V_1–V_3 are often small or absent (Figure 8–33). QS deflections also occur frequently in leads III and aV_F in the absence of MI.

Left anterior fascicular block results in relative early activation of the part of the septum supplied by the left posterior fascicle. It displaces inferiorly the initial anteriorly directed septal forces. If the right or mid-precordial leads are situated above the null point of the initial inferiorly directed QRS vector, they record a Q wave that mimics anteroseptal infarction (Figure 8–34). The same event takes place in persons with an asthenic body build or decreasing R wave amplitude during tachycardia in subjects with chronic obstructive lung disease (Figure 8–35).

Changes in cardiac orientation due to a large posterior pericardial effusion can result in a QS pattern in the right and mid-precordial leads.[200] With ventricular preexcitation the presence of delta waves may simulate inferior, anterior, lateral, or posterior infarction depending on the location of the accessory pathway.

The absence of R waves in leads V_1, V_2, and even V_3 or V_4 in persons without heart disease is often caused by relatively high placement of electrodes in relation to the heart. This means that when the diaphragm position is low, even

the correctly placed precordial electrodes may face not the ventricles but the atria or the great vessels. Figure 8–36 shows that this occurred in 13 of 18 subjects in whom roentgenograms of the chest were recorded in the supine position at a distance of 6 feet between the chest wall and the x-ray tube.[201]

The effect of low diaphragm position and the electrode position above the null point of the origin of the inferiorly directed initial QRS deflection can be recognized by recording initial R waves in leads placed below the standard position (e.g., at the level of the ensiform process or epigastrium). In the study of Surawicz et al.[201] of patients with a QS pattern in lead V_3, lead V_3 at the ensiform level (V_{3E}) showed an R wave in 24 of 25 patients without MI and in 3 of 24 patients with MI.

Vectorcardiography may be also helpful for determining whether an absent R wave in the right or mid-precordial leads is caused by a relatively high position of the electrodes or a true absence of initial, anteriorly directed force.

Q waves exceeding 30 ms in duration in leads I and aV_L and the left precordial leads may also occur in the absence of heart disease, particularly in persons with an atypical position of the heart (e.g., left-sided pneumothorax) (Figure 8–37), kyphoscoliosis, and other types of chest deformity.[200,201] A few instances of abnormal Q waves simulating inferior or anterior MI have been reported in patients with mitral valve prolapse and normal coronary arteriograms.[202]

Perpendicular orientation of the initial QRS vector to the lead axis results in an isoelectric

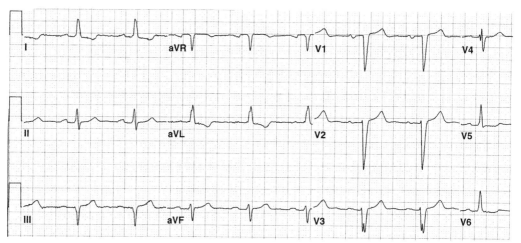

Figure 8–33 Pseudoinfarction pattern on the ECG of a 42-year-old woman with aortic valvular stenosis, severe left ventricular hypertrophy, pulmonary hypertension, normal coronary arteries, and a left ventricular ejection fraction of 55 percent. Incomplete left bundle branch block (QRS duration = 118 ms), left atrial enlargement, and first-degree AV block are present.

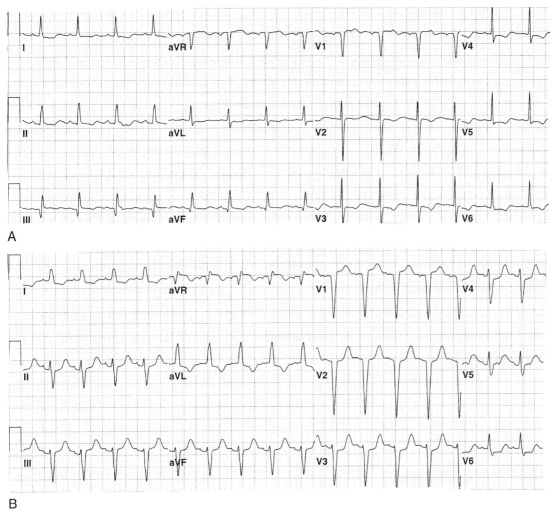

Figure 8–34   Left anterior fascicular block simulates an anteroseptal infarction and obscures an inferior infarction on the ECG of a 70-year-old man. **A,** Pattern shows inferior infarction associated with total occlusion of the right coronary artery and 90 percent occlusion of a second obtuse marginal branch of the circumflex artery. **B,** One day later a left anterior fascicular block is present: QRS duration has increased from 86 ms to 118 ms, there is a pseudoinfarction pattern in leads V_1 and V_2, and the Q wave has disappeared in leads III and aV_F.

R wave. This often creates a pseudoinfarction pattern in the presence of RBBB. Anteroseptal infarction is simulated when the isoelectric r is present in lead V_1 or V_2, and inferior infarction is simulated when the isoelectric r occurs in lead III. The diagnostic error can be avoided by comparing the timing of the onset of the QRS complex in the lead in question with a synchronously recorded lead in which the initial QRS deflection is recognizable.

PULMONARY EMBOLISM AND ACUTE COR PULMONALE

Compared with other diagnostic modalities, ECG is not a sensitive indicator of pulmonary embolism (PE). Studies in animals and humans have shown that nearly 50 percent of the arterial bed must be occluded to produce a change in the ECG; however, when present, the ECG pattern may simulate inferior MI. In 1935 McGinn and White[203] published the first clinical paper correlating ECG changes with PE. In five patients the ECG recorded within 21 hours of the clinical event showed a prominent S wave in lead I, a Q wave in lead III, and a negative T wave in lead III. Subsequent studies in patients with PE showed that the pattern described by McGinn and White occurs infrequently.[204] Other patterns simulating MI are shown in Figures 8–38 and 12–49.

Rapid disappearance of ECG abnormalities favors the diagnosis of PE and suggests that the

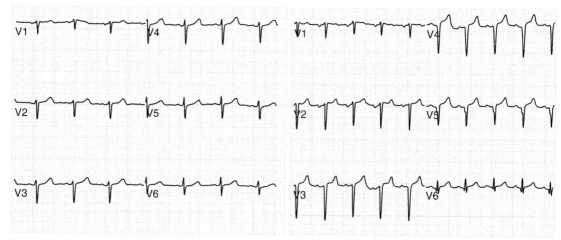

Figure 8–35 Pseudoinfarction pattern in a 56-year-old woman with chronic lung disease. Precordial leads recorded 5 days apart. On the left, the heart rate is 85 bpm; on the right, the heart rate is 128 bpm. There was no evidence of heart disease. Normal echocardiogram with left ventricular ejection fraction of 60 percent.

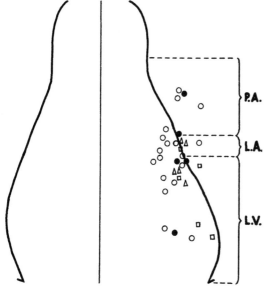

Figure 8–36 Location of the V₃ electrode on the precordium in relation to the cardiac silhouette on the chest roentgenogram. Sectors *LV*, *LA*, and *PA* correspond to the levels of the left ventricle, left atrium, and pulmonary artery, respectively. Open circles represent patients without myocardial infarction; solid circles represent patients with normal hearts and low diaphragm position; squares represent patients with normal hearts and a normal or high diaphragm position. (From Surawicz B, Van Horne RG, Urbach JR, et al: QS and QR pattern in leads V₃ and V₄ in the absence of myocardial infarction: Electrocardiographic and vectorcardiographic study. Circulation 12:391, 1955.)

pattern is caused by a change in cardiac position and perhaps an intraventricular conduction disturbance. A large PE may also cause dilatation and ischemia of the right ventricle, dilatation of the right atrium, and increased sympathetic stimulation. The corresponding ECG changes may include sinus tachycardia, atrial arrhythmias (particularly atrial flutter), axis shift in the frontal plane, inverted T waves in two or more precordial leads, "clockwise rotation," "P pulmonale," and incomplete or complete RBBB.

These nonspecific changes were present in 25 of 36 patients (69 percent) in whom the diagnosis of PE was suspected clinically.[204] However, when the electrocardiographer was the first to raise suspicion of PE on the basis of these findings, the diagnosis of PE was subsequently established in only 5 of 64 patients (8 percent). Among those without PE, however, 72 percent had other causes of acute cor pulmonale, such as pneumonia, exacerbation of obstructive airway disease, bronchial asthma, atelectasis, pneumothorax, recent pneumonectomy, or upper airway obstruction.[204]

OTHER UNCOMMON PSEUDOINFARCTION PATTERNS

Figure 8–39 shows a pseudo-Q wave simulated by an inverted P wave in the presence of an AV junctional rhythm with a short PR interval. Intraventricular conduction disturbances during advanced hyperkalemia may simulate MI, particularly when associated with a "dialyzable" injury current (Figure 8–40). Other abnormalities of ST segment simulating acute injury pattern of MI and T wave abnormalities similar to T waves associated with MI are discussed in Chapters 7 and 9.

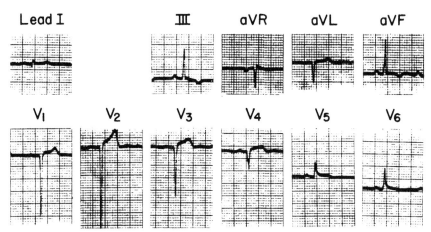

Figure 8–37   Left-sided spontaneous pneumothorax. ECG, recorded from a 26-year-old man who complained of sudden onset of chest pain and dyspnea, shows abnormal QS complexes with slight ST segment elevation in leads V_1–V_4. T waves are inverted in leads III, aV_F, and V_6. Changes in the precordial leads resemble those of acute anteroseptal myocardial infarction. The chest radiograph, however, showed massive left-sided pneumothorax with collapse of the lung. The heart and mediastinum were displaced to the right. Suction tube drainage was applied to the left pleural space. After the left lung was reexpanded, a repeat ECG showed disappearance of the Q waves in leads V_2–V_4. (From Chou TC: Pseudoinfarction. Cardiovasc Clin 5:199, 1973.)

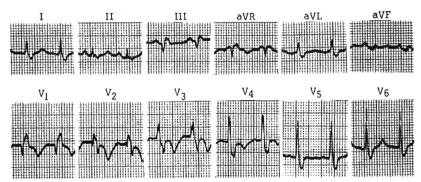

Figure 8–38   Pulmonary embolism. ECG was obtained from a 61-year-old man with massive pulmonary embolism. The diagnosis was verified by autopsy. There was minimal coronary atherosclerosis, with no evidence of myocardial infarction. Note the right bundle branch block with T wave inversion in leads V_1–V_5. A deep, wide Q wave is present in lead III, and a small QS complex appears in lead aV_F. (From Chou TC: Pseudoinfarction. Cardiovasc Clin 5:199, 1973.)

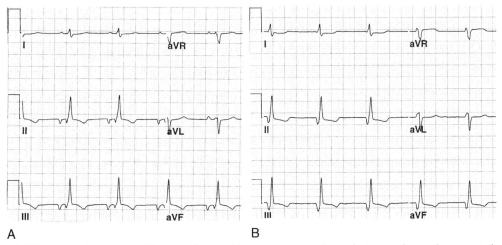

Figure 8–39   ECG limb leads on a 73-year-old man with coronary artery disease but no evidence of previous infarction. **A,** Note the atrioventricular junctional rhythm with negative P waves in leads II and III followed by an isoelectric PR segment and a small q wave. **B,** The PR segment is absent, and a negative P wave simulates a Q wave of an inferior infarction. The two ECGs were recorded on the same day.

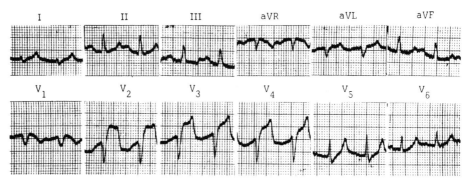

I	II	III	aVR	aVL	aVF

V$_1$	V$_2$	V$_3$	V$_4$	V$_5$	V$_6$

Figure 8–40 ECG of a patient with hyperkalemia. The serum potassium was 9.6 mEq/L. (From Chou TC: Pseudoinfarction. Cardiovasc Clin 5:199, 1973.)

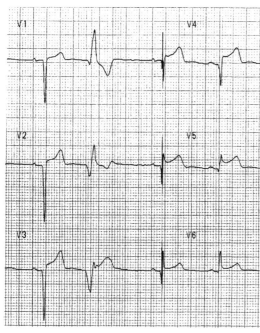

Figure 8–41 ECG precordial leads from a patient with an anterior infarction and a premature ventricular complex displaying a wide Q wave.

Q WAVES IN PREMATURE VENTRICULAR COMPLEXES

It has been reported that a QR pattern in a premature ventricular complex (PVC) with a Q wave >40 ms and a Q amplitude greater than the R amplitude in lead V$_1$ has 93 to 95 percent specificity for detection of an anterior MI[205,206] (Figure 8–41). A Q wave in leads III and aV$_F$ is of more limited value for detecting an inferior infarction.[206]

REFERENCES

1. Wilson FA, Hill IG, Johnston FD: The form of the electrocardiogram in experimental myocardial infarction. III. The later effect produced by ligation of the anterior descending branch of the left coronary artery. Am Heart J 10:903, 1935.
2. Wilson FN, Johnston FD, Hill IG: The form of the electrocardiogram in experimental myocardial infarction. IV. Additional observations on the later effects produced by ligation of the anterior descending branch of the left coronary artery. Am Heart J 10:1025, 1935.
3. Chou T-C: Electrocardiography. In: Clinical Practice, 4th ed. Philadephia, Saunders, 1996.
4. Goldberger E: Unipolar Lead Electrocardiography and Vectorcariography, 3rd ed. Philadelphia, Lea & Febiger, 1953.
5. Myers GB, Klein HA, Hiratzka T: V. Correlation of electrocardiographic and pathologic findings in posterior infarction. Am Heart J 38:547, 1949.
6. Myers GB, Klein HA, Hiratzka T: VI. Correlation of electrocardiographic and pathologic findings in posterolateral infarction. Am Heart J 38:837, 1948.
7. Johnsrude CL, Perry JC, Cecchin F, et al: Differentiating anomalous left main pulmonary artery in infants from myocarditis and dilated cardiomyopathy by electrocardiogram. Am J Cardiol 75:71, 1995.
8. Essen RV, Merz W, Efert S: QRS mapping in the evaluation of acute anterior myocardial infarction. Circulation 62:266, 1980.
9. Bar FW, Volders PGA, Hoeppener P, et al: Development of ST-segment elevation and Q- and R-wave changes in acute myocardial infarction and the influence of thrombolytic therapy. Am J Cardiol 77:337, 1996.
10. Kaplan BM, Berkson DM: Serial electrocardiograms after myocardial infarction. Ann Intern Med 60:430, 1964.
11. Kalbfleisch JM, Shadaksharappa KS, Conrad LL, et al: Disappearance of the Q-deflection following myocardial infarction. Am Heart J 76:193, 1968.
12. Coll S, Betriu AM, De Flores T, et al: Significance of Q-wave regression after transmural acute myocardial infarction. Am J Cardiol 61:739, 1988.
13. Iwasaki K, Kusachi S, Hina K, et al: Q-wave regression unrelated to patency of infarct-related artery or left ventricular ejection fraction or volume after anterior wall acute myocardial infarction treated with or without reperfusion therapy. Am J Cardiol 76:14, 1995.

14. Lyck F, Holmvang L, Grande P, et al: Effects of revascularization after first acute myocardial infarction on the evolution of QRS complex changes (the DANAMI trial). Am J Cardiol 83:488, 1999.
15. Phibbs B: "Transmural" versus "subendocardial" myocardial infarction: an electrocardiographic myth. J Am Coll Cardiol 1:561, 1983.
16. Bodenheimer MM, Banka VS, Helfant RH: Correlation of pathologic Q waves on the standard electrocardiogram and the epicardial electrogram of the human heart. Circulation 54:213, 1976.
17. Mirvis DM, Ingram L, Molly KM, et al: Electrocardiographic effects of experimental nontransmural myocardial infarction. Circulation 71:1206, 1985.
18. Baer FM, Theissen P, Voth E: Morphologic correlate of pathologic Q waves as assessed by gradient-echo magnetic resonance imaging. Am J Cardiol 74:430, 1994.
19. Kornreich F, Montague TJ, Rautaharju M: Identification of first acute Q wave and non–Q wave myocardial infarction by multivariate analysis of body surface potential maps. Circulation 84:2442, 1991.
20. Selvester RH, Wagner GS, Ideker RE: Myocardial infarction. In: MacFarlane PW, Lawrie TD (eds): Comprehensive Electrocardiology. New York, Pergamon, 1989.
21. Flowers NC, Horan LG, Johnson JC: Anterior infarctional changes occurring during mid and late ventricular activation detectable by surface mapping techniques. Circulation 54:906, 1976.
22. Solomon JC, Selvester RH: Simulation of measured activation sequence in the human heart. Am Heart J 85:518, 1973.
23. Shalev Y, Fogelman R, Oettinger M, et al: Does the electrocardiographic pattern of "anteroseptal" myocardial infarction correlate with the anatomic location of myocardial injury? Am J Cardiol 75:763, 1995.
24. Warner RA, Hill NE, Mookherjee S, et al: Diagnostic significance for coronary artery disease of abnormal Q waves in the "lateral" electrocardiographic leads. Am J Cardiol 58:431, 1986.
25. Ha D, Kraft DI, Stein PD: The anteriorly oriented horizontal vector loop: the problem of distinction between direct posterior myocardial infarction and normal variation. Am Heart J 88:408, 1974.
26. Bough EW, Boden WE, Korr KS, et al: Left ventricular asynergy in electrocardiographic "posterior" myocardial infarction. J Am Coll Cardiol 4:209, 1984.
27. Nestico PF, Hakki AH, Iskandrian AS, et al: Electrocardiographic diagnosis of posterior myocardial infarction revisited: a new approach using a multivariate discriminant analysis and thallium-201 myocardial scintigraphy. J Electrocardiol 19:33, 1986.
28. Kataoka H: Relation of T-wave polarity in precordial V_1 lead to right or left circumflex coronary pathoanatomy in acute inferior myocardial infarction. Chest 105:360, 1994.
29. Casas RE, Marriott HJL, Glancy DL: Value of leads V_7-V_9 in diagnosing posterior wall acute myocardial infarction and other causes of tall R waves in V_1-V_2. Am J Cardiol 80:508, 1997.
30. Bayes de Luna A, Cino JM, Pujadas S, et al: Concordance of electrocardiographic patterns and healed myocardial infarction location detected by cardiovascular magnetic resonance. Am J Cardiol 97:445, 2006.
31. Pearce ML, Kossowsky W, Levine R: Isolated abnormalities in high precordial leads, an infrequent sign of myocardial infarction. Am Heart J 72:442, 1966.
32. Mazzoleni A, Hagan AD, Glover MU, et al: On the relationship between Q waves in leads II and aV_F and inferior-posterior wall motion abnormalities. J Electrocardiogr 16:367, 1983.
33. Young E, Williams C: The frontal plane vectorcardiogram in old inferior myocardial infarction: criteria for diagnosis and electrocardiographic correlation. Circulation 37:604, 1968.
34. Warner RA, Hill NE, Mookherjee S, et al: Electrocardiographic criteria for the diagnosis of combined inferior myocardial infarction and left anterior hemiblock. Am J Cardiol 51:718, 1983.
35. Andersen HR, Falk E, Nielsen D: Right ventricular infarction: frequency, size and topography in coronary heart disease: a prospective study comprising 107 consecutive autopsies from a coronary care unit. J Am Coll Cardiol 10:1223, 1987.
36. Forman MB, Goodin J, Phelan B, et al: Electrocardiographic changes associated with isolated right ventricular infarction. J Am Coll Cardiol 4:640, 1984.
37. Isner JM, Robert WC: Right ventricular infarction complicating left ventricular infarction secondary to coronary heart disease. Am J Cardiol 42:885, 1978.
38. Ratliff NB, Hackel DB: Combined right and left ventricular infarction: pathogenesis and clinicopathologic correlation. Am J Cardiol 45:217, 1980.
39. Wartman WB, Hellerstein HK: The incidence of heart disease in 2,000 consecutive autopsies. Ann Intern Med 28:41, 1948.
40. Cabin HS, Clubb KS, Wackers F, et al: Right ventricular myocardial infarction with anterior wall left ventricular infarction: an autopsy study. Am Heart J 113:16, 1987.
41. Morgera T, Alberti E, Sivestri F, et al: Right precordial ST and QRS changes in the diagnosis of right ventricular infarction. Am Heart J 108:13, 1984.
42. Chou TC, Van der Bel-Kahn J, Allen J, et al: Electrocardiographic diagnosis of right ventricular infarction. Am J Med 70:1175, 1981.
43. Lopez-Sendon J, Coma-Canella I, Alcasena S, et al: Electrocardiographic findings in acute right ventricular infarction: sensitivity and specificity of electrocardiographic alterations in right precordial leads V_4R, V_3R, V_1, V_2 and V_3. J Am Coll Cardiol 6:1273, 1985.
44. Braat S, Brugada P, DeZwaan C, et al: Value of electrocardiogram in diagnosing right ventricular infarction in patients with an acute inferior wall myocardial infarction. Br Heart J 49:368, 1983.
45. Candell-Riera J, Figueras J, Valle V, et al: Right ventricular infarction: relationship between ST segment elevation in V_4R and hemodynamic, scintigraphic and echocardiographic findings in patients with acute inferior myocardial infarction. Am Heart J 101:281, 1981.
46. Zehender M, Kasper W, Kauder E, et al: Right ventricular infarction as an independent predictor of prognosis after acute inferior myocardial infarction. N Engl J Med 328:981, 1993.
47. Dabrowska B, Walczak E, Preis R, et al: Acute infarction of the left ventricular papillary muscle: electrocardiographic pattern and recognition of its location. Clin Cardiol 19:404, 1996.
48. Rothfeld B, Fleg JL, Gottlieb SH: Insensitivity of the electrocardiogram in apical myocardial infarction. Am J Cardiol 53:715, 1984.
49. Tamura A, Kataoka H, Mikuriya Y: Electrocardiographic findings in a patient with pure septal infarction. Br Heart J 65:166, 1991.
50. Zeymer U, Neuhaus KL, Wegscheider K, et al: Effects of thrombolytic therapy in acute inferior myocardial infarction with or without right ventricular involvement. J Am Coll Cardiol 32:876, 1998.
50a. McCann GP, Van Dockum WG, Beek AM, Nijveldt R, Ten Cate FJ, Ten Berg JM, Van Rossum AC. Extent of

myocardial infarction and reverse remodeling assessed by cardiac magnetic resonance in patients with and without right bundle branch block following alcohol septal ablation for obstructive hypertrophic cardiomyopathy. Am J Cardiol. 99(4):563–7, 2007.

51. Zalenski RJ, Rydman RJ, Sloan EP, et al: Value of posterior and right ventricular leads in comparison to the standard 12-lead electrocardiogram in evaluation of ST-segment elevation in suspected acute myocardial infarction. Am J Cardiol 79:1579, 1997.

52. Castle CH, Keane WM: Electrocardiographic "peri-infarction block." Circulation 31:403, 1965.

53. First SR, Bayley RH, Bedford DR: Peri-infarction block: an electrocardiographic abnormality occasionally resembling bundle-branch block and local ventricular block of other types. Circulation 2:31, 1950.

54. Grant RP: Peri-infarction. Prog Cardiovasc Dis 2:237, 1959–1960.

55. Durrer D, Van Lier AA, Buller J: Epicardial and intramural excitation in chronic myocardial infarction. Am Heart J 68:765, 1964.

56. Mayarga-Cortes A, Rozanski JJ, Sung RJ, et al: Right ventricular apical activation times in patients with conduction disturbances occurring during acute transmural myocardial infarction. Am J Cardiol 43:913, 1979.

57. Vassallo JA, Cassidy DM, Marchlinski FE, et al: Abnormalities of endocardial activation pattern in patients with previous healed myocardial infarction and ventricular tachycardia. Am J Cardiol 58:479, 1986.

58. Kadish A, Balke W, Levine JE, et al: Activation patterns in healed experimental myocardial infarction. Circ Res 65:1698, 1989.

59. Hatal R, Savard P, Tremblay G, et al: Three distinct patterns of ventricular activation in infarcted human hearts. Circulation 91:1480, 1995.

60. Langner PH, Geselowitz DB, Mansure FT: High frequency components in the electrocardiograms of normal subjects and of patients with coronary heart disease. Am Heart J 62:746, 1961.

61. Flowers NC, Horan LG, Tolleson WJ, et al: Localization of the site of myocardial scarring in man by high frequency components. Circulation 40:927, 1969.

62. Goldberger AL, Bhargava V, Froelicher V, et al: Effect of myocardial infarction on high frequency QRS potentials. Circulation 64:34, 1981.

63. Zaman AG, Morris JL, Smyllie JH, et al: Late potentials and ventricular enlargement after myocardial infarction: a new role for high-resolution electrocardiography?. Circulation 88:905, 1993.

64. Babbitt DG, Binkley PF, Schaal SF: Clinical significance of terminal QRS abnormalities in the setting of inferior myocardial infarction. J Electrocardiol 24:85, 1991.

65. Young E, Levine HD, Vokonas PS, et al: Vectorcardiogram in old inferior myocardial infarction. II. Mid-to-late QRS changes. Circulation 62:1143, 1970.

66. Warner RA, Battaglia J, Hill NE, et al: Terminal portion of the QRS in the electrocardiographic diagnosis of inferior myocardial infarction. Am J Cardiol 55:896, 1985.

67. Wagner NB, Sevilla DC, Krucoff MW, et al: Transient alterations of the QRS complex and ST segment during percutaneous transluminal balloon angioplasty of the left anterior descending coronary artery. Am J Cardiol 62:1038, 1988.

68. Barnhill JE, Wikswo JP, Dawson AK, et al: The QRS complex during transient myocardial ischemia: studies in patients with variant angina pectoris and in a canine preparation. Circulation 71:901, 1985.

69. Frink RN, James TN: Normal blood supply to the human His bundle and proximal bundle branches. Circulation 32:1020, 1973.

70. Fuchs RM, Achuff SC, Grunwald L, et al: Electrocardiographic localizations of coronary artery narrowings: studies during myocardial ischemia and infarction in patients with one-vessel disease. Circulation 60:1209, 1984.

71. Blanke H, Cohen M, Schlueter GU, et al: Electrocardiographic and coronary arteriographic correlations during acute myocardial infarction. Am J Cardiol 54:249, 1984.

72. Assali A, Sclarovsky S, Herz I, et al: Importance of left anterior hemiblock development in inferior wall acute myocardial infarction. Am J Cardiol 80:672, 1997.

73. Dunn RF, Newman HN, Bernstein L, et al: The clinical features of isolated circumflex coronary artery disease. Circulation 69:477, 1984.

74. Weinshel AM, Isner JM, Salem EN, et al: The coronary anatomy of right ventricular myocardial infarction: relationnship between the site of right coronary occlusion and origin of the right ventricular free wall branches. Circulation 68 (Suppl III):351, 1983.

75. Midgette AS, Griffith JL, Califf RM, et al: Prediction of the infarct-related artery in acute myocardial infarction by a scoring system using summary ST-segment and T-wave changes. Am J Cardiol 78:389, 1996.

75a. Bayes de Luna A, Wagner G, Birnbaum Y, Nikus K, Fiol M, Gorgels A, Cinca J, Clemmensen PM, Pahlm O, Sclarovsky S, Stern S, Wellens J, Zareba W; International Society for Holter and Noninvasive Electrocardiography. A new terminology for left ventricular walls and location of myocardial infarcts that present Q wave based on the standard of cardiac magnetic resonance imaging: a statement for healthcare professionals from a committee appointed by the International Society for Holter and Noninvasive Electrocardiography. Circulation 114:1755–1760, 2006.

76. Essen RV, Merz W, Effert S: Spontaneous course of ST-segment elevation in acute anterior myocardial infarction. Circulation 59:105, 1979.

77. Zmyslinski RW, Akiyama T, Biddle TL, et al: Natural course of S-T segment and QRS complex in patients with acute anterior myocardial infarction. Am J Cardiol 43:29, 1979.

78. Mills RM, Young E, Gorlin R, et al: Natural history of S-T segment elevation after acute myocardial infarction. Am J Cardiol 35:609, 1975.

79. Wilson FN, Macleod AG, Barker PS: The T deflection of the electrocardiogram. Trans Assoc Am Physicns 46:29, 1931.

80. Surawicz B: Electrophysiologic Basis of ECG and Cardiac Arrhythmias. Baltimore, Williams & Wilkins, 1995.

81. Deanfield JE, Davies G, Mongiardi F, et al: Factors influencing R wave amplitude in patients with ischemic heart disease. Br Heart J 49:8, 1983.

82. Feldman T, Chua KG, Childers RW: R wave of the surface and intracoronary electrogram during acute coronary artery occlusion. Am J Cardiol 58:885, 1986.

83. David D, Naito M, Michelson E, et al: Intramyocardial conduction: a major determinant of R wave amplitude during acute myocardial ischemia. Circulation 65:161, 1982.

84. Madias JE: The "giant R waves" ECG pattern of hyperacute phase of myocardial infarction. J Electrocardiol 26:77, 1993.

85. Feldman JL, Coste P, Furber A, et al: Incomplete resolution of ST-segment elevation is a marker of transient microcirculatory dysfunction after stenting for acute myocardial infarction. Circulation 107:2684, 2003.

86. Sciagra R, Parodi G, Migliorini A, et al: ST-segment analysis to predict infarct size and functional outcome in acute myocardial infarction treated with primary

coronary intervention and adjunctive Abciximab therapy. Am J Cardiol 97:48, 2006.

87. Dong J, Ndreppa G, Schmitt C, et al: Early resolution of ST-segment elevation correlates with myocardial salvage assessed by Tc-99m sestamibi scintigraphy in patients with acute myocardial infarction after mechanical or thrombolytic reperfusion therapy. Circulation 105:2496, 2002.

88. Krucoff MW, Croll MA, Pope JE, et al: Continuous 12-lead ST segment recovery analysis in the TAMI 7 study: performance of a noninvasive method for real-time detection of failed myocardial reperfusion. Circulation 88:437, 1993.

89. Poli A, Fetiveau R, Vandoni P, et al: Integrated analysis of myocardial blush and ST-segment elevation recovery after successful primary angioplasty. Circulation 106:313, 2002.

90. Veldkamp RF, Green CL, Wilkins ML, et al: Comparison of continuous ST-segment recovery analysis with methods using static electrocardiograms for noninvasive patency assessment during acute myocardial infarction. Am J Cardiol 73:1069, 1994.

91. Richardson SG, Morton P, Murtaugh JG, et al: Relation of coronary arterial patency and left ventricular function to electrocardiographic changes after streptokinase treatment during acute myocardial infarction. Am J Cardiol 61:961, 1988.

92. Shah PK, Cercek B, Lew AS, et al: Angiographic validation of bedside markers of reperfusion. J Am Coll Cardiol 21:55, 1993.

93. Schechter M, Rabinowitz B, Becker B, et al: Additional ST segment elevation during the first hour of thrombolytic therapy: an electrocardiographic sign predicting a favorable outcome. J Am Coll Cardiol 20:1460, 1992.

94. Miida T, Oda H, Toeda T, et al: Additional ST-segment elevation immediately after reperfusion and its effect on myocardial salvage in anterior wall acute myocardial infarction. Am J Cardiol 73:851, 1994.

95. Kondo M, Tamura K, Tanio H, et al: Is ST segment reelevation associated with reperfusion an indicator of marked myocardial damage after thrombolysis?. J Am Coll Cardiol 21:62, 1993.

96. Langer A, Krucoff MW, Klootwijk P, et al: Prognostic significance of ST segment shift after resolution of ST elevation with myocardial infarction treated with thrombolytic therapy: the GUSTO-I ST-segment Monitoring Substudy. J Am Coll Cardiol 31:783, 1998.

97. Somitsu Y, Nakamura M, Degawa T, et al: Prognostic value of slow resolution of ST-segment elevation following successful direct percutaneous transluminal coronary angioplasty for recovery of left ventricular function. Am J Cardiol 80:406, 1997.

98. Brodie BR, Stuckey TD, Hansen C, et al: Relation between electrocardiographic ST-segment resolution and early and late outcomes after primary percutaneous coronary intervention for acute myocardial infarction. Am J Cardiol 95:343, 2005.

99. Kircher BJ, Topol EJ, O'Neill WW, et al: Prediction of infarct coronary artery recanalization after intravenous thrombolytic therapy. Am J Cardiol 59:513, 1987.

100. McLaughlin MG, Stone GW, Aymong E, et al: Prognostic utility of comparative methods for assessment of ST-segment resolution after primary angioplasty for acute myocardial infarction. The Controlled Abciximab and device investigation to Lower Angioplastic Complications (CADILLAC) Trial. J Am Coll Cardiol 44:1215, 2004.

101. Bren GB, Wasserman AG, Ross AM: Electrocardiographic infarct evolution is accelerated by successful thrombolysis: a report from the NHIBI Thrombolysis in Myocardial Infarction (TIMI) trial. J Am Coll Cardiol 9:63A, 1987.

102. Timmis GC: Electrocardiographic effects of reperfusion. Cardiol Clin 5:427, 1987.

103. Raitt MH, Maynard C, Wagner GS, et al: Appearance of abnormal Q waves early in the course of acute myocardial infarction: implications for efficacy of thrombolytic therapy. J Am Coll Cardiol 25:1084, 1995.

104. Lee CW, Hong M-K, Suk H, et al: Determinants and prognostic implications of terminal QRS complex distortion in patients treated with primary angioplasty for acute myocardial infarction. Am J Cardiol 88:210, 2001.

105. Cercek B, Lew AS, Laramee P, et al: Time course and characteristics of ventricular arrhythmias after reperfusion in acute myocardial infarction. Am J Cardiol 60:214, 1987.

106. Gorgels APM, Vos MA, Letsch IS, et al: Usefulness of the accelerated idioventricular rhythm as a marker for myocardial necrosis and reperfusion during thrombolytic therapy in acute myocardial infarction. Am J Cardiol 61:231, 1988.

107. Myers GB, Klein HA, Stofer BE: I. Correlation of electrocardiographic and pathologic findings in anteroseptal infarction. Am Heart J 36:535, 1948.

108. Myers GB, Klein HA, Hiratzka T: II. Correlation of electrocardiographic and pathologic findings in large anterolateral infarcts. Am Heart J 36:838, 1948.

109. Myers GB, Klein HA, Hiratzka T: III. Correlation of electrocardiographic and pathologic findings in anteroposterior infarction. Am Heart J 37:205, 1949.

110. Myers GB, Klein HA, Hiratzka T: IV. Correlation of electrocardiographic and pathologic findings in infarction of the interventricular septum and right ventricle. Am Heart J 37:720, 1949.

111. Myers GB, Klein HA, Stofer BE: VII. Correlation of electrocardiographic and pathologic findings in lateral infarction. Am Heart J 37:374, 1949.

112. Levine HD, Philips E: An appraisal of the newer electrocardiography: correlations in one hundred and fifty consecutive autopsied cases. N Engl J Med 245:833, 1951.

113. Paton BC: The accuracy of diagnosis of myocardial infarction: a clinicopathologic study. Am J Med 23:761, 1957.

114. Woods JD, Laurie W, Smith WG: The reliability of the electrocardiogram in myocardial infarction. Lancet 2:265, 1963.

115. Sigurdsson E, Thorgeirsson G, Sigvaldson H, et al: Unrecognized myocardial infarction: epidemiology, clinical characteristics, and the prognostic role of angina pectoris: a Reykjavik study. Ann Intern Med 122:96, 1995.

116. Sheifer SE, Manolio TA, Gersh BJ: Unrecognized myocardial infarction. Ann Intern Med 135:801, 2001.

117. Gunnar RM, Pietras RJ, Blackaller J, et al: Correlation of vectorcardiographic criteria for myocardial infarction with autopsy findings. Circulation 35:158, 1967.

118. Horan LG, Flowers NC, Johnson JC: Significance of the diagnostic Q wave of myocardial infarction. Circulation 43:428, 1971.

118a. Das MK, Khan B, Jacob S, et al: Significance of a fragmented QRS complex versus a Q wave in patients with coronary artery disease. Circulation 113:2495, 2006.

119. Selvester RH, Solomon JC, Gillespie TL: Digital computer model of a total body electrocardiographic surface map. Circulation 38:684, 1968.

120. Wagner GS, Freye CJ, Palmeri ST, et al: Evaluation of a QRS scoring system for estimating myocardial

infarction size. I. Specificity and observer agreement. Circulation 65:342, 1982.

121. Pahlm O, Haisty WK Jr, Wagner NB, et al: Specificity and sensitivity of QRS criteria for diagnosis of single and multiple myocardial infarcts. Am J Cardiol 68:1300, 1991.

122. Ideker RE, Wagner GS, Ruth WK, et al: Evaluation of a QRS scoring system for estimating myocardial infarct size. II. Correlation with quantitative anatomic findings for anterior infarcts. Am J Cardiol 49:1604, 1982.

123. Roark SE, Ideker RE, Wagner GS, et al: Evaluation of a QRS scoring system for estimating myocardial infarct size. III. Correlation with quantitative anatomic findings for inferior infarcts. Am J Cardiol 51:382, 1983.

124. Palmeri ST, Harrison DG, Cobb FR, et al: A QRS scoring system for assessing left ventricular function after myocardial infarction. N Engl J Med 306:4, 1982.

125. Ward RM, White RD, Ideker RE, et al: Evaluation of a QRS scoring system for estimating myocardial infarct size. III. Correlation with quantitative anatomic findings for posterolateral infarcts. Am J Cardiol 53:706, 1984.

126. Sevilla DC, Wagner NB, Pegues R, et al: Correlation of the complete version of the Selvester QRS scoring system with quantitative anatomic findings for multiple left ventricular myocardial infarcts. Am J Cardiol 69:465, 1992.

127. Pahlm US, Chaitman BR, Rautaharju PM, et al: Comparison of the various electrocardiographic scoring codes for estimating anatomically documented sizes of single and multiple infarcts of the left ventricle. Am J Cardiol 81:809, 1998.

128. Cowan MJ, Bruce RA, Reichenbach DD: Validation of a computerized QRS criterion for estimating myocardial infarction size and correlation with quantitative morphologic measurements. Am J Cardiol 57:60, 1986.

129. Aldrich HR, Wagner NB, Boswick J, et al: Use of initial ST segment deviation for prediction of final electrocardiographic size of acute myocardial infarction. Am J Cardiol 61:749, 1988.

130. Wilkins ML, Maynard C, Annex BH, et al: Admission prediction of expected final myocardial infarct size using weighted ST-segment, Q wave, and T wave measurements. J Electrocardiol 30:1, 1997.

131. Mikell FL, Petrovich J, Snyder MC, et al: Reliability of Q wave formation and QRS score in predicting regional and global left ventricular performance in acute myocardial infarction with successful reperfusion. Am J Cardiol 57:923, 1986.

132. Christian TF, Clements JP, Behrenbeck T, et al: Limitations of the electrocardiogram in estimating infarction size after acute reperfusion therapy for myocardial infarction. Ann Intern Med 114:264, 1991.

133. Giannuzzi P, Giozdano A, Imparato A, et al: Reliability of standard electrocardiogram in detecting left ventricular asynergy in 315 patients with recent myocardial infarction. Clin Cardiol 10:105, 1987.

134. Fioretti P, Tijssen JG, Azar AJ, et al: Prognostic value of predischarge 12 lead electrocardiogram after myocardial infarction compared with other routine clinical variables. Br Heart J 57:306, 1987.

135. Juergens CP, Fernandes C, Hasche ET, et al: Electrocardiographic measurement of infarct size after thrombolytic therapy. J Am Coll Cardiol 27:617, 1996.

136. Conde CA, Meller J, Espinoza J, et al: Disappearance of abnormal Q waves after aortocoronary bypass surgery. Am J Cardiol 36:889, 1975.

137. Bateman TM, Czar LSS, Gray RJ, et al: Transient pathologic Q waves during ischemic events: an electrocardiographic correlate of stunned but viable myocardium. Am Heart J 106:1421, 1983.

138. Bassan MM, Oatfield R, Hoffman I, et al: New Q waves after aortocoronary bypass surgery. N Engl J Med 290:349, 1974.

139. Zeft HJ, Freedberg HD, King JF, et al: Reappearance of anterior QRS forces after coronary bypass surgery. Am J Cardiol 36:163, 1975.

140. Freedman SB, Dunn RF, Bernstein K, et al: Influence of coronary collateral blood flow on the development of exertional ischemia and Q wave infarction in patients with severe single-vessel disease. Circulation 71:681, 1985.

141. Hutchins GM, Bulkley BH: Infarct expansion versus extension: two different complications of acute myocardial infarction. Am J Cardiol 41:1127, 1978.

142. Anderson CI, Harrison DG, Stack NC, et al: Evaluation of serial QRS changes during acute inferior myocardial infarction using a QRS scoring system. Am J Cardiol 52:252, 1983.

143. Haiat R, Chiche P: Transient abnormal Q waves in the course of ischemic heart disease. Chest 65:140, 1974.

144. Nohara R, Kambara H, Suzuki Y, et al: Septal Q wave in exercise testing: evaluation by single-photon emission computed tomography. Am J Cardiol 55:905, 1985.

145. Meller J, Conde CA, Donoso E, et al: Transient Q waves in Prinzmetal's angina. Am J Cardiol 35:691, 1975.

146. Albert DE, Califf RM, Lecocq DA, et al: Comparative rates of resolution of QRS changes after operative and nonoperative acute myocardial infarcts. Am J Cardiol 51:378, 1983.

147. Krone RJ, Greenberg H, Dwyer EM, et al: Long-term prognostic significance of ST segment depression during acute myocardial infarction. J Am Coll Cardiol 22:361, 1993.

148. Stone PH, Raabe DS, Jaffe AS, et al: Prognostic significance of location and type of myocardial infarction: independent adverse outcome associated with anterior location. J Am Coll Cardiol 11:453, 1988.

149. Klein LW, Helfant RH: The Q-wave and non–Q wave myocardial infarction: differences and similarities. Prog Cardiovasc Dis 29:205, 1986.

150. Birnbaum Y, Chetrit A, Sclarovsky S, et al: Abnormal Q waves on the admission electrocardiogram of patients with first myocardial infarction: prognostic implications. Clin Cardiol 20:472, 1997.

151. Hands ME, Lloyd BL, Robinson JS, et al: Prognostic significance of electrocardiographic site of infarction after correction for enzymatic size of infarction. Circulation 73:885, 1986.

152. Willems JL, Willems RJ, Willems GM, et al: Significance of initial ST segment elevation and depression for the management of thrombolytic therapy in acute myocardial infarction. Circulation 82:1147, 1990.

153. Birnbaum Y, Sclarovsky S, Herz I: Admission clinical and electrocardiographic characteristics predicting in-hospital development of high-degree atrioventricular block in inferior acute myocardial infarction. Am J Cardiol 80:1134, 1997.

154. O'Rourke RA: Treatment of right ventricular infarction: thrombolytic therapy, coronary angioplasty, or neither?. J Am Coll Cardiol 37:882, 1998.

155. Birnbaum Y, Herz I, Sclarovsky S, et al: Prognostic significance of the admission electrocardiogram in acute myocardial infarction. J Am Coll Cardiol 27:1128, 1996.

156. Hochrein J, Sun F, Pieper KS, et al: Higher T-wave amplitude associated with better prognosis in patients receiving thrombolytic therapy for acute myocardial infarction (a GUSTO-I Substudy). Am J Cardiol 81:1078, 1998.

157. Sclarovsky-Benjaminov F, Sclarovsky S, Birnbaum Y: The predictive value of the electrocardiographic pattern of acute Q-wave myocardial infarction for recurrent ischemia. Clin Cardiol 18:710, 1995.

158. Maeda S, Imai T, Kuboki K, et al: Pathologic implications of restored positive T waves and persistent negative T waves after Q wave myocardial infarction. J Am Coll Cardiol 28:1514, 1996.

159. Tamura A, Nagase K, Mikuriya Y, et al: Significance of spontaneous normalization of negative T waves in infarct-related leads during healing of anterior wall acute myocardial infarction. Am J Cardiol 84:1341, 1999.

160. Go AS, Barron HV, Rundle AC, et al: Bundle-branch block and in-hospital mortality in acute myocardial infarction. Ann Intern Med 129:690, 1998.

161. Sgarbossa EB, Pinski SI, Topol EJ, et al: Acute myocardial infarction and complete bundle branch block at hospital admission: characteristics and outcome in the thrombolytic era. J Am Coll Cardiol 31:105, 1998.

162. Sgarbossa EB, Pinski SL, Gates KB, et al: Predictors of in-hospital bundle branch block reversion after presenting with acute myocardial infarction and bundle branch block. Am J Cardiol 82:373, 1998.

163. Simons GR, Sgarbossa E, Wagner G, et al: Atrioventricular and intraventricular conduction disorders in acute myocardial infarction: a reappraisal in the thrombolytic era. PACE 22:2651, 1998.

164. Kosuge M, Kimura K, Ishikawa T, et al: Clinical features of patients with reperfused inferior wall acute myocardial infarction complicated by early complete atrioventricular block. Am J Cardiol 88:1187, 2001.

165. Mauri F, Franzosi MG, Maggioni AP, et al: Clinical value of 12-lead electrocardiography to predict the long-term prognosis of GISSI-1 patients. J Am Coll Cardiol 39:1549, 2002.

166. Yerra L, Anevakar N, Skali H, et al: Association of QRS duration and outcomes after myocardial infarction: the VALIANT trial. Heart Rhythm 3:313, 2006.

167. Elhendy A, Hamill SC, Mahoney DW, et al: Relation of QRS duration on the surface 12-lead electrocardiogram with mortality in patients with known or suspected coronary artery disease. Am J Cardiol 96:1082, 2005.

168. Brilakis ES, Wright RS, Kopecky SL, et al: Bundle branch block as a predictor of long-term survival after acute myocardial infarction. Am J Cardiol 88:205, 2001.

168a. Wong C-K, Gao W, Stewart RAH, et al: Risk stratification of patients with acute anterior myocardial infarction and right bundle branch block. Importance of QRS duration and early ST-segment resolution after fibrinolytic therapy. Circulation 114:783, 2006.

169. Bar FW, Brugada P, Dassen WR, et al: Prognostic value of Q waves, R/S ratio, loss of R wave voltage, ST-T segment abnormalities, electrical axis, low voltage and notching: correlation of electrocardiogram and left ventriculogram. J Am Coll Cardiol 4:17, 1984.

170. Miller RR, Amsterdam EA, Bogren HG, et al: Electrocardiographic and cineangiographic correlations in assessment of the location, nature and extent of abnormal left ventricular segmental contraction in coronary artery disease. Circulation 449:447, 1974.

171. Bodenheimer MM, Banka VS, Helfant RH: Q waves and ventricular asynergy: predictive value and hemodynamic

significance of anatomic localization. Am J Cardiol 35:615, 1975.

172. Dubnow MH, Burchell HB, Titus JL: Post-infarction ventricular aneurysm: a clinicopathologic and electrocardiographic study of 80 cases. Am Heart J 70:753, 1965.

173. Frances C, Romero A, Grady D: Left ventricular pseudoaneurysm. J Am Coll Cardiol 32:537, 1998.

174. Cokkinos DV, Hallman GL, Cooley DA, et al: Left ventricular aneurysm: analysis of electrocardiographic features and postresection changes. Am Heart J 82:149, 1971.

175. Cinca J, Bardaji A, Carreno A, et al: ST segment elevation at the surface of a healed myocardial infarction in pigs: conditions for passive transmission from the ischemic peri-infarction zone. Circulation 91:1552, 1995.

176. Oliva PB, Hammill SC, Edwards WD: Cardiac rupture, a clinically predictable complication of acute myocardial infarction: report of 70 cases with clinicopathologic correlations. J Am Coll Cardiol 22:720, 1993.

177. Yoshino H, Yotsukara M, Yano K, et al: Cardiac rupture and admission electrocardiography in acute anterior myocardial infarction: implication of ST elevation in aV$_L$. J Electrocardiol 33:49, 2000.

178. Hayashi T, Hirano Y, Takai H, et al: Usefulness of ST-segment elevation in the inferior leads in predicting ventricular septal rupture in patients with anterior wall acute myocardial infarction. Am J Cardiol 96:1037, 2005.

179. Figueras J, Curos A, Cortodellas J, et al: Relevance of electrocardiographic findings, heart failure, and infarct site in assessing risk and timing of left ventricular free wall rupture during acute myocardial infarction. Am J Cardiol 76:543, 1995.

180. Solodky A, Behar S, Herz I, et al: Comparison of incidence of cardiac rupture among patients with acute myocardial infarction treated by thrombolysis versus percutaneous transluminal coronary angioplasty. Am J Cardiol 87:1105, 2001.

181. Birnbaum Y, Wagner GS, Gates KB, et al: Clinical and electrocardiographic variables associated with increased risk of ventricular septal defect in acute anterior myocardial infarction. Am J Cardiol 86:830, 2000.

182. Pfeffer MA, Braunwald E: Ventricular remodeling after myocardial infarction: experimental observations and clinical implications. Circulation 81:1161, 1990.

183. Bigi R, Mafrici A, Colombo P, et al: Relation of terminal QRS distortion to left ventricular functional recovery and remodeling in acute myocardial infarction treated with primary angioplasty. Am J Cardiol 96:1233, 2005.

184. Siilvet H, Amin J, Padmanabhan S, et al: Prognostic implications of increased QRS duration in patients with moderate and severe left ventricular systolic dysfunction. Am J Cardiol 88:182, 2001.

185. Lancellotti P, Kulbertus HE, Pierard LA: Predictors of rapid QRS widening in patients with coronary artery disease and left ventricular dysfunction. Am J Cardiol 93:1410, 2004.

186. Harding JD, Piacentino VIII, Gaughan JP, et al: Electrophysiological alterations after mechanical circulatory support in patients with advanced cardiac failure. Circulation 104:1241, 2001.

187. Perloff JK, Roberts WC, De Leon AC, et al: The distinctive electrocardiogram of Duchenne's progressive muscular dystrophy. Am J Med 42:179, 1967.

188. Sanyal SK, Johnson WW, Thapar MK, et al: An ultrastructural basis for electrocardiographic alterations

associated with Duchenne's progressive muscular dystrophy. Circulation 57:1122, 1978.

189. Hejtmancik MR, Bradfield JY, Miller GV: Myocarditis and Friedreich's ataxia. Am Heart J 38:757, 1948.

190. Goldman AM: Acute myocarditis simulating myocardial infarction. Dis Chest 41:61, 1962.

191. Buja LM, Khoi NB, Roberts WC: Clinically significant cardiac amyloidosis. Am J Cardiol 26:394, 1970.

192. Harris TR, Copeland GD, Brody DA: Progressive injury current with metastatic tumor of the heart: case report and review of the literature. Am Heart J 69:392, 1965.

193. Wigle ED, Baron RH: The electrocardiogram in muscular subaortic stenosis: effect of a left septal incision and right bundle-branch block. Circulation 34:585, 1966.

194. Braudo M, Wigle ED, Keith JD: A distinctive electrocardiogram in muscular subaortic stenosis due to ventricular septal hypertrophy. Am J Cardiol 14:599, 1964.

195. Lemery R, Kleinebenne A, Nihoyanopoulos P, et al: Q waves in hypertrophic cardiomyopathy in relation to the distribution and severity of right and left ventricular hypertrophy. J Am Coll Cardiol 16:368, 1990.

196. Savage DD, Seides SF, Clark CE, et al: Electrocardiographic findings in patients with obstructive and nonobstructive hypertrophic cardiomyopathy. Circulation 58:402, 1978.

197. Maron BF, Wolfson JK, Ciro E, et al: Relation of electrocardiographic abnormalities and patterns of left ventricular hypertrophy identified by 2-dimensional echocardiography in patients with hypertrophic cardiomyopathy. Am J Cardiol 51:189, 1983.

198. Goldberger AL: Q wave T wave vector discordance in hypertrophic cardiomyopathy: septal hypertrophy and strain pattern. Br Heart J 42:201, 1979.

199. Salem BI, Schnee M, Leatharman LL, et al: Electrocardiographic pseudo-infarction: appearance with a large posterior pericardial effusion after cardiac surgery. Am J Cardiol 42:681, 1978.

200. Surawicz B, Van Horne RG, Urbach JR, et al: QS and QR pattern in leads V_3 and V_4 in absence of myocardial infarction: electrocardiographic and vectorcardiographic study. Circulation 12:391, 1955.

201. Surawicz B: Abnormal electrocardiogram in the absence of heart disease. Proc Life Insur Med Directors Assoc 60:84, 1976.

202. Tuquan SK, Mau RD, Schwartz MJ: Anterior myocardial infarction patterns in the mitral valve prolapse systolic click syndrome. Am J Med 58:719, 1975.

203. McGinn S, White PD: Acute cor pulmonale resulting from pulmonary embolism: its clinical recognition. JAMA 104:1473, 1935.

204. Allen RD, Surawicz B: The electrocardiogram in pulmonary embolism. In: Mobin-Uddin K (ed): Pulmonary Thromboembolism. Springfield, IL, Charles C Thomas, 1973.

205. Lichtenberg SB, Schwartz MJ, Case RB: Value of premature ventricular contraction morphology in the detection of myocardial infarction. J Electrocardiol 13:167, 1980.

206. Wahl JM, Hakki AH, Iskandrian AS, et al: Limitations of premature ventricular complex morphology in the diagnosis of myocardial infarction. J Electrocardiol 19:131, 1986.

9

Non-Q Wave Myocardial Infarction, Non-ST Elevation Myocardial Infarction, Unstable Angina Pectoris, Myocardial Ischemia

Non-ST Elevation Myocardial Infarction (NSTEMI)

Non-Q Wave Myocardial Infarction (NQMI)
Variable Genesis of the NQMI Pattern
ECG Diagnosis of NQMI
Prognosis of Patients with NQMI

Unstable Angina Pectoris (UAP)
Categories of UAP
Severity and Extent of ECG Abnormalities

Repolarization Abnormalities Simulating Myocardial Ischemia
ST Segment Deviations
ST Segment Depression: Normal Variant

ST Segment Elevation in the Absence of Myocardial Ischemia
ST Segment Elevation after Myocardial Contusion

T Wave Abnormalities
Increased Amplitude of Upright T Wave
Syndrome X
Pericarditis
T Wave Abnormalities Attributed to Myocardial Damage
Variant Angina Pectoris

Silent Myocardial Ischemia

Atrial Infarction

The terms *non-Q wave myocardial infarction* (NQMI), *non-ST elevation myocardial infarction* (NSTEMI), *unstable angina pectoris* (UAP), and *myocardial ischemia* are often applied interchangeably to characterize clinical syndromes of acute ischemic heart disease. Yet each of these terms has a different meaning.

Myocardial ischemia is the substrate of NSTEMI, NQMI, and UAP. It must be documented by electrocardiographic (ECG) changes and supported by the evidence of perfusion defects or wall motion abnormalities. The ECG abnormalities during acute ischemic processes are not specific because they resemble the ECG abnormalities encountered in patients with chronic ischemic heart disease (e.g., in the presence of hibernating myocardium). Therefore the more reliable markers of instability are the changes in the ECG pattern rather than any particular fixed patterns.

The terms NQMI and NSTEMI differ from UAP by the presence of biochemically documented myocardial necrosis. In practice, it may be

difficult to determine whether the absence of cardiac enzyme or myocardial protein elevation denotes both previously and presently absent myocardial necrosis or a return to normal after a relatively recent event.

The term *angina* refers to a subjective awareness of myocardial ischemia. Yet it is well known that myocardial ischemia and MI can be painless or silent, which means that the absence of symptoms does not rule out NQMI, NSTEMI, or acute ischemia.

For these reasons, the information included in the presentation of a patient with an acute ischemic process should specify the character, duration, and stability of symptoms; the ECG findings; and the presence or absence of necrosis documented by a rise in cardiac enzyme or myocardial protein concentrations in blood. The availability of the echocardiographic, scintigraphic, or magnetic resonance imaging (MRI) data may further refine assessment of the ischemic pattern.

Non-ST Elevation Myocardial Infarction (NSTEMI)

The term NSTEMI has been applied to a subset of "coronary syndromes." The new nomenclature was introduced following the discovery of new biochemical markers of myocardial necrosis (troponins) and increasing use of new interventional approaches to treat the "unstable" coronary artery disease (CAD). The term NSTEMI defies precise electrocardiographic definition. The difference between UAP and NSTEMI is the difference between the absence and the presence of biochemical markers of myocardial necrosis, such as troponin, in the blood. A certain number of patients with NSTEMI develop Q waves.[1] Other problems defying accurate definition of NSTEMI include the inability to determine whether a transient ST elevation had preceded the first available ECG and the possibility of unrecognized ST segment elevation in some leads, particularly the lead aV_R. Moreover, it appears that new ST segment depression may be present in some patients with a diagnosis of NSTEMI, which requires the presence of ST segment elevation in some leads on the opposite side of the electrical field. Therefore NSTEMI does not describe an ECG pattern, but rather is a clinical diagnosis with variable ECG patterns. These patterns are exemplified in Figures 9–2, 9–4, 9–5, 9–6, 9–7 and 9–9 and discussed in the context of NQMI.

The reported factors affecting the prognosis of patients with NSTEMI include a.o. the extent of ST segment deviation,[2,3] ST segment depression in the lateral leads,[4] abnormal T waves,[5] and sustained ventricular arrhythmias.[6]

Non-Q Wave Myocardial Infarction (NQMI)

The term NQMI has replaced the former ECG diagnosis of subendocardial infarction because it has been amply established that the presence or absence of a Q wave does not depend on the localization of the MI. Q waves may be absent when the MI is "transmural" or, conversely, may be present when the infarction does not involve the full thickness of the ventricular wall.

Savage et al.[7] showed that even small subendocardial infarcts, involving only 10 to 20 percent of the ventricular thickness, can cause abnormal Q waves. Raunio and associates[8] described the pathologic findings in ECGs obtained 48 hours before death in 80 patients with MI. Abnormal Q waves were present in 8 of 15 patients (53 percent) with subendocardial infarction and in 42 of 65 patients (65 percent) with transmural MI. Similar findings were reported by Antaloczy et al.,[9] who correlated the ECG with pathologic data in 100 patients with MI.

With regard to coronary angiography, Kerensky et al.[10] reported that in patients with NQMI a single culprit lesion could be identified in 49 percent of patients, whereas in 37 percent of patients no angiographic culprit lesion was present; the remaining 14 percent had multiple lesions.

Similar to NSTEMI, the term NQMI correlates poorly with the clinical condition or with a defined pathologic substrate. Another drawback of the term is that it encompasses a heterogeneous group of ECG patterns (see later discussion).

Before the advent of thrombolytic therapy of MI, the reported prevalence of NQMI among patients with acute MI was in the range of 16 to 40 percent.[11–16] Roberts and Fromm[17] estimated that the proportion of patients with NQMI has been steadily increasing, with more than half of all infarctions now classified as NQMI, but the initial ECG is believed to provide a specific diagnosis in only about 5 percent of all patients presenting with chest pain to the emergency room.[17]

At the onset of MI it is difficult to predict whether a Q wave will develop. Boden et al.[18] studied serial ECGs in patients with acute NQMI confirmed by creatine kinase MB elevation to determine the percentage of patients with early ST segment elevation who would develop Q waves during the follow-up. They found that of 187 patients who exhibited ≥1 mm ST segment elevation in two or more contiguous leads, a Q wave evolved in 32 (20 percent). Of 252 patients with early ST segment depression, T wave inversion, or both, a Q wave evolved in 39 (15 percent). Thus in 80 percent of patients with and 85 percent of patients without ST segment elevation and absent Q waves on the admission ECG, Q waves did not develop during a subsequent 2-week period of observation.[18]

These findings contrast with the observations in patients undergoing thrombolytic therapy, in whom Q wave developed in about 80 percent with the initial ST segment elevation. Thus in the GUSTO study,[19] Q waves did not develop in 4601 (21.3 percent) of 21,510 patients with acute ST segment elevation. In a later GUSTO report[20] Q waves did not develop in 409 (20 percent) of 2046 patients with ST segment elevation undergoing thrombolytic therapy. The absence of Q wave development in the initial GUSTO study was associated with a lesser degree of anterior ST segment elevation.[19] Also, in the later report[20] patients who did not develop Q waves had a lesser degree of ST segment elevation in nonanterior locations, and their infarct-related artery was more likely to be nonanterior with a more distally located occlusion.

More recent correlations with cardiovascular magnetic resonance studies showed that the differentiation between Q wave and non-Q wave MI is useful in the determination of the total MI size, but not in defining whether MI is transmural or nontransmural.[21] Another study of Sievers et al.[22] also concluded that "transmural" and "nontransmural" MIs cannot be differentiated by ECG. Kaentrop et al.[23] showed that the best predictor of Q wave in the ECG was the quantified percent scar tissue. A cut-off value of 17 percent yielded a sensitivity and specificity of 90 percent to predict the presence vs. absence of Q wave.

VARIABLE GENESIS OF THE NQMI PATTERN

Some conditions responsible for the NQMI pattern include the following:

1. MI with a Q wave equivalent of R or R/S in the right precordial leads, which is an indication of posterolateral infarction, most often caused by circumflex artery disease
2. Development of a Q wave aborted by thrombolytic treatment or coronary angioplasty
3. Initial presentation of a progressive process with subsequent Q wave development

4. Resolution of coronary vasospasm
5. Subendocardial infarction
6. Other nontransmural infarcts
7. Q wave masked by left bundle branch block (LBBB) or preexcitation

Some factors responsible for the variable genesis of the NSTEMI pattern include:

1. Initial vs. recurrent event
2. Initial presentation preceded by a subsided ST segment elevation (transient normalization, or pseudonormalization) (see Figures 9–1 and 9–7)
3. Initial presentation with subsequent Q wave development
4. Predominant ST segment depression with unrecognized "reciprocal" ST elevation
5. Variable T wave changes
6. Variable preceding therapeutic interventions

ECG DIAGNOSIS OF NQMI

The ECG difference between Q wave MI and NQMI is not always clearly defined because some investigators consider cases with marked reduction of R wave amplitude to be Q wave infarctions.[24,25] Different definitions may account for some of the varying results obtained in the studies correlating the ECG with pathologic findings.[26]

The absence of universally, clearly defined QRS criteria makes it imperative to document the presence of evolutionary ST segment or T wave changes (or both). During the acute phase the ST segment may be elevated or depressed in the leads that face the epicardial surface of the infarcted area (Figures 9–1 and

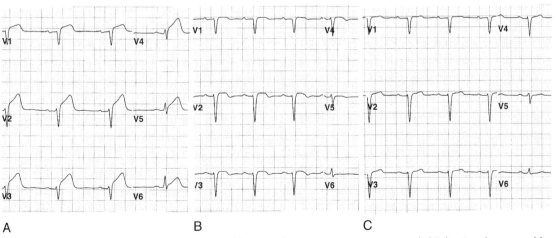

A   B   C

Figure 9–1   ECG precordial leads of a 52-year-old man with acute non-Q wave myocardial infarction documented by a rise in cardiac enzyme levels. **A,** ECG recorded on day 1 at 2:33 AM shows diffuse ST segment elevation. **B,** Next day at 6:35 AM. Note the T wave inversion in the leads with previous ST segment elevation. There was apical akinesis with an estimated left ventricular ejection fraction of 45 percent. **C,** Same day at 4:20 PM pseudonormalization of the ECG after emergency coronary angioplasty and placement of a stent into a subtotally occluded proximal left anterior descending artery.

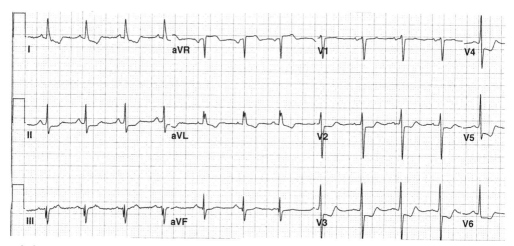

Figure 9–2 ECG of an 84-year-old woman with non-Q wave infarction documented by a rise in cardiac enzyme levels shows depression of the ST segment in leads I, II, aV$_L$, and V$_2$–V$_6$ and ST segment elevation in lead aV$_R$. Patient had severe three-vessel coronary artery disease with mild mid-anterior and distal inferior wall hypokinesis and an estimated left ventricular ejection fraction of 45 percent.

9–2). Among the 93 cases of NQMI studied by Ogawa et al.,[27] ST segment elevation was present in 35 (38 percent), ST segment depression in 49 (52 percent), and T wave changes alone in 9 (10 percent). Willich et al.[16] found ST segment elevation in 207 (61 percent) and ST segment depression in 97 (29 percent) in the initial ECG of 340 patients with NQMI.

The T wave inversion usually evolves in the leads with ST segment elevation or ST segment depression (Figures 9–3 and 9–4), and the T wave is often deeply inverted. NQMI is one of the most common causes of the so-called giant negative T waves (see Chapter 23).

The extent and magnitude of T wave abnormalities produced by NQMI correlate poorly with the extent and severity of coronary artery disease. To illustrate this, I have selected four cases of NQMI that have similar ECG abnormalities but different pathology of the coronary arteries: severe four-vessel coronary artery disease (Figure 9–5), occlusion of the proximal left anterior

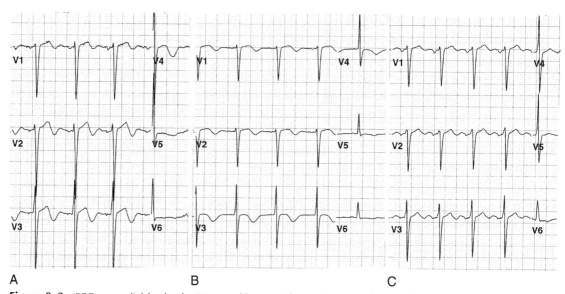

Figure 9–3 ECG precordial leads of a 72-year-old man with non-Q wave infarction documented by a rise in cardiac enzyme levels. **A,** Day of infarction. Note the slight ST segment elevation with terminal T wave inversion and a QTc of 577 ms. **B,** Following day. Note the T wave inversion without ST segment elevation. **C,** Following day. ECG is nearly normal. Patient had 90 percent ostial stenosis of the left anterior descending artery. Ventriculography was not performed because of renal insufficiency.

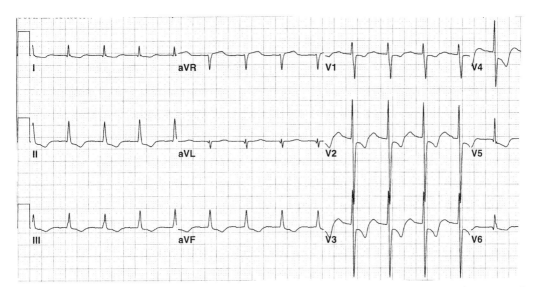

Figure 9–4   ECG of an 85-year-old woman with non-Q wave infarction documented by a rise in cardiac enzyme levels and associated with pulmonary edema on admission. Note the ST segment depression with pointed inverted T waves and prominent upright U waves in leads V_1–V_4. Echocardiogram revealed moderately severe left ventricular wall motion abnormalities, with an estimated left ventricular ejection fraction of 40 percent, moderately severe aortic stenosis, aortic regurgitation, and mitral regurgitation with a pulmonary artery pressure of 70 mmHg.

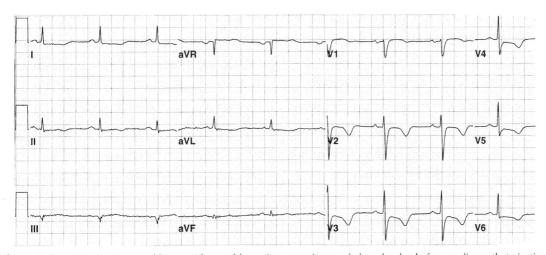

Figure 9–5   ECG of a 74-year-old man with unstable angina pectoris recorded on the day before cardiac catheterization. The latter showed extensive four-vessel disease with 95 percent distal left main stenosis, 90 percent proximal left anterior descending artery stenosis, total obstruction of the left circumflex artery at the ostium, total occlusion of the dominant right coronary artery at the mid-level, and abundant collateral circulation. Ventriculography showed mild anterior apical hypokinesis.

descending (LAD) artery (see Figure 9–3), occlusion of the LAD coronary artery at midlevel (Figure 9–6), and absence of coronary obstructive lesions (Figure 9–8). The extent of myocardial involvement cannot be predicted from the magnitude and extent of T wave abnormalities. For example, Figure 9–9 shows an ECG of a patient with severe disease of the dominant left circumflex artery causing severe hypokinesis of the inferior and lateral wall, with relatively minor T wave abnormalities limited to leads I and aV_L.

In most cases, the T wave abnormalities tend to persist longer than the ST segment deviations. Kloner reported that negative T waves became normal concurrently with the disappearance of wall motion abnormalities within 6 months after coronary angioplasty, presumably owing to

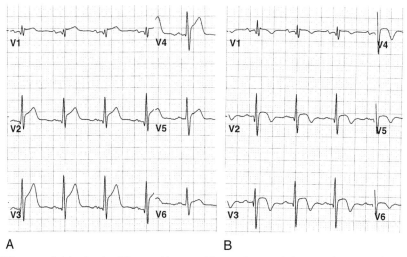

Figure 9–6   ECG precordial leads of a 75-year-old man with non-Q wave infarction documented by a rise in cardiac enzyme levels. **A,** Day of infarction. Note the ST segment elevation. QTc was 399 ms. **B,** At 1 hour 6 minutes later there was less T segment elevation and T wave inversion. QTc was 440 ms. Patient had 95 percent stenosis of the left anterior descending artery at the mid-level, with involvement of two diagonal branches, 60 percent stenosis of the right coronary artery, and anterior apical hypokinesis.

recovery of the stunned (hypoperfused) or hibernating (damaged but capable of recovery) myocardium.[28] In parallel with the advances in management of the acute coronary syndromes, one more often observes rapid regression of T wave abnormalities caused by the NQMI (see Figure 9–3).

PROGNOSIS OF PATIENTS WITH NQMI

In the past, patients with NQMI were considered potentially unstable, having late morbidity and mortality rates similar to those in patients with Q wave MI.[29] This perception has changed recently with the changing modes of treatment. It has been shown that in patients undergoing thrombolytic therapy, the 30-day and 1-year prognoses were better in those without than those with subsequent Q wave development.[19]

Unstable Angina Pectoris (UAP)

There is no sharp line that distinguishes stable from unstable forms of angina pectoris, but in most patients with symptomatic ischemic heart disease, the presence or absence of stability can be established by the history and the ECG. Angina can be defined as stable if it occurs relatively infrequently and is predictably provoked by circumstances that increase the myocardial oxygen demand above a certain threshold defined by the metabolic equivalents of task

(METs) or the product of heart rate blood pressure. The ECG changes during the episodes of stable angina pectoris are usually reproducible during a stress test and most often consist of horizontal or downsloping ST segment depression in several leads. These changes are sometimes accompanied by T wave inversion in the leads with downsloping ST segment depression. Both ST and T changes return to normal within a relatively short time during recovery from the stress.

The vector of abnormal T waves tends to be directed away from the area of abnormal (i.e., prolonged) repolarization. This means that the T wave becomes negative in leads I, aV_L, V_5, and V_6 in the presence of anterolateral ischemia; leads V_1–V_3 in the presence of a less extensive anterior ischemia; leads II, III, and aV_F in the presence of inferior ischemia; and upright in the right precordial leads in the presence of posterior ischemia. The correlation between the distribution of the T wave abnormalities and localization of myocardial ischemia, however, is not as reliable as the correlation between the distribution of Q waves and the location of the MI.

Reversible U wave inversion, if present, is a specific sign of myocardial ischemia (Figure 9–10). The QRS duration is often transiently increased during an anginal attack, and in one study[30] it was observed in 70 percent of patients in the signal-averaged ECG (see Chapter 1).

The ECG changes during the episodes of UAP tend to be more pronounced, involving more

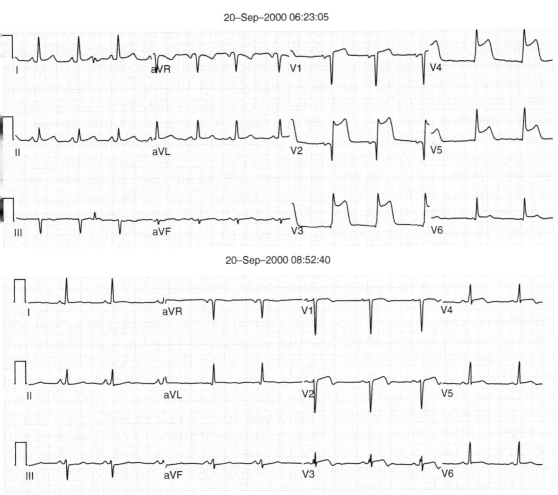

Figure 9–7   ECG of a 40-year-old woman with isolated 80% narrowing of the left anterior descending coronary artery and no other abnormalities of the major coronary artery branches. Cardiac catheterization revealed mild anterior hypokinesis with an estimated left ventricular ejection fraction of 50 percent. *Top:* Pattern of ST elevation myocardial infarction (STEMI) with Q waves in leads V_1–V_2. *Bottom:* 2.5 hours later, Q waves are absent and ST elevation is nearly subsided. Because of the elevated troponin level, the myocardial infarction was classified as NSTEMI.

leads and persisting for longer periods of time than those occurring in the presence of stable angina. In particular, the T wave inversion tends to persist after regression of the ST segment depression. Transient ST segment elevation during the ischemic episodes occurs infrequently but more often during episodes of unstable angina than stable angina. The diagnosis of UAP is supported by the occurrence of symptoms at rest, when the angina wakes the patient during sleep, and when the attacks have a repetitive pattern.

CATEGORIES OF UAP

Braunwald[31] categorized UAP on the basis of severity of symptoms and the clinical setting. In the category of symptoms, a score of 1 is assigned

to UAP with no pain at rest, a score of 2 to UAP with remote pain at rest occurring more than 48 hours before angiography, and a score of 3 to recent symptoms at rest occurring less than 48 hours before angiography. In the category of settings, the three scores, in progressive order, are UAP secondary to noncardiac condition, primary UAP, and UAP early after MI. Multivariate regression analysis identified the UAP score based on this classification as the most important predictor of intracoronary thrombus and lesion complexity.[32] Subsequently, patients with a score 3 were subclassified into troponin-positive and troponin-negative groups, with the former being at greater risk of MI and cardiac death.[34]

In terms of pathogenesis, Braunwald[33] identified the following five different, but not mutually

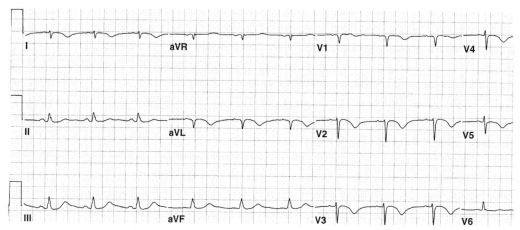

Figure 9–8   ECG of a 50-year-old woman 1 day after the onset of a non-Q wave infarction documented by a rise in cardiac enzyme levels. It shows diffuse T wave abnormalities and prolonged QTc (511 ms). Patient had normal coronary arteries and mild anterolateral wall motion abnormality, with an estimated left ventricular ejection fraction of 55 percent.

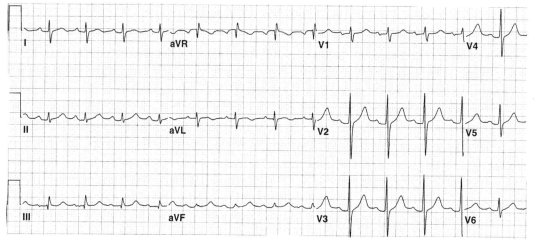

Figure 9–9   ECG of a 45-year-old man recorded 12 hours after the onset of a non-Q wave infarction documented by a rise in cardiac enzyme levels. Note the shift terminal T wave inversion in leads I and aV$_L$. Patient had single coronary artery disease with complete occlusion of the first obtuse marginal branch and 70 percent stenosis of the left circumflex artery at mid-level. There was severe hypokinesis of the inferolateral wall.

exclusive, causes of UAP: (1) nonocclusive thrombus superimposed on preexisting plaque; (2) progressive mechanical obstruction; (3) dynamic obstruction; (4) secondary to increased myocardial oxygen consumption; and (5) inflammation/infection.

SEVERITY AND EXTENT OF ECG ABNORMALITIES

Gorgels and associates[35] correlated the ECG changes during angina pectoris at rest with the findings during coronary angiography. They found that the number of leads with ST segment deviation and the magnitude of ST segment deviation during chest pain at rest showed a positive correlation with the number of diseased coronary arteries. In patients with left main or three-vessel coronary artery disease, the ST segment depression was often present in leads I, II, and V$_4$–V$_6$ and ST segment elevation in lead aV$_R$. When the sum of the ST segment deviations in these leads was >12 mm, the positive predictive accuracy for left main or three-vessel coronary artery disease was 86 percent.[35]

Klootwijk et al.[36] calculated the ischemic burden using computer-assisted monitoring during UAP in 12 ECG leads to assess the results of

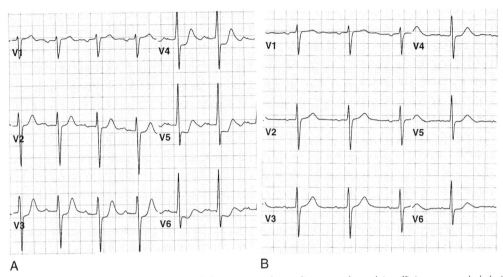

Figure 9–10 ECG of an 84-year-old man with hypertensive heart disease and renal insufficiency recorded during an attack of angina pectoris (**A**) and 7 hours later after treatment with intravenous nitroglycerin (**B**). Note the ST segment depression associated with negative U waves, best seen in leads V_5 and V_6 (**A**) and the return to normal after treatment (**B**).

the treatment of ischemia. The burden was expressed as the sum of the area under the curve of the ST vector magnitude trend of all episodes per patient or the sum of the areas under the curves of 12 leads during the episodes.[36]

The diagnosis of UAP has two contrasting aspects. On one hand, it is a frequent precursor of MI, as implied by the commonly used designation "preinfarction angina." At the same time, UAP is believed to convey some protection by promoting a collateral circulation and the phenomenon of preconditioning.[37,38] As an example of possible protection, Shiraki et al.[39] found that preinfarction angina was an independent predictor of the absence of right ventricular infarction in patients with acute inferior MI caused by right coronary artery occlusion.[39]

Repolarization Abnormalities Simulating Myocardial Ischemia

ST SEGMENT DEVIATIONS

The mechanism of ST deviation caused by the systolic and diastolic currents of injury during myocardial ischemia is discussed in Chapter 7. Injury current, however, is not the only mechanism of ST segment deviation from the baseline.[40]

Careful inspection of any normal ECG complex of large amplitude or of a sufficiently amplified complex reveals that the earliest portion of the ST segment normally deviates from the baseline. This phenomenon is explained by the various stages of ventricular repolarization during this period. The myocardial fibers depolarized during the early QRS portion are at a more advanced stage of repolarization than those depolarized during the late QRS portion. This creates potential differences after the end of the QRS complex before all fibers achieve the same level of plateau potential. This is shown in Figure 7–1A, where the ventricular complex of the ECG is derived from the potential differences between two action potentials hypothetically attributed to the first and last ventricular fibers depolarized during the recording of a single QRS complex. In this derived ECG, configuration of the ST segment and T wave is determined by the potential differences during repolarization. Small differences at the very onset of repolarization may be expected to cause deviation of the junction (i.e., J depression) and the early portion of the ST segment. For this reason it is customary to measure the magnitude of the ST segment deviation approximately 60 to 80 ms after the end of the QRS complex when all ventricular fibers are expected to be depolarized to the same level of membrane potential, forming an isoelectric ST segment followed by the onset of rapid repolarization, which initiates the T wave.

The deviation of the ST segment becomes more pronounced when the duration of the QRS complex increases. Figure 7–1C shows the postulated mechanism of repolarization abnormalities secondary to conduction delay, indicated by the increased duration of the interval between upstrokes of the two action potentials. The longer duration of the QRS complex enhances the potential differences during the entire course of repolarization because a larger number of early depolarized fibers begins to pass through the rapid phase of repolarization while the fibers that are depolarized late are still at the level of the plateau. In this diagram the potential difference (indicated by the arrow) persists throughout the repolarization phase; therefore the entire ST segment deviates from the baseline. This is known as *secondary deviation of the ST segment.* Secondary ST segment changes are most often encountered in the presence of ventricular hypertrophy and LBBB patterns and are usually accompanied by secondary T wave changes.

Another cause of abnormal ST segment deviation results from primary repolarization abnormalities at the cellular level when the slope of repolarization during the plateau is steeper than normal, as shown in Figure 7–1C. This may cause deviation of the ST segment from the baseline in the absence of ischemia or changes in the sequence of depolarization. The short ventricular action potential with a steep slope of repolarization shown in Figure 7–1C may be caused by digitalis or tachycardia. The exercise-induced ST segment depression during tachycardia in the absence of myocardial ischemia can be attributed to such a mechanism.

In addition, depression of the ST segment may be caused by a negative T wave of the P wave (Tp), which corresponds to the time period between the two arrows in Figure 7–3 (lower right). This figure shows that the negative Tp wave causes a downsloping course of the PR segment, which helps recognize the mechanism of the depressed ST junction. The same mechanism explains ST segment elevation caused by an upright Tp wave following a negative P wave[41] (see Figure 7–6).

ST SEGMENT DEPRESSION: NORMAL VARIANT

A slightly downsloping or horizontal ST segment depression may occur as a normal variant in the absence of myocardial ischemia, drugs, hypokalemia, or secondary repolarization abnormalities. On the routine ECG at rest, this occurs more commonly in women than in young or middle-aged men[42–44] (Figure 9–11). During ambulatory monitoring, however, transient ST segment depression from 0.1 to 0.4 mV, lasting 30 seconds to 2 hours, was recorded in 15 of 50 normal male volunteers aged 35 to 59 years.[45] ST segment depression in the absence of demonstrable myocardial ischemia during exercise is a common finding, with a higher prevalence in women than in young or middle-aged men (Figure 9–12). False-positive exercise tests are discussed in Chapter 10.

ST SEGMENT ELEVATION IN THE ABSENCE OF MYOCARDIAL ISCHEMIA

The most common cause of ST segment elevation unrelated to myocardial ischemia is secondary ST segment elevation in the right precordial leads in the presence of left ventricular hypertrophy or an

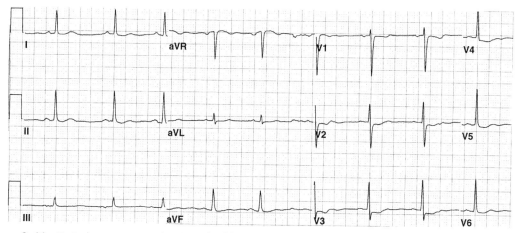

Figure 9–11   Typical common normal variant of mild ST segment depression with low T waves; this pattern is more prevalent in women than in men. ECG of a 45-year-old woman who had no evidence of heart or coronary artery disease. During treadmill exercise there was no increase in ST segment depression, but the T wave amplitude increased.

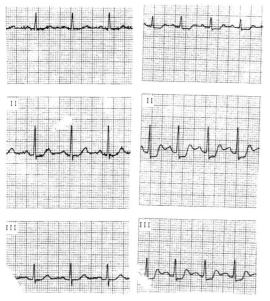

Figure 9–12 Selected ECG leads before and during exercise of a 62-year-old woman who had a normal increase of contractility in all segments of the left ventricle on the echocardiogram after exercise.

LBBB pattern. Other causes are discussed in Chapter 7.

ST SEGMENT ELEVATION AFTER MYOCARDIAL CONTUSION

Abnormal ECGs were found to correlate directly with complications of blunt cardiac trauma requiring treatment, whereas normal ECG and CPK-MB correlated with lack of clinically significant complications.[46,47] ECG changes simulating Q wave MI and NQMI have been encountered with T wave abnormalities and ST segment elevation.[48] An example of diffuse ST elevation caused by blunt chest trauma following airbag deployment in a patient with presumably normal coronary arteries is shown in Figure 9–13. Also see Chapter 12.

T Wave Abnormalities

In the differential diagnosis of an abnormal T wave, the following T wave characteristics suggest the presence of myocardial ischemia or NQMI: (1) the T wave is preceded by a horizontal ST segment; (2) the T wave is nearly symmetric and deep; (3) T wave abnormalities occur in several contiguous leads; and (4) the QT interval is prolonged. The specificity of the diagnosis increases with an increasing number of these features. Nevertheless, the diagnosis of myocardial ischemia should not be based exclusively on the characteristics of T wave changes without other supporting evidence because conditions other than myocardial ischemia can produce similar T wave abnormalities (see later discussion and Chapter 23).

INCREASED AMPLITUDE OF UPRIGHT T WAVE

Tall "hyperacute" T waves occasionally recorded at the very early stage of acute MI (see Figure 7–39A) are seldom seen during UAP. If present, they are most commonly present in the precordial leads.[49] The QT interval is usually prolonged. In the presence of myocardial ischemia

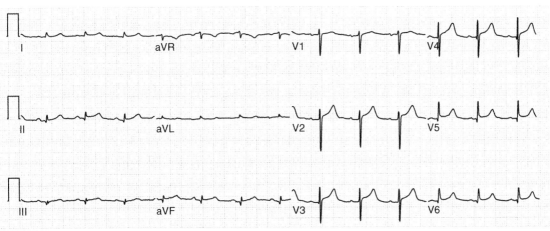

Figure 9–13 Myocardial contusion. ECG of an 84-year-old woman admitted with chest pain following a motor vehicle accident in which the airbag was released. ECG shows diffuse ST elevation, which subsided within 2 days (not shown). Echocardiogram was normal.

of the inferior wall, tall upright T waves in the precordial leads represent either reciprocal changes or myocardial ischemia of the posterior wall.

Prominent T waves are often seen as a normal variant (see Figure 1–20) in healthy individuals, predominantly at a young age, in males, and at slow heart rates, sometimes in association with ST segment elevation. To my knowledge there is no upper normal limit of T wave amplitude. Some of the other conditions associated with tall upright T waves are hyperkalemia, in which the T wave is usually pointed and narrow (see Chapter 22), and intracranial hemorrhage (see Chapter 22).

SYNDROME X

The label *syndrome X* has been pinned to several groups of patients who have in common angina-like chest pain and no evidence of obstructive disease in the large coronary artery branches. In some of these patients there is evidence of myocardial ischemia induced by stress or abnormal vasomobility of coronary microvessels. Some individuals with syndrome X have inverted T waves in many leads. In one study of such patients, the presence of symmetric inverted T waves at rest was associated with a coronary vasoconstrictor response to a cold pressor test.[50] In other studies, evidence of myocardial ischemia was present in some but not all patients with syndrome X and abnormal T waves. Also, the presence of stress-induced ST segment depression in patients with syndrome X occurs with and without evidence of myocardial ischemia. Lactate metabolism, oxygen saturation in the coronary sinus, regional myocardial perfusion, and left ventricular wall motion in these patients may be normal or abnormal.[50–55]

PERICARDITIS

Unlike myocardial ischemia, the interval between the nadir of the negative T wave and T end of the wave is usually not prolonged, and the duration of the QTc interval is normal.[56] The direction of the T wave vector in pericarditis suggests prolongation of activity in the damaged fibers. Histologic studies suggest that the damage is limited to a thin subepicardial layer of myocardium. Accordingly, pericarditis appears to represent a large T wave abnormality produced by a relatively small mass of abnormal myocardium extending over a wide surface area. Pericarditis is discussed in Chapter 11.

T WAVE ABNORMALITIES ATTRIBUTED TO MYOCARDIAL DAMAGE

The primary "coronary" or "postischemic" T wave pattern with a normal ST segment, abnormal T vector, pointed T wave, and prolonged QT interval may appear in patients with various pathologic processes including such conditions as pulmonary embolism, acute cor pulmonale, myocardial tumor, abscess, gumma, acute myocarditis caused by diphtheria, brucellosis, malaria, trichinosis, rheumatic fever, mumps, measles, scrub typhus, and various other infections. Similar T wave changes may be caused by acute and chronic cardiomyopathy of obscure etiology, Friedreich's ataxia, chest trauma, lightning stroke, various poisons (phosphorus, carbon monoxide, venoms, adder bite, scorpion sting), and certain drugs (emetine, chloroquine, plasmoquin, antimony compounds, lithium, and arsenicals).

These T wave abnormalities are probably due to transient or permanent prolongation of repolarization in certain regions of the heart. They usually regress slowly after recovery from the disease or after elimination of the noxious agent from the body. Some of these T wave abnormalities may be caused not by structural myocardial damage but rather by functional, neurogenic repolarization changes precipitated by the disease. For instance, in one patient with abnormal T waves attributed to myocardial damage produced by a scorpion sting, the autopsy did not reveal cardiac abnormalities and the ECG changes were thought to be a result of excessive catecholamine liberation.

The T wave abnormalities in patients with various cardiomyopathies are usually secondary to QRS abnormalities produced by ventricular hypertrophy. Sometimes primary T wave abnormalities precede changes of the QRS complex. The mechanism of such T wave abnormalities is unknown.

Primary T wave abnormalities frequently occur also in patients with mitral insufficiency caused by mitral valve prolapse[57] and a floppy mitral valve in Marfan syndrome.[58] The T waves are usually flat or inverted in leads II and III, and the QTc interval is prolonged. The mechanism of these T wave abnormalities is obscure. Myocardial ischemia is unlikely because these changes frequently occur in children and young adults. It is conceivable that T wave abnormalities are a result of prolonged repolarization in the abnormal left ventricular ridge described with this syndrome.[59]

VARIANT ANGINA PECTORIS

The syndrome of variant angina pectoris is caused by spasm of a normal or diseased major coronary artery. The diagnosis should not be made without ruling out the enzyme changes that indicate MI. The symptoms and ECG changes may be provoked by agents that constrict coronary arteries, such as ergonovine maleate.

In Prinzmetal's original description based on the findings in 23 cases, the variant form of angina pectoris was characterized by the development of chest pain at rest or during nonstrenuous normal activity.[60] Induction of spasm by isoproterenol during tilt test for evaluation of syncope has been reported.[61] On the ECG, transient ST segment elevation with reciprocal ST segment depression is observed during chest pain. The leads in which the ST segment elevation is present usually correspond to the distribution of a major coronary artery and are often predictive of the site of impending MI. During anginal episodes, the R wave in these leads may become taller and the S wave may decrease in amplitude or disappear. In such cases the wide RSTT complex resembles a monophasic action potential (see Figure 7–29). In some patients, continuous monitoring during the attack shows that ST segment elevation increases to a maximal level over a few minutes, remains constant for a few minutes, and then recedes.

Arrhythmias are more likely to develop when the ST segment elevation during the ischemic episode is more pronounced.[62] The most frequently observed arrhythmias include premature ventricular complexes and an accelerated ventricular rhythm, although rapid ventricular tachycardia, torsade de pointes, and ventricular fibrillation have been recorded. The atrioventricular (AV) conduction disturbances, varying from first degree to a complete AV block, occur mainly in patients in whom ST segment elevation involves the inferior leads.[26]

Silent Myocardial Ischemia

Silent myocardial ischemia is observed in patients with asymptomatic coronary artery disease, in patients with symptomatic angina and painless periods, and after MI.[63–66] ECG manifestations of silent ischemia usually consist of the horizontal or downsloping ST segment depression recorded during an exercise test or during ambulatory ECG monitoring. Silent ST segment elevation may occur but is uncommon.

In a review of literature, Rozanski and Berman[14] found that in patients known to have coronary artery disease, about one third of the episodes of ST segment depression observed during exercise testing occur silently. Ambulatory ECG monitoring in patients with histories of angina pectoris and an abnormal exercise test showed that about 75 percent of the episodes of ST segment depression are silent.[14] The frequency of myocardial ischemia, silent or symptomatic, follows a typical circadian rhythm, with most episodes occurring during the morning hours.[67,68] The prognosis of patients with chronic stable symptomatic coronary artery disease and exercise-induced silent ischemia over several years is similar to that of patients in whom the ischemia is associated with symptoms.[69,70] In patients with UAP, however, the probability of MI and death during the follow-up is reported to be higher in patients with silent ischemic episodes.[70,71] This is particularly true if the duration of the silent ischemia is more than 1 hour during each 24-hour monitoring period.[70,72] The subject is reviewed in depth by Cohn and Fox.[73]

Atrial Infarction

Atrial infarction is seldom recognized by ECG but is reported to occur in 1 to 17 percent of patients with MI.[74,75] Numerous abnormalities of the P wave and PR interval and various atrial arrhythmias have been associated with atrial (usually right) infarction,[76] but none of the findings attained a high level of specificity or sensitivity. Displacement of the PQ interval, which represents part of the atrial ST (STa) segment, is considered the most useful sign of atrial infarction. This may be best appreciated in patients with AV block (see Chapter 2). Elevation of the STa segment with or without reciprocal STa depression suggests atrial injury. STa segment elevation may produce a diagnostic monophasic pattern during the early stage of ventricular ischemia (Figure 9–14). Depression of the STa segment alone is not a reliable sign unless the degree of depression is marked.[77] The development of an abnormal P wave configuration with the shape of an M or a W during an acute episode of ischemia also arouses suspicion.[77]

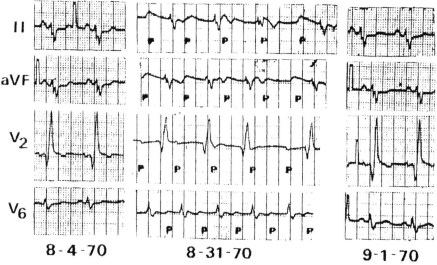

Figure 9–14 ECG pattern of atrial infarction manifested by a monophasic atrial pattern on 8/31/70. P wave is normal before (8/4/70) and after (9/1/70) the onset of infarction. (From Surawicz B: Electrophysiologic Basis of ECG and Cardiac Arrhythmias. Baltimore, Williams & Wilkins, 1995.)

REFERENCES

1. Antman EM, Braunwald E: Acute myocardial infarction. *In:* Braunwald E, Zipes DP, Libby P (eds): Heart Disease. Philadelphia, Saunders, 2001, pp 1114–1118.
2. Holvang L, Clemmensen P, Lindahl B, et al: Quantitative analysis of the admission electrocardiogram identifies patients with unstable coronary artery disease who benefit the most from early invasive treatment. J Am Coll Cardiol 41:905, 2003.
3. Kaul P, Yuling F, Chang W-C, et al: Prognostic value of ST segment depression in acute coronary syndromes: insights from Paragon-A applied to GUSTO IIB. J Am Coll Cardiol 38:64, 2001.
4. Barrabes JA, Figueras J, Moure C, et al: Prognostic significance of ST segment depression in lateral leads I, aV$_L$, V$_5$ and V$_6$ on admission electrocardiogram in patients with a first acute myocardial infarction without ST segment elevation. J Am Coll Cardiol 35:1813, 2000.
5. Jacobsen MD, Wagner GS, Holmvang L, et al: Clinical significance of abnormal T waves in patients with non-ST segment elevation acute coronary syndromes. Am J Cardiol 88:1225, 2001.
6. Al-Khatib SM, Granger CB, Huang Y, et al: Sustained ventricular arrhythmias among patients with acute coronary syndromes with no ST elevation. Circulation 106:309, 2002.
7. Savage RM, Wagner GS, Ideker RE, et al: Correlation of postmortem anatomic findings with electrocardiographic changes in patients with myocardial infarction. Circulation 55:279, 1977.
8. Raunio H, Rossanen V, Romppanen T, et al: Changes in the QRS complex and ST segment in transmural and subendocardial myocardial infarction: a clinicopathologic study. Am Heart J 98:176, 1979.
9. Antaloczy Z, Barcsak J, Magyaar E: Correlation of electrocardiographic and pathologic findings in 100 cases of Q wave and non-Q wave myocardial infarction. J Electrocardiol 21:331, 1988.
10. Kerensky RA, Wade M, Deedwania P, et al: Revisiting the culprit lesion in non-Q wave myocardial infarction: results from the VANQWISH trial angiographic core laboratory. J Am Coll Cardiol 39:1456, 2002.
11. De Wood MA, Stifter WF, Simpson CS, et al: Coronary arteriographic findings soon after non-Q wave myocardial infarction. N Engl J Med 315:417, 1986.
12. Huey BL, Gheorghiade M, Crampton RS, et al: Acute non-Q wave myocardial infarction associated with early ST segment elevation: evidence for spontaneous coronary reperfusion and implications for thrombolytic trials. J Am Coll Cardiol 9:18, 1987.
13. Maisel AS, Ahnve S, Gilpin E, et al: Prognosis after extension of myocardial infarct: the role of Q-wave or non-Q wave infarction. Circulation 71:211, 1985.
14. Rozanski A, Berman DS: Silent myocardial ischemia. I. Pathophysiology, frequency of occurrence, and approaches toward detection. Am Heart J 114:615, 1987.
15. Stimmel B, Katz AM, Donoso E: Q wave development in acute subendocardial infarction. Arch Intern Med 131:676, 1973.
16. Willich SN, Stone PH, Muller JE, et al: High-risk subgroups of patients with non-Q wave myocardial infarction based on direction and severity of ST segment deviation. Am Heart J 114:1110, 1987.
17. Roberts R, Fromm RE: Management of acute coronary syndromes based on risk stratification by biochemical markers: an idea whose time has come. Circulation 98:1831, 1998.
18. Boden WE, Gibson RS, Schechtman KB, et al: ST segment shifts are poor predictors of subsequent Q wave evolution in acute myocardial infarction: a natural history of early non-Q wave infarction. Circulation 79:537, 1989.
19. Barbagelata A, Califf RM, Sgarbossa EB, et al: Thrombolysis and Q wave versus non-Q wave first acute myocardial infarction: a GUSTO-I Substudy. J Am Coll Cardiol 29:770, 1997.
20. Goodman SG, Lange A, Ross AM, et al: Non-Q-wave versus Q-wave myocardial infarction after thrombolytic therapy: angiographic and prognostic insights from the global utilization of streptokinase and tissue plasminogen activator for occluded coronary arteries. I. Angiographic substudy. Circulation 97:444, 1998.

21. Moon JCC, Perez de Arenaza D, Elkington AG, et al: The pathologic basis of Q-wave and non-Q wave myocardial infarction. A cardiovascular magnetic resonance study. J Am Coll Cardiol 44:504, 2004.

22. Sivers B, John B, Brandts B, et al: How reliable is electrocardiography in differentiating transmural from nontransmural myocardial infarction? A study with contrast magnetic resonance imaging as gold standard. International J Cardiol 97:417, 2004,

23. Kaandorp TAM, Bax JJ, Lamb HJ, et al: Which parameters on magnetic resonance imaging determine Q waves on the electrocardiogram?. Am J Cardiol 95:925, 2005.

24. Gibson RS, Crampton RS, Watson DD, et al: Precordial ST-segment depression during acute inferior myocardial infarction: clinical, scintigraphic and angiographic correlations. Circulation 66:732, 1982.

25. Sullivan W, Vlodaver Z, Tuna N, et al: Correlation of electrocardiographic and pathologic findings in healed myocardial infarction. Am J Cardiol 42:724, 1978.

26. Chou TE-C: Electrocardiography in Clinical Practice, 4th ed. Philadelphia, Saunders, 1979, p 121.

27. Ogawa H, Hiramori K, Haze K, et al: Classification of non-Q-wave myocardial infarction according to electrocardiographic changes. Br Heart J 54:473, 1985.

28. Kloner RA: Inverted T waves: an electrocardiographic marker of stunned or hibernating myocardium in man?. Circulation 82:1060, 1990.

29. Berger CJ, Murabito JM, Evans JC, et al: Prognosis after first myocardial infarction: comparison of Q-wave and non-Q wave myocardial infarction in the Framingham Heart Study. JAMA 268:1545, 1992.

30. Michaelides AP, Dilaveris PE, Psomadaki ZD, et al: QRS prolongation on the signal-averaged electrocardiogram versus ST-segment changes on the 12-lead electrocardiogram; which is the most sensitive electrocardiographic marker of myocardial ischemia? Clin Cardiol 22:403, 1999.

31. Braunwald E: Unstable angina: a classification. Circulation 80:410, 1989.

32. Ahmed WH, Bittl JA, Braunwald E: Relation between clinical presentation and angiographic findings in unstable angina pectoris, and comparison with that in stable angina. Am J Cardiol 72:544, 1993.

33. Braunwald E: Unstable angina: an etiologic approach to management. Circulation 98:2219, 1998.

34. Hamm CW, Braunwald E: Classification of unstable angina revisited. Circulation 102:118, 2000.

35. Gorgels APM, Vos MA, Mulleneers R, et al: Value of electrocardiogram in diagnosing the number of severely narrowed coronary arteries in rest angina pectoris. Am J Cardiol 72:999, 1993.

36. Klootwijk P, Meij S, Melkert R, et al: Reduction of recurrent ischemia with Abciximab during continuous ECG-ischemia monitoring in patients with unstable angina refractory to standard treatment (CAPTURE). Circulation 98:1358, 1998.

37. Yoshikawa T, Inoue S, Abe S, et al: Acute myocardial infarction without warning: clinical characteristics and significance of preinfarction angina. Cardiology 82:42, 1993.

38. Ottani E, Galvani M, Ferrinin D, et al: Prodromal angina limits infarct size: a role for ischemic preconditioning. Circulation 91:291, 1995.

39. Shiraki H, Yoshikawa T, Anzai T, et al: Association between preinfarction angina and a lower risk of right ventricular infarction. N Engl J Med 338:941, 1998.

40. Surawicz B: Electrophysiologic Basis of ECG and Cardiac Arrhythmias. Baltimore, Williams & Wilkins, 1995, p 569.

41. Surawicz B, Saito S: Exercise testing for myocardial ischemia in patients with abnormal electrocardiogram at rest. Am J Cardiol 41:943, 1978.

42. Gubner R: Determinants of ischemic electrocardiographic abnormalities and chest pain. Part II. The exercise electrocardiogram test. J Occup Med 3:110, 1961.

43. Surawicz B: QRS, ST segment, T wave, and U wave specificity for myocardial ischemia and infarction. In: Corday E, Swan HJ (eds): Clinical Strategies in Ischemic Heart Disease. Baltimore, Williams & Wilkins, 1979.

44. Lepeschkin E, Surawicz B: Characteristics of true-positive and false-positive results of electrocardiographic Master two-step exercise test. N Engl J Med 258:511, 1958.

45. Armstrong WF, Jordan JW, Morris SN, et al: Prevalence and magnitude of ST and T wave abnormalities in normal men during continuous ambulatory electrocardiography. Am J Cardiol 49:1638, 1982.

46. Maenza RL, Seaberg D, D'Amico F: A meta-analysis of blunt cardiac trauma: ending myocardial confusion. Am J Emergency Med 14:237, 1996.

47. Litmathe J, Boeken U, Gramsch-Zabel H, et al: The incidence of myocardial contusion in 123 patients with blunt chest trauma: diagnostic criteria and outcome. Intensivmedizin und Notfallmedizin 40:585, 2003.

48. Nagarajan DV, Wilde M, Papouchado M: Reversible acute myocardial injury following air bag deployment. Emergency Med J 22:382, 2005.

49. Montorsi P, Fabbiochi F, Loaldi A, et al: Coronary adrenergic hyperactivity in patients with syndrome X and abnormal electrocardiogram at rest. Am J Cardiol 68:1698, 1991.

50. Camici PG, Marraccini P, Lorenzoni R, et al: Coronary hemodynamics and myocardial metabolism in patients with syndrome X: response to pacing stress. J Am Coll Cardiol 17:1461, 1991.

51. Cannon RO, Camici PG, Epstein SE: Pathophysiological dilemma of syndrome X. Circulation 85:883, 1992.

52. Nihoyannopoulos P, Kaski JC, Crake T, et al: Absence of myocardial dysfunction during stress in patients with syndrome X. J Am Coll Cardiol 18:1463, 1991.

53. Tousoulis D, Crake T, Lefroy DC, et al: Left ventricular hypercontractility and ST segment depression in patients with syndrome X. J Am Coll Cardiol 22:1607, 1993.

54. Tweddel AC, Martin W, Hutton I: Thallium scans in syndrome X. Br Heart J 68:48, 1992.

55. Surawicz B, Lasseter KC: Electrocardiogram in pericarditis. Am J Cardiol 26:471, 1970.

56. Barlow JB, Bosman CK, Pocock WA, et al: Late systolic murmurs and nonejection ("mid-late") systolic clicks: analysis of 90 patients. Br Heart J 30:203, 1968.

57. Bowers D: An electrocardiographic pattern associated with mitral valve deformity in Marfan's syndrome. Circulation 23:303, 1961.

58. Ehlers KH, Engle MA, Levin AR, et al: Left ventricular abnormality with late mitral insufficiency and abnormal electrocardiogram. Am J Cardiol 26:3333, 1970.

59. Prinzmetal M, Kennamer R, Merliss R, et al: Angina pectoris. I. A variant form of angina pectoris: preliminary report. Am J Med 27:375, 1959.

60. Wang C-H, Lee C-C, Cherng W-J: Coronary vasospasm induced during isoproterenol head-up tilt test. Am J Cardiol 80:1508, 1997.

61. Kerin NZ, Rubenfire M, Naimi M, et al: Arrhythmias in variant angina pectoris: relationship of arrhythmias to ST segment elevation and R-wave change. Circulation 60:1343, 1979.

62. Chierchia S, Lazzari M, Friedman B, et al: Impairment of myocardial perfusion and function during painless myocardial ischemia. J Am Coll Cardiol 1:924, 1983.

63. Deanfield JE, Shea M, Ribiero P, et al: Transient ST-segment depression as a marker of myocardial ischemia during daily life. Am J Cardiol 54:1195, 1984.

64. Maseri A: Role of coronary artery spasm in symptomatic and silent myocardial ischemia. J Am Coll Cardiol 9:249, 1987.

65. Von Arnim T, Hoffling B, Schreiber M, et al: Characteristics of episodes of ST elevation or ST depression during ambulatory monitoring in patients subsequently undergoing coronary angiography. Br Heart J 54:484, 1985.

66. Quyumi A, Wright CM, Mockus LJ, et al: How important is a history of chest pain in determining the degree of ischemia in patients with angina pectoris? Br Heart J 54:22, 1985.

67. Rocco MB, Barry J, Campbell S, et al: Circadian variation of transient myocardial ischemia in patients with coronary artery disease. Circulation 75:395, 1987.

68. Falcone C, de Servi S, Poma E, et al: Clinical significance of exercise-induced silent myocardial ischemia in patients with coronary artery disease. J Am Coll Cardiol 9:295, 1987.

69. Weiner DA, Ryan TJ, McCabe CH, et al: Significance of silent myocardial ischemia during exercise testing in patients with coronary artery disease. Am J Cardiol 59:725, 1987.

70. Gottlieb SO, Weisfeldt ML, Ouyang P, et al: Silent ischemia as a marker for early unfavorable outcomes in patients with unstable angina. N Engl J Med 314:1214, 1986.

71. Gottlieb SO, Weisfeldt ML, Ouyang P, et al: Silent ischemia predicts infarction and death during 2 year follow-up of unstable angina. J Am Coll Cardiol 10:756, 1987.

72. Nademanee K, Intarachot V, Josephson MA, et al: Prognostic significance of silent myocardial ischemia in patients with unstable angina. J Am Coll Cardiol 10:1, 1987.

73. Cohn PF, Fox KM: Silent myocardial ischemia. Circulation 108:1263, 2003.

74. Gardin JM, Singer DH: Atrial infarction: importance, diagnosis, and localization. Arch Intern Med 141:1345, 1981.

75. Zimmerman HA, Bersano E, Dicosky C: The Auricular Electrocardiogram. Springfield, IL, Charles C Thomas, 1968.

76. Sivertssen E, Hoel B, Bay G, et al: Electrocardiographic atrial complex and acute atrial myocardial infarction. Am J Cardiol 31:450, 1973.

77. Liu CK, Greenspan P, Piccirillo RT: Atrial infarction of the heart. Circulation 23:331, 1961.

10 Stress Test

BORYS SURAWICZ • MORTON TAVEL

Introduction

The principal clinical indication for the electrocardiographic (ECG) stress test is the detection and assessment of myocardial ischemia in patients with known or suspected coronary artery disease (CAD). In the past, the accuracy of detection of myocardial ischemia could be verified only by means of coronary angiography or at autopsy. Currently, however, noninvasive technologies are available for accurate detection of myocardial ischemia by means of nuclear scintigraphy, echocardiography, and the emerging application of magnetic resonance imaging (MRI).

The terms *true positive* and *true negative stress tests* are now applied when the ECG findings are confirmed by the results of the previously mentioned tests, which are considered to represent a "gold standard." The term *false positive* is applied when the ECG findings fulfill the diagnostic criteria of myocardial ischemia that is not detected by nuclear imaging or echocardiography.

Because the diagnostic accuracy of the detection of myocardial ischemia by nuclear and echocardiographic imaging tests is only in the neighborhood of 75 to 90 percent,[1-4] it is possible that the ECG diagnosis of ischemia may be correct when the presence of ischemia was not detected by the imaging. The term *false-negative test* is used when the ECG fails to detect myocardial ischemia diagnosed by imaging techniques. The sensitivity, specificity, and predictive accuracy of the stress test are discussed later. The results of the stress test play a large role in supporting the indication for diagnostic coronary angiography.

The yield of exercise testing is not limited to the information derived from the ECG. Important information is derived from the blood pressure response and the character of the stress-induced discomfort, particularly the chest pain. The performance of the test is helpful in revealing the patient's conditioning and functional capacity. The test can be also useful in the evaluation of cardiac therapy and the assessment of cardiac arrhythmias and conduction disturbances.

Indications and Contraindications

Table 10–1 lists the guidelines for the performance of the ECG stress test, adapted from those recommended by the American College of Cardiology/American Heart Association (ACC/AHA) Task Force in 1997[5] and updated in 2002.[6] Table 10–2 lists the most important contraindications to exercise testing.

Safety of the Exercise Test

In a survey of 500,000 stress tests, the mortality was 1 in 20,000 tests.[7] Nonfatal complications, such as myocardial infarction (MI), requiring hospitalization within 1 week of the test occur at the rate of about 8 per 10,000 tests. In subjects with histories of ventricular tachycardia (VT) or fibrillation, serious but nonfatal arrhythmia complications occurred during 2.3 percent of the tests.[8] In contrast, the incidence of such complications in subjects without histories of sustained ventricular arrhythmias is approximately 0.05 percent. More recently, the TIMI STUDY group[9] reported 1 death and 1 MI among 494 patients with unstable angina pectoris or non-ST elevation MI (NSTEMI) subjected to exercise test. A symptom-limited exercise test performed 1 day after coronary artery stenting was reported to be free of untoward complications in a study involving 1000 patients.[10]

Although patients undergoing exercise testing are generally at low risk, the occasional occurrence of serious complications, as shown later in Figure 10–15, make it mandatory to have an immediate access to a resuscitation kit including an external automatic defibrillator. Adherence to

TABLE 10–1	Reasons for Stress Testing

1. Patients undergoing initial evaluation with suspected or known coronary artery disease (CAD), including those with complete right bundle branch block or less than 1 mm of ST depression at rest
2. Patients with suspected or known CAD, previously evaluated, now presenting with significant change in status
3. Low-risk unstable angina patients 2 to 3 days after presentation who have been free of active ischemic or heart failure symptoms
4. Intermediate-risk unstable angina patients 2 to 3 days after presentation who have been free of active ischemic or heart failure symptoms
5. Before hospital discharge for prognostic assessment, activity prescription, and evaluation for medical therapy
6. Early after hospital discharge for prognostic assessment, activity prescription, evaluation of medical therapy, and cardiac rehabilitation if the predischarge test was not done
7. Late after hospital discharge for prognostic assessment, activity prescription, evaluation of medical therapy, and cardiac rehabilitation if the early exercise test was submaximal
8. To evaluate functional capacity of selected patients with congenital or valvular heart disease
9. Periodic monitoring in patients who continue to participate in exercise training or cardiac rehabilitation
10. To evaluate asymptomatic males over the age of 40 with special occupations (e.g., airline pilots, bus drivers)
11. Evaluation of asymptomatic subjects with diabetes mellitus who plan to start vigorous exercise
12. Evaluation of subjects with multiple risk factors as a guide to risk-reduction therapy
13. Evaluation of asymptomatic men older than 45 years and women older than 55 years who plan to start vigorous exercise, and who are at high risk for CAD due to other diseases such as peripheral vascular disease or chronic renal failure
14. To evaluate the functional capacity and response to therapy with cardiovascular drugs in patients with CAD or heart failure
15. To evaluate the blood pressure response of patients being treated for systemic arterial hypertension who wish to engage in vigorous dynamic or static exercise
16. Identification of appropriate settings in patients with rate-adaptive pacemakers
17. Evaluation of congenital complete atrioventricular (AV) block in patients considering increased physical activity or participation in competitive sports
18. Evaluation of patients with known or suspected exercise-induced arrhythmias
19. Evaluation of medical, surgical, or ablative therapy in patients with exercise-induced arrhythmias (including atrial fibrillation)

TABLE 10–2	Contraindications to Stress Testing

1. Very recent acute myocardial infarction (generally <6 days)
2. Angina pectoris that is unstable or present at rest, excluding conditions listed in Table 10–1
3. Severe symptomatic and unstable left ventricular dysfunction
4. Potentially life-threatening cardiac dysrhythmias
5. Acute pericarditis, myocarditis, or endocarditis
6. Acute pulmonary embolus or infarction
7. Non-cardiac illness that precludes physical exertion (i.e., acute thrombophlebitis or deep vein thrombosis), serious general illness, neuromuscular or arthritic conditions, and inability or lack of desire or motivation to perform the test
8. Severe aortic stenosis
9. Severe hypertension

the guidelines proposed by the Joint Committee of the ACC/AHA[5,6] may be expected to minimize the risk of this procedure.

Graded Exercise Test

The most prevalent method of stressing the patient is the graded exercise test using either the treadmill or the bicycle ergometer. These tests replaced the earlier two-step exercise test introduced by Master more than 60 years ago.[11] Cardiac output and myocardial oxygen consumption are increased during exercise. In the presence of obstructive CAD, the increased demand may exceed the reserve capacity of the coronary blood flow, causing myocardial ischemia. The latter may also occur in other types of heart disease if the heart cannot meet the increased demand of myocardial oxygen consumption during exercise.

In the graded exercise test (GXT), the patient begins to exercise with a low workload that is increased in small increments during continuous ECG monitoring until the target heart rate is reached or the patient is unable to continue. Other reasons for interrupting the test often include worrisome symptoms, an excessively high or low blood pressure, serious arrhythmias, or ECG changes suggestive of myocardial ischemia.

The protocol used for treadmill testing varies among different medical centers. Perhaps the most widely used is that of Bruce and Hornsten.[12] The test is performed at least 2 hours after a meal. Baseline ECGs in the resting state are recorded in the supine and upright position. The exercise consists of increasing workloads at 2- or 3-minute intervals. Table 10–3 presents the stages of a "modified Bruce" protocol employed in many clinics. It is especially useful because it facilitates extrapolation from maximum treadmill performance to levels of work and recreational activity and allows the determination of the presence

TABLE 10–3	Relationship among Treadmill Workloads, General Activities, and Cardiac Classification (New York Heart Association)		
Treadmill Level	METs (approx.)	Functional Class (NYHA)	Equivalent Environmental Activities
1.7 mph, 0% grade	1.8	4	Minimal: wash/shave, dress, desk work, writing, sewing, piano playing, walk 1.5 mph
1.7 mph, 5% grade	3	3	Very light: drive car, clerical and assembly work, shuffleboard, billiards, walk 2 mph
1.7 mph, 10% grade	5	2	Light: clean windows, rake, wax floors, paint, stock shelves, light welding and carpentry, golf, dancing (waltz), table tennis, walk 3 mph
2.5 mph, 12% grade	7	1	Moderate: light gardening, lawn mowing (level), slow stair climbing, exterior carpentry, doubles tennis, badminton, walk 3.5 mph
3.4 mph, 14% grade	9–10	0	Heavy: saw wood, heavy shoveling, tend furnace, moderate stair climbing, canoeing, fencing, singles tennis, jogging 4–5 mph
4.2 mph, 16% grade	11–12	0	Very heavy: carry loads upstairs, rapid stair climbing, heavy labor, lumberjack, raquetball, basketball, ski touring, run 6 mph

and extent of impaired cardiac function (graded by New York Heart Association Classes).

The test begins with the subject walking at a speed of 1.7 miles per hour (mph) on a flat surface (0 percent grade [stage 1]) and involves progressive increases in grade and speed. The estimated workload is reported in metabolic equivalents (METs), a convention that facilitates comparison of different exercise protocols as well as comparison with work or recreation effort requirements. The term *MET* signifies the energy cost of activity in multiples of resting oxygen consumption. One MET, representing the energy consumption at rest, is approximately equal to an oxygen uptake of 3.5 mL/kg/min. Thus 2 METs would indicate an uptake of 7 mL/kg/min, and so on. Because oxygen consumption is determined primarily by cardiac output in the absence of pulmonary or skeletal limitations, this information allows for rough estimates of functional cardiac capacity. Although oxygen uptake is not actually measured in most clinical laboratories, an approximate value can be estimated by consulting published information derived from the various treadmill workloads. Such information can provide reasonably accurate estimates of functional cardiac status. Depending on the state of physical conditioning, a healthy individual can usually attain 10 or more METs, although increasing age and deconditioning may modestly reduce this maximum.[13] In many clinics the test is stopped at an arbitrary target point of 85 percent of the predicted maximal heart rate (MHR) for the subject's age. The MHR is derived by subtracting the subject's age from 220.* This practice is customary when the stress test is combined with scintigraphy or echocardiography, but in a purely electrographic test it is often advisable to reach 100 percent of MHR or to exercise to the point of exhaustion or warning signs.

During the exercise the ECG is monitored continuously with an oscilloscope, and short strips of selected leads are recorded at prescribed intervals. We use leads II, aV_F, and V_5 recorded simultaneously every minute. The blood pressure is measured every 3 minutes during the exercise. At the end of the exercise, a complete 12-lead ECG is recorded immediately and then every 1 to 2 minutes for at least 6 minutes or until the tracing returns to the resting pattern. The blood pressure is measured at 2, 4, and 6 minutes after exercise. Examination of the ECG changes that occur during the recovery period

is also important because in some patients abnormalities appear only after the cessation of the exercise[15,16] (see later discussion).

For safety and proper assessment of the test performance, a physician or a trained physician's assistant should be in attendance during the test.

Blood Pressure Response to Exercise

In response to the increased stroke volume and contractile force, the systolic blood pressure normally rises progressively with increasing workloads and heart rates, reaching about 160 to 220 mmHg with maximum effort. Because exercise lowers overall peripheral vascular resistance, the diastolic pressure exhibits little or no change (less than 10 mmHg). The failure of the systolic pressure to rise to at least 130 mmHg or a systolic blood pressure fall by 10 mmHg or more during exercise may indicate left ventricular dysfunction caused by myocardial ischemia, which may expose the presence of severe CAD.[17,18] Alternatively, an abnormal fall in blood pressure may result from a fall in systemic vascular resistance caused by an abnormal vasodilator response in non-exercising vascular beds.[19] In this case, the response may be also triggered by myocardial ischemia through a neurogenic reflex mechanism and may be associated with increased cardiac output during exercise.

An abnormal rise in exercise systolic pressure to a level >214 mmHg in a subject with a normal resting pressure predicts an increased risk for future sustained hypertension at rest (estimated to occur in approximately 10 to 26 percent of subjects) and a slightly greater propensity for total cardiovascular events over the next 5 to 10 years.[20]

Normally the systolic pressure falls rapidly after cessation of exercise, dropping by an average of 15 percent or more at 3 minutes after stopping. Myocardial ischemia may reduce the rate at which blood pressure falls. At 3 minutes postexercise, blood pressure ≥90 percent of the peak systolic level during exercise suggests the presence of ischemia.[21–23] Although the mechanism for this abnormal pressure response is uncertain, it may result from ischemic impairment of left ventricular function during exercise followed by the subsequent recovery of contractility. This response has been found to signal profound and extensive ischemia, with the difference between the maximum systolic blood pressure during exercise and the blood pressure 3 minutes after exercise decreasing proportionally with the extent of coronary artery disease.[22]

---

*It has been suggested to derive MHR from a regression equation: MHR = 208 − 0.7 × age.[14] However, this has not been widely adopted.

Heart Rate Response to Exercise

In general, the heart rate rises proportionally with the workload, reaching its maximal level at peak workload. The rapidity of the rate increase with increasing workloads depends primarily upon the left ventricular stroke volume, which, among other factors, depends upon the degree of physical conditioning and functional capacity of the heart. Thus, if the stroke volume is limited by either of these factors, the heart rate rises excessively in response to workload, peaking relatively early and reducing maximum exercise capacity. The degree of limitation is roughly proportional to the limitation of cardiac output and stroke volume.

Another abnormal condition, chronotropic incompetence, is an attenuated heart rate response in the absence of rate-limiting atrioventricular block or rate-depressing drug action. Patients exhibiting this response often have significant organic heart disease. Their condition is independently predictive of all-cause mortality among patients with known or suspected CAD,[24] including those treated with beta blockers.[25] Unfortunately, the varying definition of chronotropic incompetence limits its diagnostic usefulness.[26] The various definitions include: the inability to achieve 85 percent of maximum heart rate, the failure to achieve 100 beats/min at maximum exercise,[27] and heart rate response in terms of percentage of standard deviations around a mean heart rate for each stage of the treadmill exercise.[24,28]

The rate of heart recovery after exercise also provides important information about ventricular function and prognosis that extends beyond such factors as effort tolerance and rate response during exercise. A study by Cole et al.[28] showed that if the heart rate falls by 12 beats/min or less at 1 minute after peak exercise during the cooldown phase in early recovery (while walking 1.5 mph at 2.5 percent grade), the subsequent 6-year mortality rate was two to four times greater in comparison with those experiencing a more rapid fall in heart rate after adjusting for common risk factors, including nuclear perfusion defects. A similar outcome was reported in the study of 2935 consecutive patients by Vivekananthan et al.[29] Elhendy et al.[30] studied 3221 patients who underwent treadmill exercise echocardiography. Of these, target rate (85 percent) was not achieved in 15 percent, and low chronotropic index was observed in 25 percent of patients. Both conditions were associated with increased mortality and increased cardiac events after adjusting for left ventricular function and severity of induced myocardial ischemia.

Nissinen et al.[31] found that impaired heart rate recovery predicts mortality in the survivors of acute MI when cardiac medication is optimized according to contemporary guidelines. In the study of Shetler et al.,[32] heart rate recovery at 2 minutes after exercise outperformed other time points in prediction of death. Bhatheja et al.[33] assessed the rate response as the ratio of the heart rate at the peak response to heart rate at rest and found that a blunted heart rate response was predictive of a marked increase in risk of death after adjusting for age, gender, and standard cardiovascular risk factors. Another study[34] found that a heart rate profile during exercise that encompasses changes during both exercise and recovery is a predictor of sudden death. It has been reported that rapid initial heart rate rise was associated with improved survival.[34a]

The retarded heart rate drop during recovery probably signifies reduced vagal tone, which is often associated with impaired myocardial function and decreased exercise capacity. Desai et al.[35] observed that the main portion of the abnormal heart rate recovery could be explained by the chronotropic incompetence. After a period of training, the heart rate response improves,[36] a finding suggestive of enhanced vagal tone. Consistent with these findings, the Framingham study investigators found that rapid heart recovery immediately after exercise was associated with a lower risk of cardiac events.[37] This opinion, however, is not uniformly shared, because an abnormal heart recovery rate failed to affect the survival benefit after early cardiac revascularization in a study of patients with myocardial ischemia.[38]

Cardiac Auscultation

Cardiac auscultation before and after exercise may be rewarding in terms of recognition of murmurs and third and fourth heart sounds. The appearance of third heart sound and diastolic gallop sound after exercise is usually indicative of impaired left ventricular function. Certain murmurs, such as that of aortic stenosis, may increase in intensity after exercise, and in some conditions, such as obstructive cardiomyopathy, systolic murmur may become manifest only after exercise.[39]

Recording Techniques

The results of exercise testing are affected by the recording technique. The conventional 12-lead ECG is the most widely chosen for the GXT.

When the conventional 12 leads are recorded nearly simultaneously, almost all the ST segment changes are demonstrated in leads II, aV_F, and V_3–V_6; 89 percent of that information is contained in lead V_5 and 94 percent in leads V_3–V_6.[28,40,41] It has been suggested[41–43] that the addition of right precordial leads (i.e., leads V_{1R}–V_{4R}) may improve the diagnostic accuracy of ischemia detection in the distribution of the right and circumflex left coronary arteries. In the study of 2021 treadmill tests, however, the addition of both right and posterior precordial leads (16-lead system) did not increase detection of positive responses during exercise testing.[44]

In order to eliminate baseline artifacts, most modern recording systems include computerized methods to average multiple cardiac cycles to provide a "smoothed-out" version of each complete PQRST complex. Although attractive, this method can introduce its own artifacts; therefore the clinician should examine all original recordings before forming conclusions.

Diagnostic Accuracy of the Exercise Test in CAD: Sensitivity and Specificity of the Conventional Criteria

Sensitivity is the percentage of patients with myocardial ischemia resulting from significant coronary obstructive disease (usually one or more coronary vessels with segments of >50 percent narrowing) manifesting an abnormal test. It is represented by the following formula:

$$\text{Sensitivity} = \frac{\text{Positive test responders}}{\text{Total number of subjects with disease}} \left(\begin{array}{c} \times 100\,\text{for} \\ \text{percentage}[\%] \end{array} \right)$$

Specificity is the percentage of patients free of disease who demonstrate a negative test response. It is expressed in the following formula:

$$\text{Sensitivity} = \frac{\text{Negative test responders}}{\text{Total number of subjects without disease}} \left(\begin{array}{c} \times 100\,\text{for} \\ \text{percentage}[\%] \end{array} \right)$$

Both sensitivity and specificity define intrinsic qualities of a test as derived from "pure" populations; in other words, those known to have disease and those known to be free of disease.

Predictive Value of a Test Result

When one is testing mixed populations that contain subjects with and without coronary artery disease, the concept most often employed is the "predictive value" of a positive or negative test. The predictive value of a positive test is the proportional likelihood of the disease being present after a positive test result is found in a given individual. For instance, a predictive value of 0.7 (or 70 percent) would simply mean that a given subject who displays a positive test result would have a 70 percent likelihood of having disease. Conversely, the predictive value of a negative test expresses the likelihood that a subject is free of disease after a test is found to be negative. In contrast to sensitivity and specificity, which are derived from homogenous populations with or without disease, predictive value is strongly influenced by disease prevalence (pre-test probability) within the population to be tested, as well as by the sensitivity and specificity of the test itself. The relationship among these factors is expressed by the following formulas:

Predictive value of a positive test(PVPT) :

$$\text{PVPT} = \frac{(\text{Sensitivity} \times \text{Probability of disease})}{\begin{array}{c}(\text{Sensitivity} \times \text{Probability of disease})+ \\ \{(1 - \text{Specificity}) \times (1 - \text{Probability of diseases})\}\end{array}}$$

Where *Probability of disease* represents the proportion of the pre-test population harboring the disease.

From this formula, one sees that the predictive value is affected by both the sensitivity/specificity of the test itself and the pre-test probability. It is, however, most strongly influenced by the values in the latter part of the denominator (i.e., 1 – Specificity and 1 – Probability of disease in the pre-test population). The higher the values of specificity and prior probability of disease, the lower are these two numbers (and their product), and the closer the predictive value approaches 1 (or 100 percent), the highest value obtainable. Thus, both high test specificity and/or the pre-test disease prevalence play equal roles in allowing a given test—when positive—to predict with greater likelihood the presence of disease.

Predictive value of a negative test (PVNT) :

$$\text{PVNT} = \frac{\text{Specificity} \times (1 - \text{Probability of disease})}{\begin{array}{c}\{\text{Specificity} \times (1 - \text{Probability of disease})\} + \\ \{(1 - \text{Sensitivity}) \times (\text{Probability of diseases})\}\end{array}}$$

In this instance, one sees that the PVNT is most strongly influenced by the test sensitivity as well as the pretest prevalence, i.e. the higher the sensitivity and the lower the pretest disease prevalence, the greater is the resulting PVNT value, therefore the greater is the opportunity to *exclude* the likelihood of disease, given a negative test result.

These concepts are frequently referred to as *Bayes' theorem,* which expresses the idea that the post-test likelihood of disease depends upon the qualities of both the test itself as well as the composition of the population subjected to this test. This is useful in understanding the meaning of test results in general, as well as in test selection. For instance, if one wishes to select the proper test to provide the greatest chance of excluding a disease (high predictive value of a negative test), one would best select a test with the highest possible sensitivity and apply it to a population with the lowest possible prevalence of disease. On the other hand, if one wishes to select a test to provide the greatest chance of positively identifying a disease while minimizing the number of false-positive responders (high predictive value of a positive test), one would select a test with the highest possible specificity and apply it to a population that harbors a high initial prevalence of the disease in question.

Criteria for a Positive Exercise Test

CONVENTIONAL CRITERIA

1. *Horizontal or downsloping ST segment depression of 1 mm (0.1 mV) or more with a duration of 0.08 second or more (Figure 10–1, D and E)*

   Whenever possible, the PR segment is the reference line with which the ST segment is compared. Although not an ideal reference, this segment is usually less distorted during tachycardia than the TP segment.

   The criterion of ≥ 1 mm horizontal or downsloping segment depression has been most often accepted as an abnormal response to exercise. Junctional ST depression with slowly upsloping ST segment depression also is considered to be an abnormal response[44–49] when using the criterion of 1.5-mm ST depression about 60 to 80 ms after the J point (see Figure 10–1C). Less upsloping ST deviation is not abnormal (Figure 10–2).

   In our opinion, the criterion of horizontal 1- to 2.5-mm ST depression lacks sufficient discriminatory power between true- and false-positive stress tests. In our unpublished study of 288 consecutive subjects who completed the test with post

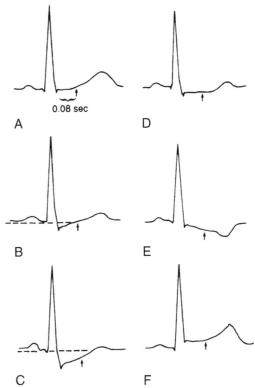

Figure 10–1   Schematic representation of various ST segment patterns potentially produced by exercise. **A,** Normal. **B,** Junctional depression that returns to the baseline (PR segment) within 0.08 second (arrow). **C,** Junctional depression that remains below the baseline at 0.08 second. **D,** Horizontal ST depression. **E,** Downsloping ST depression. **F,** ST elevation. See text for explanation.

exercise ST depression ≥ 1 mm, 100 subjects had evidence of ischemia by nuclear imaging or echocardiography (true positive) and 188 had no evidence of myocardial ischemia (false-positive response). ST depression > 1 mm but < 1.5 mm was present in 2 percent of subjects with true-positive tests and in 14 percent of subjects with false-positive tests. ST depression between 1.5 and 2.5 mm was present in 82 percent of subjects with true-positive responses and in 80 percent of subjects with false-positive responses. ST depression > 2.5 mm was present in 16 percent of patients with true-positive responses and in 6 percent of patients with false-positive responses (the latter small difference was statistically significant). The average ST depression was 1.7 mm in both men and women in the false-positive group compared with 1.9 mm in women and 2.2 mm in men in the true-positive group. In 5 percent of patients with true-positive

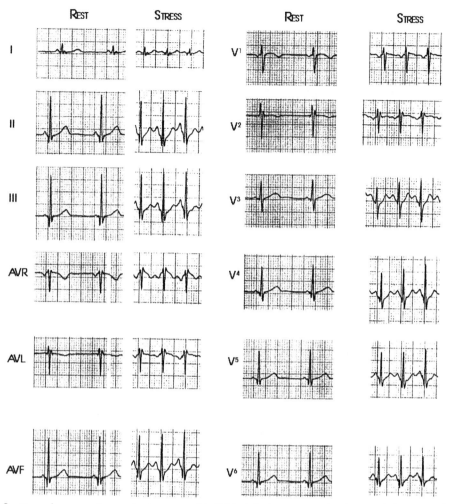

Figure 10–2   Normal response to exercise in a normal individual. In the poststress leads, recorded 10 seconds after peak exercise, there is slight junctional depression with upsloping ST segment in several leads.

responses and 2 percent of patients with false-positive responses, depression of the ST segment was present only during recovery.

The results of this unpublished study show that the level of ST segment depression per se was not helpful in diagnosing ischemia, and they suggest that the threshold for abnormal response should be raised from the level of 1.0 mm to 1.5 mm.

In this regard, we concur with the suggestion of Ellestad[50] that 1.5-mm ST depression is a more helpful discriminator than 1.0-mm ST depression, because in our study only 2 of 100 subjects with a true-positive test developed ST depression less than 1.5 mm. Earlier, Rifkin and Hood[51] pointed out that for the ST depression within range of 1 to 1.5 mm, the risk difference is rather small over the entire range of pre-test risk factors.

It may be that the criteria for the abnormal level of ST depression to detect myocardial ischemia in a population of subjects with risk factors and/or symptoms are more stringent than criteria for estimating long-term prognosis in apparently healthy volunteers because in a study of 1083 volunteers without CAD who enrolled into the Baltimore Study of Aging, ST depression ≥ 1 mm predicted distant future coronary events, whereas an upsloping ST depression and a horizontal ST depression < 1 mm were of no prognostic significance.[52]

The magnitude of ST deviation from the baseline may be influenced by the overall amplitude of the ECG signal. Hollenberg et al.[53] reported that increased R wave amplitude may exaggerate ST depression during exercise. Accuracy was improved by normalizing the R wave amplitude to

12 mm for V_5 and to 8 mm for aV_F and then correcting the ST depression by the derived percentage difference. Ellestad et al.[54] noted that the correction of ST depression for R wave amplitude is especially useful in patients with a low R wave in V_5. This group[55] subsequently found that if the R wave decreases by >1 mm in V_5 at the end of exercise, ST depression $\geq$0.5 mm constitutes a positive ischemic response and thereby increases the sensitivity of the ECG stress test. These observations differ from those of Froelicher et al.,[56] who found no improvement in test accuracy by adjusting for R wave amplitude. (The role of QRS amplitude is further discussed later.)

The review of literature shows that the sensitivity of ST depression for the detection of obstructive CAD and myocardial ischemia varies widely in published reports,[57–59] undoubtedly reflecting various confounding factors such as referral bias and severity of disease in the selected population. In general, there is a decrease in sensitivity but an increase in specificity as the level of ST segment depression required for a positive response is increased.[56,60] In studies in which referral bias was minimized, sensitivity values of abnormal ST segment depression were in the range of 45 to 60 percent.[58,62] The likelihood of a positive response increases progressively with increasing severity and extent of CAD. Most investigators reported sensitivities in the range of 40, 66, and 76 percent for one-, two-, and three-vessel disease, respectively.[61,62] Consistently with these observations, Tavel and Schaar[60] found that ST depression was more often encountered with large perfusion defects in response to stress imaging, and that large areas of hypoperfusion were associated with increased average depth of ST depression.[60] This was confirmed in a study of 1006 patients in whom the extent of myocardial ischemia was assessed by computed tomographic (CT) myocardial perfusion imaging.[63]

The specificity of ST depression in the evaluation of myocardial ischemia has been found to vary considerably, with a mean value derived from a meta-analysis reported to be 72 percent.[57] Referral bias might have reduced these values spuriously because when this type of bias is minimized, these values generally approach or exceed 90 percent.[56,64,65]

In general, the distribution of leads manifesting ST depression is not helpful for localizing obstructive coronary artery disease[56,60,61,66–68] because, as pointed out earlier, lead V_5 alone is most apt to reflect this change when ischemia is present. Some investigators, however, found that ST depression in lead V_1 (isolated or associated with changes in other leads) suggests the presence of ischemia in the posterior regions representing a reciprocal depression to ST elevation in the posterior wall.[69,70] As noted earlier, the inclusion of posterior and right-sided leads has not been helpful uniformly.

In contrast to the almost universal changes produced in the left precordial leads (V_4–V_6), myocardial ischemia seldom produces ST depression confined to the inferior leads (II, III, aV_F), and the presence of such limited distribution usually denotes a false-positive test,[71,72] attributable in some cases to P wave repolarization. (See later discussion.)

2. *Time of onset and regression of the depressed ST segment*

Early appearance of depressed segment has important diagnostic significance.[72] Two- or three-vessel disease or main left obstruction was present in about 90 percent of patients who had depressed, downsloping ST segments or ischemic changes appearing early (in the first 3 minutes of exercise) or persisting for more than 8 minutes after exercise. Most studies indicate that more than 90 percent of those who have positive responses at Bruce stage I or II had significant and extensive CAD as evident by subsequent events[73] or the extent of arteriographic or scintigraphic abnormalities.[74]

Several studies showed that the pattern of regression of ST changes in the recovery period may be useful in distinguishing ischemic responses from false-positive responses. In true ischemia, the major ST depression tends to coincide with the termination of exercise and continues—often intensifying—for at least 2 to 3 minutes after cessation. The persistence of this depression in recovery usually parallels its onset; in other words, when it begins early at low workloads, it is more persistent during recovery. When it reaches a maximum later in the exercise phase, it often regresses relatively late in recovery (i.e., >3 minutes). In contrast, false-positive ST depression tends to reach its maximum immediately before or at the peak exertion but regresses quickly upon cessation, frequently returning to normal within 1 to 3 minutes of recovery. In the latter instance, as the heart rate slows during recovery, ST depression is less deep when compared with corresponding cycle lengths during the exercise, whereas subjects with true ischemia usually show equal or greater ST displacement at comparable cycle lengths during recovery.[75]

The presence of ST depression during recovery has been correlated with echocardiographic wall motion abnormalities and with perfusion defects outlined with dual-isotope single photon emission tomography[76] (see later discussion).

In our experience, the duration of ST abnormalities after the end of exercise was the most helpful discriminator between false-positive and true-positive tests. In patients with false-positive tests, recovery of ST depression occurred in 69 percent after less than 1 minute and persisted for more than 4 minutes in only 10 percent of cases. Conversely, in patients with true-positive tests ST segment recovery persisted for less than 1 minute in 19 percent of women and 29 percent of men but lasted more than 4 minutes in 70 percent of both men and women.

The ST depression during recovery often changed from horizontal to downsloping, resulting in a negative T wave, which in our unpublished study was present during recovery in 62 percent of patients with true-positive tests and in only 6 percent of patients with false-negative tests. Figure 10–3 shows an example of two typical responses to exercise, one of which is true positive and the other is false positive. The depth of ST depression is similar in both, but the difference is evident in the pattern of recovery. Earlier studies also showed that the longer duration of ST abnormalities during recovery supports the diagnosis of myocardial ischemi.[15,63,73,77,78] Chahine et al.[78] found that prolonged postexercise ST depression, designated as post-exercise "evolutionary pattern," was a more specific predictor of coronary atherosclerosis and was usually associated with more severe CAD. Our results differ from those of Bogaty et al.,[74] who reported an incidence of <2 minutes of recovery time of ST segment depression in 50 percent of patients with significant CAD.

ST segment depression occasionally begins only after cessation of exercise.

The diagnostic and prognostic significance of such a delayed response is generally similar to those occurring during exercise[79–81] (i.e., some had true- and some had false-positive tests), consistent with the previously reported findings in such patients.[15,82] However, the onset of such change delayed by more than 2 to 3 minutes into recovery suggests a false-positive response.[83,84] When ST changes during exercise are equivocal, the finding of progressively greater downsloping ST depression during recovery is a fairly specific sign of severe ischemia, signaling a greater incidence of cardiac events in follow-up.[85,86]

3. *Deep T wave inversion*

In the study of Chikamori et al.,[80] T wave inversion exceeding 5 mm during recovery was present in 13 percent of patients with ST segment depression >1 mm during stress and was correlated with the presence of left main or three-vessel coronary artery disease. In our experience, the incidence of this finding is lower.

4. *Gender differences and resting ST depression*

It has been known for a long time that the incidence of false-positive tests is higher in women than in men.[11,87] Both Bayesian and non-Bayesian factors have been cited to explain this gender difference,[88–93] but no uniformly acceptable explanation has been found. Based on the Bayes theorem, the lower prevalence of CAD among women results in a lower predictive value of a positive test in this gender.

The possible contribution of female hormones to the generation of false-positive tests in women is inconclusive because of conflicting results in different studies. Morise et al.[94] found that administration of estrogen alone was not an independent predictor of false-positive tests, whereas an estrogen/progesterone combination or progesterone alone does play a role in the generation of false-positive tests. In the study of Rovang et al.,[95] 20 percent of postmenopausal women had a false-positive exercise response during treatment with oral exogenous estrogen alone or with a combination of estrogen and progesterone. Bokhari and Bergman[96] found also that estrogen administration increased the rate of false-positive tests, but the decreased specificity imparted by estrogen was counteracted in part by the co-administration of progesterone.

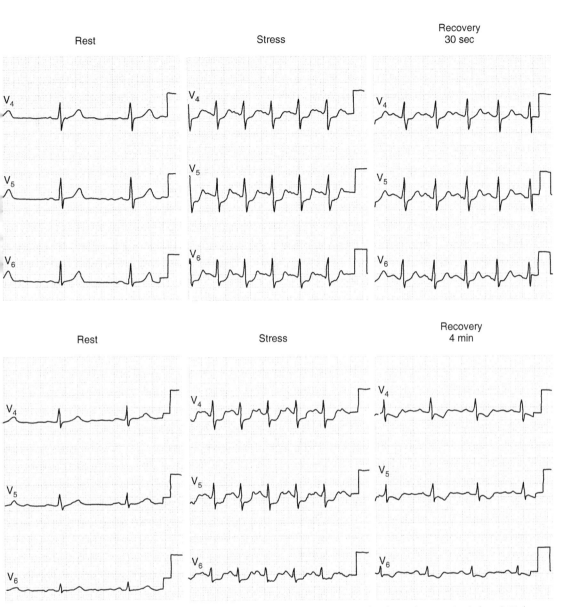

Figure 10–3 Example of a false-positive test *(top)* and true-positive test *(bottom)* with similar exercise-induced ST depression but different changes during recovery. The patient whose ECG is shown at the bottom was a 68-year-old man with abnormal myocardial perfusion and three-vessel, 50 to 70 percent coronary obstruction who had no symptoms during exercise. The patient whose ECG is shown at the top was a 63-year-old man who had no chest pain during exercise and whose nuclear imaging showed no perfusion defects.

In our opinion, the gender difference in response to exercise between men and women is caused by the gender difference in the basic pattern at rest.

It has been reported[97,98] that the baseline ECG in women and in most men at advanced age displays a so-called female pattern, characterized by the absence of J point elevation and a slow ascent of the ST segment into the T wave in the precordial leads. Earlier studies have shown that the incidence of false-positive ECG stress tests is increased in the presence of pre-existing ST depression at rest.[99–104] We assumed that a similar increase in false-positive tests may be expected to take place in the presence of a non-depressed but flat ST segment that is characteristic of the female pattern. Indeed, in our unpublished study, the incidence of false-positive tests was greater in both women and men with female pattern than in subjects with male pattern, but the difference tended to disappear when we substituted ST displacement (i.e., the difference between ST levels before and after exercise) for absolute level of ST depression, which does not consider the pre-exercise level of ST segment. Our measurements were made in lead V_5 and will require confirmation by other investigators.

Earlier, Okin et al.[89] found that the gender difference in the incidence of false-positive tests decreased after examination of the rate recovery loop of ST segment depression (see later discussion).

5. *Association with chest pain*

Exercise-induced myocardial ischemia manifested by significant and protracted ST depression may be associated with chest pain or may be silent. The latter was reported to be a strong predictor of coronary morbidity and mortality in middle-aged men with any conventional risk factors.[105]

The development of typical anginal chest pain during the test generally signifies fairly extensive ischemia and adds significantly to test sensitivity.[60] Moreover, typical chest pain during testing is almost as predictive of ischemia as is ST segment depression. Tavel and Schaar[60] found that, independent of ST changes, the appearance of typical angina pectoris during treadmill exercise–induced stress signifies a greater extent of ischemia than in subjects without symptoms. Several other studies found that history of angina signals a poorer prognosis,[106–108] but in some other studies there was no correlation between the symptoms and prognosis.[109–111] In a recent study from Denmark,[112] the sensitivity and specificity of exercise ECG changes for reversible perfusion defects in patients with angina pectoris were 72 percent and 87 percent, respectively, but Jeetley et al.[107] reported that stress echocardiography was superior to ECG in diagnosing ischemia in patients with chest pain and negative troponin.

Unfortunately, the interpretation of chest pain as a typical angina pectoris is a domain of clinical judgment, and the differentiation between typical angina and non-typical discomfort is not always clear. In our study of 288 patients with post-exercise ST

depression ≥1 mm, some type of chest discomfort was reported by 56 percent of patients with true-positive tests and by 79.5 percent of patients with false-positive tests.

Amsterdam et al.[113] studied 1000 patients presenting to the emergency room with chest pain "suggestive of cardiac etiology." A symptom-limited ECG stress test was positive for ischemia in 12 percent, negative in 64 percent, and nondiagnostic in 23 percent of patients. All patients with a negative test were discharged from the emergency room without additional studies to rule out myocardial ischemia and suffered no deaths, with 1 non-Q wave MI at 30-day follow-up. This study emphasizes the importance of clinical judgment in the evaluation of chest discomfort in low-risk populations.

6. *ST segment elevation*

When the ST segment is depressed in some leads, ST elevation will occur in the leads on the opposite side of the electrical field. Thus, in the presence of ST segment depression in the anterior precordial leads, there is usually detectable ST segment elevation in leads aV_R and V_1 (and occasionally in V_2 and aV_L). This finding is probably of no independent significance (Figure 10–4).

The appearance of ST segment elevation in the leads I-III and/or V_2–V_6 is uncommon in the absence of previous MI but, when present, implies a more severe, possibly transmural myocardial ischemia exceeding that occurring with ST depression alone.[114] In two studies evaluated by Bruce et al.,[115] ST segment elevation emerged as a useful predictor of untoward events when exercise test was performed before diagnostic invasive studies.

The reported incidence of ST segment elevation among patients with chest pain and no previous MI ranged from 0.2 to 1.7 percent.[114,115] High-grade proximal coronary stenosis is usually found in these cases (Figure 10–5), a combination associated with ominous prognosis.[116] The correlation between the site of ST segment elevation and the artery involved is usually good.[69,116–119]

Additionally, an isolated transient increase in the amplitude of positive T wave in the anterior leads V_1–V_3 is believed to represent a variant of ST elevation and strongly suggests narrowing of left anterior descending (LAD) coronary artery, a finding said to be highly specific for this lesion.[69,120]

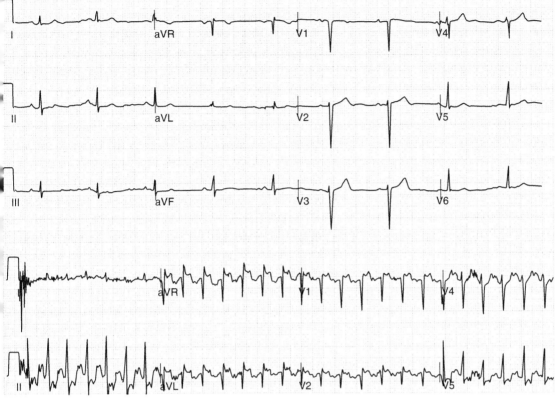

Figure 10–4 ECG of a 53-year-old man with 70 percent left anterior descending (LAD) and 50 percent right coronary artery (RCA) occlusion before and after exercise. The ECG is normal at rest *(top)*. The ECG immediately after the end of exercise shows a heart rate of 169 beats/min, horizontal ST depression in leads II, III, aV$_F$, and V$_5$–V$_6$, and reciprocal ST elevation in leads aV$_R$, aV$_L$, and V$_1$–V$_3$ *(bottom)*. Note that ST elevation in aV$_R$ is greater in V$_1$—a sign frequently ascribed in the literature to left main disease.

Exercise-induced ST segment elevation is seen most commonly in patients who have had previous myocardial infarction, and it can be likened to an "anamnestic response." The reported incidence ranges from 14 to 27 percent,[121–127] with greater incidence in patients with previous anterior MI than in those with previous inferior MI.[117,128] In patients with acute Q wave infarctions, ST elevation induced during routine pre-discharge treadmill exercise test was reported to be associated with larger infarctions.[129]

The ST elevation almost always occurs in the leads with abnormal Q waves.[130,131] It is usually associated with poor left ventricular function[124,132] and, in more than 90 percent of cases, with the presence of akinesis or dyskinesis.[117,129,132,133]

Although some studies suggest that such ST changes reveal residual myocardial viability in the infarct area,[134,135] a more likely mechanism in most cases is a passive segmental wall motion abnormality.[136]

Findings reported in one study,[137] however, suggested that residual viability could be found only in the presence of reciprocal ST depression in leads reflecting the opposite side of the heart. In this context, therefore, reciprocal ST depression may not signal the presence of ischemia.

In cases of prior inferior MI, the ST elevation accompanying the Q waves in the leads II, III, and aV$_F$ is often associated with reciprocal ST depression in leads I and aV$_L$,[134] which does not signify an additional area of ischemia. However, ST depression in lateral precordial leads remains a useful marker of ischemia. In the study of Taniei et al.,[137a] increased viability and reversible myocardial ischemia in subjects with healed anterior MI was suggested by a counterclockwise rotation of the ST/HR loop (see later discussion).

Ten to thirty percent of patients with variant angina may exhibit exercise-induced ST elevation,[117] usually in the same leads that record ST elevation during

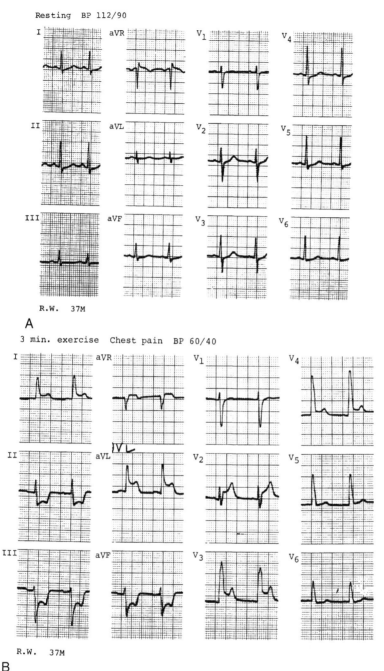

Resting BP 112/90

R.W. 37M

A

3 min. exercise Chest pain BP 60/40

R.W. 37M

B

Figure 10–5 Severe left main coronary artery disease in a 37-year-old man with a history of chest pain. **A,** In the resting ECG, there is a slight ST depression in some of the leads. His blood pressure before the exercise was 112/90. Three minutes after beginning the treadmill exercise, he had chest pain and hypotension, with a blood pressure of 60/40. The exercise was discontinued immediately. **B,** The 12-lead ECG reveals ST segment elevation in leads I, aV$_L$, and V$_2$–V$_4$, with ST segment depression in leads II, III, and aV$_F$. Coronary arteriogram revealed 90 percent occlusion of the left main artery.

angina at rest. In studies reporting on the occurrence of spasm of a major coronary artery,[116,135,138] the site of ST elevation corresponded to the myocardial area supplied by the artery undergoing spasm (Figure 10–6). Most patients with variant angina and exercise-induced ST elevation, however, also have fixed lesions.[139]

Transient, exercise-induced ST elevation has been reported in cases of acute pericarditis[140] and may be mistaken for myocardial ischemia in the acute care setting.

One study[141] suggested that exercise test could aid in the distinction between the so-called "early repolarization" and pericarditis, as the ST elevation subsided in the former but often remained unchanged in the latter. These correlations, however, are not without exception.[142]

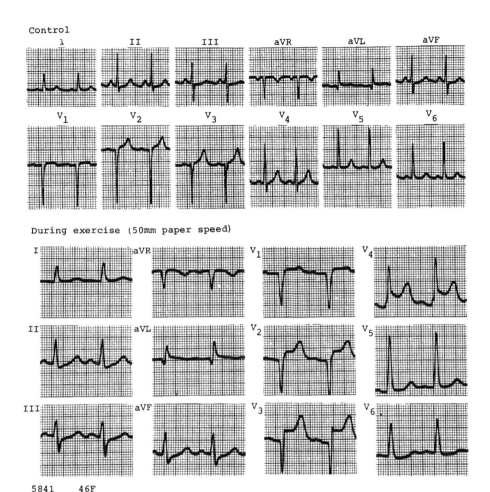

Control

During exercise (50mm paper speed)

5841   46F

Figure 10–6 Positive graded treadmill exercise test with ST segment elevation. The patient is a 46-year-old woman with a typical history of angina pectoris. The resting ECG shows Q wave in aV_L and QS pattern in V_1–V_3, suggesting possible old anterior myocardial infarction. The exercise ECG shows marked ST segment elevation in leads V_1–V_4. Two minutes after beginning the exercise, the patient had chest pain. Coronary arteriogram revealed only 30 percent narrowing of the left anterior descending coronary artery. The left ventricular cineangiogram was normal. Exercise-induced coronary spasm was believed to be the cause of the ST segment elevation. (Courtesy of Dr. Donald Romhilt.)

7. *U wave abnormalities*

Gerson and associates[143] found that in patients with chest pain, exercise-induced U wave inversion had a sensitivity of 21 percent and a specificity of 99 percent for the diagnosis of severe stenosis of the proximal LAD or left main coronary artery (Figure 10–7). The latter finding was disputed by Jain et al.[144] In some cases, the U wave inversion occurred in the absence of abnormal ST segment response. Chikamori et al.[145,146] reported that exercise-induced increase in U wave amplitude in the precordial leads (>0.05 mV) was a highly specific finding in detection of ischemia in the distribution of the left circumflex and/or right coronary arteries. These were assumed to represent reciprocal changes for U wave inversion in the leads with inferoposterior myocardial ischemia.

LESS COMMONLY USED OR CONTROVERSIAL CRITERIA

1. *The ST segment/heart rate (ST/HR) slope and ST/HR index*

The degree of ST segment displacement in relation to the increase in heart rate (ST/HR index) and rotation of ST/HR loop with exercise have been introduced as more accurate indicators of myocardial ischemia and severity of CAD.[147–150] This method requires manual or computerized construction of plots of ST segment deviation and heart rate throughout treadmill exercise and recovery and is independent

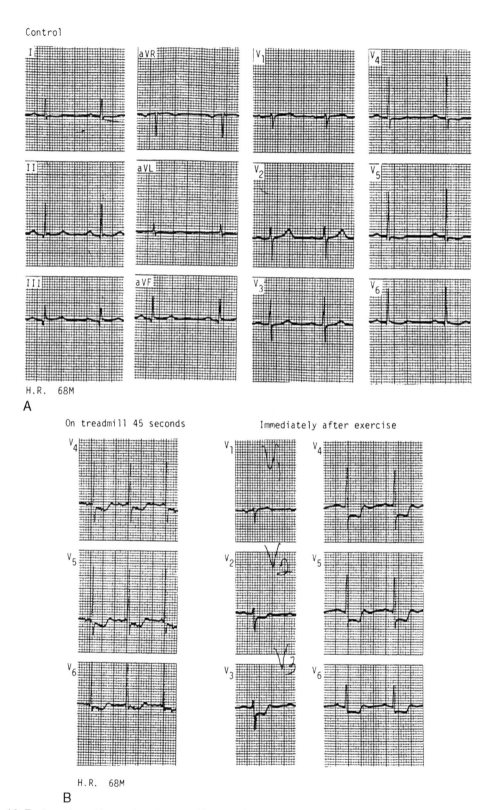

Figure 10–7   Strongly positive test in a 68-year-old man with a history of myocardial infarction 10 years ago, followed for exertional angina. **A,** Resting ECG shows slight ST depression in several leads. **B,** 45 seconds after the onset of exercise on the treadmill, the patient complained of chest pain, with the ECG showing marked horizontal ST segment depression and negative U waves. The exercise was stopped.

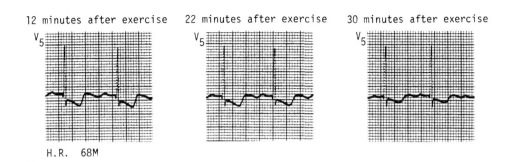

12 minutes after exercise   22 minutes after exercise   30 minutes after exercise

H.R.   68M

C

Figure 10–7 cont'd. C, 30 minutes after exercise, the ECG shows negative T waves and U waves. Coronary arteriogram showed 80 percent occlusion of the left main coronary artery and complete occlusion of the proximal left anterior descending coronary artery. The first marginal branch of the left circumflex artery was also occluded.

of the absolute magnitude of ST depression at the end of exercise. The advantages of this method have not been uniformly confirmed,[151–154] and the usefulness of the heart rate–adjusted   ST segment changes in the detection of CAD therefore remains uncertain[155] and, at best, may add only limited incremental diagnostic value.[156] Thus, this method has not gained wide acceptance in practice.

2. *Increase in R wave amplitude*

The ventricular dilation resulting from akinesis or dyskinesis may increase the proximity of the left ventricular wall to the site of precordial lead recording, and thereby increase the QRS amplitude in patients with myocardial ischemia.

Bonoris and co-workers[157] reported an increase in the R wave amplitude immediately after exercise in patients with severe multivessel coronary artery narrowing and ventricular dysfunction. The results of later studies varied, with some supporting and others not supporting the original observation.[158–163] Nevertheless, although the sensitivity of this finding is low, the R wave amplitude increase by over 2 mm at peak exercise has been said to strongly suggest ischemia.[164] In general, however, analysis of R wave amplitude is rarely employed in clinical practice.

3. *Decrease in the Q wave amplitude in lead V$_5$*[165,166]

Normally the Q wave increases in response to exercise, presumably because of septal thickening in response to inotropic stimulation. A decrease or no change in this wave has been observed in conjunction with CAD with involvement of the LAD coronary artery, usually in association with multi-vessel disease. Although it is a relatively insensitive (15 to 17 percent)

indicator of such disease, Q wave reduction in lead V$_5$ has been said to be a highly specific finding (100 percent)[166]; this latter observation requires confirmation. A possible mechanism in some cases may be the development of an incomplete left bundle branch block (LBBB).

4. *P wave prolongation*[167]

As ischemia develops during exercise, compliance of the left ventricle decreases, resulting in increased diastolic left ventricular and atrial filling pressures. This may transiently increase the P wave duration. Normally the P wave shortens by about 0.02 second in response to exercise; in the presence of ischemia, the P wave may lengthen slightly or remain unchanged. This observation requires confirmation.

5. *Transient axis shifts and intraventricular conduction disturbances*

Normally the axis in the frontal plane shifts to the right during exercise. Exercise-induced leftward shift of the mean QRS axis or left anterior fascicular block may occur in patients with narrowing of the LAD coronary artery, possibly caused by ischemia of the left anterior fascicle.[168,169] Although occurring in only about 10% of those with LAD narrowing, any leftward axis shift is said to be highly specific of this condition. Even in those who show no exercise-induced rightward axis shift, LAD disease is commonly found (sensitivity 66 percent), although it is a less specific finding (78 percent).[168]

Transient left posterior fascicular block occurs seldom but is said to be highly specific for coronary artery disease.[170] It is presumably a consequence of septal ischemia but apparently does not implicate an involvement of any specific coronary artery.

Exercise-induced complete LBBB was present in 1.1 percent of 2584 consecutive patients who underwent both treadmill tests and coronary angiography. Coronary artery disease was absent in patients in whom LBBB appeared at a heart rate >125 beats/min, but was present in 50 percent of patients in whom LBBB appeared at a heart rate <125 beats/min.[171] In the study of Grady et al.,[172] exercise-induced LBBB independently predicted a higher rate of deaths and major cardiac events.

Transient complete right bundle branch block (RBBB) probably has no predictive value per se unless associated with typical angina and/or exercise-induced ST depression in the anterior precordial leads,[173,174] but even the latter finding can occur in the absence of coronary artery disease.[16]

Normally the QRS duration remains unchanged or shortens slightly in response to exercise. It has been reported that in the presence of ischemia, the QRS may lengthen slightly (i.e., >3 to 5 ms) and

may allow for detection of ischemia with greater sensitivity and specificity than ST segment changes alone,[175–178] even in patients with recent MI.[178] Michaelides et al.[176] found that the QRS prolongation correlated with extent of ischemia, becoming progressively longer with one (9.7 ms), two (13.6 ms), and three (16.3 ms) ischemic areas as in the nuclear scans. QRS prolongation also correlated to a lesser extent with the number of stenotic coronary arteries. In our opinion, the specificity of QRS widening after exercise has not been adequately tested, as we have encountered several cases with transient QRS widening in absence of myocardial ischemia (Figure 10–8). Also, selective prolongation of S waves (10 to 12 ms) has been noted in a few subjects with resting RBBB or left anterior fascicular block and, in this context, is believed to be highly suggestive of LAD coronary artery stenosis.[179] Signal-averaged ECG recording techniques have been used to assess minor

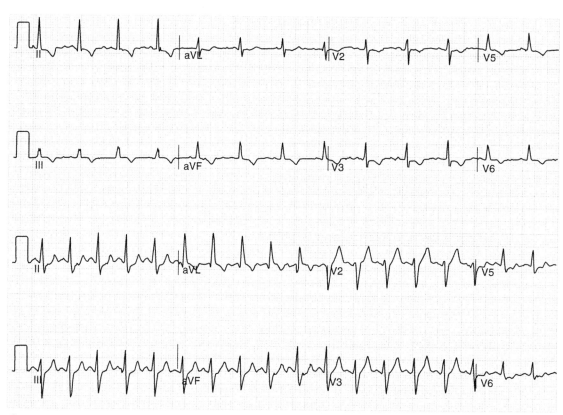

Figure 10–8 ECG at rest *(top)* and after exercise *(bottom)* of a 52-year-old man referred for stress ECG because of abnormal T waves at rest. After exercise, ST depression <0.1 mV, T wave normalization occurred, and QRS duration increased from 92 ms at rest to 110 ms after exercise. Nuclear imaging showed no evidence of myocardial ischemia.

increases in QRS duration, which commonly occur in conjunction with spontaneous episodes of angina pectoris.[177]

7. *Changes in the QT interval*

The baseline QTc (i.e., QT interval corrected for heart rate) is about 5 to 10 ms longer in women and older men than in younger men,[98] but no significant gender differences were found at faster rates.[179] Normally the QTc interval shortens with exercise. Some investigators found that this interval either fails to shorten or lengthens when ischemia is present.[180–182] Others[183] have suggested that abnormal exercise-induced QT dispersion (i.e., the difference between shortest and longest QT intervals when multiple leads are compared) is increased in the presence of ischemia.[184] Unfortunately, measurement of QT dispersion is difficult in the absence of steady state during tachycardia, limiting the potential clinical value of this measurement.

SUGGESTED CRITERIA FOR EXTENSIVE ISCHEMIA AND LEFT MAIN OR SEVERE THREE-VESSEL DISEASE

Several studies reported changes that are most predictive of left main or three-vessel CAD,[90–92,111–115] as follows:

1. ST depression ≥ 2 mm in five or more leads (see Figure 10–7)
2. Downsloping ST depression during recovery
3. Early positive response (Bruce stage 1 or 2)
4. Persistence of ST depression for more than 6 minutes during recovery
5. Exertional hypotension.

When two or more of these changes are observed, extensive myocardial ischemia is usually present with high-grade left main or severe three-vessel occlusive lesions.[16,72,185–188]

Positive Exercise Tests in the Absence of Obstructive CAD

Exercise-induced ST depression in the absence of obstruction to the major coronary arteries occurs in many circumstances. The examples of structural lesions causing this by placing a greater burden on left ventricular dynamics and oxygen requirements include: mitral or aortic valvular disease (Figure 10–9), hypertension, other causes of left ventricular hypertrophy (LVH), and pericardial constriction.[189]

In the absence of heart disease, an abnormal exercise response may occur after glucose ingestion in subjects who otherwise had normal exercise ECGs,[190] which is a reason for performing exercise testing at least 2 hours after a meal.

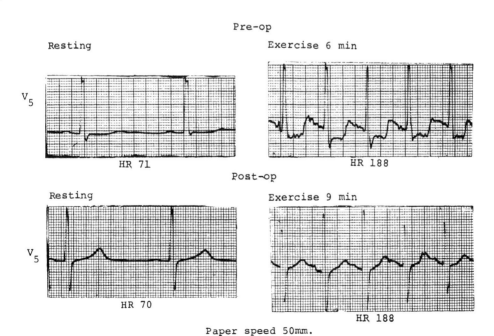

Figure 10–9   False-positive exercise in aortic stenosis. The patient is an 11-year-old boy with severe congenital aortic stenosis. A systolic pressure gradient of 110 mmHg across the aortic valve was demonstrated during cardiac catheterization. In the ECG, ischemic ST segment depression is present during exercise prior to surgery but is not after aortic valvectomy. (Courtesy of Dr. Frederick James.)

Although usually causing changes primarily confined to the T waves, hyperventilation is known to produce ST segment changes that mimic those of myocardial ischemia. False-positive ECG responses to exercise secondary to hyperventilation have been demonstrated in up to 15 percent of patients with normal coronary arteriograms.[191–193] In our experience, the incidence of ST depression after hyperventilation is not as high. The mechanism for the false-positive response during hyperventilation is unclear. If the abnormal response to hyperventilation is suspected, the individual with such changes may be instructed to voluntarily hyperventilate for a period of 2 to 3 minutes with ECG monitoring before the stress test in order to compare the effects of hyperventilation and exercise. This maneuver, however, should be performed only in selected cases when necessary. It may produce dizziness and discomfort and interfere with the proper execution of the ensuing standard test.

ST segment depression and (more frequently) T wave changes can occur while standing. This is especially common in limb leads. In a study of 200 normal subjects between the ages of 15 and 30 years, 16 percent of subjects showed such a postural change.[194] A high incidence of false-positive responses on standing in healthy subjects with labile ST and T wave changes also was reported by McHenry and associates.[195] Such patients may demonstrate exaggerated exercise-induced increases in heart rate.[196,197] They have no chest pain, and the ST changes may disappear as exercise proceeds. Propranolol tends to abolish these changes.

Exercise test is often abnormal in subjects with a so-called syndrome X (see Chapter 9). The symptoms and the ECG changes have been attributed to coronary spasm[196] or microvascular disease.[197] Therefore, the abnormal ECG stress test may not be truly false-positive.

Patients with mitral valve prolapse syndrome and normal coronary arteriograms may have false-positive exercise responses.[198] This phenomenon is clinically important because chest pain and vasoregulatory abnormalities[198] are often encountered in these patients. Mitral valve prolapse also was found to be common in patients with hyperventilation-induced ST changes.[199]

Atrial repolarization waves may produce spurious depression of the ST segment[200–202] (see Chapter 2). The atrial repolarization polarity is directed opposite to that of the P wave and can extend well into the ST segment. Thus with exercise-induced tachycardia, the amplitude of both P wave and atrial repolarization wave increases, and the PR segment shortens, thus shifting the atrial repolarization wave toward the ST segment. This will cause upsloping ST depression in leads with upright P wave and ST elevation in leads with inverted P wave (see Figures 2–17 and 10-10). In practice, this phenomenon may be suspected when there is a prominent P wave together with a short PR segment. The effect of atrial repolarization tends to be most prominent in the "inferior" leads and seldom mimics ST changes caused by myocardial ischemia.

Digitalis is known to cause a false-positive test in subjects with and without heart disease.[203,204] In a study of 98 healthy men treated with digitalis, 25 percent had positive submaximal GXT.[204] A direct relation was found between increasing age and a high incidence of digoxin-induced positive responses to exercise. The effects of the long-lasting digitoxin can cause changes that may persist for as long as 3 weeks after discontinuation of the drug. The effect of digoxin can persist for as long as 1 week after discontinuation of the drug. Hamasaki et al.[205] found that digitalis-induced ST segment depression occurs gradually as the heart rate increases in response to exercise, a pattern differing from that seen during myocardial ischemia in which the ST depression progresses more rapidly as the peak heart rates are approached.

Although the exercise testing in subjects with abnormal potassium concentration is believed to be safe,[205a] the presence of hypokalemia is

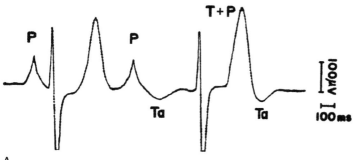

Figure 10–10 The effect of atrial repolarization (Ta) on the ST segment. This was derived from a patient with atrioventricular dissociation and demonstrates the negative deflection produced by the Ta and its negative influence on the ST segment in the first complex at the left. (Modified from Froelicher VF, Morrow K, Brown M, et al: Prediction of atherosclerotic cardiovascular death in men using a prognostic score. Am J Cardiol 73:133, 1994.)

A

often associated with abnormal exercise responses,[206] causing changes that can be abolished after potassium repletion. Therefore, caution is advised in interpreting the test results of patients receiving diuretic therapy.

Causes of False-Negative Responses

Drugs that limit the heart rate response to exercise (beta-adrenergic blocking agents, diltiazem, and verapamil) reduce the heart rate and maximum systolic arterial blood pressure during exercise, thus decreasing the left ventricular work and myocardial oxygen requirements. This can reduce or prevent the ST segment depression.[207] These drugs should be discontinued 72 hours before the test. In the process of increasing exercise capacity, nitrates may prevent or minimize changes in exercise ECG.[208] Quinidine and phenothiazines have been reported to cause false-negative responses.[102] Additionally, RBBB has been reported to "mask" exercise-induced ST segment depression.[209]

Exercise Testing in Patients with Abnormal Resting ECGs

A number of reports suggest that exercise testing may be of value even when the resting ECG is abnormal.[58,59,100,210] In practice, most abnormal resting ECG changes consist of nonspecific ST segment and T wave changes. In general, additional ST depression of 1 mm or more with exercise has a diagnostic accuracy approaching that found in the absence of resting changes. Such changes also have been found to have prognostic significance similar to those found in patients with a normal resting ECG.[104,211] However, in a study of 1122 patients with depressed ST segment at rest undergoing myocardial perfusion (SPECT) and followed for an average of 3.4 years, additional ST depression conferred no prognostic value unless it was ≥ 3 mm.[58]

Secondary ST segment and T wave changes in patients with LVH, intraventricular conduction disturbances, such as LBBB or Wolff-Parkinson-White (WPW) syndrome, tend to interfere with proper interpretation of exercise responses. False-positive and false-negative responses may be seen in the presence of LBBB, although Ibrahim et al.[212] reported that additional exercise-induced J point depression in the leads II, aV_F, and V_5 was suggestive of ischemia. Most useful in their study was a change of ≥ 0.5 mm in lead II. False-positive changes are common in patients with WPW pattern.[213,214]

As a rule, we do not advocate ECG stress alone in patients with LBBB, WPW pattern, LVH, right ventricular hypertrophy (RVH), and deep T wave inversions at rest, but in patients with slight or moderate T abnormalities, T wave normalization is likely to occur as a result of increased sympathetic stimulation in the absence of ST segment changes.[215] An example is shown in Figure 10–11.

Normalization of resting T wave inversion in response to exercise may occur in different clinical settings.[100,215–217] In some studies, T wave normalization suggested preservation of myocardial viability,[218–220] but in other studies it did not help to identify either viability or ischemia.[129,216]

Aravindakshan et al.[215] evaluated the results of stress test in 185 patients with documented ischemic heart disease (IHD) and 28 patients without evidence of myocardial ischemia. The test was positive in 88 percent of patients with and in 4 percent of patients without IHD. In the majority of patients in both groups, the T wave either did not change or became more positive or less negative; that is, "less abnormal" after exercise. The pattern of exercise-induced T wave changes was similar in patients with and without IHD and was influenced predominantly by the physiologic effects of exercise. T wave normalization after exercise occurred frequently in patients with and without IHD, as well as in patients with positive and negative exercise tests. These results indicate that T wave abnormalities that are not caused by hypertrophy, conduction disturbances, drugs, or electrolyte imbalance do not modify the results of the ECG stress test, and that behavior of the T wave after exercise does not alter the interpretation of the postexercise ECG. The independent behavior of the ST segment and the T wave after exercise is consistent with the theory that ST segment and the T wave are generated by different components of the ventricular action potential.[102,215,221] The study of Daoud et al.[222] suggests that T wave normalization is a physiologic effect of increased sympathetic stimulation that causes a more synchronous ventricular repolarization.

ST segment elevation may be seen in the resting ECGs of healthy subjects as a feature of a normal male pattern, which is often called an "early repolarization." In a study involving a relatively small number of subjects with so-called early repolarization, the ST segment returned to the isoelectric baseline in patients with normal coronary arteriograms, whereas those with significant CAD had horizontal ST segment depression.[223] In our experience,[98] elevated J

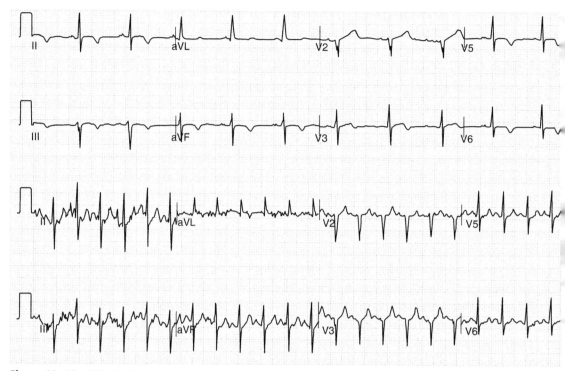

Figure 10–11   ECG of a 50-year-old man referred for stress test because of abnormal resting ECG with negative T wave in several leads *(top)*. Note the T wave normalization immediately after exercise *(bottom)*. Nuclear imaging showed no evidence of myocardial ischemia.

point in subjects with male pattern descends during tachycardia but still remains >1 mm above baseline in the right precordial leads. ST elevation is less pronounced in the leads V_4–V_6, both at rest and after exercise, and therefore the pattern seldom interferes with evaluation of the exercise test in these leads.

Pharmacologic Stress Tests

Drugs are delivered intravenously in two types of pharmacologic tests. In one type, dobutamine causes an effect resembling that of exercise by increasing heart rate and contractility, but with variable effects on blood pressure. In the other type, administration of adenosine or dipyridamole has no appreciable chronotropic or inotropic effect, but increases coronary blood flow by lowering coronary resistance and provoking myocardial ischemia in the regions supplied by diseased and hypoperfused coronary arteries, which cannot further dilate in response to the drug.

The ECG interpretation of these tests is the same as that of treadmill tests. In comparison with the latter, dobutamine more frequently causes sustained supraventricular and ventricular ectopic activity.

Personal experience suggests that the sensitivity and predictive value of the ECG in response to dipyridamole is lower compared with the treadmill test, but false-positive tests appear to be less frequent. Figure 10–12 shows ECG changes indicative of ischemia associated with chest pain in a patient with marked myocardial perfusion defect after dipyridamole administration in the setting of three-vessel coronary artery disease.

Prognostic Value of Exercise Testing

The results of exercise testing have significant prognostic implications, but in most studies referenced in this section, the therapy differed from the contemporary approach to management of patients with coronary syndromes and documented myocardial ischemia. This makes it difficult to assess the relevance of past observations.

ASYMPTOMATIC AND UNSELECTED SUBJECTS

Studies in which large groups of unselected individuals are screened with stress tests consistently

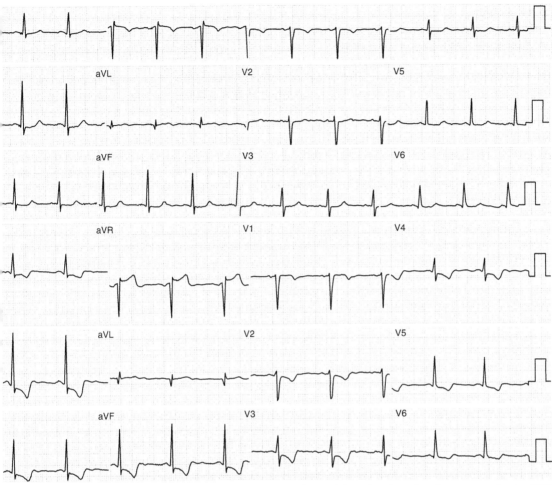

Figure 10–12   ECG of a 63-year-old woman with extensive perfusion defect after dipyridamole stress test. Resting ECG shows horizontal ST depression <0.1 mV in several leads *(top)*. Administration of dipyridamole-induced hypotension, pain in the chest and jaw, and diffuse downsloping ST depression with T wave inversion in several leads *(bottom)*.

show that subjects manifesting abnormal ST responses are at greater risk for subsequent cardiovascular events (e.g., angina, acute MI, sudden death).[224–231] In general, after a follow-up period of 5 to 13 years, those with positive ECG responses show approximately a four- to sixfold greater incidence of such events in comparison with those responding normally to stress. Inability to exercise more than 6 minutes (approximately 6 METs) and inability to increase the heart rate to 85 percent of age-predicted normal maximum values also are significant indicators of increased risk of coronary events.[232] Individuals demonstrating high exercise tolerance (>10 METs) generally enjoy an excellent prognosis, regardless of the ECG response and even in the presence of known coronary artery disease.[233–235]

As mentioned previously, practical significance of these studies is limited because of the greater ability to detect myocardial ischemia by means of nuclear and echocardiographic imaging and a growing trend to apply interventional therapy in asymptomatic or mildly symptomatic patients with diagnosis of obstructive CAD.

The combination of various exercise test variables has allowed for estimation of long-term prognosis.[229,236] Variables found to be independently associated with time to cardiovascular death were weighted to create an equation that calculates a numeric score. The Duke Test Score (DTS),[233] which is the most widely employed and endorsed by other investigators,[234] is based on three exercise variables: exercise tolerance in METs, the largest measured ST segment depression during exercise, and a treadmill angina pectoris score. These are summarized in the nomogram in Figure 10–13. The Long Beach Veteran's Administration Score[236] incorporates

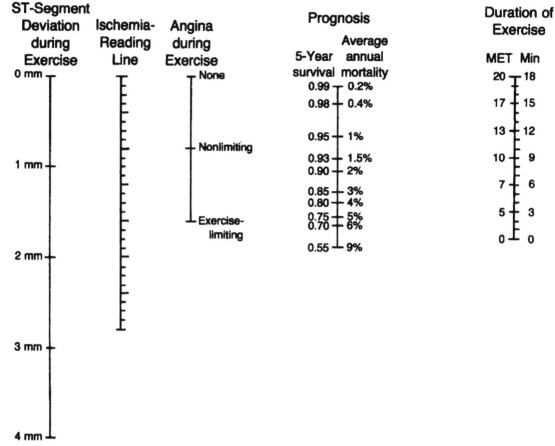

Figure 10–13   Nomogram of the prognostic information derived from treadmill data. Determination of prognosis proceeds in five steps. First, the observed amount of exercise-induced ST segment deviation (the largest depression after resting changes have been subtracted) is marked on the line at the left for ST segment deviation during exercise. Second, the observed degree of angina during exercise is marked on the line for angina. Third, the marks for ST segment deviation and degree of angina are connected with a straight edge. The point where this line intersects the ischemia-reading line is noted. Fourth, the total number of minutes achieved on the treadmill according to the Bruce protocol (or the equivalent number of metabolic equivalents [METs] achieved from an alternative protocol) is marked on the exercise-duration line at the right. Fifth, the mark for ischemia is connected with that for exercise duration. The point at which this line intersects the line for prognosis indicates the average 5-year survival rate and annual mortality for patients with these characteristics. (Reprinted with permission from Mark DB, Shaw L, Harrell FE Jr, et al: Prognostic value of a treadmill exercise score in outpatients with suspected coronary artery disease. N Engl J Med 325:849, 1991.)

slightly different variables: the presence of congestive heart failure or need for digitalis glycosides, exercise-induced ST segment depression, change in systolic blood pressure, and exercise capacity in METs. The Framingham Risk Score evaluated three exercise test variables: ST segment depression ≥1 mm, failure to achieve target heart rate, and exercise capacity.[232,237] Gulati et al.[237] tested the prognostic value of a nomogram developed for symptomatic and asymptomatic women based on predicted exercise capacity, in which predicted MET = 14.7 – (0.13 × age).

In general, DTS and other scores incorporating other variables provide a more accurate prognosis than single components of the score. In several studies, the role of exercise-induced ST depression was subservient. Thus, in a large study of younger and elderly veterans,[238] specific diagnostic score provided significantly better discrimination than exercise ST measurements alone. In another large study of residents of Olmsted County, MN, workload was the only treadmill exercise testing variable associated with outcome.[239] In asymptomatic women, DTS was not a better predictor of cardiac mortality than exercise capacity alone.[240] In this study, ST segment changes and symptoms failed to provide additional prognostic information. In a study of 4640 patients without known CAD, Morise et al.[241] found that the recently revised ACC/ AHA pre-test risk specified guidelines[6] were more useful in predicting cardiac mortality than DTS.

In a multicenter study of 1678 patients after successful revascularization,[242] exercise parameters did not improve prediction of mortality after the 1- and 3-year tests prescribed by the ACC/AHA guidelines for routine testing in stable patients.

Exercise Testing after MI

PATIENTS WITH OLD MI

The GXT in patients with MI that occurred 2 or more months previously may be useful in assessing the presence of ischemia and left ventricular dysfunction. In the ECG leads with abnormal Q waves of infarction, exercise often causes transient ST elevation of 1 mm or more; the significance of this change has been previously discussed. Earlier studies indicate that exercise-induced ST depression after a single previous MI identifies presence of myocardial ischemia resulting from multivessel coronary disease.[124,127,243] Stone and co-workers[244] performed submaximal treadmill exercise 6 months after MI in 473 patients and followed them for 12 months. The mortality was significantly greater in patients who exhibited any of the following: inability to exercise beyond stage 1 of the modified Bruce protocol (2 to 3 METs), development of ST segment elevation of 1 mm or greater during exercise, failure to increase the systolic blood pressure by at least 10 mmHg from rest to peak exercise, and the development of any ventricular ectopic complexes during exercise or the recovery period. The estimated risk for mortality ranged from 1 percent if none of these features were present to 17 percent if three or more were present.

PATIENTS WITH RECENT MI

Limited exercise testing soon after an uncomplicated MI may be useful in evaluating the patient's prognosis and in guiding therapy.[243,244–248] Testing may be done as early as 1 week or even earlier after infarction[244,246] but is often deferred for as long as 2 or 3 weeks after this event. Exercise on the treadmill is usually stopped when the subject reaches an arbitrary heart rate, which is generally 120 or 130 beats/min, or 70 percent of predicted maximum heart rate for age. However, several investigators[242–244] found that symptom-limited testing could be done safely and could be more informative in subjects after uncomplicated MIs before hospital discharge (average 6 to 7 days after MI). In patients with uncomplicated MI who are free of angina

and congestive heart failure, the risk of the limited exercise testing is low, but recurrent acute MI and ventricular fibrillation have been reported.[248,249]

Exercise-induced angina, ST segment displacement, falling blood pressure or failure to increase blood pressure to 110 mmHg or higher, ventricular tachyarrhythmias, poor exercise tolerance (<6 METs), and inability to reach exercise heart rate of 120/min off beta blockers are predictive of higher risk for future cardiac events such as unstable angina, recurrent MI, and cardiac death.[245–256] A poor blood pressure response during limited exercise also is suggestive of reduced left ventricular function.[243] The predictive value of early testing, especially when symptom-limited, is similar to that of testing performed 6 weeks after infarction.[249,257] This applies to patients with both Q wave and non-Q wave infarction[250,251,258,259] and in the presence or absence of thrombolytic treatment.[251] In one study in patients with uncomplicated MI, cardiac death was predicted by heart rate adjusted ST segment analysis.[255] The significance of exercise-induced ST elevation[260] was the same as in the studies previously discussed.

With maximal testing, the ability to reach a high heart rate–systolic pressure product of 21,700 or more implies good myocardial perfusion and a good prognosis (6-month mortality 0.8 percent vs. 2% in those failing to reach this product).[251]

Can the ECG Stress Test Rule Out Presence of Significant CAD?

The appeal of the GXT without echocardiographic or scintigraphic addition is the relative simplicity and the relative low cost. However, such a test cannot rule out the presence of CAD with absolute certainty. Nevertheless, there is a large segment of the adult population in whom the negative ECG stress test alone can be reassuring to the patient by conferring a very low probability of significant CAD. The factors supporting such low probability include: (1) younger age, (2) lack of coronary risk factors, (3) absence of symptoms or presence of atypical symptoms, and (4) ability to perform a strenuous test (e.g., at >10 METs) with normal heart rate and blood pressure response.

Exercise Testing and Arrhythmias

ATRIAL ARRHYTHMIAS

Among 5735 patients studied at the Mayo Clinic,[261] exercise-induced atrial ectopic complexes occurred

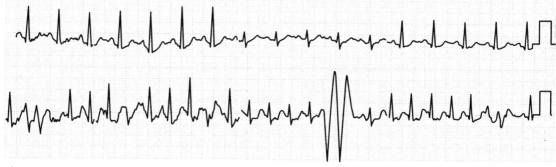

Figure 10–14 ECG strips of lead 3. Exercise-induced ventricular arrhythmia. The patient is known to have coronary artery disease. No arrhythmia is seen in the resting ECG before *(top)* or during the treadmill exercise test. Repetitive ventricular ectopic complexes are present in the tracing 1 minute after the exercise was terminated *(bottom)*.

in 24 percent, supraventricular tachycardia in 3.4 percent, and atrial fibrillation in 0.8 percent of patients. Atrial arrhythmias did not influence the rate of long-term adverse cardiac events after adjustment for clinical and exercise variables known to predict such events.

VENTRICULAR ARRHYTHMIAS

Premature ventricular complexes (PVCs) are often induced by exercise in subjects both with and without heart disease. In the general population, the incidence of PVCs increases with increasing age and strenuousness of exercise and can be as high as 50 percent at the top workload, often including the new appearance of repetitive forms.[262–265] In some studies, exercise-induced ventricular arrhythmias—including non-sustained ventricular tachycardia—recorded in large groups of asymptomatic subjects who were followed for 5 to 10 years were found to be benign.[266] However, in other studies, PVCs during exercise increased the risk of cardiovascular death,[267,268] even in the absence of ischemia demonstrable by nuclear techniques.[268] In the Framingham Heart Study, the presence of PVCs was associated with increased all-cause mortality, but at a much lower threshold than previously reported.[269] Elhendy et al.[270] found a 10 percent incidence of exercise-induced ventricular arrhythmia in patients with suspected CAD. This was associated with greater risk of fatal and non-fatal MI. The risk was attributed to a relation between ventricular arrhythmia and the severity of LV dysfunction. In the study of Frolkis et al.,[271] increased mortality was predicted by ventricular "ectopy" after but not during exercise. This was also reported by others,[262,263] particularly in patients with heart failure.[263]

In patients with CAD, the reported incidence of exercise-induced ventricular arrhythmias

ranges from 38 to 65 percent[264,272] (Figures 10–14 and 10-15). Several studies suggest decreased survival rate of patients with CAD, including those with recent MI, if they have exercise-induced ventricular arrhythmias.* Some reports dispute such an association, however,[275,276] at least in low-risk patients with stable coronary disease.[277]

In patients with angina and ST abnormalities, the presence of exercise-induced ventricular arrhythmias adds to the association with significant multi-vessel disease.[278] The importance of the ischemic ST segment changes in association with the ventricular arrhythmias is exemplified by the study of Udall and Ellestad,[279] who followed for 5 years 1327 patients with known or suspected heart disease who had ventricular ectopic complexes before or during exercise and/or during recovery phase of treadmill exercise test. The annual incidence of new coronary events (MI, angina, cardiac deaths) was 6.4 percent in patients with ventricular ectopic complexes alone, 9.5 percent in patients with ischemic ST segment changes alone, and 11.4 percent in those with both premature ventricular complexes and ST segment changes. In their laboratory, the ST depression in ventricular premature complexes was found to be useful in predicting myocardial ischemia.[280]

In the presence of isolated coronary spasm, exercise-induced VT occurs rarely, but appears to be associated with a more favorable prognosis than VT in patients with the usual varieties of ischemic heart disease.[281]

Cardiac diseases other than CAD with increased incidence of ventricular arrhythmias related to exercise include mitral valve prolapse, cardiomyopathy (dilated and hypertrophic), aortic stenosis, and long QT syndromes.

---

*References 131, 251, 256, 262, 263, and 272–274.

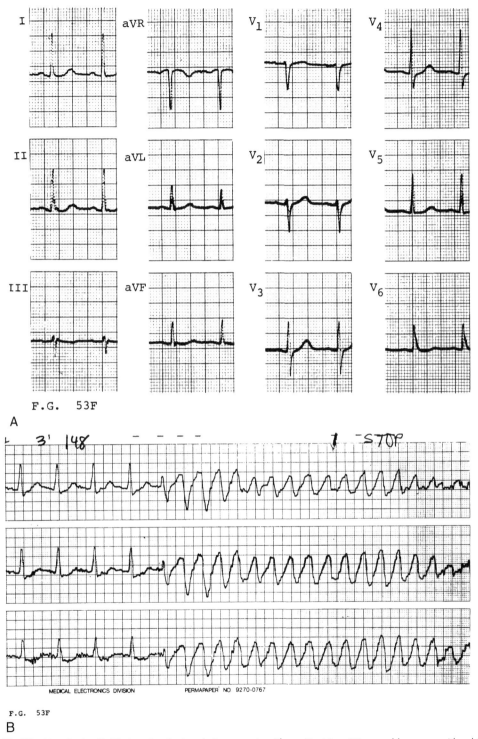

F.G.   53F

A

3' 148   — — — —   ↑ STOP

MEDICAL ELECTRONICS DIVISION   PERMAPAPER NO. 9270-0767

F.G.   53F

B

Figure 10–15 Ventricular fibrillation developing during exercise. The patient is a 53-year-old woman with a history of hypertension, diabetes, and chest pain. **A,** The resting ECG shows minor nonspecific ST and T wave abnormalities. Three minutes after beginning the treadmill exercise, she had a sensation of tightness in her chest. **B,** The ECG revealed ventricular tachycardia followed by ventricular fibrillation. The patient underwent successful defibrillation.

Exercise-induced idiopathic ventricular tachycardia[282] is discussed in Chapter 17.

In conclusion, the prevailing evidence suggests that appearance of ventricular arrhythmias in response to exercise in subjects without heart disease has no diagnostic or prognostic implications. However, in association with known CAD, heart failure, or with markers of ischemia, such as ST depression or angina-type symptoms, ventricular arrhythmias tend to be predictive of subsequent cardiac events.

REFERENCES

1. Ryan T, Segar DS, Sawada SG, et al: Detection of coronary artery disease with upright bicycle exercise echocardiography. J Am Soc Echocardiogr 6:186, 1993.
2. Marwick TH, Nemec JJ, Paskow FJ, et al: Accuracy and limitation of exercise echocardiography in a routine clinical setting. J Am Coll Cardiol 19:74, 1992.
3. Galassi AR, Azzarelli S, Lupo L, et al: Accuracy of exercise testing in the assessment of the severity of myocardial ischemia as determined by means of technetium-99m tetrofosmin SPECT scintigraphy. J Nucl Cardiol 7:575, 2000.
4. Hachamowitz R, Berman DS, Kiat H, et al: Exercise myocardial perfusion SPECT in patients with known coronary artery disease. Incremental prognostic value and use in risk stratification. Circulation 93:905, 1996.
5. Gibbons RJ, Balady GJ, Beasley JW, et al: ACC/AHA Guidelines for exercise testing. A report of the ACC/AHA task force on practice guidelines. J Am Coll Cardiol 30:260, 1997.
6. Gibbons RJ, Balady GJ, Bricker JM, et al: ACC/AHA 2002 Guideline Update for Exercise Testing. A report of the American College of Cardiology/American Heart Association Task Force on Practice Guidelines (Committee to update the 1997 exercise testing guidelines). Circulation 106;1883, 2002.
7. Stuart LJ, Ellestad MH. National survey of exercise stress testing facility. Chest 77:94, 1980.
8. Young DZ, Lampert S, Graboys TB, et al: Safety of maximal exercise testing in patients at high risk for ventricular arrhythmia. Circulation 70:184, 1984.
9. Karha J, Gibson CM, Murphy SA, et al for the TIMI Study Group: Safety of stress testing during the evolution of unstable angina pectoris or non-ST elevation myocardial infarction. Am J Cardiol 94:1537, 2004.
10. Roffi M, Wenaweser P, Windecker S, et al: Early exercise after coronary stenting is safe. J Am Coll Cardiol 42:1569, 2003.
11. Master AM: The Master two-step test. Am Heart J 75:809, 1966.
12. Bruce RA, Hornsten TR: Exercise stress testing in evaluation of patients with ischemic heart disease. Prog Cardiovasc Dis 11:371, 1969.
13. Fletcher GG, Froelicher VF, Hartley LH, et al. Exercise standards: a statement for health professionals from the American Heart Association. Circulation 82:2286, 1990.
14. Tanaka H, Monahan KD, Seals DR: Age-predicted maximal heart rate revisited. J Am Coll Cardiol 37:153, 2001.
15. Soto JR, Watson DD, Beller GA: Incidence and significance of ST segment depression occurring solely during recovery after exercise testing. Am J Cardiol 88:670, 2001.
16. Froelicher VF, Myers JN: Interpretation of ECG responses In: Exercise and the Heart. Philadelphia, Saunders, 2000, pp 121–160.
17. Sanmarco ME, Pontius S, Selvester RH: Abnormal blood pressure response and marked ischemic ST segment depression as predictors of severe coronary artery disease. Circulation 61:572, 1980.
18. Weiner DA, McCabe CH, Cutler SS, et al: Decrease in systolic blood pressure during exercise testing: reproducibility, response to coronary bypass surgery and prognostic significance. Am J Cardiol 49:1627, 1982.
19. Lele SS, Scalia G, Thomson H, et al: Mechanism of exercise hypotension in patients with ischemic heart disease. Circulation 90:2701, 1994.
20. Allison TG, Cordeiro MAS, Miller TD, et al: Prognostic significance of exercise-induced systemic hypertension in healthy subjects. Am J Cardiol 83:371, 1999.
21. Taylor AJ, Beller GA: Postexercise systolic blood pressure response: association with the presence and extent of perfusion abnormalities on thallium-201 scintigraphy. Am Heart J 129:227, 1995.
22. Tsuda M, Hatano K, Hayashi H, et al: Diagnostic value of postexercise systolic blood pressure response for detecting coronary artery disease in patients with or without hypertension. Am Heart J 125:718, 1993.
23. Hashimoto M, Okamoto M, Yamagata T, et al: Abnormal systolic blood pressure response during exercise recovery in patients with angina pectoris. J Am Coll Cardiol 22:659, 1993.
24. Lauer MS, Francis GS, Okin PM, et al: Impaired chronotrophic response to exercise stress testing as a predictor of mortality. JAMA 281:524, 1999.
25. Khan MN, Pothier CE, Lauer MS: Chronotropic incompetence as a predictor of death among patients with normal electrograms taking beta blockers (metoprolol or atenolol). Am J Cardiol 96:1328, 2005.
26. Dreifus LS, Fisch C, Griffin JC, et al: Guidelines for implantation of cardiac pacemakers and antiarrhythmic devices: a report of the ACC/AHA task force on assessment of diagnostic and therapeutic cardiovascular procedures. Circulation 84:455, 1991.
27. Ellestad MH, Wan M: Predictive implications of stress testing: follow-up of 2700 subjects after maximum treadmill stress testing. Circulation 51:363, 1975.
28. Cole CR, Blackstone EH, Pashkow MJ, et al: Heart-rate recovery immediately after exercise as a predictor of mortality. N Engl J Med 341:1351, 1999.
29. Vivekananthan DP, Blackstone EH, Pothier CE, et al: Heart rate recovery after exercise is a predictor of mortality, independent of the angiographic severity of coronary artery disease. J Am Coll Cardiol 42:831, 2000.
30. Elhendy A, Mahoney DW, Khanderia BK, et al: Prognostic significance of impairment of heart rate response to exercise. Impact of left ventricular function and myocardial ischemia. J Am Coll Cardiol 42:823, 2003.
31. Nissinen SI, Makikallio TH, Seppanen T, et al: Heart rate recovery after exercise as a predictor of mortality among survivors of acute myocardial infarction. Am J Cardiol 91:711, 2003.
32. Shetler K, Marcus R, Froelicher VF, et al: Heart rate recovery: validation and methodological issues. J Am Coll Cardiol 38:1980, 2001.
33. Bhatheja R, Francis GS, Pothier CE, et al: Heart rate response during dipyridamole stress as a predictor of mortality in patients with normal myocardial perfusion and normal electrocardiograms. Am J Cardiol 95:1159, 2005.
34. Jouven X, Empana J-P, Schwartz PJ, et al: Heart-rate profile during exercise as a predictor of sudden death. N Engl J Med 352:1951, 2005.

34a.Leeper NJ, Dewey FE, Ashely EA, et al: Prognostic value of heart rate increase at onset of exercise testing. Circulation 115:468, 2007.

35. Desai MY, De la Pena-Almaguer E, Mannting F: Abnormal heart rate recovery after exercise as a reflection of an abnormal chronotropic response. Am J Cardiol 87:1164, 2001.

36. Kligfield P, McCormick A, Chai A, et al: Effect of age and gender on heart recovery after submaximal exercise during cardiac rehabilitation in patients with angina pectoris, recent acute myocardial infarction, or coronary bypass surgery. Am J Cardiol 92:601, 2003.

37. Marshed-Meibodi A, Larson MG, Levy D, et al: Heart rate recovery after treadmill exercise testing and risk of cardiovascular disease events (The Framingham Heart Study). Am J Cardiol 90:848, 2002.

38. Chen MS, Blackstone EH, Pohier CE, et al: Heart rate recovery and impact of myocardial revascularization on long-term mortality. Circulation 110:2851, 2004.

39. Tavel ME: Stress testing in cardiac evaluation. Current concepts with emphasis on the ECG. Chest 119:907, 2001.

40. Blackburn H, Taylor HL, Okamoto N, et al: The exercise electrocardiogram: a systematic comparison of chest lead configurations employed for monitoring during exercise. In: Karvonen M, Barry A (eds): Physical Activity and the Heart. Springfield, IL, Charles C Thomas, 1966.

41. Mahmood K, Higham D: Does the routine use of the lead aV$_{4R}$ increase prognostic yield in exercise electrocardiography?. Brit J Cardiol 9:106, 2002.

42. Braat SH, Kingma JH, Brugada P, et al: Value of lead V$_{4R}$ in exercise testing to predict proximal stenosis of the right coronary artery. J Am Coll Cardiol 5:1308, 1985.

43. Michaelides AP, Psomadaki ZD, Dilaveris PE, et al: Improved detection of coronary artery disease by exercise electrocardiography with the use of right precordial leads. N Engl J Med 340:340, 1999.

44. Sabapathy R, Bloom HL, Lewis WR, et al: Right precordial and posterior chest leads do not increase detection of positive response in electrocardiogram during exercise treadmill testing. Am J Cardiol 91:75, 2001.

45. McHenry PL, Fisch C: Clinical applications of the treadmill exercise test. Mod Concepts Cardiovasc Dis 46:21, 1977.

46. Rijneke AD, Ascoop CA, Talmon JL: Clinical significance of upsloping ST segments in exercise electrocardiography. Circulation 61:671, 1980.

47. Sheffield LT: Upsloping ST segments. Easy to measure, hard to agree upon. Circulation 84:426, 1991.

48. Sansoy V, Watson DD, Beller GA: Significance of slow upsloping ST segment depression on exercise stress testing. Am J Cardiol 79:709, 1997.

49. Stuart RJ, Ellestad MH: Upsloping ST segments in exercise testing. Am J Cardiol 37:19, 1976.

50. Ellestad MH: Stress Testing. Principles and Practice, ed 5. New York, Oxford University Press, 2003, pp 202.

51. Rifkin RD, Hood WB Jr: Bayesian analysis of electrocardiographic exercise testing. N Engl J Med 297:681, 1977.

52. Rywik TM, O'Connor FC, Gittings NS, et al: Role of non-diagnostic exercise exercise-induced ST segment abnormalities in predicting future coronary events in asymptomatic volunteers. Circulation 106:2787, 2002.

53. Hollenberg MBM, Wisneski JA, Gertz ED: Influence of R-wave amplitude on exercise-induced ST depression: need for a "gain factor" correction when interpreting stress electrocardiograms. Am J Cardiol 56:13, 1985.

54. Ellestad MH, Crump R, Surber M: The significance of lead strength on ST change during treadmill stress test. J Electrocardiol 25:31, 1992.

55. Cheng S, Ellestad MH, Selvester RH, Gianrossi R, Detrano R, Mulvihill D, et al. Exercise-induced ST depression in the diagnosis of coronary artery disease: a meta-analysis. Circulation 80:87, 1989.

56. Froelicher VF, Lehmann KG, Thomas R, et al: The electrocardiographic exercise test in a population with reduced workup bias: diagnostic performance, computerized interpretation, and multivariable prediction. Ann Int Med 128:965, 1998.

57. Gianrossi R, Detrano R, Mulvihill D, et al: Exercise-induced ST depression in the diagnosis of coronary artery disease: a meta-analysis. Circulation 80:87, 1989.

58. De Lorenzo A, Hachamovitch R, Kang X, et al: Prognostic value of myocardial perfusion SPECT versus exercise electrocardiography in patients with ST segment depression on resting electrocardiography. J Nucl Cardiol 12:655, 2005.

59. Kwok Y, Kim C, Grady D, et al: Meta-analysis of exercise testing to detect coronary artery disease in women. Am J Cardiol 83:660, 1999.

60. Tavel ME, Shaar C: Relation between the electrocardiographic stress test and degree and location of myocardial ischemia. Am J Cardiol 84:119, 1999.

61. Bartel AG, Behar VS, Peter RH, et al: Graded exercise stress tests in angiographically documented coronary artery disease. Circulation 49:348, 1974.

62. McHenry PL, Phillips JF, Knoebel SB: Correlation of computer-quantitated treadmill exercise electrocardiogram with arteriographic location of coronary artery disease. Am J Cardiol 30:747, 1972.

63. Hauser TH, Dorbala S, Sulaiman A, et al: Quantitative relation of ST segment depression during exercise to the magnitude of myocardial ischemia as assessed by single-photon emission computed tomographic myocardial perfusion imaging, Am J Cardiol 94:703, 2004.

64. Tavel ME: Specificity of electrocardiographic stress test in women versus men. Am J Cardiol 70:545, 1992.

65. Morise AP, Diamond GA: Comparison of the sensitivity and specificity of exercise electrocardiography in biased and unbiased populations of men and women. Am Heart J 130:741, 1995.

66. Dunn RF, Freedman B, Bailey IK, et al: Localization of coronary artery disease with exercise electrocardiography: correlation with thallium-201 myocardial perfusion scanning. Am J Cardiol 48:839, 1981.

67. Fox RM, Hakki AH, Iskandrian AS: Relation between electrocardiographic and scintigraphic location of myocardial ischemia during exercise in one-vessel coronary artery disease. Am J Cardiol 53:1529, 1984.

68. Kaplan MA, Harris CM, Aronow WS, et al: Inability of the submaximal treadmill stress test to predict the location of coronary disease. Circulation 47:250, 1973.

69. Halon DA, Mevorach D, Rodeanu M, et al: Improved criteria for localization of coronary artery disease from the exercise electrocardiogram. Noninvasive Cardiol 84:331, 1994.

70. Michaelides A, Psomadaki ZD, Richter DJ, et al: Exercise-induced ST segment changes in lead V1 identify the significantly narrowed coronary artery in patients with single-vessel disease. J Electrocardiol 32:7, 1999.

71. Miranda CP, Liu J, Kadar A, et al: Usefulness of exercise-induced ST segment depression in the inferior leads during exercise testing as a marker for coronary artery disease. Am J Cardiol 69:303, 1992.

72. Goldschlager N, Selzer A, Cohn K: Treadmill stress tests as indicators of presence and severity of coronary artery disease. Ann Intern Med 85:277, 1976.

73. Cohn PF, Vokonas PS, Herman MV, et al: Postexercise electrocardiogram in patients with abnormal resting electrocardiograms. Circulation 43:648, 1971.

74. Bogaty P, Guimond J, Robitaille NM, et al: A reappraisal of exercise electrocardiographic indexes of the severity of ischemic heart disease: angiographic and scintigraphic correlates. J Am Coll Cardiol 29:1497, 1997.

75. Okin PM, Ameisen O, Kligfield P: Recovery-phase patterns of ST segment depression in the heart rate domain. Circulation 80:533, 1989.

76. Akutsu Y, Shinozuka A, Nishimura H, et al: Significance of ST segment morphology noted on electrocardiography during the recovery phase after exercise in patients with ischemic heart disease as analyzed with simultaneous dual-isotope single photon emission tomography. Am Heart J 144:335, 2002.

77. Patel D, Baman TS, Beller GA: Comparison of the predictive value of exercise-induced ST depression versus exercise technetium-99m sestamibi single photon emission computed tomographic imaging for detection of coronary artery disease in patients with left ventricular hypertrophy. Am J Cardiol 93:333, 2004.

78. Chahine RA, Awder MR, Mnayer M, et al: The evolutionary pattern of exercise-induced ST segment depression. J Electrocardiol 12:235, 1979.

79. Podrid PJ, Graboys TB, Lown B: Prognosis of medically treated patients with coronary artery disease with profound ST segment depression during exercise testing. N Engl J Med 305:1111, 1981.

80. Chikamori T, Doi YL, Furuno T, et al: Diagnostic significance of deep T-wave inversion induced by exercise testing in patients with suspected coronary artery disease. Am J Cardiol 70:403, 1992.

81. Karnegis JN, Matts J, Tuna N, et al: Comparison of exercise-positive with recovery-positive treadmill graded exercise test. Am J Cardiol 60:544, 1987.

82. Lachterman B, Lehmann KG, Abrahamson D, et al: "Recovery only" ST segment depression and the predictive accuracy of the exercise test. Ann Int Med 112:11, 1990.

83. Rywik TM, Zink NS, Gittings AA, et al: Independent prognostic significance of ischemic ST segment response limited to recovery from treadmill exercise in asymptomatic subjects. Circulation 97:2117, 1998.

84. Savage MP, Squires LS, Hopkins JT, et al: Usefulness of ST segment depression as a sign of coronary artery disease when confined to the recovery period. Am J Cardiol 60:1405, 1987.

85. Barlow JB: The "false positive" exercise electrocardiogram: value of time course patterns in assessment of depressed ST segments and inverted T waves. Am Heart J 110:1328, 1985.

86. Rodriguez M, Moussa I, Froning J, et al: Improved exercise test accuracy using discriminant function analysis and "recovery ST slope." J Electrocardiol 26:207, 1993.

87. Surawicz B, Lepeschkin E: Characteristics of true-positive and false-positive results of the electrocardiographic Master two-step test. N Engl J Med 285:211, 1958.

88. Chaitman BR: Exercise stress testing. In: Braunwald E, Zipes DP, Libby P (eds): Heart Disease, ed 6. Philadelphia, Saunders, 2001, pp 129–154.

89. Okin PM: Exercise electrocardiography. In: Topol EJ (ed): Textbook of Cardiovascular Medicine, ed 2. Baltimore, Lippincott, Willams & Wilkins, 2002 pp 1075–1087.

90. Weiner DA, Ryan TJ, McCabe SH, et al: Exercise stress testing: correlation among history of angina, ST segment response and prevalence of coronary artery disease in the Coronary Artery Surgical Study (CASS). N Engl J Med 301:230, 1979.

91. Barolsky SM, Gilbert CA, Faruqui H, et al: Differences in electrocardiographic response to exercise of women and men: a non-Bayesian factor. Circulation 60:1021, 1979.

92. Miller TD, Roger VL, Milavetz JJ, et al: Assessment of the exercise electrocardiogram in women versus men using tomographic myocardial perfusion imaging as the reference standard. Am J Cardiol 87:868, 2001.

93. Morise AP: Exercise electrocardiography in women with suspected coronary disease. In: Ellestad MH, Amsterdam EA (eds): Exercise Testing: New Concepts for the New Century. Boston, Kluwer Academic, 2002, pp 57–70.

94. Morise AP: Progestin therapy as a viable auxillary to established predictors of positive exercise test in women. J Nonivas Cardiology Vol:27, 1997.

95. Rovang KS, Arouni AJ, Mohiuddin SM: Effect of estrogen on exercise electrocardiogram in healthy postmenopausal women. Am J Cardiol 86:477, 2000.

96. Bokhari S, Bergmann SR: The effect of estrogen compared to estrogen plus progesterone on the exercise electrocardiogram. J Am Coll Cardiol 40:1092, 2002.

97. Bidoggia H, Maciel JP, Capalozza N, et al: Sex-dependent electrocardiographic pattern of cardiac repolarization. Am Heart J 140:430, 2000.

98. Surawicz B, Parikh SR: Prevalence of male and female patterns of early ventricular repolarization in the normal ECG of males and females from childhood to old age. J Am Coll Cardiol 40:1870, 2002.

99. Roitman D, Jones WB, Sheffield CT: Comparison of submaximal exercise test with coronary cineangiogram. Ann Int Med 72:641, 1970.

100. Linhart JW, Turnoff HB: Maximum treadmill exercise test in patients with abnormal control electrocardiogram. Circulation 49:667, 1974.

101. Erikssen J, Enge Forfang K, Storstein O: False positive electrocardiographic tests in 105 presumably healthy males. Circulation 54:371, 1976.

102. Surawicz B, Saito S: Exercise testing for detection of myocardial ischemia in patients with abnormal electrocardiograms at rest. Am J Cardiol 41:943, 1978.

103. Elhendy A, von Domburg RT, Baz JJ, et al: Gender differences in the relation between ST T wave abnormalities at baseline electrocardiogram and stress myocardial perfusion abnormalities in patients with suspected coronary artery disease. Am J Cardiol 84:865, 1999.

104. Fearon WF, Lee DP, Froelicher VF: The effect of resting ST segment depression on the diagnostic characteristics of the exercise treadmill test. J Am Coll Cardiol 35:1206, 2000.

105. Laukkanen JA, Kurl S, Lakka TA, et al: Exercise-induced silent myocardial ischemia and coronary morbidity and mortality in middle-aged men. J Am Coll Cardiol 38:72, 2001.

106. Cole J, Ellestad MG: Significance of chest pain during treadmill exercise. Am J Cardiol 41:227, 1978.

107. Jeetley P, Burden L, Senior R: Stress echocardiography is superior to exercise ECG in the risk stratification of patients presenting with acute chest pain with negative troponin. Eur J Echocardiogr 7:155, 2006.

108. Bigi R, Galati A, Curti G, et al: Different clinical and prognostic significance of painful and silent myocardial ischemia detected by exercise electrocardiography and dobutamine stress echocardiography after uncomplicated myocardial infarction. Am J Cardiol 81:75, 1998.

109. Weiner DA, Ryan TJ, McCabe CH, et al: Risk of developing an acute myocardial infarction or sudden coronary death in patients with exercise-induced silent myocardial ischemia. A report from the Coronary

Artery Surgery Study (CASS) registry. Am J. Cardiol 62:1155, 1988.

110. Bonow RO, Bacharach ST, Green MV, et al: Prognostic implications of symptomatic versus asymptomatic (silent) myocardial ischemia induced by exercise in mildly symptomatic and in asymptomatic patients with angiographically documented coronary artery disease. Am J Cardiol 60:778, 1987.

111. Weiner DA, Ryan TJ, McCabe CH, et al: Significance of silent myocardial ischemia during exercise testing in patients with coronary artery disease. Am J Cardiol 59:725, 1987.

112. Flemming Hoilund-Carlsen P, Johansen A, Christensen HW, et al: Usefulness of the electrocardiogram in diagnosing ischemic or coronary heart disease in patients with chest pain. Am J Cardiol 95:96, 2005.

113. Amsterdam EA, Kirk JD, Diercks DB, et al: Immediate exercise testing to evaluate low-risk patients presenting to the emergency department with chest pain. J Am Coll Cardiol 40:251, 2002.

114. Sriwattanakomen S, Ticzon AR, Zubritzky SA, et al: S-T segment elevation during exercise:electrocardiographic and arteriographic correlation in 38 patients. Am J Cardiol 45:762, 1980.

115. Bruce RA, Fisher LD, Pettinger M, et al: ST segment elevation with exercise: a marker for poor ventricular function and poor prognosis. Coronary artery surgery study (CASS) confirmation of Seattle Heart Watch results. Circulation 77:897, 1988.

116. Galik DM, Mahmarian JJ, Verani MS: Therapeutic significance of exercise-induced ST segment elevation in patients without previous myocardial infarction. Am J Cardiol 72:1, 1993.

117. Chaitman BR, Waters DD, Theroux P, et al: S-T segment elevation and coronary spasm in response to exercise. Am J Cardiol 47:1350, 1981.

118. Dunn RF, Freedman B, Kelly DT, et al: Exercise-induced ST segment elevation in leads V_1 or aV_L: a predictor of anterior myocardial ischemia and left anterior descending coronary artery disease. Circulation 63:1357, 1981.

119. Longhurst JC, Kraus WL: Exercise-induced ST elevation in patients without myocardial infarction. Circulation 60:616, 1979.

120. Lee JH, Crump R, Ellestad MH: Significance of precordial T-wave increase during treadmill stress testing. Am J Cardiol 76:1297, 1995.

121. Stiles GL, Rosati RA, Wallace AG: Clinical relevance of exercise-induced S-T segment elevation. Am J Cardiol 46:931, 1980.

122. Waters DD, Chaitman BR, Bourassa MG, et al: Clinical and angiographic correlates of exercise-induced ST segment elevation: Increased detection with multiple ECG leads. Circulation 61:286, 1980.

123. Lahiri A, Balasubramanian V, Millar-Craig MW, et al: Exercise-induced ST segment elevation: electrocardiographic, angiographic, and scintigraphic evaluation. Br Heart J 43:582, 1980.

124. Paine RD, Dye LE, Roitman DI, et al: Relation of graded exercise test findings after myocardial infarction to extent of coronary artery disease and left ventricular dysfunction. Am J Cardiol 42:716, 1978.

125. Smith JW, Dennis CA, Gassmann A, et al: Exercise testing three weeks after myocardial infarction. Chest 75:12, 1979.

126. Tubau JF, Chaitman BR, Bourassa MG, et al: Detection of multivessel coronary disease after myocardial infarction using exercise stress testing and multiple ECG lead systems. Circulation 61:44, 1980.

127. Weiner DA, McCabe CH, Klein MD, et al: ST segment changes post infarction: predictive value for multivessel coronary disease and left ventricular aneurysm. Circulation 58:887, 1978.

128. de Feyter PJ, Majid PA, van Eenige MJ, et al: Clinical significance of exercise-induced ST segment elevation. Br Heart J 46:84, 1981.

129. Hahalis G, Stathopoulos C, Apostopoulos D, et al: Contribution of the ST elevation/T wave normalization, predischarge treadmill exercise test to patient management and risk stratification after acute myocardial infarction. J Am Coll Cardiol 40:62, 2002.

130. Dunn RF, Bailey IK, Uren R, et al: Exercise-induced ST segment elevation: correlation of thallium-201 myocardial perfusion scanning and coronary arteriography. Circulation 61:989, 1980.

131. Henry RL, Kennedy GT, Crawford MH: Prognostic value of exercise-induced ventricular ectopic activity for mortality after acute myocardial infarction. Am J Cardiol 59:1251, 1987.

132. Ho JL, Lin LC, Yen RF, et al: Significance of dobutamine-induced ST segment elevation and T-wave pseudonormalization in patients with Q-wave myocardial infarction: simultaneous evaluation by dobutamine stress echocardiographhy and thallium-201 SPECT. Am J Cardiol 84:125, 1999.

133. Ricci R, Bigi R, Galati A, et al: Dobutamine-induced ST segment elevation in patients with acute myocardial infarction and the role of myocardial ischemia, viability, and ventricular dyssynergy. Am J Cardiol 79:733, 1997.

134. Elhendy A, van Domburg RT, Bax JJ, et al: The significance of stress-induced ST segment depression in patients with inferior Q wave myocardial infarction. J Am Coll Cardiol 33:1909, 1999.

135. Specchia G, de Servi S, Falcone C, et al: Significance of exercise-induced ST segment elevation in patients without myocardial infarction. Circulation 63:46, 1981.

136. Margonato A, Ballarotto C, Bonetti F, et al: Assessment of residual tissue viability by exercise testing in recent myocardial infarction: comparison of the electrocardiogram and myocardial perfusion scintigraphy. J Am Coll Cardiol 19:948, 1992.

137. Nakano A, Lee JD, Shimizu H, et al: Reciprocal ST segment depression associated with exercise-induced ST segment elevation indicates residual viability after myocardial infarction. J Am Coll Cardiol 33:620, 1999.

137a. Taniai S, Koide Y, Yotsukura M, et al: A new application of the ST HR loop to evaluate exercise-induced reversible ischemia in healed anterior myocardial infarction. Am J Cardiol 98:346, 2006.

138. Yasue H, Omote S, Takizawa A, et al: Circadian variation of exercise capacity in patients with Prinzmetal's variant angina: role of exercise-induced coronary arterial spasm. Circulation 59:938, 1979.

139. de Servi S, Falcone C, Gavazzi A, et al: The exercise test in variant angina: results in 114 patients. Circulation 64:684, 1981.

140. Do TM, Campos-Esteve MA, Berry MA, et al: Pericarditis causing exercise test induced ST elevations. Am J Cardiol 78:251, 1996.

141. Chapman DW, Overholt E: Acute benign idiopathic pericarditis: a report of twenty cases. Arch Intern Med 99:708, 1957.

142. Saviolo R, Spodick DH: Electrocardiographic responses to maximal exercise during acute pericarditis and early repolarization. Chest 90:460, 1986.

143. Gerson MC, Phillips JF, Morris SN, et al: Exercise-induced U-wave inversion as a marker of stenosis of

the left anterior descending coronary artery. Circulation 60:1014, 1979.

144. Jain A, Jenkins MG, Gettes LS: Lack of specificity of negative U wave for anterior myocardial ischemia as evidenced by intracoronary electrogram during ballon angioplasty. J Am Coll Cardiol 15:1007, 1990.

145. Chikamori T, Yamada M, Takata J, et al: Exercise-induced prominent U waves as a marker of significant narrowing of the left circumflex or right coronary artery. Am J Cardiol 74:495, 1994.

146. Chikamori T, Takata J, Furuno T, et al: Usefulness of U-wave analysis in detecting significant narrowing limited to a single coronary artery. Am J Cardiol 75:508, 1995.

147. Elamin MS, Boyle R, Kardash MM, et al: Accurate detection of coronary heart disease by new exercise test. Br Heart J 48:311, 1982.

148. Finkelhor RS, Newhouse KE, Vrobel TR, et al: The ST segment/heart rate slope as a predictor of coronary artery disease: comparison with quantitative thallium imaging and conventional ST segment criteria. Am Heart J 112:296, 1986.

149. Okin PM, Gergman G, Kligfield P: Effect of ST segment measurement point on performance of standard and heart rate-adjusted ST segment criteria for the identification of coronary artery disease. Circulation 84:57, 1991.

150. Okin PM, Kligfield P, Ameisen O, et al: Identification of anatomically extensive coronary artery disease by the exercise ECG ST segment/heart rate slope. Am Heart J 115:1002, 1988.

151. Bobbio M, Detrano R, Schmid JJ, et al: Exercise-induced ST depression and ST/heart rate index to predict triple-vessel of left main coronary disease: a multicenter analysis. J Am Coll Cardiol 19:11, 1992.

152. Morise AP, Duval RD: Accuracy of ST/heart rate index in the diagnosis or coronary artery disease. Am J Cardiol 69:603, 1992.

153. Lachterman B, Lehmann KG, Detrano R, et al: Comparison of ST segment/heart rate index to standard ST criteria for analysis of exercise electrocardiogram. Circulation 82:44, 1990.

154. Thwaites BC, Quyyumi AA, Raphael MJ, et al: Comparison of the ST/heart rate slope with the modified Bruce exercise test in the detection of coronary artery disease. Am J Cardiol 57:554, 1986.

155. Bobbio M, Detrano R: A lesson from the controversy about heart rate adjustment of ST segment depression. Circulation 84:1410, 1991.

156. Hsu TS, Lee CP, Chern MS, et al: Critical appraisal of exercise variables: a treadmill study. Coronary Art Dis 10:15, 1999.

157. Bonoris PE, Greenberg PS, Christison GW, et al: Evaluation of R wave amplitude changes versus ST segment depression in stress testing. Circulation 57:904, 1978.

158. Baron DW, Ilsley C, Sheiban I, et al: R wave amplitude during exercise: relation to left ventricular function and coronary artery disease. Br Heart J 44:512, 1980.

159. Battler A, Froelicher V, Slutsky R, et al: Relationship of QRS amplitude changes during exercise to left ventricular function and volumes and the diagnosis of coronary artery disease. Circulation 60:1004, 1979.

160. Berman JL, Wynne J, Cohn PF: Multiple-lead QRS changes with exercise testing: diagnostic value and hemodynamic implications. Circulation 61:53, 1980.

161. Fox K, England D, Jonathan A, et al: Inability of exercise-induced R wave changes to predict coronary artery disease. Am J Cardiol 49:674, 1982.

162. Hopkirk JA, Uhl GS, Hickman JR, et al: Limitation of exercise-induced R wave amplitude changes in

163. detecting coronary artery disease in asymptomatic men. J Am Coll Cardiol 3:821, 1984.

163. Wagner S, Cohn S, Selzer A: Unreliability of exercise-induced R wave changes as indexes of coronary artery disease. Am J Cardiol 44:1241, 1979.

164. Ellestad MH, Lerman S, Thomas L: The limitations of the diagnostic power of exercise testing. Am J Noninvas Cardiol 3:139, 1989.

165. Nohara R, Kambara H, Suzuki Y, et al: Septal Q wave in exercise testing: evaluation by single-photon emission computed tomography. Am J Cardiol 55:905, 1985.

166. Furuse T, Mashiba H, Jordan JW, et al: Usefulness of Q-wave response to exercise as a predictor of coronary artery disease. Am J Cardiol 59:57, 1987.

167. Pandya A, Ellestad MH, Crump R: Time course of changes in P-wave duration during exercise. Cardiology 87:343, 1996.

168. Shiran A, Halon DA, Merdler A, et al: Exercise-induced left-axis deviation of the QRS complex in left anterior descending coronary artery disease and reversal after revascularization. Am J Cardiol 74:1277, 1994.

169. Boran KJ, Oliveros RA, Boucher CA, et al: Ischemia-associated intraventricular conduction disturbances during exercise testing as a predictor of proximal left anterior descending coronary artery disease. Am J Cardiol 51:1098, 1983.

170. Madias JE, Knez P: Transient left posterior hemiblock during myocardial ischemia–eliciting exercise treadmill testing. J Electrocardiol 32:57, 1999.

171. Vasey CG, O'Donnell J, Morris SN, et al: Exercise-induced left bundle branch block and its relation to coronary artery disease. Am J Cardiol 82:832, 1985.

172. Grady TA, Chiu AC, Snader CE, et al: Prognostic significance of exercise-induced left bundle branch block. JAMA 279:153, 1998.

173. Whinnery JE, Froelicher VF, Stuart AJ: The electrocardiographic response to maximal treadmill exercise in asymptomatic men with right bundle branch block. Chest 71:335, 1977.

174. Tanaka T, Friedman MJ, Okada RD, et al: Diagnostic value of exercise-induced ST segment depression in patients with rights bundle branch block. Am J Cardiol 41:670, 1978.

175. Cantor A, Goldfarb B, Mai O, et al: Ischemia detection in women: the diagnostic value of exercise QRS duration changes. J Electrocardiology 31:271, 1998.

176. Michaelides AP, Dilaveris PE, Psomadaki ZD, et al: QRS prolongation on the signal-averaged electrocardiogram versus ST segment changes on the 12-lead electrocardiogram: which is the most sensitive electrocardiographic marker of myocardial ischemia?. Clin Cardiol 22:403, 1999.

177. Cantor A, Goldfarb B, Aszodi A, et al: Ischemia detection after myocardial infarction. J Electrocardiol 31:9, 1998.

178. Michaelides A, Boudoulas H, Vyssoulis GP, et al: Exercise-induced S-wave prolongation in left anterior descending coronary artery stenosis. Am J Cardiol 70:1407, 1992.

179. Mayuga KA, Parker M, Sukthanker ND, et al: Effect of age and gender on the QT response to exercise. Am J Cardiol 87:163, 2001.

180. Macieira-Coelho E, Garcia-Alves M, Lacerda AP, et al: Postexercise changes of the QTc interval in patients with recent myocardial infarction. J Electrocardiol 26:125, 1993.

181. Egloff C, Merola P, Schiavon C, et al: Sensitivity, specificity, and predictive accuracy of the Q wave, QX/QT

ratio, QTc interval and ST depression during exercise testing in men with coronary artery disease. Am J Cardiol 60:1006, 1987.

182. Arab D, Valeti V, Schuenemann HJ, et al: Usefulness of the QTc interval in predicting myocardial ischemia in patients undergoing exercise stress testing. Am J Cardiol 85:764, 2000.

183. Koide Y, Yotsukura M, Yashino H, et al: Usefulness of QT dispersion immediately after exercise as an indicator of coronary stenosis independent of gender or exercise-induced ST segment depression. Am J Cardiol 86:1312, 2000.

184. Stoletniy LN, Pai RG: Value of QT dispersion in the interpretation of exercise stress test in women. Circulation 96:904, 1997.

185. Colby J, Hakki AH, Iskandrian AS, et al: Hemodynamic, angiographic and scintigraphic correlates of positive exercise electrocardiograms: emphasis on strongly positive exercise electrocardiograms. J Am Coll Cardiol 2:21, 1983.

186. McNeer JF, Margolis JR, Lee KL, et al: The role of the exercise test in the evaluation of patients for ischemic heart disease. Circulation 57:64, 1978.

187. Blumenthal DS, Weiss JL, Mellits ED, et al: The predictive value of a strongly positive stress test in patients with minimal symptoms. Am J Med 70:1005, 1981.

188. Schneider RM, Seaworth JF, Dohrmann ML, et al: Anatomic and prognostic implications of an early positive treadmill exercise test. Am J Cardiol 50:682, 1982.

189. Smith RH, Le Petri B, Moisa RB, et al: Association of increased left ventricular mass in the absence of electrocardiographic left ventricular hypertrophy with ST depression during exercise. Am J Cardiol 76:973, 1995.

190. Riley CP, Oberman A, Sheffield LT: Electrocardiographic effects of glucose ingestion. Arch Intern Med 130:703, 1972.

191. Jacobs WF, Battle WE, Ronan JA: False-positive ST-T wave changes secondary to hyperventilation and exercise. Ann Intern Med 81:479, 1974.

192. Lary D, Goldschlager N: Electrocardiographic changes during hyperventilation resembling myocardial ischemia in patients with normal coronary arteriograms. Am Heart J 87:383, 1974.

193. McHenry PL, Cogan OJ, Elliott WC, et al: False positive ECG response to exercise secondary to hyperventilation: cineangiographic correlation. Am Heart J 79:683, 1970.

194. Lachman AB, Semler HJ, Gustafson RH: Postural ST-T changes in the electrocardiogram simulating myocardial ischemia. Circulation 31:557, 1965.

195. McHenry PL, Richmond HW, Weisenberger BL, et al: Evaluation of abnormal exercise electrocardiogram in apparently healthy subjects: Labile repolarization (ST T) abnormalities as a cause of false-positive responses. Am J Cardiol 47:1152, 1981.

196. Likoff W, Segal BL, Kasparian H: Paradox of normal selective coronary arteriograms in patients considered to have unmistakable coronary heart disease. N Engl J Med 276:1063, 1967.

197. Epstein SE, Cannon RO, Bonow RO: Exercise testing in patients with microvascular angina. Circulation 83 (Suppl II):III-73, 1991.

198. Engel PJ, Alpert BL, Hickman JR Jr: The nature and prevalence of the abnormal exercise electrocardiogram in mitral valve prolapse. Am Heart J 98:716, 1979.

199. Gardin JM, Isner JM, Ronan JA, et al: Pseudoischemic "false positive" S-T segment changes induced by hyperventilation in patients with mitral valve prolapse. Am J Cardiol 45:952, 1980.

200. Sapin PM, Koch GG, Blauwet MB, et al: Identification of false positive exercise tests with use of electrocardiographic criteria: a possible role for atrial repolarization waves. J Am Coll Cardiol 18:127, 1991.

201. Sapin PM, Blauwet MB, Koch GG, et al: Exaggerated atrial repolarization waves as a predictor of false positive exercise tests in an unselected population. J Electrocardiol 28:313, 1995.

202. Hayashi H, Okajima M, Yamade K: Atrial T (Ta) wave and atrial gradient in patients with AV block. Am Heart J 91:689, 1976.

203. Nordstrom-Ohrberg G: Effect of digitalis glycosides and exercise test in healthy subjects. Acta Med Scand 176 (Suppl 420):1, 1984.

204. Sketch MH, Mooss AN, Butler ML, et al: Digoxin-induced positive exercise tests: their clinical and prognostic significance. Am J Cardiol 48:655, 1981.

205. Hamasaki S, Nakano F, Arima S, et al: A new criterion combining ST/HR slope and (ST/(HR) index for detection of coronary artery disease in patients on digoxin therapy. Am J Cardiol 81:1100, 1998.

205a.Modesto KM, Moller JE, Freeman WK, et al: Safety of exercise testing in patients with abnormal concentrations of serum potassium. Am J Cardiol 97:1247, 2006.

206. Soloff LA, Fewell JW: Abnormal electrocardiographic responses in exercise in subjects with hypokalemia. Am J Med Sci 242:724, 1961.

207. Gianelly RE, Treister BL, Harrison DC: The effect of propranolol on exercise induced ischemic S-T depression. Am J Cardiol 24:161, 1969.

208. Goldstein RF, Rosing DR, Redwood DR, et al: Clinical and circulatory effects of isosorbide dinitrate: comparison with nitroglycerin. Circulation 43:629, 1971.

209. Chacko KA, Jacob A, Bhat KVR: Right bundle branch block masks exercise-induced ST segment depression. Am J Noninvas Cardiol 8:391, 1994.

210. Kansal S, Roitman D, Sheffield LT: Stress testing and ST segment depression at rest. Circulation 54:636, 1976.

211. Giorgetti A, Sambuceti G, Neglia D, et al: Myocardial blood flow and perfusion reserve in infarcted patients with stress-induced normalization of previously negative T waves: a positron emission tomography study. J Nucl Cardiol 6:11, 1999.

212. Ibrahim NS, Selvester RS, Hagar JM, et al: Detecting exercise-induced ischemia in left bundle branch block using the electrocardiogram. Am J Cardiol 82:832, 1998.

213. Gazes PC: False-positive exercise test in the presence of the Wolff-Parkinson-White syndrome. Am Heart J 78:13, 1969.

214. Strasberg B, Ashley WW, Wyndham CRC, et al: Treadmill exercise testing in the Wolff-Parkinson-White syndrome. Am J Cardiol 45:742, 1980.

215. Aravindakshan V, Surawicz B, Allen RD: Electrocardiographic exercise test in patients with abnormal T waves at rest. Am Heart J 93:706, 1977.

216. Frais MA, Hoeschen RJ: Exercise-induced T wave normalization is not specific for myocardial ischemia detected by perfusion scintigraphy. Am Heart J 119:1225, 1990.

217. Noble RJ, Rothbaum DA, Knoebel SB, et al: Normalization of abnormal T waves in ischemia. Arch Int Med 136:391, 1976.

218. Mobilia G, Zanco P, Desideri A, et al: T wave normalization in infarct-related electrocardiographic leads during exercise testing for detection of residual viability. J Am Coll Cardiol 32:75, 1998.

219. Rambaldi R, Bigi R, Desideri A, et al: Prognostic usefulness of dobutamine-induced ST segment elevation and

T-wave normalization after uncomplicated acute myocardial infarction. Am J Cardiol 86:786, 2000.

220. Marin JJ, Heng MK, Sevrin R, et al: Significance of T wave normalization in the electrocardiogram during exercise stress test. Am Heart J 114:1342, 1994.

221. Surawicz B: The pathogenesis and clinical significance of primary T-wave abnormalities. In: Schlant RC, Hurst JW (eds): Advances in Electrocardiography. New York, Grune and Stratton, 1972, pp 381, 397.

222. Daoud FS, Surawicz B, Gettes LS: Effect of isoproterenol on the abnormal T wave. Am J Cardiol 30:810, 1972.

223. Alimurung BN, Gilbert CA, Felner JM, et al: The influence of early repolarization variant on the exercise electrocardiogram: a correlation with coronary arteriograms. Am Heart J 99:739, 1980.

224. Kwok JMF, Miller TD, Christian TF, et al: Prognostic value of a treadmill exercise score in symptomatic patients with nonspecific ST T abnormalities on resting ECG. JAMA 282:1047, 1999.

225. Bruce RA, DeRouen TA, Hossack KF: Value of maximal exercise tests in risk assessment of primary coronary artery disease events in healthy men: five years' experience of the Seattle Heart Watch Study. Am J Cardiol 46:371, 1980.

226. Froelicher VF, Thomas MM, Pillow C, et al: Epidemiologic study of asymptomatic men screened by maximal treadmill testing for latent coronary artery disease. Am J Cardiol 34:770, 1974.

227. Giagnoni E, Secchi M, Wu SC, et al: Prognostic value of exercise EKG testing in asymptomatic normotensive subjects: a prospective matched study. N Engl J Med 309:1085, 1983.

228. McHenry PL, O'Donnell J, Morris SN, et al: The abnormal exercise electrocardiogram in apparently healthy men: a predictor of angina pectoris as an initial coronary event during long-term follow-up. Circulation 70:547, 1984.

229. Doyle JT, Kinch SH: The prognosis of an abnormal electrocardiographic stress test. Circulation 41:545, 1970.

230. Ellestad MH, Wan MKC: Predictive implications of stress testing: follow-up of 2700 subjects after maximum treadmill stress testing. Circulation 51:363, 1975.

231. Rautaharju PM, Princas RJ, Eifler WJ, et al: Prognostic value of exercise electrocardiogram in men at high risk of future coronary heart disease: multiple risk factor intervention trial experience. J Am Coll Cardiol 8:1,1986.

232. Balady GJ, Larson MG, Ramachandran SV, et al: Usefulness of exercise testing in the prediction of coronary disease risk among asymptomatic persons as a function of the Framingham risk score. Circulation 110:1920, 2004.

233. Mark DB, Shaw L, Harrell FE Jr, et al: Prognostic value of a treadmill exercise score in outpatients with suspected coronary artery disease. N Engl J Med 325:849, 1991.

234. Chatziioannou SN, Moore WH, Ford PV, et al: Prognostic value of myocardial perfusion imaging in patients with high exercise tolerance. Circulation 99:867, 1999.

235. Roger V, Jacobsen SJ, Pellikka PA: Prognostic value of treadmill exercise testing. Circulation 98:2836, 1998.

236. Froelicher VF, Morrow K, Brown M, et al: Prediction of atherosclerotic cardiovascular death in men using a prognostic score. Am J Cardiol 73:133, 1994.

237. Gulati M, Black HR, Shaw LJ, et al: The prognostic value of a nomogram for exercise capacity in women. New Engl J Med 353:468, 2005.

238. Lai S, Kaykha A, Yamazaki T, et al: Treadmill scores in elderly men. J Am Coll Cardiol 43:606, 2004.

239. Goraya TY, Jacobsen SJ, Pelikka PA, et al: Prognostic value of treadmill exercise testing in elderly persons. Ann Int Med 132:862, 2000.

240. Gulati M, Arnsdorf MF, Shaw LJ, et al: Prognostic value of the Duke treadmill score in asymptomatic women. Am J Cardiol 96:369, 2005.

241. Morise AP, Jalisi F: Evaluation of pretest and exercise test scores to assess all-cause mortality in unselected patients presenting for exercise testing with symptoms of suspected coronary artery disease. J Am Coll Cardiol 42:842, 2003.

242. Krone RJ, Hardison RM, Chaitman BR, et al: Risk stratification after successful coronary revascularization: the lack of a role for routine exercise testing. J Am Coll Cardiol 38:136, 2001.

243. Starling MR, Crawford MH, Richards KL, et al: Predictive value of early postmyocardial infarction modified treadmill exercise testing in multivessel coronary artery disease detection. Am Heart J 102:169, 1981.

244. Stone PH, Turi ZG, Muller JE, et al: Prognostic significance of the treadmill exercise test performance 6 months after myocardial infarction. J Am Coll Cardiol 8:1007, 1986.

245. Davidson DM, DeBusk RF: Prognostic value of a single exercise test 3 weeks after uncomplicated myocardial infarction. Circulation 61:236, 1980.

246. Starling MR, Crawford MH, Henry RL, et al: Prognostic value of electrocardiographic exercise testing and noninvasive assessment of left ventricular ejection fraction soon after acute myocardial infarction. Am J Cardiol 57:532, 1986.

247. Theroux P, Water DD, Halphen C, et al: Prognostic value of exercise testing soon after myocardial infarction. N Engl J Med 301:341, 1979.

248. Weld FM, Chu KL, Bigger JT, et al: Risk stratification with low-level exercise testing 2 weeks after acute myocardial infarction. Circulation 64:306, 1981.

249. Pederson A, Grande P, Saunamaki K, et al: Exercise testing after myocardial infarction (Letter). N Engl J Med 302:174, 1980.

250. Jain A, Myers GH, Sapin PM, et al: Comparison of symptom-limited and low-level exercise tolerance test early after myocardial infarction. J Am Coll Cardiol 22:1816, 1993.

251. Juneau M, Colles P, Theroux P, et al: Symptom-limited versus low-level exercise testing before hospital discharge after myocardial infarction. J Am Coll Cardiol 20:927, 1992.

252. Villella M, Villella A, Barlera S, et al: Prognostic significance of double product and inadequate double product response to maximal symptom-limited exercise stress testing after myocardial infarction in 6296 patients treated with thrombolytic agents. Am Heart J 137:443, 1999.

253. Koppes GM, Kruyer W, Beckmann CH, et al: Response to exercise early after uncomplicated acute myocardial infarction in patients receiving no medication: long-term follow-up. Am J Cardiol 46:764, 1980.

254. Krone RJ, Gillespie JA, Weld FM, et al: Low-level exercise testing after myocardial infarction: usefulness in enhancing clinical risk stratification. Circulation 71:80, 1985.

255. Bigi R, Cortigiani L, De Chiara B, et al: Exercise versus recovery electrocardiography in predicting mortality in patients with uncomplicated myocardial infarction. Eur Heart J 25:558, 2004.

256. Waters DD, Bosch X, Bouchard A, et al: Comparison of clinical variables and variables derived from a limited predischarge exercise test as predictors of early and late

mortality after myocardial infarction. J Am Coll Cardiol 5:1, 1985.

257. Senaratne MPJ, Hsu L, Rossall RE, et al: Exercise testing after myocardial infarction: relative values of the low level predischarge and post discharge exercise test. J Am Coll Cardiol 12:1416, 1988.

258. Miranda CP, Herbert WH, Dubach P, et al: Post myocardial infarction exercise testing. Non-Q wave versus Q wave correlation with coronary angiography and long-term prognosis. Circulation 84:2357, 1991.

259. Sia STB, MacDonald PS, Horowitz JD, et al: Usefulness of early exercise testing after non-Q-wave myocardial infarction in predicting prognosis. Am J Cardiol 57:738, 1986.

260. Haines DE, Beller GA, Watson DD, et al: Exercise-induced ST segment elevation 2 weeks after uncomplicated myocardial infarction: contributing factors and prognostic significance. Am J Cardiol 9:996, 1987.

261. Bunch TJ, Chandrasekaran K, Gersh BJ, et al: The prognostic significance of exercise-induced atrial arrhythmias. J Am Coll Cardiol 43:1236, 2004.

262. Meine TJ, Patel MR, Shaw LK, et al: Relation of ventricular premature complexes during recovery from a myocardial perfusion exercise stress test to myocardial ischemia. Am J Cardiol 97:1570, 2006.

263. O'Neill JO, Young JB, Pothier CE, et al: Severe frequent ventricular ectopy after exercise is a predictor of death in patients with heart failure. J Am Coll Cardiol 44:820, 2004.

264. McHenry PL, Morris SN, Kavalier M, et al: Comparative study of exercise-induced ventricular arrhythmias in normal subjects and patients with documented coronary artery disease. Am J Cardiol 37:609, 1976.

265. Faris JV, McHenry PL, Jordan JW, et al: Prevalence and reproducibility of exercise-induced ventricular arrhythmias during maximal exercise testing in normal men. Am J Cardiol 37:617, 1976.

266. Busby MJ, Shefrin EA, Fleg JL: Prevalence and long-term significance of exercise-induced frequent or repetitive ventricular ectopic beats in apparently healthy volunteers. J Am Coll Cardiol 14:1659, 1989.

267. Jouven X, Zureik M, Desnos M, et al: Long-term outcome in asymptomatic men with exercise-induced premature ventricular depolarizations. N Engl J Med 343:826, 2000.

268. Marieb MA, Beller GA, Gibson RS, et al: Clinical relevance of exercise-induced ventricular arrhythmias in suspected coronary artery disease. Am J Cardiol 66:172, 1990.

269. Morshedi-Meibodi A, Evans JC, Levy D, et al: Clinical correlates and prognostic significance of exercise-induced ventricular premature beats in the community. The Framingham Heart Study. Circulation 109:2417, 2004.

270. Elhendy A, Chandrasekaran K, Gersh BJ, et al: Functional and prognostic significance of exercise-induced ventricular arrhythmias in patients with suspected coronary artery disease. Am J Cardiol 90:95, 2002.

271. Folkis JP, Pothier CE, Blackstone EH, et al: Frequent ventricular ectopy after exercise as a predictor of death. N Engl J Med 348:781, 2003.

272. Goldschlager N, Cake D, Cohn K: Exercise-induced ventricular arrhythmias in patients with coronary artery disease: their relationship to angiographic findings. Am J Cardiol 31:434, 1973.

273. Califf RM, McKinnis RA, McNeer JF, et al: Prognostic value of ventricular arrhythmias associated with treadmill exercise testing in patients studied with cardiac catheterization for suspected ischemic heart disease. J Am Coll Cardiol 2:1060, 1983.

274. Margonato A, Mailhac A, Bonetti F, et al: Exercise-induced ischemic arrhythmias in patients with previous myocardial infarction: role of perfusion and tissue viability. J Am Coll Cardiol 27:593, 1996.

275. Nair CK, Aronow WS, Sketch MH, et al: Diagnostic and prognostic significance of exercise-induced premature ventricular complexes in men and women: a four year follow-up. J Am Coll Cardiol 1:1201, 1983.

276. Sami M, Chaitman B, Fisher L, et al: Significance of exercise-induced ventricular arrhythmia in stable coronary artery disease: a Coronary Artery Surgery Study project. Am J Cardiol 54:1182, 1984.

277. Schweikert RA, Pashkow FJ, Snader CE, et al: Association of exercise-induced ventricular ectopic activity with thallium myocardial perfusion and angiographic coronary artery disease in stable, low-risk populations. Am J Cardiol 83:530, 1999.

278. Goldschlager N, Cohn K, Goldschlager A: Exercise-related ventricular arrhythmias. Mod Concepts Cardiovasc Dis 48:67, 1979.

279. Udall JA, Ellestad MH: Predictive implications of ventricular premature contractions associated with treadmill stress testing. Circulation 56:985, 1977.

280. Rasouli ML, Ellestad MH: Usefulness of ST depression in ventricular premature complexes to predict myocardial ischemia. Am J Cardiol 87:891, 2001.

281. Chevalier P, Dacosta A, Defaye P, et al: Arrhythmic cardiac arrest due to isolated coronary artery spasm: long-term outcome of seven resuscitated patients. J Am Coll Cardiol 31:57, 1998.

282. Mont L, Seixas T, Brugada P, et al: Clinical and electrophysiologic characteristics of exercise-related idiopathic ventricular tachycardia. Am J Cardiol 68:897, 1991.

11 Pericarditis and Cardiac Surgery

Pericarditis
Pericardial Effusion
Effect of Pressure Produced by Fluid or
 Fibrin
Changes Attributed to Superficial
 Myocarditis
QTc Inteval
Evolution of ECG Changes

Cardiac Arrhythmias
Differentiation from MI, Normal Variant,
 and Myocarditis
Incidence and Magnitude of ECG
 Abnormalities

ECG Changes after Cardiac Surgery

Pericarditis

The electrocardiographic (ECG) abnormalities caused by pericarditis evolve through several distinct stages that reflect different clinical and pathologic stages of the disease.[1] The abnormalities can be attributed to three factors: (1) the presence of effusion; (2) "injury" of the superficial myocardium by the pressure of fluid or fibrin; and (3) superficial myocarditis.

PERICARDIAL EFFUSION

Pericardial effusion has two effects: low voltage and cyclic variations in the amplitude of ECG complexes (electrical alternans).

Low Voltage

The low voltage is usually due to the short-circuiting effect of the pericardial fluid. The low amplitude of the ventricular complex is frequently associated with normal amplitude of the P wave in the limb leads. It may be explained by the absence of effusion over the posterior surface of the atria, which is in part devoid of pericardial duplication.[2] The relation between the amount of fluid and the decrease in voltage, however, is not consistent.[3] Echocardiographic studies have shown that low QRS voltage is a weak predictor of pericardial effusion.[4] In most instances the amplitude of the ventricular complex increases after pericardiocentesis (Figure 11–1). If this fails to occur, the low voltage probably is the result of the insulating effect of fibrin deposits.[5] A commonly used definition of low voltage requires the QRS amplitude to be less than 0.5 mV in each of the limb leads and less than 1.0 mV in each of the precordial leads (Figure 11–2). The requirements in some computer programs are less strict, which creates confusing reports.

Low voltage of the QRS complex may be seen in pathologic states other than pericardial effusion. For instance, with hypothyroidism the low voltage appears to result from myxedematous myocardial involvement. Low QRS voltage also is commonly seen with chronic constrictive pericarditis and various types of diffuse myocardial disease such as amyloidosis, scleroderma, and cardiac neoplasm. Myocardial fibrosis in chronic ischemic heart disease may reduce the QRS amplitude. The most common extracardiac causes of low voltage are pleural effusion, emphysema, pneumothorax, and excess epicardial or subcutaneous fat overlying the heart.

Electrical Alternans

Variations in the amplitude of the ventricular complex may resemble the "electrical alternans" produced by alternating changes in ventricular repolarization or intraventricular conduction (see Chapter 24). With pericarditis, however, the "alternans" is caused by changes in cardiac position that result from the rotational, pendular motion of the heart. Normal rotation of the heart along the axis is attributed to the contraction of spiral muscle and uncoiling of the large vessels. This motion is normally restrained by the relaxation, filling, and gentle pressure of the lung and mediastinum. The presence of effusion removes these normal restraints, and the heart has more freedom of rotation during systole and less

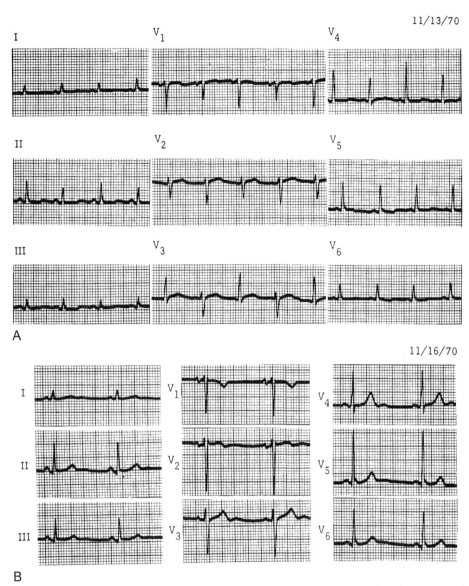

Figure 11-1 Electrical alternans in a 50-year-old woman with pericardial effusion and cardiac tamponade due to a neoplasm. **A,** Tracing made on 11/13/70 demonstrates alternation of the QRS complex during cardiac tamponade. **B,** Electrical alternans is no longer present in the tracing of 11/16/70 after the tamponade was relieved. The voltage of the QRS complex is increased, and the T waves have a more normal appearance. (From Fowler NO: The electrocardiogram in pericarditis. Cardiovasc Clin 5:256, 1973.)

tendency to complete restoration during diastole.[6,7] This motion was termed *cardiac nystagmus* by Littman.[7] The variations in amplitude differ from the typical alternans pattern in that they occur gradually over more than two consecutive complexes, although true alternans may be present (Figure 11–3). Such alternans occurs when the natural frequency of pendular motion is approximately half the heart rate.[6]

Subtle variations in the amplitude of the ventricular and occasionally the atrial complexes occur in most cases with large effusion, but the alternans involving the P wave, QRS complex, and T wave together, called "total electrical alternans," is highly suggestive of cardiac tamponade in patients with pericarditis.[8] This phenomenon has low sensitivity for recognizing pericardial effusion, however, as total electrical alternans was found in only 4 of 56 patients with cardiac tamponade reported by Guberman and associates.[9] An additional 7 patients had alternans of the QRS complex alone. Of the 11 patients with total alternans or only QRS alternans, 6 had malignant pericardial effusion (see Figure 11–1).

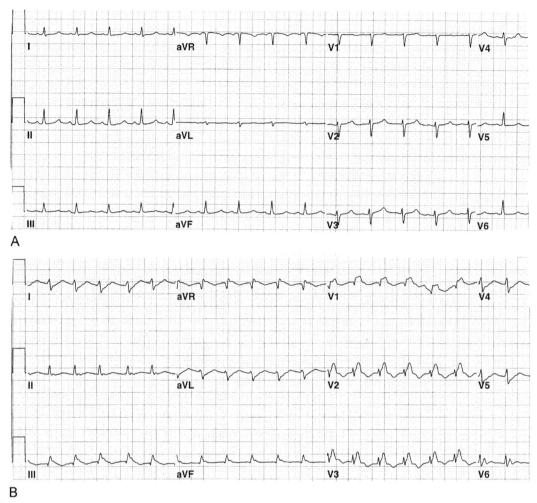

Figure 11–2 ECG of a 51-year-old woman with pericardial effusion due to metastatic carcinoma of the breast. **A,** Note the sinus rhythm at a rate of 109 beats/min and low voltage in all leads except lead II. **B,** Three days later, with clinical and echocardiographic evidence of cardiac tamponade requiring removal of a hemorrhagic effusion, the ECG shows a slightly irregular tachycardia of uncertain mechanism at a rate of 141 beats/min, further decrease in voltage, and a right bundle branch block pattern with ST segment elevation in the right precordial leads, possibly caused by compression of the right ventricle.

EFFECT OF PRESSURE PRODUCED BY FLUID OR FIBRIN

ST Segment Deviation

Pressure on the myocardium produces a "current of injury" manifested by deviation of the ST segment from the baseline. The resulting ST vector is directed inferiorly and anteriorly. In horizontal hearts the ST vector tends to be parallel to the lead II axis and in vertical hearts to the lead III axis. The direction is therefore similar to that of the normal ST vector as well as to that of the mean QRS vector.

Surawicz and Lassiter[1] analyzed ST segment changes in 12 standard leads in serial tracings from 31 patients with proved acute pericarditis.

The ST segment was elevated in 90 percent of patients. ST elevation was present in more than 70 percent of patients in leads I, II, V_5, and V_6; in 32 to 55 percent of patients in leads III, aV_L, a_F, V_3, and V_4; in 26 percent of patients in lead V_2; and only in one patient (3 percent) in lead V_1. Reciprocal ST segment depression occurred in 64 percent of the patients, usually in leads aV_R and V_1. In one patient the ST segment was depressed in lead III.

PR Segment Changes

Spodick[10–12] and others[13] described a PR segment (STa) shift with acute pericarditis in as many as 82 percent of patients. The PR segment

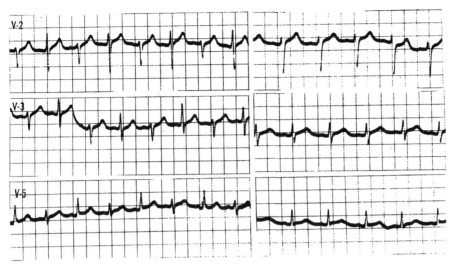

Figure 11–3   **Left,** Alternans of the QRS complex and T wave in the presence of a large pericardial effusion causing cardiac tamponade. **Right,** Alternans ceases after removal of the pericardial fluid. (From Surawicz B, Fisch C: Cardiac alternans: diverse mechanisms and clinical manifestations. J Am Coll Cardiol 20:483, 1992.)

was depressed in all leads except lead aV_R and occasionally lead V_1. In lead aV_R the PR segment was always elevated. PR segment displacement is seen best in leads II, aV_R, aV_F, and V_4–V_6. In a more recent study of 50 consecutive patients with acute pericarditis, Baljepally and Spodick[14] found that 11 patients had PR segment deviation without ST segment displacement, 20 had both PR segment and ST segment changes, 7 had ST segment changes without PR segment changes, and 12 had neither PR nor ST segment changes. In these studies[11,14] the PR segment deviation was the earliest ECG abnormality at the time when the ST segment was elevated or was returning to the baseline but before the T waves became inverted in patients with acute pericarditis. Charles et al.[13] proposed that any PR segment depression > 0.8 mV or elevation > 0.5 mV suggests the presence of atrial injury. Figure 11–4 is the ECG of a 19-year-old man with idiopathic pericarditis. In 40 asymptomatic patients with pericardial effusion of varying etiology, PR segment depression was observed in 23 patients.[15]

It should be noted that recognition of PR segment depression requires establishment of a reference line (i.e., isoelectric baseline), assumed to be represented by the TP segment. This is sometimes difficult in the presence of tachycardia or ST segment elevation.

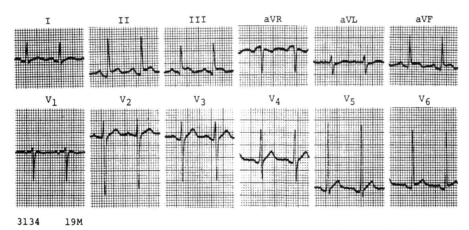

3134   19M

Figure 11–4   PR segment depression in acute pericarditis in a 19-year-old man with acute idiopathic pericarditis. The PR segment depression is seen best in leads II, aV_F, and V_1–V_6. PR segment is elevated in lead aV_R. ST segment elevation is seen best in the inferior and left precordial leads.

CHANGES ATTRIBUTED TO SUPERFICIAL MYOCARDITIS

Transient abnormalities of the ST segment without subsequent T wave changes occur in some patients with pericarditis, but most patients develop T wave abnormalities. They are attributed to superficial myocarditis (epicarditis) and can usually be differentiated from the T wave abnormalities of myocardial infarction (MI) because: (1) the myocardial surface responsible for the abnormal T waves is more extensive with pericarditis than with MI; (2) the muscle mass of fibers with abnormal repolarization responsible for the T wave changes is smaller with pericarditis than with MI; and (3) the inflammatory changes associated with pericarditis appear to produce myocardial damage more slowly and insidiously than the ischemic changes associated with acute MI.

Characteristically, the T wave vector in pericarditis is directed to the right, superiorly, and posteriorly. T wave inversion is therefore observed in leads that normally display upright T waves.

In typical cases of pericarditis the T wave becomes inverted in all standard leads except aV_R and V_1, but the amplitude of negative T waves is usually relatively low, and the T waves are often incompletely inverted (Figure 11–5). An incompletely inverted T wave, such as a diphasic (positive-negative) wave or a notched T wave, is a characteristic feature of the ECG pattern of pericarditis.[16,17] Surawicz and Lassiter[1] found a notched summit of the T wave before the return of the ST segment to baseline in 40 percent of patients.

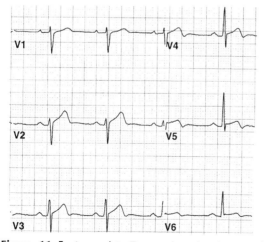

Figure 11–5 Incomplete T wave inversion in several leads on the ECG of a 37-year-old man recorded 4 days after the onset of chest pain associated with a pericardial friction rub. ST segment is still slightly elevated in leads V_4–V_6.

QTc INTERVAL

Surawicz and Lassiter[1] compared the QTc interval from the same lead in 16 patients with pericarditis when the T wave was inverted and shortly after recovery when the T wave became upright. The difference between the QTc interval in these two conditions was negligible, and in most cases the QTc interval was normal. These series did not include patients with postoperative pericarditis (see later discussion) in whom the QTc interval is usually prolonged, most likely as a result of surgery and not pericarditis per se.

EVOLUTION OF ECG CHANGES

Spodick[10] described four stages of evolutionary ST and T wave changes. During stage 1 there is ST segment elevation in leads that face the epicardial surface of the ventricles. In stage 2 the ST junction returns to baseline, and the T wave amplitude begins to decrease. During this transitional stage, different leads frequently reflect different stages of ST segment and T wave abnormalities. Thus the ECG may appear normal when the ST segment elevation disappears before the appearance of T wave abnormalities. Surawicz and Lassiter[1] observed such normalization in 20 percent of patients for periods ranging from 1 day or less to 5 days (average 2.3 days). During stage 3 the T waves are inverted. Stage 4 represents ECG resolution with a return to the normal pattern. One or more stages of the ECG changes may be absent, depending on the time of the recording relative to the disease process, the frequency of observation, and the severity of the disease. The typical ST changes were reported in 90 percent or more of the patients with acute pericarditis[1,11] (Figures 11–6 and 11–7).

CARDIAC ARRHYTHMIAS

Cardiac arrhythmias are not common with acute pericarditis, but if present they usually are supraventricular in origin. In a prospective study of 100 consecutive cases, Spodick[18] found arrhythmias (all atrial) in seven patients, all of whom had underlying heart disease. Of these seven patients, five had atrial fibrillation, one had junctional tachycardia, and one had atrial flutter. In the experience of Chou,[19] atrial flutter is encountered almost as often as atrial fibrillation. The pathologic studies of James[20] revealed involvement of the sinoatrial node in patients who had pericarditis associated with atrial arrhythmias.

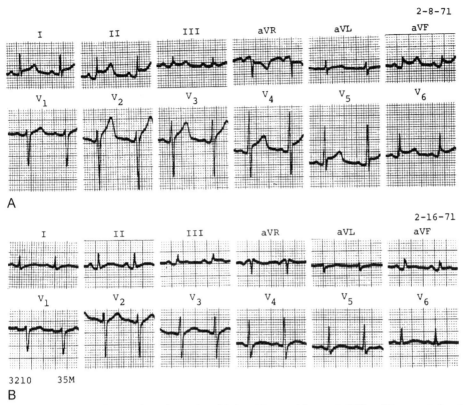

2-8-71

A

2-16-71

B

3210   35M

Figure 11–6 Serial changes of acute idiopathic pericarditis in a 36-year-old man. **A,** Diffuse ST segment elevation involving all leads except aV$_R$ and aV$_L$. In lead aV$_R$ the ST segment is depressed. The QRS complex is normal. **B,** The ST segment is almost isoelectric, and T waves are flattened or notched.

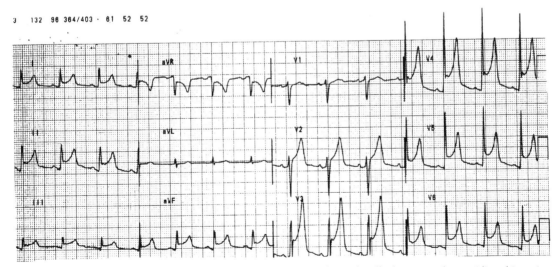

Figure 11–7 ECG of a 37-year-old man with clinically and echocardiographically documented acute idiopathic pericarditis. Note the large amplitude of the ST segment elevation, a finding seen more commonly with acute ischemia than with acute pericarditis; the reciprocal ST segment depression is seen only in lead aV$_R$. PR segment depression is apparent in lead II.

DIFFERENTIATION FROM MI, NORMAL VARIANT, AND MYOCARDITIS

Myocardial Infarction

The ST segment deviation in pericarditis is usually less pronounced than during the early stages of MI. Elevation > 0.5 mV (see Figure 11–7) is uncommon. These observations suggest that the injury current is probably smaller with pericarditis than with acute MI. However, the ventricular surface area generating the ST vector is usually more extensive with typical pericarditis than with MI. Therefore with pericarditis, the elevation of the ST segment is recorded in more standard leads than it is during MI. At the same time, reciprocal depression of the ST segment with pericarditis is recorded in fewer standard leads than with infarction.

The T wave in pericarditis is inverted in more standard leads than in most cases of MI. With pericarditis, however, the T waves are usually less deeply or less completely inverted than with MI.

The absence of QTc lengthening in pericarditis may help differentiate pericarditis from subacute or chronic ischemia. During the acute injury stage of MI the elevated ST segment is typically convex, and the terminal portion of the QRS complex is frequently obliterated and incorporated into the ST segment. During the acute stage of pericarditis the elevated ST segment is usually concave, and no component of the QRS complex is obliterated, which means that when the S wave is pulled up by the elevated ST segment, the J point is clearly discernible. However, the same configuration can be observed in patients with acute MI and in subjects without heart disease.

Evolution of ST segment and T wave abnormalities during pericarditis usually occurs more slowly and more asynchronously than during acute MI. With pericarditis the T wave remains upright until the ST segment returns to the isoelectric line, whereas with MI the T wave often begins to invert when the ST segment is still elevated, resulting in an upward convexity of the ST segment. Fusion of the ST segment and T wave into a single monophasic curve practically rules out acute pericarditis as the sole cause of ST segment elevation.

Normal Variant

Diffuse ST segment elevation often is seen in healthy young individuals in the normal male pattern, often called "early repolarization" (see Chapter 1). Unlike that seen with pericarditis, this is a stable pattern, unchanged on serial observations.

Similar to acute pericarditis, the ST segment changes are most marked in the precordial leads, but ST depression in lead V_1, if present, favors a diagnosis of acute pericarditis.[21] The normal variant is usually associated with tall T waves in the same leads in which the ST segment is elevated, and the ratio of the amplitude of ST elevation to the amplitude of the T waves (ST/T ratio) in lead V_6 is <0.25.[22] It has been reported[22] that with pericarditis the PR segment depression is seen in the limb leads and the precordial leads, whereas in normal subjects with ST elevation the PR segment depression is confined to either the limb leads or the precordial leads.

Myocarditis

The most common finding associated with myocarditis is diffuse T wave inversion without ST segment shift, although ST segment displacement, usually depression, occurs occasionally. Often myocarditis and pericarditis coexist. Chou[19] observed acute myocarditis in children with the ECG findings of marked ST segment elevation and reciprocal ST segment depression resembling that seen in patients with acute MI. The presence of ventricular arrhythmias or an atrioventricular (AV) or intraventricular conduction defect supports the diagnosis of myocarditis.

INCIDENCE AND MAGNITUDE OF ECG ABNORMALITIES

The incidence and severity of the ECG abnormalities of pericarditis depend on the etiology of the disease. Patients with chronic effusion may have no signs of pericarditis except low voltage and low T wave amplitude.[23] The typical pattern with ST segment and T wave changes occurs in almost all children and in all patients with traumatic and idiopathic (viral) pericarditis.

The characteristic ST segment elevation occurred in about 64 percent of the 325 cases of idiopathic pericarditis reviewed by Soffer,[24] and normal ECGs were recorded in only 6 percent. In 35 patients with tuberculous pericarditis reported by Rooney and co-workers,[25] only 9 percent had ST elevation typical of pericarditis, but 84 percent had T wave inversion compatible with the diagnosis. The classic changes are present in most patients with purulent pericarditis.[26]

The changes appear less frequently with rheumatic, uremic, and neoplastic pericarditis. For instance, among 33 patients with uremic pericarditis reported by Bailey and associates,[27] only 1 had the typical changes. The lower incidence of typical

ECG abnormalities in these conditions may be caused by masking of the pericarditis pattern by concomitant ECG changes due to other processes.

An ECG diagnosis of pericarditis complicating acute MI—for which Spodick[28] suggested the term "infarct pericarditis" to avoid potential confusion with the post-MI syndrome—is difficult. In the study of Kainin et al.,[29] 31 of 423 patients admitted to the coronary care unit had pericardial friction rub, but only 1 had diagnostic ST segment changes on the ECG. Such rarity of typical diagnostic criteria may be attributed to the regional character of pericarditis, which is usually limited to the area of transmural infarction. This makes it difficult to distinguish the changes due to pericarditis from those due to the acute infarction. Sometimes pericarditis is suspected when the ST segment is isoelectric or elevated in the leads in which reciprocal ST segment depression is usually expected to take place (see Figure 7–29).

According to Oliva and associates,[30] the behavior of the T wave is more helpful. Based on a study of 43 patients with postinfarction pericarditis diagnosed clinically, these investigators established that regional pericarditis is recognizable (in the absence of reinfarction or unless the infarct is small) by the presence of positive T waves in the leads in which the T waves would be expected to be inverted within 48 hours after the infarction. Similar significance is attached to a premature reversal of negative T waves to positive deflections. Oliva and associates[31] suggested that these changes, designated "atypical T wave evolution," represent a reliable indicator of a transmural process.

The diagnosis of pericarditis in post-MI syndrome is less difficult because usually the ST and T changes recur after the acute changes of the infarct have subsided.[23,32] In Dressler's series,[23] half of the 44 cases had ECG changes compatible with pericarditis. The ECG is less helpful than expected for postpericardiotomy syndrome.[32,33] With postpericardiotomy syndrome after traumatic hemopericardium, however, the typical changes are seen in two thirds of patients.[34] Subepicardial hemorrhage, an uncommon cause of diffuse ST and T wave changes simulating pericarditis, is illustrated in Figure 11–8. The subepicardial hemorrhage was the result of a dissecting aneurysm.

Transient ECG changes associated with pericarditis, lasting 1 to a few days, are seen frequently during the early postoperative period after cardiac surgery. They represent the most common cause of the ECG pattern of pericarditis in hospitals with a large volume of cardiac surgery. With pericarditis due to radiation therapy, the symptoms and signs are commonly delayed for a few months to several years (generally less than 1 year) after treatment. The ECG shows either ST and T wave changes of acute pericarditis or findings associated with pericardial effusion. With rheumatic, rheumatoid, or neoplastic pericarditis, the ECG changes are observed only occasionally.[1,35] In six cases of documented pericarditis after percutaneous transluminal coronary angioplasty, a typical ECG pattern was present in only one patient.[36]

The *duration* of the ECG changes in pericarditis also depends on the cause of the pericarditis and the extent of the associated myocardial damage. Persistent ECG abnormalities occur most often with purulent, tuberculous, and neoplastic pericarditis. With idiopathic pericarditis the ST segment changes usually return to normal within 1 week, whereas T wave inversion may

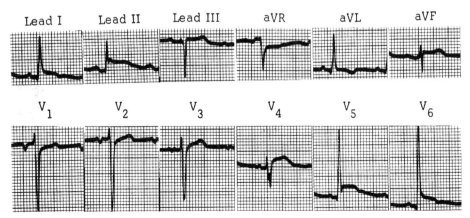

Figure 11–8 Subepicardial hemorrhage in a 61-year-old man who had a dissecting aneurysm. At autopsy it was found that the dissection had extended subepicardially. ECG shows abnormal P waves consistent with left atrial enlargement and left ventricular hypertrophy. Note the diffuse ST segment elevation with T wave inversion in some of the leads.

persist for weeks or months. In a review of 234 patients who had follow-up examinations,[37] only 13 had persistent changes lasting more than 3 months. In some cases the inverted T wave varied in depth and contour from day to day despite the absence of other evidence of active disease.

ECG Findings in Chronic Constrictive Pericarditis

The ECG abnormalities of constrictive pericarditis are nonspecific, although some abnormalities usually are present. If the ECG is normal, the diagnosis of constrictive pericarditis should be reconsidered.[19]

The ECGs of patients with constrictive pericarditis usually show low voltage. In reported series, an abnormally low-amplitude QRS complex was seen in 55 to 90 percent of cases,[38–40] possibly reflecting myocardial atrophy.[41]

Flattening, notching, or inversion of the T waves in many standard leads is the most common finding with constrictive pericarditis (Figures 11–9 and 11–10). In the larger reported series, these changes were present in 90 to 100 percent of cases.[38,39,42,43] Patients with sinus rhythm frequently have intraatrial conduction disturbances that produce P wave abnormalities resembling the pattern of left atrial enlargement (Figure 11–11). Abnormal Q waves suggestive of MI may be seen in patients with constrictive pericarditis and normal coronary arteries due to the presence of myocardial fibrosis.[44] Right axis deviation or a right ventricular hypertrophy pattern is seen occasionally in patients with constrictive pericarditis.[45] In some cases it can be explained by the presence of severe fibrotic annular subpulmonary

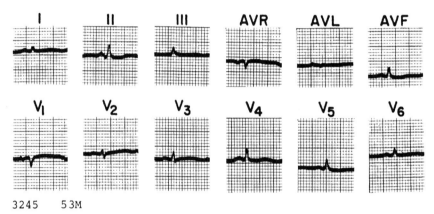

3245   5 3M

Figure 11–9 Constrictive pericarditis proved by surgery. ECG shows low voltage of the QRS complex in all leads. Diffuse ST segment and T wave abnormalities are also present.

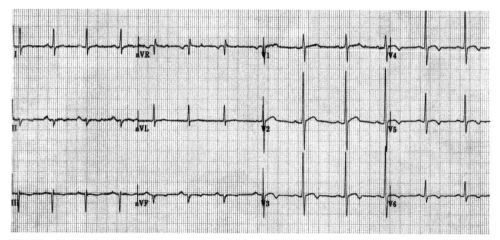

Figure 11–10 Pseudoinfarction in a 58-year-old man with calcific constrictive pericarditis due to histoplasmosis. Coronary arteriogram was normal. In the ECG, abnormal Q waves are present in leads III and aV_F, resembling inferior myocardial infarction. The T waves are inverted in the inferior leads and leads V_3–V_6.

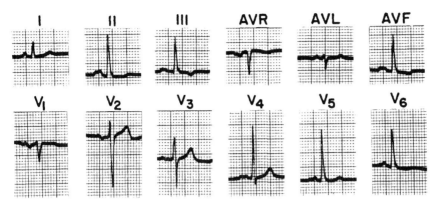

Figure 11–11   Abnormal P waves in constrictive pericarditis in a 58-year-old man who has a severely calcified pericardium. "P mitrale" type of P waves are seen best in leads II and aV$_F$ and in some of the precordial leads. Abnormal T waves are present in the inferior and left precordial leads.

constriction resulting in anatomic right ventricular hypertrophy. More often the pathophysiology of the right axis deviation is unclear.

In contrast to acute pericarditis, atrial arrhythmias are common in advanced stages of disease. In several series, atrial fibrillation was reported in 23 to 36 percent and atrial flutter in 6 to 10 percent of the cases.[38,42,43,46]

Congenital Defect of the Pericardium

Congenital defect or absence of the pericardium is uncommon. The left side of the pericardium is usually affected.[47] The ECG findings may mimic those of right ventricular hypertrophy or anterior MI (Figure 11–12). In a review of the ECG

findings of 41 cases of uncomplicated complete defect of the left pericardium, Inoue and associates[48] found right axis deviation in 56 percent, incomplete right bundle branch block in 47 percent, clockwise rotation in 47 percent, and tall and peaked P waves in the right precordial leads in 26 percent of the cases. These changes are attributed to marked clockwise rotation of the heart along its longitudinal axis.

ECG Changes after Cardiac Surgery

In the United States the most commonly performed open heart operation is coronary artery bypass grafting (CABG). Even though the

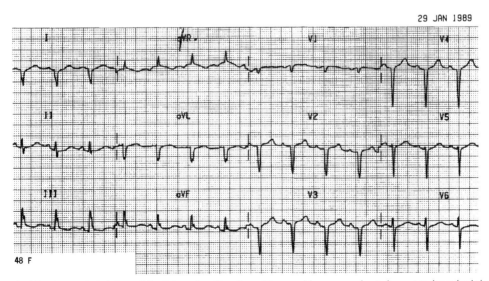

29 JAN 1989

48 F

Figure 11–12   Congenital defect of the left pericardium in a 48-year-old woman who is known to have had the defect since the age of 20 years. Diagnosis was confirmed by the appearance of air in the pericardial space after intrapleural injection. Clinical examination and right heart catheterization revealed no evidence of any other cardiac abnormality. The patient was previously reported. (From Fowler NO: Congenital defect of the pericardium: its resemblance to pulmonary artery enlargement. Cardiovasc Clin 26:114, 1962.)

operation does not require incision of the myocardium, transient postoperative ECG changes are nearly always present. It has been reported that new Q waves developed in as many as 10 percent of patients after CABG but were attributed to MI in only one third of the cases.[49,50] The incidence of postoperative MI appears to decline in centers with a large operative volume. In some cases the appearance of new Q waves after operation is caused by cessation of electrical cancellation and unmasking of a preexisting MI.[51,52] Disappearance of abnormal Q waves after CABG has also been reported.[53]

The ECG is affected by a host of factors, such as changes in the autonomic nervous tone, effects of cardioplegia ("warm" or "cold"), and manipulation of the heart. The most consistent change (if sought) is deviation of the ST segment (i.e., elevation, or lessened depression attributed to postoperative pericarditis [discussed earlier]) (Figures 11–13 and 11–14). Nonspecific T wave abnormalities are also common. They frequently

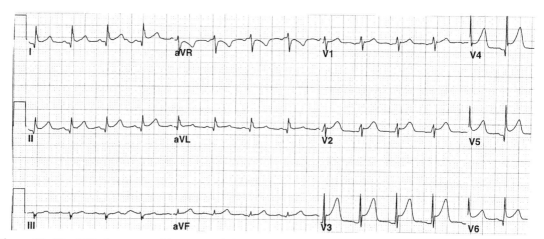

Figure 11–13   ECG of a 65-year-old man recorded 2 days after a coronary artery bypass operation. It shows a pattern of acute pericarditis with ST segment elevation in leads I, II, aV$_L$, and V$_2$–V$_6$. Reciprocal ST segment depression is present only in lead aV$_R$. PR segment appears depressed in leads I and II. ECG was normal before the operation and returned to normal within a few days after surgery.

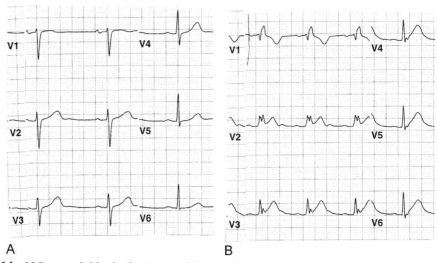

A   B

Figure 11–14   ECG precordial leads of a 61-year-old man with single–vessel coronary artery disease manifested by 90 percent narrowing of the proximal left anterior descending coronary artery and 80 percent narrowing at the origin of the diagonal branch. **A,** Preoperative ECG is normal. **B,** One day after coronary artery bypass graft (CABG) there is right bundle branch block with ST segment elevation in leads I, aV$_L$, and V$_2$–V$_4$. It is most likely caused by pericarditis, because reciprocal ST segment depression was present only in lead aV$_R$ (not shown). Pattern returned to normal within a few days.

accompany tachycardia or represent evolution of the pericarditis pattern. Unlike pericarditis of other etiologies, postoperative pericarditis is accompanied by lengthening of the QTc interval, which immediately after operation may be related to hypothermia. More often, QTc lengthening is caused by other factors because it persists usually for more than 1 day.

Not uncommonly, transient ST segment elevation after surgery is caused by recurrence of the acute injury pattern in the region of a previous MI. It can be differentiated from pericarditis by

an amplitude of the ST segment deviation larger than that induced by pericarditis and by the presence of reciprocal ST segment depression accompanying the ischemia-induced ST segment elevation (Figures 11–15 and 11–16). Rare ECGs simulating acute MI have been seen after cardiac valve replacement (see Chapter 7). Figure 11–17 shows such a case in a patient who had no coronary artery disease.

Changes in the frontal plane axis are probably related to changes in the position of the heart but may be also caused by commonly occurring

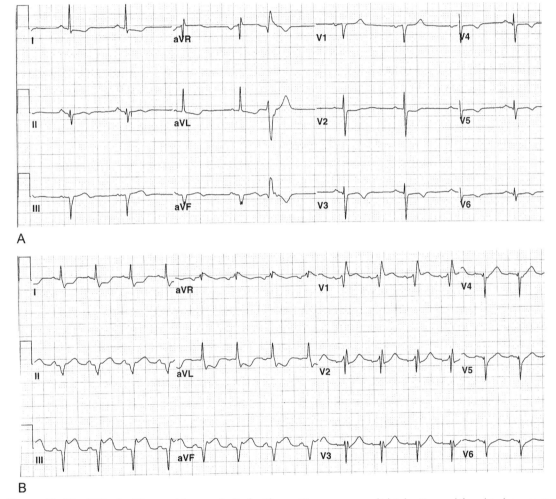

Figure 11–15   ECG of a 78-year-old man admitted with non-Q wave myocardial infarction and found to have severe obstructive disease of the left anterior descending and right coronary arteries with marked hypokinesis of the inferior wall. **A,** Preoperative ECG shows sinus rhythm with a single premature ventricular complex, inferior infarction, and symmetric inverted T waves in leads V_3–V_6. **B,** Ten hours after saphenous vein grafting and endarterectomy of the distal right coronary artery, saphenous vein grafting of the intermediate ventricular branch, and implantation of the left internal mammary artery into the left anterior descending coronary artery. ECG shows an acute injury pattern with ST segment elevation in leads II, III, aV_F, and V_1 and reciprocal ST segment depression in leads I and aV_L. QRS duration increased from 102 ms in **A** to 142 ms in **B,** with a terminal delay that may be caused by inferior periinfarction block or right bundle branch block. Preoperative pattern returned within a few days.

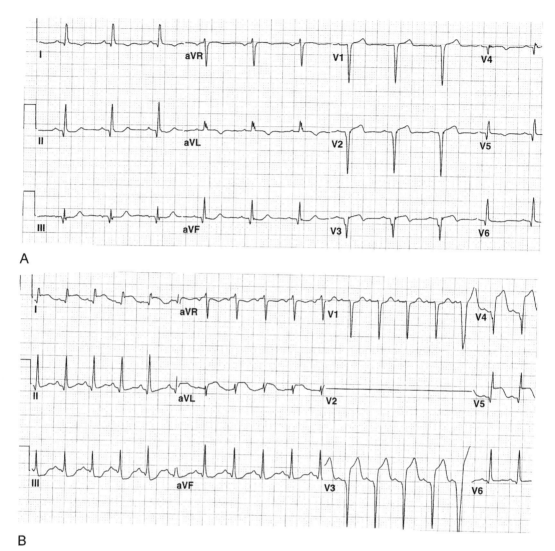

Figure 11–16 ECG of a 50-year-old man with three–vessel coronary artery disease 1 day before (**A**) and 1 day after (**B**) surgical revascularization. **A,** Pattern of a previous anterolateral myocardial infarction, which according to the history is about 2 years old. **B,** Acute injury pattern with ST segment elevation in leads I, aV$_L$, and V$_3$–V$_5$. Reciprocal ST segment depression is seen in leads III and aV$_F$. Lead V$_2$ is absent because of the surgical dressing. ECG returned to the preoperative pattern within 3 days.

intraventricular conduction disturbances. The latter consist of nonspecific widening of the QRS complex, fascicular blocks, and complete and incomplete right bundle branch block (RBBB) and left bundle branch block (LBBB). AV conduction disturbances, however, are seldom more advanced than prolongation of the PR interval.

Common rhythm disturbances include sinus tachycardia, supraventricular ectopic complexes and rhythms such as ectopic atrial tachycardia, AV junctional tachycardia, atrial fibrillation, atrial flutter, ventricular ectopic complexes, and

nonsustained ventricular tachycardia. Atrial arrhythmias develop in 11 to 40 percent of patients after CABG and in more than 50 percent of patients after valvular surgery.[54] They are usually transient, but atrial flutter and atrial fibrillation may require cardioversion. Atrial fibrillation after CABG occurred in 43 percent of patients with proximal or mid-artery stenosis of the right coronary artery and in only 19 percent of patients without significant right coronary disease.[55] Figure 11–18 shows rhythm strips of six types of postoperative supraventricular arrhythmia in six patients. Common arrhythmias are

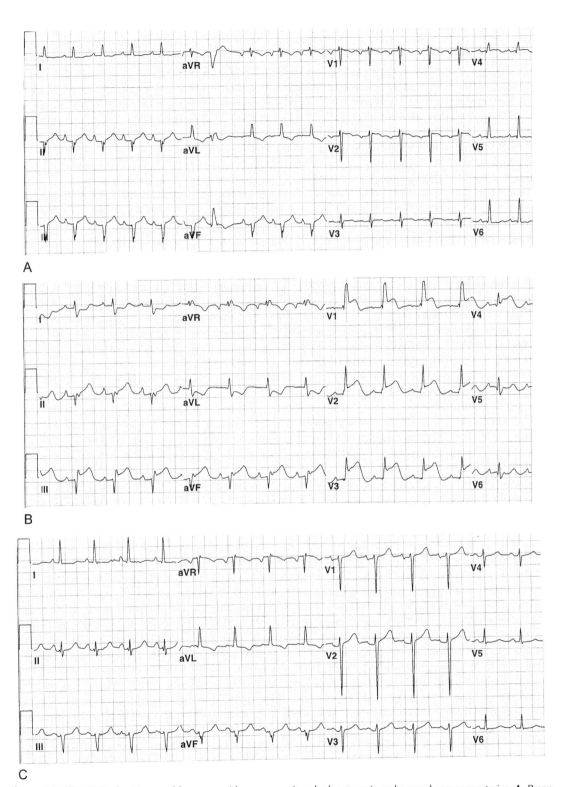

Figure 11–17   ECG of a 61-year-old woman with severe aortic valvular stenosis and normal coronary arteries. **A,** Preoperative ECG shows a sinus rhythm with a QRS duration of 80 ms, left axis deviation, and a mildly abnormal T wave in leads I and aV$_L$. **B,** Three days later, on the first day after replacement of the aortic valve with a St. Jude prosthetic valve, the QRS pattern suggests an inferoposterior infarction with a QRS duration of 118 ms. ST segment elevation suggests an acute inferior and right ventricular injury pattern. Cardiac enzymes were not diagnostic of infarction. **C,** The following day, the ECG shows complete regression of the infarction and the acute injury pattern. Postoperative course was uneventful, and the transient ECG abnormality was attributed to a coronary spasm or to a rapidly resolving coronary embolus.

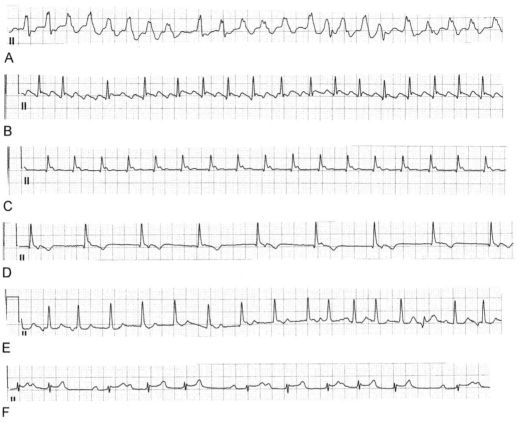

Figure 11–18 ECG strips of lead II from six patients recorded within the first few days after coronary artery bypass operations. All patients had sinus rhythm, normal PR, and normal QRS duration before operation. From top to bottom: **A,** Atrial fibrillation with aberrant ventricular conduction in a 70-year-old man. **B,** Atrial flutter with variable ventricular response in a 53-year-old man. **C,** Atrioventricular (AV) junctional tachycardia at a rate of 132 beats/min in a 54-year-old woman. **D,** AV junctional rhythm at a rate of 63 beats/min with variable VA conduction in a 53-year-old woman. **E,** Multifocal atrial tachycardia in a 71-year-old woman. **F,** Second-degree AV block with 4 to 5 Wenckebach conduction in a 69-year-old man with a previous inferior infarction.

atrial fibrillation, atrial flutter, and AV junctional rhythms. Less common arrhythmias are multifocal atrial tachycardia and second-degree AV block. Sustained ventricular tachycardia and ventricular fibrillation are unusual complications in the absence of recurrent myocardial ischemia or MI. The long-term postoperative prognosis is not affected by the presence of advanced postoperative conduction disturbances[56] or nonsustained ventricular tachycardia.[57]

Operations to correct congenital heart defects often result in the appearance of RBBB because of damage to the moderator band and distal right bundle branch from the ventriculotomy.[58] Occasionally RBBB is associated with a left fascicular block (mostly anterior). Postoperative LBBB is becoming more common as more complex congenital lesions are being corrected.[58] The ECG pattern of congenital heart disease in adults is discussed in Chapter 12.

REFERENCES

1. Surawicz B, Lassiter KC: Electrocardiogram in pericarditis. Am J Cardiol 26:471, 1970.
2. Holzmannn M: Klinische Elektrokardiographie. Stuttgart, Georg Thieme, 1965, pp 511–525.
3. Harvey AN, Whitehill MR: Tuberculous pericarditis. Medicine 16:45, 1937.
4. Casale PN, Devereux RB, Kligfield P, et al: Pericardial effusion: relation of clinical echocardiographic and electrocardiographic finding. J Electrocardiol 17:115, 1984.
5. Nizet PM, Marriott HJL: Electrocardiogram and pericardial effusion. JAMA 198:169, 1966.

6. McGregor M, Baskind E: Electric alternans in pericardial effusion. Circulation 11:837, 1955.
7. Littman D: Alternation of the heart. Circulation 27:280, 1963.
8. Littman D, Spodick DH: Total electrical alternation in pericardial disease. Circulation 17:912, 1958.
9. Guberman BA, Fowler NO, Engel PJ, et al: Cardiac tamponade in medical patients. Circulation 64:633, 1981.
10. Spodick DH: The electrocardiogram in acute pericarditis: distributions of morphologic and axial changes in stages. Am J Cardiol 33:470, 1974.
11. Spodick DH: Diagnostic electrocardiographic sequences in acute pericarditis: significance of PR segment and PR vector changes. Circulation 48:575, 1973.
12. Spodick DH: Differential diagnosis of acute pericarditis. Prog Cardiovasc Dis 14:192, 1971.
13. Charles MA, Bensinger TA, Glasser SP: Atrial injury current in pericarditis. Arch Intern Med 131:657, 1973.
14. Baljepally R, Spodick DH: PR-segment deviation as the initial electrocardiographic response in acute pericarditis. Am J Cardiol 82:1505, 1998.
15. Kudo Y, Yamasaki F, Doiy, et al: Clinical correlates of PR-segment depression in asymptomatic patients with pericardial effusion. J Am Coll Cardiol 39:2000, 2002.
16. Winternitz M, Langendorf R: The electrocardiogram in pericarditis. Acta Med Scand 94:141, 1938.
17. Stewart JR, Fajardo LF: Radiation-induced heart disease: an update. Prog Cardiovasc Dis 27:173, 1984.
18. Spodick DH: Arrhythmias during acute pericarditis: a prospective study of 100 consecutive cases. JAMA 235:39, 1976.
19. Chou TE-C: Electrocardiography. In: Clinical Practice: Adult and Pediatric, 4th ed. Philadelphia, Saunders, 1996, pp 240–246.
20. James TN: Pericarditis and the sinus node. Arch Intern Med 110:305, 1962.
21. Spodick DH: Differential characteristics of the electrocardiogram in early repolarization and acute pericarditis. N Engl J Med 295:523, 1976.
22. Ginzton LE, Laks MM: The differential diagnosis of acute pericarditis from the normal variant: new electrocardiographic criteria. Circulation 65:1004, 1982.
23. Dressler W: The post-myocardial infarction syndrome. Arch Intern Med 103:28, 1959.
24. Soffer A: Electrocardiographic abnormalities in acute, convalescent and recurrent stages of idiopathic pericarditis. Am Heart J 60:729, 1960.
25. Rooney JJ, Crocco JA, Lyons HA: Tuberculous pericarditis. Ann Intern Med 72:73, 1970.
26. Sagrista-Sauleda J, Barrabes JA, Permanyer-Miralda G, et al: Purulent pericarditis: review of a 20-year experience in a general hospital. J Am Coll Cardiol 22:1661, 1993.
27. Bailey GL, Hampers CL, Hager EB, et al: Uremic pericarditis: clinical features and management. Circulation 38:582, 1968.
28. Spodick DH: Definition of postinfarction pericarditis [letter]. Circulation 91:1609, 1995.
29. Kainin PM, Flessan A, Spodick DH: Infarction-associated pericarditis: rarity of diagnostic electrocardiogram. N Engl J Med 311:1211, 1984.
30. Oliva PB, Hammill SC, Edwards WD: Electrocardiographic diagnosis of postinfarction regional pericarditis. Circulation 88:896, 1993.
31. Oliva PB, Hammill SC, Talano JV: T wave changes consistent with epicardial involvement in acute myocardial infarction. J Am Coll Cardiol 24:1073, 1994.
32. Engle MA, Ito T: The postpericardiotomy syndrome. Am J Cardiol 7:73, 1961.
33. McGuinness JB, Taussig HB: The postpericardiotomy syndrome: its relationship to ambulation in the presence of "benign" pericardial and pleural reaction. Circulation 26:500, 1962.
34. Tabatznik B, Isaacs JP: Postpericardiotomy syndrome following traumatic hemopericardium. Am J Cardiol 7:83, 1961.
35. Franco AE, Levine HD, Hall AP: Rheumatoid pericarditis: report of 17 cases diagnosed clinically. Ann Intern Med 77:837, 1972.
36. Slack JD, Pinkerton CA: The electrocardiogram often fails to identify pericarditis after percutaneous transluminal coronary angioplasty. J Electrocardiol 19:399, 1986.
37. McGuire J, Helm RA, Iglauer A, et al: Nonspecific pericarditis and myocardial infarction. Circulation 14:874, 1956.
38. Dalton JC, Pearson RJ, White PD: Constrictive pericarditis: a review and long-term follow-up of 78 cases. Ann Intern Med 45:445, 1956.
39. Gimlette TMD: Constrictive pericarditis. Br Heart J 21:9, 1959.
40. Portal RW, Besterman EMM, Chambers RJ, et al: Prognosis after operation for constrictive pericarditis. BMJ 1:563, 1966.
41. Dines DE, Edwards JE, Burchell HB: Myocardial atrophy in constrictive pericarditis. Proc Staff Meet Mayo Clin 33:93, 1958.
42. Chamblis JR, Jaruszewski EJ, Brofman BL, et al: Chronic cardiac compression. Circulation 4:816, 1951.
43. Wood P: Chronic constrictive pericarditis. Am J Cardiol 7:48, 1961.
44. Levine HD: Myocardial fibrosis in constrictive pericarditis. Circulation 48:1268, 1973.
45. Chesler E, Mitha AS, Matisonn RE: The ECG of constrictive pericarditis: pattern resembling right ventricular hypertrophy. Am Heart J 91:420, 1976.
46. Bashi VV, John S, Ravikumar E, et al: Early and late results of pericardiectomy in 118 cases of constrictive pericarditis. Thorax 43:637, 1988.
47. Nasser WK, Helmen C, Tavel ME, et al: Congenital absence of the left pericardium: clinical, electrocardiographic, radiographic, hemodynamics, and angiographic findings in six cases. Circulation 41:469, 1970.
48. Inoue H, Fujii J, Mashima S, et al: Pseudo right atrial overloading pattern in complete defect of the left pericardium. J Electrocardiol 14:413, 1981.
49. Mirvis DM: Electrocariography. A Physiologic Approach. St Louis, Mosby, 1993, p 250.
50. Taylor GJ, Bourland M, Mikell FI, et al: Dubious reliability of Q wave formation in predicting new regional left ventricular akinesis after coronary artery bypass grafting. Am J Cardiol 62:1299, 1998.
51. Zeft HJ, Friedberg HD, King JF, et al: Reappearance of anterior QRS forces after coronary bypass surgery. Am J Cardiol 38:163, 1975.
52. Bassan MM, Oatfield R, Hoffman I, et al: New Q waves after aortocoronary bypass surgery: unmasking of an old infarction. N Engl J Med 290:349, 1974.
53. Conde CA, Meller J, Espinoza J, et al: Disappearance of abnormal Q waves after aortocoronary bypass surgery. Am J Cardiol 36:889, 1975.
54. Ommen SR, Odell JA, Stanton MS: Atrial arrhythmias after cardiothoracic surgery. N Engl J Med 338:1429, 1997.

55. Mendes LA, Connelly GF, McKenney PA, et al: Right coronary artery stenosis: an independent predictor of atrial fibrillation after coronary artery bypass surgery. J Am Coll Cardiol 25:198, 1995.

56. Mustonen P, Hippelainen M, Vanninen E, et al: Significance of coronary artery bypass grafting-associated conduction defects. Am J Cardiol 81:558, 1998.

57. Pinto R, Romerill DB, Nasser WK, et al: Prognosis of patients with frequent premature ventricular complexes and nonsustained ventricular tachycardia after coronary artery bypass graft operation. Clin Cardiol 19:321, 1996.

58. 58. Liebman J: Electrocardiography in congenital heart disease. *In:* Macfarlane PW, Lawrie TDV (eds): Comprehensive Electrocardiology. New York, Pergamon, pp 796–797.

12 Diseases of the Heart and Lungs

Valvular Heart Disease

Electrocardiographic (ECG) changes produced by valvular disease reflect the morphologic abnormalities of cardiac chambers caused by the disease (discussed in Chapters 2 and 3). Mitral stenosis is one of the few valvular lesions in which the ECG can lead to the diagnosis: The pattern of left atrial enlargement is associated with right ventricular hypertrophy (RVH) or right axis deviation in the frontal plane (see Figures 2–10 and 3–11). Sometimes in patients with severe mitral stenosis the pattern of left atrial enlargement occurs in the absence of any other ECG abnormality (Figure 12–1).

Pure mitral regurgitation produces no specific ECG pattern. The pattern of left atrial enlargement is usually less distinct than that of mitral stenosis, and the pattern of RVH that may develop secondary to pulmonary hypertension is seldom seen. In some cases RVH is suspected when the amplitude of the S wave in lead V_1 is lower than one would expect to find in a patient with left ventricular hypertrophy (LVH), suggested by the tall R wave in the left precordial leads (Figure 12–2).

Severe aortic valvular disease is usually associated with varying degrees of LVH (see Figure 4–1). Figure 12–3 shows a typical LVH pattern in an adult with congenital aortic stenosis. In elderly patients with sclerotic or calcific aortic valvular stenosis, the ECG may remain normal even when the stenosis is critical (Figure 12–4). In patients with aortic regurgitation, the T waves in the left precordial leads may remain upright even with advanced stages of the disease (Figure 12–5).

Cardiomyopathies

The ECG is of limited usefulness for the differential diagnosis of ischemic vs. nonischemic cardiomyopathy because (1) common to both are the patterns of ventricular hypertrophy and intraventricular conduction disturbances; (2) patterns of remote myocardial infarction (MI) are often obscured by the ECG changes resulting from ventricular hypertrophy and intraventricular conduction disturbances; and (3) QRS changes simulating MI (pseudoinfarction patterns) commonly occur in patients with various types of nonischemic cardiomyopathy. Despite the low specificity of the ECG patterns encountered in patients with cardiomyopathies, cases exist when certain anatomic or pathologic characteristics of the disease produce similar ECG patterns that may become valuable markers in the differential diagnosis of the clinical problem.

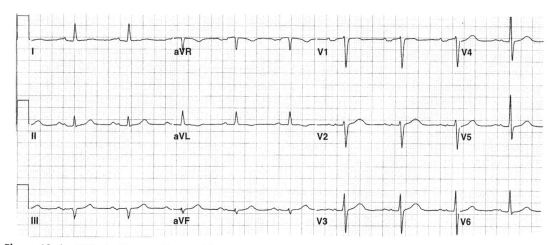

Figure 12–1   ECG of a 76-year-old man with severe mitral stenosis, moderately severe aortic regurgitation, and intermittent atrial fibrillation. ECG recorded after electrical cardioversion shows a PR interval of 234 ms and a pattern of left atrial enlargement but no other abnormalities. Prolongation of the PR interval is caused by increased P wave duration.

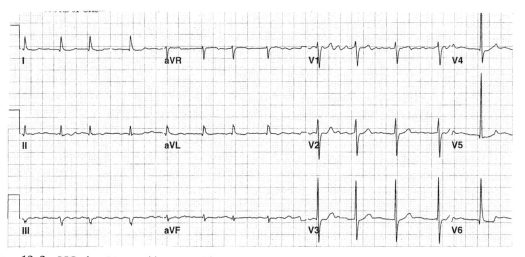

Figure 12–2   ECG of an 84-year-old woman with severe mitral regurgitation caused by myxomatous degeneration of the valve. Left ventricular function was good, and coronary arteries were normal. ECG recorded 1 day after surgical valve replacement with porcine prosthesis shows atrial fibrillation, minor ST segment and T wave abnormalities attributed to digitalis, increased (2.0 mV) R amplitude in lead V_6, and relatively low S amplitude in leads V_1 and V_2 (0.7 and 1.0 mV, respectively).

DILATED CARDIOMYOPATHY

In patients with sinus rhythm, P wave abnormalities consistent with left atrial or biatrial enlargement are often present.[1,2] The most common ECG abnormality is caused by LVH or dilation[3] (Figure 12–6). The typical LVH pattern may be obscured by low-voltage intraventricular conduction disturbances (IVCDs) or the concomitant presence of RVH. Atrioventricular (AV) and intraventricular conduction disturbances are present in most patients with advanced dilated cardiomyopathy and are manifested by first-degree AV block, left fascicular block, diffuse nonspecific QRS widening, and incomplete or complete left bundle branch block (LBBB).[3–6] The incidence of LBBB ranged in various series from 9 to 44 percent,[1] which is probably higher than in patients with ischemic cardiomyopathy of comparable clinical severity. In a patient with cardiomegaly of unknown cause, the presence of LBBB supports the diagnosis of primary myocardial disease.[1] The presence of right bundle branch block (RBBB) is less common.[7,8] IVCDs are often atypical or complex (Figures 12–7 and 12–8; see also Figure 6–13) and resemble

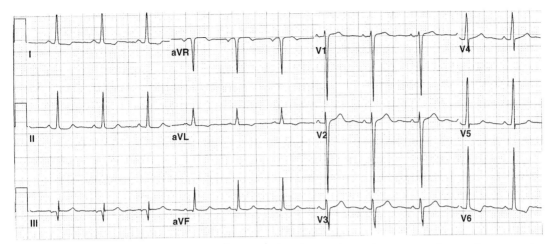

Figure 12–3 ECG of a 25-year-old woman with congenital aortic stenosis, previous open aortic commissurotomy at age 2.5, and aortic valve repair at age 9. Echocardiogram showed marked left ventricular hypertrophy, aortic stenosis with a 100-mmHg pressure gradient across the valve, and estimated aortic valve area of 0.9 cm². Patient underwent replacement of the aortic valve by the pulmonary valve and replacement of the right ventricular outflow tract with a cadaver homograft (Ross procedure). Preoperative ECG shows a left ventricular hypertrophy pattern with a Q wave in lead III (pseudoinfarction pattern).

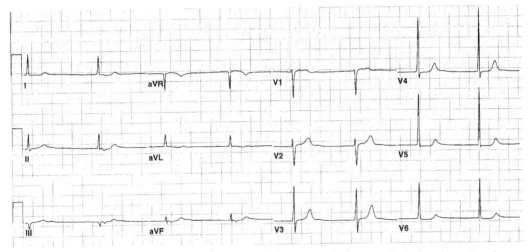

Figure 12–4 ECG of a 94-year-old man with severe calcific aortic valvular stenosis (estimated aortic valve area is 0.6 cm²). Pattern is normal except for an atrioventricular junctional rhythm at a rate of 46 beats/min.

nonspecific complex IVCDs in patients with advanced ischemic cardiomyopathy (Figure 12–9).

Abnormal Q waves mimicking anterior or inferior MI may be present as a result of myocardial fibrosis, IVCD, or changes in the direction of the initial QRS vector resulting from changes in cardiac position.[4,9,10] Compared with hypertrophic cardiomyopathy, dilated cardiomyopathy is characterized by significantly more abnormal Q waves, greater prolongation of the QRS duration, and lower amplitude of the sum of R in V_5 or V_6 plus S in V_1.[11] In some cases the predominant changes consist of the left atrial enlargement pattern alone (see Figure 2–11), diffuse T wave abnormalities (Figure 12–10), or sinus tachycardia without other ECG abnormalities (Figure 12–11). A high incidence of supraventricular and ventricular arrhythmias has been reported in most series of patients with dilated cardiomyopathy.[6] Atrial fibrillation tends to develop late,[6,12,13] and complete AV block is rare.[1] It has been reported that QRS duration ≥120 ms is a significant predictor of ventricular arrhythmias.[14]

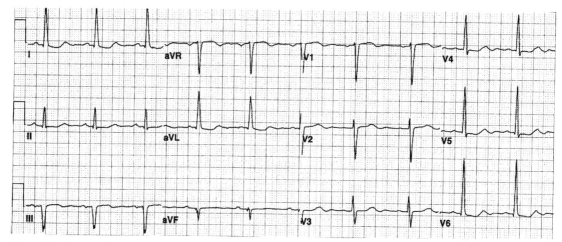

Figure 12–5   ECG of an 82-year-old woman with long-standing severe aortic regurgitation, mild mitral regurgitation, left ventricular ejection fraction of 40 percent, and normal coronary arteries. The preoperative pattern (before aortic valve replacement) shows left ventricular hypertrophy with slight ST segment depression and an upright T wave of low amplitude in leads I, aV$_L$, V$_5$, and V$_6$. In lead III the S wave is preceded by a small r deflection.

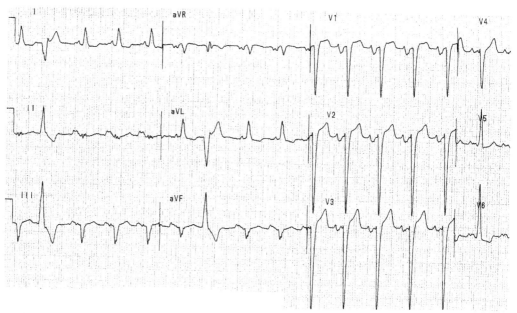

Figure 12–6   ECG of a 33-year-old man with end-stage dilated cardiomyopathy recorded 2 weeks before cardiac transplantation.

HYPERTROPHIC CARDIOMYOPATHY

The role of ECG in the diagnosis of hypertrophic cardiomyopathy (HC) has been disputed. In one study of 134 patients the ECG was normal in only 7 percent; the most frequent ECG abnormality was an LVH pattern with or without abnormal Q waves.[15] In a study of 448 consecutive patients with HC, the power of ECG to assess the clinical condition was challenged because of the weak correlation between ECG

voltage and the anterior wall LV wall thickness. Of 55 patients with LV wall thickness ≥30 mm, only 44 percent showed greatly increased QRS voltage. However, of 44 patients with HC-related death, ECG was normal only in 1.[16]

Idiopathic obstructive cardiomyopathy became a subject of intense investigation during the early 1960s. During this period many investigators encountered the characteristic ECG pattern simulating MI with a deeper-than-normal Q wave in

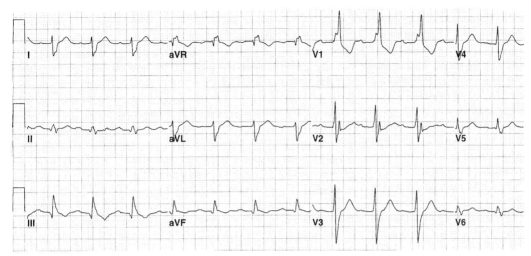

Figure 12–7   ECG of a 76-year-old patient admitted after an episode of syncope. Patient had severe dilated cardiomyopathy, left ventricular ejection fraction of 20 percent, and normal coronary arteries. ECG shows sinus rhythm, PR interval of 250 ms, QRS duration of 144 ms, right bundle branch block, and left posterior fascicular block. Atrial flutter and ventricular flutter were induced in the electrophysiology laboratory.

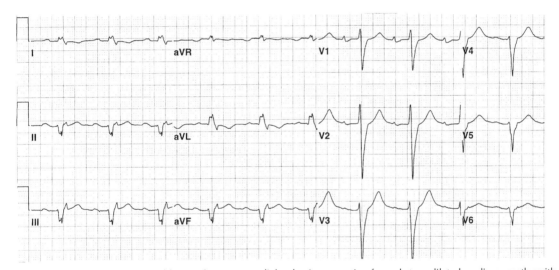

Figure 12–8   ECG of a 45-year-old man after a myocardial reduction operation for end-stage dilated cardiomyopathy with pulmonary hypertension and implanted automatic cardioverter-defibrillator. Note the sinus rhythm, left atrial enlargement, PR interval of 252 ms, QRS duration of 180 ms with an atypical left bundle branch block, and rS pattern in leads V_4–V_6.

the "lateral" and "inferior" leads and a taller-than-normal R wave in the right precordial leads (Figure 12–12; see also Figures 4–14 and 8–31).[16–20] This ECG pattern is discussed in Chapter 8.

Abnormal Q waves may be present in both obstructive and nonobstructive types of HC.[21,22] The abnormal Q waves may develop during the course of the disease, and if present, may increase or decrease in amplitude,[22] but none of these changes correlates well with the clinical characteristics of the disease or its prognosis. However, cardiac magnetic resonance study revealed that abnormal Q waves were associated with greater upper anterior septal thickness.[23a]

The coexistence of HC and the Wolff-Parkinson-White (WPW) pattern appears to be more than coincidental. Frank and Braunwald[23] reported that the WPW pattern was present in 40 of 123 patients. In another study, among 105 consecutive patients with the WPW pattern, 8 had associated HC.[24]

Primary and secondary T wave abnormalities are present in most patients with symptomatic HC. Giant inverted T waves (>1.0 mV) are believed to occur more often in patients with apical-type HC[26] (Figure 12–13). This is apparently true of the experience in Japan, but not in the West.[27] In the study of Keren et al.,[26] giant

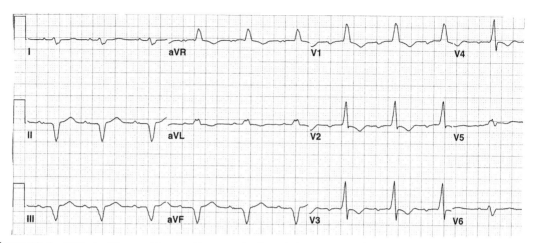

Figure 12–9 ECG of a 73-year-old man with congestive heart failure, severe ischemic cardiomyopathy, global akinesis, anterior apical dyskinesis, and an estimated left ventricular ejection fraction of 5 percent. The left anterior descending and left circumflex arteries were totally occluded. Note the sinus rhythm with PR interval of 252 ms, QRS duration of 124 ms, right bundle branch block with low R waves in leads V_5 and V_6, and superior axis in the frontal plane.

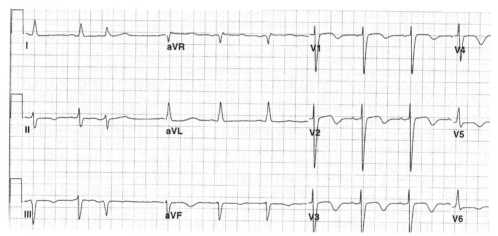

Figure 12–10 ECG of a 63-year-old woman who underwent cardiac catheterization after suffering a cardiac arrest. The study showed a poorly contracting left ventricle, left ventricular ejection fraction of 10 percent, normal coronary arteries, and no valvular lesions. Note the diffuse T wave abnormalities of the type encountered in patients with myocardial ischemia and a prolonged QTc (609 ms).

T waves were present in 5 of 23 patients with apical hypertrophy, and patients with the deepest T waves tended to have the least degree of septal apical thickening. In seven patients with apical hypertrophic cardiomyopathy, Maron et al.[28] found T wave inversion of <0.6 mV but no giant T waves. Koga et al.[29] found that giant negative T waves disappeared concomitant with a decrease in R wave amplitude during a 10-year or longer follow-up of patients with the Japanese form of apical hypertrophy characterized by giant negative T waves and tall R waves in the left precordial leads. In another subtype of HC (predominant hypertrophy of the posterior wall), 2 of 17 patients had deeply inverted T waves in the left precordial leads.[30]

The incidence and severity of supraventricular and ventricular arrhythmias appear to increase with the progression of the disease. The occurrence of atrial fibrillation is associated with worsening of symptoms, whereas the presence of ventricular tachyarrhythmias was reported to be associated with an increased incidence of sudden and nonsudden cardiac death.[30–34] A recent study by Adabag et al.,[35] however, found that ventricular tachyarrhythmias had a low positive and a relatively high negative predictive value in their study of 178 patients with HC.

Takotsubo cardiomyopathy is characterized by transient left ventricular apical ballooning that most often affects postmenopausal women and is

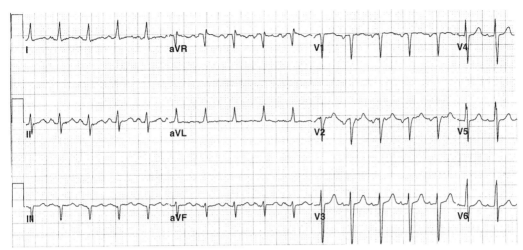

Figure 12–11 ECG of a 44-year-old man with severe dilated cardiomyopathy, left ventricular ejection fraction of 15 percent, and normal coronary arteries. Pattern is normal except for sinus tachycardia.

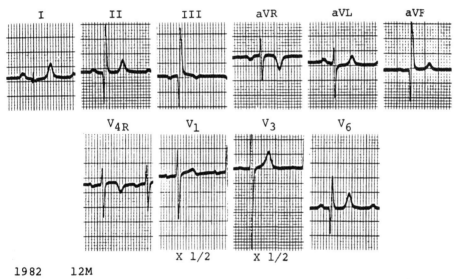

Figure 12–12 Idiopathic hypertrophic cardiomyopathy, nonobstructive, in a 12-year-old boy. The diagnosis was based on clinical and angiographic findings. No intraventricular pressure gradient was demonstrable during cardiac catheterization. ECG shows left ventricular hypertrophy. Abnormal Q waves are present in leads II, III, aV$_F$, and V$_6$. (Courtesy of Dr. Samuel Kaplan.)

often associated with ST-segment elevation in precordial leads and chest pain simulating MI. However, it is not often associated with ventricular arrhythmias and sudden death, even though the QT interval is significantly prolonged.[36,37]

RESTRICTIVE CARDIOMYOPATHY

Restrictive cardiomyopathy is discussed in association with the specific cardiomyopathies in which the restrictive component plays a dominant role, although in many cases the etiology is not clear. The ECG is usually abnormal, with a predominance of left, right, or biventricular hypertrophy.[38]

ARRHYTHMOGENIC RIGHT VENTRICULAR DYSPLASIA

The typical ECG pattern of patients with symptomatic arrhythmogenic right ventricular dysplasia (ARVD) resembles that of incomplete or complete RBBB with a negative T wave in the right precordial leads, but the terminal QRS deflection (r' or R') may be "focal," which means it is not represented by a synchronous terminal QRS delay in other leads. In a large study of patients with ARVD, the presence of isolated QRS prolongations in leads V1 through V3 was associated with significantly higher RV end-

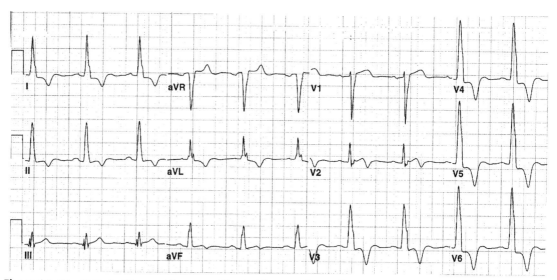

Figure 12–13   ECG of a 59-year-old woman with apical hypertrophic cardiomyopathy documented by echocardiography. A high-velocity jet in the area of the left ventricular apex was associated with a pressure gradient of 36 mmHg. ECG shows left bundle branch block with pointed and deeply inverted T waves, most prominently in the left precordial leads.

diastolic volume.[38a] In some patients the delayed terminal QRS deflection differs in shape from r′ and resembles the Greek letter epsilon (Figure 12–14). This epsilon wave corresponds to a late potential.[39,40] Several investigators have considered the epsilon wave a major diagnostic criterion of dysplasia, but it is probably a marker of a more advanced disease because its overall incidence in 75 cases reported by Bender et al.[40] was only 5.5 percent. At the same time a late potential in the shape of an epsilon appears sometimes in patients with other cardiomyopathies, probably corresponding to the underlying sites of slow conduction (Figure 12–14). The presence of a negative T wave in the right and

mid-precordial leads is another characteristic ECG abnormality.[41] In some cases T wave changes appear to be primary, and the extension of T wave negativity in the precordial leads has a direct relation to right ventricular enlargement. In a study of 20 patients with ARVD reported by Metzger et al.,[42] ECG abnormalities were present in 90 percent of cases, but serial ECG recordings provided no information about anatomic progression of the disease monitored by echocardiography.

In 50 patients with ARVD reported by Nasir et al.,[43] RBBB was present in 22 percent and T wave inversion in leads V_1–V_3 in 88 percent of patients. The most prevalent ECG criterion was prolonged S wave upstroke in leads V_1–V_3, measuring ≥55 ms. This criterion correlated with severity of the disease and induction of VT on electrophysiological study.

Ventricular arrhythmias usually have an LBBB configuration.[44] The abnormal signal-averaged ECG and low right ventricular ejection fraction were predictive of serious ventricular arrhythmias.[45] Body surface mapping suggested that the substrate of arrhythmia was the delayed depolarization in the structurally abnormal right ventricle.[46] Abnormalities of the signal-averaged ECG have been found in the pedigrees of patients with ARVD.[47]

NEUROLOGIC AND NEUROMUSCULAR DISORDERS

Friedreich's Ataxia

Cardiac lesions in patients with Friedreich's ataxia consist of diffuse interstitial fibrosis, which may explain the similarity between the

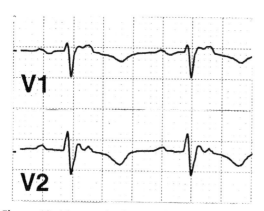

Figure 12–14   ECG leads V_1 and V_2 of a 64-year-old man with severe ischemic cardiomyopathy, episodes of sustained monomorphic ventricular tachycardia (left bundle branch block and superior axis morphology), history of coronary artery bypass surgery, and aortic valve replacement. Note an indentation on the early portion of the ST segment in the shape of a Greek epsilon.

QRS abnormalities of this condition and of MI. Hypertrophy of one or both ventricles with thickening of papillary muscles is often present.

The ECG is abnormal in 75 to 92 percent of cases[48–53]; the most common abnormalities consist of T wave changes and right or left axis deviation in the frontal plane.[50,51] Abnormal Q waves in the inferior and lateral leads, usually with tall R waves in the right precordial leads, simulating MI of the inferior and posterolateral wall (see Figure 8–29), are present in 14 to 20 percent of the cases.[48,50] These changes also resemble the pseudoinfarction patterns in patients with HC. An association of Friedreich's ataxia and HC has been reported.[50,52] In one study approximately one third of patients with Friedreich's ataxia had HC.[52] Charcot-Marie-Tooth disease (peroneal muscular atrophy) clinically resembles Friedreich's ataxia, but the incidence of cardiac involvement in this condition is low.[53]

Muscular Dystrophies

Progressive pseudohypertrophic muscle dystrophy (Duchenne type) affects the myocardium of most symptomatic patients, and ECG abnormalities are present in up to 95 percent.[54] The most typical pattern simulates posterior, lateral, or posterolateral MI, with deep Q waves in the lateral leads and tall R waves in the right precordial leads (see Figure 8–28). These abnormalities were attributed by Perloff et al.[55] to myocardial fibrosis of the posterolateral wall of the left ventricle. Both the fibrosis and the corresponding QRS changes are encountered most frequently in older patients with more advanced disease.[56] In some cases the pattern resembles that of anterior MI (Figure 12–15).

Arrhythmias and conduction disturbances are often present. The abnormalities in 20 patients studied by Perloff[57] included persistent or labile sinus tachycardia, sinus pauses, ectopic atrial and ventricular complexes and rhythms, atrial flutter, intraatrial conduction disturbances, Mobitz I type AV block, short PR interval, IVCDs, and rightward axis deviation compatible with left posterior fascicular block.

The myocardium is also affected in a juvenile form of progressive muscular atrophy (Kugelberg-Welander syndrome). Atrial arrhythmias and AV conduction disturbances are the most frequent ECG abnormalities.[58]

Unlike the Duchenne type, ECG abnormalities are usually absent in the fascioscapular type of muscular dystrophy,[59] but ECG abnormalities may be present in the limb-girdle type of cardiomyopathy, and right ventricular conduction delay has been reported in a number of cases.[60] It is believed, however, that the ECG does not necessarily mirror the presence of significant myocardial involvement.[60]

Myotonic Dystrophy

Myotonic dystrophy is the most common familial muscular dystrophy affecting adults. The most prominent cardiac abnormality is fibrosis and fatty infiltration of the entire conducting system from the sinoatrial node to the bundle branches.[61–64] ECG abnormalities are present in 45 to 85 percent of patients. The most frequently mentioned changes are first-degree AV block, abnormal left axis deviation, bundle branch block, abnormal Q waves, and various ST segment and T wave abnormalities.[65–68] Both PR lengthening to >240 ms and older age identified individuals at risk of cardiac events[68]; sudden cardiac death has been linked to the presence of advanced AV block and ventricular arrhythmias.[69] Bundle branch reentry appears to be a common mechanism of sustained

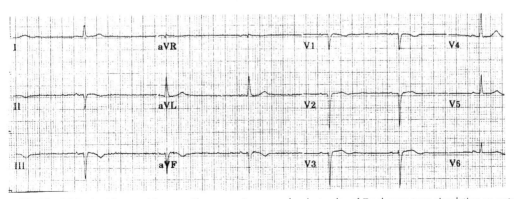

Figure 12–15   ECG of a 37-year-old man with progressive muscular dystrophy of Duchenne type simulating an anterior myocardial infarction.

ventricular tachycardia.[69] Additionally, QT-prolongation associated with torsade de pointes has been reported.[70] Figure 12–16 shows an abnormal ECG from a patient with cardiomegaly.

In the largest reported study, Groh et al.[71] examined ECGs in 385 patients in whom the diagnosis of myotonic dystrophy was confirmed by the genetic abnormality of cytosine-thymine-guanine (CTG) repeat expansion, ECGs were abnormal in 64.9 percent of patients, and the presence of conduction abnormalities correlated with age and CTG repeat length.

Kearns-Sayre Syndrome

Kearns-Sayre syndrome is an uncommon mitochondrial myopathy associated with progressive external ophthalmoplegia and pigmentary retinopathy. The myocardium is spared, but the cardiac conduction system is selectively affected. The AH interval tends to be short, and the infranodal conduction is often impaired (Figure 12–17). As a net effect the duration of the PR interval may remain normal or may be only slightly prolonged. The original description of the syndrome by

Kearns and Sayre included complete AV block. Advanced conduction disturbances such as bifascicular and trifascicular block may be present.[72–74]

Myasthenia Gravis

It has been reported that nonspecific T wave abnormalities, prolonged QT interval, and RBBB occur significantly more often in patients with myasthenia gravis than in the normal population.[75]

Quadriplegia and Paraplegia

Paraplegic and quadriplegic individuals have a higher incidence of right axis deviation than the normal population, probably resulting from decreased left ventricular mass.[76]

Connective Tissue Diseases

SCLERODERMA HEART DISEASE

In patients with systemic sclerosis, the heart may be involved directly owing to myocardial fibrosis.

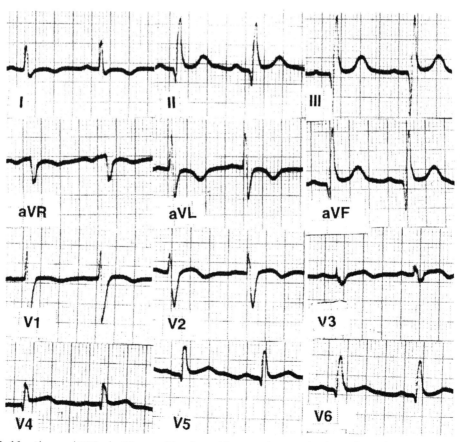

Figure 12–16 Abnormal ECG of a 30-year-old patient with myotonic muscular dystrophy and cardiomegaly.

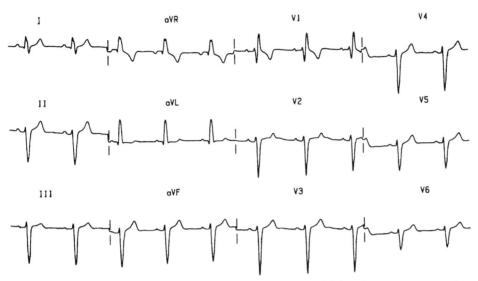

Figure 12–17 Kearns-Sayre syndrome in a 22-year-old man with external ophthalmoplegia, pigmentary retinopathy, and complete right bundle branch block with left anterior fascicular block as seen on the ECG.

It may also be involved indirectly as a result of systemic hypertension secondary to renal involvement or pulmonary hypertension as a result of pulmonary vascular abnormalities or pulmonary fibrosis.[1,77] The ECG changes reflect these anatomic abnormalities. Myocardial fibrosis can cause low QRS voltage.[77] In a series of 60 patients, the ECG showed signs of RVH in 27 percent and LVH in 15 percent.[77]

Systemic Lupus Erythematosus

The most common ECG abnormalities in patients with systemic lupus erythematosus are caused by pericarditis or systemic hypertension.[78,79] MI can occur as a result of coronary vasculitis.[78] In about 20 percent of women affected by the disease during their pregnancy, infants are born with congenital AV block.

Polyarteritis

ECG abnormalities were reported in 85 percent of patients with polyarteritis documented at autopsy.[80] Changes are attributed to hypertension, myocardial ischemia, or ventricular hypertrophy. Coronary arteritis is a common manifestation of the disease, and aneurysms of the coronary arteries are observed occasionally.[1,80,81]

Polymyositis and Dermatomyositis

Polymyositis-dermatomyositis may be associated with myocarditis, myocardial fibrosis including conduction system involvement, and coronary vasculitis.[82–85] The incidence and severity of ECG abnormalities vary among series. In one study,[83] ECG abnormalities were present in 52 percent of patients and consisted of variable degrees of AV block, bundle branch block, left axis deviation, abnormalities of ventricular repolarization, and supraventricular and ventricular arrhythmias. In another study the ECG was abnormal in 25 of 77 patients with polymyositis; the two most common abnormalities were RBBB and left anterior fascicular block.[85]

Rheumatoid Heart Disease

Rheumatoid granulomas may be seen in the myocardium, but the ECG abnormalities are more often related to pericarditis.[1,86]

Reiter Syndrome

Clinical and pathologic changes in the heart of patients with Reiter syndrome are analogous to those with ankylosing spondylitis. The most common ECG abnormality reported in one series was transient first-degree AV block.[87] Other abnormalities included second-degree AV block, fascicular block, and bundle branch block. Complete AV block is a rare manifestation of Reiter syndrome.

Acute Rheumatic Fever and Rheumatic Carditis

The outstanding ECG manifestation of rheumatic carditis is a prolonged PR interval.[89,90] Other frequent abnormalities include type I second-degree AV block and diffuse T wave inversion. Complete

AV block may occur (Figure 12–18). The most characteristic rhythm disturbance is accelerated AV junctional rhythm with or without AV dissociation.[88,90] Left or right bundle branch block is seen also (see Figure 12–18).

MYOCARDIAL TUMORS

ECG changes in patients with primary or metastatic tumors depend on the location and extent of the space-occupying lesion.[1] Atrial myxomas may cause P wave abnormalities and atrial arrhythmias, including atrial flutter and atrial fibrillation. In one personally observed case of a large left atrial myxoma, the ECG showed a pattern of incomplete RBBB with ST segment elevation in the right precordial leads, similar to the pattern observed in patients with Brugada syndrome (see Chapter 7) (Figure 12–19). Some tumors, such as mesothelioma, tend to affect

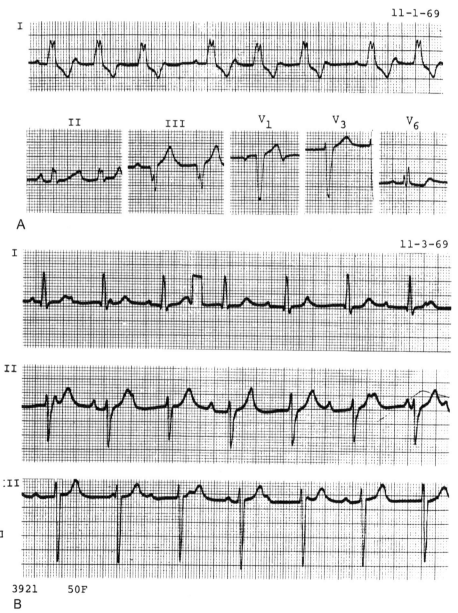

Figure 12–18 Acute rheumatic fever and carditis in a 50-year-old woman with rheumatic heart disease, aortic insufficiency, and recurrence of acute rheumatic fever with carditis. **A,** Note the development of second-degree atrioventricular (AV) block with Wenckebach phenomenon and complete left bundle branch block. **B,** Two days later the patient had complete AV block and idioventricular rhythm. She was treated with steroids.

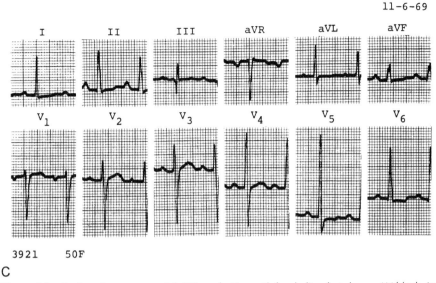

11-6-69

3921   50F

C

Figure 12–18 cont'd   C, There is a return to 1:1 AV conduction with borderline first-degree AV block. Intraventricular conduction is now normal. The morphology of the ventricular complexes is consistent with left ventricular hypertrophy.

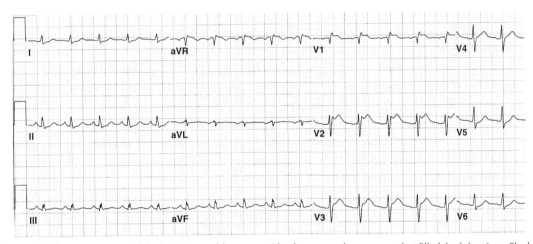

Figure 12–19   Preoperative ECG of a 65-year-old woman with a large vascular myxoma that filled the left atrium. She had normal coronary arteries and no other abnormalities. Note the sinus tachycardia and incomplete right bundle branch block with an elevated ST segment in leads V_1 and V_2, a pattern often seen in patients with Brugada syndrome (see Chapter 7). This pattern was no longer present after the tumor was resected.

the AV node. Tumor invasion of the intraventricular septum may cause bundle branch block or complete AV block. Low voltage may result from extensive destruction of the myocardium or pericardial effusion.[91] Persistent acute injury pattern with ST segment elevation may simulate an MI or a ventricular aneurysm[92] (Figure 12–20). Q waves indistinguishable from those seen with MI occur in patients with primary or secondary tumors. The most common abnormalities, however, consist of nonspecific ST segment or T wave changes[1,93] (Figure 12–21).

Carcinoid heart disease involving right-sided cardiac valves may cause P wave abnormalities, incomplete or complete RBBB, and an RVH pattern.[94]

Endocrine Disorders

Endocrine disorders can produce many changes in the function and structure of the cardiovascular system. Such changes may have various direct and indirect effects on the electrical activity of the heart, thereby inducing ECG changes.

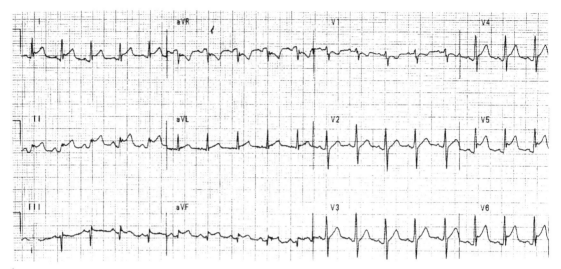

Figure 12–20   ECG of a 67-year-old man with a mesothelioma encircling the heart. It shows an acute injury pattern, probably due to compression by the tumor.

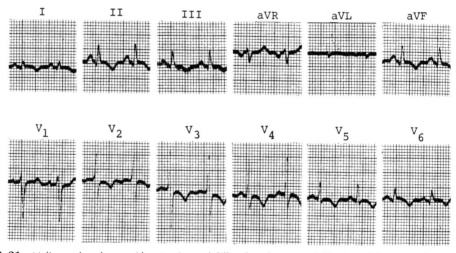

Figure 12–21   Malignant lymphoma with extensive and diffuse lymphomatous infiltration of the pericardium and myocardium in a 37-year-old man. Diagnosis was confirmed at autopsy. About 80 percent of the myocardium was replaced by the tumor tissue. ECG shows that the amplitude of the R waves in the left precordial leads is reduced. Diffuse symmetric T wave inversion involves most of the leads.

THYROID DISEASES

Hyperthyroidism

Sinus tachycardia or atrial fibrillation is commonly present in patients with hyperthyroidism and may precede other clinical manifestations of the disease. In one study of 123 hyperthyroid patients,[95] sinus tachycardia was present in 37.4 percent and atrial fibrillation in 12.2 percent. In another study of 466 patients with hyperthyroidism, sinus tachycardia was present in 45.7 percent and atrial fibrillation in 10.9 percent.[96]

The incidence of atrial fibrillation increases with age. Among 170 patients with thyrotoxicosis whose ages ranged from 37 to 77 years, atrial fibrillation was present in 39 (23 percent). It seldom occurred in patients younger than age 55.[97] In another study, atrial fibrillation was absent in all patients younger than 40 years who had no associated heart disease of other etiology.[96] Spontaneous reversion to sinus rhythm occurred after treatment in 19 of 39 in one follow-up study[97] and in 11 of 13 in another.[96] The frequency of atrial fibrillation may be higher in patients with triiodothyronine (T_3) toxicosis than in those in whom the serum concentration of both T$_3$ and thyroxine (T$_4$) are increased.[98]

In patients with sinus rhythm, the severity of tachycardia parallels the severity of disease. In contrast to atrial fibrillation, the highest incidence of sinus tachycardia is in the youngest age group.[96] The incidence of atrial flutter in patients with hyperthyroidism ranges from 1.5 to 2.0 percent.[96,99] Paroxysmal supraventricular tachycardia and ventricular tachycardia are uncommon in patients with hyperthyroidism. Intraatrial conduction disturbances, manifested by prolongation (>0.10 second) or notching of the P wave, occurred in 81 (17.4 percent) of 542 patients and was more common in women than in men.[96] The PR interval of patients with hyperthyroidism is frequently prolonged even in the absence of heart disease or treatment with digitalis.[100] The incidence of first-degree AV block ranges from 3.2 to 8.9 percent.[95,96,101] In some patients, PR prolongation precedes atrial fibrillation (Figure 12–22). The PR interval duration usually returns to normal when the patient becomes euthyroid. Second- and third-degree AV block are encountered less commonly than first-degree block.[100]

IVCDs occurred in 13.1 percent of 466 hyperthyroid patients without associated heart disease of other etiology.[96] The IVCD usually disappeared when the patient became euthyroid. The most common conduction disturbance was incomplete RBBB (9.2 percent) followed by left anterior fascicular block.[96] Some investigators reported that the incidence of the WPW pattern was higher in patients with hyperthyroidism than in the general population.[100]

The amplitude of the P wave and QRS complex is frequently increased. The tall P waves simulate "P pulmonale," and the QRS complexes of large amplitude simulate LVH.[100] Various nonspecific ST segment and T wave abnormalities have been reported in about 25 percent of patients with hyperthyroidism.[100] In some patients with abnormal T waves the ST segment was elevated, simulating the pattern of pericarditis.[95] The ST segment and T wave changes varied from day to day and, unlike the changes seen with myocarditis or pericarditis, were usually evanescent.[95] In most cases ST segment and T wave changes returned to normal after treatment.[95,98,102] In thyrotoxic periodic paralysis,

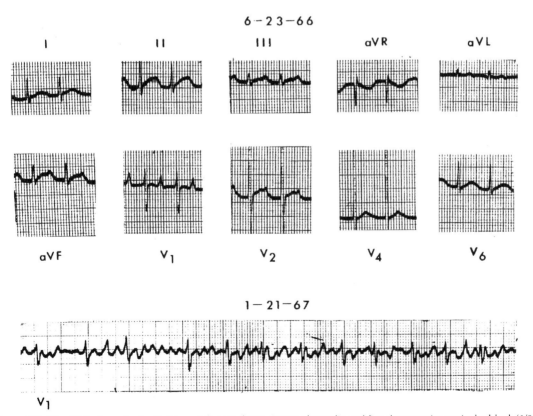

Figure 12–22   ECG of a patient with Graves' disease shows sinus tachycardia and first-degree atrioventricular block (6/23/66) about 7 months before the onset of chronic atrial fibrillation (1/21/67). (From Surawicz B, Mangiardi ML: Electrocardiogram in endocrine and metabolic disorders. Cardiovasc Clin 8:243, 1977.)

ECG changes are caused mainly by hypokalemia.[103] (See Chapter 22.)

Hypothyroidism

Wood suggested that the combination of sinus bradycardia, low-voltage QRS complexes, and lowering or inversion of the T wave was pathognomonic of myxedema[104] (Figure 12–23). The low voltage and the T wave changes are most likely due to the short-circuiting effect of intracardiac and extracardiac myxedematous material and perhaps to associated pericarditis.[105] The QT interval is prolonged, but because the T wave amplitude is low, precise measurement of this interval is often impossible.[100] Three repolarization abnormalities occur with myxedema: flat T wave; T wave or ST segment changes typical of pericarditis; and deeply inverted T waves possibly related to myocardial ischemia. It has been pointed out that there is usually good correlation between ECG signs (bradycardia, low voltage, T wave changes) and the radiologic manifestations of cardiac myxedema.[106]

The P wave amplitude is usually low, and in some patients an unrecognizable P wave simulates atrial fibrillation. Sinus bradycardia is common. In one series of 44 untreated patients, the heart rate was less than 90 beats/min in all.[107] The incidence of AV and intraventricular conduction disturbances is about three times higher in patients with myxedema than in the general population.[97] Among a group of 42 patients, 5 had first-degree AV block, 6 had left anterior fascicular block, 2 had left posterior fascicular block, 1 had LBBB, and 1 had RBBB.[108]

Syncope caused by ventricular tachyarrhythmia, predominantly torsade de pointes, has been reported in patients with myxedema coma. It is probably precipitated by a long QT interval rather than hypothermia.[109,110]

PARATHYROID DISORDERS

Hypoparathyroidism

No changes in the heart rate, duration of the PR interval, or the QRS complex were found in 22 patients with hypoparathyroidism, and no significant rhythm disturbances occurred.[111] The interval from the onset of QRS to the onset of the T wave (Q-oTc interval) was prolonged in all but three patients. In patients with hypocalcemia, the Q-oTc interval expresses the duration of the ST segment because the QRS duration does not change. In the absence of other electrolyte disturbances, the duration of the ST segment is roughly inversely proportional to the plasma calcium concentration.[111,112] Hypocalcemia does not change the duration of the T wave.[108,109] Therefore the durations of the Q-oTc and QTc intervals change in the same manner as those of the Q-oTc intervals.[108] In many patients with hypocalcemia due to hypoparathyroidism, the polarity of the T wave remains unchanged, but sometimes the T waves become low, flat, or sharply inverted in leads with an upright QRS complex.[100,113] Intravenous calcium administration restores normal polarity transiently in patients with negative T waves (Figure 12–24). Long-term therapy results in permanent normalization of the ECG. In patients with a prolonged QT interval due to hypocalcemia, the U wave is

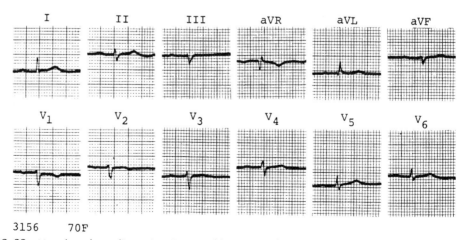

3156   70F

Figure 12–23 Myxedema heart disease in a 70-year-old woman with a 15-year history of myxedema. She had a recurrence of the symptoms and signs of myxedema after she stopped taking her medication for 1 year. She has no symptoms of coronary artery disease. The heart is not enlarged on radiographic examination. ECG shows first-degree atrioventricular block. There is low voltage of the P waves and QRS complexes with abnormal left axis deviation. T waves are inverted in leads V₁–V₃.

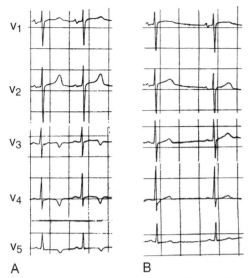

A   B

Figure 12–24 ECG of a patient with hypocalcemia caused by hypoparathyroidism. **A,** Note the prolonged ST segment, prolonged QT, and T wave inversion. **B,** After administration of 10 mL of 10 percent calcium chloride solution intravenously, the QT interval has shortened and the T wave has normalized. (From Surawicz B, Mangiardi ML: Electrocardiogram in endocrine and metabolic disorders. Cardiovasc Clin 8:243, 1977.)

usually absent or not recognizable.[108,109] Prolonged hypocalcemia may lead to cardiomyopathy with QRS abnormalities attributed to LVH.[114]

Hyperparathyroidism

In 12 patients with hyperparathyroidism the plasma calcium concentration ranged from 12.4

to 16.0 mg/dL.[115] There was no correlation between the plasma calcium concentration and the heart rate. The Q-oTc interval was inversely proportional to the plasma calcium concentration. Measurement of the Q-oTc is sometimes more helpful in the diagnosis of hypercalcemia than is measurement of the QTc interval, probably because of the slight prolongation of the QRS complex (Figure 12–25). First- and second-degree AV block are occasionally present,[100] but rhythm disturbances and other conduction disturbances are infrequent.[116] Arrhythmias are believed to occur frequently during hypercalcemic crises,[117] but I have found no documented cases of such events.[100]

DISEASES OF THE HYPOTHALAMUS AND PITUITARY

As the center of autonomic activity, the hypothalamus plays an important role in the sympathetic and vagal control of cardiac activity. Hypothalamic injury was believed to be responsible for the neurogenic T wave changes observed in patients with subarachnoid hemorrhage.[105] The "cardiovascular accident (CVA) pattern" that appeared in several patients after cryohypophysectomy[105] was also attributed to hypothalamic injury.

Abnormal T waves and a prolonged QTc interval have been reported in most patients with untreated pituitary insufficiency.[100,118] ECG abnormalities usually disappear within several months after the onset of hormonal replacement. The T wave abnormalities may be transiently

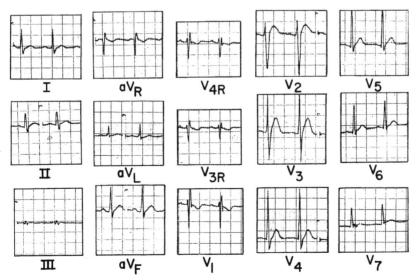

Figure 12–25 ECG of a 46-year-old man with hypercalcemia caused by hyperparathyroidism shows absence of the ST segment, PR of 150 ms, and QRS of 100 ms. (From Surawicz B, Mangiardi ML: Electrocardiogram in endocrine and metabolic disorders. Cardiovasc Clin 8:243, 1977.)

reversed by intravenous administration of small doses of isoproterenol[119] (Figure 12–26).

Hypertrophy of the heart and congestive heart failure are frequently present in patients with acromegaly, but there is no characteristic ECG pattern in patients who have acromegaly and heart disease. In seven groups of patients totaling 116 subjects with documented or suspected heart disease, the incidence of ECG abnormalities ranged from 50 to 80 percent.[100] The most common abnormalities, in order of decreasing frequency, were ST segment depression with or without T wave abnormalities, LVH pattern, bundle branch block or other intraventricular conduction disturbances, remote MI pattern, and supraventricular or ventricular ectopic complexes. Atrial fibrillation, atrial flutter, and first-degree AV block seldom occurred in these patients, and higher-degree AV block was not reported.

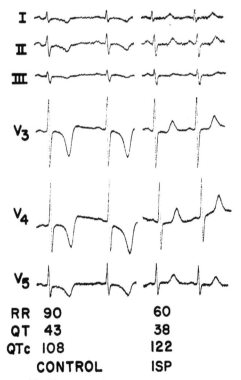

RR	90	60
QT	43	38
QTc	108	122
CONTROL		**ISP**

Figure 12–26 ECG of a patient with hypopituitarism before the start of therapy with prednisone and thyroid *(left)*. Note the deeply inverted T waves, which become normal after administration of a small intravenous isoproterenol (ISP) dose *(right)*. (From Daoud FS, Surawicz B, Gettes LS: Effect of isoproterenol on the abnormal T wave. Am J Cardiol 30:810, 1972. Copyright 1972 Excerpta Medica, Inc., with permission.)

ADRENAL DISEASE

Adrenal Insufficiency

The ECG is abnormal in about one half of patients with Addison's disease. The most common abnormalities are low or inverted T waves, prolonged QTc, low voltage in limb leads, and sinus bradycardia.[100,120] These abnormalities occurred more frequently in women than in men. The ECG abnormalities regressed within variable time after replacement therapy. The average PR interval was reported to be longer than in a normal control population.[121] First-degree AV block was present in 14.5 to 20.0 percent of patients.[100] During an addisonian crisis the ECG may show signs of hyperkalemia.[100,104]

Cushing's Disease and Hyperaldosteronism

In patients with Cushing's disease or hyperaldosteronism, the ECG changes and arrhythmias are related to hypertension and electrolyte imbalance. The average PR interval was reported to be shorter in patients with Cushing's disease than in the normal population.[121]

Pheochromocytoma

The ECG abnormalities in patients with pheochromocytoma may be due to hypertension, myocardial ischemia, or "catecholamine myocarditis," attributed to excess circulating catecholamines.[122] In one series, the ECG was abnormal in 18 of 23 patients.[123] The most common ECG abnormalities during the chronic phase are sinus tachycardia, LVH pattern, and T wave inversion in lead I and in left precordial leads.[122,123]

During hypertensive crisis the ECG may show one of the following patterns: (1) depression of the ST segment in limb and precordial leads attributed to subendocardial ischemia; (2) transient elevation of the ST segment; (3) giant T wave inversion similar to the "CVA pattern" with prolonged QTc,[105] and (4) various tachyarrhythmias. Sudden death was mentioned in most large series, and ventricular fibrillation was recorded during crises.[124]

Turner Syndrome Phenotype and Sex Chromosome Abnormalities

The ECG abnormalities in patients with Turner syndrome usually are related to associated congenital cardiac lesions. However, patients with Noonan syndrome or the "Ullrich-Turner" phenotype with pulmonary valve stenosis had characteristic ECG patterns different from those in other patients with pulmonary stenosis. These ECGs were characterized by extreme right axis deviation and minimal initial leftward and anterior force attributed to abnormal anatomy of the conducting system.[100] Prolonged PR was found in 47,XYY males and shortened PR in 45,X females.[125] Intraventricular conduction disturbances occurred more frequently in 47,XYY males than in the general population.[125] No significant ECG abnormalities were found in men with a 47,XXY karyotype or in 47,XXX women.[125]

Metabolic Disturbances

The ECG abnormalities in patients with metabolic disturbances are commonly caused by abnormal electrolyte concentrations. Certain patterns occur characteristically in various clinical disorders: hyperkalemia and hypocalcemia in patients with uremia (Figure 12–27); hypokalemia and hypocalcemia in patients with hypochloremic alkalosis due to hepatic coma (Figure 12–28); and hypokalemia with hypercalcemia in patients with multiple myeloma (see Chapter 22). Changes in blood pH within a range compatible with life do not produce any recognizable changes in electrolyte concentration.

DIABETES MELLITUS

ECG abnormalities are common in patients with diabetes even in the absence of hypertension, myocardial ischemia, or MI. In one study the ECG was abnormal in 50 percent of adult diabetic patients.[126] I have seen frequently unexplained diffuse T wave abnormalities in diabetic patients without symptoms of heart disease or cardiomegaly. An association between diabetes and left axis deviation has been described.[127]

In patients with diabetic ketoacidosis, the ECG reflects the presence of hyperkalemia even when total body potassium is depleted. Treatment of acidosis shifts potassium into the cells and produces hypokalemia. The ECG reflects the changes in extracellular potassium and is helpful for monitoring the treatment of diabetic ketoacidosis.[128] However, the ECG pattern does not always correlate with the plasma potassium concentration.[100] Some of the discrepancies are attributed to rapid changes in the extracellular potassium concentration and differences between potassium concentration in the peripheral venous blood and the interstitial fluid in the myocardium.

Abnormalities of central nervous system function may be responsible for some of the repolarization abnormalities. Henderson[129] described a pattern in which T waves were deeply inverted in the left precordial leads but tall and peaked in the right precordial leads.[129] Several publications include examples of deeply inverted, symmetric T waves during treatment of diabetic acidosis at a time when the potassium abnormalities were no longer present.[129–131] I analyzed serial ECG changes during treatment of acidosis in 17 patients and found typical patterns of hyperkalemia or hypokalemia in 10 patients and symmetric T wave inversions in 13. In 4 patients the ST segment was elevated in several leads. Acute pericarditis was suspected in these patients, but only 1 had pericardial friction rub. Various arrhythmias have been reported during treatment of diabetic acidosis, usually in the presence of hypokalemia.

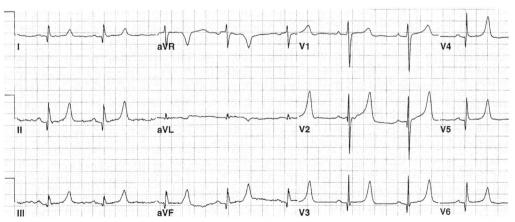

Figure 12–27   ECG of an 87-year-old patient with renal insufficiency, hyperkalemia (potassium 6.2 mEq/L), and hypocalcemia (calcium 3.3 mEq/L). Note the prolonged ST segment (and QT interval) and the narrow, pointed T wave.

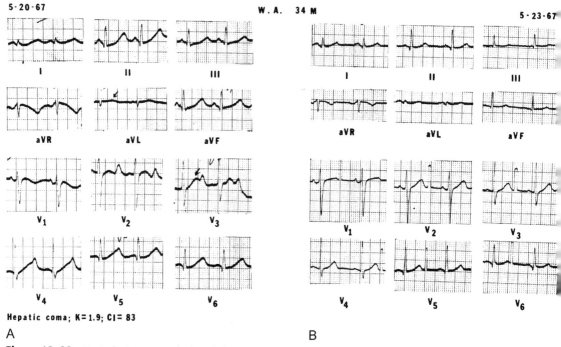

Figure 12–28   Typical ECG pattern for hypokalemia and hypocalcemia before (A) and after (B) treatment with KCl solution in a patient in hepatic coma with metabolic alkalosis. (From Surawicz B, Mangiardi ML: Electrocardiogram in endocrine and metabolic disorders. Cardiovasc Clin 8:243, 1977.)

Hypoglycemia causes tachycardia and occasional ectopic rhythms. Administration of large doses of glucose may produce slight transient ST segment depression and decreased T wave amplitude.

Cardiac Glycogenosis

The following ECG changes occur frequently in patients with glycogen storage disease: short PR interval, high-voltage QRS, and the LVH pattern.[132]

Amyloidosis

The ECG pattern associated with amyloidosis depends on the extent and distribution of amyloid deposits in the myocardium, conducting system, coronary arteries, or cardiac nerves.[100] For 98 cases from 13 studies, the incidence of conduction disturbances and arrhythmias was as follows: RBBB in 10 percent, LBBB in 6 percent, first- and second-degree AV block in 26 percent, complete AV block in 9 percent, AV junctional rhythm in 7 percent, atrial fibrillation in 19 percent, and ectopic atrial tachycardia with 2:1 block in 1 percent.

Figure 12–29 shows an ECG of a patient with an apparent pan-conduction disease manifested by sinus bradycardia, first-degree AV block, and LBBB. Other common ECG abnormalities include low voltage and patterns similar to that of an old inferior or anterior infarction. In a review of 339 cases reported in the literature, Buja and colleagues[133] found low voltage in 50 percent, left axis deviation in 59 percent, and a pseudoinfarction pattern (most displaying small or absent R deflection in leads V_1–V_3) in 64 percent (Figure 12–30). The ECGs in 127 patients with primary systemic amyloidosis and biopsy-proven cardiac involvement showed low voltage in 46 percent, pseudoinfarction pattern in 97 percent, and criteria for LVH in 16 percent of patients.[134] Falk et al.[135] found a high incidence of complex ventricular arrhythmias during ambulatory monitoring of patients with primary or familial amyloidosis. The presence of arrhythmias correlated with heart failure and an abnormal echocardiogram.

Symptomatic disease of the conducting system may be a manifestation of primary, senile, or familial forms of amyloidosis.[136] Prolongation of the HV interval is common and may be suspected from the surface ECG in the presence of a narrow QRS complex caused by an equal conduction delay in both bundle branches.[137] Among 23 autopsy cases of cardiac amyloidosis,[138] conduction or rhythm abnormalities were present in 21 during life (91 percent), although direct amyloid infiltration of the

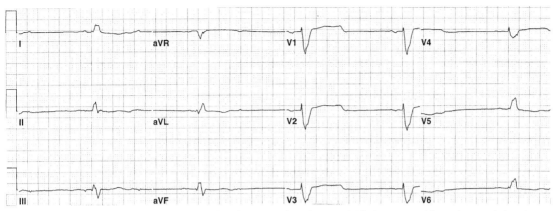

Figure 12–29   ECG of a 76-year-old man with a diagnosis of cardiac amyloidosis supported by a characteristic echocardiographic pattern. Note the sinus bradycardia, PR interval of 242 ms, and left bundle branch block with QRS duration of 202 ms.

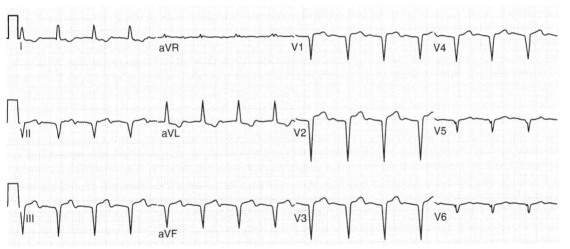

Figure 12–30   ECG of a 48-year old man with primary amyloidosis and pseudoinfarction ECG pattern. First-degree atrioventricular block is also present. At autopsy the heart was infiltrated with amyloid. The coronary arteries were normal, and there was no myocardial infarction.

specialized conducting system did not account for most of these disturbances.

In patients with secondary amyloidosis, ST segment and T wave abnormalities attributed to myocardial ischemia have been found in association with occlusion of small coronary vessels by the amyloid deposits.[139] The ECG changes are similar to those seen with primary amyloidosis and include low voltage in the limb leads, pseudoinfarction patterns, and first-degree AV block.[140]

Hemochromatosis

Deposits of iron in the heart are usually more extensive in the contracting myocardium than in the conducting myocardium.[141] The most common ECG changes in patients with hemochromatosis are low voltage, T wave abnormalities,

bundle branch block, and various supraventricular arrhythmias.[141,142] The latter have been correlated with the iron deposits in the atrial myocardium.[142] AV and intraventricular conduction disturbances were present in the cases that revealed iron deposition in the AV node and His bundle.[143,144] Figure 12–31 is an ECG of a patient with hemochromatosis.

Lipid Storage Disease

Lipid infiltration is responsible for conduction abnormalities and chamber enlargement in patients with Fabry's disease and other storage disorders. Among 32 patients with Fabry's disease, the most frequent abnormalities were a short PR interval and various arrhythmias; AV block and intraventricular conduction disturbances

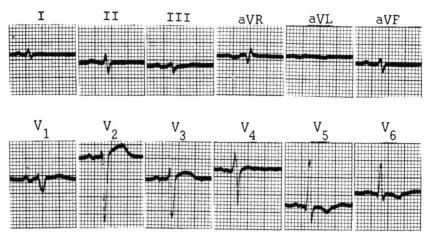

Figure 12–31 Autopsy-proven hemochromatosis with extensive involvement of the myocardium. The heart weighed more than 500 g. There was minimal atherosclerosis of the coronary arteries. ECG shows low voltage of the QRS complex in the limb leads. The frontal plan QRS axis is indeterminate. T wave abnormalities are present in the limb leads and leads V_4–V_6.

(usually RBBB) were present in 22 patients.[145] The ECG seen with Fabry's disease and other lipid storage disorders may also simulate patterns of MI.[100]

Miscellaneous Conditions

Minor repolarization abnormalities in patients with Tay-Sachs disease were attributed to ganglioside deposits in the heart.[146] In patients with thrombotic thrombocytic purpura, microthrombi and localized hemorrhages can cause localized lesions in the conducting system, resulting in ECG changes.[147] Bundle branch block and complete AV block have been reported in patients with generalized lentigo.[148]

TOXIC AGENTS

ECG abnormalities can occur in patients with various cardiomyopathies induced by drugs, toxins, and venoms. A common cause of cardiomyopathy is chemotherapy with doxorubicin, daunomycin, and bleomycin. ECG changes associated with doxorubicin-induced cardiomyopathy are not specific but most often include sinus tachycardia, flattening of the T wave, prolonged QT interval, and low voltage.[149]

Serious ECG abnormalities, including acute injury pattern and ventricular tachyarrhythmias, have been reported in patients with carbon monoxide poisoning.[150] Changes simulating acute myocardial ischemia and MI have been reported after scorpion stings[151] and secondary to anaphylactic shock induced by bee and wasp stings.[152]

Granulamatous and Infectious Cardiomyopathies

Myocardial Sarcoidosis

Myocardial involvement occurs in 20 to 25 percent of patients with sarcoidosis.[153] The disease frequently involves the interventricular septum and the conduction system.[1,154,155] Among 47 cases summarized from the literature, complete AV block occurred in 22 patients and a less advanced AV block in 12 patients.[156] Supraventricular and ventricular arrhythmias are common, and sudden death has been reported[157,158] (Figure 12–32). Pulmonary involvement may lead to cor pulmonale manifested by an RVH pattern on the ECG.

Viral Myocarditis

Patients with severe myocarditis often have sinus tachycardia, diffuse T wave abnormalities, prolonged QT interval, and occasionally Q waves simulating MI. Figure 12–33 shows the ECG abnormalities most often encountered in patients with myocarditis. Matsuura et al.[159] studied 29 patients with suspected myocarditis using antimyosin scintigraphy to assess the severity of the myocardial necrosis. They found a high correlation between intraventricular conduction disturbances and severe myocardial necrosis in 16 patients. In many countries, infections such as mumps, hepatitis, infectious mononucleosis, and coxsackie virus myocarditis[160,161] have been surpassed in terms of frequency of cardiac

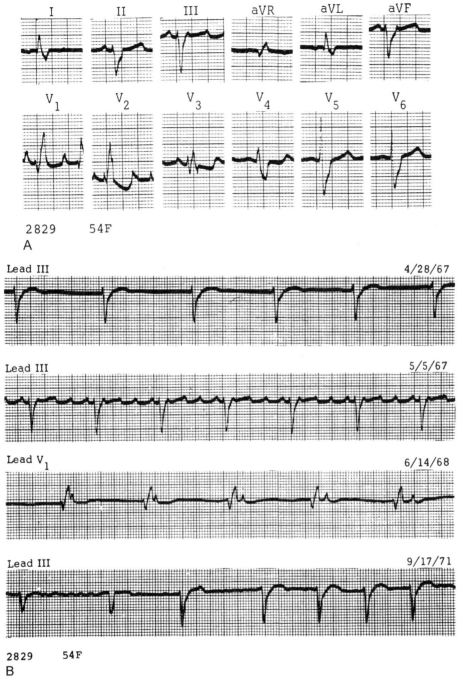

Figure 12–32   Myocardial sarcoidosis in a 54-year-old woman who was known to have had sarcoidosis for 5 years. She died suddenly, and no autopsy was performed. The diagnosis of myocardial sarcoidosis was based on clinical data. **A,** Abnormal P waves are suggestive of right atrial enlargement. Left anterior fascicular block and complete right bundle branch block also are present. **B,** Tracing illustrating some of her arrhythmias, including atrioventricular (AV) junctional escape rhythm (4/28/67), atrial flutter (5/5/67), junctional escape rhythm with AV dissociation (6/14/68), and atrial fibrillation (9/17/71).

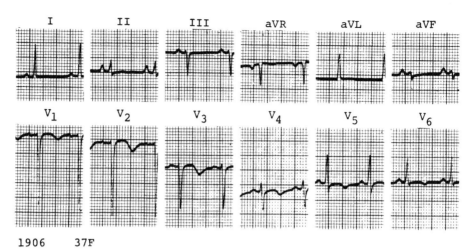

1906   37F

Figure 12–33   Acute myocarditis in a 37-year-old woman with a history of flu-like symptoms followed by the development of cardiomegaly, S_3 and S_4 gallops, and congestive heart failure. ECG shows diffuse T wave abnormalities with symmetric T wave inversion in the precordial leads. There is poor progression of the R wave in the precordial leads. The presence of anterior myocardial damage cannot be determined.

involvement by the retrovirus causing acquired immune deficiency syndrome (AIDS).[162–164] ECG changes occur in 35 to 58 percent of AIDS patients[1,160] and consist mostly of ST segment and T wave abnormalities attributed to myocarditis (see Figure 7–39). Other factors include pericarditis, ventricular hypertrophy, and toxic effects of drugs used to treat the disease. Bundle branch block and ventricular tachycardia may occur.[1]

Various ECG abnormalities have been reported in patients with peripartum cardiomyopathy, which in some cases has been attributed to a viral infection. None of these abnormalities, however, are characteristic of the disease.[165]

Other Infections

Diphtheria often affects the heart, particularly the conducting system, causing AV block and intraventricular conduction disturbances.[105] The most common manifestation of *Lyme carditis* is first-degree AV block.[166] In one series of 20 patients, 8 developed transient complete AV block, and 13 had diffuse QRS and T wave abnormalities compatible with myopericarditis.[167] In another series of 52 patients, 45 (87 percent) had AV block; in 28 of these patients the AV block was advanced or complete. In most cases the block was at the level of the AV node.[168] Myocardial involvement is the dominant feature of *Chagas disease,* and the ECG is abnormal in nearly all symptomatic patients. The most characteristic abnormality is RBBB with or without left fascicular block.[169]

Heart Transplantation

Considering the fact that in most cases the ECG of a heart donor is not expected to be abnormal antemortem, it is surprising to encounter a high incidence of ECG abnormalities in patients with transplanted hearts. In most cases the ECG abnormalities appear early, which suggests that they are related to the preoperative and operative handling of the heart and possibly to the altered neurohormonal milieu, cardiac denervation, increased pulmonary vascular resistance, and other unidentified factors in the host.

The donor heart is implanted by suturing its atria to the corresponding structures of the recipient residual atria. This procedure frequently results in the presence of two sets of P waves (Figures 12–34 and 12–35). Activation of the atria by the preserved sinoatrial (SA) node of the recipient heart generates P waves of small amplitude, whereas excitation of the donor heart by its SA node usually produces P waves of normal amplitude and configuration. The rate of the denervated donor heart is usually faster than that of the recipient.[170,171] The two sets of P waves are usually dissociated from each other (see Figure 12–35, *top*) but in some cases become synchronized[172] (see Figure 12–35, *bottom*). The mechanism of synchronization is uncertain, as the two sets of atria are anatomically separated by the suture line. In many cases the P waves from the recipient atria are not discernible because of their small amplitude or the presence of sinus node dysfunction or atrial fibrillation before transplantation.[170]

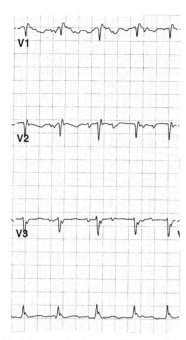

Figure 12–34   ECG leads V_1–V_3 from a recipient of a cardiac transplant. Note the incomplete right bundle branch block with two types of P waves and irregular RR intervals. In lead V_2, one of the P waves is W-shaped (before the second QRS complex and after the third QRS complex), and the other P wave is mostly negative (before and after the third QRS complex and between the fourth and the fifth QRS complex). The two P waves appear to be dissociated, but their relation to the QRS complex is not obvious.

Dissociation between two sets of P waves creates unusual atrial rhythms, particularly when one of the two atrial components develops ectopic activity, atrial flutter, or atrial fibrillation.[173] Arrhythmias caused by atrioatrial interactions in the presence of electrical conduction across the suture line can be cured by radiofrequency ablation.[174,175]

A complete or incomplete RBBB is present in more than 80 percent of ECGs after transplantation[170] (Figures 12–36 and 12–37). In many cases the complete RBBB pattern changes to an incomplete RBBB pattern within a few months.[170] The pathogenesis of the RBBB after cardiac transplantation is inadequately understood but the prognosis is benign.[170a]

Next in frequency is the persistent left anterior fascicular block, which occurs in 7 to 25 percent of patients after transplantation[170,176] (Figure 12–38). It has been reported that stable or progressive conduction disturbances indicate a worse prognosis.[177] The frequently recorded rhythm disturbances during the postoperative period include sinus bradycardia, SA conduction disturbances, atrial tachyarrhythmias (Figure 12–39), AV junctional rhythms, first-degree AV block, and premature ventricular complexes.[176–179] During a long-term follow-up, intermittent atrial tachyarrhythmias were recorded in 50 percent of patients (Figure 12–40), and late atrial fibrillation was associated with an increased all-cause mortality[180] whereas increased incidence of atrial flutter was associated with rejection.[181]

Minor ST segment or T wave changes are often present, caused in many cases by postoperative pericarditis. Sometimes, however, deeply inverted symmetric T waves are indistinguishable from T wave changes caused by myocardial ischemia or non-Q wave MI (see Figure 12–37). A Q wave infarction pattern is also known to occur after heart transplantation. The QT and QTc intervals in the transplanted hearts are usually within normal limits.[182]

The ECG appears to be of limited use in the diagnosis of acute rejection. The decrease in QRS amplitude occurs during rejection (Figure 12–41) but is not a reliable indicator of rejection.[176]

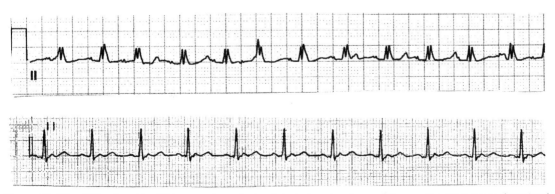

Figure 12–35   ECG strips of lead II from two transplant recipients show two types of P wave. *Top,* P waves are dissociated. *Bottom,* The relation between the two P wave types (one immediately after the QRS complex and the other before the following QRS complex) is constant.

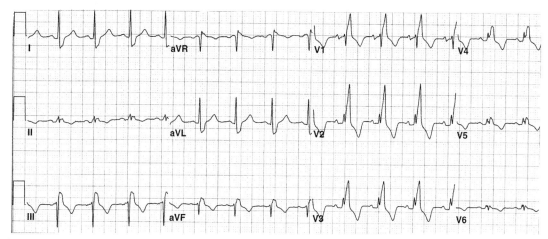

Figure 12–36 Complete right bundle branch block (QRS duration 144 ms) in a 61-year-old recipient of a cardiac transplant 1.5 years previously.

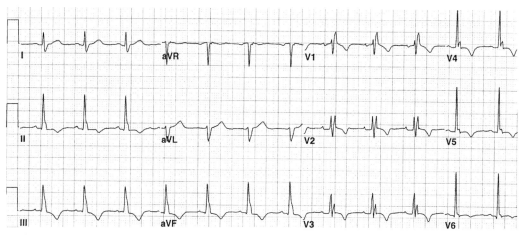

Figure 12–37 Incomplete right bundle branch block (QRS duration 110 ms) in a 45-year-old recipient of a cardiac transplant 6 years previously. Diffuse T wave abnormalities are present.

Neither are T wave inversion and atrial arrhythmia.[170] It has been reported that during acute rejection the sudden appearance of first-degree AV block suggests severe involvement of the conduction system with impending cardiac arrest.[183] Because recipients of the transplanted hearts who had coronary artery disease often maintain their coronary risk factors, it is not surprising that severe coronary artery disease can develop in the transplanted hearts within a relatively short time (see Figures 12–38 and 12–42).

TRAUMA TO THE HEART

Cardiac trauma may be caused by a penetrating wound or a blunt injury. Most of the nonpenetrating cardiac injuries result from a motor vehicle impact, specifically compression by the steering wheel. There are numerous other causes of blunt trauma to the chest, including cardiac resuscitation procedures.[170] The most frequently encountered ECG changes that occur shortly after trauma or following a delay of 1 to 2 days consist of ST segment and T wave changes similar to those produced by myocardial ischemia or myocarditis[184] (Figure 12–43; see also Figure 8–36). The ECG may indicate pericarditis and in some cases a pattern of acute MI. Intraventricular conduction disturbances occur fairly frequently, particularly RBBB[185–187] (Figure 12–44). AV conduction disturbances and various types of supraventricular and ventricular ectopic activity are often present but tend to be transient[188] (Figure 12–45).

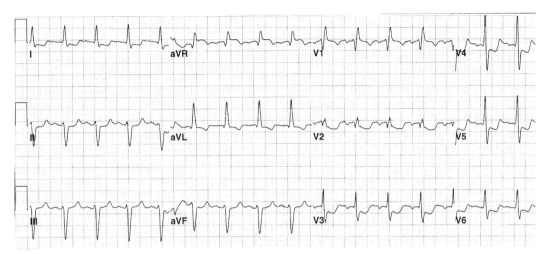

Figure 12–38 ECG of a 68-year-old man who has severe diffuse coronary artery disease not amenable to revascularization 11 years after cardiac transplantation. Note the sinus tachycardia (105 beats/min), right bundle branch block, left anterior fascicular block, and apparent subendocardial ischemia with ST segment depression in leads I, II, and V_2–V_6 and ST segment elevation in leads aV_R and V_1.

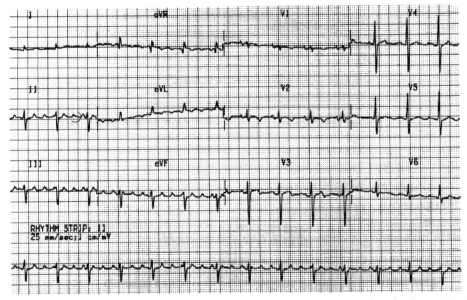

Figure 12–39 Atrial flutter originating from the recipient atrial remnants. Sinus P waves from the donor atria can best be seen preceding the QRS complexes in leads V_1 and V_2. In the other leads they are distorted or masked by the flutter waves generated from the recipient atrial remnants. Note also the left anterior fascicular block and nonspecific T wave changes.

ELECTRICAL INJURY

Electricity can both kill and revive. Sudden death from electrocution is usually caused by ventricular fibrillation or cardiac arrest. In survivors of electrical accidents by high-tension alternating current, lightning, or other causes, ECG changes have been reported in 10 to 46 percent of afflicted individuals.[170] The abnormalities include various supraventricular and ventricular arrhythmias, ST segment and T wave changes simulating acute injury and myocardial ischemia

(Figure 12–46), prolonged QT interval, and bundle branch block.[170,188–190]

Pulmonary Diseases

CHRONIC OBSTRUCTIVE PULMONARY DISEASE

The characteristic ECG pattern in patients with chronic obstructive pulmonary disease (COPD) is attributed to changes in the spatial orientation of

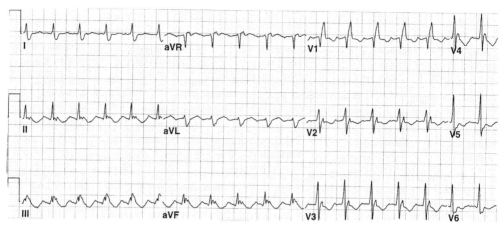

Figure 12–40 ECG of a 51-year-old recipient of a cardiac transplant 6 years earlier. Note the atrial tachycardia with 2:1 response and right bundle branch block (QRS 126 ms).

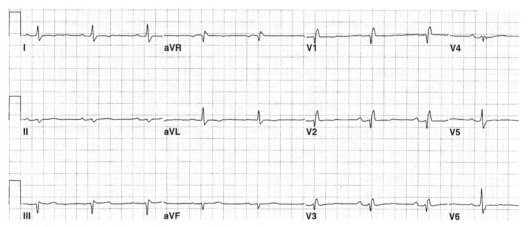

Figure 12–41 ECG of a 65-year-old man recorded 6 weeks after cardiac transplantation and with suspected rejection. Note the low-voltage right bundle branch block (QRS 122 ms) and flat T waves.

the heart, the insulating effect of the overaerated lungs, and the low position of the diaphragm. Typical ECG changes include peaked P waves in leads II, III, and aV$_F$; low R wave amplitude in all leads; posterior displacement of the QRS forces in the horizontal plane; and late QRS vector oriented superiorly and to the right, resulting in a wide slurred S wave in leads I, II, III, V$_4$, V$_5$, and V$_6$[191,192] (Figure 12–47; see also Figures 2–5, 3–19, and 8–40). Pathognomonic of emphysema, in the absence of MI, is low voltage with a posteriorly and superiorly oriented QRS vector and a P wave axis >60 degrees in the limb leads.[193] Atrial repolarization may become more prominent, as evidenced by depression of the Ta wave in lead II.[194] The QRS duration tends to be shorter in patients with COPD than in patients with any other

disease.[195] Chou listed the following findings that suggest the presence of COPD:

1. P waves >0.25 mV in lead II, III, or aV$_F$
2. P wave axis to the right of 80 degrees in the frontal plane
3. Lead I sign with an isoelectric P wave, QRS amplitude <0.15 mV, and T wave amplitude <0.05 mV
4. QRS amplitude in all limb leads <0.5 mV
5. QRS axis to the right of 90 degrees in the frontal plane
6. QRS amplitude <0.5 mV in lead V$_5$ or V$_6$; or R wave <0.7 mV in lead V$_5$ or R wave <0.5 mV in lead V$_6$
7. R/S ratio <1 in lead V$_5$ or V$_6$
8. S$_1$S$_2$S$_3$ pattern with R/S ratio <1 in leads I, II, and III

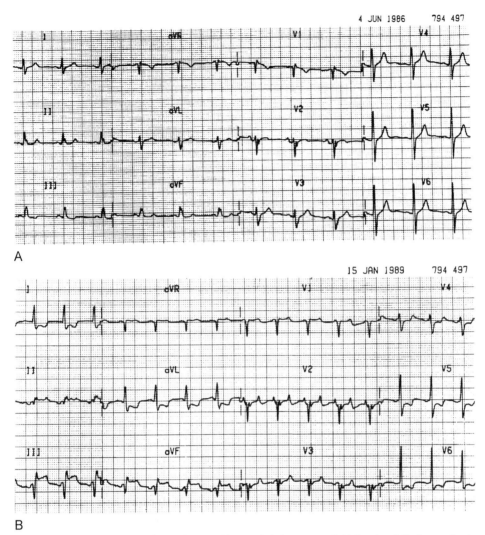

Figure 12–42   Accelerated coronary atherosclerosis with acute inferior myocardial infarction (MI) after cardiac transplantation in a 28-year-old man with a history of idiopathic dilated cardiomyopathy. Cardiac transplantation was performed 2 years before the recording of tracing **(A),** which shows two sets of P waves and incomplete right bundle branch block. Coronary arteriogram performed at that time was normal. In June 1988 a repeat coronary arteriogram revealed 20 percent narrowing in the proximal portion of the dominant right coronary artery. The left coronary artery was normal. The patient complained of shortness of breath 2 days before the tracing was recorded **(B)**. ECG revealed atrial flutter with changes of acute inferior MI. Tracing also shows poor R wave progression in the right precordial leads. ST segment depression and T wave inversion in the anterolateral leads probably represent reciprocal changes of the acute inferior infarction. Coronary arteriogram obtained 4 days later revealed complete occlusion of the right coronary artery in its midportion. Patient died 25 days later. At autopsy the heart weighed 685 g, with dilatation of both atria and ventricles and left ventricular hypertrophy. The coronary arteries showed atherosclerosis. The right coronary artery was occluded at its proximal portion. A transmural inferior MI was found extending from the apex to the base. Microscopic examination revealed acute cellular and chronic vascular rejection of the allograft.

According to Chou,[194] chronic lung disease is likely to be present if one or more of these P wave changes and one or more of these QRS changes is present.

Correlation with Severity of Lung Disease

Spodick and associates analyzed the ECGs of 301 patients with various degrees of pulmonary emphysema.[196] In 77 percent of patients the P axis was between +70 and +90 degrees. The presence of tall peaked P waves >0.25 mV in the inferior leads was associated with moderately severe or severe disease, but the presence of peaked P waves of normal amplitude (found in 54 percent of cases) had no relation to the degree of functional impairment. Other investigators found that the rightward shift of the

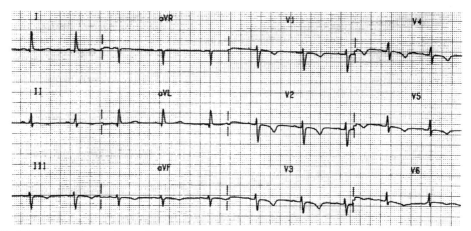

Figure 12–43 T wave abnormalities after nonpenetrating trauma in a 30-year-old woman involved in a motor vehicle accident during which her chest hit the dashboard of the car. ECG recorded immediately after the accident showed diffuse T wave changes that became more marked by the next day, when this tracing was obtained. T wave inversion is most pronounced in the precordial leads.

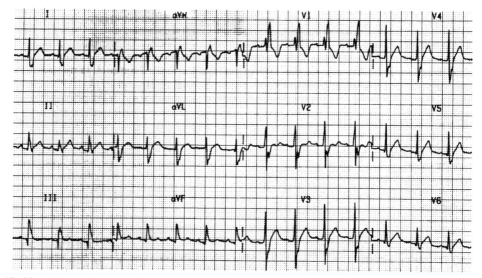

Figure 12–44 Right bundle branch block (RBBB) due to nonpenetrating trauma in a 21-year-old man who was involved in a motor vehicle accident during which his chest hit the steering column. He sustained multiple injuries including laceration of the liver and spleen. ECG shows complete RBBB, which resolved 4 days later.

P axis is helpful for estimating the severity of the lung disease.[197] Occasionally the negative component of the biphasic P wave in the right precordial leads is quite prominent; but unlike that with left atrial enlargement, the slope of the line connecting the peak of the positive and the nadir of the negative P deflection is normal (i.e., fairly steep). Baljepally and Spodick[198] confirmed in a study of 100 patients with vertical P wave axis (>70 degrees) that such an axis is a highly sensitive (89 percent) and highly specific (96 percent) sign of pulmonary emphysema.

A frontal plane QRS axis to the right of +60 degrees is present in about 60 percent of patients with emphysema.[192] The degree of right axis deviation is significantly related to the degree of airway obstruction.[198] The $S_1S_2S_3$ pattern is present in about one fourth of the patients.[192] This pattern has been attributed to the conduction delay in the right ventricle.[199] Leftward displacement of the transitional zone with an R/S ratio of <1 in leads V_5 and V_6 is also a frequent finding in patients with severe COPD.[194]

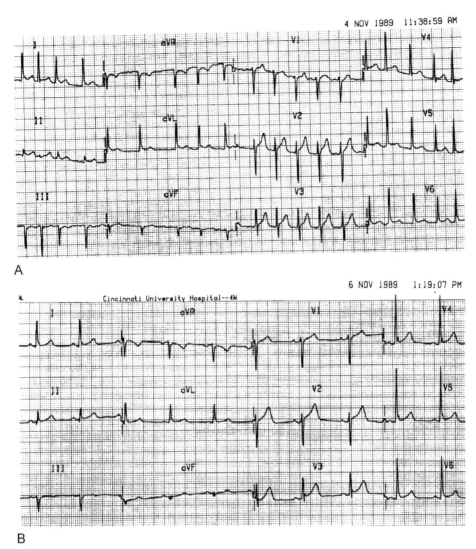

Figure 12–45 Atrial fibrillation due to nonpenetrating trauma in a 32-year-old man who was involved in a head-on motor vehicle collision. He had external evidence of chest injury and no history of cardiac disease. **A,** ECG obtained shortly after the accident shows atrial fibrillation with rapid ventricular response. There is slight flattening of the T waves in the left precordial leads. Later tracings proved the slight diffuse ST segment elevation to be due to early repolarization instead of pericarditis. No pericardial rub was heard. Cardiac enzymes and an echocardiogram were normal. Atrial fibrillation converted to normal sinus rhythm the next day. **B,** Tracing obtained on the third day shows diffuse ST segment elevation attributed to "early repolarization".

In patients with chronic bronchitis, a rightward shift of the axis, increased P amplitude, and a QRS pattern suggestive of RVH are seldom present until the 1-second forced expiratory volume (FEV$_1$) is less than 45 percent of the predicted normal value.[200] In a study of 112 patients, a rightward P wave axis was present in 29 percent and an RVH pattern in only 10 percent.[194,201]

The best criteria for judging the severity of COPD are: (1) an R amplitude in V$_6$ of <0.5 mV; (2) R/S amplitude in V$_6$ of ≤1.0 mV; and (3) increased P wave amplitude in leads II and III.[202] The best indicators of deteriorating

pulmonary function in patients with COPD are reported to be (1) progressive reduction of the R wave and R/S ratio in the orthogonal lead x (also lead I and left precordial leads); (2) progressive shift of the QRS axis in the superior direction; and (3) rightward shift of the P wave axis.

In 150 patients with severe emphysema, the presence of advanced disease was suggested by: (1) increased P wave amplitude in leads II, III, and aV$_F$; (2) Ta wave >0.1 mV in leads II, III, and aV$_F$; (3) vertical heart position; (4) deep S waves in the left precordial leads; and (5) tendency to

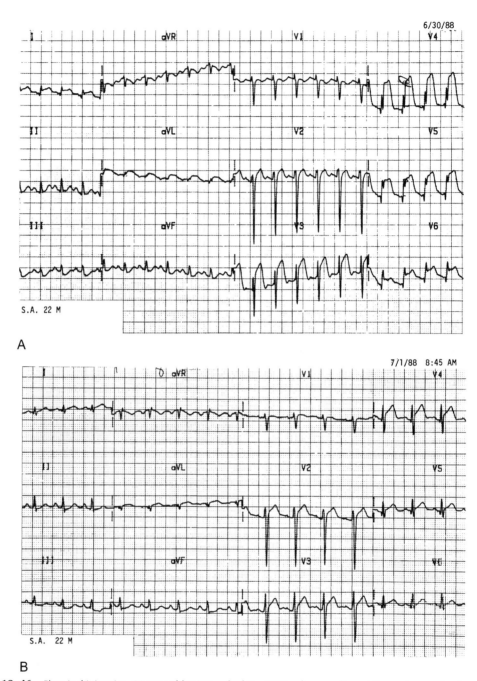

Figure 12–46 Electrical injury in a 22-year-old painter who hit a 4400-volt power line while moving an aluminum ladder. He lost consciousness, and cardiopulmonary resuscitation was applied within a few minutes. After he was transported to a nearby hospital, he was found to have ventricular tachycardia and ventricular fibrillation. Normal sinus rhythm resumed after direct-current countershock. **A,** The 12-lead ECG shows sinus tachycardia with marked ST segment elevation in the antero-lateral leads, suggesting myocardial injury. Anterolateral myocardial infarction may be present. **B,** One day later, the heart rate is slower. ST segment elevation in the anterolateral leads is less pronounced.

low voltage.[203] A study of 126 patients with severe COPD was reported by Smit et al.[204] Of the initial 25 ECG variables, only the P wave amplitude in lead II and the S wave amplitude in lead V_6 were predictive of 5-year survival.

Transient changes during exacerbations of pulmonary insufficiency in patients with incipient or overt cor pulmonale include T wave inversion in the right precordial leads, ST segment depression in leads II, III, and aV_F, and transient RBBB.[205]

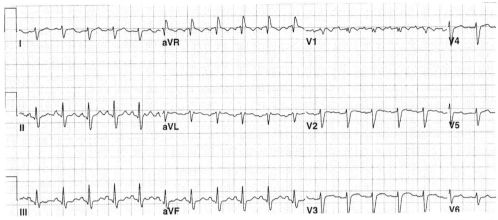

Figure 12–47   ECG of a 57-year-old man with severe chronic obstructive airway disease shows sinus tachycardia, right axis deviation, incomplete right bundle branch block, and deep S waves in the left precordial leads.

Diagnosis of RVH in the Presence of COPD

Autopsy correlations in 46 patients with chronic lung disease showed that the most reliable sign of RVH was right axis deviation and dominant S waves in the left precordial leads.[206] Other findings suggestive of RVH include signs of right atrial enlargement, an RSR′ or QR pattern in lead V_1, or an inverted T wave in the right precordial or inferior leads[194] (Figure 12–48). In the presence of an rSr′ pattern in the right precordial leads,[193] a slurred S wave in the left precordial leads and a prominent R wave in lead aV_R may indicate the presence of RVH. The ECG was of little value in the diagnosis of RVH in the presence of coexisting LVH or myocardial ischemia.[204]

Arrhythmias and COPD

Other than sinus tachycardia, the arrhythmias in patients with pulmonary insufficiency tend to be transient and occur predominantly during exacerbation of disease, respiratory failure, infection, or pulmonary embolism. The arrhythmias are mostly supraventricular in origin. Multiform atrial tachycardia is almost pathognomonic of the presence of pulmonary insufficiency. Other atrial tachyarrhythmias are ectopic uniform atrial tachycardia, atrial flutter, and (less often) atrial fibrillation. Among 1482 patients with severe COPD, arrhythmias were present in 7 percent.[207] Most of the patients also had evidence of RVH.[194,207] An increased incidence of ventricular ectopic

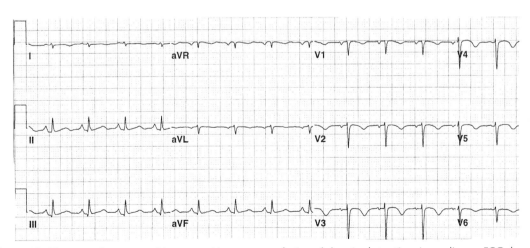

Figure 12–48   ECG of a 67-year-old woman with acute exacerbation of chronic obstructive airway disease. ECG shows a pattern of chronic lung disease with a vertical QRS axis in the frontal plane and deep S waves in the left precordial leads. T wave inversion occurred transiently during exacerbation of the disease and regressed within 4 days in leads V_3–V_6 (not shown). Right ventricle was dilated, left ventricle was of normal size, and there was no evidence of myocardial ischemia in the nuclear scan after infusion of dobutamine.

frequency in patients with COPD was observed during sleep in the presence of oxygen desaturation.[208]

PNEUMOTHORAX

The ECG changes in patients with pneumothorax are caused chiefly by displacement of the heart, resulting most often in right axis deviation, regardless of whether the pneumothorax occurs on the left or the right.[194] Insulation by the air often causes low voltage, and QS deflections may be present in several precordial leads. There may also be ST segment elevation and T wave inversion simulating a pattern of MI. Some of these changes may be partially normalized when the ECG is recorded with the patient in the upright position.[209] The incidence of the pseudoinfarction pattern, however, is low relative to the common occurrence of the rightward shift of the QRS axis, diminution of the precordial R voltage, decrease in QRS amplitude, and precordial T wave inversion.[210] A large spontaneous pneumothorax may produce a pattern of acute cor pulmonale (see Figure 8–37).

SCOLIOSIS

Among 802 patients (586 younger than 18 years) with isolated scoliosis followed or operated on (or both), the data for such variables as heart rate, QTc, P wave amplitude, PR interval, and QRS amplitude were similar to the data reported for the population without scoliosis.[211] The QRS axis in the frontal plane was normal in 94 percent of patients under 18 years of age and in 87 percent of patients older than 18 years. Right axis deviation was present in 5 percent and RVH in 2 percent; they were equally frequent in younger and older age groups. Left axis deviation was present in 1 percent of the younger age group and in 8 percent of the older age group. In this study, only 1.3 percent of patients had associated congenital heart disease.

ACUTE PULMONARY EMBOLISM

ECG Findings

Acute pulmonary embolism can produce an ECG pattern of acute cor pulmonale (see Chapter 8). Table 12–1 lists ECG changes suggestive of pulmonary embolism. The changes listed can be attributed to the following four factors: (1) increased sympathetic stimulation; (2) change in cardiac position; (3) dilation of the right ventricle; and (4) possible ischemia of the right ventricle. The last two factors, in turn, can be attributed to acute pulmonary hypertension.[212–215]

TABLE 12–1	ECG Changes Suggestive of Pulmonary Embolism
Negative T$_3$	Clockwise rotation
S$_I$ Sinus tachycardia	"P pulmonale"
Q$_{III}$ Recent axis shift	Complete or incomplete right bundle branch block
Negative T in two or more right precordial leads	Atrial arrhythmias

Allen and Surawicz[216] evaluated the usefulness of the ECG for (1) supporting evidence of a clinically suspected pulmonary embolism and (2) the ability to detect clinically unsuspected pulmonary embolism. The study included 100 patients with the ECG pattern identified by the code number based on the signs listed in Table 12-1. The researchers found that, among 36 patients in whom pulmonary embolism was suspected by the referring physician, the ECG provided evidence to support the diagnosis in 69 percent of cases. However, among 64 patients in whom the electrocardiographer suggested the diagnosis of pulmonary embolism to the clinician, the ECG contributed to the detection of pulmonary embolism in only 8 percent (5 patients). In 20 percent of this group no diagnosis was found to explain the ECG pattern, and in 72 percent the clinical diagnosis simulating pulmonary embolism was consistent with acute cor pulmonale caused by pneumonia (12 patients), COPD (15 patients), postpneumonectomy (2 patients), pneumothorax and atelectasis (5 patients), pleural effusion (3 patients), upper airway obstruction (2 patients), and other conditions (7 patients). This study underscores the lack of specificity of ECG changes produced by acute cor pulmonale of different etiologies.

The incidence of the various ECG abnormalities in 30 patients with proven pulmonary embolism in this study was as follows: sinus tachycardia in 73 percent, "P pulmonale" in 33 percent, RBBB in 20 percent, axis shift in 23 percent, S$_I$ in 60 percent, Q$_{III}$ in 53 percent, negative T$_{III}$ in 20 percent, negative T in two or more precordial leads in 50 percent, supraventricular arrhythmia in 13 percent, and "clockwise rotation" in 56 percent. In 49 consecutive patients with pulmonary embolism reported by Sreeram et al.,[217] the incidence of these variables was as follows: (1) incomplete or complete RBBB ($n = 33$) associated with ST segment elevation in lead V$_1$ ($n = 17$); (2) S waves in leads

I and aV_L of >0.15 mV ($n = 36$); (3) a shift in the transition zone in the precordial leads to V_5 ($n = 25$); (4) Q waves in leads III and aV_F but not in lead II ($n = 24$); (5) right axis deviation ($n = 15$); (6) a low-voltage QRS complex in limb leads ($n = 10$); and (7) T wave inversion in leads III and aV_F ($n = 16$) or leads V_1 to V_4 ($n = 13$). In three other studies in which the number of patients with pulmonary embolism ranged from 50 to 90,[218,219] the incidence of ECG abnormalities was similar to those in the personal study: sinus tachycardia, 48 to 68 percent; S_IQ_{III} or $S_IQ_{III}T_{III}$ pattern, 12 to 25 percent; RBBB, 14 to 25 percent; T inversion in right precordial leads, 10 to 46 percent; ST segment elevation in lead III, 16 to 28 percent; clockwise rotation, 7 to 60 percent; P pulmonale, 6 to 28 percent; atrial tachyarrhythmias (atrial tachycardia, atrial flutter, atrial fibrillation), 14 to 38 percent; and no significant abnormalities, 20 to 24 percent.

The large variability of results is not surprising because the incidence and severity of the ECG pattern depends on the timing and magnitude of the obstruction in the pulmonary arterial tree. Most observers have emphasized the transient nature of the ECG abnormalities. Patients with a normal ECG generally have a small perfusion defect and low pulmonary arterial pressure.[219] When pulmonary embolism is sufficently large to produce marked hypoxemia, severe hypotension, or shock, ECG changes are present in nearly all cases.[194] In a group of patients with massive pulmonary embolism, T wave inversion or RBBB was present in 62 percent of patients; only 3 patients had normal tracings.[220] T wave inversion in leads V_1–V_4 is the most persistent of all ECG abnormalities, lasting an average of 41 days (range 16–120 days)[210] (Figure 12–49). A global T wave inversion with QT prolongation has been reported.[221]

ECG Differentiation of MI from Pulmonary Embolism and Chronic Cor Pulmonale

The ECG changes associated with pulmonary embolism may simulate acute inferior infarction and, to a lesser degree, anterior infarction (Figure 12–50; see also Figure 8–38). In patients with pulmonary embolism, a significant Q wave may appear in leads III and aV_F, and the ST segment may be slightly elevated in these leads. The degree of ST elevation is usually less than would be expected in the presence of an acute inferior infarction. Similar to right ventricular infarction, the ST segment may be elevated in leads V_{4R}–V_{6R}.[222] With pulmonary embolism the T wave is frequently negative in lead III and less frequently negative in lead aV_F. Rapid regression of these changes, particularly disappearance of the Q wave in serial tracings, favors a diagnosis of pulmonary embolism rather than MI. When the ECG changes in the inferior leads are accompanied by T wave inversion in the right precordial leads, the ECG pattern erroneously suggests an inferior infarction (Figure 12–51).

In some cases the ECG is of no help in the differential diagnosis between myocardial ischemia and non-Q wave MI of the anterior wall and chronic cor pulmonale. The latter can be recognized on the ECG by the presence of

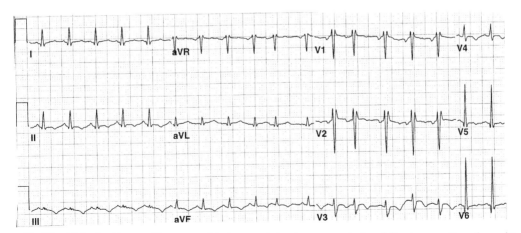

Figure 12–49 ECG of a 46-year-old woman with documented pulmonary embolism following resection of a malignant thymoma. Echocardiogram showed normal left ventriclar function and right atrial enlargement; the estimated right ventricular pressure was 30 mmHg. ECG shows sinus tachycardia, premature atrial complexes, and T wave abnormalities, which regressed within 4 weeks (not shown).

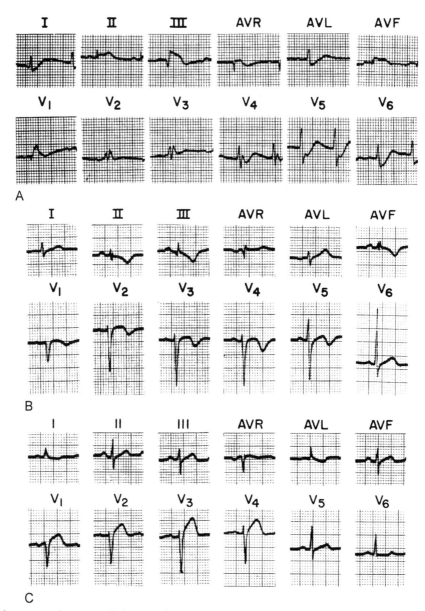

Figure 12–50 Acute pulmonary embolism simulating acute inferior myocardial infarction (MI) in a 67-year-old man who was brought to the hospital because of syncope and shock. **A,** ECG obtained on arrival shows complete right bundle branch block (RBBB). Q wave is present in lead III, with ST segment elevation in all the inferior leads. ST segment depression is present in leads I, aV$_L$, and V$_4$–V$_6$. Acute inferior MI was diagnosed. On the same day, repeated ECGs show disappearance of the RBBB pattern. A definite Q wave also has developed in leadaV$_F$, with T wave inversion in the inferior leads. **B,** Tracing recorded 2 days later shows that the Q wave in lead III is smaller, and the Q wave in lead aV$_F$ is no longer present. In the precordial leads, there is leftward displacement of the transitional zone, with T wave inversion from leads V$_1$–V$_5$. Radioisotope lung scan revealed large perfusion defects. Serial enzymes were not consistent with MI. The tracing gradually returned to normal. **C,** Tracing made 2 weeks later shows no Q wave in the inferior leads. QRS complexes are within normal limits. Minor ST and T changes are consistent with a digitalis effect.

various RVH patterns (Figures 12–52 and 12–53; see also Figures 3–16 and 3–20). In patients with pickwickian syndrome, RVH and right axis deviation (see Figure 3–22) or right axis deviation alone (Figure 12–54) is often present.

Congenital Heart Disease in Adults

Adult patients with congenital heart disease belong in two categories: those who have undergone

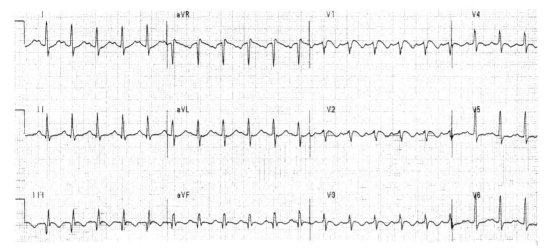

Figure 12–51 ECG of a 35-year-old woman with a pulmonary embolism simulating inferior myocardial infarction. The negative T waves in leads V_1–V_3 are attributed to right ventricular "strain" or ischemia.

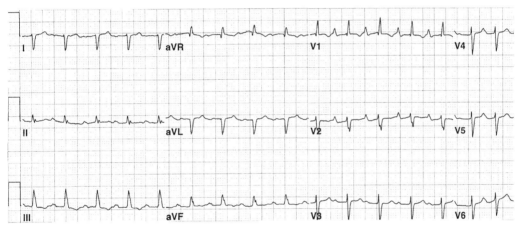

Figure 12–52 ECG of an 87-year-old woman with chronic cor pulmonale simulating posterolateral myocardial infarction. Echocardiogram showed massive dilation of the right atrium and right ventricle with an estimated pulmonary artery pressure >100 mmHg. ECG shows sinus tachycardia, premature atrial complex, PR interval of 220 ms, right axis deviation, right atrial enlargement, and right ventricular hypertrophy pattern.

corrective or palliative surgical intervention and those who have not. In both categories, the ECG may reveal certain specific characteristics that provide helpful clues to the clinical diagnosis of various congenital defects.

Atrial Septal Defect

Most adult patients with atrial septal defect (ASD) maintain a sinus rhythm for a long time; but with the advanced stages of the disease, which are usually associated with marked atrial enlargement, one frequently encounters atrial tachycardia, atrial flutter, or atrial fibrillation. The latter was found in 13 to 19 percent of adult patients.[223,224] The arrhythmias tend to persist after surgical correction of the defect and in some cases appear for the first time after operation.[225,226] This was attributed to right atrial stretch and persisting conduction delay at the crista terminalis after closure of ASD.[227]

In the study of Brandenburg et al.,[228] the incidence of paroxysmal atrial tachyarrhythmias in 188 patients age 44 years or older was 14 percent (16 patients had atrial fibrillation, 2 atrial flutter, and 9 atrial tachycardia). During the postoperative period, attacks of atrial fibrillation tended to increase in severity, and atrial fibrillation became sustained in 88 percent of patients with paroxysmal atrial fibrillation, whereas paroxysmal supraventricular tachycardia gradually diminished or disappeared.

The P wave may show signs of right atrial enlargement,[229] and the PR interval may be

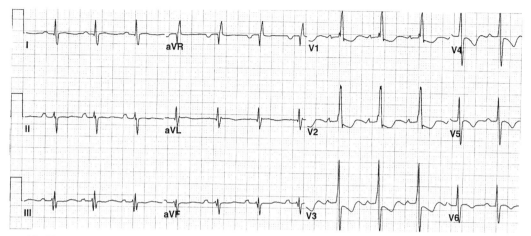

Figure 12–53   ECG of a 32-year-old man with familial pulmonary hypertension (pulmonary artery pressure 70/46 mmHg). Note the right ventricular hypertrophy pattern with inverted T waves in the precordial leads.

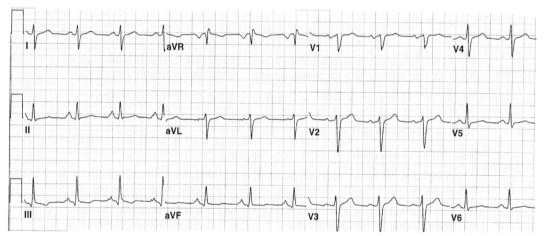

Figure 12–54   ECG of a 30-year-old man with sleep apnea and morbid obesity (height 5 feet, 7 inches; weight 377 pounds). Left ventricular dimensions and function were normal, and there was no evidence of stress-induced ischemia. Note the right axis deviation.

prolonged. The incidence of a prolonged PR interval and advanced AV block is higher in patients with ASD primum than in those with ASD secundum. The frontal plane QRS axis is most helpful in the differential diagnosis between secundum and primum ASD. With the secundum defect, the mean QRS axis is (with few exceptions) between 0 and +180 degrees and in most cases to the right of 100 degrees[223,230] (Figure 12–55).

In one study of 910 patients with a secundum-type ASD defect, left axis deviation was present in only 2 to 3 percent. In contrast, most patients with ASD primum have left axis deviation superior to –30 degrees (Figure 12–56). Pryor et al.[230] found that in 91 percent of patients with ostium primum defect, the mean frontal axis was superior to 0 degrees, and no patient had true right axis deviation.

The right axis in the secundum defect can be attributed to right ventricular overload, whereas the superior axis (as in left anterior fascicular block) is believed to be caused by preexcitation of the posterobasal region of the left ventricle resulting from an abnormal anatomic structure of the conducting system and not being counterbalanced by the excitation front in the anterior wall.[231] In support of this hypothesis, Feldt et al. found a marked posteroinferior displacement of the left bundle branch system and relative hypoplasia of the anterior left bundle branch fascicle in hearts with a partial or complete form of AV canal.[232]

With the sinus venosus type of ASD defect, which comprises 12 percent of all ASDs, the frontal QRS axis is similar to that of the ASD secundum type. In 50 cases of sinus venosus

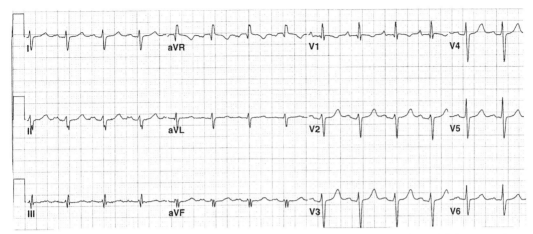

Figure 12–55 Preoperative ECG of a 27-year-old woman with a large (6-cm diameter) atrial septal defect, secundum type, and mild pulmonary hypertension. Note the right axis deviation, incomplete right bundle branch block, and a pattern suggestive of left atrial enlargement and right ventricular hypertrophy.

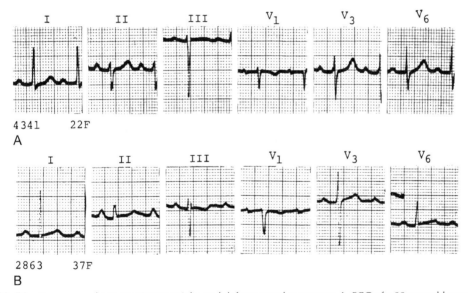

Figure 12–56 Two cases of ostium primum atrial septal defect proved at autopsy. **A**, ECG of a 22-year-old woman with a large left-to-right shunt and normal pulmonary arterial pressure. Note the marked abnormal left axis deviation. The morphology of the QRS complex in lead V₁ is normal and is not typical of an atrial septal defect. **B**, The tracing from this 37-year-old woman shows first-degree atrioventricular block. The frontal plane QRS axis is about +20 degrees, which is atypical for an ostium primum defect. Lead V_1 shows a normal rS complex.

defect the QRS axis in the frontal plane ranged from +45 to +135 degrees in all but 3 patients, in whom the axis was directed leftward; in 44 percent of patients the axis was to the right of +90 degrees.[233]

The most characteristic ECG finding in patients with all types of ASD is incomplete RBBB with an rSR′ or rSr′ pattern in lead V_1 (Figures 12–55 and 12–57). It was present in 60 percent of 370 patients from four studies reviewed by Chou.[223] Complete RBBB occurs in 5 to 19 percent of cases[223] and is more prevalent in older patients. Other morphologies of the QRS complex in lead V_1 include RS, Rs, qR, qRS, monophasic R, RSR′S′, or a normal rS or QS pattern.[223] In the presence of increased pulmonary artery pressure, the ECG shows an RVH pattern manifested by increased amplitude of R (or R′) or a qR pattern in lead V_1.[219,229]

A frequently observed pattern in patients with secundum or sinus venosus ASD, independent of the RBBB, is a notched R wave in the inferior limb leads.[234] This pattern, called "crochetage," was observed in 73.1 percent of patients with

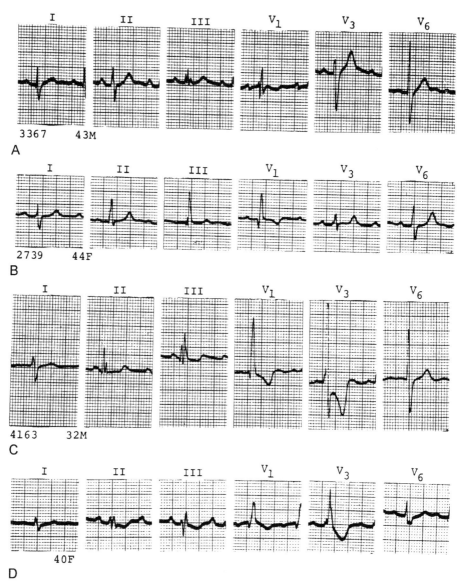

Figure 12–57   Four proved cases of ostium secundum atrial septal defect with different QRS morphology in lead V_1 and different hemodynamic findings. **A,** A 43-year-old man had a small left-to-right shunt and normal pulmonary arterial pressure. He had paroxysmal atrial flutter. ECG shows sinus rhythm and an rSR′s′ pattern in lead V_1. Frontal plane QRS axis is indeterminate. **B,** A 44-year-old woman had a pulmonary arterial pressure that was moderately elevated and a pulmonary-to-systemic flow ratio of 3:1. Lead V_1 shows a qR pattern. **C,** A 32-year-old man had autopsy-proven ostium secundum atrial septal defect, anomalous pulmonary venous return to the right atrium, and severe pulmonary hypertension. ECG showed abnormal right axis deviation and an rSR′ pattern in lead V_1 with tall R′. There are also secondary ST and T wave changes in the right and mid-precordial leads. **D,** A 40-year-old woman had a secundum-type defect proved at surgery. Pulmonary arterial pressure was normal. She had a large left-to-right shunt, with a pulmonary-to-systemic flow ratio of 6:1. The PR interval on the ECG is 0.22 second. Frontal plane QRS axis is indeterminate. QRS duration is 0.12 second, and there is an rSR′ pattern in lead V_1 consistent with complete right bundle branch block. Some of the ST and T wave changes probably are due to a digitalis effect.

ASD.[234] The incidence of "crochetage" was lower in patients with a ventricular septal defect, pulmonary stenosis, or mitral stenosis and in normal subjects.[232] In patients with ASD the incidence increased in the presence of greater left-to-right shunt; and early disappearance was observed in 35.1 percent after surgical closure of the defect. The sensitivity and specificity of the notch for diagnosis of ASD are fairly high when it is associated with incomplete RBBB or when present in all three "inferior" leads. The cause of this pattern remains unexplained.

With the advent of echocardiography it became evident that the classic ECG criteria for diagnosing primum, secundum, and sinus venosus ASD have limited sensitivity compared with echocardiography and should not be relied on to exclude the diagnosis of ASD in practice.[235]

Ventricular Septal Defect

The ECG reflects the hemodynamic characteristics of the ventricular septal defect (VSD).[233–235] A normal ECG suggests a small VSD. The pattern of LVH associated with signs of left atrial enlargement[236] indicates a moderate left-to-right shunt without pulmonary hypertension. The pattern of combined left and right ventricular hypertrophy with large biphasic QRS complexes in the standard limb and mid-precordial leads, as described by Katz and Wachtel,[237] is often present in patients with a large defect and variable degree of pulmonary hypertension (see Figure 3–8). In patients with marked pulmonary hypertension (i.e., Eisenmenger syndrome), RVH predominates. The two most commonly encountered ECG patterns in adults with VSD are a normal ECG associated with a small left-to-right shunt and an RVH pattern indicating severe pulmonary hypertension.[223]

The sinus rhythm is usually maintained in patients with Eisenmenger syndrome; right atrial enlargement is often present, and the frontal QRS axis is deviated to the right (except in some cases of VSD associated with an endocardial cushion defect). There is also evidence of RVH with or without LVH[238] (see Figure 3–13).

During the stage preceding irreversible pulmonary hypertension, the ECG of patients with large defects and bidirectional shunts often shows a fairly characteristic $S_1S_2S_3$ pattern. In the study of Burch and DePasquale,[239] this pattern was present in 35 percent of 110 patients.[239] In another 36 percent of these patients, a deep S wave was present in leads I and II but not in lead III.[238] The presence of deep S waves in the standard limb leads is often associated with R' in lead V_1, deep S waves in leads V_5 and V_6, and a deep Q wave in lead V_6. These ECG changes were attributed to hypertrophy of the crista supraventricularis caused by the volume overload of the right ventricle analogous to the abnormalities in patients with ASD.[223,239]

Aorticopulmonary Septal Defect

Aorticopulmonary septal defect is seldom encountered in adults. The prevalent ECG pattern is that of biventricular hypertrophy.[240]

Patent Ductus Arteriosus

Among those with patent ductus arteriosus, the ECG is usually normal when the ductus is small. In patients with a large left-to-right shunt, an LVH pattern is usually present (Figure 12–58), sometimes with upright T waves in the left precordial leads ("diastolic overload pattern"). In the presence of pulmonary hypertension and a bidirectional or reversed shunt, the ECG usually shows either RVH or combined ventricular hypertrophy. Sinus rhythm is usually maintained, and

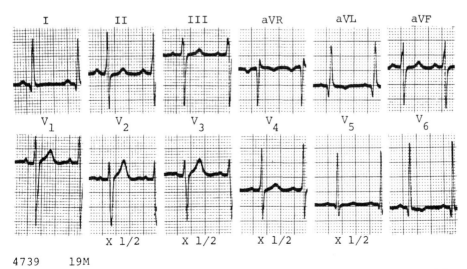

4739   19M

Figure 12–58   Patent ductus arteriosus in a 19-year-old man, with the diagnosis proven at surgery. A 3:1 left-to-right shunt was demonstrated at cardiac catheterization, and the pulmonary arterial pressure was normal. ECG shows a frontal plane QRS axis of −15 degrees. The QRS voltage and ST and T wave changes are consistent with left ventricular hypertrophy.

the PR interval is prolonged in about 10 percent of patients.[241]

Discrete Subaortic Stenosis

The ECG findings in patients with discrete subaortic stenosis are similar to those in patients with aortic valvular stenosis.[242]

Coarctation of the Aorta

The predominant ECG abnormality in patients with coarctation of the aorta is an LVH pattern caused by hypertension. In a series of 200 cases, increased QRS voltage with normal T waves was present in 22 percent and with secondary ST and T wave abnormalities in 18 percent (Figure 12–59).[243] The latter occurred usually in patients who had associated abnormalities, such as aortic valve disease or VSD.[223] In one study of 234 patients, the incidence of additional congenital heart lesions was 34 percent.[244]

In about half of patients with coarctation of the aorta, the ECG is normal. Signs of left atrial enlargement are seen in about 20 percent of patients[223] and first-degree AV block in about 10 percent.[245]

RBBB is present in 10 to 20 percent of patients with coarctation of the aorta without other associated congenital anomalies.[223,245] The high incidence of this pattern is incompletely understood.

Pulmonary Stenosis

The ECG of patients with isolated pulmonary stenosis reflects the presence of concentric RVH and right atrial enlargement. The frequency and severity of the ECG abnormalities depend on the severity of the obstruction.[246,247] In patients with mild pulmonary stenosis the ECG is usually normal.[245] When the pulmonary stenosis is moderately severe, an rSR' pattern in lead V_1 may be present, but most patients with moderately severe pulmonary stenosis have a monophasic R, qR, or RS complex with depressed ST segment and inverted T wave,[223] similar to the ECG of children (Figure 12–60; see also Figure 3–18). In a study of 105 patients, Cayler et al.[248] found that the presence of an R wave >2 mV in lead V_1 was usually associated with a right ventricular pressure of >100 mmHg (see Figure 3–14). In another study of 539 patients with isolated valvular pulmonary stenosis, an RSR' pattern in lead V_1 was found in 20 percent. On average, patients with an RSR' pattern had lower right ventricular systolic pressure and a lower gradient across the valve than patients with a QR, R, or RS pattern. An R' wave of a given voltage was associated with generally lower right ventricular systolic pressure than an R wave of equal amplitude.[249] The PR interval and the QRS duration are usually normal in patients with isolated pulmonary stenosis.

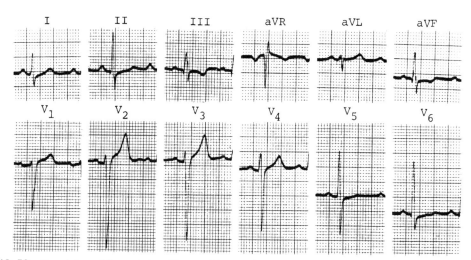

Figure 12–59 Coarctation of the aorta in a 19-year-old man. The coarctation is located just beyond the origin of the left subclavian artery. During catheterization there was a gradient of 67 mmHg across the area of constriction. On the ECG, ST and T wave abnormalities are seen in the left precordial leads. Left ventricular hypertrophy could not be definitely diagnosed, as the voltage of the QRS complex is within the normal range for the patient's age.

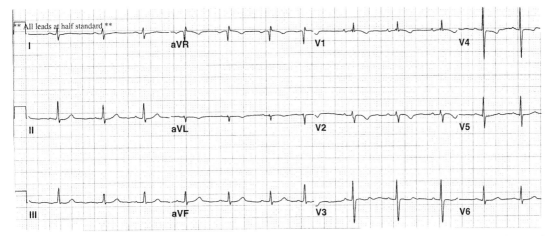

Figure 12–60 ECG of a 5-year-old child with moderately severe valvular pulmonary stenosis (right ventricular systolic pressure 50 mmHg) shows right ventricular hypertrophy. Note the half-normal standardization.

Tetralogy of Fallot

Tetralogy of Fallot and the related trilogy and pentalogy manifest in many anatomic forms and hemodynamic patterns. The ECG is nearly always abnormal, and the abnormality sometimes indicates the hemodynamic status caused by the anomaly.[223]

Right atrial enlargement is seen in about 30 to 50 percent of patients.[223,250,251] The most commmon other abnormality is right axis deviation and an RVH pattern (see Figure 3–10). R or rR', rSR', rs or RS, and qR patterns in lead V_1 are seen, in descending order of frequency.[223] In a study of 25 adult patients not previously operated on, an rSR' pattern in lead V_1 was present

in 58 percent.[252] In patients who have undergone corrective surgery, RBBB with or without left anterior fascicular block is the most prevalent ECG pattern[253,254] (Figure 12–61). In one study[255] a QRS duration >150 ms was significantly associated with postoperative right ventricular dysfunction and significant regurgitation of the pulmonary valve.

Ventricular arrhythmias, including nonsustained ventricular tachycardia, are frequently present in adults after repair of tetralogy. In a retrospective study of 359 postoperative patients with tetralogy of Fallot, 48 percent had ventricular ectopic activity during 24-hour ambulatory monitoring, and in 17 percent ventricular tachycardia was inducible during programmed

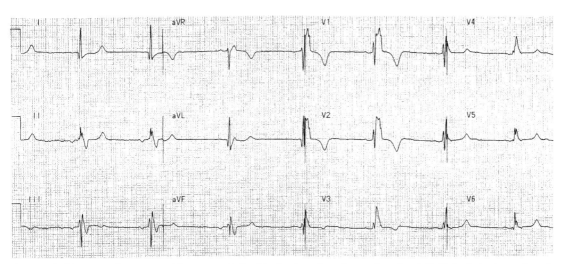

Figure 12–61 ECG of a 43-year-old woman admitted for implantation of a cardioverter-defibrillator to treat symptomatic ventricular tachycardia. She underwent operative treatment for tetralogy of Fallot (probably a Blalock procedure) during childhood, followed by complete repair at age 38. Note the right bundle branch block with a QRS duration of 172 ms.

electrical stimulation.[255] Supraventricular arrhythmias, including SA conduction disturbances, atrial fibrillation, and atrial flutter, were found in one third of the adult patients in whom tetralogy was surgically repaired[257] (Figure 12–62). The incidence of arrhythmic sudden cardiac death in patients after repair of tetralogy is estimated to be 1 to 5 percent, but the cause is unknown.[258,259] Late sudden death was associated with transient complete AV block that persisted beyomd the third postoperative day.[260]

Ebstein's Anomaly

The wide spectrum of anatomic anomalies associated with downward displacement of the tricuspid valve ranges from the mild form of "form fruste" to severe disabling conditions with severe tricuspid regurgitation.[261] In typical cases the ECG shows a characteristic pattern that sometimes provides the first clue to the diagnosis.

Abnormal P waves suggestive of right atrial enlargement are present in 60 to 95 percent of patients.[262,263] Before the advent of surgical treatment for this condition, high-amplitude P waves suggested a poor prognosis.[263] The PR interval is prolonged in 16 to 34 percent of patients.[261,264,265]

RBBB is present in most cases, but the pattern is atypical because the QRS amplitude is low and the QRS complex in the right precordial leads tends to be polyphasic (i.e., rSR′, rSrs′, or RS) (Figures 12–63 and 12–64). In one series a low-voltage, polyphasic, notched and slurred QRS complex in right-sided precordial leads

was present in 47 percent of cases. Q waves in lead V_1 are often present in association with tricuspid regurgitation.[266] Deep wide Q waves with a negative T wave are often present also in leads II and III.[256,261] A QR or Qr pattern with T wave inversion in leads V_1–V_4 has been considered by some authors to be almost pathognomonic of Ebstein's anomaly.[223,266] The presence of notched r′ or R′ is attributed to delayed activation of the "atrialized" right ventricular wall.[261] An RVH pattern is not observed in uncomplicated Ebstein's anomaly.

A right-sided AV accessory pathway is present in 7 to 25 percent of patients with Ebstein's anomaly.[261,262,265] The WPW pattern and RBBB seldom coexist; but if the co-existence occurs, an RBBB of low amplitude is almost diagnostic of Ebstein's anomaly[223] (see Figures 12–63 and 12–65). The most common serious arrhythmia is the orthodromic or antidromic AV circus movement tachycardia utilizing the bypass tract. Supraventricular tachycardia, atrial fibrillation, or ventricular tachycardia was found in 34 of 52 patients preoperatively.[267] After operation for repair of Ebstein's anomaly, more than one half of patients had symptomatic supraventricular or ventricular tachycardias during follow-up.[268]

Intracardiac electrograms may be useful for documenting atrialization of a portion of the right ventricle. Some ECG findings encountered in patients with Ebstein's anomaly may be misleading. A wide P wave of 0.12 to 0.19 second's duration may lead to a false diagnosis of left atrial enlargement,[261] and RBBB with a qR or qRs pattern in lead V_6 may falsely suggest LVH.

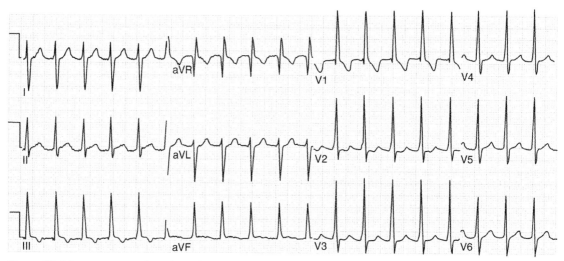

Figure 12–62 Supraventricular tachycardia, probably ectopic atrial tachycardia, with a prolonged PR interval in a 26-year old woman who underwent surgical correction of tetralogy of Fallot in early childhood. The QRS duration is increased (124 ms), possibly due to flecainide, and there is right axis deviation and right ventricular hypertrophy.

3/24/69

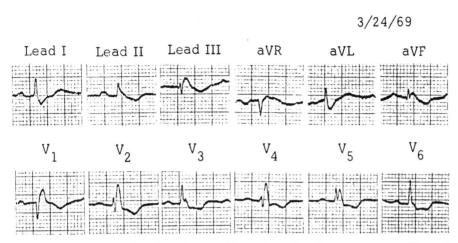

Figure 12–63 Ebstein's anomaly with Wolff-Parkinson-White syndrome in a 35-year-old woman. Diagnosis of Ebstein's anomaly was confirmed at surgery. PR interval is 0.20 second. There is a complete right bundle branch block with a QR pattern in lead V_1. Some of the ST and T wave changes are probably due to digitalis effects.

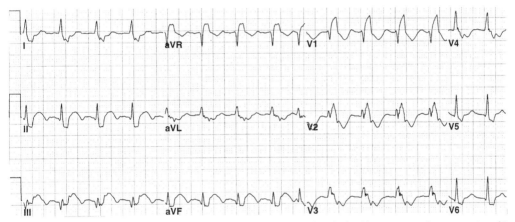

Figure 12–64 ECG of a 29-year-old woman born with Ebstein's anomaly. She had been operated on at age 2 and is now admitted to the hospital with atrial flutter and severe tricuspid regurgitation. Note the atrial flutter with a predominant 2:1 response and right bundle branch block with a characteristic wide terminal QRS portion of relatively low amplitude. QRS duration is 196 ms.

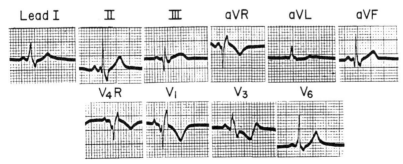

Figure 12–65 Ebstein's anomaly with Wolff-Parkinson-White pattern in a 7-year-old girl. PR interval is 0.09 second. QRS duration measures 0.12 second. Delta waves are present and are inscribed downward in leads V_{4R} and V_1. Signs of right bundle branch block are also present, with an R' in leads V_{4R} and V_1. (Courtesy of Dr. Samuel Kaplan.)

The ECG findings in patients with partial parchment of the right ventricular wall (i.e., Uhl's anomaly) may be similar. In one reported case of this anomaly with an inexcitable right ventricle, examination of the conducting system revealed destruction of both bundle branches; and the ECG showed bilateral bundle branch block.[269]

Dextrocardia

In the presence of dextrocardia with situs inversus, the ECG has the appearance of a tracing in which the right and left arm electrodes are reversed, the precordial lead in V_1 position corresponds to lead V_2, and the lead in V_2 position corresponds to lead V_1, whereas the leads in V_{3R} to V_{6R} positions correspond to leads V_3–V_6 and leads V_3–V_6 correspond to leads V_{3R}–V_{6R}. Leads aV_R and aV_L are reversed. Dextrocardia is suspected when the P wave is negative in lead I. Reversal of the right and left arm electrodes results in the same pattern in the limb leads, but, unlike dextrocardia, the morphology of the precordial leads is practically unaffected.

Proper interpretation of the ECG in the presence of dextrocardia requires recording precordial leads on the right side of the chest. Dextrocardia with situs inversus should be differentiated from dextroposition, which means displacement of the heart, most often an acquired condition (Figure 12–66). Dextrocardia without situs inversus is nearly always associated with other congenital anomalies and is rarely encountered in adults.

Tricuspid Atresia

Tricuspid atresia is one of the few congenital cyanotic heart diseases in which the ECG shows left or superior axis deviation that meets the criterion for left anterior fascicular block (Figure 12–67). This pattern was present in a series of 18 adults with tricuspid atresia, most of whom underwent palliative surgery during childhood.[270]

Survivors of the Fontan operation for tricuspid atresia or other forms of functional single ventricle are reaching adulthood in increasing numbers.[271] Atrial tachycardia, atrial flutter, and fibrillation occur in 10 to 20 percent of these patients.[272]

Survivors of Switch Operation for Complete Transposition of Great Vessels

Flinn et al.[273] studied 372 patients with complete transposition of the great vessels who survived the Mustard operation, which was performed at a mean age of 2 years. The most important observation consisted of a decreasing prevalence of normal sinus rhythm and the appearance of supraventricular tachyarrhythmias. Second- and third-degree AV block was present in 3 percent of patients. Sudden cardiac death was weakly associated with the presence of dominant ectopic tachyarrhythmias. More recently, Puley et al.[274] reported that, of 86 consecutive adults who had undergone the Mustard procedure as children, only 39 percent were

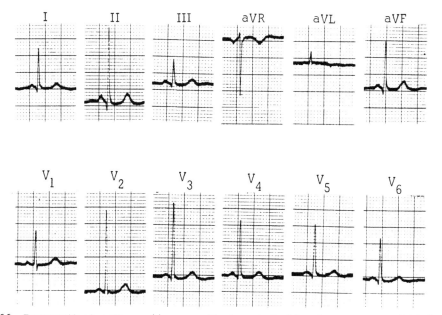

Figure 12–66   Dextroposition in a 40-year-old woman with a hypoplastic right pulmonary artery and right lung, probably of congenital origin. Heart and mediastinum are displaced to the right chest. On the ECG, the limb leads are normal except for a relatively large R wave in lead II and S wave in lead aV_R. Precordial leads show tall R waves in leads V_1–V_3; the amplitude of the R waves decreases from V_2 to V_6.

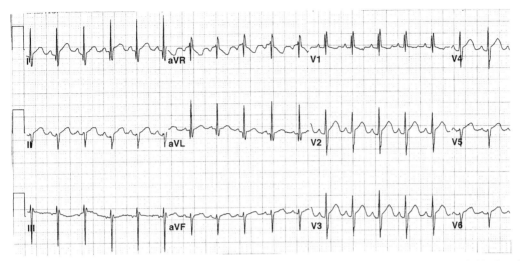

Figure 12–67 ECG of a 1-year-old male child with tricuspid atresia shows incomplete right bundle branch block and left anterior fascicular block.

arrhythmia free; 2 died suddenly, and pacemakers were implanted in 19 (22 percent).

Corrected Transposition of Great Vessels

The position of the AV node is abnormal and AV conduction disturbances are common in the presence of ventricular inversion and corrected transposition of the great vessels. Complete AV block may be present.[275] The initial QRS deflection has the same direction as in LBBB because the ventricular conduction system is inverted (Figure 12–68). In the absence of other abnormalities, the duration of the QRS complex and other conduction intervals is normal.[276] An abnormal Q wave in leads V_1 and V_2 may mimic an anterior infarction, and an abnormal Q wave in lead III may mimic an inferior infarction.[277,278]

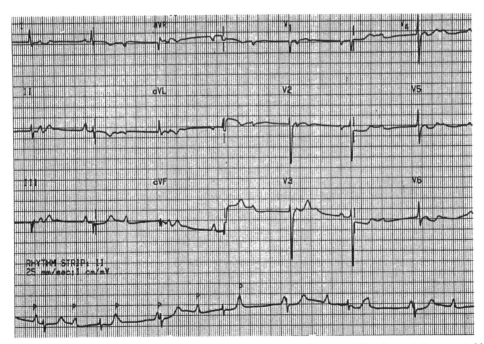

Figure 12–68 Corrected transposition of the great arteries in a 43-year-old woman. The diagnosis is supported by echocardiographic findings. No other anatomic cardiac lesion was found. ECG shows complete atrioventricular block with junctional escape rhythm at the rate of 50 beats/min. A QS deflection is apparent in lead V_1, and an absence of Q waves can be seen in leads V_5 and V_6. Q waves are present in leads III and aV_F. P waves are abnormal.

REFERENCES

1. Chou T-C: Myocardial diseases. *In:* Electrocardiography in Clinical Practice. Adult and Pediatric, 4th ed. Philadelphia, Saunders, 1966, pp 257–280.

2. Flowers NV, Horan LG: Electrocardiographic and vector-cardiographic features of myocardial disease. *In:* Fowler NO (ed): Myocardial Diseases, Orlando, Grune & Stratton, 1973.

3. Hamby RI, Raia F: Electrocardiographic aspects of primary myocardial disease in 60 patients. Am Heart J 76:316, 1968.

4. Marriott HJ: Electrocardiographic abnormalities, conduction disorders and arrhythmias in primary myocardial disease. Prog Cardiovasc Dis 7:99, 1964.

5. Stapleton JF, Segal JP, Harvey WP: The electrocardiogram of myocardiopathy. Prog Cardiovasc Dis 13:217, 1970.

6. Dec WG, Fuster V: Idiopathic dilated cardiomyopathy. N Engl J Med 331:1564, 1994.

7. Roberts WC, Siegel RJ, McManus BM: Idiopathic dilated cardiomyopathy: analysis of 152 necropsy patients. Am J Cardiol 60:1340, 1987.

8. Wilensky RL, Yudelman P, Cohen AI, et al: Serial electrocardiographic changes in idiopathic dilated cardiomyopathy confirmed at necropsy. Am J Cardiol 62:276, 1988.

9. Pruitt RD, Curd GW, Leachman R: Simulation of electrocardiogram of apicolateral myocardial infarction by myocardial destructive lesions of obscure etiology (myocardiopathy). Circulation 25:506, 1962.

10. Tavel ME, Fisch C: Abnormal Q waves simulating myocardial infarction in diffuse myocardial disease. Am Heart J 68:534, 1964.

11. Kamiyama N, Nezuo S, Sawayama T, et al: Electrocardiographic features differentiating dilated cardiomyopathy from hypertrophic cardiomyopathy. J Electrocardiol 3:301, 1997.

12. Fuster V, Gersh BJ, Giuliani ER, et al: The natural history of idiopathic dilated cardiomyopathy. Am J Cardiol 47:525, 1981.

13. Likoff MJ, Chandler SL, Kay HR: Clinical determinants of mortality in chronic congestive heart failure secondary to idiopathic dilated or ischemic cardiomyopathy. Am J Cardiol 59:634, 1987.

14. Guttigoli AB, Wilner BF, Stein KM, et al: Usefulness of prolonged QRS duration to identify high-risk ischemic cardiomyopathy patients with syncope and inducible ventricular tachycardia. Am J Cardiol 95:391, 2005.

15. Savage DD, Seides SP, Clark CE: Electrocardiographic findings in patients with obstructive and nonobstructive hypertrophic cardiomypathy. Circulation 58:402, 1978.

16. Montgomery JV, Harris KM, Casey SA, et al: Relation of electrocardiographic pattern to phenotypic expression and clinical outcome in hypertrophic cardiomyopathy. Am J Cardiol 96:270, 2005.

17. Wigle ED, Baron RH: The electrocardiogram in muscular subaortic stenosis: effect of a left septal incision and right bundle branch block. Circulation 34:585, 1966.

18. Lemery R, Kleinebenner A, Nihoyannopoulos P, et al: Q waves in hypertrophic cardiomyopathy in relation to the distribution and severity of right and left ventricular hypertrophy. J Am Coll Cardiol 16:368, 1990.

19. Maron BF, Wolfson JK, Ciro E, et al: Relation of electrocardiographic abnormalities and patterns of left ventricular hypertrophy identified in 2-dimensional echocardiography in patients with hypertrophic cardiomyopathy. Am J Cardiol 51:189, 1983.

20. Goldberger AL: Q wave T wave vector discordance in hypertrophic cardiomyopathy: septal hypertrophy and strain pattern. Br Heart J 42:201, 1979.

21. Chen CH, Nobuyoshi M, Kawai C: ECG pattern of left ventricular hypertrophy in nonobstructive hypertrophic cardiomyopathy: the significance of mid-precordial changes. Am Heart J 97:687, 1979.

22. Hollister RM, Goodwin JF: The electrocardiogram in cardiomyopathy. Br Heart J 25:357, 1963.

23. Frank S, Braunwald E: Idiopathic hypertrophic subaortic stenosis: clinical analysis of 126 patients with emphasis on natural history. Circulation 37:759, 1968.

23a. Dumont CA, Monserrat L, Soler R, et al: Interpretation of electrocardiographic abnormalities in hypertrophic cardiomyopathy with cardiac magnetic resonance. Europ Heart J 27:1725, 2006.

24. Perosio AM, Suarez LD, Bunster AM, et al: Pre-excitation syndrome and hypertrophic cardiomyopathy. J Electrocardiol 16:29, 1983.

25. Yamaguchi H, Ishimura T, Nishiyama S, et al: Hypertrophic nonobstructive cardiomyopathy with giant negative T waves (apical hypertrophy): ventriculographic and echocardiographic features in 30 patients. Am J Cardiol 44:401, 1979.

26. Keren G, Belhassen B, Sherez B, et al: Apical hypertrophic cardiomyopathy: evaluation by noninvasive and invasive techniques in 23 patients. Circulation 71:45, 1985.

27. Alfonso F, Nihoyannpoulos P, Stewart J, et al: Clinical significance of giant negative T waves in hypertrophic cardiomyopathy. J Am Coll Cardiol 15:965, 1990.

28. Maron BJ, Bonow RO, Seshagiri TNR, et al: Hypertrophic cardiomyopathy with ventricular septal hypertrophy localized to the apical region of the left ventricle (apical hypertrophic cardiomyopathy). Am J Cardiol 49:1838, 1982.

29. Koga Y, Katoh A, Matsuyama K, et al: Disappearance of giant negative T waves in patients with Japanese form of apical hypertrophy. J Am Coll Cardiol 26:1672, 1995.

30. Lewis JF, Maron BJ: Hypertrophic cardiomyopathy characterized by marked hypertrophy of the posterior left ventricular free wall: significance and clinical implications. J Am Coll Cardiol 18:421, 1991.

31. McKenna WJ, Chetty S, Oakley CM, et al: Arrhythmia in hypertrophic cardiomyopathy: exercise and 48 hour ambulatory electrocardiographic assessment with and without beta adrenergic blocking therapy. Am J Cardiol 45:1, 1980.

32. Maron BJ, Savage DD, Wolfson JK, et al: Prognostic significance of 24 hour ambulatory electrocardiographic monitoring in patients with hypertrophic cardiomyopathy: a prospective study. Am J Cardiol 48:252, 1981.

33. Glancy DI, O'Brien KP, Gold HL, et al: Atrial fibrillation in patients with idiopathic hypertrophic subaortic stenosis. Br Heart J 32:652, 1970.

34. Nicod P, Rolikar R, Peterson KL: Hypertrophic cardiomyopathy and sudden death. N Engl J Med 318:1255, 1988.

35. Adabag AS, Casey SA, Kuskowski MA, et al: Spectrm and prognostic significance of arrhythmias on ambulatory Holter electrocardiogram in hypertrophic cardiomyopathy. J Am Coll Cardiol 45:697, 2005.

36. Bybee KA, Kara T, Prasad A, et al: Systematic review: transient left ventricular apical ballooning: a syndrome that mimics ST-segment elevation myocardial infarction. Ann Intern Med 141:858, 2004.

37. Matsuoka K, Okubo S, Fuji E, et al: Evaluation of the arrhythmogenicity of stress-induced "Takotsube-

cardiomyopathy" from the time course of the 12-lead surface electrocardiogram. Am J Cardiol 92:230, 2003.

38. Benotti JR, Grossman W, Cohn PF: Clinical profile of restrictive cardiomyopathy. Circulation 61:1286, 1980.

38a. Sen-Choudhry S, Syrris P, Ward D, et al: Clinical and genetic characterization of families with arrhythmogenic right ventricular dysplasia/cardiomyopathy provides novel insights into patterns of disease expression. Circulation 115:1710, 2007.

39. Fontaine G, Frank R, Fontaine F, et al: Right ventricular tachycardias. In: Parmley WW, Chatterjee K (eds): Cardiology, vol 1. Philadelphia, JB Lippincott, 1991, pp 1–17.

40. Bender V, Vauthier M, Mabo P, et al: Characteristics and outcome in arrhythmogenic right ventricular dysplasia. Am J Cardiol 75:411, 1995.

41. Nava A, Canciani B, Buja G, et al: Electrocardiographic study of negative T waves on precordial leads in arrhythmogenic right ventricular dysplasia: relationship with right ventricular volumes. J Electrocardiol 21:239, 1988.

42. Metzger JT, de Chillou C, Cheriex E, et al: Value of the 12–lead electrocardiogram in arrhythmogenic right ventricular dysplasia, and absence of correlation with echocardiographic findings. Am J Cardiol 72:964, 1993.

43. Nasir K, Bomma C, Tandri H, et al: Electrocardiographic features of arrhythmogenic right ventricular dysplasia/cardiomyopathy according to disease severity. A need to broaden diagnostic criteria. Circulation 110:1527, 2004.

44. Daliento L, Turrini P, Nava A, et al: Arrhythmogenic right ventricular cardiomyopathy in young versus adult patients: similarities and differences. J Am Coll Cardiol 25:655, 1995.

45. Turrini P, Angelini A, Thiene G, et al: Late potentials and ventricular arrhythmias in arrhythmogenic right ventricular cardiomyopathy. Am J Cardiol 83:1214, 1999.

46. Peeters HAP, Sippens-Groenewegen A, Schoonderwoerd EFD, et al: Body surface QRST integral mapping. Arrhythmogenic right ventricular dysplasia versus idiopathic right ventricular tachycardia. Circulation 95:2668, 1997.

47. Yoshioko N, Tsuchihashi K, Yuda S, et al: Electrocardiographic and echocardiographic abnormalities in patients with arrhythmogenic right ventricular cardiomyopathy and in their pedigrees. Am J Cardiol 85:885, 2000.

48. Child JS, Perloff JK, Bach PM, et al: Cardiac involvement in Friedreich's ataxia: a clinical study of 75 patients. J Am Coll Cardiol 7:1370, 1986.

49. Harding AE, Hewer RI: The heart disease of Friedreich's ataxia: a clinical and electrocardiographic study of 115 patients, with an analysis of serial electrocardiographic changes in 30 cases. Q J Med 208:489, 1983.

50. Gach JV, Andriange M, Franck G: Hypertrophic obstructive cardiomyopathy and Friedreich's ataxia: report of a case and review of literature. Am J Cardiol 60:436, 1971.

51. Albouras ET, Shub C, Gomez MR, et al: Spectrum of cardiac involvement in Friedreich's ataxia: clinical, electrocardiographic and echocardiographic observations. Am J Cardiol 58:518, 1986.

52. Smith ER, Sangalang VE, Heffernan LR: Hypertrophic cardiomyopathy: the heart diesease of Friedreich's ataxia. Am Heart J 94:428, 1977.

53. Isner JM, Hawley RJ, Weintraub AM, et al: Cardiac findings in Charcot-Marie-Tooth disease. A prospective study of 68 patients. Arch Intern Med 139:1161, 1979.

54. Slucka C: The electrocardiogram in Duchenne progressive muscular dystrophy. Circulation 38:933, 1968.

55. Perloff JK, Roberts WC, DeLeon AC, et al: The distinctive electrocardiogram of Duchenne's progressive muscular dystrophy: an electrocardiographic-pathologic correlative study. Am J Med 42:179, 1967.

56. Gilroy J, Calahan JL, Berman KL, et al: Cardiac and pulmonary complications in Duchenne's progressive muscular dystrophy. Circulation 27:484, 1963.

57. Perloff JK: Cardiac rhythm and conduction in Duchenne's muscular dystrophy: a prospective study of 20 patients. J Am Coll Cardiol 3:1263, 1984.

58. Tanaka H, Uemura N, Toyama Y: Cardiac involvement in the Kugelberg-Welander syndrome. Am J Cardiol 38:528, 1978.

59. Welsh JD, Lynn TN, Haase GR: Cardiac findings in 73 patients with muscular dystrophy. Arch Intern Med 112:199, 1963.

60. Mascarenhas DAN, Spodick DH, Chad DA, et al: Cardiomyopathy of limb-girdle muscular dystrophy. J Am Coll Cardiol 24:1328, 1994.

61. Moorman JR, Coleman RE, Packer DL, et al: Cardiac involvement in myotonic muscular dystrophy. Medicine 64:371, 1985.

62. Nguyen HH, Wolfe JT, Holmes DR, et al: Pathology of the cardiac conduction system in myotonic dystrophy: a study of 12 cases. J Am Coll Cardiol 11:662, 1988.

63. Perloff JK, Stevenson WG, Roberts NK, et al: Cardiac involvement in myotonic muscular dystrophy (Steinert's disease): a prospective study of 25 patients. Am J Cardiol 54:1074, 1984.

64. Tokgozoglu LS, Ashizawa T, Pacifico A, et al: Cardiac involvement in a large kindred with myotonic dystrophy. JAMA 274:813, 1995.

65. Olofsson B, Forsberg H, Andersson S, et al: Electrocardiographic findings in myotonic dystrophy. Br Heart J 59:47, 1988.

66. Payne CA, Greenfield JC: Electrocardiographic abnormalities associated with myotonic dystrophy. Am Heart J 65:436, 1963.

67. Grigg LE, Chan W, Mond HG, et al: Ventricular tachycardia and sudden death in myotonic dystrophy: clinical, electrophysiologic and pathologic features. J Am Coll Cardiol 6:254, 1985.

68. Colleran JA, Hawley RJ, Pinnow EE, et al: Value of the electrocardiogram in determining cardiac events and mortality in myotonic dystrophy. Am J Cardiol 80:1494, 1997.

69. Merino JL, Carmona JR, Fernandez-Lozano I, et al: Mechanisms of sustained ventricular tachycardia in myotonic dystrophy. Implications for catheter ablation. Circulation 98:541, 1998.

70. Umeda Y, Ikeda U, Yamamoto J, et al: Myotonic dystrophy associated with QT prolongation and torsade de pointes. Clin Cardiol 22:136, 1999.

71. Groh WJ, Lowe MR, Zipes DP: Severity of cardiac conduction involvement and arrhythmias in myotonic dystrophy Type I correlates with age and CGT repeat length. J Card Electrophysiol 13:444, 2002.

72. Petty RKH, Harding EA, Morgan-Hughes JA: The clinical features of mitochondrial myopathy. Brain 109:915, 1986.

73. Gallastegui J, Hariman RJ, Handler B, et al: Cardiac involvement in the Kearns-Sayre syndrome. Am J Cardiol 60:385, 1987.

74. Roberts NK, Perloff JK, Kark RAP: Cardiac conduction in the Kearns-Sayre syndrome (a neuromuscular disorder associated with progressive external ophthalmoplegia and pigmentary retinopathy). Am J Cardiol 44:1396, 1979.

75. Buyukozturk K, Ozdemir C, Kohen D: Electrocardiographic findings in 24 patients with myasthenia gravis. Acta Cardiol 31:301, 1976.

76. Kessler KM, Pina I, Green B, et al: Cardiovascular findings in quadriplegic and paraplegic patients and in normal subjects. Am J Cardiol 58:525, 1988.

77. Escudero J, McDevitt E: The electrocardiogram in scleroderma: analysis of 60 cases and review of the literature. Am Heart J 56:846, 1958.
78. DuBois EL: Lupus Erythematosus, ed 2. Los Angeles, University of Southern California Press, 1974.
79. Hejtmancik MR, Wright JC, Quint R, et al: The cardiovascular manifestations of systemic lupus erythematosus. Am Heart J 68:119, 1964.
80. Holsinger DR, Osmundson PJ, Edwards JE: The heart in periarteritis nodosa. Circulation 25:610, 1962.
81. Schrader ML, Hochman JS, Bulkley BH: The heart in polyarteritis nodosa: a clinicopathologic study. Am Heart J 109:1353, 1985.
82. Denbow CE, Lie JT, Tancredi RG, et al: Cardiac involvement in polymyositis: a clinicopathologic study of 20 autopsied patients. Arthritis Rheum 22:1088, 1979.
83. Gottdiener JS, Sherber HS, Hawley RJ, et al: Cardiac manifestations in polymyositis. Am J Cardiol 41:1141, 1978.
84. Haupt HM, Hutchins GM: The heart and cardiac conduction system in polymyositis-dermatomyositis: a clinicopathologic study of 16 autopsied patients. Am J Cardiol 50:998, 1982.
85. Stern R, Godbold JH, Chess Q, et al: ECG abnormalities in polymyositis. Arch Intern Med 144:2185, 1984.
86. Bonfiglio T, Atwater TC: Heart disease in patients with seropositive rheumatoid arthritis. Arch Intern Med 124:714, 1969.
87. Ruppert GB, Lindsay J, Barth WF: Cardiac conduction abnormalities in Reiter's syndrome. Am J Med 73:335, 1982.
88. Clarke M, Keith JD: Atrioventricular conduction in acute rheumatic fever. Br Heart J 34:472, 1972.
89. Feinstein AR, Wood HF, Spagnuolo M, et al: Rheumatic fever in children and adolescents: a long term epidemiologic study of subsequent prophylaxis, streptococcal infections and clinical sequelae. VII. Cardiac changes and sequelae. Ann Intern Med 60(Suppl):87, 1964.
90. Bates RC: Acute rheumatic fever: a study of 132 cases in young adults. Ann Intern Med 48:1017, 1958.
91. Biran S, Hochman A, Levij AS, et al: Clinical diagnosis of secondary tumors of the heart and pericardium. Dis Chest 55:202, 1969.
92. Harris TR, Copeland GD, Brody DA: Progressive injury current with metastatic tumor of the heart. Am Heart J 69:392, 1965.
93. Cates CI, Virmani R, Vaughn WK, et al: Electrocardiographic markers of cardiac metastasis. Am Heart J 112:1297, 1985.
94. Trell E, Rausing A, Ripa J, et al: Carcinoid heart disease. Am J Med 54:433, 1973.
95. Hoffman L, Lowrey RD: The electrocardiogram in thyrotoxicosis. Am J Cardiol 6:893, 1960.
96. Staffurth JS, Gibberd MB, Hilton PS: Atrial fibrillation in thyrotoxicosis treated with radioiodine. Postgrad Med J 41:663, 1965.
97. Benker VG, Preiss H, Kreuser H, et al: EKG Veraenderungen bei Hyperthyreose: Untersuchungen an 542 Patienten. Z Kardiol 63:799, 1974.
98. Woeber KA: Thyrotoxicosis and the heart. N Engl J Med 392:94, 1992.
99. Goss JE, Shmock CL, Pryor R, et al: Cardiac arrhythmias with thyrotoxicosis. Rocky Mountain Med J 64:31, 1967.
100. Surawicz B, Mangiardi ML: Electrocardiogram in endocrine and metabolic disorders. Cardiovasc Clin North Am 8:243, 1977.
101. Blizzard JJ, Rupp JJ: Prolongation of the PR interval as a manifestation of thyrotoxicosis. JAMA 173: 1845, 1960.
102. Jost VF: Kammerendteilveraenderungen im EKG bei Thyreotoxicosis factitia. Z Kardiol 62:864, 1974.
103. Boccalandro C, Lopez L, Boccalandro F, et al: Electrocardiographic changes in thyrotoxic periodic paralysis. Am J Cardiol 91:775, 2003.
104. Wood P: Diseases of the Heart and Circulation. London, Eyre & Spottiswoode, 1968, p 1024.
105. Surawicz B: The pathogenesis and clinical significance of primary T wave abnormalities. In: Hurst JW, Schlant R (eds): Advances in Electrocardiography. Orlando, Grune & Stratton, 1972, p 377.
106. Bricaire H, Joly J: Manifestations cardiovasculaires de l'hypothyroidie. Rev Prat (Paris) 18:2147, 1968.
107. Douglas S: Analysis of ECG patterns in hypothyroid heart disease. NY State J Med 60:2227, 1960.
108. Lardoux H, Cenac E, Perlemuter L, et al: Troubles de conduction intracardiaque et hypothyroidie de le'adulte: etude systematique de 42 cas. Nouv Press Med 25:1859, 1975.
109. Fredlund BO, Olsson SB: Long QT interval and ventricular tachycardia of torsade de pointe type in hypothyroidism. Acta Med Scand 213:213, 1983.
110. Kumar A, Bhandari AK, Rahimtoola SH: Torsade de pointes and marked QT prolongation in association with hypothyroidism. Ann Intern Med 106:712, 1987.
111. Bronsky D, Dubin A, Waldstein SS, et al: Calcium and the electrocardiogram. I. The electrocardiographic manifestations of hypoparathyroidism. Am J Cardiol 7:823, 1961.
112. Surawicz B: Relationship between electrocardiogram and electrolytes. Am Heart J 73:814, 1967.
113. Rimailho A, Bouchard P, Schaison G, et al: Improvement of hypocalcemic cardiomyopathy by correction of serum calcium level. Am Heart J 109:611, 1980.
114. Dobra M, Wayneberge M, Lardy P, et al: A cardiopathie hypocalcemique: etude clinique; premieres experimentales sur les arrets cardiaques par dissociation electromecanique. Presse Med 30:1381, 1971.
115. Bronsky D, Dubin A, Waldstein SS, et al: Calcium and the electrocardiogram. II. The electrocardiographic manifestations of hyperparathyroidism and of marked hypercalcemia from various other etiologies. Am J Cardiol 7:833, 1961.
116. Voss EM, Drake EH: Cardiac manifestations of hyperparathyroidism with presentation of a previously unreported arrhythmia. Am Heart J 73:235, 1967.
117. Chodack P, Attie JN, Groder MG: Hypercalcemic crisis coincidental with hemorrhage in parathyroid adenoma. Arch Intern Med 116:416, 1965.
118. Bernart WF, De Andino AM: Electrocardiograpohic changes in hypopituitarism of pregnancy. Am Heart J 55:231, 1958.
119. Daoud FS, Surawicz B, Gettes LS: Effects of isoproterenol on the abnormal T wave. Am J Cardiol 30:810, 1972.
120. Sommerville W, Levine HD, Thorn GW: The electrocardiogram in Addison's disease. Medicine 30:43, 1951.
121. Lown B, Arons WL, Ganong WF, et al: Adrenal steroids and atrioventricular conduction. Am Heart J 50:760, 1955.
122. Van Vliet PD, Burchell HB, Titus J: Focal myocarditis associated with pheochromocytoma. N Engl J Med 274:1102, 1966.
123. Moorhead EL, Caldwell JR, Kelly AR, et al: The diagnosis of pheochromocytoma. JAMA 196:1107, 1966.
124. Northfield TC: Cardiac complications of pheochromocytoma. Br Heart J 29:588, 1967.
125. Price WH, Lauder IJ, Wilson J: The electrocardiogram and sex chromosome aneuploidy. Clin Genet 6:1, 1974.

126. Maaz E: EKG-Veraenderungen bei Langzeitdiabetikern. Z Ges Inn Med 27:1073, 1972.
127. Medaile JH, Papier C, Hezman JB, et al: Diabetes mellitus among 10,000 adult men. I. Five years incidence and associated variables. Israel J Med Sci 10:681, 1984.
128. Soler NG, Bennett MA, Fitzgerald MG, et al: Electrocardiogram as a guide to potassium replacement in diabetic ketoacidosis. Diabetes 23:610, 1974.
129. Henderson CB: Potassium and the cardiographic changes in diabetic acidosis. Br Heart J 15:87, 1953.
130. Gibbs P: Three cases of acute ketotic diabetes mellitus with myocarditis: a common viral origin? BMJ 3:781, 1974.
131. Harte O, Cladi PH: EKG Veraenderungen im diabetischem Koma. Wien Med Klin Wochenschr 35:858, 1973.
132. Ehlers KH, Hagstrom JWC, Lukas DS, et al: Glycogen-storage disease of the myocardium with obstruction to left ventricular outflow. Circulation 25:96, 1962.
133. Buja LM, Khoi NB, Roberts WC: Clinically significant cardiac amyloidosis. Arch Intern Med 26:394, 1970.
134. Murtagh B, Hammill SC, Gertz MA, et al: Electrocardiographic findings in primary systemic amyloidosis and biopsy-proven cardiac involvement Am J Cardiol 95:535, 2005.
135. Falk RH, Rubinow A, Cohen AS: Cardiac arrhythmias in systemic amyloidosis: correlation with echocardiographic abnormalities. J Am Coll Cardiol 3:107, 1984.
136. Mathew V, Olson KJ, Gertz MA, et al: Symptomatic conduction system disease in cardiac amyloidosis. Am J Cardiol 79:1491, 1997.
137. Reisinger J, Dubrey SW, Lavalley M, et al: Electrophysiologic abnormalities in AL (primary) amyloidosis with cardiac involvement. J Am Coll Cardiol 30:1046, 1997.
138. Ridolfi RL, Bulkley BH, Hutchins GM: The conduction system in cardiac amyloidosis: clinical and pathologic features of 23 patients. Am J Med 62:677, 1977.
139. Hango M, Yamamoto H, Kohda T, et al: Comparison of electrocardiographic findings in patients with AL (primary) amyloidosis and in familial amyloid polyneuropathy and anginal pain and their relation to histopathologic findings. Am J Cardiol 85:849, 2000.
140. Dubrey SW, Cha K, Simms RW: Electrocardiography and Doppler echocardiography in secondary (AA) amyloidosis. Am J Cardiol 77:313, 1996.
141. Buja LM, Roberts WC: Iron in the heart: etiology and clinical significance. Am J Med 51:209, 1971.
142. Easley RM Jr, Schreiner B, Yu PN: Brief recordings: reversible cardiomyopathy associated with hemochromatosis. N Engl J Med 387:866, 1972.
143. Vigorita VJ, Hutchins GM: Cardiac conduction system in hemochromatosis: clinical and pathologic features of six patients. Am J Cardiol 44:418, 1979.
144. Petit DW: Hemochromatosis with complete heart block. Am Heart J 29:253, 1945.
145. Mehta J, Tuna N, Moller JH, et al: Electrocariographic and vectorcardiographic abnormalities in Fabry's disease. Am Heart J 93:699, 1977.
146. Torres RR, Schneck L, Kleinberg W: Electrocardiographic and biochemical abnormalities in Tay-Sachs disease. Bull NY Acad Med 47:717, 1971.
147. Ridolfi RL, Hutchins GM, Bell WR: The heart and cardiac conduction system in thrombotic thrombocytopenic purpura: a clinicopathologic study of 17 autopsied patients. Ann Intern Med 91:357, 1979.
148. Smith RF, Pulicichio LU, Holmes AV: Generalized lentigo: electrocardiographic abnormalities, conduction disorders and arrhythmias in three cases. Am J Cardiol 25:501, 1970.
149. Singal PK, Iluskovic N: Doxorubicin-induced cardiomyopathy. N Engl J Med 339:900, 1998.
150. Anderson RF, Allenswort DC, De Groot WJ: Myocardial toxicity from carbon monoxide poisoning. Ann Intern Med 67:1172, 1967.
151. Gueron M, Stern J, Cohen W: Severe myocardial damage and heart failure in scorpion sting: report of five cases. Am J Cardiol 19:719, 1967.
152. Levine HD: Acute myocardial infarction following wasp sting: report of two cases and clinical survey of the literature. Am Heart J 91:365, 1976.
153. Wilkins CE, Barron T, Lowrimore MG, et al: Cardiac sarcoidosis: two cases with ventricular tachycardia and review of cardiac involvement in sarcoid. Texas Heart Inst J 12:377, 1988.
154. Bashour FA, McConnell T, Skinner W, et al: Myocardial sarcoidosis. Dis Chest 53:413, 1968.
155. Porter GH: Sarcoid heart disease. N Engl J Med 263:1350, 1960.
156. Gold JA, Cantor PJ: Sarcoid heart disease: a case with an unusual electrocardiogram. Arch Intern Med 104:101, 1959.
157. Roberts WC, McAllister HA, Ferrans VJ: Sarcoidosis of the heart: a clinicopathologic study of 35 necropsy patients (group I) and review of 78 previously described necropsy patients (group II). Am J Med 63:86, 1977.
158. Winters SL, Cohen M, Greenberg S, et al: Sustained ventricular tachycardia associated with sarcoidosis: assessment of the underlying cardiac anatomy and the prospective utility of programmed ventricular stimulation, drug therapy, and an implantable antitachycardia device. J Am Coll Cardiol 181:937, 1991.
159. Matsuura H, Palacios IF, Dec GW, et al: Intraventricular conduction abnormalities in patients with clinically suspected myocarditis are associated with myocardial necrosis. Am Heart J 127:1290, 1994.
160. Hoagland RJ: Cardiac involvement in infectious mononucleosis. Am J Med Sci 232:252, 1956.
161. Smith WG: Coxsackie B myopericarditis in adults. Am Heart J 80:34, 1970.
162. Acierno IJ: Cardiac complications in acquired immunodeficiency syndrome (AIDS): a review. J Am Coll Cardiol 13:1144, 1989.
163. Cammarosano C, Lewis W: Cardiac lesions in acquired immunodeficiency syndrome (AIDS). J Am Coll Cardiol 5:703, 1985.
164. Levy WS, Simon GI, Rios JC, et al: Prevalence of cardiac abnormalities in human immunodeficiency virus infection. Am J Cardiol 63:86, 1989.
165. Homans DC: Peripartum cardiomyopathy. N Engl J Med 312:1431, 1985.
166. Greenberg YJ, Brennan JJ, Rosenfeld LE: Lyme myocarditis presenting as fascicular tachycardia with underlying complete heart block. J Card Electrophysiol 8:323, 1997.
167. Steere AC, Batsford WP, Weinberg M, et al: Lyme carditis: abnormalities of Lyme disease. Ann Intern Med 93 (Part I):8, 1980.
168. McAllister HF, Klementowicz PT, Andrews C, et al: Lyme carditis: an important cause of reversible heart block. Ann Intern Med 110:339, 1989.
169. Rosenbaum MB: Chagasic myocardiopathy. Prog Cardiovasc Dis 7:199, 1964.
170. Chou TC: Electrocardiography in Clinical Practice. Adult and Pediatric, 4th ed. Philadelphia, Saunders, 1996, pp 585–600.
170a. Marcus GM, Hoang KL, Hunt SA, et al: Prevalence, patterns of development, and prognosis of right bundle branch block in heart transplant recipients. Am J Cardiol 98:1288, 2006.

171. Alexopoulos D, Yusuf S, Bostock J, et al: Ventricular arrhythmias in long-term survivors of orthotopic and heterotopic cardiac transplantation. Br Heart J 59: 648, 1988.

172. Bexton R, Nathan AW, Hellestrand KJ, et al: Electrophysiologic abnormalities in the transplanted human heart. Br Heart J 50:555, 1983.

173. Stinson EB, Schroeder JS, Griepp RB, et al: Observations on the behavior of recipient atria after cardiac transplantation in man. Am J Cardiol 30:615, 1972.

174. Saoudi N, Redonnet M, Anseleme F, et al: Catheter ablation of atrioatrial conduction as a cure for atrial arrhythmia after orthotopic heart transplantation. J Am Coll Cardiol 32:1048, 1998.

175. Lefroy DC, Fang JC, Stevenson LW, et al: Recipient-to-donor atrioatrial conduction after orthotopic heart transplantation: surface electrocardiographic features and estimated prevalence. Am J Cardiol 82:444, 1998.

176. Sandhu JS, Curtiss EJ, Follansbee WP, et al: The scalar electrocardiogram of the orthotopic heart transplant recipient. Am Heart J 119:197, 1990.

177. Leonelli FM, Dunn JK, Young JB, et al: Natural history, determinants, and clinical relevance of conduction abnormalities following orthotopic heart transplantation. Am J Cardiol 77:47, 1996.

178. Bexton RS, Nathan AW, Hellestrand KJ, et al: The electrophysiologic characteristics of the transplanted human heart. Am Heart J 107:1, 1984.

179. Locke TJ, Karnik R, McGregor CGA, et al: The value of the electrocardiogram in the diagnosis of acute rejection after orthotopic heart transplantation. Transplant Int 2:143, 1989.

180. Pavri BD, O'Nunaun SS, Newell JB, et al: Prevalence and prognostic significance of atrial arrhythmias after orthotopic cardiac transplantation. J Am Coll Cardiol 25:1673, 1995.

181. Cui G, Tung T, Kobashigawa J, et al: Increased incidence of atrial flutter associated with the rejection of heart transplantation. Am J Cardiol 88:280, 2001.

182. Surawicz B: Electrophysiologic Basis of ECG and Cardiac Arrhythmias. Baltimore, Williams & Wilkins, 1995, p 196.

183. Calzolari V, Angelini A, Basso C, et al: Histologic findings in the conduction system after cardiac transplantation and correlation with electrocardiographic findings. Am J Cardiol 84:756, 1999.

184. Liedtke AJ, De Muth WE: Nonpenetrating cardiac injuries: a collective review. Am Heart J 86:687, 1973.

185. Dolara A, Morando P, Pampaloni M: Electrocardiographic findings in 98 consecutive non-penetrating chest injuries. Dis Chest 52:50, 1967.

186. Kumpuris AG, Casale TB, Mokotoff DM, et al: Right bundle branch block: occurrence following nonpenetrating chest trauma without evidence of cardiac contusion. JAMA 242:172, 1979.

187. Attenhofer C, Vuilliomenet A, Richter M, et al: Heart contusions: pathological findings and clinical course. Schweiz Med Wochenschr 122:1593, 1992.

188. Di Vincenti PC, Moncrief JA, Pruitt BA: Electrical injuries: a review of 65 cases. J Trauma 9:497, 1969.

189. Jackson SHD, Parry DJ: Lightning and the heart. Br Heart J 43:454, 1980.

190. Jensen PJ, Thomsen P, Bagger J, et al: Electrical injury causing ventricular arrhythmias. Br Heart J 57:279, 1987.

191. Burch GE, DePasquale NP: The electrocardiographic diagnosis of pulmonary heart disease. Am J Cardiol 11:622, 1963.

192. Schmock CL, Pomerantz B, Mitchell RS, et al: The electrocardiogram in emphysema with and without chronic airway obstruction. Chest 60:328, 1971.

193. Selvester RH, Rubin HB: New criteria for the electrocardiographic diagnosis of emphysema and cor pulmonale. Am Heart J 69:437, 1965.

194. Chou TC: Electrocardiography in Clinical Practice. Adult and Pediatric. Philadelphia, Saunders, 1996, pp 281–295.

195. Zambrano SS, Moussavi MS, Spodick DH: QRS duration in chronic obstructive lung disease. J Electrocardiol 7:35, 1974.

196. Spodick DH, Hauger-Klevine JH, Tyler JM, et al: Electrocardiogram in pulmonary emphysema. Am Rev Respir Dis 88:14, 1963.

197. Catalayud JB, Abad JM, Khoi NH, et al: P-wave changes in chronic obstructive pulmonary disease. Am Heart J 79:444, 1970.

198. Baljepally R, Spodick DH: Electrocardiographic screening for emphysema: the frontal P axis. Clin Cardiol 22:226, 1999.

199. Bayes de Luna A, Carrio I, Subirana MT, et al: Electrophysiological mechanisms of the SI, SII, SIII electrocardiographic morphology. J Electrocardiol 20:38, 1987.

200. Caird FI, Wilcken DEL: The electrocardiogram in chronic bronchitis with generalized obstructive lung disease. Am J Cardiol 10:5, 1962.

201. Chappell AG: The electrocardiogram in chronic bronchitis and emphysema. Br Heart J 28:517, 1966.

202. Silver HM, Calatayud JB: Evaluation of QRS criteria in patients with chronic obstructive pulmonary disease. Chest 59:153, 1971.

203. Wasserburger RH, Kelly JR, Rasmussen HK, et al: The electrocardiographic pentalogy of pulmonary emphysema. Circulation 20:831, 1969.

204. Smit JM, Burema J, May JF, et al: Prognosis in severe chronic obstructive pulmonary disease with regard to the electrocardiogram. J Electrocardiol 16:77, 1983.

205. Kilcoyne MM, Davis AL, Ferrer MI: A dynamic electrocardiographic concept useful in the diagnosis of cor pulmonale: result of a survey of 200 patients with chronic obstructive pulmonary disease. Circulation 42:903, 1970.

206. Millar FJC: The electrocardiogram in chronic lung disease. Br Heart J 29:43, 1967.

207. Thomas AJ, Valahbji P: Arrhythmia and tachycardia in pulmonary heart disease. Br Heart J 31:491, 1969.

208. Shepard JW, Garrison MW, Grither DA, et al: Relationship of ventricular ectopy to nocturnal oxygen desaturation in patients with chronic obstructive pulmonary disease. Am J Med 78:28, 1985.

209. Copeland RB, Omenn GS: Electrocardiogram changes suggestive of coronary artery disease in pneumothorax. Arch Intern Med 125:151, 1970.

210. Walston A, Brewer DL, Kitchens CD, et al: The electrocardiographic manifestations of spontaneous left pneumothorax. Arch Intern Med 80:375, 1974.

211. Hwang B, Simon G, Keim HA: The electrocardiogram in patients with scoliosis. J Electrocardiol 15:131, 1982.

212. McGinn S, White PD: Acute cor pulmonale resulting from pulmonary embolism: its clinical recognition. JAMA 104:1473, 1935.

213. Love WS Jr, Brugler GW, Winslow N: Electrocardiographic studies in clinical and experimental pulmonary embolization. Ann Intern Med 11:2109, 1938.

214. Durant TM, Ginsburg IW, Roesler H: Transient bundle branch block and other electrocardiographic changes in pulmonary embolism. Am Heart J 17:423, 1939.

215. Szucs MM Jr, Brooks HL, Grossman W, et al: Diagnostic sensitivity of laboratory findings in acute pulmonary embolism: diagnosis by chest lead electrocardiography. Br Heart J 3:21, 1941.

216. Allen RD, Surawicz B: The electrocardiogram in pulmonary embolism. In: Mobin-Uddin K (ed): Pulmonary Thromboembolism. Springfield, IL, Charles C Thomas, 1973, pp 199–211.

217. Sreeram N, Cheriex EC, Smeets JLRM, et al: Value of the 12-lead electrocardiogram at hospital admission in the diagnosis of pulmonary embolism. Am J Cardiol 73:298, 1994.

218. Cutforth RH, Oram S: The electrocardiogram in pulmonary embolism. Br Heart J 20:41, 1958.

219. Stein PD, Dalen JE, McIntyre KM, et al: The electrocardiogram in acute pulmonary embolism. Prog Cardiovasc Dis 17:247, 1975.

220. Sutton GC, Honey M, Gibson RV: Clinical diagnosis of acute massive pulmonary embolism. Lancet 1:271, 1969.

221. Lui CY: Acute pulmonary embolism as the cause of global T wave inversion and QT prolongation. J Electrocardiol 26:91, 1993.

222. Chia BL, Tan H-C, Lim YT: Right sided chest lead electrocardiographic abnormalities in acute pulmonary embolism. Intern J Cardiol 61:43, 1997.

223. Chou TC: Congenital heart disease in adults. In: Electrocardiography in Clinical Practice. Adult and Pediatric, 4th ed. Philadelphia, Saunders, 1996.

224. Tikoff G, Schmidt AM, Hecht HH: Atrial fibrillation in atrial septal defect. Arch Intern Med 121:402, 1968.

225. Popper RW, Knott JMS, Selzer A, et al: Arrhythmias after cardiac surgery. I. Uncomplicated atrial septal defect. Am Heart J 64:455, 1962.

226. Wolf PS, Vogel JHK, Pryor R, et al: Atrial septal defect in patients over 45 years of age. Br Heart J 30:115, 1968.

227. Morton JB, Sanders P, Vohra JK, et al: Effect of chronic right atrial stretch on atrial electricardiographic remodeling in patients with an atrial septal defect. Circulation 107:1775, 2003.

228. Brandenburg RO Jr, Holmes DR Jr, Brandenburg RO, et al: Clinical follow-up study of paroxysmal supraventricular tachyarrhythmias after operative repair of a secundum type atrial septal defect in adults. Am J Cardiol 51:273, 1983.

229. Toscano-Barboza E, Brandenburg RO, Swan HJC: Atrial septal defect: the electrocardiogram and its hemodynamic correlation in 100 proved cases. Am J Cardiol 2:698, 1958.

230. Pryor R, Woodwork MB, Blount SG: Electrocardiographic changes in atrial septal defects: ostium secundum defect versus ostium primum (endocardial cushion) defect. Am Heart J 58:689, 1959.

231. Durrer D, Roos JP, Van Dam RI: The genesis of the electrocardiogram of patients with ostium primum defects (ventral atrial septal defects). Am Heart J 71:642, 1966.

232. Feldt RH, DuShane JW, Titus JL: The atrioventricular conduction system in persistent common atrioventricular canal defect: correlations with electrocardiogram. Circulation 42:437, 1970.

233. Davia JE, Cheitlin MD, Bedynek JL: Sinus venosus atrial septal defect: analysis of fifty cases. Am Heart J 85:177, 1973.

234. Heller J, Hagege AA, Besse B, et al: "Crochetage" (notch) on R wave in inferior limb leads: a new independent electrocardiographic sign of atrial septal defect. J Am Coll Cardiol 27:877, 1996.

235. Greenstein R, Naaz G, Armstrong WF: Usefulness of electrocardiographic abnormalities for detection of atrial septal defect in adults. Am J Cardiol 88:1054, 2001.

236. Papadopoulos C, Lee YC, Scherlis L: Isolated ventricular septal defect: electrocardiographic, vectorcardiographic, and catheterization data. Am J Cardiol 16:359, 1965.

237. Katz LN, Wachtel H: The diphasic QRS type of electrocardiogram in congenital heart disease. Am Heart J 13:202, 1937.

238. Brammell HL, Vogel JHK, Pryor R, et al: The Eisenmenger syndrome: a clinical and physiologic reappraisal. Am J Cardiol 28:679, 1972.

239. Burch GE, DePasquale N: The electrocardiogram, spatial vectorcardiogram and ventricular gradient in congenital ventricular septal defect. Am Heart J 60:195, 1960.

240. Blieden LC, Moller JH: Aorticopulmonary septal defect: an experience with 17 patients. Br Heart J 36:630, 1974.

241. Mirowski M, Arevalo F, Medrano GA, et al: Conduction disturbances in patent ductus arteriosus: a study of 200 cases before and after surgery with determination of P-R index. Circulation 25:807, 1962.

242. Sung C-S, Price EC, Cooley DA: Discrete subaortic stenosis in adults. Am J Cardiol 42:283, 1978.

243. Wood P: Disease of the Heart and Circulation, 3rd ed. Philadelphia, JB Lippincott, Philadelphia, 1968, p 379.

244. Liberthson RR, Pennington DG, Jacobs ML, et al: Coarctation of the aorta: review of 234 patients and clarification of management problems. Am J Cardiol 43:835, 1979.

245. Burch GE, DePasquale N: Electrocardiography in the Diagnosis of Congenital Heart Disease. Philadelphia, Lea & Febiger, 1967.

246. Scherlis L, Koenker RJ, Lee Y: Pulmonary stenosis: electrocardiographic, vectorcardiographic and catheterization data. Circulation 28:288, 1963.

247. Bentivoglio LG, Medrano GA, Munoz L, et al: The electrocardiogram in pulmonary stenosis with intact septa. Am Heart J 59:347, 1960.

248. Cayler GG, Ongley P, Nadas AS: Relation of systolic pressure in the right ventricle to the electrocardiogram. N Engl J Med 258:979, 1958.

249. Ellison RC, Miettinen OS: Interpretation of RSR1 in pulmonary stenosis. Am Heart J 88:7, 1974.

250. Bender SR, Dreifus LS, Downing D: Anatomic and electrocardiographic correlation in Fallot's tetralogy. Am J Cardiol 7:475, 1961.

251. Pileggi F, Bocanegra J, Tranchesi J, et al: The electrocardiogram in tetralogy of Fallot: a study of 142 cases. Am Heart J 59:667, 1960.

252. Higgins CB, Mulder DG: Tetralogy of Fallot. Am J Cardiol 29:837, 1972.

253. Okoroma EO, Guller B, Maloney JD, et al: Etiology of right bundle branch block pattern after surgical closure of ventricular septal defects. Am Heart J 90:14, 1975.

254. Downing JW, Kaplan S, Bove KE: Postsurgical left anterior hemiblock and right bundle branch block. Br Heart J 34:263, 1972.

255. Chandar JS, Wolff GS, Garson A, et al: Ventricular arrhythmias in postoperative tetralogy of Fallot. Am J Cardiol 65:655, 1990.

256. Book WM, Parks WJ, Hoplins K, et al: Electrocardiographic predictors of right ventricular volume measured by magnetic resonance imaging late after total repair of tetralogy of Fallot. Clin Cardiol 22:740, 1999.

257. Roos-Hesselink J, Perlroth MG, McGhie J, et al: Atrial arrhythmias in adults after repair of tetralogy of Fallot: correlations with clinical, exercise and echocardiographic findings. Circulation 91:2214, 1995.

258. Quattlebaum TG, Varghese J, Neill CA, et al: Sudden death among postoperative patients with tetralogy of Fallot: a follow-up study of 243 patients for an average of twelve years. Circulation 54:289, 1976.

259. Garson A, Porter CJ, Gillette PC, et al: Induction of ventricular tachycardia during electrophysiologic study after repair of tetralogy of Fallot. J Am Coll Cardiol 6:1493, 1983.

260. Hakanson JS, Moller JH: Significance of early transient complete heart block as a predictor of sudden death late after operative correction of tetralogy of Fallot. Am J Cardiol 87:1271, 2001.

261. Bialostozky D, Horwitz S, Espino-Vela J: Ebstein's malformation of the tricuspid valve. Am J Cardiol 29:826, 1972.

262. Genton E, Blount SG: The spectrum of Ebstein's anomaly. Am Heart J 73:395, 1967.

263. Kumar AE, Fyler DC, Miettinen OS, et al: Ebstein's anomaly: clinical profile and natural history. Am J Cardiol 28:84, 1971.

264. Lowe KG, Emslie-Smith D, Robertson PGC, et al: Scalar, vector, and intracardiac electrocardiogram in Ebstein's anomaly. Br Heart J 30:617, 1968.

265. Vacca JB, Bussmann DW, Mudd JG: Ebstein's anomaly: complete review of 108 cases. Am J Cardiol 2:210, 1958.

266. Sodi-Pallares D, Marsico F: The importance of electrocardiographic patterns in congenital heart disease. Am Heart J 49:202, 1955.

267. Sodi-Pallares D: New Bases of Electrocardiography. St Louis, Mosby, 1956, p 270.

268. Oh JK, Holmes DR Jr, Hayes DL, et al: Cardiac arrhythmias in patients with surgical repair of Ebstein's anomaly. J Am Coll Cardiol 6:1351, 1985.

269. Bharati S, Ciraulo DA, Bilitch M, et al: Inexcitable right ventricle and bilateral bundle branch block in Uhl's diseae. Circulation 57:636, 1978.

270. Patterson W, Baxley WA, Karp RB, et al: Tricuspid atresia in adults. Am J Cardiol 49:141, 1982.

271. Mair DD, Hagler DJ, Julsrud PR, et al: Early and late results of the modified Fontan procedure for double inlet left ventricle: the Mayo Clinic experience. J Am Coll Cardiol 18:1727, 1991.

272. Porter CJ, Garson A: Incidence and management of dysrhythmias after Fontan procedure. Herz 18:318, 1993.

273. Flinn CJ, Wolff GS, Dick MII, et al: Cardiac rhythm after the Mustard operation for complete transposition of the great arteries. N Engl J Med 310:1635, 1984.

274. Puley G, Siu S, Connelly M, et al: Arrhythmia and survival in patients >18 years of age after the Mustard procedure for complete transposition of the great arteries. Am J Cardiol 83:1080, 1999.

275. Daliento L, Corrado D, Buja G, et al: Rhythm and conduction disturbances in isolated, congenitally corrected transposition of the great arteries. Am J Cardiol 58:314, 1986.

276. Gillette PC, Busch U, Mullins CE, et al: Electrophysiologic studies in patients with ventricular inversion and "corrected transposition." Circulation 60:939, 1979.

277. Ruttenberg HD, Elliott LP, Anderson RC, et al: Congenital corrected transposition of the great vessels: correlation of electrocardiograms and vectorcardiograms with associated cardiac malformations and hemodynamic states. Am J Cardiol 17:339, 1966.

278. Friedberg DZ, Nadas AS: Clinical profile of patients with congenital corrected transposition of the great arteries. N Engl J Med 282:1053, 1970.

13 | Sinus Rhythms

The sinoatrial (SA) node is a small structure measuring about $5 \times 15 \times 1$ mm. Its task is to sort out various inputs regulating the heart rate, assume control of the heart rate, and suppress other automatic activity outside the SA node. The SA node is strategically located in the lateral part of the sulcus terminalis at the junction of the superior vena cava and the atrium. It is spindle shaped with a tail (cauda) running down the sulcus terminalis toward the orifice of the inferior vena cava. Usually, but not universally, a single SA node artery passes through the node, but in some cases there are multiple small arteries. The sinus node artery arises in 55 percent of individuals from the right coronary artery and in 45 percent from the left circumflex artery.[1]

The main cellular elements of the SA node are small, densely packed, round, pale cells with sparse myofibrils and rare gap junctions. The pacemaker (p) cells are arranged in elongated clusters and make contact with each other but not with the ordinary working myocardium. The latter communication is maintained via "transitional" cells, which form a narrow zone at the borders of the node, most abundantly in the crista terminalis. Numerous autonomic ganglia and nerves are in close proximity to the SA node. Pacemaker cells are sensitive to stretch, temperature, pressure, and various tactile, osmotic, and chemical stimuli. These properties enable them to serve as receptors for sensing time, pressure, volume, and chemical signals in the circulatory system.[2]

The SA node is located superficially just underneath the epicardium; therefore it can be readily damaged during cardiac surgery (e.g., cannulation of great veins) or during surgical correction of congenital anomalies (e.g., Mustard's procedure). The nodal cells are set in dense fibrous tissue. During normal aging the amount of fibrous tissue increases relative to the space occupied by the p cells.[3] At an advanced age the connective tissue tends to become predominant; and in extreme cases, contact is lost between the nodal cells and the atrial myocardium, a presumable substrate of the sick sinus syndrome and SA block. The sinus node electrogram recorded with transvenous electrodes shows two low-frequency, low-amplitude deflections that precede the P wave of the electrocardiogram (ECG).[4,5] Direct recording of sinus node potentials using the electrode catheter technique can be achieved in 50 to 86 percent of patients,[6] but obtaining stable recordings is often difficult. There is a wide range in SA intervals (30 to 150 ms), and the values overlap for patients with normal and abnormal SA node function.[6]

The P wave during sinus rhythm is always upright in leads I and II and inverted in lead aV_R; it is variable in leads III and aV_L. In the precordial leads the sinus P wave is upright in leads V_4–V_6 and is either upright, inverted, or most often biphasic (positive-negative) in leads V_1 and V_2. In sinus rhythm the morphology of the P wave in the same lead usually does not change from beat to beat, but minor variations in shape related to the respiratory cycles may be seen, especially in leads III and aV_F.

Initiation of the Sinus Impulse

High-resolution mapping in humans has shown that initiation of the sinus impulse is dynamic and can be multicentric, with more than one focus initiating a single impulse.[7] Shifts in the site of origin correlate with changes in rate and are consistent with minor P wave changes observed on the surface ECG.[7] The term "wandering atrial pacemaker" is used sometimes in the presence of varying P wave morphology. With rare exceptions, the assumed wandering of the pacemaker in the sinus node is seen only in the presence of sinus arrhythmia. At fast rates, the P wave in the inferior leads is taller and the PR interval is longer because the location of the pacemaker is higher. At slow rates the P wave in the inferior leads decreases in amplitude, and the PR becomes shorter as the pacemaker is shifted toward the tail of the sinus node. As long as the pacemaker is confined within the sinus node or its vicinity, the P waves remain upright in leads I, II, V_5, and V_6. This relationship between the location of the pacemaker and the morphology of the P waves was documented during electrophysiologic studies in which the sinus node electrograms were correlated with the body surface ECGs.[8,9] In everyday practice, however, it is difficult to determine whether the fluctuating P wave morphology is caused by the shift of the pacemaker within the sinus node, differences in the propagation of the impulse in the atria, or respiratory variations. For this reason the term "wandering pacemaker" is not useful.

Sinus Rate

It is well known that the sinus rate decreases with age, both at rest and during exercise. In adults, sinus bradycardia and sinus tachycardia cannot be defined precisely because the values depend not only on age and gender but also on many other variables, such as ambient temperature, altitude, and physical fitness. Most cardiologists agree that the operational limits for a normal sinus heart rate in adults range from 50 to 90 beats/min.[10]

Spodick et al.[11] tabulated data from 500 consecutive asymptomatic men and women, aged 50 to 80 years, and found that within the span of these 30 years the average heart rate declined in men from 75 to 69 beats/min but rose in women from 71 to 73 beats/min. In the same cohort the minimum rate in men ranged from 43 to 48 beats/min and in women from 47 to 54 beats/min. These low limits agree with earlier findings showing that in elderly men a heart rate of less than 50 beats/min does not indicate depressed cardiac performance.[12] In a more recent study,[13] a heart rate of less than 50 beats/min was present in 4 percent of subjects older than 40 years and did not signify chronotropic incompetence during exercise.

Sinus tachycardia is attributed to increased sympathetic activity and usually can be explained by the conditions resulting in increased sympathetic activity (e.g., fever, congestive heart failure, bleeding). There is also a nonreentrant type of automatic chronic nonparoxysmal sinus tachycardia that may occur in otherwise healthy persons. It is termed "inappropriate sinus tachycardia" (see later discussion).

Sinus Arrhythmias

Minor variation in the PP intervals is present in most subjects. The differences between the longest and shortest intervals, however, usually do not exceed 0.16 second except with sinus arrhythmia.

With sinus arrhythmias, the P wave morphology is normal but the PP interval varies by more than 0.16 second. There are two types of sinus arrhythmia. The more common type is respiratory sinus arrhythmia, in which the variation in heart rate is related to the respiratory cycle. The sinus rate increases gradually during inspiration and decreases with expiration. The variation is attributed to changes in vagal tone as a result of reflex mechanisms arising from the pulmonary and systemic vascular systems during respiration. The arrhythmia is a normal phenomenon that is usually prevalent in infants and children and tends to decrease with age (Figure 13–1, *top*).

The nonrespiratory sinus arrhythmia is more likely to be seen in elderly individuals in association with heart disease (Figure 13–1, *bottom*). In many instances the mechanism is unknown, but in some cases the sinus arrhythmia is a manifestation of sinus node dysfunction (e.g., after acute inferior infarction) or in patients with SA block. It is seen also in the presence of an increase in intracranial pressure.

As a rule, both types of sinus arrhythmia (respiratory and nonrespiratory) are seen more commonly when the sinus rate is slow. The rhythm tends to become regular when the rate is increased with exercise or atropine. Sinus arrhythmia is often simulated by premature sinus or atrial complexes, sinoatrial block, or sinus pauses.

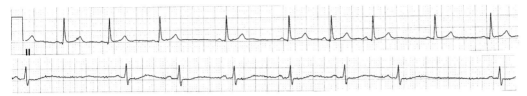

Figure 13–1 Electrocardiograpic lead II. *Top,* Physiologic respiratory arrhythmia in a 14-year-old girl. *Bottom,* Similar asymptomatic sinus arrhythmia in a 93-year-old woman is more likely to result from sinus node malfunction.

VENTRICULOPHASIC SINUS ARRHYTHMIA

Ventriculophasic sinus arrhythmia is seen in patients with partial or complete atrioventricular (AV) block. The PP interval containing the QRS complex is shorter than the PP interval not containing the QRS complex.[14,15] This phenomenon was observed in about 30 to 40 percent of cases with complete AV block and less often with second-degree AV block (Figure 13–2). Changes in intracardiac pressure and volume and in stroke volume are probably responsible for the reflex-mediated changes in the sinus cycle. Differences in perfusion of the sinus node may also play a role in this phenomenon.

SINUS BRADYCARDIA

Sinus bradycardia is usually not considered clinically significant unless the rate is less than 50 beats/min. Such a rate, however, is frequently seen in healthy adults, especially in athletes and regularly exercising subjects at all ages. A rate as slow as 35 beats/min or less may be seen, but in healthy individuals (Figure 13–3) the rate is usually more than 40 beats/min, especially during the waking hours. If the sinus rate is less than 40 beats/min, the possibility of SA block should be considered. During sleep the heart rate may be close to 35 beats/min in the absence of symptomatic bradycardia during waking hours. Many elderly individuals have sinus bradycardia without apparent cause.[12] Increased vagal tone is often responsible for sinus rate slowing. Transient sinus bradycardia occurs with the Valsalva maneuver, carotid sinus massage, or vomiting. Increased intracranial pressure may be accompanied by significant bradycardia. Other causes include hypothyroidism, hypothermia, hyperkalemia, Cheyne-Stokes respiration during the apneic phase (Figure 13–4), and some episodes of myocardial ischemia. Commonly used drugs that cause sinus bradycardia are β-adrenergic blockers, verapamil, diltiazem, digitalis, amiodarone, and clonidine.

In the presence of organic heart disease, sinus bradycardia is seen in 11 to 14 percent of patients with acute myocardial infarction (MI).[16] Its incidence is even higher during the early phase of inferior infarction.[18] Sinus bradycardia is also encountered in patients with ischemic and nonischemic cardiomyopathy and in patients with primary disease of the cardiac conduction system. Familial sinus bradycardia has been reportedly

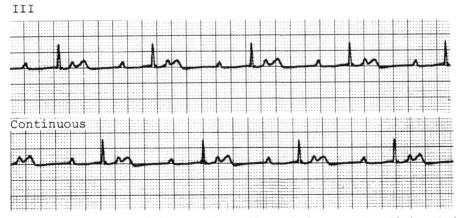

Figure 13–2 Ventriculophasic sinus arrhythmia in a 36-year-old man who has no symptoms. Rhythm strip shows a second-degree atrioventricular block with 2:1 conduction. PP intervals that contain the QRS complexes are shorter than those without the QRS complexes. No other evidence of heart disease was found.

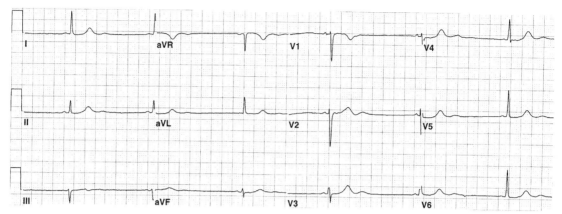

Figure 13–3   Asymptomatic sinus bradycardia (36 beats/min) in a 54-year-old woman who had no evidence of heart disease. Note the prominent U waves. QTc is 438 ms.

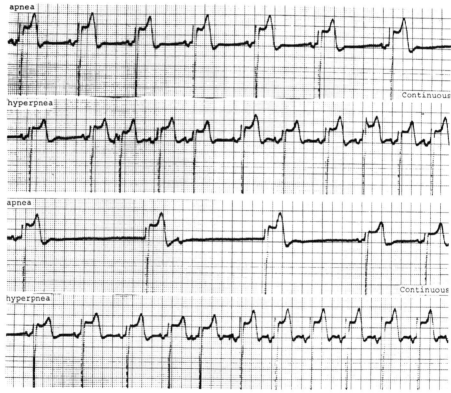

Figure 13–4   Bradycardia during the apneic phase of Cheyne-Stokes respiration in a 64-year-old man with chronic renal failure. Sinus bradycardia is present during apnea (first strip). In the third strip there is sinus arrest or sinoatrial block with junctional escape complexes.

caused by a mutation of the cardiac pacemaker channel.[17]

SINUS TACHYCARDIA

As a general guideline, the maximum heart rate is considered to be 220 beats/min minus years of age. This rate, however, is often exceeded during vigorous exercise or intense sympathetic stimulation. Therefore sinus tachycardia must often be included in the differential diagnosis of tachycardias of uncertain mechanism. The recognition of sinus tachycardia may become difficult when the P wave is superimposed on the preceding T wave. The differentiation of various narrow QRS tachycardias is discussed in Chapter 16.

During sinus tachycardia the T wave amplitude is often decreased (Figure 13–5), although it may be increased as a result of increased sympathetic stimulation (Figure 13–6). (Also see Chapter 10.) The PR interval is usually shortened but may be unchanged or prolonged. Junctional-type ST segment depression may be present, part of which is the result of an increased amplitude of the negative atrial T wave. A previously upright T wave may be flattened or even inverted. Conversely, a previously inverted T wave may become upright, presumably as a result of increased sympathetic stimulation. The QT interval is shortened, but most of the decrease of the RR interval is at the expense of the TP segment.

Sinus tachycardia occurs under a variety of circumstances. In healthy individuals it may be induced by exercise, anxiety, and other situations associated with increased sympathetic stimulation as well as by the use of alcohol, caffeine-containing beverages, and drugs such as β-adrenergic agonists and anticholinergic agents. Among disease states, the precipitating conditions include fever, hypotension, hypoxia, congestive heart failure, bleeding, anemia, hyperthyroidism, AV fistula, pheochromocytoma, and myocarditis. Sinus tachycardia is seen in about one third of patients with acute MI.[19]

INAPPROPRIATE SINUS TACHYCARDIA

"Inappropriate" sinus tachycardia, also known as *nonparoxysmal sinus tachycardia* or *permanent sinus tachycardia*, is characterized by an increased sinus rate at rest and exaggerated acceleration of the heart rate during physiologic

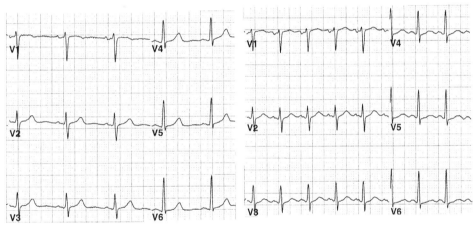

Figure 13–5   ECG precordial leads of a 43-year-old woman with nonangina-type chest pain. *Left,* Heart rate is 71 beats/min. *Right,* Heart rate is 124 beats/min. Note the decreased T wave amplitude in several leads during sinus tachycardia.

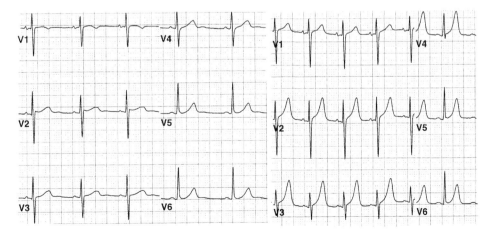

Figure 13–6   ECG precordial leads of a 30-year-old woman with nonangina-type chest pain. The two tracings were recorded on the same day. *Left,* Heart rate is 73 beats/min. *Right,* Heart rate is 100 beats/min. T wave amplitude is increased during sinus tachycardia.

stress. The P wave morphology suggests an origin in or close to the sinus node.[20,21] The mechanism leading to an exaggerated response of the sinus node to minimal physiologic stress is incompletely understood.[22] It has been shown that the usual negative chronotropic response to adenosine is impaired in these patients.[23] The condition is most common in young women, with a disproportionate number employed in the health care field.[24]

A study of six female patients by Morillo et al.[22] suggested that the mechanism is related to a primary sinus node abnormality characterized by a high intrinsic heart rate, depressed efferent cardiovagal reflex, and β-adrenergic hypersensitivity. Chronic sinus tachycardia at rest may result from an excessive resting sympathetic influence mediated through β-adrenergic receptors or from deficient resting vagal nerve influences. In most cases, β-adrenergic blockade slows the rate of tachycardia, but sometimes tachycardia is resistant to drug therapy. Sinus node modification using radiofrequency catheter ablation has been employed successfully to reduce the maximal heart rate significantly.[25,26]

The neuropathic postural tachycardia syndrome, also known as *chronic idiopathic orthostatic intolerance*, primarily affects young women. The symptoms include lightheadedness, dimming of vision, confusion, and anxiety, which are relieved by lying or sitting down. The remarkable increase in heart rate upon standing is not associated with a decrease in blood pressure. Patients with this syndrome frequently have high plasma catecholamine concentrations and evidence of sympathetic denervation of the legs.[27,28]

PREMATURE IMPULSES ORIGINATING IN THE SINUS NODE

"Sinus node extrasystoles" were described by Wenckebach in 1908.[2] Their presence is suspected when the contour of the premature P wave on the ECG is the same as during regular sinus rhythm, as well as when the postextrasystolic interval is equal to the sinus cycle (Figure 13–7). A slight difference in P wave contour and slight shortening of the postextrasystolic cycle may be present.[29] However, the similarity of morphology

between the premature and nonpremature P wave does not rule out the origin of the premature impulse in the atrium near the SA node. In some cases it can be shown that the premature sinus impulses are parasystolic in origin, and that the parasystolic focus is modulated in the same manner as other automatic foci (see Chapter 17).

POSTEXTRASYSTOLIC PAUSE

If the premature impulse reaches the sinus node and resets the sinus impulse formation, the postextrasystolic pause, although shorter than compensatory, is longer than the spontaneous cycle. The lengthening of the postextrasystolic pause, which tends to increase with increasing prematurity, can be attributed to several mechanisms: conduction time into and out of the SA node, decreased slope of diastolic depolarization, and shift to a site at which the intrinsic rate is slower.[30] The postextrasystolic pause can also be shorter than the spontaneous cycle, as with complete or incomplete interpolation or due to a pacemaker shift.[31]

SINUS NODE REENTRY AND REENTRANT TACHYCARDIA

Reentry within the SA node, resulting in single reciprocal echo complexes and reentrant reciprocating tachycardia, is more difficult to demonstrate than reentry within the AV node. Proof of the reentrant circuit by mapping was obtained first in the rabbit SA node by Allessie and Bonke.[32] Using a combination of 192 intracardiac electrodes to map the right atrium and several intracellular electrodes to explore the SA node, these investigators were able to record an echo complex and show that the reentrant circuit was located completely within the SA node, which means that the atrium was not an essential link in the reentrant circuit.

The suggested diagnostic criteria for sinus node reentry are as follows: (1) initiation of atrial echo complexes is independent of the atrial relative refractory period; (2) the echo

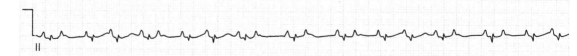

Figure 13–7 ECG strip of lead II in a 69-year old man with previous inferior myocardial infarction and premature complexes exhibiting the same P wave morphology as the sinus rhythm, and therefore suspected to be of sinus origin. The rhythm is, in part, bigeminal.

nterval should be shorter than the spontaneous cycle length; (3) the activation pattern of the echo complex is the same as that of the sinus complex; (4) reentry should be independent of the delay in the AV node; (5) tachycardia can be terminated by appropriately timed atrial premature stimulus or carotid massage; (6) reentry should be reproducible at different sites of atrial stimulation; (7) the entrance block into the sinus node should be excluded by demonstrating that the reentrant complex resets the sinus node; and (8) a right-sided accessory pathway that could mimic the sequence of activation of the atrial premature complex should be excluded.[33-35]

SA node reentry has been induced by programmed electrical stimulation in both healthy subjects and patients with SA node dysfunction. The incidence of inducibility varies from 4.0 percent[36] to 9.4 percent[37] and 11 percent.[38] SA node and AV node reentry can coexist,[39] probably coincidentally. In patients with sinus node reentry, there is usually no relation between the rate of induced sinus reentrant tachycardia and the spontaneous heart rate.[35] Episodes of sinus node reentry are usually brief, and symptoms

are mild or absent. Symptoms may be more serious when the rate is rapid.

Among 65 men undergoing electrophysiologic studies for symptomatic paroxysmal supraventricular tachycardia over a 4-year period, 11 had sustained sinus node reentrant tachycardia at cycle lengths ranging from 250 to 590 ms.[40] These tachycardias are frequently associated with organic heart disease but are not manifestations of SA node dysfunction. In the study of Gomes et al.,[40] 9 of 11 patients had coronary artery disease, and 5 of these patients had had a previous inferior MI. In general, sinus node reentrant tachycardia teminates spontaneously or abruptly during carotid sinus massage.[41] Criteria for differentiating sinus node reentrant tachycardia from inappropriate sinus tachycardia and atrial tachycardia are shown in Table 13–1.

In some individuals with sinus node reentry, spontaneous variations of cycle length are wider (e.g., 140 and 180 ms) than in those with other forms of supraventricular tachycardia.[40] The correct mechanism may remain undetected for long periods. The incidence of sinus node reentrant tachycardia was reported to range from as

TABLE 13–1	Criteria for Differentiating Sinus Node Reentrant Tachycardia from Other Tachycardias					
Tachycardia	P wave	Onset	Rate Stability	Termination	Induction	CSM
SNRe-T or SARe-T	Upright leads II, III, aV$_F$; similar to or identical to sinus P wave	Sudden, initiated by APDs	CL variation common	Abrupt	Easily inducible	Abrupt termination
Inappropriate sinus tachycardia	Same	Gradual	Warm-up effect	Gradual deceleration	Noninducible	Slowing, no termination
Atrial tachycardia	Usually inverted in leads II, III, aV$_F$, unless originating in the HRA; however, P wave morphology usually different from sinus	Sudden, initiated by APDs	Stable CL	Abrupt	Variable	Usually no effect

From Gomes A, Mehta D, Langan MN: Sinus node reentrant tachycardia. PACE 18(Part I):1045, 1995, by permission.
APD = atrial premature depolarization; CL = cycle length; CSM = carotid sinus massage; SARe-T = sinoatrial reentrant tachycardia; SNRe-T = sinus node reentrant tachycardia; HRA = high right atrium.

low as 1.8 percent in 379 patients with tachycardias referred for electrophysiologic studies[42] to 16.9 percent of symptomatic paroxysmal supraventricular tachycardias.[40] Figure 13–8 shows an assumed sinus node reentrant tachycardia that developed during exercise. Figure 13–9 shows the termination of an assumed sinus node reentrant tachycardia at the end of exercise in another patient.

SINUS PAUSE, SINUS ARREST

Sinus pause is the result of transient failure of impulse formation within the SA node or impulse propagation from the SA node. When the postulated sinus inactivity, manifested by absent P waves, is prolonged, the condition is called *sinus arrest*. No precise definition distinguishes these two entities.

Sinus pause should be differentiated from: (1) SA block; (2) marked sinus arrhythmia; (3) blocked premature atrial impulses; (4) single reciprocating ("echo") P waves; (5) suppression of sinus activity after conducted premature (usually atrial) complexes; and (6) overdrive suppression after ectopic tachycardia. With SA block the long cycle may be recognized as a multiple of the basic PP interval, but no such relation is demonstrable with sinus pause. With sinus arrhythmia, the lengthening of the PP interval is usually gradual and phasic. The blocked premature P waves and the retrogradely conducted "echo" P waves can be usually detected as distortions of the preceding T wave, at least in some leads. Suppression of sinus activity after a conducted premature complex is an uncommon phenomenon with a poorly understood mechanism; the resulting sinus pauses can be long, causing syncope (Figure 13–10). Overdrive suppression of sinus activity after a prolonged (usually supraventricular) tachycardia is a better understood phenomenon that can be demonstrated at the cellular level.[2] Depending on the duration of the pause, it may be terminated by an ectopic atrial, AV junctional, or ventricular escape complex. If the sinus arrest is prolonged, a slow AV junctional or ventricular escape rhythm may be present. Under such circumstances it is impossible to determine whether the underlying mechanism is sinus arrest or SA block. When the ventricular rhythm is regular and the P wave is absent, the possibility of sinoventricular conduction with atrial standstill and conduction through the internodal tract should be considered. This mechanism has been demonstrated during hyperkalemia (see Chapter 22).

Sinus pauses are occasionally seen in normal individuals with increased vagal tone or a hypersensitive carotid sinus.[43] In one case, a prolonged AV asystole was associated with hiccups.[44] Locatelli et al.[45] reported three cases of asystole and severe bradycardia as a manifestation of left temporal lobe complex partial seizure. Sinus pauses or arrest may be caused by digitalis and other drugs mentioned during the discussion of sinus bradycardia. Among patients with MI, sinus pauses or arrests are usually seen in those with infarction of the inferior wall.

SINOATRIAL BLOCK

Sinoatrial block may be caused by impaired automaticity, impaired conduction, or both.[46] These two mechanisms cannot be distinguished from each other without a direct recording of SA node activity. Figure 13–11 shows the assumed mechanisms for the various types of SA block. A first-degree SA block cannot be recognized on the surface ECG. Second-degree SA blocks are recognized frequently because of their effect on the atrial rhythm. Analogous to second-degree AV block, there are two types of second-degree SA block: type I (Wenckebach periodicity) and type II, manifested by dropped P waves during sinus rhythm (Figure 13–12). Type I block is clinically more prevalent than type II block. The former is suspected when there is a sequence of progressively shorter PP intervals followed by a longer PP interval that includes a blocked sinus impulse.[47] In the case of Wenckebach periodicity, in which only one impulse at the end of the period is blocked, the duration of the presumed sinus cycle can be calculated by dividing the total duration of the period by the number of visible cycles +1. The Wenckebach phenomenon was reported to occur in 17 percent of 219 SA blocks reviewed by Greenwood and Finkelstein.[48] Figure 13–13 shows the repetitive sequence of normal, delayed, and blocked SA conduction caused by 3:2 SA block and resulting in a bigeminal rhythm.

With type II block, the long cycle between the P waves is a multiple of the basic PP intervals. The duration of the long cycle may be the equivalent of two, three, or more beats. In some cases the duration of the long cycle is less than the exact multiple of the basic PP intervals. This is especially true in patients who have sinus arrhythmia. The precise limit of the differences is difficult to define, but an interval of 0.10 second was suggested by one author.[49]

SA block is often associated with escape rhythms from subsidiary foci. When the effective sinus rhythm is slightly slower than the AV junctional escape rhythm, a bigeminal rhythm known

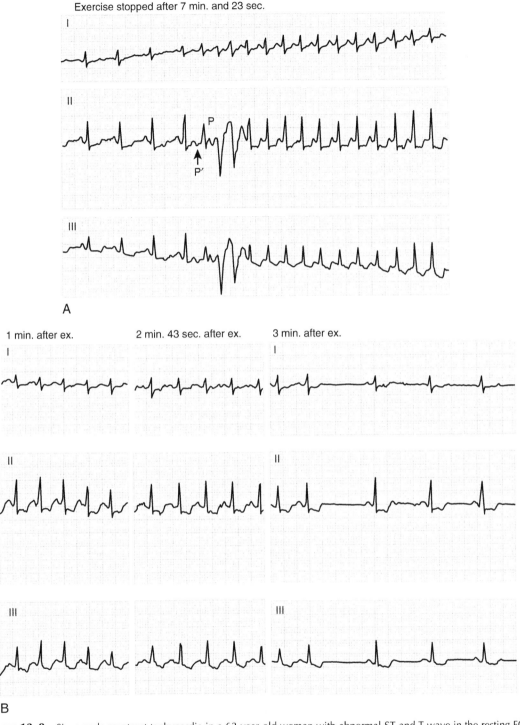

Figure 13–8 Sinus node reentrant tachycardia in a 62-year-old woman with abnormal ST and T wave in the resting ECG (not shown). **A,** Sinus node reentrant tachycardia immediately after the exercise was stopped. Tracing shows initiation of the tachycardia by a premature atrial beat (P′). The three wide QRS complexes are due to aberrant ventricular conduction. The heart rate is 210 beats/min at the beginning of the tachycardia and gradually decreases to 134 beats/min approximately 3 minutes after the exercise when the tachycardia terminates suddenly. **B,** Appearance of the P waves in the three simultaneously recorded leads during the tachycardia is identical to that during normal sinus rhythm. Radionuclide ventriculography revealed hypokinesis of the posterobasal wall of the left ventricle. The left ventricular ejection fraction was normal.

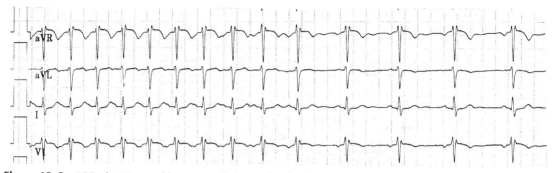

Figure 13–9 ECG of a 54-year-old man recorded immediately after completion of a treadmill exercise test. It shows no evidence of myocardial ischemia on the nuclear scan. A nearly abrupt termination of tachycardia with the same sinus P wave morphology suggests that tachycardia resulted from sinus node reentry.

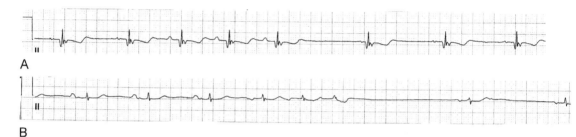

Figure 13–10 ECG lead II rhythm strips in two patients with sick sinus syndrome. **A,** This 71-year-old woman had presyncopal episodes. Note the three sinus complexes with upright P waves and a PR interval of 220 ms (third, fourth, and fifth complexes). The preceding complex and the three following complexes appear to be ectopic atrial or atrioventricular junctional escape complexes preceded by a low notched P wave. This pattern suggests high-degree sinus exit block. **B,** A 73-year-old woman with symptomatic bradycardia. The sinus P wave is wide and notched, which suggests an intraatrial conduction disturbance. After the first three sinus complexes (52 beats/min) there are three atrial premature complexes with a progressively increasing PR interval, followed by a 2.5-second pause and two atrial escape complexes. This is an example of marked suppression of sinus activity by premature atrial complexes.

as "escape capture bigeminy" can occur[3,50–52] (Figure 13–14). Monir et al.[51] analyzed mechanisms of escape capture bigeminy in 14 patients. In one case they identified SA entrance and exit block. Digitalis, β adrenergic–blocking, or calcium channel–blocking drugs were identified as culprits in eight instances.

SA block is often intermittent, as the patient may have normal sinus rhythm for days or weeks between episodes. Patients with SA block often have additional rhythm disturbances, including AV block and supraventricular tachycardias, an association called *tachycardia-bradycardia syndrome* (see later discussion). Before the established practice of digitalis blood level measurements, transient SA block was commonly seen as a manifestation of digitalis toxicity. Other conditions are administration of drugs causing bradycardia, acute MI, acute myocarditis, and increased vagal tone (e.g., carotid sinus stimulation). Chronic SA block is most commonly seen in elderly subjects with idiopathic degeneration of the SA node.

The technique of recording SA node electrograms disclosed the existence of diverse mechanisms of SA block, such as bidirectional SA entrance and exit block, unidirectional SA exit block, and the absence of a recordable SA node electrogram attributed to failure of the SA node impulse formation.[52] Histopathologic correlations have shown that: (1) the amount of nodal cells is inversely proportional to age; (2) a chronic SA block may be associated with extensive fibrosis of the SA node[53,54] or perinodal tissue[54,55]; (3) ischemia of the SA node is an infrequent cause of SA conduction disturbances, and obstructive disease of the SA node artery seldom results in sick sinus syndrome (SSS)[56]; and (4) the most common cause of SSS in children is probably an aftereffect of corrective surgery for congenital heart disease.[57]

Sick Sinus Syndrome

Two types of SSS are recognized: one with and one without associated tachyarrhythmia. The term *sick sinus syndrome* was used by Lown[58] to describe bradycardia and associated supraventricular

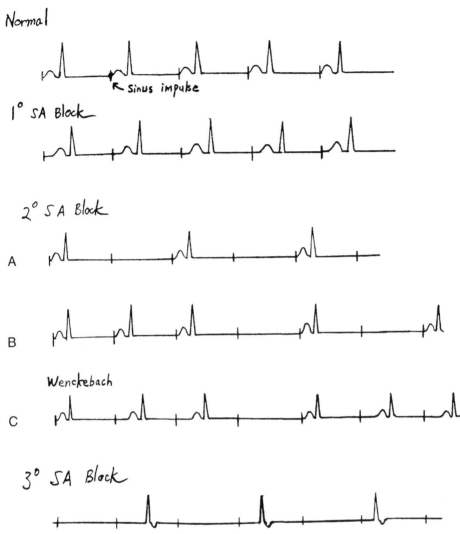

Figure 13–11   Normal sinus rhythms with various degrees of sinoatrial (SA) block. Sinus impulses not seen on the body surface ECG are represented by the vertical lines. With first-degree SA block, although there is prolongation of the interval between the sinus impulses and the P wave, such a delay cannot be detected on the ECG. The diagnosis of second-degree SA block depends on the presence of pause or pauses that are the multiple of the basic PP interval (**B**). Persistent 2:1 SA block cannot be distinguished from marked sinus bradycardia (**A**). A feature of the Wenckebach phenomenon is gradual shortening of the PP interval before the pause (**C**). With third-degree SA block, the ECG records only the escape rhythm.

arrhythmias following an electrical cardioversion of atrial fibrillation. Subsequently, Ferrer[59] applied this term to patients with the following manifestations: (1) persistent, severe, unexplained sinus bradycardia; (2) sinus arrest, brief or sustained, with an escape atrial or AV junctional rhythm (see Figure 13–10); (3) prolonged sinus arrest with failure of the subsidiary pacemaker, resulting in total cardiac asystole; (4) chronic atrial fibrillation with a slow ventricular response not due to drug therapy; and (5) an inability of the heart to resume sinus rhythm following electroconversion for atrial fibrillation.

Many patients with the syndrome have more than one of these mechanisms. In a series of 56 cases reported by Rubenstein et al.,[60] sinus bradycardia was seen in 39 percent, sinus arrest or SA block in 60 percent, and tachycardia-bradycardia syndrome (see later discussion) in 60 percent. Among the 46 patients with sinus bradycardia reported by Eraut and Shaw,[61] 35 also had sinus arrest or SA block and 76 percent had tachyarrhythmias. Sutton and Kenny[62] reviewed the literature on the natural history of SSS. Among the 1805 patients included in 37 studies, 300 (16.6 percent) patients also had AV block or bundle branch block at the initial

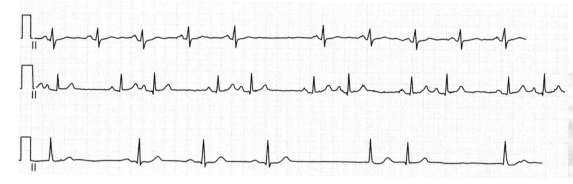

Figure 13–12   Three ECG strips of lead II from three different patients with different types of sinoatrial (SA) block. *Top strip:* Probable type 2 block manifested by a dropped P wave without change in rhythm. *Middle strip:* Type 1 SA block with 3:2 conduction and prolonged P-R in each second conducted sinus complex. *Lower strip:* Long periods of absent P waves (probably high-degree SA block) with junctional escape complexes. The first and the last junctional complexes conduct retrogradely to the atria, and there is probable AV nodal reentry after the second AV junctional escape complex.

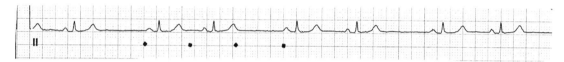

Figure 13–13   Calculation of the sinus rate is based on the assumption that the illustrated arrangement represents a 3:2 sinoatrial (SA) block, the sinus discharge is regular, the first sinus impulse after the pause coincides with the onset of the P wave, the second sinus impulse after the pause is conducted with a delay, and the third sinus discharge is blocked. The interval between the first two postpause complexes is 2200 ms. Assuming that this interval contains four regular sinus discharges, the sinus cycle length is 550 ms. Assumed times of sinus discharges are marked by dots.

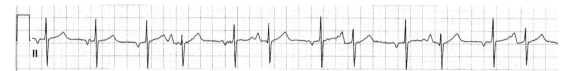

Figure 13–14   ECG lead II. Pattern represents a so-called sinus capture bigeminy in a 67-year-old man who had no evidence of heart disease. See text discussion.

diagnosis of SSS. Furthermore, AV block developed in 8.4 percent of the patients during the follow-up period of 34 months.

The causes of SSS may be summarized as follows[60–64]: (1) idiopathic; (2) ischemic heart disease; (3) primary nonischemic cardiomyopathy; (4) hypertensive heart disease; (5) secondary cardiomyopathy including those resulting from connective tissue disease, syphilis, metastatic tumor, amyloidosis, myxedema, hemochromatosis, Friedreich's ataxia, muscular dystrophy, and scleroderma; (6) mitral valve prolapse; (7) rheumatic heart disease; (8) acute myocarditis; (9) congenital heart disease; (10) familial sinus node disease; (11) surgical injury to the SA node, especially following repair of transposition of the great vessels[65]; and (12) after the Cox-Maze III procedure for management of chronic medically refractory atrial fibrillation.[65] In some reported series, patients without an apparent cause constitute the

largest group of cases[60,64] (Figure 13–15), whereas others found coronary artery disease in a large number of patients.[66,67]

Detailed pathologic studies of the SA node in patients with SSS have been carried out in a limited number of cases.[49,60,67] Degenerative changes of the SA node were found.[54,67] Engel et al.[56] suggested that SSS in patients with coronary artery disease is probably not related to involvement of the sinus node artery; however, in a postmortem angiographic study of 25 patients with SSS reported by Shaw et al.,[69] 5 had reduced filling of the sinus node artery.

TACHYCARDIA-BRADYCARDIA SYNDROME

The tachycardia-bradycardia syndrome has been observed in 54 to 76 percent of patients with SSS.[59,60,66] It is not a pure clinical or ECG entity

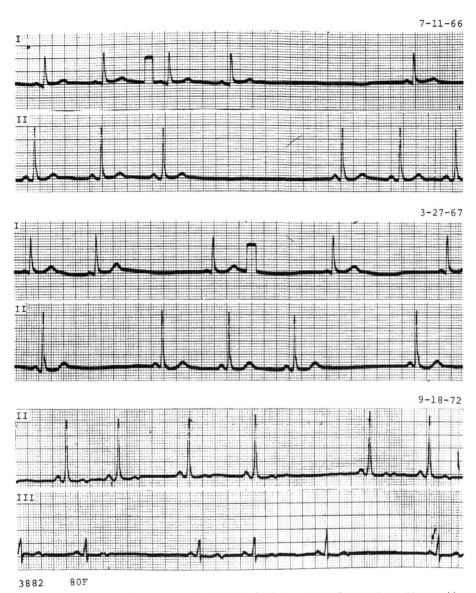

7-11-66

3-27-67

9-18-72

3882   80F

Figure 13–15   Intermittent second-degree sinoatrial (SA) block of many years' duration in an 80-year-old woman with heart disease of unknown cause. The diagnosis of second-degree SA block was first made in 1964. She has intermittent second-degree SA block with 4:1 or 2:1 conduction as illustrated. She remained symptom-free from the SA block in 1977.

but rather is a conglomerate of combinations of cardiac rhythm disturbances and their clinical manifestations.[70] The syndrome occurs in all age groups but is more common in the elderly. The etiology of arrhythmias responsible for the tachycardia-bradycardia syndrome is frequently obscured by difficulty distinguishing between conditions directly causing arrhythmias and those coexisting with them. Nevertheless, in many cases the cause and effect can be established. Thus certain MIs, usually those involving the inferior wall, are complicated by a combination of SA block and paroxysmal atrial fibrillation. Other conditions listed in various series include diseases of the mitral or aortic valve, hypertensive heart disease, cardiomyopathy, cardiac amyloidosis, diphtheria, hyperthyroidism, and digitalis toxicity.

The incidence of atrial fibrillation in 958 unpaced patients with SSS from 21 studies[62] was 8.2 percent. Moreover, during an average follow-up of 38 months, atrial fibrillation developed in 15.8 percent of patients.

Familial occurrence of the tachycardia-bradycardia syndrome has been reported. In one such family followed by Surawicz and Hariman,[71] a slow heart rate in several generations of family members was attributed to absent sinus node function. The inheritance was autosomal dominant. In these subjects, tachycardia was caused by a paroxysmal AV nodal reentry or, more often, by paroxysmal atrial fibrillation. The tachycardia-bradycardia syndrome can occur after surgical procedures, such as repair of complete transposition of the great vessels or other complex congenital anomalies. Postoperative tachycardia-bradycardia syndrome may also occur after repair of atrial septal defects. These arrhythmias have been attributed to injury of intranodal conducting pathways.

Possible mechanisms responsible for the tachycardia-bradycardia syndrome can be divided into the following categories: (1) tachycardia initiated by bradycardia; (2) bradycardia initiated by tachycardia; (3) bradycardia and tachycardia resulting from a common mechanism or a common cause; and (4) bradycardia and tachycardia coexisting through operation of unrelated mechanisms (Figure 13–16).

Bradycardia may initiate tachycardia by facilitating supraventricular reentrant tachycardia. This occurs when an AV junctional or atrial escape complex that follows a long sinus pause conducts retrogradely to the atria. If this retrograde conduction is sufficiently delayed, the impulse may return to the ventricles through another pathway and may initiate reciprocating AV nodal tachycardia (see Chapter 16).

Long pauses are commonly seen following the cessation of supraventricular tachycardia, atrial flutter, or atrial fibrillation. They may be due to depression of the sinus pacemaker and concomitant failure of the escape pacemakers. The latter may be caused by depressed automaticity, exit block, or a combination of the two. An interesting although relatively uncommon rhythm disturbance is tachycardia-dependent AV block associated with depression of the escape pacemakers.[72] This phenomenon has been attributed to the overdrive suppression of conduction.[73] A more common mechanism of bradycardia caused by tachycardia is the overdrive suppression of automaticity. Another mechanism of bradycardia initiated by tachycardia is an exit block that occurs during a normal or accelerated escape rhythm.[74] In some cases bradycardia is assumed to be caused by repetitive concealed conduction within the diseased conducting system (Figure 13–17).

Tachycardias and bradycardias with a common cause include arrhythmias induced by drugs, electrolyte imbalance, endocrine disorders, and perhaps vagal stimulation. Toxic doses of digitalis

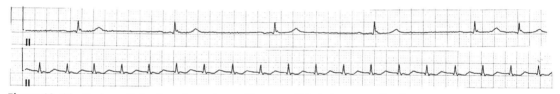

Figure 13–16   Tachycardia-bradycardia syndrome. These two ECG rhythm strips of lead II were recorded 1 day apart in an 81-year-old man who had normal ventricular function. *Top,* Sinus rhythm at a rate of 36 beats/min with a single premature atrioventricular (AV) junctional complex. The small, wide biphasic P wave suggests intraatrial conduction disturbance; QRS duration is 100 ms. *Bottom,* Supraventricular tachycardia of uncertain mechanism without recognizable P waves or flutter waves at a rate of 127 beats/min.

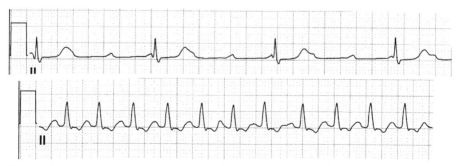

Figure 13–17   Tachycardia-bradycardia syndrome. ECGs from a 93-year-old woman recorded about 3 hours apart without intervening medication. *Top,* Sinus rhythm (128 beats/min), complete atrioventricular (AV) dissociation, and an escape rhythm with right bundle branch block morphology (39 beats/min). *Bottom,* Sinus tachycardia (140 beats/min) with a PR interval of 160 ms, left bundle branch block, and premature supraventricuar complexes (seventh and ninth complexes in the rhythm strip). The normal PR interval suggests that the AV dissociation in the upper strip was caused by a functional block distal to the AV node, perhaps as a result of repeated concealed conduction.

cause frequently alternating bradycardia and tachycardia because digitalis impairs SA and AV conduction and enhances automaticity of ectopic pacemakers. The mere presence of atrial premature complexes can induce the tachycardia-bradycardia syndrome. Tachycardias occur when premature complexes induce atrial flutter or fibrillation, whereas bradycardia appears when premature complexes are blocked or are followed by depression of the sinus pacemaker. In an unusual variant of the tachycardia-bradycardia syndrome, tachycardia was caused by rapid antidromic impulse conduction through an accessory pathway and bradycardia by a high-degree AV block during sinus rhythm.[75]

Detection of Sinus Node Dysfunction

Ambulatory ECG monitoring, particularly event monitoring, is one of the most useful tools for evaluating patients suspected of having SSS. Although sinus pauses longer than 2 to 3 seconds on the ambulatory ECG are generally considered to suggest sinus node dysfunction, they are seen in healthy individuals, especially during sleeping hours. Clinically significant SA node disease can be definitively diagnosed only if the rhythm disturbance is observed at the time of symptom occurrence. In the electrophysiology laboratory, intravenous administration of atropine and measurements of SA conduction time and sinus node recovery time have been used to detect sinus node dysfunction.

SA CONDUCTION TIME

An interval believed to represent the SA conduction time (SACT) has been determined by the method of premature atrial stimulation[76] or by constant atrial pacing.[77] Both techniques measure the reset sinus return cycle and interpret this interval as the sum of the spontaneous cycle, the anterograde conduction time into the SA node, and the retrograde conduction time from the SA node. Thus the difference between the return cycle and the spontaneous cycle represents the sum of the anterograde and retrograde conduction times. Assuming that these two conduction times are equal, the SACT is obtained by dividing the combined time by 2. The validity of this measurement rests on a variety of assumptions: (1) that the paced premature impulses or runs do not change the sinus rate; (2) that the SA node pacemaker does not shift; and (3) that

the conduction times into and out of the SA node are indeed equal.

Judging by the number of factors that can affect the duration of the return cycle, there is little certainty that the interval believed to be the SACT is an exact measure of this process. Reiffel et al.[78] have shown that the SACT varies predictably inversely with the duration of the sinus cycle; that is, the SACT decreases when the cycle length increases, an effect explained by refractoriness. However, potential errors caused by electrotonic interaction among the SA node and the atrial impulse and shifts of the pacemaker sites are more difficult to detect. Thus it is not surprising that the calculated SACT values in subjects without apparent sinus node disease have varied considerably among studies, ranging from 40 to 153 ms[35] and 46 to 116 ms[5] to 108 to 272 ms.[79] These values may not represent the pure SACT because when SA node electrograms were recorded intraoperatively,[80] SACT measured directly was 30 to 40 ms at cycle lengths of about 600 to 700 ms.

SINUS NODE RECOVERY TIME

The sinus node recovery time (SNRT) tests the integrity of the automaticity of the SA node following an attempted overdrive by rapid pacing. The test is based on the assumption that automaticity suppressed by overdrive recovers less rapidly when the SA node is diseased than when it is functioning normally. Hence the postpacing pause, which is the time interval between the last paced atrial beat and the subsequent sinus escape beat, is measured. Because the postpacing interval is influenced by the prepacing rate, the SNRT must be corrected for the sinus rate. The rate-corrected SNRT is obtained by subtracting the duration of the sinus cycle from the duration of the postpacing interval.[81,82] The results are also influenced by the rate and duration of pacing,[81,83] which makes it difficult to define normal values. In one study[84] the ratio of the uncorrected SNRT to the basic cycle length in patients with documented SSS ranged from 1.38 to 4.86.

The intrinsic heart rate and the intrinsic corrected SNRT can be obtained by eliminating the effects of the autonomic nervous input. This is measured following β-adrenergic blockade and administration of atropine.[85] The clinical usefulness of this test has been disputed. It has been reported that the intrinsic SNRT lengthens with increasing age, whereas the basic SNRT is not affected by age.[86]

The sensitivity of the corrected SNRT and SACT for detecting sinus node dysfunction is 54 percent and 51 percent, respectively. Assessment of SNRT after pharmacologic blockade of the autonomic nervous system using atropine and propranolol increases the sensitivity of the method in patients with suspected sinus node dysfunction and normal baseline results.[87] In a consensus statement on the state of the art of electrophysiologic testing,[88] the sensitivity of combined SACT and SNRT in patients with symptomatic sinus node disease was estimated to be about 68 percent and the specificity 88 percent.

SINUS NODE DURING ATRIAL FIBRILLATION

Clinical observations suggest that spontaneous pharmacologically or electrically induced termination of atrial fibrillation is usually followed by a prompt resumption of sinus rhythm. This suggests the absence of appreciable overdrive suppression of the SA node by rapid atrial discharges. A study of Kirchhof and Allesssie[89,90] addressed this problem by studying transmembrane action potentials in isolated perfused rabbit hearts during induced atrial fibrillation. These investigators found that the SA node was protected by a high-degree (about 5:1) entrance block. Therefore pacemakers in the center of the SA node were activated at a rate that was only slightly higher than the average rate during sinus rhythm, a phenomenon designated "concealed automaticity."

In contrast to the protected center of the node, the SA border was activated at a rapid rate with an exit block that dissipated upon termination of the atrial fibrillation. The sinus rhythm resumed promptly without evidence of overdrive suppression. In human subjects, Gomes et al.[91] recorded regular SA node electrograms with extracellular electrodes during atrial fibrillation, which was taken as evidence of SA node entrance block.[2]

CHRONOTROPIC INCOMPETENCE

Chronotropic incompetence is an attenuated heart rate response to exercise that has been shown to be independently predictive of mortality and coronary heart disease risk in healthy populations even after adjusting for age, physical fitness, standard cardiovascular risk factors, and ST segment changes with exercise.[92,93] It has been assessed in three ways: (1) failure to achieve 85 percent of the age-predicted maximum heart rate; (2) measurement of the actual increase in rate from rest to exercise; and (3) a low chronotropic index, a heart rate response measure that accounts for effects of age, resting heart rate, and physical fitness.[94,95]

Heart Rate Variability

"Heart rate variability" has become the conventionally accepted term to describe variations of both instantaneous heart rate and RR intervals.[96] The development of computer-based methods to analyze heart rate variability has provided an opportunity to assess the prognostic significance of the fluctuating activity of the cardiac autonomic system in healthy individuals and in patients with various cardiovascular and noncardiovascular disorders. Among the many methods to evaluate heart rate variability, the simplest to perform are the time domain measures. Generally, three main components can be detected: (1) a high-frequency component (around 0.25 Hz) related to respiratory activity; (2) a low-frequency component with a peak frequency around 0.1 Hz; and (3) a very-low-frequency component at around or below frequencies of 0.03 to 0.05 Hz.[97] For information about the methodology and clinical significance, the reader is referred to the report of a special task force.[96]

Heart Rate Turbulence

See Chapter 17.

REFERENCES

1. James TN: Anatomy of the coronary arteries in health and disease. Circulation 32:1020, 1965.
2. Surawicz B: Electrophysiologic Basis of ECG and Arrhythmias. Baltimore, Williams & Wilkins, 1995, pp 268–279.
3. Pick A, Langendorf R: Interpretation of Complex Arrhythmias. Philadelphia, Lea & Febiger, 1979.
4. Hariman RJ, Krongrad E, Boxer R, et al: Method for recording electrical activity of the sinoatrial node and automatic atrial foci during cardiac catheterization in human subjects. Am J Cardiol 45:775, 1980.
5. Reifel JA, Gang E, Gliklich J, et al: The human sinus node electrogram: a transvenous catheter technique and a comparison of directly measured and indirectly estimated sinoatrial conduction time in adults. Circulation 62:1324, 1980.
6. Levy S, Lekieffre J: Direct recording of sinus node potentials using electrode catheter techniques. Clin Cardiol 17:203, 1994.
7. Schuessler RB, Boineau JP, Bromberg BI: Origin of the sinus impulse. J Cardiovasc Electrophysiol 7:263, 1996.
8. Boineau JP, Canavan TE, Schuessler RB, et al: Demonstration of a widely disturbed atrial complex in the human heart. Circulation 77:1221, 1988.

9. Gomes JA, Winter SL: The origin of the sinus complex in man: demonstration of dominant and subsidiary foci. J Am Coll Cardiol 9:45, 1987.

10. Spodick DH: Survey of selected cardiologists for an operational definition of normal sinus heart rate. Am J Cardiol 72:487, 1993.

11. Spodick DH, Raju P, Bishop RL, et al: Operational definition of normal sinus heart rate. Am J Cardiol 69:1245, 1992.

12. Agruss NS, Rosin EY, Adolph RJ, et al: Significance of chronic sinus bradycardia in elderly people. Circulation 66:924, 1972.

13. Tresch DD, Fleg JL: Unexplained sinus bradycardia: clinical significance and long-term prognosis in apparently healthy persons older than 40 years. Am J Cardiol 58:1009, 1986.

14. Rosenbaum MB, Lepeschkin E: The effect of ventricular systole on auricular rhythm in auriculoventricular block. Circulation 43:836, 1971.

15. Schamroth L: Ventriculophasic atrial extrasystoles associated with complete atrioventricular block. Am J Cardiol 21:593, 1968.

16. Meltzer LE, Kitchell JB: The incidence of arrhythmias associated with acute myocardial infarction. Prog Cardiovasc Dis 9:50, 1966.

17. Milanesi R, Baruscotti M, Gnocchi-Ruscone Y, et al: Familial sinus bradycardia associated with a mutation in the cardiac pacemaker channel. N Engl J Med 354:151, 2006.

18. Adgey AAJ, Geddes JS, Webb SW, et al: Acute phase of myocardial infarction. Lancet 2:501, 1971.

19. DeSanctis RW, Block P, Hutter AM: Tachyarrhythmias in myocardial infarction. Circulation 45:681, 1972.

20. Bauernfeind RA, Amat-y-Leon F, Dhingra RC, et al: Chronic nonparoxysmal sinus tachycardia in otherwise healthy persons. Ann Intern Med 91:702, 1979.

21. Yee R, Guiraudon GM, Gardner MJ, et al: Refractory paroxysmal sinus tachycardia: management by subtotal right atrial excision. J Am Coll Cardiol 3:400, 1984.

22. Morillo CA, Klein GJ, Thakur RK, et al: Mechanism of "inappropriate" sinus tachycardia. Circulation 90:873, 1994.

23. Still A-M, Hikuri HV, Airaksinen KEJ, et al: Impaired negative chronotropic response to adenosine in patients with inappropriate sinus tachycardia. J Cardiovasc Electrophysiol 13:557, 2002.

24. Krahn AD, Yee R, Klein GJ, et al: Inappropriate sinus tachycardia: evaluation and therapy. J Cardiovasc Electrophysiol 6:1124, 1995.

25. Lee RJ, Kalman JM, Fitzpatrick AP, et al: Radiofrequency catheter modification of the sinus node for "inappropriate" sinus tachycardia. Circulation 92:2919, 1995.

26. Marrouche NF, Beheiry S, Tomassoni G, et al. Three-dimensional nonfluoroscoping mapping and ablation of inappropriate sinus tachycardia. J Am Coll Cardiol 39:1046, 2002.

27. Low PA, Opfer-Gehrking TL, Textor SC, et al: Postural tachycardia syndrome (POTS). Neurology 45(Suppl 5):519, 1995.

28. Jacob G, Costa F, Shannon JR, et al: The neuropathic postural tachycardia syndrome. N Engl J Med 343:1008, 2000.

29. Langendorf R, Mintz S: Premature systoles originating in the sinoauricular node. Br Heart J 8:178, 1946.

30. Bonke FI, Bouman LN, van Rijn HE: Change of cardiac rhythm in the rabbit after an atrial premature beat. Circ Res 24:533, 1968.

31. Steinbeck G, Luderitz B: Sinoatrial pacemaker shift following atrial stimulation in man. Circulation 56:402, 1977.

32. Allessie MA, Bonke FI: Direct demonstration of sinus node reentry in the rabbit heart. Circ Res 44:557, 1979.

33. Narula OS: Sinus node reentry: a mechanism for supraventricular tachycardia. Circulation 50:1114, 1974.

34. Wu D, Amat-y-Leon F, Denes P, et al: Demonstration of sustained sinus and atrial reentry as a mechanism of paroxysmal supraventricular tachycardia. Circulation 51:234, 1975.

35. Breithardt G, Seipel L: Role of sinus node reentry in the genesis of supraventricular arrhythmias. In: Masoni A, Alboni P (eds): Cardiac Electrophysiology Today. London, Academic, 1982.

36. Josephson ME, Seides SF: Clinical Cardiac Electrophysiology: Techniques and Interpretations. Philadelphia, Lea & Febiger, 1979.

37. Wellens HJ: Role of sinus node reentry in the genesis of sustained cardiac arrhythmias. In: Bonke FI (ed): The Sinus Node: Structure, Function and Clinical Relevance. The Hague, Martinus Nijhoff, 1978.

38. Dhingra RC, Wyndham C, Amat-y-Leon F, et al: Sinus nodal responses to atrial extrastimuli in patients without apparent sinus node disease. Am J Cardiol 36:445, 1975.

39. Paulay KL, Ruskin JN, Damato AN: Sinus and atrioventricular nodal reentrant tachycardia in the same patient. Am J Cardiol 36:810, 1975.

40. Gomes JA, Hariman RJ, Kang PS, et al: Sustained symptomatic sinus node reentrant tachycardia: incidence, clinical significance, electrophysiologic observations and the effects of antiarrhythmic agents. J Am Coll Cardiol 5:45, 1985.

41. Gomes JA, Mehta DA, Langan MN: Sinus node reentrant tachycardia. PACE 18(Part I):1045, 1995.

42. Wellens HJJ: Role of sinus node re-entry in the genesis of sustained cardiac arrhythmias. In: Bonke FI (ed): The Sinus Node: Structure Function and Clinical Relevance. The Hague, Martinus Nijhoff, 1978, pp 422–427.

43. Gang ES, Oseran DS, Mandel WJ, et al: Sinus node electrogram in patients with the hypersensitive carotid sinus syndrome. J Am Coll Cardiol 5:1484, 1985.

44. Malhotra S, Schwartz MJ: Atrioventricular asystole as a manifestation of hiccups. J Electrocardiol 28:59, 1995.

45. Locatelli ER, Varghese JP, Shuaib A, et al: Cardiac asystole and bradycardia as a manifestation of left temporal lobe complex partial seizure. Ann Intern Med 130:581, 1999.

46. Bigger JT, Reiffel JA: Sick sinus syndrome. Annu Rev Med 30:91, 1979.

47. Schamroth L, Dove E: The Wenckebach phenomenon in sinoatrial block. Br Heart J 28:350, 1966.

48. Greenwood RJ, Finkelstein D: Sinoatrial Heart Block. Springfield, IL, Charles C Thomas, 1964.

49. Rasmussen K: Chronic sinoatrial heart block. Am Heart J 81:38, 1971.

50. Bradley SM, Marriott HJL: Escape-capture bigeminy: report of a case of A-V dissociation initiated by 2:1 S-A block with resulting bigeminal rhythm. Am J Cardiol 1:640, 1958.

51. Monir G, Dreifus LS, Gursoy AS, et al: Escape capture bigeminy. A manifestation of sinoatrial conduction block. J Electrocardol 32:51, 1999.

52. Wu D, Yeh S-J, Lin F-C, et al: Sinus automaticity and sinoatrial conduction in severe symptomatic sick sinus syndrome. J Am Coll Cardiol 19:355, 1992.

53. Thery C, Gosselin B, Lekieffre J, et al: Pathology of sinoatrial node: correlations with electrocardiographic findings. Am Heart J 93:735, 1977.

54. Demoulin JC, Kulbertus HE: Histopathological correlates of sinoatrial disease. Br Heart J 60:1384, 1978.

55. Bharati S, Nordenberg A, Bauernfeind R, et al: The anatomic substrate for the sick sinus syndrome in adolescence. Am J Cardiol 46:163, 1980.

56. Engel TR, Meister SG, Feitosa GS, et al: Appraisal of
sinus node artery disease. Circulation 52:286, 1975.

57. Greenwood RD, Rosenthal A, Sloss LJ, et al: Sick sinus
syndrome after surgery for congenital heart disease.
Circulation 52:208, 1975.

58. Lown B: Electrical reversion of cardiac arrhythmias.
Br Heart J 29:469, 1967.

59. Ferrer MI: The sick sinus syndrome in atrial disease.
JAMA 206:645, 1968.

60. Rubenstein JJ, Shulman CL, Yurchak PM, et al: Clinical
spectrum of the sick sinus syndrome. Circulation 46:5,
1972.

61. Eraut D, Shaw DB: Sinus bradycardia. Br Heart J 33:742,
1971.

62. Sutton R, Kenny RA: The natural history of sick sinus
syndrome. PACE 9:1110, 1986.

63. Ferrer MI: The Sick Sinus Syndrome. Mt Kisco, NY,
Futura, 1974.

64. Fowler NO, Fenton JC, Conway GF: Syncope and cerebral dysfunction caused by bradycardia without atrioventricular block. Am Heart J 80:303, 1970.

65. Hayes CJ, Gersony WM: Arrhythmias after the Mustard
operation for the transposition of the great arteries: a
long term study. J Am Coll Cardiol 71:33, 1986.

66. Pasic M, Musci M, Siniawski H, et al: Transient sinus
node dysfunction after the Cox-Maze III procedure in
patients with organic heart disease and chronic fixed
atrial fibrillation. J Am Coll Cardiol 32:10, 1989.

67. Kaplan BM, Langendorf R, Lev M, et al: Tachycardia-
bradycardia syndrome (so-called "sick sinus syndrome").
Am J Cardiol 34:363, 1974.

68. Moss AJ, Davis RJ: Brady-tachy syndrome. Prog Cardiovasc Dis 16:439, 1974.

69. Shaw DB, Linker NJ, Heaver PA, et al: Chronic sinoatrial
disorder (sick sinus syndrome): a possible result of
cardiac ischemia. Br Heart J 58:598, 1987.

70. Surawicz B, Reddy CP: Tachycardia-bradycardia syndrome. In: Surawicz B, Reddy CP, Prystowsky EN (eds):
Tachycardias. Boston, Martinus Nijhoff, 1984.

71. Surawicz B, Hariman RS: Follow-up of the family with
congenital absence of sinus rhythm. Am J Cardiol
61:487, 1988.

72. Aravindakshan V, Surawicz B, Daoud FS: Depression of
escape pacemakers associated with rapid supraventricular rate in patients with atrioventricular block. Circulation 50:255, 1974.

73. Takahashi N, Gilmour RF Jr, Zipes DP: Overdrive suppression of conduction in the canine His-Purkinje system after occlusion of the anterior septal artery.
Circulation 70:495, 1984.

74. Wellens HJ, Wesdorp JC, Dueren DR, et al: Second
degree block during reciprocal atrioventricular nodal
tachycardia. Circulation 53:595, 1976.

75. Castellanos A, Agha AS, Mendoza LJ, et al: Intermittent
AV conduction disturbances in patients with AV nodal
bypass tracts. Br Heart J 39:1, 1977.

76. Strauss HC, Saroff AL, Bigger JT, et al: Premature atrial
stimulation as a key to the understanding of sinoatrial
conduction in man. Circulation 67:86, 1973.

77. Narula OS, Shantha N, Vasquez M, et al: A new method
for measurement of sinoatrial conduction time. Circulation 58:706, 1978.

78. Reiffel JA, Bigger JT, Konstam MA: The relationship
between sinoatrial conduction time and sinus cycle

length during spontaneous sinus arrhythmia in adults.
Circulation 50:924, 1974.

79. Kirkorian G, Touboul P, Attalah G, et al: Premature atrial
stimulation during regular atrial pacing: a new approach
to the study of the sinus node. Am J Cardiol 54:109,
1984.

80. Hariman RJ, Krongrad E, Boxer R, et al: Methods for
recording electrograms of the sinoatrial node during cardiac surgery in man. Circulation 61:1024, 1980.

81. Mandel W, Hayakawa H, Danzig R, et al: Evaluation of
sinoatrial node function in man by overdrive suppression. Circulation 44:59, 1971.

82. Narula OS, Samet P, Javier RP: Significance of the sinus-
node recovery time. Circulation 45:140, 1972.

83. Kulbertus HE, de Leval-Rutten F, Mary L, et al: Sinus
node recovery time in the elderly. Br Heart J 37:420,
1975.

84. Gann D, Tolentino A, Samet P: Electrophysiologic evaluation of elderly patients with sinus bradycardia. Ann
Intern Med 90:24, 1979.

85. Jordan JL, Yamaguchi I, Mandel WJ: Studies on the
mechanism of sinus node dysfunction in the sick sinus
syndrome. Circulation 57:217, 1978.

86. Kuga K, Yamaguchi I, Sugishita Y, et al: Assessment by
autonomic blockade of age-related changes of the sinus
node function and autonomic regulation in sick sinus
syndrome. Am J Cardiol 61:361, 1988.

87. Bergfeldt L, Vallin H, Rosenqvist M, et al: Sinus node
recovery time assessment revisited: role of pharmacologic blockade of the autonomic nervous system. J Cardiovasc Electrophysiol 7:95, 1996.

88. McGuire MA, Johnson DC, Nunn GR, et al: Surgical
therapy for atrial tachycardia in adults. J Am Coll Cardiol 14:1777, 1989.

89. Kirchhof CJ, Allessie MA: Sinus node automaticity during atrial fibrillation in isolated rabbit hearts. Circulation
86:263, 1992.

90. Kirchhof CJ: The sinus node and atrial fibrillation. Doc-
toral thesis, Datawyse Maastricht, 1989.

91. Gomes JA, Kang PS, Matheson M, et al: Coexistence of
sick sinus rhythm and atrial flutter-fibrillation. Circulation 63:80, 1981.

92. Ellestad MH: Chronotropic incompetence: the implications of heart rate response to exercise (compensatory
parasympathetic hyperactivity?). Circulation 93:1485,
1996.

93. Lauer MS, Mehta R, Pashkow FJ, et al: Association of
chronotropic incompetence with echocardiographic
ischemia and prognosis. J Am Coll Cardiol 32:1280,
1998.

94. Lauer MS, Okin PM, Larson MG, et al: Impaired heart
rate response to graded exercise: prognostic implications
of chronotropic incompetence in the Framingham study.
Circulation 93:1520, 1996.

95. Lauer MF, Francis GS, Okin PM, et al: Impaired chronotropic response to exercise stress testing as a predictor of
mortality. JAMA 281:524, 1999.

96. Task Force of the European Society of Cardiology and
the North American Society of Pacing and Electrophysiology: Heart rate variability: standards of measurement,
physiological interpretation and clinical use. Circulation
93:1043, 1996.

97. Hedman A, Hartikainen J, Hakumaki M: Physiological
background underlying short-term heart rate variability.
J Autonom Nerv Syst 3:267, 1998.

14 | Atrial Rhythms

The existence of pacemaker fibers in the atria outside the sinoatrial (SA) node helps explain ectopic atrial impulses, whereas the existence of specialized continuous internodal pathways helps explain the phenomenon of sinoventricular conduction in the presence of SA block during hyperkalemia. The presence of continuous anatomic pathways, however, has not been universally accepted. No insulated tracts such as bundle branches have been found in the atrial myocardium, although cells with characteristics of conduction system cells appear to exist. The interatrial tract (Bachman bundle) is a structure connecting the two atria ventrally. In the dog it contains rapidly conducting specialized fibers that enable rapid impulse propagation between the atria. The possible role of this pathway in clinical electrocardiography or atrial arrhythmias is not known.[1]

Premature Atrial Impulses: Atrial Extrasystoles, Premature Atrial Depolarizations

Premature atrial complexes originate from ectopic complexes in the atria. The P wave morphology differs from that of the sinus P wave, although the differences may be slight (Figure 14–1). The prematurity of the ectopic atrial complex varies. It may be early, superimposed on the ventricular complex of the preceding sinus impulse; or it may be late, occurring just before the next sinus impulse. In the latter instance, an atrial fusion complex may result if part of the atrial activation originates from the ectopic focus and part from the sinus node. Such a fusion complex has an intermediate morphology, between that of the sinus and the ectopic complex (see Figure 14–1). The premature atrial complexes, either unifocal or multifocal, may appear at random intervals or after one, two, or three sinus complexes, resulting in a bigeminal, trigeminal, or quadrigeminal rhythm (Figure 14–2). They may occur in pairs (see Figure 14–2). In some cases repetitive atrial premature complexes are caused by reciprocation (Figure 14–3, bottom strip).

The site of the ectopic focus can be established accurately using a large array of intracardiac and surface electrodes. On the surface electrocardiogram (ECG), however, analysis of P wave morphology is less helpful for defining the source of ectopic activity. This is because foci located at divergent sites can produce similar P wave patterns,[2,3] and different P wave patterns can be caused by impulses originating at the same site owing to differences in intraatrial or interatrial conduction. Notwithstanding these limitations, certain correlations have been established. If the focus is near the sinus node, the premature P wave simulates the sinus P wave closely. If the focus is in the vicinity of the atrioventricular (AV) junction, the premature ectopic P wave is inverted in the inferior leads. Such a P wave differs from the premature AV junctional complex in that the PR interval is usually 0.12 second or longer. Clinical correlations suggest that a negative P wave in lead I usually indicates a left atrial focus[4,5]

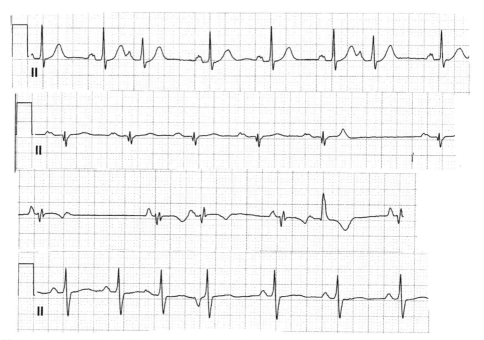

Figure 14–1 Strips of ECG lead II. *Top row,* Premature atrial complexes with a slightly longer PR interval than that in the sinus complexes are conducted with slight aberration. *Second row,* Early blocked premature atrial complex recognizable by the altered shape of the T wave. *Third row,* Three premature atrial complexes. The first is blocked; the second is normally conducted; and the third, being more premature, is conducted with aberration. *Fourth row,* Two atrial premature complexes in a row. The first is a fusion P wave between the positive sinus P wave and the negative atrial ectopic P wave.

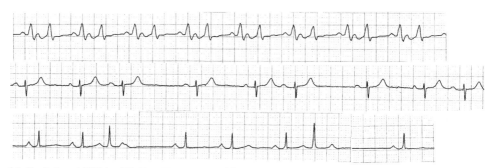

Figure 14–2 Strips of ECG lead II. *Top,* Bigeminy. *Middle,* So-called trigeminy. *Bottom,* Two premature atrial complexes in a row; the second is blocked.

unless it is associated with dextrocardia or dextroversion.[6] A negative P wave in leads II, III, and aV$_F$ can signify a focus in the left atrium,[4,5] coronary sinus, or low right atrium.[4,7] In the right precordial leads, the normal P wave or an ectopic P wave arising near the sinus node is usually positive-negative, although it may be positive if the late negative component is isoelectric or negative if the early positive component is isoelectric. In contrast, the left atrial or low right atrial ectopic P wave is usually negative-positive, but it may be positive if the early negative component is isoelectric.

The term "dome-and-dart P wave" was introduced[5,8] to describe the configuration of an ectopic P wave in lead V$_1$ in certain types of left atrial rhythms in patients with congenital heart disease. A dome-and-dart P wave consists of a broad, rounded initial portion and a sharp, peaked late portion. The term has been applied only rarely in the more recent literature.

Limited insight into the sequence of atrial activation can be obtained by recording esophageal or intracavitary leads simultaneously with surface ECG.[9–11] In the esophageal lead the P wave is upright at the level of the ventricles,

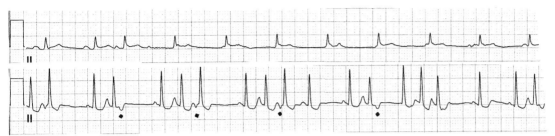

Figure 14–3 Strips of ECG lead II illustrating certain sequelae of the atrial premature complexes. *Top,* Prolonged sinus node depression after two atrial premature complexes, of which the second is blocked; the rhythm becomes atrioventricular (AV) junctional with a sinus P wave recognizable after the seventh QRS complex, in the eighth and ninth complexes, and before the last two complexes of the accelerated AV junctional escape rhythm. *Bottom,* Complex arrhythmia initiated by atrial premature complexes. The basic rhythm is sinus; atrial premature complexes are recognizable as positive P waves superimposed on the sinus T waves. The dots indicate negative P waves attributed to reciprocation (echo complexes). The morphology of T wave without the superimposed negative P wave can be recognized in the third-from-last ventricular complex (sinus). The negative P waves marked by the first and the fourth dot are not followed by QRS complexes, whereas the negative P waves marked by the second and the third dot are followed each by an aberrantly conducted ventricular complex attributed to AV nodal reentry. The two complexes after the fourth dot are AV junctional (the second is probably reentrant), and the third is an atrial premature complex, followed by two sinus complexes and an atrial premature complex.

inverted above the level of the heart, and diphasic at the atrial level. The point at which there is a change of direction in the biphasic (positive-negative) electrogram marks the onset of the intrinsicoid deflection (ID)[12] (see Chapter 1). It has been shown that the onset of the ID is nearly simultaneous at all levels of the posterior left atrium and the posteroinferior wall of the right atrium. This reflects the tangential spread of atrial excitation. Consequently, the onset of posterior atrial ID can be recorded in any atrial esophageal electrogram displaying an RS complex.

The onset of ID on the anterior wall of the right atrium can be recorded in the right atrial intracardiac leads. On the surface ECG, the onset of ID corresponds to the peak of the initial upright P wave in the right precordial leads displaying a diphasic P wave. The relation between the anterior and posterior IDs establishes the sequence of atrial depolarization. In 60 unpublished cases of simultaneously recorded right precordial and esophageal leads, Surawicz[1] found that the posterior wall was depolarized before the anterior wall in 80 percent of ectopic atrial complexes, the walls were depolarized simultaneously in about 10 percent, and the anterior wall was depolarized before the posterior wall in the remaining 10 percent.

The PR interval of the premature atrial complexes may be normal, shorter than normal, or longer than in normal sinus complexes (see Figure 14–1). Waldo et al.[13] showed that the PR interval was longer when atria were paced from epicardial sites than when paced from endocardial sites. The PR interval is usually similar to the PR interval of the basic sinus complex when the ectopic impulse appears relatively late and the

pacemaker is near the SA node. The PR becomes shorter if the focus is near the AV node. The PR tends to lengthen when the coupling interval is short. An early premature complex may not be conducted to the ventricles, resulting in a blocked premature atrial complex (see Figure 14–1). A blocked premature atrial complex should not be mistaken for a second-degree AV block. In the latter case the PP interval remains constant, and the P wave morphology is unchanged.

As a rule, the ventricular complex of a premature atrial complex does not differ from that of the basic sinus complex, but aberrant intraventricular conduction is common (see Figure 14–1 and 14–4). In most instances the aberrant ventricular conduction has right bundle branch block (RBBB) pattern morphology because of the relatively longer refractory period of the right branch. The left bundle branch block (LBBB) pattern may be seen especially in patients with heart disease, and various QRS morphologies may be encountered in the same individual. Aberrancy is more likely to occur when the premature impulse appears early (a short RP′ interval) and the preceding RR interval is long.

POSTEXTRASYSTOLIC PAUSE

The ectopic atrial impulses that reach and depolarize the SA node reset the sinus cycle. Therefore the cycle length after the premature atrial complex is longer than the basic sinus cycle. Additional lengthening of the postextrasystolic cycle occurs when the premature discharge of the SA node depresses the rhythmicity of the sinus node[14] (Figure 14–5). Unlike that after premature ventricular impulses, however, the

Atrial Arrhythmias

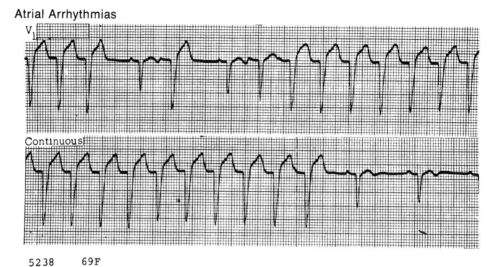

5238   69F

Figure 14–4 Ectopic atrial tachycardia with aberrant ventricular conduction. An isolated premature atrial complex with aberrant ventricular conduction is seen in the top strip. The rhythm simulates ventricular tachycardia.

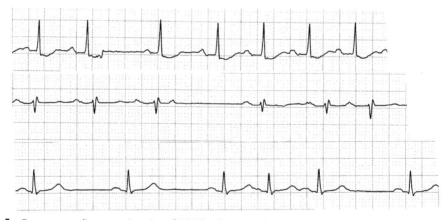

Figure 14–5 Postextrasystolic pauses in strips of ECG lead II. *Top,* The pause after the atrial premature complex is nearly equal to the preceding sinus pause, which suggests that the sinus node is undisturbed. *Middle,* The pause after the premature atrial complex is 150 ms longer than the preceding or subsequent PP interval, which suggests that the sinus node is reset. *Bottom,* Atrial premature complex is interpolated.

pause is usually not fully compensatory. In the presence of a retrograde SA block, the SA nodal rhythmicity is undisturbed; and when the sinus rate is slow, the premature atrial impulse may be interpolated between two normally occurring sinus P waves (see Figure 14–5). In some cases, premature atrial complexes cause prolonged depression of sinus activity (see Figure 14–3, top strip) (see Chapters 13 and 16).

CLINICAL SIGNIFICANCE

Most individuals with premature atrial complexes have no organic heart disease. Among 100 healthy young men and women monitored by ambulatory ECGs for a 24-hour period, supraventricular ectopic complexes were observed in 64 percent.[15,16] Fewer than 2 percent of these subjects, however, had more than 100 such ectopic complexes during the 24-hour period. In some patients without heart disease, the premature complexes appear to be related to emotional stress, mental and physical fatigue, excessive smoking, or alcohol or coffee intake.

The incidence of premature atrial complexes increases with increasing age and in patients with organic heart disease. The premature complexes tend to occur more often when atrial disease or atrial enlargement is present. They are known to precede the establishment of atrial flutter or atrial fibrillation.

Ectopic Atrial Rhythm, Accelerated Atrial Rhythm

During *ectopic atrial rhythm* (often called "ectopic atrial pacemaker"), the atrial rate is less than 100 beats/min and the PR interval is within the normal range. The P wave morphology varies, depending on the location of the ectopic focus. Considerations of the origin of the ectopic focus are the same as those for single atrial premature complexes.

Ectopic atrial rhythm is often transient and is seen in subjects with and without structural heart disease. It can be easily recognized if the premature P wave morphology can be compared with that of the P waves during sinus rhythm (Figure 14–6). When the ectopic pacemaker is located in the lower atrium, the P waves in the inferior leads are inverted and the rhythm may be mistaken as AV junctional. It has been customary, although without any firm support by experimental data, to consider the rhythm as AV junctional when the PR interval is less than 0.12 second.

An ectopic atrial rhythm may be called *accelerated atrial rhythm* when the atrial rate is faster than the patient's sinus rate but is less than 100 to 110 beats/min (see Figures 14–6 and 14–7). Accelerated atrial rhythm is most commonly recognized on ambulatory ECGs when the onset and termination of the ectopic rhythm can be identified.

Automatic Ectopic Atrial Tachycardia

Automatic atrial tachycardia (sometimes described as focal) may be transient, recurrent, sustained, or incessant. The tachycardia is considered sustained when it lasts longer than 30 seconds. The transient and recurrent forms, believed to arise in an ectopic atrial focus,[17-19] are the most common paroxysmal supraventricular arrhythmias, recorded in as many as one fourth of older patients undergoing ambulatory ECG monitoring. They occur in a wide variety of subjects without heart disease and in patients with various types of heart disease. These tachycardias often appear during sleep or in the presence of sinus bradycardia. This form of atrial tachycardia

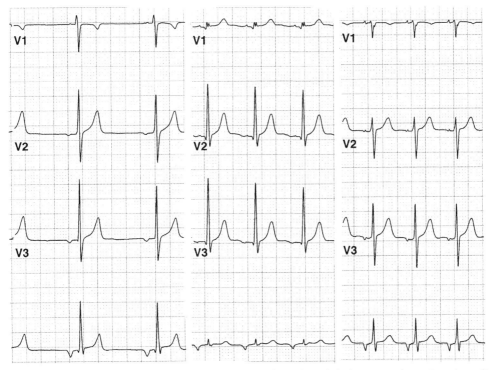

Figure 14–6   ECG leads V_1–V_3 and II in three patients with accelerated atrial rhythm or atrial ectopic tachycardia. Rates are 60 beats/min *(left)*, 91 beats/min *(middle)*, and 102 beats/min *(right)*. In each case the ectopic origin of the P wave is most recognizable in lead II (at the bottom of each vertical column).

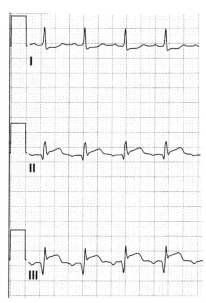

Figure 14–7 ECG leads I through III show ectopic atrial tachycardia at a rate of 106 beats/min in a 40-year-old man with an acute inferior myocardial infarction. Ectopic rhythm was transient.

of nonsustained ectopic atrial tachycardia that is probably automatic because the P wave morphology during tachycardia is the same as in the premature atrial complex initiating the run.

Chronic persistent atrial tachycardias are less common but are frequently disabling. Tachycardia tends to be incessant with rare, short bouts of intermittent sinus rhythm. Many patients with this type of tachycardia have no evidence of underlying heart disease, although heart disease may eventually develop, apparently as a result of the incessant tachycardia.[22]

The sustained and potentially disabling automatic atrial tachycardias occur more often in pediatric patients,[26] apparently caused by remnants of automatic tissues in the atrium. The automatic mechanism is rare in geriatric patients because automaticity decreases with aging.[23] The distributions of right and left atrial tachycardias were approximately equal in pediatric patients.[23] The most common location in the left atrium is near the orifice of the pulmonary veins.[23] Other locations include the inferior left atrium, base of the left atrial appendage, high lateral left atrium,[24] mitral annulus,[25] and septum.[26] In the right atrium, two thirds of tachycardias are located along the crista terminalis (cristal atrial tachycardias).[27] Tachycardias arising in the interatrial septum and not involving the AV node are termed *septal atrial tachycardias*.[28] Other right atrial locations include the right atrial appendage, lateral wall, tricuspid annulus, and near the coronary sinus.[27] According to Kistler et al.,[29] the most useful ECG leads for distinguishing the right atrial from the left atrial ectopic locations are leads aV_L and V_1. A positive or biphasic P wave in lead aV_L was associated with right atrial focus

also has been called *benign slow paroxysmal atrial tachycardia*.[23] Paroxysms are usually of short duration, and the rate tends to be slow (i.e., <150 beats/min). In the study of Stemple et al.,[20] the median number of complexes was seven and the average heart rate was 116 beats/min. In the experience of Chou and Ceaser,[21] one or more transient episodes of transient ectopic atrial tachycardia were observed in 582 (21.6 percent) of 2670 consecutive adults in 12- to 24-hour ambulatory ECGs. Figure 14–8 shows three examples of short runs

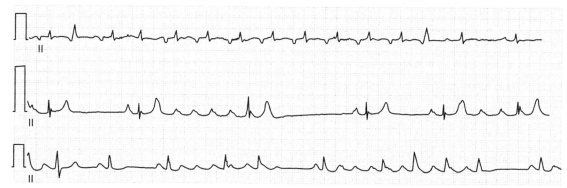

Figure 14–8 Three ECG strips of lead II in three different patients with short runs of ectopic atrial tachycardia recognizable by P wave morphology different from that in sinus complexes. *Top,* The rate of atrial tachycardia is 96 beats/min, and the run of atrial tachycardia is interrupted by a ventricular premature complex (third complex from the end). *Middle,* The rate of ectopic atrial tachycardia (P waves are notched at the peak) is 200 beats/min; there is high-degree atrioventricular (AV) block. The tachycardia begins with a premature atrial complex (PAC) and ends after a nonducted PAC. *Bottom,* The rate of atrial tachycardia (ectopic P waves are lower than sinus P waves) is 160 beats/min; there is a high-degree AV block during atrial tachycardia, which terminates after a P wave conducted to the ventricle with a prolonged PR interval.

with a sensitivity of 88 percent and a specificity of 79 percent. In the lead V_1, 100 percent specificity for right atrial focus was present with a positive-negative P wave and for left atrial focus with a negative-positive P wave.[29a]

In patients with recurrent forms of automatic atrial tachycardias, the tachycardia is usually initiated by a late atrial premature impulse during sinus rhythm. The P wave configuration of a tachycardia-initiating complex is identical to that of succeeding complexes.[30] Tang et al.[27] found that analysis of P wave configuration in leads aV_L and V_1 was helpful for distinguishing right from left atrial loci. The sensitivity and specificity of a positive or biphasic P wave in lead aV_L to predict a right atrial focus were 88 percent and 79 percent, respectively. The sensitivity and specificity of a positive (not specified whether preceded by a negative deflection) P wave in lead V_1 for predicting a left atrial focus were 93 percent and 88 percent, respectively.[27]

In contrast to reentrant tachycardia, the PR interval of the tachycardia initiating a premature atrial complex is usually not prolonged.[30] After onset, the cycle length of tachycardia shortens progressively (warm-up phenomenon) for several cycles, but once established the PP intervals do not vary by more than 50 ms unless an exit block from the focus of tachycardia is present (Figure 14–9). During tachycardia, P waves are visible. The configuration and axis of P waves are usually abnormal but sometimes resemble P waves of sinus origin. The rate of tachycardia tends to vary from day to day and from hour to hour and is influenced by a variety of physiologic factors modifying autonomic tone. During sleep the rate of tachycardia slows or AV block occurs. Atropine and isoproterenol increase the tachycardia rate. The automatic ectopic atrial tachycardia is not affected by vagal stimulation such as carotid sinus massage or the Valsalva maneuver, although these maneuvers may produce AV block.[21,31,32] In the study of 80 cases of focal tachycardia, 67 (84 percent) were adenosine-sensitive.[32a]

During electrophysiologic studies the initiation of automatic tachycardia does not depend on the coupling interval of the premature stimulus or conduction delay. At short coupling intervals the response of automatic supraventricular tachycardia differs from that of reentrant supraventricular tachycardia because it does not terminate but is "reset" without cessation of the tachycardia. Overdrive pacing captures the atrium but, upon cessation of the pacing, the tachycardia immediately resumes without an intervening sinus complex. This suggests that the focus of automatic tachycardia is "protected." Chronic, persistent atrial tachycardia is quite resistant to treatment, including direct-current countershock. In a growing number of cases the treatment of choice has become ablation or excision of ectopic atrial foci responsible for tachycardia.[26,28,33,34] Ablation was also successful in rare patients with 2 or 3 simultaneous focal atrial tachycardias.[34a]

ECG FINDINGS

The ECG criteria are as follows:
1. There are three or more successive abnormal P waves whose morphology is different from that of the sinus P waves.

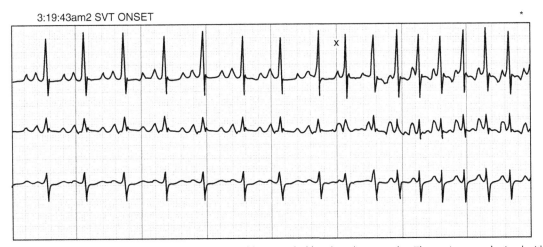

3:19:43am2 SVT ONSET

Figure 14–9 Ectopic atrial tachycardia in a 55-year-old man with dilated cardiomyopathy. The tracing was obtained with a Holter monitor. Tachycardia is initiated with a premature atrial complex (marked with an x), and the morphology of the P waves during the tachycardia is similar to that of the initiating premature complex. There is a short "warm-up" period until the heart rate reaches 166 beats/min. The episode lasted 13 minutes 30 seconds (the end of the episode is not shown). Note the T wave changes during the tachycardia.

2. The atrial rate is generally between 100 and 180 beats/min.
3. The rhythm is regular (after the first few complexes).
4. The paroxysm consists of three or more complexes in succession.
5. There is a QRS complex after each P wave, and the QRS complex usually resembles that of the sinus complex unless there is aberrant ventricular conduction.
6. The PR interval tends to be normal or prolonged.
7. Tachycardia-induced ST segment and T wave changes may occur.

If the atrial rate is rapid, the AV junction may be only partially recovered when the successive atrial impulses arrive. The PR interval may therefore be longer than that of the sinus complex. In some cases, some of the P waves are not followed by a QRS complex, resulting in ectopic atrial tachycardia with block, a rhythm commonly known as *paroxysmal atrial tachycardia with block* (discussed later in the chapter).

The QRS complex in ectopic atrial tachycardia usually resembles that of the patient's sinus complex. A prolonged QRS complex may be the result of aberrant ventricular conduction. In most cases the aberrant QRS complex has an RBBB pattern, although an LBBB pattern also is seen. Occasionally, aberrant ventricular conduction is present at the onset of a paroxysm, and normal QRS configuration returns as the tachycardia continues. The QRS complex may also be abnormal because of a preexisting ventricular conduction defect. In either case, the rhythm may mimic paroxysmal ventricular tachycardia and present a difficult but important diagnostic problem.

As with sinus tachycardia, ST segment depression and T wave inversion may be seen during the tachycardia. Furthermore, T wave abnormalities may be present for hours or even days after the cessation of long-lasting tachycardia. This is called *posttachycardia T wave abnormality* (see Chapter 23).

Intraatrial Reentry Tachycardia

Allessie et al.[35] showed that reentrant activity can be induced by early premature stimuli in small pieces of rabbit atria. As a specific mechanism of tachycardia in humans, atrial reentry was recognized by several groups of investigators.[36-39] With intraatrial reentrant tachycardia, a reentry circuit confined to the atrium consists of two functionally distinct pathways with different conduction velocities and refractory periods.[22,36,40,41]

The diagnostic criteria include (1) regular ectopic supraventricular tachycardia; (2) an activation sequence differing from that in sinus rhythm; (3) tachycardia that does not require participation of the AV node; and (4) a rate slower than that of atrial flutter.[42] Demonstration of second-degree AV block is helpful for documenting the mechanism.[42]

According to Josephson,[31] reentrant atrial tachycardia accounted for about 6 percent of the 280 cases of paroxysmal supraventricular tachycardia studied in their electrophysiology laboratory. The heart rate may range from 120 to 240 beats/min. As a rule, the tachycardia is initiated by a premature atrial complex.

The morphology of the P wave varies depending on the location of the reentry circuit in the atrium and the pathway of the activation impulse. Unlike the automatic (ectopic) type of atrial tachycardia, the P wave morphology during the tachycardia differs from that of the initiating premature complex.[20,21] Furthermore, the morphology of the P wave during the episode also may vary because the impulse exiting from the reentry circuit may be conducted along different pathways in the atria from beat to beat.[32] The tachycardia rhythm is regular without a warm-up. The changes in the PR interval and the QRS duration, if present, are rate related and similar to those seen with the automatic type.

Differentiation of intraatrial reentry tachycardia from ectopic atrial tachycardia is difficult from the body surface ECG, especially if the onset of the tachycardia is not recorded. They can be distinguished in the electrophysiology laboratory because, in contrast to ectopic automatic tachycardia, intraatrial reentry tachycardia can be induced by programmed stimulation[43] (Figure 14–10).

In a series of nine patients reported by Haines and DiMarco,[42] the cycle length of tachycardia ranged from 260 to 460 ms; 89 percent of patients had underlying structural heart disease, and 68 percent had concomitant atrial flutter or atrial fibrillation. Intraatrial reentrant tachycardia is a common complication of cardiac surgery, especially after surgery for congenital heart disease.[44-46] It is believed that surgical scars and patches serve as boundaries of reentrant circuits.[45] This was also the case for a patient after orthotopic heart transplantation in whom the right atrial free-wall suture line[47] was the site of the acquired interatrial conduction path from the recipient atria to the donor atria.[47] A rare case of incessant tachycardia using a concealed

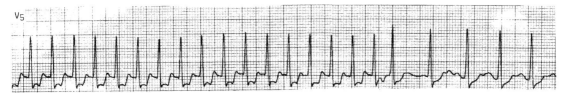

Figure 14–10 ECG lead V_5 in a 50-year-old man with exercise-induced paroxysmal supraventricular tachycardia. Electrophysiologic study established a diagnosis of inducible atrial tachycardia by demonstrating a "high-low" sequence of propagation. Note the atrial tachycardia at a rate of 193 beats/min with positive P waves; the tachycardia is terminated by a premature atrial complex with a negative P wave. These findings suggest atrial reentrant tachycardia.

atrionodal bypass tract and continuing despite AV block was reported.[48]

As an alternative mechanism to reentry, triggered activity could not be ruled out in patients with atrial tachycardias but appeared unlikely because verapamil or β-adrenergic blocking drugs were therapeutically ineffective. Engelstein et al.[49] found that atrial reentrant tachycardias were not affected by adenosine administration and thus could be differentiated from the automatic tachycardias. Similarly, Markowitz et al.[50] found that adenosine-sensitive tachycardia is usually focal in origin. In contrast, Chen et al.[51] found that a relatively high dose of adenosine could terminate intraatrial reentrant tachycardia in 24 of 27 patients. Iesaka et al.[52] found that focal reentry at the low anteroseptal right atrium site adjacent to the AV junction (presumably within the approaches to the AV node), but not involving AV nodal pathways, could be terminated by small doses of adenosine in 11 patients.[52] It has been reported that focal reentry can be differentiated from focal automaticitry using high-density mapping.[53]

Foci of macro-reentrant atrial tachycardia can be successfully ablated by radiofrequency energy applied to a critical area in the atrial reentrant circuit.[44–46,54] The increasing number of procedures of isolating pulmonary veins in patients with atrial fibrillation has led to the discovery of both focal and macro-reentrant atrial tachycardias originating in the pulmonary veins diagnosed before and after ablation.[55,56] Pacing from each of the pulmonary veins established useful criteria for localizing the site of tachycardia.[29,57]

REPETITIVE PAROXYSMAL ATRIAL TACHYCARDIA

Repetitive paroxysmal atrial tachycardia is characterized by recurring short runs of atrial tachycardia that are almost constantly present for months or years and only occasionally interrupted by normal sinus rhythm[54] (Figure 14–11). Using the more stringent definition, the individual paroxysms of this dysrhythmia should not be

separated by more than two normal beats. The tachycardia often has a slightly irregular rhythm whose mechanism is unknown. Similar repetitive behavior also is seen with other types of tachyarrhythmias such as atrial flutter, atrial fibrillation, paroxysmal junctional tachycardia, and ventricular tachycardia.[58,59] Repetitive atrial tachycardia is rare; it may be seen in patients with or without organic heart disease.

Paroxysmal Atrial Tachycardia with Block

Paroxysmal atrial tachycardia (PAT) with block is currently often called *ectopic atrial tachycardia with block*. The early term has remained in use, mainly because of tradition.

The clinical importance of PAT with block was brought to attention mainly by Lown et al.,[60] who proposed the following criteria.
1. Abnormal P (or P′) waves whose morphology is different from that of the sinus P waves
2. Atrial rate generally between 150 and 250 beats/min
3. Isoelectric intervals between P waves in all leads
4. Second-degree or more advanced AV block

PAT with block generally is believed to be due to increased automaticity of an ectopic atrial focus associated with impaired AV conduction. Triggered activity due to the presence of delayed afterpotentials may be responsible for some cases, especially those due to digitalis intoxication.[61]

As with other ectopic atrial rhythms, the morphology of the P waves depends on the location of the ectopic atrial pacemaker. The P waves frequently are small and not easily identifiable. In some cases, lead V_1 is the best one to use to search for the blocked P waves. Although the atrial rate may range from 150 to 250 beats/min, it is less than 200 beats/min in most cases and occasionally as low as 110 beats/min. The atrial rhythm is generally regular. Some variation

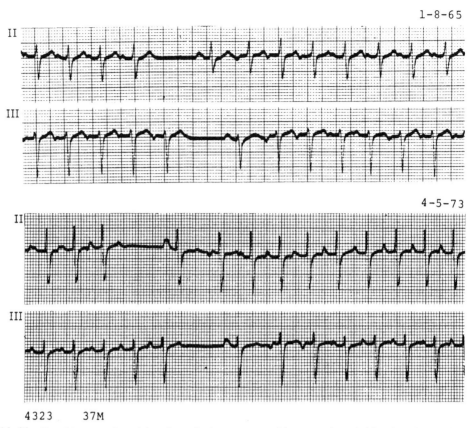

Figure 14–11   Repetitive ectopic atrial tachycardia in a 37-year-old man with probable idiopathic cardiomyopathy. Repetitive ectopic atrial tachycardia has been noted for at least 8 years.

of the PP interval, however, was seen in nearly half of the series reported by Lown et al.[62] The AV block in this dysrhythmia usually is second degree with 2:1 conduction, but 3:1 conduction or the Wenckebach phenomenon may be observed (Figures 14–12 to 14–15). Complete AV block is uncommon. PAT with block cannot be diagnosed when there is 1:1 AV conduction with prolongation of the PR interval. The PR prolongation in such cases may be physiologic because of the rapid atrial impulses. In some cases with 1:1 conduction, however, second-degree AV block develops during carotid sinus massage.

DIFFERENTIAL DIAGNOSIS

Because the P waves in PAT with block are often small and superimposed on the ventricular complexes, this rhythm frequently is mistaken for AV nodal reentrant tachycardia, atrial tachycardia without block, or sinus tachycardia. When the block varies, the irregular ventricular rhythm may be mistaken for atrial fibrillation. The arrhythmia that most closely simulates PAT with block is atrial flutter. The differentiation may be important

because PAT with block frequently results from digitalis toxicity, but atrial flutter does not. With atrial flutter, the atrial rate is usually more than 250 beats/min, and there is constant oscillation of the baseline. If the atrial rate is between 200 and 250 beats/min and the flutter waves are atypical, differentiation of these arrhythmias is often impossible based on the ECG.

CLINICAL SIGNIFICANCE

Digitalis intoxication is the predominant cause of PAT with block. Among the 112 episodes of this arrhythmia reviewed by Lown and Levine in 1958,[58] 73 percent were attributed to digitalis. Other reports implicated digitalis toxicity in 40 to 82 percent of cases.[63,64] In recent years the digitalis dosage used generally has been reduced, resulting in a marked decline of this arrhythmia. In patients not receiving digitalis, this arrhythmia has diverse etiology; it is found usually in patients with advanced heart disease. Body potassium depletion from the use of diuretics was often the precipitating factor, although the serum potassium level was not necessarily below normal. In one reported series of

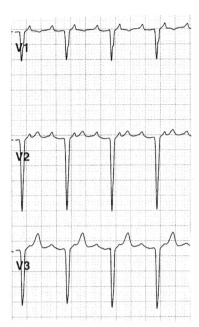

Figure 14–12   ECG leads V_1–V_3 in an 82-year-old man with a previous anterior myocardial infarction show ectopic atrial tachycardia at a rate of 208 beats/min with 2:1 ventricular response.

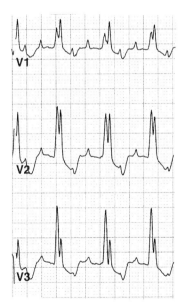

Figure 14–13   ECG leads V_1–V_3 in a 66-year-old man with right bundle branch block and left anterior fascicular block show ectopic atrial tachycardia at a rate of 288 beats/min and 3:1 ventricular response. Atrial rate is within the range of atrial flutter, but no flutter waves were recognizable in any of the leads (not shown).

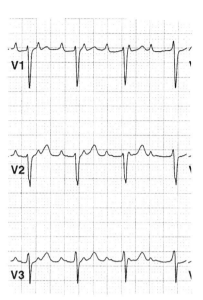

Figure 14–14   EC leads V_1–V_3 in a 76-year-old man with a history of palpitations show ectopic atrial tachycardia at a rate of 175 beats/min with 2:1 ventricular response and Wenckebach periodicity of the conducted P wave.

patients with this arrhythmia, chronic pulmonary disease was found in more than half of the patients treated with digitalis.[65]

Atrial Standstill

Experimental atrial standstill has been induced by drugs, chilling of the SA node, CO_2 poisoning, or anoxia.[66] In humans, atrial standstill has been categorized as: (1) temporary (caused usually by the sick sinus syndrome, vagal action, drugs, hyperkalemia, or following open heart surgery)[67]; (2) terminal; or (3) persistent.

The recent study of Makita et al.[68] suggests that genetic defects in cardiac sodium channel SCN5A underlie the congenital atrial standstill.

Bloomfield and Sinclair-Smith[66] described the first case of atrial standstill documented by cardiac catheterization and proposed the following criteria for its diagnosis, also known as "silent atrium": (1) absent P wave on surface and intracardiac ECGs; (2) absent a wave in the intracardiac pressure record; (3) regular rhythm; and (4) angiographic evidence of an immobile atrium. An additional requirement is unresponsiveness to atrial pacing.[69] The standstill may involve both atria or be confined to the right atrium with a normally functioning left atrium.[65] It may be associated with idiopathic atrial enlargement as the only pathologic abnormality, but usually the atrial myocardium is damaged

I

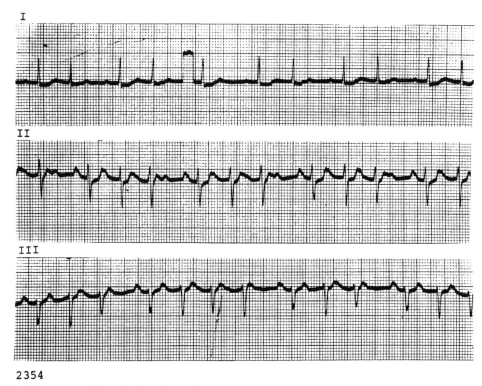

2354

Figure 14–15   Paroxysmal atrial tachycardia with block. A Wenckebach phenomenon is present. There is gradual lengthening of the PR interval and shortening of the RR interval before the block occurs.

and underlying depolarization is suspected.[70] The regular rhythm may be caused by an AV junctional escape pacemaker or sinoventricular conduction.[71] The absence of P waves alone is not sufficient to establish the diagnosis because P waves may be absent also on the surface ECG in cases of atrial tachycardia in which atrial activity is limited to small regions of the atrium.[72]

Multifocal Atrial or Chaotic Tachycardia

Multifocal atrial tachycardia also is known as *chaotic atrial tachycardia* or *chaotic atrial mechanism*.[73-75] This tachycardia is characterized by P waves of varying morphology (Figure 14–16). It is assumed that distinct P waves originate from different foci, although one cannot rule out the

possibility that the focus is single and the changes in P wave morphology are caused by variable intraatrial conduction or variable degrees of fusion with the sinus P wave. Neither P wave morphology nor the duration of the PR interval is decisive when differentiating multifocal rhythms from multiform rhythms (i.e., rhythms originating from the same focus but having a different spread of excitation). The term *multiform* is preferred because it does not commit the ECG interpreter to an uncertain mechanism. The condition usually occurs in seriously ill patients, often with chronic lung disease and respiratory failure; it usually resolves following successful management of the underlying clinical disorder. Most patients with multifocal atrial tachycardia are elderly. Treatment with theophylline and β-adrenergic agonists may be a contributing factor. In most

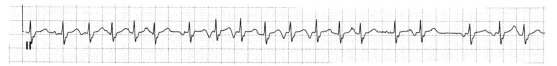

Figure 14–16   ECG lead II strip shows multifocal atrial tachycardia at a rate of 154 beats/min in a 79-year-old man with chronic obstructive lung disease. Note the irregular rhythm and at least four P wave shapes.

cases the arrhythmia is resolved within days, although it may persist for longer periods. There is a close relation between multifocal atrial tachycardia and either atrial flutter or atrial fibrillation. The tachycardia can be postural.[76] In one case, pathologic studies revealed a mesenchymal tumor at the site of an automatic focus near the lip of the fossa ovalis.[77]

The ECG is characterized by: (1) three or more morphologically distinct P waves in the same lead; (2) the absence of one dominant atrial pacemaker (in distinction to sinus rhythm with frequent premature atrial complexes); (3) an isoelectric baseline; and (4) varying PP, PR, and RR intervals. Some P waves may be nonconducted, and some may be conducted to the ventricles with aberration. The ventricular rate is usually 100 to 150 beats/min but may be as low as 90 beats/min[78] or as high as 250 beats/min. It can be diagnosed only with an ECG because the physical examination findings clinically resemble atrial fibrillation when the rhythm is irregular.[79] In several reported series, multifocal atrial tachycardia was seen in 0.2 to 0.4 percent of the ECGs from the institutions where the studies were performed.[73–75,80–82]

The rhythm is often preceded or followed by frequent premature atrial complexes, sinus tachycardia, atrial fibrillation, atrial flutter, ectopic atrial tachycardia, or PAT with block. In one series it was preceded by or progressed to atrial fibrillation or flutter in 55 percent of cases.[79] Many of the patients had diabetes mellitus.[74,82]

The role of digitalis relative to this rhythm has been debated.[73,81] Electrolyte imbalance (e.g., hypokalemia and hypomagnesemia) has been reported as the etiology of this arrhythmia. Multifocal atrial tachycardia implies a poor prognosis in patients with infection or with pulmonary insufficiency and congestive heart failure. However, the direct cause of death is not the arrhythmia but rather is the underlying disease. Arrhythmia may be present in children without underlying heart disease.[83] The ventricular rate may be reduced by administration of verapamil, an indication that abnormal atrial activity represents a form of triggered tachycardia (see Chapter 17).

Atrial Parasystole

Atrial parasystole is encountered less frequently than ventricular parasystole. With atrial parasystole, the ectopic P waves (P′) are independent of the sinus activity. The morphology of the ectopic P waves is often similar to that of the sinus complexes. The coupling intervals vary. The interectopic (P′P′) intervals have a common denominator (Figure 14–17). In most instances the ectopic atrial impulse can be conducted to the ventricles whenever the latter are not in the refractory phase.[84,85] Atrial parasystole may be seen in individuals with or without heart disease.

The reported range of the parasystolic rate ranges from 33 to 56 beats/min.[84] The parasystolic focus can be fully protected from sinus impulses without evidence of modulation,[86] but more often it is electrotonically modulated by the sinus pacemaker, as evidenced by the PP intervals fitting a phase-response curve (see Chapter 17).[86] The SA node pacemaker may remain undisturbed, but more often it is interfered with, discharged, or blocked.[84,87,88]

Atrial Dissociation

Atrial dissociation has been seen more commonly in recent years because of cardiac transplantation. In those occasional cases not associated with cardiac transplantation, the ectopic depolarization always is limited to an area of one atrium; the ectopic P (P′) waves are small and bizarre and are never conducted to the ventricles (Figure 14–18). The interectopic intervals are more variable than are those of atrial parasystole. Atrial dissociation is usually a manifestation of advanced heart disease and often occurs a few hours before death.[89]

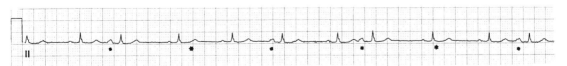

Figure 14–17 Atrial parasystole at a rate of about 40 beats/min. Note the variable coupling. Dots mark the manifested parasystolic P waves, and stars mark the assumed concealed discharges that are unable to propagate because of atrial refractoriness after the preceding P wave of the dominant sinus rhythm.

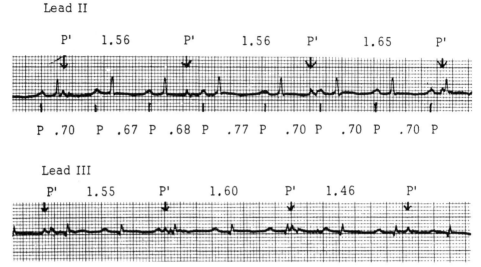

Figure 14–18 Atrial dissociation. The ectopic P waves are indicated by P′ waves. None of the P′ waves are conducted to the ventricle. The length of the P′P′ interval is more variable than that seen with atrial parasystole. The patient had an acute anterior myocardial infarction and died a few hours after this tracing was recorded.

In patients who have undergone cardiac transplantation, the recipient's atrial remnant, which includes the sinus node, generates regular impulses that depolarize the atrial remnant, resulting in a second set of P waves (see Chapter 12). Because of the small size of the atrial remnant and its electrical isolation from the donor's heart by the surrounding scar tissue, the P waves are generally small and are dissociated from the P waves and QRS complexes of the donor's heart. Complex atrial arrhythmias can occur when one part of the atrium develops atrial flutter or fibrillation. Cases have been reported with atrial flutter in one atrium and atrial fibrillation in another.[90]

REFERENCES

1. Surawicz B: Electrophysiologic Basis of ECG and Cardiac Arrhythmias. Baltimore, Williams & Wilkins, 1995, pp 18, 306.
2. Puech P: The P wave: correlation of surface and intra-atrial electrograms. Cardiovasc Clin 2:43, 1974.
3. Wu D, Denes P, Amat-y-Leon F, et al: Limitations of the surface electrocardiogram in diagnosis of atrial arrhythmias. Am J Cardiol 336:91, 1975.
4. MacLean WA, Karp RB, Kouchoukos NT, et al: P-wave changes during ectopic atrial rhythms in man: a study utilizing atrial pacing with fixed electrodes. Circulation 52:426, 1975.
5. Beder SD, Gillette PC, Garson A, et al: Clinical confirmation of ECG criteria for left atrial rhythm. Am Heart J 103:848, 1982.
6. Mirowski M, Neill CA, Bahnson HT, et al: Negative P waves in lead I in dextroversion: differential diagnosis from mirror-image dextrocardia. Circulation 26:413, 1962.
7. Leon DF, Lancaster JF, Shaver JA, et al: Right atrial ectopic rhythms: experimental production in man. Am J Cardiol 25:6, 1970.
8. Mirowski M, Neill CA, Taussig HB: Left atrial ectopic rhythm in mirror-image dextrocardia and in normally placed malformed hearts. Circulation 27:864, 1963.
9. Hecht HH: The electrocardiogram of the human auricle: an analysis of simultaneous standard, precordial, and esophageal leads. Clin Res 16:56, 1943.
10. Levine MD, Hellems HK, Willenborg MR, et al: Studies in intracardiac electrocardiography in man: the potential variations in the right atrium. Am Heart J 37:46, 1949.
11. Massumi R, Tawakkol AA: Direct study of left atrial P waves. Am J Cardiol 20:331, 1967.
12. Hecht HH, Woodbury LA: Excitation of human auricular muscle and the significance of the intrinsicoid deflection of the auricular electrocardiogram. Circulation 2:37, 1950.
13. Waldo AL, Vitikainen KJ, Harris PD, et al: The P wave and the P-R interval: effects of the site of origin of atrial depolarization. Circulation 42:653, 1970.
14. Pick A, Langendorf R, Katz LN: Depression of cardiac pacemakers by premature impulses. Am Heart J 41:478, 1949.
15. Brodsky M, Wu D, Denes P, et al: Arrhythmias documented by 24 hour continuous electrocardiographic monitoring in 50 male medical students without apparent heart disease. Am J Cardiol 39:390, 1977.
16. Sobotka PA, Mayer JH, Bauernfeidn RA, et al: Arrhythmia documented by 24-hour continuous ambulatory electrocardiographic monitoring in young women without apparent heart disease. Am Heart J 101:753, 1981.
17. Gilette PC, Garson A: Electrophysiologic and pharmacologic characteristics of automatic ectopic atrial tachycardia. Circulation 56:571, 1977.
18. Goldreyer BN, Gallagher JJ, Damato AN: The electrophysiologic demonstration of atrial ectopic tachycardia in man. Am Heart J 85:205, 1973.
19. Josephson ME, Kastor JA: Supraventricular tachycardia: mechanisms and management. Ann Intern Med 87:346, 1977.
20. Stemple DR, Fitzgerald JW, Winkle RA: Benign slow paroxysmal atrial tachycardia. Ann Intern Med 87:44, 1977.
21. Chou TC, Ceaser JH: Ambulatory electrocardiogram: clinical applications. Cardiovasc Clin 13:321, 1983.

22. Garson A, Gillette PC: Junctional ectopic tachycardia in children: electrocardiography, electrophysiology and pharmacologic response. Am J Cardiol 44:298, 1979.

23. Chen S-A, Tai C-T, Chiang C-E, et al: Focal atrial tachycardia: reanalysis of the clinical and electrophysiologic characteristics and prediction of successful radiofrequency ablation. J Cardiovasc Electrophysiol 9:355, 1998.

24. Tang CW, Scheinman MM, Van Hare GF, et al: Use of P wave configuration during atrial tachycardia to predict site of origin. J Am Coll Cardiol 26:1315, 1995.

25. Kistler PM, Sanders P, Hussin A, et al: Focal atrial tachycardia arising from the mitral annulus. J Am Coll Cardiol 41:2212, 2003.

26. Marrouche NF, Sippens Groenewegen A, Yang Y, et al: Clinical and electrophysiologic characteristics of left septal atrial tachycardia. J Am Coll Cardiol 40:1133, 2002.

27. Kalman JM, Olgin JE, Karch MR, et al: "Cristal tachycardias": origin of right atrial tachycardias from the crista terminalis identified by intracardiac echocardiography. J Am Coll Cardiol 31:451, 1998.

28. Lesh MD, Kalman JM: To fumble flutter or tackle "tach"? Toward updated classifiers for atrial tachyarrhythmias. J Cardiovasc Electrophysiol 7:460, 1996.

29. Kistler PM,Kalman JM: Locating focal atrial tachycardias from P-wave morphology. Heart Rhythm 2:561, 2004.

29a. Kistler PM, Roberts-Thomson KC, Haqqani HM, et al: P-wave morphology in focal atrial tachycardia. Development of an algorithm to predict the anatomic site of origin. J Am Coll Cardiol 48:1010, 2006.

30. Reddy CP: Supraventricular ectopic tachycardias due to mechanisms other than reentry. In: Surawicz B, Reddy CP, Prystowsky EN (eds): Tachycardias. Boston, Martinus Nijhoff, 1984.

31. Josephson ME: Clinical Cardiac Electrophysiology, 2nd ed. Philadelphia, Lea & Febiger, 1993.

32. Morady F, Scheinman MM: Paroxysmal supraventricular tachycardia. Mod Concepts Cardiovasc Dis 51:107, 1982.

32a. Markowitz SM, Nemirovsky D, Stein KM, et al: Adenosine-insensitive focal atrial tachycardia. J Am Coll Cardiol 49:1324, 2007.

33. Pappone C, Stabile G, Di Simone A, et al: Role of catheter-induced mechanical trauma in localization of target sites of radiofrequency ablation in automatic atrial tachycardia. J Am Coll Cardiol 27:1090, 1996.

34. Kottkampf H, Hindricks G, Breithardt G, et al: Three dimensional electromagnetic catheter technology: electroanatomical mapping of right atrium and ablation of ectopic atrial tachycardia. J Cardiovasc Electrophysiol 8:1332, 1997.

34a. Hillock RJ, Kalman JM, Roberts-Thomson Kc, et al: Multiple focal tachycardia in a healthy adult population: Characterization and description of successful radiofrequency ablation. Heart Rhythm 4:434, 2007.

35. Allessie MA, Bonke FI, Schopman F: Circus movement in rabbit atrial muscle as a mechanism of tachycardia. Circ Res 33:54, 1973.

36. Wu D, Amat-y-Leon F, Denes P, et al: Demonstration of sustained sinus and atrial reentry as a mechanism of paroxysmal supraventricular tachycardia. Circulation 51:234, 1975.

37. Wellens HJ: Unusual examples of supraventricular reentrant tachycardia. Circulation 51:997, 1975.

38. Akhtar M, Caracta AR, Lau SH, et al: Demonstration of intra-atrial conduction delay, block, gap and reentry: a report of two cases. Circulation 58:947, 1978.

39. Coumel P, Flammang D, Attuel P, et al: Sustained intraatrial reentrant tachycardia: electrophysiologic study of 20 cases. Clin Cardiol 2:167, 1979.

40. Coumel P: Supraventricular tachycardias. In: Krikler DM, Goodwin JF (eds): Cardiac Arrhythmias: The Modern Electrophysiological Approach. Philadelphia, Saunders, 1975, p 116.

41. Goldreyer BN, Bigger JT: Site of re-entry in paroxysmal supraventricular tachycardia in man. Circulation 43:15, 1971.

42. Haines DE, DiMarco JP: Sustained intraatrial reentrant tachycardia: clinical, electrocardiographic and electrophysiologic characteristics and long-term follow up. J Am Coll Cardiol 15:1345, 1990.

43. Chen SA, Chiang CE, Yang CJ, et al: Radiofrequency catheter ablation of sustained intra-atrial reentrant tachycardia in adult patients. Circulation 88:578, 1993.

44. Kalman JM, Van Hare GF, Olgin JE, et al: Ablation of "incisional" reentrant atrial tachycardia complicating surgery for congenital heart disease. Circulation 93:502, 1006.

45. Baker BM, Lindsay BD, Bromberg BI, et al: Catheter ablation of clinical intraatrial reentrant tachycardias resulting from previous atrial surgery: localizing and transecting its critical isthmus. J Am Coll Cardiol 28:411, 1996.

46. Triedman JK, Bergau DM, Saul P, et al: Efficacy of radiofrequency ablation for control of intraatrial reentrant tachycardia in patients with congenital heart disease. J Am Coll Cardiol 30:1032, 1997.

47. Rothman SA, Miller JM, Hsia HH, et al: Radiofrequency ablation of a supraventricular tachycardia due to interatrial conduction from the recipient to donor atria in an orthotopic heart transplant recipient. J Cardiovasc Electrophysiol 6:544, 1995.

48. Zivin A, Morady F: Incessant tachycardia using a concealed atrionodal bypass tract. J Cardiovasc Electrophysiol 9:191, 1998.

49. Engelstein ED, Lippman N, Stein KM, et al: Mechanism-specific effects of adenosine on atrial tachycardia. Circulation 89:2645, 1994.

50. Markowitz SM, Stein KM, Mittal S, et al: Differential effects of adenosine on focal and macroreentrant atrial tachycardia. J Cardiovasc Electrophysiol 10:489, 1999.

51. Chen S-A, Chiang C-E, Yang C-I, et al: Sustained atrial tachycardia in adult patients: electrophysiological characteristics, pharmacological response, possible mechanisms, and effects of radiofrequency ablation. Circulation 90:1262, 1994.

52. Iesaka Y, Takahashi A, Goya M, et al: Adenosine-sensitive atrial reentrant tachycardia originating from the atrioventricular nodal transitional area. J Cardiovasc Electrophysiol 8:854, 1997.

53. Sanders P, Hocini M, Jais P, et al: Characterization of focal arial tachycardia using high-density mapping. J Am Coll Cardiol 46:2088, 2005.

54. Chen S-A, Chiang C-E, Yang C-I, et al: Radiofrequency catheter ablation of sustained intra-atrial reentrant tachycardia in adult patients: identification of electrophysiological characteristics and endocardial mapping techniques. Circulation 88:578, 1993.

55. Mesas CE, Pappone C, Lang CCE: Left atrial tachycardia after circumferential pulmonary vein ablation for atrial fibrillation. J Am Coll Cadiol 44:1071, 2004.

56. Gerstenfeld EP, Callans DJ, Dixit S, et al: Mechanisms of organized left atrial tachycardias occurring after pulmonary vein isolation. Circulation 110:1351, 2004.

57. Yamane T, Shah DC, Peng J-T, et al: Morphological characteristics of P waves during selective pulmonary vein pacing. J Am Coll Cardiol 38:1505, 2001.

58. Parkinson J, Papp C: Repetitive paroxysmal tachycardia. Br Heart J 9:241, 1947.

59. Levine HD, Smith C: Repetitive paroxysmal tachycardia in adults. Cardiology 55:2, 1970.
60. Lown B, Wyatt NF, Levine HD: Paroxysmal atrial tachycardia with block. Circulation 21:129, 1960.
61. Waldo AL: Mechanism of atrial fibrillation, atrial flutter, and ectopic atrial tachycardiaa brief review. Circulation 75(Suppl III):37, 1987.
62. Lown B, Levine HD: Atrial Arrhythmias, Digitalis and Potassium. New York, Landsberger, 1958.
63. El-Sherif N: Supraventricular tachycardia with AV block. Br Heart J 32:46, 1970.
64. Freiermuth LJ, Jick S: Paroxysmal atrial tachycardia with atrioventricular block. Am J Cardiol 1:584, 1958.
65. Chou T-C: Electrocardiography in Clinical Practice. Adult and Pediatric, 4th ed. Philadelphia, Saunders, 1996, p 3.
66. Bloomfield DA, Sinclair-Smith C: Persistent atrial standstill. Am J Med 39:335, 1965.
67. Waldo AL, Vitikainen KJ, Kaiser GA, et al: Atrial standstill secondary to atrial inexcitability (atrial quiescence): recognition and treatment following open heart surgery. Circulation 67:690, 1972.
68. Makita N, Dasaki K, Gronewegen WA, et al: Congenital atrial standstill associated with coinheritance of a novel SCN4A mutation and connexin 40 polymorphism. Heart Rhythm 2:1128, 2005.
69. Patton RD, Damato AN, Berkowitz WD, et al: The electrically silent right atrium. J Electrocardiol 3:239, 1970.
70. Harley A: Persistent right atrial standstill. Br Heart J 38:646, 1976.
71. Jacobson LB: Sinoventricular conduction during atrial arrest. J Electrocardiol 5:385, 1972.
72. Zipes DP, Gaum WA, Genetos BC, et al: Atrial tachycardia without P waves masquerading as an AV junctional tachycardia. Circulation 55:253, 1977.
73. Lipson MJ, Naimi S: Multifocal atrial tachycardia (chaotic atrial tachycardia). Circulation 42:397, 1970.
74. Phillips J, Spano J, Burch G: Chaotic atrial mechanism. Am Heart J 78:171, 1969.
75. Shine KI, Kastor JA, Yurchak PM: Multifocal atrial tachycardia: clinical and electrocardiographic features in 32 patients. N Engl J Med 279:344, 1968.
76. Saksena S, Siegel P, Rathyen W: Electrophysiologic mechanisms in postural supraventricular tachycardia. Am Heart J 106:151, 1983.
77. Josephson ME, Spear JF, Harken AH, et al: Surgical excision of automatic atrial tachycardia: anatomic and electrophysiologic correlates. Am Heart J 104:1076, 1982.
78. Kothari S, Apiyasawa S, Asad N, et al: Evidence supporting a new rate threshold for multifocal atrial tachycardia. Clin Cardiol 28:561, 2005.
79. Strickberger SA, Miller CB, Levine JH: Multifocal atrial tachycardia from electrolyte imbalance. Am Heart J 115:680, 1988.
80. Berlinerblau R, Feder W: Chaotic atrial rhythm. J Electrocardiol 5:135, 1972.
81. Chung EK: Appraisal of multifocal atrial tachycardia. Br Heart J 33:500, 1971.
82. Kones RJ, Phillips JH, Hersh J: Mechanism and management of chaotic atrial mechanism. Cardiology 59:92, 1974.
83. Bisset GS, Seigel SF, Gaum WE, et al: Chaotic atrial tachycardia in childhood. Am Heart J 101:268, 1981.
84. Chung KY, Walsh TJ, Massie E: Atrial parasystole. Am J Cardiol 14:255, 1964.
85. Friedberg HD, Schamroth L: Atrial parasystole. Br Heart J 32:172, 1970.
86. Kinoshita S, Takahashi K, Nakagawa K: Influence of early nonparasystolic impulses on the atrial parasystolic rhythm. Am J Cardiol 53:1455, 1984.
87. Oreto G, Luzza F, Satrillo G, et al: Sinus modulation of atrial parasystole. Am J Cardiol 58:1097, 1986.
88. Langendorf R, Lesser ME, Plotkin P, et al: Atrial parasystole with interpolation: observations on prolonged sinoatrial conduction. Am Heart J 63:649, 1962.
89. Chung KY, Walsh TJ, Massie E: A review of atrial dissociation, with illustrative cases and critical discussion. Am J Med Sci 250:72, 1965.
90. O'Donnell J: Dissimilar atrial rhythm. ACC Curr J Rev May/June:63, 1999.

15 Atrial Flutter and Atrial Fibrillation

Atrial Flutter
Clinical Correlation
Relation of Atrial Flutter to Other Atrial
   Arrhythmias and Differential Diagnosis
Mechanisms of Atrial Flutter
Implications for Treatment
Classification

Atrial Fibrillation
Ventricular Response

Pharmacologic and Mechanical Slowing
   of Ventricular Response
Morphology of Fibrillatory Waves
Clinical Correlations
Mechanism of Atrial Fibrillation
Implications for Treatment
Focal Atrial Fibrillation and Role of
   Pulmonary Veins
Diagnosis of Premature Ventricular
   Complexes in the Presence of Atrial
   Fibrillation

Atrial Flutter

Atrial flutter is characterized by a rapid, regular atrial rhythm at a rate of 200 to 400 beats/min. There are usually no isoelectric segments between the regular, uniformly shaped, biphasic, sawtooth-like oscillations. Most commonly the ventricular response in the absence of treatment is 2:1 but may be 4:1, 3:1, 3:2, or any other manifestation of a second-degree atrioventricular (AV) block (Figure 15–1). When the AV conduction varies, Wenckebach-type conduction is often recognized if there is gradual lengthening of the flutter-to-R interval until the expected conduction fails (Figure 15–2).

A higher-degree AV block usually results from impaired AV conduction or drug treatment. In the presence of complete AV block, the RR intervals are regular but the flutter waves have no constant relation to the QRS complexes (see Figure 15–1). The escape pacemaker may be located in the AV junction or in the ventricles. Atrial flutter with complete AV block may also be associated with AV junctional tachycardia.

One-to-one conduction during atrial flutter is one of the most hemodynamically perilous and life-threatening arrhythmias. It may occur when the impulse is conducted through an AV accessory pathway with a short refractory period or when the impulse is conducted through the AV node but the rate of flutter is slowed by an antiarrhythmic drug, particularly types IA and IC sodium channel–blocking antiarrhythmic drugs.

One-to-one conduction may be also precipitated by increased sympathetic stimulation (e.g., excitement, exercise, induction of anesthesia)[1] (Figures 15–3 to 15–5). Additionally, intravenous administration of atropine may result in 1:1 conduction. In two well-studied cases of 1:1 conduction, histologic examination revealed a bundle connecting the atrium with the His bundle.[2]

The flutter waves are usually best seen in leads II, III, aV_F, and V_1 (Figure 15–6). If the flutter waves are superimposed on the QRS complex and T waves, the rhythm may be difficult to recognize. Often small, sharp deflections in lead V_1 are helpful for determining the atrial rate, leading to a correct diagnosis[2] (see Figure 15–4B). Other methods for visualizing atrial flutter include recording the intraatrial or esophageal leads.[3,4]

Vagal maneuvers and adenosine administration are used to decrease the ventricular rate and to reveal the sawtooth appearance of the flutter (Figure 15–7). Vagal stimulation sometimes precipitates atrial fibrillation.[5]

CLINICAL CORRELATION

Atrial flutter may be chronic or paroxysmal. In general, flutter is a less stable rhythm than atrial fibrillation and frequently converts to atrial fibrillation or to sinus rhythm.[6] Atrial flutter usually occurs in association with atrial pathology, and most patients with atrial flutter have structural heart disease. The predisposing factors are atrial distension and atrial conduction disturbances, frequently manifested by a prolonged

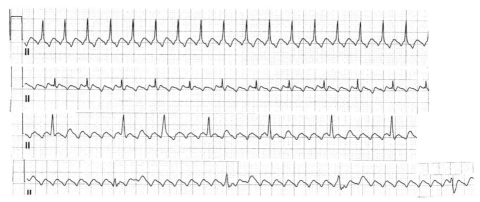

Figure 15–1 ECG strips of lead II showing atrial flutter with 2:1 response *(top row)*; 3:1 response *(second row)*; and varying response 6:1, 3:1, 4:1, 5:1, 5:1, 5:1 in six consecutive cycles *(third row)*, as well as complete AV block with an escape rhythm at a rate of 30 beats/min *(bottom row)*. The diagnosis of block is confirmed by the regular rate of the escape pacemaker and the absence of a constant relation between the flutter waves and the QRS complex.

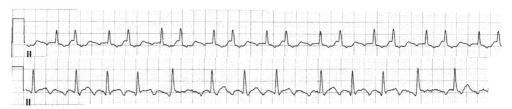

Figure 15–2 ECG strips of lead II show atrial flutter with Wenckebach-type conduction to the ventricles. *Top,* Constant 3:2 conduction. *Bottom,* Constant 2:1 block with progressive lengthening of each following conducted flutter–QRS duration. Arrangements are 4:3, 5:3, and 4:3 in three consecutive groups separated by a pause. The flutter rate and rhythm are unchanged, and the apparent absence of the flutter wave during the pause after the fifth and twelfth QRS complexes is explained by fusion of the negative flutter wave with the upright T wave.

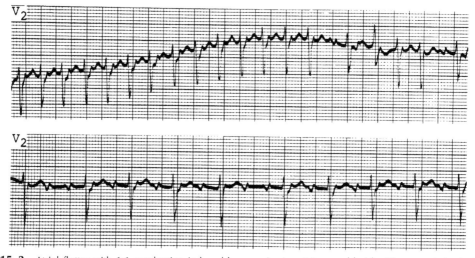

Figure 15–3 Atrial flutter with 1:1 conduction induced by exercise in a 16-year-old girl with congenital mitral insufficiency. A mitral valve prosthesis had been inserted 3 years previously. She was receiving digitalis and quinidine at the time this tracing was recorded. There is atrial flutter with 2:1 to 3:1 atrioventricular (AV) conduction at rest. Typical flutter wave morphology is seen in the inferior leads (not shown here). Atrial rate is 200 beats/min. The tracing taken immediately after exercise shows 1:1 AV conduction.

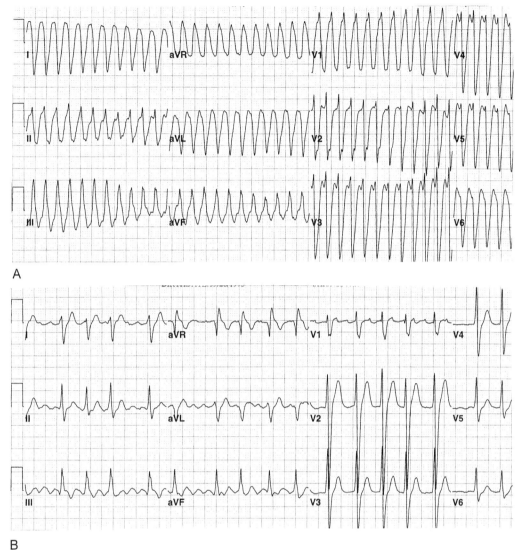

Figure 15–4   Atrial flutter in a 23-year-old man with alcoholic cardiomyopathy and intraventricular conduction disturbance. **A,** ECG in the emergency room shows atrial flutter with 1:1 response at a rate of 278 beats/min. **B,** Sixteen minutes later, the ventricular response varies from 2:1 to 3:1 with an average ventricular rate of 116 beats/min. Note the similar pattern of intraventricular conduction disturbance, with the QRS duration decreasing from 172 ms to 132 ms at a slower ventricular rate, apparently due to a lesser degree of aberrancy. The diagnosis of 1:1 flutter was confirmed in the electrophysiology laboratory. Patient had several episodes of 1:1 flutter during follow-up, usually precipitated by alcohol intake.

interatrial conduction time and prolonged P wave duration.[7]

Atrial flutter may be transient, lasting for minutes or hours, or it may persist for months or even years. In the study of Castellanos et al.,[8] 55 percent of the episodes in 49 patients lasted less than 7 days and 10 percent lasted longer than 1 year. In patients with acute myocardial infarction (MI), the incidence of atrial flutter in several studies ranged from 0.8 to 5.3 percent.[1] Atrial flutter can be seen in patients with acute and chronic cor pulmonale,[9,10] pulmonary embolism,[10] pericarditis,

or hyperthyroidism; after cardiac surgery; and in patients with atrial septal defect, both before and after surgical repair.[11] No evidence of organic heart disease is found in a small percentage of patients.[12]

RELATION OF ATRIAL FLUTTER TO OTHER ATRIAL ARRHYTHMIAS AND DIFFERENTIAL DIAGNOSIS

Atrial premature complexes are frequent precursors of atrial flutter. Epicardial mapping at the

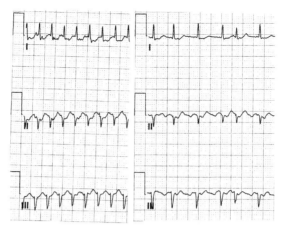

Figure 15–5   ECG leads I through III show atrial flutter in an 80-year-old patient with chronic lung disease. *Left,* 1:1 response with a ventricular rate of 254 beats/min, apparently precipitated by excitement. *Right,* At 96 seconds later, a varying ventricular response with an average ventricular rate of 163 beats/min.

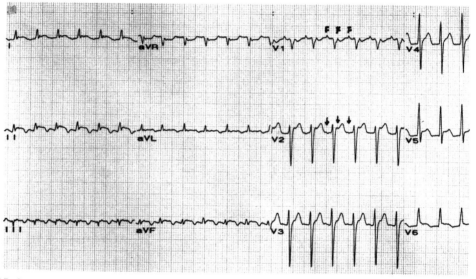

Figure 15–6   Acute pericarditis with atrial flutter in a 28-year-old woman with acute pericarditis and moderate pericardial effusion. The flutter waves can be seen in lead V₁ at a rate of 300 beats/min. There is 2:1 atrioventricular conduction. QRS voltage is low in the limb leads. The diffuse ST segment elevation is consistent with acute pericarditis.

onset of atrial flutter during the postoperative period showed that the typical flutter was initiated by a premature atrial complex followed by a transitional irregular atrial rhythm of variable duration (mean 9.35 seconds).[13] Atrial flutter and fibrillation occur often in the same person. They can appear on the same electrocardiogram (ECG) as atrial flutter-fibrillation, also known as "impure atrial flutter" (Figure 15–8). Treatment with digitalis shortens the atrial refractory period and often converts atrial flutter to atrial fibrillation. Conversely, treatment with sodium channel–blocking drugs such as quinidine or procainamide often converts atrial fibrillation to atrial flutter as a transitional stage before restoration of sinus

rhythm. During transition the flutter cycle tends to be slightly irregular, with variable morphology of the flutter waves.

Rytand et al.[14] found an apparent relation between atrial size and the rate of flutter. Patients with markedly enlarged atria tended to have a slower rate, and massive dilatation of the atria was accompanied by increased duration of the flutter cycle, resulting in rates of less than 200 beats/min in some patients. Also, sodium channel–blocking antiarrhythmic drugs decrease the rate of flutter waves, whereas digitalis tends to increase the rate.

Repetitive atrial flutter is an unusual form of atrial flutter in which episodes of atrial flutter

Control

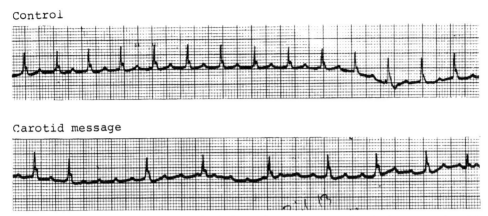

Carotid message

Figure 15–7   Atrial flutter with 2:1 conduction. The rhythm in the upper strip may be mistaken as ectopic atrial tachycardia with a rate of 133 beats/min. On carotid sinus massage, flutter waves at a rate of 266 beats/min are demonstrated during the period of increased atrioventricular block.

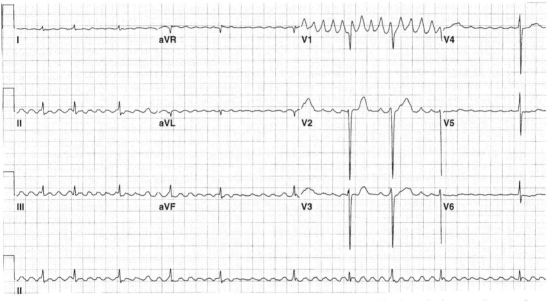

Figure 15–8   Variable morphology of flutter waves, best seen in the rhythm strip of lead II at the bottom. The term *flutter-fibrillation* is used to describe such a rhythm.

are interrupted by a few sinus complexes (Figure 15–9). Ectopic atrial tachycardia and atrial flutter seldom coexist in the same patient, but the attacks of atrial flutter may be followed by sinus bradycardia in patients with the tachycardia-bradycardia syndrome.

Atrial flutter must be considered in the differential diagnosis of narrow QRS tachycardias; it is one of the most common causes of such arrhythmias in the elderly and patients with structural heart disease. Unlike sinus tachycardia, the ventricular rate during atrial flutter tends to remain stable. More difficult is the differential diagnosis among atrial flutter with a 2:1 response, AV

nodal reentrant tachycardia, AV reentrant tachycardia, and AV junctional automatic and ectopic atrial tachycardia because of the similar ventricular rates in all of these tachycardias. The uncertainty arises when only half of the flutter waves are visible. It may be helpful in such cases to measure the distance between the two visible atrial deflections and project one half of this distance onto the ECG. This may reveal whether the morphology of the ECG at that point in time is compatible with the presence of a disguised second flutter deflection.

Abnormally wide QRS complexes during atrial flutter may be due to a preexisting intraventricular

II

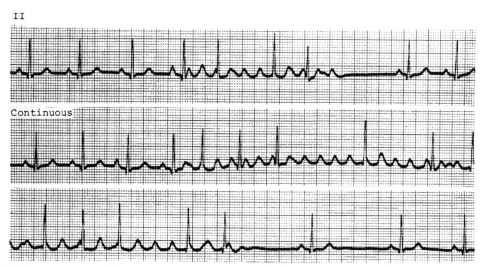

Figure 15–9 Repetitive atrial flutter in a 32-year-old woman who has no symptoms and shows no other evidence of organic heart disease. Flutter rate varies during different episodes. Flutter waves are of the uncommon type, in that they are upright in lead II.

conduction disturbance, ventricular preexcitation, aberrant conduction, or the effect of antiarrhythmic (particularly IC type) drugs (Figure 15–10). Atrial flutter with a wide QRS complex and 2:1 response may be indistinguishable from ventricular tachycardia when the flutter waves are masked by ventricular complexes.

MECHANISMS OF ATRIAL FLUTTER

The proposed mechanisms of atrial flutter include (1) a large reentrant loop, (2) a small reentrant loop, and (3) a single focus or multiple foci of automaticity.[14,15] Lewis et al.[16] favored the mechanism of circus movement, with the main wave traveling around the orifices of the venae cavae and providing tangential offshoots to excite the remainder of the atria. Studies of Allessie et al.[17] in the rabbit atria demonstrated

reentry of the leading-circle type without an anatomic obstacle and without an excitable gap. Boineau[18] carried out extensive mapping of the atria in a dog with spontaneous atrial flutter and observed two forms of flutter. Both forms resulted from circus movement reentry with zones of fast and slow conduction: one type due to clockwise and the other due to counterclockwise motion in the right atrium. This study emphasized the importance of a large anatomic obstacle in the maintenance of flutter and suggested that the difference between the polarity of flutter waves was due to different activation patterns.

Waldo's group developed a model of sterile pericarditis for studying experimental flutter in dogs.[19] In this model,[20] in which a diffuse inflammatory reaction involved 50 to 80 percent of the atrial wall, atrial flutter was associated

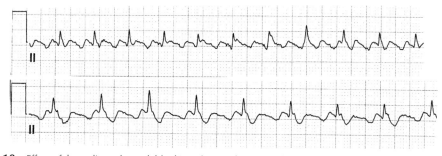

Figure 15–10 Effect of the sodium channel–blocking class IC drug propafenone on the rate of atrial flutter in a 73-year-old woman with chronic obstructive lung disease. ECG strips are from lead II before treatment *(top)* and after 1 week of treatment with 300 mg propafenone twice daily *(bottom)*. Before treatment the flutter rate is 250 beats/min with 2:1 ventricular response. After treatment the flutter rate is 186 beats/min with 2:1 ventricular response. Thus the ventricular rate decreased from 125 to 93 beats/min, and QRS duration increased after propafenone treatment from 94 ms to 106 ms.

with a single loop of reentry that included a region of slow conduction. These observations in a model with an inflicted lesion were in agreement with the findings of Boineau in a dog with a naturally acquired lesion and suggested that atrial flutter is sustained by the presence of two barriers, one formed by the normal anatomic structures (e.g., the vena cava) and the other by a pathologic obstacle to conduction (e.g., a scar). The experimental and clinical studies of Waldo and co-workers[15] established that type I flutter involved a large reentrant circuit with an excitable gap.

The existence of automatic foci in rare cases of atrial flutter was recognized by Wellens et al.[21] In some cases, atrial flutter coexists with typical automatic atrial tachycardias. In most cases, however, atrial flutter is a reentrant arrhythmia with an excitable gap in the right atrium and a wave of excitation traveling up the septum and down the free wall of the right atrium. The site of slow conduction in the reentrant circuit is located inferiorly and posteriorly in the right atrium, but individual variations in the zone of block occur because the ascending medial septal activation does not follow a consistent pattern.[22]

The evidence in support of reentry include (1) initiation and termination by pacing (Watson and Josephson[23] induced atrial flutter by programmed electrical stimulation in about 80 percent of patients with documented atrial flutter); (2) patterns of entrainment by overdrive pacing; (3) demonstration of fragmented electrical activity covering 36 to 100 percent of the flutter cycle, predominantly in the right atrium, with disappearance or marked decrease of fragmentation after reestablishing the sinus rhythm[24]; and (4) patterns of resetting by premature stimuli[25] similar to those seen with reentrant ventricular tachycardia (see Chapter 17).

With typical human atrial flutter, the crista terminalis, eustachian ridge, and tricuspid annulus have been identified as barriers to conduction.[26] The tricuspid annulus constitutes a continuous anterior barrier constraining the reentrant wavefront of counterclockwise atrial flutter.[27] A fully excitable gap is present in all portions of the circuit.[28] The upper turnover site of the reentry circuit of a common atrial flutter is anterior to the orifice of the superior vena cava.[29]

IMPLICATIONS FOR TREATMENT

Experimental studies suggest that the region of slow conduction may represent the proper target of interventions. In humans, Puech et al.[30]

described an isthmus of slow conduction in the posteroseptal part of the right atrium between the orifices of the inferior vena cava, the coronary sinus, and the tricuspid ring. Frequent involvement of this area in circus movement atrial flutter suggests that it could represent a promising target of ablation to interrupt atrial flutter.[2] Subsequent studies have shown that atrial flutter can be abolished permanently by radiofrequency pulses delivered at the narrowest part in the tissue between the tricuspid valve ring and the orifices of the inferior vena cava and proximal coronary sinus, respectively.[31–36] The most common area of ablation is in the cavotricuspid isthmus flanked by the inferior vena cava, the tricuspid valve, and the coronary sinus ostium. The effectiveness of ablation requires demonstration of "isthmus block"[37,38] (Figure 15–11). The success rate of the abolition of bidirectional transisthmus conduction is 95 percent.[35,39] Recurrences are rare and in most cases represent recovery of isthmus conduction after a complete block.[36]

Rational pharmacologic treatment of atrial flutter may consist of (1) slowing conduction to block the propagation within the circuit or (2) lengthening the refractory period to prolong the wavelength of the tachycardia.[40]

CLASSIFICATION

Atrial flutter exemplifies a macro-reentrant tachycardia. Wells et al.[3] classified atrial flutter into two types.[3] In type I the atrial rate is 240 to 350 beats/min (although it can be faster or slower, particularly during treatment with antiarrhythmic drugs) (see Figure 15–10), and the flutter can be entrained by atrial pacing. In type II the rate of flutter is 340 to 430 beats/min, and the flutter cannot be entrained by rapid pacing.

Type I atrial flutter is more often called *common* or *typical atrial flutter* and is subdivided into a more prevalent counterclockwise (cephalad) type with the flutter wave axis directed superiorly (i.e., inverted deflection in leads II, III, and aV$_F$) (see Figure 15–1) and a less prevalent clockwise type (cranial to caudal) with flutter waves upright in leads II, III, and aV$_F$ (Figure 15–12). In lead V$_1$ the flutter waves are upright in the common type but are either upright or inverted in the uncommon type. It has been suggested that in a clockwise atrial flutter the left atrium is activated predominantly over Bachmann's bundle and in a counterclockwise flutter predominantly over coronary sinus.[41] The clockwise pattern includes a so-called upper loop involving the upper portion of the right atrium.[42]

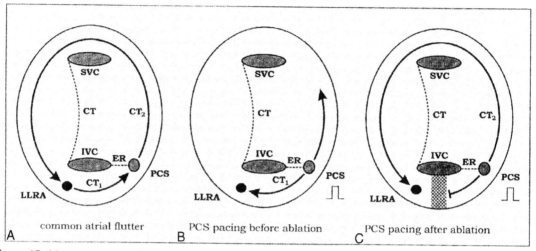

Figure 15–11 Measurement of isthmus conduction before and after isthmus ablation for treatment of atrial flutter. CT = crista terminalis; CT_1 = conduction across the isthmus; CT_2 = conduction time over roof of right atrium; ER = eustachian ridge; IVC = inferior vena cava; LLRA = low lateral right atrium; PCS = proximal coronary sinus; SVC = superior vena cava. (From Johna R, Eckardt L, Fetsch T, et al: A new algorithm to determine complete isthmus conduction block after radiofrequency catheter ablation for typical atrial flutter. Am J Cardiol 94:1666, 1999. Copyright 1999 Excerpta Medica, Inc., by permission.)

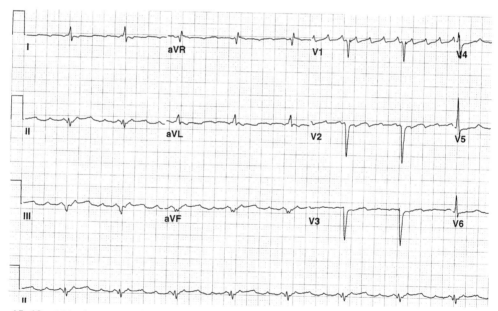

Figure 15–12 ECG of a 65-year-old man with coronary artery disease shows clockwise-type typical atrial flutter with upright flutter waves in leads II and III. Rate of flutter is 244, and ventricular response is 4:1.

Most right atrial flutters with positive flutter wave on surface ECG may be supported by a reentrant circuit around the inferior vena cava or a figure-eight, double-loop reentry involving both the inferior vena cava and tricuspid annulus.[43] Rarely, both clockwise and counterclockwise flutter types are present in the same person on different occasions (Figure 15–13).

Type II atrial flutter is also known as *atypical* or *uncommon atrial flutter*. It comprises a heterogeneous group of unstable arrhythmias that are transitional to atrial fibrillation.[4] This arrhythmia is not infrequently induced in the electrophysiology laboratory by atrial pacing.[4] The sequence of activation is usually incompatible with clockwise or counterclockwise atrial flutter.

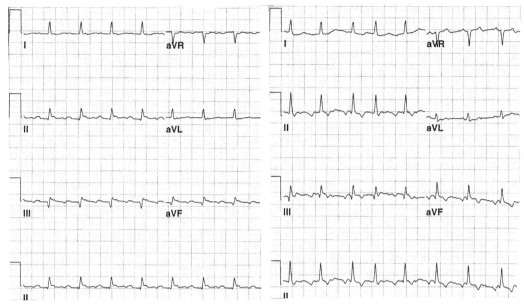

Figure 15–13   Two variants of typical atrial flutter in the same patient on two occasions at a 1-month interval. *Left,* ECG recorded on June 15 shows atrial flutter at a rate of 222 beats/min with 2:1 ventricular response and upright flutter waves in leads II and III. *Right,* ECG recorded on July 14 shows atrial flutter at a rate of 236 beats/min with a variable ventricular response and inverted flutter waves in leads II and III.

TABLE 15–1	Atrial Flutter (Rapid [250 to 350 beats/min] Macro-Reentrant Atrial Rhythm)

Right atrial flutter

  I. Isthmus dependent
    A. Clockwise and counterclockwise
    B. Double wave reentry
    C. Lower loop reentry (single break or multiple breaks)
 II. Nonisthmus dependent
    A. Upper loop reentry
    B. "Scar" reentry
    C. Critical flutter circuits
III. Surgical circuits
    A. Incisional scar
    B. Isthmus dependent
    C. Complex circuits

Left atrial circuits

    A. Mitral annular circuits
    B. "Scar" related
    C. Left membranous circuits

The inability to entrain most such arrhythmias suggests a leading circle mechanism[5] without a fully excitable gap[4] or a focal mechanism. It has been shown that atypical atrial flutter may exhibit variable periodicity, making it difficult to distinguish from atrial fibrillation.[43a] Gomes et al.[44] defined uncommon atrial flutter as a heterogeneous

entity involving more than one circuit, localized atrial fibrillation, or both. Left atrial circuits may be recognized in the ECG because of flat or low-amplitude forces in the inferior leads.[45] Slowing of conduction in the left atrial septum due to antiarrhythmic drugs or atrial myopathy appears to cause left septal atrial flutter.[46]

Table 15–1 shows the classification of atrial flutter proposed by Scheinman[47] and based on specific circuits.

Atrial Fibrillation

Atrial fibrillation is a disorganized, asynchronous fractionated activity recognizable by the absence of P waves and the presence of small irregular oscillations, so-called fibrillatory waves. Atrial fibrillation may be acute or chronic, paroxysmal, or established. The paroxysmal episodes occur suddenly and last for seconds, minutes, or days. They terminate spontaneously but tend to recur and eventually may become established. The predictors of recurrence include advanced age, increased left atrial size, impaired left ventricular function, and heart failure.[48,49]

Permanent atrial fibrillation signifies the presence of a permanent anatomic or electrophysiologic disturbance leading to propagation of chaotic impulses. Electrophysiologic abnormalities found in patients with atrial fibrillation include sinoatrial

(SA) node dysfunction, a short atrial refractory period, intraatrial conduction disturbances, and a wide zone of fragmented activity.[2]

Electrocardiographically, fibrillation may be fine or coarse, without evidence of organized activity on the surface ECG or in the endocavitary leads. In patients with paroxysmal recurrent atrial fibrillation with or without heart disease, the fibrillatory process may begin as atrial flutter or may be precipitated by one or more atrial premature complexes (Figures 15–14 to 15–16). In a number of patients with paroxysmal supraventricular tachycardia, atrial fibrillation evolves during an attack of tachycardia.[50]

Paroxysmal atrial fibrillation ends spontaneously after some seconds (see Figure 15–14), minutes, hours, or days. This means that the electrophysiologic matrix is not permanently abnormal. This conclusion is usually supported by the normal pattern of P waves during sinus rhythm and the inability to initiate permanent atrial fibrillation by rapid pacing or premature atrial stimulation. Because both sympathetic and vagal stimulation shorten the refractory

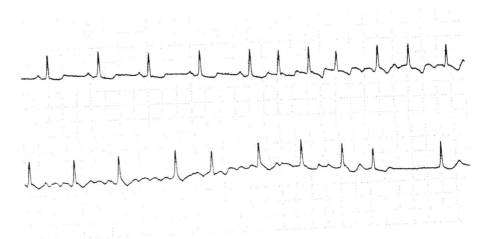

Figure 15–14   Continuous record during ambulatory monitoring shows onset and termination of a short episode of atrial fibrillation.

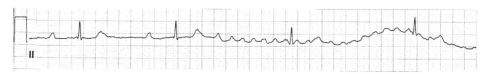

Figure 15–15   ECG strip of lead II shows transition from sinus rhythm with 2:1 atrioventricular block to atrial flutter, followed by atrial fibrillation.

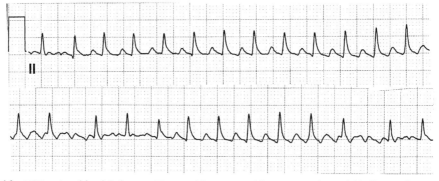

Figure 15–16   ECG strip of lead II from a 60-year-old woman with paroxysmal atrial fibrillation shows a continuous tracing sequence of atrial fibrillation, sinus tachycardia, atrial flutter, atrial fibrillation, sinus rhythm, atrial flutter, and atrial fibrillation.

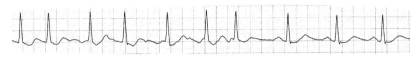

Figure 15–17   ECG strip of lead II shows termination of atrial fibrillation and resumption of sinus rhythm.

period of the atrial muscle, atrial fibrillation can be induced experimentally and clinically by sympathetic and vagal stimulation. It is believed that the autonomic nervous system plays a major role in precipitating paroxysmal atrial fibrillation, and it has been observed that in some patients the attacks occur preferentially at night or at rest when the heart rate is slow and in others preferentially when the heart rate is rapid (e.g., during exercise).[51] Shortening the atrial refractory period plays an important role not only in the initiation but also the maintenance of atrial fibrillation, a phenomenon called *electrical remodeling*.[52] Spontaneous termination of atrial fibrillation is often preceded by atrial flutter, although it may occur suddenly (Figure 15–17). Transition of atrial fibrillation to ventricular tachycardia, as seen in Figure 15–18, is a rare event.

An international consensus on nomenclature and classification of atrial fibrillation[53] proposed a subdivision of this arrhythmia into the following four categories: (1) initial (first-detected) event that may be symptomatic or asymptomatic and may or may not recur; (2) paroxysmal that terminates spontaneously within 48 hours and may be recurrent; (3) persisting, not self-terminating and lasting >7 days, or after prior cardioversion; and (4) permanent (established) that may or may not be terminated, or that relapses after cardioversion. The main purpose of this subdivision is to establish guidelines for therapy.

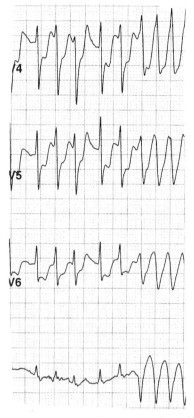

Figure 15–18   ECG leads V_4–V_6 and II show the transition from atrial fibrillation to ventricular tachycardia in a 79-year-old man with an acute inferior myocardial infarction.

VENTRICULAR RESPONSE

The ventricular rate in patients with atrial fibrillation is determined by the number of impulses that manage to reach the ventricles by overcoming both the time-dependent refractoriness of the AV node and the voltage-dependent refractoriness of the His-Purkinje system. An important role in the control of the ventricular rate during atrial fibrillation is attributed to concealed conduction of impulses in the AV node. The concept of concealed conduction is supported by the observations that the RR interval usually increases after a premature ventricular complex, which means that the retrograde penetration of the AV node by the ventricular impulse prolongs the refractory period and interferes with the

anterograde transmission of atrial impulses. Other factors contributing to rate control are the basic characteristics of the refractory period and the conductivity of the AV node,[54] electrotonic modulation,[55,56] the function of the AV junctional escape pacemakers,[57] and the strength and direction of atrial impulses reaching the AV node from the atria. As is evident from the frequent occurrence of aberrant intraventricular conduction, particularly right bundle branch block (RBBB), the long-lasting, voltage-dependent refractoriness of the conducting system distal to the AV node is a factor controlling the ventricular rate during atrial fibrillation and other atrial tachyarrhythmias.[2]

In the presence of incomplete AV block, the rate of impulses transmitted to the ventricles decreases and the irregularity of the responses tends to lessen. In the presence of high-degree AV block, the ventricles are driven by AV junctional or ventricular escape rhythms (Figures 15–19 to 15–22). When a degree of AV conduction remains preserved, the rate of these escape pacemakers may be influenced by concealed conduction of atrial impulses. When the escape pacemaker is in the ventricles, the QRS complex is usually wide. An accelerated AV junctional rhythm or AV junctional tachycardia causes regular narrow QRS tachycardias in the presence of atrial fibrillation (Figure 15–23, top strip). Wenckebach periodicity during AV junctional rhythm is not uncommon (see Figure 15–23, bottom strip). Regular ventricular response can also occur by changing to atrial flutter or by treatment with antiarrhythmia class IC drugs.[58]

During pacing-induced atrial fibrillation in humans, three responses have been observed: types I, II, and III. The irregularity, complexity, and incidence of continuous electrical activity and reentry increase from type I to type III.[59] With type I, which resembles atrial flutter, a single broad wave propagates uniformly across the right atrium. Local capture is often possible with this type owing to the presence of an excitable gap in the right and left atria.[60]

In patients with untreated atrial fibrillation the ventricular rate is often faster than 150 beats/min (Figure 15–24) and is typically accelerated by exercise, even if it is well controlled at rest (Figure 15–25). Myocardial ischemia may be exposed during a rapid rate analogous to a positive stress test (see Figure 15–25). At rapid rates, the QRS duration may increase

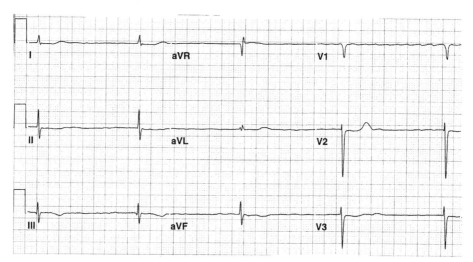

Figure 15–19   Atrial fibrillation with complete atrioventricular (AV) block and slow AV junctional escape rhythm at a rate of 34 beats/min.

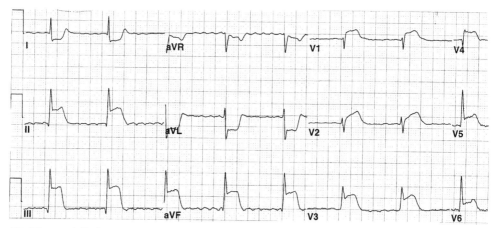

Figure 15–20   Atrial fibrillation with complete atrioventricular (AV) block and AV junctional escape rhythm at a rate of 58 beats/min from a 49-year-old man with acute inferior and right ventricular myocardial infarction.

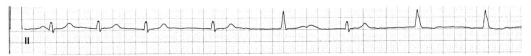

Figure 15–21 ECG strip of lead II from a 90-year-old woman with chronic atrial fibrillation. Note the slow ventricular response caused by high-degree atrioventricular block. Fifth, seventh, and eighth complexes are ventricular escape complexes.

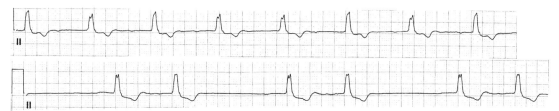

Figure 15–22 ECG strips of lead II from a 69-year-old man with coronary artery disease, mitral and aortic valve prostheses, chronic atrial fibrillation, and escape rhythm with left bundle branch block morphology. *Top,* Regular escape rhythm at a rate of 53 beats/min. *Bottom,* On the same-day ECG strip, note the same rhythm with pauses that are exactly twice as long as the cycle length, indicating an exit block.

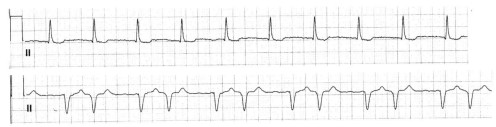

Figure 15–23 ECG strips of lead II show atrial fibrillation in two patients treated with digitalis. *Top,* Regular, presumably atrioventricular junctional rhythm at a rate of 79 beats/min. *Bottom,* Group beating suggests a 3:2 response of the escape pacemaker with right bundle branch block and left anterior fascicular block morphology.

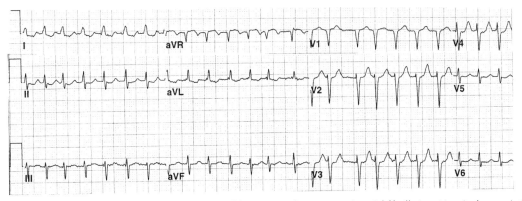

Figure 15–24 ECG strip of lead II from an 84-year-old woman with symptomatic atrial fibrillation. Ventricular rate is 165 beats/min.

owing to aberrant intraventricular conduction or a tachycardia-dependent bundle branch block, creating a wide QRS tachycardia (Figure 15–26).

Atrial fibrillation is one of the most serious arrhythmias in patients with preexcitation syndromes. In the presence of a bypass tract, rapid transmission of impulses through the accessory AV pathway to the ventricles can result in ventricular fibrillation and sudden cardiac death.

Patients with Wolff-Parkinson-White (WPW) syndrome appear to be predisposed to atrial fibrillation, with an incidence ranging from 10 to 30 percent. Langendorf et al.[61] pointed out that preexcitation should be suspected if the

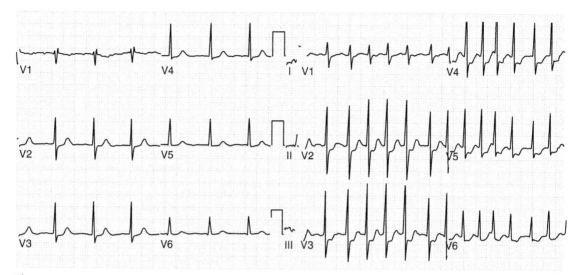

Figure 15–25   Chronic atrial fibrillation in a 79-year old woman. ECGs are recorded on 2 consecutive days. When the rate is controlled (94 beats/min), the ventricular complex is normal. At a rapid rate (172 beats/min), diffuse ST segment depression suggests myocardial ischemia; the patient was dyspneic but had no chest pain.

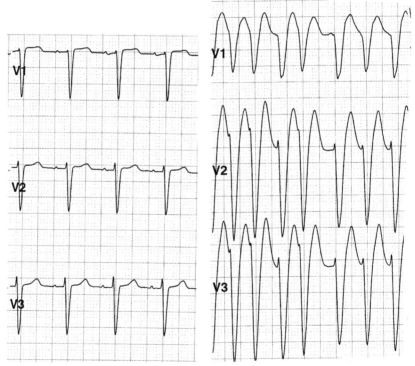

Figure 15–26   ECG leads V_1-V_3 from a 70-year-old man during sinus rhythm at a rate of 97 beats/min and during atrial fibrillation with a ventricular rate of 176 beats/min. QRS duration increased from 100 ms to 130 ms at a rapid rate.

ventricular rate during atrial fibrillation is unusually rapid (i.e., >200 beats/min). Castellanos et al.[62] demonstrated that the rapid ventricular rate is associated with a short effective refractory period of the accessory pathway. This association was confirmed by Wellens and Durrer during atrial fibrillation induced in patients with WPW syndrome.[63] A short effective refractory period (i.e., ≤250 ms) increases the risk of ventricular fibrillation in the presence of atrial fibrillation,

W.-P-W syndrome with atrial fibrillation
Lead Ⅱ   Vent. rate 230

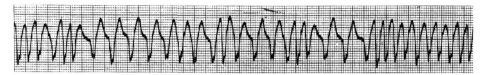

Simultaneous intracardiac lead and limb lead

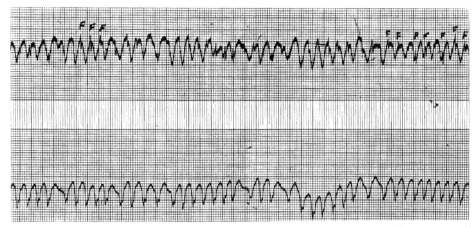

Figure 15–27 Atrial fibrillation in a patient with Wolff-Parkinson-White syndrome. Ventricular rate is 230 beats/min. Intracardiac electrogram shows the fibrillatory waves (F).

atrial flutter, or other rapid atrial tachycardia. Figure 15–27 shows rapid conduction through an accessory pathway with a short refractory period during atrial fibrillation. The incidence of atrial fibrillation is also increased in the presence of multiple accessory pathways and slow intra-atrial conduction.[2] Factors contributing to a rapid ventricular rate during atrial fibrillation other than the refractory period of the accessory pathway are concealment of impulses in the AV node, supernormal conduction through the accessory pathway, and the pattern of atrial input into the accessory pathway.[64,65]

Unlike the AV node, the refractory period of the accessory pathway tends to decrease as the rate increases. Fillette and Fontaine[66] studied RR histograms of patients with atrial fibrillation and found that the range of RR intervals distinguished patients with and without preexcitation. The conduction properties through the accessory pathway vary depending on the frequency of impulses reaching the atrial pole of the pathway and the influences of the autonomic nervous system. In the presence of accessory pathways with short refractory periods, ventricular responses may reach rates up to 300 beats/min. The tachycardias are usually irregular, with polymorphic configuration of the

ventricular complexes, as the ventricular activation reflects fusion of the complexes conducted through the accessory and normal AV pathways. The assessment of risk is facilitated by testing the effects of transient atrial fibrillation, exercise, and isoproterenol infusion.[2]

The incidence of atrial fibrillation in patients with preexcitation appears to be increased by the presence of reentrant tachycardia. This is suggested by the low recurrence rate of atrial fibrillation after ablation of the accessory pathways.[67] The probable mechanism of atrial fibrillation is stimulation during the atrial vulnerable period by the impulse returning to the atria. In patients with WPW syndrome and atrial fibrillation, retrograde conduction over the accessory pathway contributed up to 9 percent of the total atrial wavefront near the accessory pathway, indicating the presence of an excitable gap during human atrial fibrillation.[65]

PHARMACOLOGIC AND MECHANICAL SLOWING OF VENTRICULAR RESPONSE

Slowing the ventricular response in clinical practice can be accomplished by decreasing the number of impulses traversing the AV node. The categories of drugs capable of accomplishing this include: (1) digitalis by means of vagal stimulation and a direct effect; (2) β-adrenergic blockade; (3) subset of calcium channel–blocking agents acting on the AV node (e.g., verapamil, diltiazem); (4) class III antiarrhythmic drugs; and (5) adenosine. Slowing the ventricular response adequately may be difficult when the drug effect is counteracted by increased sympathetic stimulation (e.g., during exercise or with fever, infection, or anemia).

Atrioventricular conduction during atrial fibrillation can be modified by radiofrequency ablation of the right mid-septal and posteroseptal region of the tricuspid annulus, a procedure that eliminates the posterior atrionodal input,[68] or by ablation of the slow AV nodal pathway.[69,70] It has been shown that in patients with dual AV nodal pathways, the slow pathway plays the dominant role in determining the ventricular rate.[71] Observations during ambulatory monitoring[72] suggest that dual AV node physiology could be recognized by the presence of bimodal distribution of RR intervals.

MORPHOLOGY OF FIBRILLATORY WAVES

Studies have shown that atrial activation during atrial fibrillation is not entirely random, because the activation front follows the receding tail of refractoriness.[73] The tendency of wavefronts to follow paths of previous excitation is termed *linking*. Examination of intraatrial electrograms during atrial fibrillation showed transient similarities in the direction of wavelet propagation in most patients with atrial fibrillation, a finding consistent with the presence of transient linking.[73]

The atrial rate during atrial fibrillation ranges from 400 to 700 beats/min. The fibrillatory (f) waves are best seen in the inferior and right precordial leads V_{3R} and V_1. In some cases, however, f waves are not seen in any leads, and the diagnosis of atrial fibrillation is based on the irregularity of the ventricular rhythm. Depending on their amplitude, f waves are called *fine* or *coarse*. Some authors consider f waves of >0.05 mV amplitude as coarse, whereas others use 0.1 mV amplitude as the dividing line[1] (Figure 15–28). Exploration of the atria with multiple catheter electrodes in 16 patients showed that the amplitude of f waves in lead V_1 averaged 0.128 mV (coarse f waves) in the presence of cranio-caudal direction of activation and 0.06 mV (fine f waves) during disorganized activity.[74] In earlier studies the coarse waves

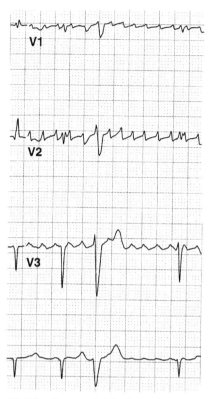

Figure 15–28   Coarse atrial fibrillation in an 84-year-old man with coronary artery disease. The wide QRS complex is probably caused by aberrant conduction. From top to bottom: leads V_1, V_2, V_3, and II.

were found more often in patients with rheumatic valvular heart disease and the fine waves in patients with other cardiomyopathies.[75] This etiologic association may no longer be valid in this era of declining incidence of rheumatic valvular disease and early surgery or valvuloplasty of valvular lesions. Several earlier studies reported that the conversion to sinus rhythm is more difficult in patients with fine waves than in those with the coarse variety.[1]

Today, separation of atrial fibrillation into coarse or fine is difficult to justify from a clinical point of view because the amplitude of fibrillatory waves on the ECG differs among leads and is not constant in any single lead. This may explain contradictory results of the correlations between the amplitude of the fibrillatory waves vs. atrial size and other clinical variables such as the etiology of heart disease or duration of arrhythmia.

Leier and Schaal[76] recorded right and left atrial electrograms in patients with coarse atrial fibrillation and atrial flutter-fibrillation. In those patients with the coarse type, the atrial fibrillation was biatrial. Flutter-fibrillation, however, signified the presence of regular tachycardia or flutter some-where in the atria and was usually associated with dissimilar atrial rhythms in the two atria. In some cases the researchers found dissimilar atrial flutter rates or fragmented flutter in two different parts of the right atrium. Earlier, Puech[77] showed that the rates of local activity in the atria varied at different recording sites and that regular and irregular depo-larizations coexisted in some cases. Zipes and De Joseph[78] recorded simultaneously right atrial and esophageal electrograms in patients with dis-similar atrial rhythms and concluded that the change from fibrillation in one atrium into more regular activity in the contralateral atrium was caused by a longer, more uniform refractory period in the latter than in the former. Simultaneous occurrence of atrial fibrillation and atrial flutter in different parts of the atria has been confirmed in patients undergoing ablation of atrial flutter and has been attributed to a possible functional interatrial block as the mechanism.[79]

CLINICAL CORRELATIONS

Most patients with established atrial fibrillation have evidence of structural heart disease with increased left atrial pressure or volume (e.g., hypertensive, ischemic, dilated, hypertrophic, or restrictive cardiomyopathy) or both. In the absence of symptomatic heart disease, the most important etiologic factor is age. In a prospective study of 5201 persons age 65 or older followed for an average period of 3.28 years, the inci-dence of atrial fibrillation was 19.2 per 1000 person-years, increasing with age, male gender, and the presence of clinical cardiovascular disease.[80] The incidence of atrial fibrillation in subjects aged >100 years was 30%.[81] Atrial fibril-lation is the most common atrial tachyarrhythmia in patients with acute MI, and its presence pre-dicts an increased incidence of stroke and a higher mortality rate.[82,83] Atrial fibrillation tends to occur in the presence of right coronary occlu-sion when there is coexistent occlusion of the left circumflex artery proximal to its left atrial cir-cumflex branch, resulting in impaired perfusion of the AV nodal artery and left atrial ischemia.[84] The overall incidence of atrial fibrillation in 3254 patients enrolled in the GUSTO-I trial was 10.4 percent.[83] In one study, left ventricular function was more impaired in patients who developed atrial fibrillation later than 24 hours after the onset of infarction than in those in whom atrial fibrillation appeared earlier.[85]

In patients with hyperthyroidism, the inci-dence of paroxysmal or established atrial fib-rillation is about 10 to 15 percent.[86] Atrial fibrillation is relatively uncommon in patients with acute pericarditis[1] but is common in those with constrictive pericarditis.[87]

Atrial fibrillation occurs transiently often after coronary artery bypass surgery. In one study the incidence was 27 percent.[88] Independent pre-dictors of this complication were advanced age, male gender, history of atrial fibrillation, history of congestive heart failure, and surgical practices such as a long cross-clamping time and pulmo-nary vein venting.[88] In a collaborative study of 106,780 Medicare beneficiaries over 65 years of age treated for acute MI between 1994 and 1996, atrial fibrillation was present in 22.1 percent (about half of subjects presented with it, and the other half developed it during hospitali-zation). Atrial fibrillation was an independent predictor of in-hospital and 1-year mortality. Patients who developed atrial fibrillation during hospitalization had a worse prognosis than those who had it on admission.[89]

Idiopathic or lone atrial fibrillation in the absence of heart disease is usually paroxysmal and frequently recurrent, often precipitated by the consumption of alcoholic beverages[90–93]; the sustained form seldom develops in these subjects.[94] The vagally mediated form of parox-ysmal lone atrial fibrillation is preferentially observed in young male adults in whom an ECG pattern of common atrial flutter alternates with atrial fibrillation.[95]

MECHANISM OF ATRIAL FIBRILLATION

Induction of atrial fibrillation requires a critical tissue mass. West and Lauda[96] showed that there is a critical weight of the tissue below which fibrillation cannot be induced. In their study the critical weight was 32 mg for the left atrium and 28 mg for the right atrium. Just as there is a critical mass below which fibrillation cannot occur, there is also a critical rate above which regular organized activity cannot continue. Thus at a certain rate, atrial flutter progresses to atrial fibrillation, provided there is critical tissue mass available to sustain fibrillation. In the laboratory, atrial fibrillation can be induced by stimulation during the vulnerable period, rapid pacing, local application of aconitine, isoproterenol infusion, acetylcholine infusion, and strong vagal stimuli.[2]

Atrial fibrillation can be started from a single, presumably automatic focus (e.g., by topical application of aconitine to the atrial appendage). Such atrial fibrillation disappears when the atrium is isolated from the focus.[2] In this case, the mechanism of fibrillation differs from atrial fibrillation initiated by rapid pacing, which remains self-sustaining when pacing is discontinued. This type of atrial fibrillation is attributed to a multitude of reentrant wavelets, a mechanism simulated in a computer model by Moe et al.[97] In this model, fibrillation was sustained by a number of independent wavelets coursing around islands of refractory tissue. Each wavelet may accelerate or decelerate as it encounters elements at different stages of excitability. The wavelets may divide, coalesce, or become extinguished. The greater the number of independent wavelets, the less chance there is of spontaneous termination. In dogs with sterile pericarditis, changes of the functional block in the right atrial wall were critical for conversion of atrial flutter to atrial fibrillation and atrial fibrillation to atrial flutter.[98] The absence of degeneration of established atrial flutter to atrial fibrillation has been attributed to the stabilizing effect of the anatomic barriers that define the substrate of atrial flutter.[99] Atrial fibrillation occurs in about 12 percent of paroxysmal reentrant AV nodal tachycardias.[100] In such cases the AV nodal reentrant impulse acts as a trigger for atrial fibrillation.

Allessie et al.[101] confirmed the validity of Moe's model using 192 electrode terminals to follow the spread of excitation during atrial fibrillation induced by rapid pacing and acetylcholine in a blood-perfused dog heart. Maps of human atria during atrial fibrillation have been similar to those in experimental animals. Atrial fibrillation was sustained by multiple wandering wavelets, and various areas were reexcited from different sites; thus there was little opportunity for any of the wavelets to complete reentry.[98] However, extensive mapping studies by Ferguson and Cox[102] revealed the presence of complete macro-reentrant loops in some instances and partial reentrant loops in others. This may explain cases in which regional entrainment of chronic atrial fibrillation was feasible in humans[103] and cases in which atrial fibrillation originated in a single right or left atrial focus firing irregularly, with the arrhythmias being eliminated by radiofrequency pulses[104] (see later discussion).

The discovery that focal ablation could eliminate paroxysmal atrial fibrillation revived the theory that atrial fibrillation could originate from a rapidly firing focus.[105] Weiss et al.[106] proposed that fibrillation is initiated by wavebreak occurring when an emerging wavefront encounters refractory tissue and splits into daughter waves. The wavebreak might produce reentry around a fixed anatomic site or might produce a vortex-like micro-reentry (rotors) around very small cores, with high-frequency

periodic activity, a mechanism discovered by Jalife et al.[107,108] in isolated heart preparations. Rapid electrical impulses emanating from these mother rotors may propagate throughout the atria and interact with functional and/or anatomical barriers, causing fragmentation and wavelet formation. These considerations fit into explanations of both the multiwave and the focal activity. The newer techniques of high-resolution optical mapping allow the examination of electrical wave propagation in greater detail. Using the noncontact mapping, Lin et al.[109] found during focal atrial fibrillation induced by atrial pacing the existence of atrial channels through lines of block that acted as mother rotors, giving rise to daughter waves and fibrillatory conduction. Thus atrial fibrillation increasingly is being recognized as a deterministic process resulting from the rapidly firing foci and fibrillatory conduction, rather than a fundamentally turbulent and self-sustaining breakdown of organized conduction.[105]

Yang et al.[105a] attempted to determine the mechanism of atrial fibrillation by examining the premature atrial complexes (PACs) during the 5 minutes preceding the onset of paroxysmal atrial fibrillation. They reported that subjects with high PAC activity had fewer episodes and shorter-duration atrial fibrillation episodes compared with those who had low PAC activity but greater burden of atrial fibrillation. It was assumed that the latter were "substrate fibrillators" and the former were "trigger fibrillators." There is an increasing evidence that in some cases atrial fibrillation can be a heritable disease due to gene mutations.[109a,109b]

IMPLICATIONS FOR TREATMENT

The concept that atrial fibrillation begets atrial fibrillation is of practical importance. Several experimental and clinical studies have established that atrial fibrillation contributes to electrical remodeling of atrial myocardium, which consists of changes in various membrane currents that control action potential duration; it results in shortening the atrial effective refractory period and decreasing the wavelength,[110] which facilitates continuation of the atrial fibrillation. A similar effect is enlargement of the atria caused by atrial fibrillation.[111,112]

Understanding the electrophysiologic substrate of atrial fibrillation has contributed to the development of two surgical procedures for maintenance of sinus rhythm: the corridor procedure introduced by Giraudon and the maze introduced by Ferguson and Cox.[102] In both procedures, the conduction pathway leading from the SA node to the AV node is isolated from the rest of the atria. With the corridor procedure the left atrial attachment of the septum and most of the right atrium are disconnected, leaving a corridor consisting of a cuff of right atrium around the superior vena cava, including the SA node, a strip of atrial septum anterior to the fossa ovalis, and the triangle of Koch with the AV node and the orifice of the coronary sinus.[113]

The maze procedure provides for only one entrance site (the SA node) and one exit site (the AV node), with multiple blind alleys along the route between the entry and exit sites. The purpose of these alleys is to depolarize the remaining atrial tissue without providing an opportunity for reentry. Both procedures are based on the premise that atrial fibrillation cannot be sustained in a small tissue mass.

It has been suggested that the effect of the maze procedure can be simulated by creating linear lesions in the right atrium or left atrium (or both) using a radiofrequency energy pulse.[114,115]

Drugs used to accomplish pharmacologic conversion to sinus rhythm have an antifibrillatory effect by slowing conduction, which prevents reexcitation, and by helping smaller units coalesce. Drugs that lengthen the refractory period may be beneficial by increasing the wavelength of the tachycardia, although a longer duration of the relative refractory period may facilitate reentrant activity.

FOCAL ATRIAL FIBRILLATION AND ROLE OF PULMONARY VEINS

Most cases of atrial fibrillation fit the model of multiple wavelets and are not amenable to ablation. Focal atrial fibrillation is a fairly recently discovered mechanism of sustained atrial fibrillation that is amenable to ablation of the initiating focus. The focal activity may be triggered, or caused, by enhanced automaticity or microreentry.[116] (See earlier discussion.) Many of the successfully ablated foci have been located in the pulmonary veins,[104,117] although right atrial foci have been mapped and ablated successfully.[116] Also, localized foci of activity alleged to initiate chronic atrial fibrillation have been found in the left atria,[118] the ostium of the inferior vena cava,[119] and the persistent left superior vena cava.[120]

There is evidence that pulmonary veins possess structures capable of generating reentrant ectopic activity. These structures are implicated not only as a trigger of atrial fibrillation in patients with appropriate substrate, but also as a source of "venous wave drivers" that are capable of maintaining atrial fibrillation.[121] This is facilitated by marked abbreviation of the action potential duration and shortened refractoriness by acetylcholine.[122] It has been amply demonstrated that the pulmonary veins are electrically connected to the left atrium by discrete fascicles, which explains how the isolation of pulmonary veins by ostial ablation can eliminate atrial fibrillation in a substantial number of patients. Haissaguerre et al.[123] were not able to re-induce atrial fibrillation using aggressive electrical stimulation in 57% of patients after pulmonary vein isolation. In some patients who had unsuccessful ablation, sources of localized atrial activation could be mapped and ablated.[123] Good results were reported in patients after pulmonary vein isolation combined with linear ablation of the cavotricuspid isthmus and mitral isthmus.[124]

DIAGNOSIS OF PREMATURE VENTRICULAR COMPLEXES IN THE PRESENCE OF ATRIAL FIBRILLATION

Differentiation of premature ventricular complexes from aberrant conduction may be difficult. A constant coupling interval favors the diagnosis of ventricular ectopy. The presence of the Ashman phenomenon favors aberrancy, but a long preceding cycle also favors precipitation of premature ventricular complexes (rule of bigeminy). A longer (pseudocompensatory) pause after a wide QRS complex favors a ventricular origin because retrograde penetration of the AV node by the ventricular ectopic impulse prolongs the AV nodal refractoriness and delays anterograde transmission of the subsequent atrial impulse. Polymorphism, particularly that manifested by various forms of incomplete RBBB, favors aberrancy but may also be caused by different degrees of fusion between the atrial and ventricular ectopic complex.

Because single, wide QRS aberrant complexes are caused almost exclusively by the Ashman phenomenon, a plot of the RR interval terminating the wide QRS complex vs. the preceding RR interval can establish the domain of the aberrantly conducted complexes. A wide QRS complex not fitting into this domain is not likely to be caused by the Ashman phenomenon and therefore is probably a ventricular ectopic complex. Because the aberrant conduction during atrial fibrillation results from the difference in refractory periods between the AV node and the bundle branches, it has a specific distribution on the RR interval scattergram. If a large number of points are available (e.g., during ambulatory monitoring), the computer-generated scatter-gram makes it possible to differentiate between aberrant ventricular conduction and ventricular ectopy with great accuracy.[125]

REFERENCES

1. Chou TC: Electrocardiography in Clinical Practice, 4th ed. Philadelphia, Saunders, 1996, pp 351–370.
2. Surawicz B: Electrophysiologic Basis of the ECG and Cardiac Arrhythmias. Baltimore, Williams & Wilkins, 1995.
3. Wells JL, MacLean WA, James TN, et al: Characterization of atrial flutter: studies in man after open heart surgery using fixed atrial electrodes. Circulation 60:665, 1979.
4. Kalman JM, Olgin JE, Saxon LA, et al: Electrocardiographic and electrophysiologic characterization of atypical atrial flutter in man: use of activation and entrainment mapping and implications for catheter ablation. J Cardiovasc Electrophysiol 8:121, 1997.
5. Allessie MA, Lammers WJ, Bonke F, et al: Intraatrial reentry as a mechanism for atrial flutter induced by acetylcholine and rapid pacing in the dog. Circulation 70:123, 1984.
6. Rytand DA, Onesti SJ, Bruns DI: The atrial rate in patients with flutter: a relationship between atrial enlargement and slow rate. Stanford Med Bull 16:169, 1958.
7. Leier CV, Meacham JA, Schaal SF: Prolonged atrial conduction. A major predisposing factor for the development of atrial flutter. Circulation 57:213, 1978.
8. Castellanos A, Lemberg L, Gosselin A, et al: Evaluation of countershock treatment of atrial flutter. Arch Intern Med 115:426, 1965.
9. Corazza IJ, Pastor BH: Cardiac arrhythmias in chronic cor pulmonale. N Engl J Med 259:862, 1958.
10. Johnson JC, Flowers NC, Horan LG: Unexplained atrial flutter: a frequent herald of pulmonary embolism. Am J Cardiol 25:105, 1970.
11. Craig RJ, Selzer A: Natural history and prognosis of atrial septal defect. Circulation 37:805, 1968.
12. Fowler NO, Gueron M: Conversion of atrial flutter with digoxin alone. Circulation 27:716, 1962.
13. Waldo AL, Cooper TB: Spontaneous onset of type I atrial flutter in patients. J Am Coll Cardiol 28:707, 1996.
14. Rytand DA: The circus movement (entrapped circuit wave) hypothesis and atrial flutter. Ann Intern Med 63:125, 1966.
15. Waldo AL, Plumb VJ, Henthorn RW: Observations on the mechanism of atrial flutter. In: Surawicz B, Reddy CP, Prystowsky E (eds): Tachycardias. Boston, Martinus Nijhoff, 1984.
16. Lewis T, Drury AN, Iliescu CC: A demonstration of circus movement in clinical flutter of the auricles. Heart 8:341, 1921.
17. Allessie MA, Bonke FI, Schopman FJ: Circus movement in rabbit atrial muscle as a mechanism of tachycardia. The "leading circle" concept. A new model of circus movement in cardiac tissue without the involvement of an anatomical obstacle. Circ Res 41:9, 1977.
18. Boineau JP: Atrial flutter: a synthesis of concepts. Circulation 72:249, 1985.
19. Page PL, Plumb VJ, Okumura K, et al: A new animal model of atrial flutter. J Am Coll Cardiol 8:872, 1986.
20. Schoels W, Gough WB, Restivo M, et al: Circus movement atrial flutter in the canine sterile pericarditis model. Circ Res 67:35, 1990.
21. Wellens HJJ, Janse MJ, van Dam RT, et al: Epicardial excitation of the atria in a patient with atrial flutter. Br Heart J 33:233, 1971.
22. Shah DC, Jais P, Haissaguerre M, et al: Three-dimensional mapping of the common atrial flutter circuit in the right atrium. Circulation 96:3904, 1997.
23. Watson RM, Josephson MR: Atrial flutter: electrophysiologic substrates and modes of initiation and termination. Am J Cardiol 45:732, 1980.
24. Cosio FG, Lopez Gil M, Arribas F, et al: Mechanisms of entrainment of human common atrial flutter studied with multiple endocardial recordings. Circulation 89:2117, 1994.
25. Niwano S, Abe H, Gonzalez X, et al: Characterization of the excitable gap in a functionally determined reentrant circuit: studies in the sterile pericarditis model of atrial flutter. Circulation 90:1997, 1994.
26. Olgin JE, Kalman JM, Lesh MD: Conduction barriers in human atrial flutter: correlation of electrophysiology and anatomy. J Cardiovasc Electrophysiol 7:1112, 1996.
27. Kalman JM, Olgin JE, Saxon LA, et al: Activation and entrainment mapping defines the tricuspid annulus as the anterior barrier in typical atrial flutter. Circulation 94:398, 1996.
28. Callans DJ, Schwartzman D, Gottlieb CD, et al: Characterization of the excitable gap in human type I atrial flutter. J Am Coll Cardiol 30:1793, 1997.
29. Tsuchiya T, Okumura K, Tabuchi T, et al: The upper turnover site in the reentry circuit of common atrial flutter. Am J Cardiol 78:1439, 1996.
30. Puech P, Latour M, Grolleau R: Le flutter et ses limites. Arch Mal Coeur 63:166, 1970.
31. Klein GJ, Guiraudon GM, Sharma AD, et al: Demonstration of macroreentry and feasibility of operative therapy in the common type of atrial flutter. Am J Cardiol 57:587, 1986.
32. Cosio FG, Lopez-Gil M, Giocolea A, et al: Radiofrequency ablation of the inferior vena cava-tricuspid valve isthmus in common atrial flutter. Am J Cardiol 71:705, 1993.
33. Feld GK, Fleck RP, Chen PS, et al: Radiofrequency catheter ablation for the treatment of human type I atrial flutter: identification of a critical zone in the reentrant circuit by endocardial mapping techniques. Circulation 86:1233, 1992.
34. Lesh MD, Van Hare GF, Epstein LM, et al: Radiofrequency catheter ablation of atrial arrhythmias. Circulation 89:1074, 1994.
35. Fischer B, Jais P, Shah D, et al: Radiofrequency catheter ablation of common atrial flutter in 200 patients. J Cardiovasc Electrophysiol 7:1225, 1996.
36. Tai C-T, Chen S-A, Chiang C-E, et al: Long-term outcome of radiofrequency catheter ablation for typical atrial flutter: risk prediction of recurrent arrhythmias. J Cardiovasc Electrophysiol 9:115, 1998.
37. Shah DC, Haissaguerre M, Jais P, et al: Atrial flutter: contemporary electrophysiology and catheter ablation. PACE 22:344, 1999.
38. Johna R, Eckardt L, Fetsch T, et al: A new algorithm to determine complete isthmus conduction block after radiofrequency catheter ablation for typical atrial flutter. Am J Cardiol 83:1666, 1999.
39. Barold SS, Shah D, Jais P, et al: Nomenclature and characterization of transisthmus conduction after ablation of typical atrial flutter. PACE 20:1751, 1997.
40. Inoue H, Yamashita T, Nozaki A, et al: Effects of antiarrhythmic drugs on canine atrial flutter due to reentry: role of prolongation of refractory period and depression

of conduction to excitable gap. J Am Coll Cardiol 18:1098, 1991.

41. Marine JE, Korley VJ, Obioha-Ngwu O, et al: Different patterns of interatrial conduction in clockwise and counterclockwise atrial flutter. Circulation 104:1153, 2001.

42. Yuniadi Y, Tai C-T, Lee K-T, et al: A new electrocardiographic algorithm to differentiate upper loop re-entry from reverse typical atrial flutter. J Am Coll Cardiol 46:524, 2005.

43. Zhang S, Younis G, Hariharan R, et al: Lower loop reentry as a mechanism of clockwise right atrial flutter. Circulation 109:1630, 2004.

43a. Krummen DE, Feld GK, Narayan SM: Diagnostic accuracy of irregularly irregular RR intervals in separating atrial fibrillation from atrial flutter. Am J Cardiol 98:209, 2006.

44. Gomes JA, Santoni-Rugiu F, Mehta D, et al: Uncommon atrial flutter: characteristics, mechanisms and results of ablative therapy. PACE 21:2029, 1998.

45. Bochoeyer A, Yang Y, Cheng J, et al: Surface electrocardiographic characteristics of right and left atrial flutter. Circulation 108:60, 2003.

46. Marrouche NF, Natale A, Wazni OM, et al: Left septal atrial flutter. Electrophysiology, anatomy and results of ablation. Circulation 109:2449, 2004.

47. Scheinman MM: Catheter ablation: a personal perspective. J Cardiovasc Electrophysiol 12:1083, 2001.

48. Vaziri SM, Larson MG, Benjamin EJ, et al: Echocardiographic predictors of nonrheumatic atrial fibrillation: the Framingham study. Circulation 89:724, 1994.

49. Flaker GC, Fletcher KA, Rothbart RM, et al: Clinical and echocardiographic features of intermittent atrial fibrillation that predict recurrent atrial fibrillation. Am J Cardiol 76:355, 1995.

50. Roark SF, McCarthy E, Lee KL, et al: Observations on the occurrence of atrial fibrillation in paroxysmal supraventricular tachycardia. Am J Cardiol 57:571, 1986.

51. Coumel PH: Atrial fibrillation. In: Surawicz B, Reddy CP, Prystowsky EN (eds): Tachycardias. Boston, Martinus Nijhoff, 1984.

52. Allessie MA: Atrial electrophysiologic remodeling: another vicious circle? J Cardiovasc Electrophysiol 9:1378, 1998.

53. Levy S, Camm AJ, Saksena S, et al: International consensus on nomenclature and classification of atrial fibrillation. J Cardiovasc Electrophysiol 14:443, 2003.

54. Toivonen L, Kadish A, Kou W, et al: Determinants of the ventricular rate during atrial fibrillation. J Am Coll Cardiol 16:1194, 1990.

55. Meijler FL, Jalife J, Beaumont J, et al: AV nodal function during atrial fibrillation: the role of electrotonic modulation of propagation. J Cardiovasc Electrophysiol 7:843, 1996.

56. Meijler F, Jalife J: On the mechanism(s) of atrioventricular nodal traansmission in atrial fibrillation. Cardiologia 42:375, 1997.

57. Hwang W, Langendorf R: Auriculoventricular nodal escape in the presence of auricular fibrillation. Circulation 1:930, 1950.

58. Weiner HL, McCarthy EA, Pritchett ELC: Regular ventricular rhythms in patients with symptomatic paroxysmal atrial fibrillation. J Am Coll Cardiol 17:1283, 1991.

59. Konings KT, Kirchhof CJ, Smeets JR, et al: High-density mapping of electrically induced atrial fibrillation in humans. Circulation 89:1665, 1994.

60. Daoud EG, Pariseau B, Niebauer M, et al: Response of type I atrial fibrillation to atrial pacing in humans. Circulation 94:1036, 1996.

61. Langendorf R, Lev M, Pick R: Auricular fibrillation with anomalous AV excitation (WPW syndrome) imitating ventricular paroxysmal tachycardia. Acta Cardiol (Brux) 2:241, 1952.

62. Castellanos A, Myerburg RJ, Craparo K, et al: Factors regulating ventricular rates during atrial flutter and fibrillation in pre-excitation (Wolff-Parkinson-White) syndrome. Br Heart J 35:811,1973.

63. Wellens HJ, Durrer D: Wolff-Parkinson-White syndrome and atrial fibrillation. Am J Cardiol 34:777, 1974.

64. Chen PS, Prystowsky EN: Role of concealed and supernormal conduction during atrial fibrillation in the pre-excitation syndrome. Am J Cardiol 68:1329, 1991.

65. Ong JJC, Kriett JM, Feld GK, et al: Prevalence of retrograde accessory pathway conduction during atrial fibrillation. J Cardiovasc Electrophysiol 8:377, 1997.

66. Fillette F, Fontaine G: Ventriclar response in atrial fibrillation: effects of AV nodal refractory periods atrioventricular block, and pre-excitation syndromes. In: Surawicz B, Reddy CP, Prystowsky EN (eds): Tachycardias. Boston, Martinus Nijhoff, 1984.

67. Sharma AD, Klein GJ, Guiraudon GM, et al: Atrial fibrillation in patients with Wolff-Parkinson-White syndrome: Incidence after surgical ablation of the accessory pathway. Circulation 72:161, 1985.

68. Chen S-A, Lee S-H, Chiang C-E, et al: Electrophysiological mechanisms in successful radiofrequency catheter modification of atrioventricular junction for patients with medically refractory paroxysmal atrial fibrillation. Circulation 93:1690, 1996.

69. Strickberger SA, Weiss R, Daoud EG, et al: Ventricular rate during atrial fibrillation before and after slow-pathway ablation: effects of autonomic blockade and beta-adrenergic stimulation. Circulation 94:1023, 1996.

70. Blanck Z, Dhala AA, Sra J, et al: Characterication of atrioventricular nodal behavior and ventricular response during atrial fibrillation before and after a selective slow-pathway ablation. Circulation 91:1086, 1995.

71. Asano Y, Saito J, Yamamoto T, et al: Electrophysiologic determinants of ventricular rate in human atrial fibrillation. J Cardiovasc Electrophysiol 6:343, 1995.

72. Rokas S, Gainitadou S, Chatzidou S, et al: A noninvasive method for detection of dual atrioventricular physiology in chronic atrial fibrillation. Am J Cardiol 84:1442, 1999.

73. Gerstenfeld EP, Sahakian AV, Swiryn S: Evidence for transient linking of atrial excitation during atrial fibrillation in humans. Circulation 86:375, 1992.

74. Roithinger FX, Sippens-Groenewegen A, Karch MR, et al: Organized activation during atrial fibrillation in man: endocardial and electrocardiographic manifestations. J Cardiovasc Electrophysiol 9:451, 1998.

75. Thurmann M, Janney JG Jr: The diagnostic importance of fibrillatory wave size. Circulation 25:991, 1962.

76. Leier CV, Schaal SF: Biatrial electrograms during coarse atrial fibrillation and flutter-fibrillation. Am Heart J 99:331, 1980.

77. Puech P: Lactivite Electrique Auriculaire Normale et Pathologique. Paris, Masson, 1956.

78. Zipes DP, De Joseph RL: Dissimilar atrial rhythms in man and dog. Am J Cardiol 32:618, 1973.

79. Horvath G, Goldberger JJ, Kadish AH: Simultaneous occurrence of atrial fibrillation and atrial flutter. J Cardiovasc Electrophysiol 11:849, 2000.

80. Psaty BM, Manolio TA, Kuller LH, et al: Incidence and risk factors for atrial fibrillation in older adults. Circulation 96:2455, 1997.

81. Lakireddy DR, Clark RA, Mohiuddin SM: Electrocardiographic findings in patients >100 years of age without clinical evidence of cardiac disease. Am J Cardiol 92:1249, 2003.

82. Surawicz B, Slack JD: Treatment of supraventricular arrhythmias in acute myocardial infarction. *In:* Francis GS, Alpert JS (eds): Coronary Care. Boston, Little, Brown, 1995, pp 217–236.

83. Crenshaw BS, Ward SR, Granger CB, et al: Atrial fibrillation in the seting of acute myocardial infarction: the GUSTO-I experience. J Am Coll Cardiol 30:406, 1997.

84. Hod H, Lew AS, Keltai M, et al: Early atrial fibrillation during evolving myocardial infarction: a consequence of impaired left atrial perfusion. Circulation 75:146, 1987.

85. Sakata K, Kurihara H, Iwamori K, et al: Clinical and prognostic significance of atrial fibrillation in acute myocardial infarction. Am J Cardiol 80:1522, 1997.

86. Silver S, Delit C, Eller M: The treatment of thyrocardiac disease with radioactive iodine. Prog Cardiovasc Dis 5:64, 1962.

87. Levine HD: Myocardial fibrosis in constrictive pericarditis: electrocardiographic and pathologic observations. Circulation 48:1268, 1973.

88. Mathew JP, Parks R, Savino JS, et al: Atrial fibrillation following coronary artery bypass graft surgery. JAMA 276:300, 1996.

89. Rathore SS, Berger AK, Weinfurt KP, et al: Acute myocardial infarction complicated by atrial fibrillation in the elderly: prevalence and outcomes. Circulation 101:969, 2000.

90. Lamb LE, Pollard LW: Atrial fibrillation in flying personnel. Circulation 29:694, 1964.

91. Peter RH, Gracey JG, Beach TB: A clinical profile of idiopathic atrial fibrillation: a functional disorder of atrial rhythm. Ann Intern Med 68:1288, 1968.

92. Brand FN, Abbott RD, Kannel WB, et al: Characteristics and prognosis of lone atrial fibrillation. JAMA 254:34, 1985.

93. Kopecky SL, Gersh BJ, McGoon MD, et al: The natural history of lone atrial fibrillation. N Engl J Med 317:669, 1987.

94. Rostagno C, Bacci F, Martelli M, et al: Clinical course of lone atrial fibrillation since first symptomatic arrhythmia episode. Am J Cardiol 76:837, 1995.

95. Coumel PH: Autonomic influences in atrial tachyarrhythmias. J Cardiovasc Electrophysiol 7:999, 1996.

96. West TC, Lauda JF: Minimal mass required for induction of a sustained arrhythmia in isolated atrial segments. Am J Physiol 202:232, 1962.

97. Moe GK, Rheinboldt WC, Abildskov JA: A computer model of atrial fibrillation. Am Heart J 67:200, 1964.

98. Ortiz J, Niwano S, Abe H, et al: Mapping the conversion of atrial flutter to atrial fibrillation and atrial fibrillation to atrial flutter. Circ Res 74:882, 1994.

99. Roithinger FX, Karch MR, Steiner PR, et al: Relationship between atrial fibrillation and typical atrial flutter in humans: activation sequence changes during spontaneous conversion. Circulation 96:3484, 1997.

100. Hamer ME, Wilkinson WE, Clair WK, et al: Incidence of symptomatic atrial fibrillation in patients with paroxysmal supraventricular tachycardia. J Am Coll Cardiol 25:984, 1995.

101. Allessie MA, Rensma PL, Brugade J, et al: Pathological physiology of atrial fibrillation. *In:* Zipes DP, Jalife J (eds): Cardiac Electrophysiology from Cell to Bedside. Philadelphia, Saunders, 1990, pp 548–558.

102. Ferguson TB, Cox JL: Surgical therapy for cardiac arrhythmias. Update. *In:* Fisch C, Surawicz B (eds): Cardiac Electrophysiology and Arrhythmias. New York, Elsevier, 1991, pp 425–448.

103. Kalman JM, Olgin JE, Karch MR, et al: Regional entrainment of atrial fibrillation in man. J Cardiovasc Electrophysiol 7:867, 1996.

104. Jais P, Haissaguerre M, Shah DC, et al: A focal source of atrial fibrillation treated by discrete radiofrequency ablation. Circulation 95:572, 1997.

105. Mansour M: Highest dominant frequencies in atrial fibrillation. A new target for ablation. J Am Coll Cardiol 47:1407, 2006.

105a. Yang A, Ruiter J, Pfeifer D, et al: Identification of "substrate fibrillators" and "trigger" fibrillators by pacemaker diagnostics. Heart Rhythm 3:682, 2006.

106. Weiss JN, Chen PS, Qu Z, et al: Ventricular fibrillation: how do we stop the waves from breaking? Circ Res 87:1103, 2000.

107. Jalife J, Berenfeld O, Skane AC, et al: Mechanisms of atrial fibrillation: mother rotors, or multiple daughter wavelets, or both? J Cardiovasc Electrophysiol 9:S2, 1998.

108. Jalife J, Berenfeld O, Mansour M: Mother rotors and fibrillatory conduction: a mechanism of atrial fibrillation. Cardiovasc Res 54:204, 2002.

109. Lin YJ, Tai CT, Kao T, et al: Electrophysiological characteristics and catheter ablation in patients with paroxysmal right atrial fibrillation. Circulation 112:1692, 2005.

109a. Fatkin D, Otway R, Vandenberg JI: Genes and atrial fibrillation. A new look at an old problem. Circulation 116:782, 2007.

109b. Volders PGA, Zhu Q, Timmermans C, et al: Mapping a novel locus for familial atrial fibrillation on chromosome 10p11-q21. Heart Rhythm 4:469, 2007.

110. Gaspo R, Bosch RF, Talajic M, et al: Functional mechanisms underlying tachycardia-induced sustained atrial fibrillation in a chronic dog model. Circulation 96:4027, 1997.

111. Daoud EG, Bogun F, Goyal R, et al: Effect of atrial fibrillation on atrial refractoriness in humans. Circulation 94:1600, 1996.

112. Franz MR, Karasik PL, Li C, et al: Electrical remodeling of the human atrium: similar effects in patients with chronic atrial fibrillation and atrial flutter. J Am Coll Cardiol 30:1785, 1997.

113. Leitch JW, Klein G, Yee R, et al: Sinus node-atrioventricular node isolation: long term results with the "corridor" operation for atrial fibrillation. J Am Coll Cardiol 17:970, 1991.

114. Haissaguerre M, Jais P, Shah DC, et al: Right and left radiofrequency catheter therapy of paroxysmal atrial fibrillation. J Cardiovasc Electrophysiol 7:1132, 1996.

115. Olgin JE, Kalman JM, Chin M, et al: Electrophysiological effects of long, linear atrial lesions placed under intracardiac ultrasound guidance. Circulation 6:2715, 1997.

116. Chen S-A, Tai T-C, Yu W-C, et al: Right atrial focal atrial fibrillation: electrophysiologic characteristics and radiofrequency catheter ablation. J Cardiovasc Electrophysiol 10:328, 1999.

117. Haissaguerre M, Jais P, Shah DC, et al: Spontaneous initiation of atrial fibrillation by ectopic beats originating in the pulmonary veins. N Engl J Med 339:659, 1998.

118. Sahadean J, Ryu K, Peltz L, et al: Epicardial mapping of chronic atrial fibrillation in patients. Preliminary observations. Circulation 110:3293, 2004.

119. Mansour M, Ruskin J, Keane D: Initiation of atrial fibrillation by ectopic beats originating from the ostium of the inferior vena cava. J Cardiovasc Electrophysiol 13:1292, 2002.

120. Hsu L-F, Jais P, Keane D, et al: Atrial fibrillation originating from persistent left superior vena cava. Circulation 109:828, 2004.

121. Haissaguerre M, Sanders P, Hocini M, et al: Pulmonary veins in the substrate for atrial fibrillation. J Am Coll Cardiol 43:2280, 2004.

122. Po SS, Li Y, Tang D, et al: Rapid and stable re-entry within the pulmonary vein as a mechanism initiating paroxysmal atrial fibrillation. J Am Coll Cardiol 45:1871, 2005.
123. Haissaguerre M, Hocini M, Sanders P, et al: Localized sources maintaining atrial fibrillation organizes by prior ablation. Circulation 113:616, 2006.
124. Jais P, Hocini M, Hsu L-F, et al: Technique and results of linear ablation at the mitral isthmus. Circulation 110:2996, 2004.
125. Suyama AC, Sunagawa K, Sugimachi M, et al: Differentiation between aberrant ventricular conduction and ventricular ectopy in atrial fibrillation using RR interval scattergram. Circulation 88:2308, 1993.

16 Atrioventricular Junctional Rhythms

Coronary Sinus Rhythm
Ectopic Impulses and Rhythms
   Originating in the AVJ

Passive AV Junctional Impulses and Rhythms
AV Junctional Escape Impulses
AV Junctional Escape Rhythms

Active-Type AV Junctional Rhythm and Junctional Tachycardia
Premature Junctional Complexes
Automatic Junctional Tachycardia

Accelerated AV Junctional Rhythm
   (Nonparoxysmal Junctional
   Tachycardia)

AV Dissociation

AV Nodal Reentry
AV Nodal Reentrant Tachycardia
Differential Diagnosis of AVNRT

Reciprocal Impulses
Reciprocal Impulses of Junctional Origin
Reciprocal Impulses of Atrial Origin
Reciprocal Impulses of Ventricular
   Origin

The atrioventricular junction (AVJ) extends from the approaches to the atrioventricular (AV) node, which are composed of transitional cells, to the bifurcation of the His bundle. There are two tracts of approaches: the anterosuperior tracts are located in the anterior intertarial septum near the apex of the Koch's triangle, and the posterior inferior approaches extend from the coronary sinus.[1]

The AV node is situated in the base of the atrial septum at the apex of Koch's triangle. Koch's triangle is delineated by the tendon of Towaro, the annulus of the tricuspid valve, and the coronary sinus, forming the base of the triangle. The average length of the triangle is 17 mm, and the average height is 13 mm.[2]

The AV node is made up of small, densely packed cells identical to p cells in the sinoatrial (SA) node, with an admixture of slender transitional cells and scattered Purkinje and myocardial cells at the margins. Like the SA node, the AV node is an epicardial structure receiving a rich autonomic nervous supply. Automatic activity can arise in the proximal part of the AVJ (AN region), the area of transition from the AV node to the His bundle (NH region), and the His bundle itself. The central part of the AV node (N region) is believed to lack automatic properties, although this point is debatable.

The His bundle penetrates the central fibrous body underneath the noncoronary cusp of the aortic valve; it reaches the crest of the trabecular septum underneath the membranous septum and begins to branch underneath the commissure between the right and noncoronary cusps of the aortic valve. The His bundle is insulated from the myocardium. Intraventricular conduction begins at the sites at which the insulation disappears.

The rhythm disturbances arising in the AVJ fall into two distinct categories: (1) ectopic impulses and rhythms originating in the AVJ; and (2) reciprocal (reentrant) impulses and rhythms dependent on slow conduction and unidirectional block in the AVJ.[3] The reentrant circuit nearly always involves the AVN, but intra-Hisian reentrant tachycardias also are known to occur.

It is often difficult to determine the origin of the impulses arising in the AVJ from the body surface electrocardiogram (ECG). Therefore the broader term *AV junctional rhythm* has replaced the formerly used term "AV nodal rhythm."

Coronary Sinus Rhythm

Rhythm that originates from the coronary sinus is characterized by retrograde P waves with a normal PR interval. Although these findings have been reproduced experimentally in humans by pacing the interior of the coronary sinus,[4,5] the term "coronary sinus rhythm" is no longer in use. It has been replaced by the terms *ectopic atrial rhythm* (sometimes designated low or left atrial) or *AV junctional rhythm*. This is because inverted P waves in leads II, III, and aV$_F$ with normal PR intervals can be elicited by stimulating sites other than the coronary sinus[6] and because the PR duration may be normal when a junctional impulse conducted anterogradely is delayed.

ECTOPIC IMPULSES AND RHYTHMS ORIGINATING IN THE AVJ

The AVJ may become the site of impulse formation when the ventricular rate becomes slower than the inherent rate of the junctional pacemaker (35 to 60 beats/min) (Figure 16–1). Such an AV junctional rhythm is an escape phenomenon and represents the slow or passive type of junctional rhythm, in contrast to the active type of AV junctional rhythm or junctional tachycardia. The latter is caused by an abnormal increase in the automaticity of the junctional pacemaker, with the resulting rhythm generally at a rate faster than 60 beats/min.

When the ectopic pacemaker is junctional in origin, activation of the atria proceeds in a retrograde direction unless there is AV dissociation or block. Therefore the P waves are inverted in leads II, III, and aV$_F$ and are usually isoelectric or upright in leads aV$_R$ and I. In the precordial leads, P wave morphology is variable.

The retrograde P wave of a junctional impulse may precede, be superimposed on, or follow the QRS complex (Figure 16–2). These P–QRS relations gave rise to the terms upper, middle, and lower nodal complexes, respectively. It has been recognized, however, that the PR or RP interval

depends not only on the location of the pacemaker in the junction but also on the relative speed of conduction in the anterograde and retrograde directions. If the pacemaker is located at the upper part of the AVJ but the retrograde conduction is delayed, the P wave may appear after, rather than before, the QRS complex. Therefore these descriptive terms may not correspond to the actual location of the pacemaker and should no longer be used when interpreting the body surface ECG.[3]

In junctional complexes with the P wave preceding the QRS complex, the PR interval is usually less than 0.11 second. If the P wave is inscribed after the QRS complex, the RP interval varies and may be as long as 0.20 second or longer.

Passive AV Junctional Impulses and Rhythms

AV JUNCTIONAL ESCAPE IMPULSES

Supraventricular escape impulses readily occur when the activity of the SA node becomes slow or when conduction below the SA node is blocked. Even transient slowing of SA nodal activity may precipitate an atrial or AV junctional escape rhythm. Single supraventricular escape impulses are usually precipitated by long pauses (e.g., sinus bradycardia), the slow phase of sinus arrhythmia, intermittent SA block, sinus arrest, partial AV block, atrial fibrillation with slow ventricular response (Figure 16–3), and conducted or blocked supraventricular premature impulses.

Occurrence of two escape impulses in a row following a single premature impulse is not

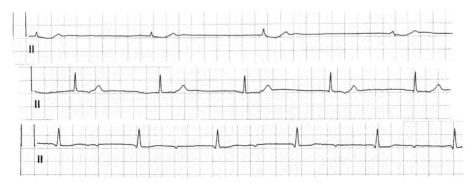

Figure 16–1   ECG strips of lead II showing slow atrioventricular (AV) junctional rhythms. *Top*, AV junctional rhythm (32 beats/min) in a 79-year-old man with apparent sinus arrest. P waves are not visible. *Middle*, ECG of an 80-year-old woman who has no evidence of heart disease. Note the AV junctional rhythm (49 beats/min) with an RP interval of 240 ms. *Bottom*, This 80-year-old woman had had a previous inferior myocardial infarction. Note the AV junctional rhythm at a rate of 47 beats/min with an RP interval of 600 ms. Another possibility is that the negative P wave is caused by an AV junctional complex that is blocked to the ventricles.

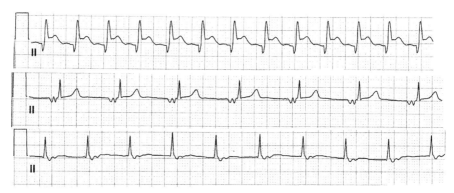

Figure 16–2 ECG strips of lead II showing accelerated atrioventricular (AV) junctional rhythms and various P/QRS relations. *Top,* AV junctional tachycardia without visible P waves and right bundle branch block (present during sinus rhythm) in a 75-year-old woman with acute inferior myocardial infarction (MI). *Middle,* AV junctional rhythm at a rate of 63 beats/min with negative P waves preceding the QRS complex in a 73-year-old man with acute anterior MI. *Bottom,* AV junctional rhythm at a rate of 88 beats/min with negative P waves after the QRS complex in a 74-year-old man with acute anterior MI.

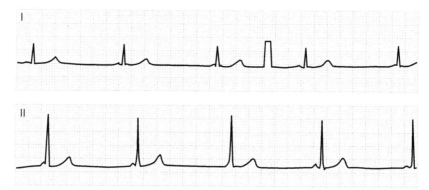

Figure 16–3 Atrioventricular junctional escape complexes occurring during the slow phase of sinus arrhythmia. The junctional QRS complexes are superimposed on the sinus P waves. The escape interval is 1.13 seconds.

uncommon. Escape impulses occasionally occur after premature ventricular impulses. If an escape complex follows a premature ventricular impulse, the escape interval may be longer than the escape interval following a conducted supraventricular impulse because the premature ventricular impulse tends to conduct retrogradely into the AV junction and discharge the escape pacemaker.[7] An escape impulse from the AV junction does not always activate both the atrium and the ventricle. The spread of excitation in one of the two directions may be blocked, and no P or QRS complex is recorded. In the absence of intracardiac electrograms, the presence of such a concealed junctional impulse can be detected only by its effect on the formation or conduction of the subsequent impulse.

Dissociated activation of the ventricles by the AV junctional escape impulse and of the atria by the SA node sinus impulse occurs often (see later discussion). Fusion P waves are relatively frequent when one part of the atrium is activated by one pacemaker and another part by another pacemaker. These fusion P waves can be recognized on the ECG when the shape of the P wave is intermediate between that of the sinus P wave and the P wave of the escape pacemaker (see Figure 14–1). In the presence of atrial fibrillation, escape impulses may signify impaired AV conduction, a common manifestation of digitalis toxicity (Figure 16–4). Because the morphology of the ventricular complexes during atrial fibrillation is frequently variable owing to varying degrees of aberrant intraventricular conduction in the conducted supraventricular complexes, differentiation between supraventricular and ventricular complexes during atrial fibrillation may be difficult, even without ventricular escape impulses.

An interesting junctional escape pattern is escape-capture bigeminy. The junctional beat is followed by a sinus capture that presents a group beating phenomenon (see Figure 13–14).

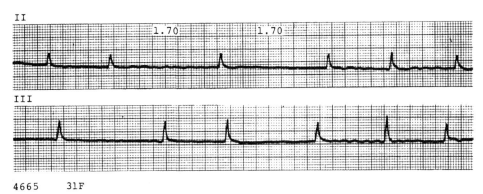

Figure 16–4   Atrial fibrillation in a 31-year-old woman with rheumatic mitral disease. The long pauses in lead II of identical cycle length suggest that the two ventricular complexes that terminate the pauses are junctional escape complexes.

AV JUNCTIONAL ESCAPE RHYTHMS

Single escape impulses are more common than escape rhythms. A succession of escape impulses can occur when the ectopic impulse conducted retrogradely discharges the SA node and delays its impulse formation, providing an opportunity for the subsequent escape impulse to become repetitive. Appropriate timing of the escape pacemaker and a slow inherent rate of the sinus pacemaker may cause an AV junctional (or an atrial) escape rhythm to last for some time. An *escape rhythm* is defined as at least three escape impulses in a row. The RR interval of the junctional escape complexes is usually constant and varies less than 0.04 second, although exceptions do occur.

The QRS complex of AV junctional origin is similar to that of the basic sinus or supraventricular complex. It is usually narrow, but its morphology may differ slightly from that of the sinus complex. The QRS complexes may be wide if there is a preexisting intraventricular conduction defect. If the tracing during sinus rhythm is not available and the AV junctional rhythm is associated with an abnormally wide QRS complex, it may simulate ventricular rhythm. Such a differentiation is often impossible from the body surface ECG alone unless some conducted supraventricular complexes are recorded (Figure 16–5).

Incomplete suppression of the activity of the SA node sets the stage for dissociation between two supraventricular rhythms. Commonly, the sinus pacemaker activates the atria, whereas the AV junctional pacemaker activates the ventricle; one or the other of the two pacemakers intermittently "captures" activation of both chambers for a varying period of time (Figures 16–6 and 16–7). The rate of AV junctional escape pacemakers is usually 40 to 60 beats/min in adults and is frequently more rapid in children.

Scherlag et al.[8] divided AV junctional pacemakers into two types. With the first type, the rate ranged from 45 to 60 beats/min and increased after atropine administration. These pacemakers are located proximal to the His bundle. With the second type, located in the His bundle, the rate ranged from 35 to 45 beats/min and did not change significantly after atropine administration.

When the rate of an ectopic supraventricular pacemaker is 100 beats/min or more, it is referred to as *ectopic tachycardia*. There remains an intermediate range of AV junctional rate of 60 to 100 beats/min, which is neither an escape rhythm nor ectopic tachycardia. A dissociation between two pacemakers is almost invariably present in this situation if the sinus node activity is not disturbed. Dissociation is often isorhythmic (Figure 16–8).

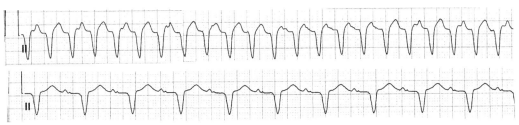

Figure 16–5   ECG rhythm strip of lead II. *Top,* Junctional tachycardia in the presence of an intraventricular conduction disturbance with atrioventricular dissociation. Regularly spaced upright P waves are best seen at the end of the strip. *Bottom,* Record obtained during sinus rhythm 2 days later shows the same QRS morphology.

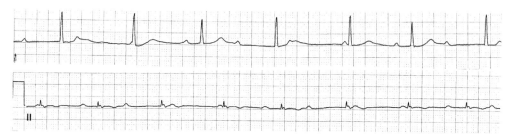

Figure 16–6 Atrioventricular (AV) dissociation caused by impaired AV conduction shown in ECG strips of lead II. *Top,* This 73-year-old woman with hypertensive heart disease shows dissociation between the sinus rhythm at a rate of 70 beats/min and the AV junctional rhythm at a rate of 48 beats/min. The dissociation is caused by partial AV block. There are two sinus capture complexes with a PR interval of 320 ms (third and sixth complexes) both preceded by long (900 and 800 ms, respectively) RP intervals. After shorter RP intervals, sinus impulses are not conducted to the ventricles. *Bottom,* A 50-year-old woman with inferior and septal myocardial infarction shows dissociation between the sinus rhythm at a rate of 75 beats/min and the AV junctional rhythm at a rate of 55 beats/min. The dissociation is caused by partial AV block. PR interval of the conducted sinus complexes (second, fifth, and probably eighth complexes) is 320 to 380 ms, and the preceding RP intervals are 620 to 700 ms.

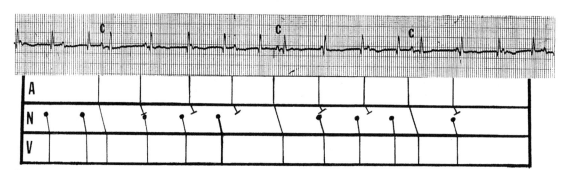

Figure 16–7 Atrioventricular (AV) dissociation caused by accelerated AV junctional rhythm at a rate of 100 beats/min. Sinus rate is 75 beats/min. AV conduction is not impaired. A = atrium; C = sinus captures; N = AV junction; V = ventricle. (Courtesy of Brendan Phibbs, MD.)

The *clinical significance* of the escape mechanisms depends on the conditions precipitating their occurrence. They often occur in healthy persons with sinus bradycardia and become suppressed when the sinus rate is increased by exercise or other maneuvers. They may be seen in patients with various heart diseases that affect the SA or AV node and in the presence of drugs that suppress the SA node or impair AV conduction. In most instances, AV junctional rhythm is a transient phenomenon, although the fast rate can precipitate myocardial ischemia (Figure 16–9).

Active-Type AV Junctional Rhythm and Junctional Tachycardia

PREMATURE JUNCTIONAL COMPLEXES

ECG Findings

Premature junctional complexes are less common than premature ventricular or atrial complexes. They may be seen in normal subjects and patients with structural heart disease.

Single junctional impulses may be parasystolic, with variable coupling and a common denominator of interectopic intervals, or extrasystolic, with a fixed coupling interval. In most instances the postextrasystolic pause is not fully compensatory because the impulse conducted retrogradely discharges the sinus node and resets its rhythmicity (Figure 16–10). The pause may be fully compensatory, however, if there is retrograde SA block and the sinus node is not reset. A fully compensatory pause may also occur if the sinus discharge occurs before arrival of the retrograde impulse from the AVJ. If the sinus impulse occurs relatively early and depolarizes part of the atria before it meets with the junctional impulse, an atrial fusion complex is produced. An AV junctional premature complex may be also interpolated (see Figure 16–10). The sinus rhythm therefore is not disturbed. Similarly, the sinus impulse may activate the entire atria and interfere with retrograde conduction of the junctional impulse. In such a case the junctional pacemaker activates only the ventricles. Temporary AV dissociation occurs, and the sinus rhythm is not

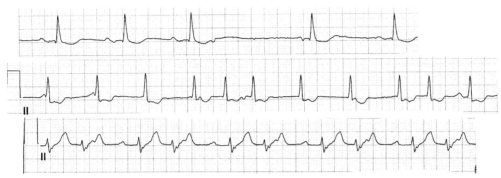

Figure 16–8   Reciprocal complexes preceded by lengthening of the PR interval in ECG strips of lead II. *Top,* Gradual lengthening of the PR interval; a negative P wave follows the third complex with the longest PR interval. This is an atrial echo complex. In this case the atrial echo causes sinus depression, similar to the depression after premature atrial complexes, a "post-echo" depression. *Middle,* Nearly isorhythmic dissociation between sinus and atrioventricular (AV) junctional rhythm. The sinus P wave after the fourth AV junctional complex is conducted with a long PR interval and is followed by a negative P wave (an atrial echo) that is conducted to the ventricles. Subsequently, there are three AV junctional complexes followed by a sinus capture with a long PR interval but without manifest reciprocation; the next sinus impulse is conducted with a normal PR interval. *Bottom,* Bigeminal rhythm caused by reciprocal atrial complexes. PR interval of the complex after the pause is 300 ms; the subsequent PR interval may be longer, but it cannot be measured because the P wave is superimposed on the T wave (the difference between the shape of two T waves is clearly seen). The negative P wave causing indentation of the second T wave is attributed to retrograde conduction (atrial echo) without conduction to the ventricles, which allows resumption of the sinus rhythm. An alternative explanation of negative P waves is an atrial premature complex, but it is less likely in this case.

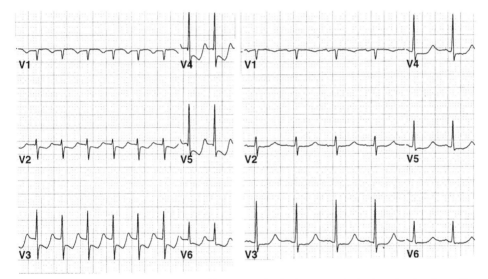

Figure 16–9   ECG precordial leads of a 66-year-old woman who had atrioventricular junctional tachycardia associated with ST segment depression and anginal pain after an operation on the lumbar spine *(left).* After cessation of tachycardia 40 minutes later the pattern was normal *(right).* Nuclear scan showed normal perfusion at rest and after exercise.

reset. As with the premature atrial complex, premature junctional complexes may appear in the constellations of bigeminy, trigeminy, and quadrigeminy or as couplets.

Differential Diagnosis

As discussed earlier, when the normal QRS complex is preceded by a negative P wave in leads II and III, a PR interval of less than 0.12 second favors a junctional origin. A negative P wave in these leads with a PR interval more than 0.12 second may indicate either an ectopic atrial or a junctional origin.

Premature junctional complexes with aberrant ventricular conduction resemble premature ventricular complexes. A junctional origin can be assumed if a retrograde P wave with a short PR interval precedes the QRS complex or if the retrograde P wave appears after the QRS and

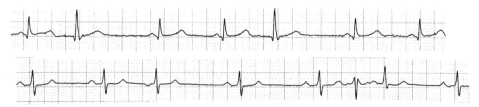

Figure 16–10   Premature junctional complexes. *Top,* Two premature junctional complexes conducted with slight aberration, no visible P waves, and a shorter than compensatory postextrasystolic pause. *Bottom,* Two premature junctional complexes, the first of which is preceded by a negative P wave and followed by a shorter than compensatory postextrasystolic pause. The second (sixth complex) is interpolated without a visible P wave and is conducted with aberration.

the RP interval is less than 0.11 second. The premature complex with an RP interval less than 0.12 second is unlikely to be ventricular in origin, as the interval is too short for ventriculoatrial (VA) conduction unless an accessory pathway is present. A longer RP interval, however, does not exclude a junctional origin of the ectopic complex.

AUTOMATIC JUNCTIONAL TACHYCARDIA

Tachycardia due to increased automaticity of the AVJ in adults is nearly always associated with structural heart disease. The ECG findings are as follows[9–11]:

1. The heart rate is 120 to 220 beats/min, but the rate may vary from minute to minute.
2. The QRS duration is normal unless aberrant ventricular conduction or bundle branch block is present.
3. The rhythm is generally regular, but occasionally it is grossly irregular, mimicking atrial fibrillation or multifocal atrial tachycardia.[10]
4. A retrograde P wave may be seen following the QRS, but AV dissociation with or without sinus capture is more common.

In the presence of retrograde atrial capture, automatic junctional tachycardia is difficult to differentiate from reentrant AV or AV nodal tachycardia on the body surface ECG. Some irregularity of the rhythm and varying of the heart rate favor the automatic mechanism rather than the reentrant mechanism. Automatic junctional tachycardia does not respond to vagal stimulation, which may or may not terminate an AV nodal or AV reentrant tachycardia. Figure 16–11 illustrates simultaneous ectopic atrial tachycardia and junctional tachycardia (double tachycardia) documented by intraatrial electrography.

Automatic junctional tachycardia may assume a configuration of bidirectional tachycardia in which the junctional impulses depolarize the ventricles through alternate pathways (fascicles),

resulting in QRS complexes of opposite polarities.[12–14] In the presence of ventricular aberrancy the alternating QRS complexes are wide, but in some cases the bidirectional tachycardia is ventricular in origin.[15]

ACCELERATED AV JUNCTIONAL RHYTHM (NONPAROXYSMAL JUNCTIONAL TACHYCARDIA)

Nonparoxysmal junctional tachycardia was first described by Pick and Dominguez.[16] It is now called *accelerated AV junctional rhythm* and is believed to be automatic with the following characteristics:

1. The rate of junctional discharge is only moderately increased, being about 70 to 130 beats/min (see Figure 16–7).
2. The ectopic rhythm lacks the sudden onset and termination that are characteristic of the paroxysmal type of AV node reentrant tachycardia.
3. The relation between the sinus rhythm and the accelerated AV junctional rhythm depends on the state of anterograde and retrograde conduction at the AVJ and on the atrial and ventricular rates. If retrograde activation of the atria occurs, a constant relation exists between the P wave and the QRS complex. If retrograde conduction is impaired, the atria remain under control of the sinus impulse, resulting in AV dissociation. The ventricular rate is generally faster than the atrial rate except when an accelerated junctional rhythm develops in the presence of atrial tachycardia, atrial fibrillation, or atrial flutter.

An accelerated junctional rhythm is seen predominantly in patients with heart disease. Common causes include digitalis intoxication, acute myocardial infarction (MI), intracardiac surgery, or myocarditis. Only in rare instances does the cause of the arrhythmia remain unexplained. In the series described by Pick and Dominguez, digitalis was responsible for more than half of

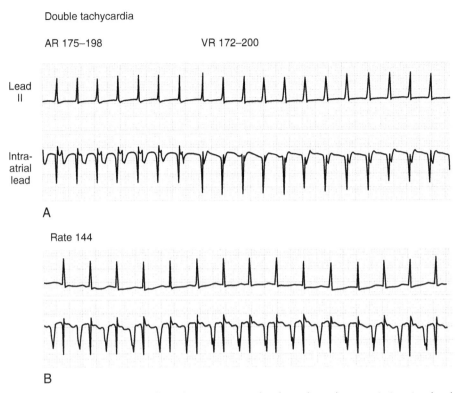

Figure 16–11   Double tachycardia. **A,** Independent ectopic atrial tachycardia and automatic junctional tachycardia are demonstrated by the intraatrial lead. **B,** Ectopic atrial tachycardia alone.

the cases.[16] MI and intracardiac surgery are probably the more common causes in recent years. The arrhythmia was reported in up to 10 percent of patients with acute MI.[17] It is more commonly associated with inferior than anterior MI. In the latter case, it is said to be a poor prognostic sign.

Occasionally there is anterograde exit block of the junctional impulse, and the ventricular rate becomes slow. On the ECG, type I exit block can be suspected in the presence of "group beating" (suggestive of Wenckebach periodicity), and type II exit block can be suspected in the presence of a long cycle that is a multiple of the basic interectopic interval[18] (Figure 16–12).

If the QRS complex is wide, an accelerated junctional rhythm resembles an accelerated ventricular rhythm. The rate of the ectopic ventricular rhythm is usually 70 to 110 beats/min. The ventricular origin of the rhythm can be recognized if capture complexes with narrow QRS or fusion complexes are present (see Chapter 17).

AV Dissociation

There is considerable disagreement and confusion about the definition of AV dissociation. It can be avoided if one remembers to ask two questions: What is dissociated from what? Why? In most cases, the term *AV dissociation* is applied when atrial and ventricular rhythms are independent of each other.

AV dissociation may be caused by default or usurpation. The cause of default may be sinus bradycardia, sinus arrest, or SA block. The atrial rate becomes slower than the inherent rate of the subsidiary pacemaker, which acts by default as an AV junctional or idioventricular escape mechanism. Usurpation is defined by increased automaticity of the subsidiary pacemaker, resulting in junctional or ventricular tachycardia. In each case the relation between the two dissociated rhythms depends on the state of the anterograde and retrograde AV conduction.

AV dissociation may be complete or incomplete. With complete AV dissociation, the atrial and ventricular rates (PP and RR intervals) remain constant, although the PR interval varies. None of the atrial impulses are conducted to the ventricles. With incomplete AV dissociation, some of the atrial impulses arrive at the AVJ at a time when the junction is no longer refractory and are conducted to the ventricles. Ventricular captures occur, and the basic ventricular rhythm

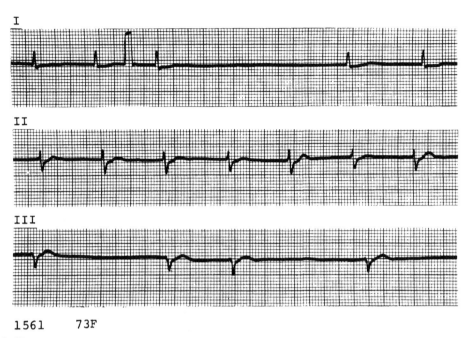

Figure 16–12   Accelerated atrioventricular junctional rhythm resulting from digitalis toxicity. There is sinus arrest. The basic ventricular rate is 72 beats/min. Retrograde P waves are seen as slight slurring at the end of the QRS in leads II and III. The long pause in lead I has a duration approximately three times that of the basic RR interval. In lead III the two long pauses have durations approximately twice that of the basic RR interval. These long pauses are probably due to exit block of the junctional impulse, both anterograde and retrograde.

is disturbed and reset. This phenomenon also has been called *AV dissociation with interference*, *AV dissociation with ventricular capture*, or *interference dissociation*.

The term *interference dissociation* has been defined differently by different authors.[19] In my opinion, the term is superfluous. If interference stands for interaction between impulses of different origin, the only condition without interference is a complete bidirectional block between the dissociated propagation ways. Under all other circumstances, some form of "interference" takes place; as such it can be defined specifically based on the observed or deduced manifestations, such as suppression, resetting, reciprocation, synchronization, altered refractoriness, concealed conduction, fusion, or capture, among others.

The broad definition of AV dissociation includes also all cases of AV block because the atrial and ventricular rhythms are dissociated from each other. However, when the cause of the dissociation is an AV block, the use of the term *dissociation*, even if technically correct, is considered unnecessary because it may lead to confusion.

With *isorhythmic AV dissociation,* the rates of the dissociated pacemakers are nearly the same (see Figure 16–8). The two rhythms appear to chase each other, which prompted Marriott and Menendez[20] to describe it as a "flirtatious"

relationship. When the relationship is persistent, it is called *synchronization*; if it is transient, it is called *accrochage*.

One of the proposed mechanisms of isorhythmic dissociation[21] (based on experimental findings) is the juxtaposition of two pacemaker sites that synchronize their discharges by some undefined interaction; this is likened to the interaction of two independent oscillators. Observation of patients with isorhythmic AV dissociation during surgery suggested that this phenomenon might be due also to AV junctional rhythm with retrograde capture of the atria; such a mechanism cannot be assumed, however, when the retrograde P waves are not inverted in the inferior leads.[22]

AV Nodal Reentry

AV NODAL REENTRANT TACHYCARDIA

One of the major contributions of programmed intracardiac electrical stimulation was the discovery that so-called paroxysmal supraventricular tachycardia not associated with accessory pathways could be induced and terminated in most afflicted patients by premature stimuli

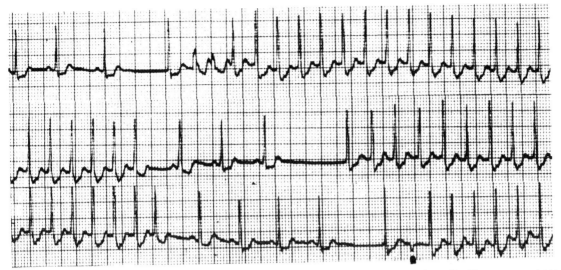

Figure 16–13 ECG of a patient with intermittent atrioventricular (AV) nodal reentrant tachycardia. The presence of AV block (a negative P wave, marked by a dot, not followed by a QRS complex) during tachycardia shows that ventricles do not participate in the tachycardia circuit.

applied during a relative refractory period of the AV node. This suggested that the tachycardia was reentrant.[23] The prerequisite for induction was appropriate lengthening of the AH interval, which in most cases resulted from Wenckebach periodicity.[24] A similar critical delay in VA conduction was required to induce ventricular echo in the presence of a retrograde Wenckebach period.[25] Lack of participation of tissues distal to the His bundle recording site was confirmed in patients with reentry continuing in the presence of AV block[26] (Figure 16–13).

Dual AV Nodal Pathways

Studies by Rosen and his colleagues[27–31] have firmly linked AV nodal reentrant tachycardia with the presence of dual AV nodal pathways. The application of premature atrial stimuli at progressively shorter coupling intervals allows generation of an AV nodal function curve that represents a plot of H_1H_2 responses as a function of A_1A_2 (coupling) intervals. A continuous curve suggests a single AV nodal pathway. The curve becomes discontinuous when minor shortening of the A_1A_2 interval (i.e., ≤ 10 ms) results in a sudden increase ("jump") of 50 ms or more in the H_1H_2 interval (Figure 16–14). After the onset of discontinuity, continuing extrastimulation generates a second continuous curve or precipitates AV nodal reentrant tachycardia (AVNRT). This may be associated with the presence of two PR intervals or RP intervals (see Figures 19–4 and 19–5). In patients with AVNRT the curve is usually discontinuous, revealing the presence of a fast and a slow anterograde pathway. Reentrant supraventricular tachycardia can be induced by atrial premature stimuli that block in the anterograde fast pathway and conduct through the anterograde slow pathway. Subsequently,

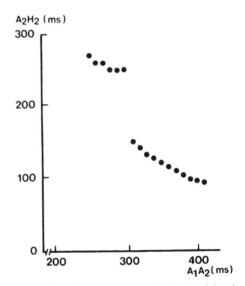

Figure 16–14 Dual atrioventricular (AV) nodal pathway curve. When the atrial premature complex interval is shortened minimally (10 ms), an abrupt increase in the anterograde conduction time occurs. Shown are the AV nodal conduction times (A_2, H_2) of atrial premature beats (A_1, A_2). (From Brugada P, Wellens HJ: Electrophysiology, mechanisms, diagnosis, and treatment of paroxysmal recurrent atrioventricular nodal reentrant tachycardia. *In:* Surawicz B, Reddy CP, Prystowsky EN (eds): Tachycardias. Boston, Martinus Nijhoff, 1984.)

the previously blocked fast pathway becomes available for retrograde conduction toward the atrium. Thus the usual circus movement consists of slow anterograde and fast retrograde pathway conduction with proximal and distal common pathways.

Shen et al.[32] reported that in 40 consecutive patients who underwent slow pathway ablation, the characteristics of fast pathway conduction were not affected, which supports the concept that fast and slow pathways are functionally distinct. Until recently these pathways were believed to be located in the AV node, but experience with ablation of these pathways is no longer consistent with this hypothesis. It has been shown that lesions that ablate nodal reentry are in atrial muscle fibers in the area of the triangle of Koch rather than in the histologically specialized AV node.[33] Moreover, ablation of the slow pathway to cure AV nodal reentrant tachycardia does not produce histologic damage to the AV node.[34]

Common AV Nodal Tachycardia

The occurrence of spontaneous AVNRT in patients with dual AV nodal pathways hinges on the appropriate relation between the conduction of these pathways. The refractory period of the slow pathway is shorter than that of the fast pathway, allowing demonstration of the discontinuous curves. The rate at which the conduction in the slow pathway becomes blocked defines the limit of slow pathway participation during reentry. In most patients with AVNRT, the slow pathway conducts as fast as 170 to 180 beats/min and in some cases up to 250 beats/min.[29] The rate at which retrograde conduction in the fast pathway is blocked defines the limits of fast pathway participation in reentry. In most patients with AVNRT, the fast retrograde pathway conducts as fast as 180 beats/min and in some cases 250 beats/min or more.[29]

The cycle length of supraventricular tachycardia is determined predominantly by the conduction time through the slow pathway because retrograde conduction is more similar among patients, although variations exist. It has been shown that the retrograde conduction time through the fast pathway tends to parallel the anterograde conduction time through this pathway (i.e., the AH interval). Rosen and coworkers found that 17 percent of patients with dual AV nodal pathways had short PR (AH) intervals associated with appropriately fast retrograde conduction through the fast pathway. This explained the facilitation of reentry in patients with short PR intervals (Lown-Ganong-Levine syndrome)[30] (Figure 16–15). It should be noted, however, that reentrant tachycardia with a short PR interval may be caused by other mechanisms, including AV reentry utilizing a concealed accessory pathway.[35]

Dual pathways in the AV node have been found in 10 to 35 percent of patients studied by programmed electrical stimulation for reasons other than paroxysmal supraventricular tachycardia and in 35 percent of children with acquired or congenital heart disease but no evidence of spontaneous or inducible supraventricular tachycardia.[36] Thus finding a dual AV nodal pathway in either anterograde or retrograde direction appears to be of no clinical significance in the absence of suspected supraventricular tachycardia.

Observations suggest that the matrix of a single dual pathway fails to explain all the clinical observations.[37] Thus it has been shown that the classic clinical definition of the AV nodal dual pathway physiology (i.e., the 50-ms "jump" in the A_2H_2 interval for a 10-ms change in the A_1A_2 interval) is applicable to only 60 to 85 percent of cases with AVNRT.[38,39] The remaining patients have smooth conduction curves. Another series of observations showed that atrial

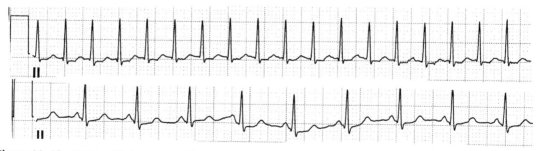

Figure 16–15   ECG lead II of a 42-year-old woman with ovarian carcinoma and a history of paroxysmal, most likely atrioventricular nodal reentrant tachycardia since childhood and a short PR interval during sinus rhythm. *Top,* Supraventricular tachycardia at a rate of 198 beats/min without a recognizable P wave. *Bottom,* Sinus rhythm, recorded 20 minutes later after treatment with adenosine intravenously. PR interval is 88 ms.

activation over the fast pathway is heterogeneous within Koch's triangle, a finding that argues against the concept of an anatomically discrete retrograde fast pathway.[40] Careful mapping techniques[41] revealed that multiple AV nodal pathways are not uncommon.[42] In the study of Chen et al.[41] the incidence of anterograde pathways with multiple AH "jumps" was about 5.2 percent. Thus the prevailing concept suggests that the AVNRT takes place in a highly complex, three-dimensional model with nonuniform anisotropy and discontinuous conduction in the AV junctional area. It has been reported that in one third of all typical AVNRT cases, a concealed atriohisian tract bypassing the A-V node constitutes the retrograde pathway.[42a]

Regardless of the circuit's exact location, radiofrequency ablation produces satisfactory results and is currently the procedure of choice for treating symptomatic AV node reentrant tachycardia. Although in many cases the fast pathways of the His bundle recording site can be successfully ablated,[43,44] slow pathway ablation is performed more frequently and appears to be more successful than ablation of the fast pathway.[45,46] Figure 16–16 demonstrates the sites used for ablation of fast and slow pathways.[47]

Atrioventricular nodal reentrant tachycardia is the most common form of paroxysmal supraventricular tachycardia, comprising approximately 50 percent of all regular supraventricular tachycardias.[48] It is seen most often in healthy individuals without organic heart disease and has the following characteristics:

1. The onset and termination of the tachycardia are abrupt. The episode may last seconds, minutes, hours, or days.
2. The episode is often initiated by a premature atrial impulse with prolonged PR interval (Figures 16–17 and 16–18).
3. The heart rate is usually 140 to 220 beats/min, and the rhythm is regular (see Figures 16–13, 16–17, 16–18, and 16–19).
4. The P-QRS complex has the morphologic characteristics of a junctional complex described previously. The P waves are inverted in leads II, III, and aV_F. The P waves may superimpose on, follow, or (rarely) precede the QRS complex.
5. The QRS complex may be normal or abnormally wide because of aberrant ventricular conduction or a preexisting intraventricular conduction defect.

In the common, or typical, form of AVNRT, which is seen in 90 to 95 percent of cases, the retrograde P waves are either totally or partially masked by the QRS complexes.[48] The P waves

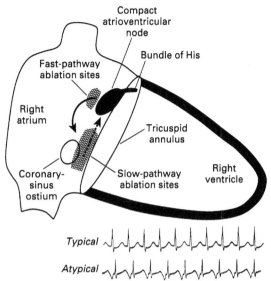

Figure 16–16 Reentry circuit of typical atrioventricular (AV) nodal tachycardia. Posterior input to the AV node (dashed arrow) serves as the anterograde slow pathway of the reentry circuit, and anterior input to the AV node (solid arrow) serves as the retrograde fast pathway. Shaded areas indicate the target sites for radiofrequency ablation of the fast and slow pathways. Also shown are typical and atypical AV nodal reentrant tachycardias, at rates of 188 and 170 beats/min, respectively, recorded in lead II. Discrete P waves are not present with typical AV nodal reentrant tachycardia. With atypical AV nodal reentrant tachycardia, inverted P waves precede the QRS complex. With this type of tachycardia the anterior input to the AV node serves as the anterograde fast pathway of the reentry circuit, and the posterior input serves as the retrograde slow pathway. (From Morady F: Radio-frequency ablation as treatment for cardiac arrhythmias. N Engl J Med 340:534, 1999. Copyright 1999 Massachusetts Medical Society, with permission.)

cannot be detected on the surface ECG in about 50 percent of the typical form (Figure 16–20). In the other near 50 percent, the P waves distort the terminal portion of the QRS complex (see Figure 16–12) and may appear as "pseudo-S" waves in the inferior leads or "pseudo-R" waves in lead V_1.[48]

Uncommon AV Nodal Tachycardia

In an uncommon variant of AVNRT (uncommon AVNRT) the anterograde limb is the fast pathway and the retrograde limb the slow pathway, resulting in a long RP' interval and a short P'R interval.[31] However, in many cases the P'R interval is still longer than the RP' interval (Figure 16–21). Tachycardia may be initiated by a premature ventricular complex.[49] The ECG pattern is indistinguishable from that of AV reentrant tachycardia, utilizing a slowly conducting accessory pathway in the retrograde direction (see later discussion). Because of

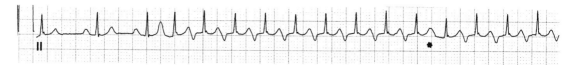

Figure 16–17   ECG lead II of a 68-year-old woman after coronary artery bypass operation shows the onset of tachycardia at a rate of 132 beats/min after an atrial premature complex with a long PR interval. It suggests atrioventricular nodal reentrant tachycardia. The tachycardia is not interrupted by the normal-appearing sinus P wave (marked by a star). This shows that atrial tissue forming the P wave does not participate in the reentrant circuit.

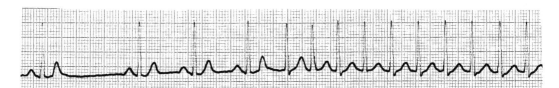

Figure 16–18   ECG strip of lead II shows the onset of atrioventricular nodal reentrant tachycardia after an atrial premature complex with a long PR interval.

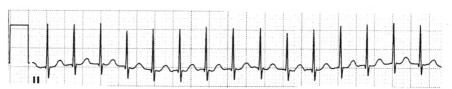

Figure 16–19   ECG lead II of a 2-year-old child with atrioventricular nodal reentrant tachycardia at a rate of 204 beats/min.

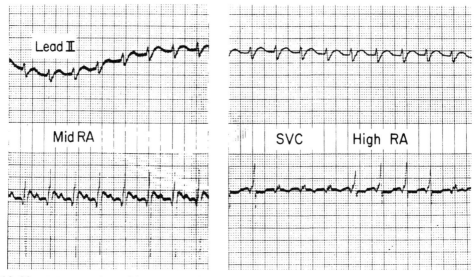

Figure 16–20   Atrioventricular nodal reentrant tachycardia. P waves are superimposed on the QRS complexes. They are demonstrated by an intraatrial electrogram obtained simultaneously with lead II. Their amplitude is largest in the mid-right atrium. (From Chou TC: Atrial and AV junctional tachycardia. *In:* Fowler NO (ed): Cardiac Arrhythmias. New York, Harper & Row, 1977.)

this similarity, the existence of a slow intranodal retrograde pathway was questioned in the earlier literature, but it was shown that tissues distal to His bundle did not participate in the reentrant circuit in patients with such tachycardias, implying that reentry indeed occurred in the AV node.[28] This type of tachycardia has been ablated selectively. Common and uncommon variants can coexist in the same patient.[50] Some patients have three or more pathways, and both AV nodal pathways forming a reentrant circuit may be "slow," giving rise to a slow-slow type of AVNRT.

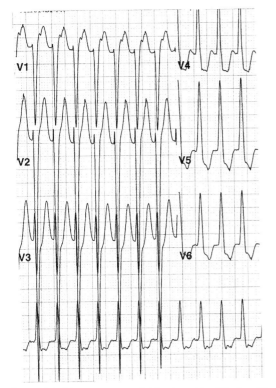

Figure 16–21 ECG precordial leads and lead II of an 80-year-old woman with atypical atrioventricular (AV) nodal reentrant tachycardia, documented in the electrophysiology laboratory and successfully ablated. RP interval is longer than in the typical AV nodal reentrant tachycardia.

Incessant Tachycardia

The tachycardia utilizing accessory pathways with AV node–like properties and long retrograde conduction times tends to manifest clinically as an incessant (or permanent) supraventricular tachycardia with a P'R interval shorter than the RP' interval. It is described here because it resembles AVNRT. Enhanced anterograde AV nodal conduction (short AH interval) and slow retrograde conduction in the accessory pathway are considered necessary to maintain the tachycardia.[51,52] The P wave is usually negative in leads II, III, aV$_F$, and V$_4$–V$_6$.[51] Its onset is generally during early childhood, and the tachycardia is characterized by age-related prolongation of the tachycardia cycle length mediated by a conduction delay in the concealed, retrogradely conducting accessory pathway, which in 76 percent of cases is posteroseptal.[51,53] Incessant tachycardia, also known as Gallavardin-type tachycardia, is present most of the time, with only a few sinus cycles interposed between episodes of tachycardia. The tachycardia is uncommon. In the study of Brugada et al.[54] the P'R was shorter than

the RP' in 28 of 300 patients with AV nodal echoes. Among patients presenting with supraventricular tachycardia to the Pediatric Arrhythmia Clinic at the University of Michigan, 1 percent had this type of tachycardia.[53] Catheter ablation is an effective treatment.[51,53]

It has been postulated that there are two slowly conducting accessory pathways. With one, conduction is suppressed by adenosine but not by verapamil; with the other, conduction is suppressed by both adenosine and verapamil.[55] The assumption underlying these differences is that the former type represents conduction dependent on the "depressed" fast channel, and the latter represents conduction dependent on the slow channel.[55]

The ECG findings of this rhythm include the following.

1. A narrow complex tachycardia that is regular with a rate of 120 to 200 beats/min
2. Retrograde P waves (superior P axis) with long RP interval and RP interval longer than the PR interval

On the body surface ECG the rhythm resembles the uncommon type of AVNRT and ectopic atrial tachycardia. It is resistant to drug therapy and may result in tachycardia-induced cardiomyopathy.

DIFFERENTIAL DIAGNOSIS OF AVNRT

In the absence of aberrant ventricular conduction or a preexisting intraventricular conduction defect, the AVNRT is diagnosed by excluding the following types of "supraventricular" (narrow QRS) tachycardias with a regular rhythm[11,48,49,56–58]:

1. Sinus tachycardia and SA nodal reentry tachycardia
2. Ectopic atrial tachycardia
3. Intraatrial reentry tachycardia
4. Atrial flutter with 2:1 conduction
5. Automatic junctional tachycardia
6. Permanent form of junctional reciprocating tachycardia
7. AV reentry tachycardia through a bypass tract

The differentiation of these supraventricular tachycardias from AVNRT is difficult at times on the body surface ECG. In most instances, however, a diagnosis of the tachycardia can be reasonably established by observing (1) whether the P waves are the result of anterograde or retrograde atrial impulse conduction and (2) the characteristics of the P-QRS relation (Figure 16–22).

If the P wave is normal and precedes the QRS complex with a normal PR interval, the tachycardia is either sinus or SA nodal reentry. The onset

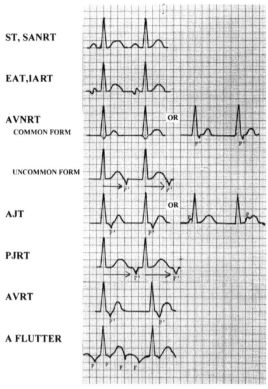

ST, SANRT

EAT, IART

AVNRT
COMMON FORM

UNCOMMON FORM

AJT

PJRT

AVRT

A FLUTTER

Figure 16–22 Morphology of the P wave in the inferior leads and its relation to the QRS complex in the various types of supraventricular tachycardia. See text discussion. A FLUTTER = atrial flutter; AJT = automatic junctional tachycardia; AVNRT = atrioventricular nodal reentrant tachycardia; AVRT = atrioventricular reentry tachycardia; EAT = ectopic atrial tachycardia; IART = intraatrial reentrant tachycardia; PJRT = permanent form of junctional reciprocating tachycardia.

and termination of sinus tachycardia are gradual, whereas those of SA nodal reentry tachycardia are sudden.[59–61] Ectopic atrial and intraatrial reentry tachycardias are characterized by an abnormal P wave followed by the QRS complex, with the PR interval being shorter than the RP interval. If the P waves are inverted in the inferior leads and the PR interval is shorter than the RP interval, the rhythm may be ectopic atrial tachycardia originating from a low atrial focus, the uncommon form of AVNRT, or the permanent form of junctional reciprocating tachycardia.

Atrial tachycardia can be excluded by showing that the atria are not required to initiate and perpetuate the tachycardia (see Figure 16–17). The following findings argue against an atrial origin: (1) initiation of supraventricular tachycardia by atrial premature pacing only after a critical delay in AV node conduction time; (2) initiation of supraventricular tachycardia by ventricular pacing only following retrograde conduction to the atria

and anterograde return of the atrial impulse through the AV node; (3) a similar atrial activation pattern during retrograde conduction over the fast AV nodal pathway during ventricular pacing and during tachycardia; (4) persistence of tachycardia in the absence of atrial activation or in the presence of atrial fibrillation; and (5) termination of supraventricular tachycardia by a ventricular premature impulse that is not conducted retrogradely to the atria.

Atrial tachycardia can be differentiated from AVNRT and orthodromic AV tachycardia by means of ventricular pacing associated with 1:1 VA conduction.[62] Upon cessation of pacing, the electrogram sequence during atrial tachycardia is atrial–atrial–ventricular, whereas with the other two tachycardia types the response is characteristically atrial–ventricular.[62]

During the "uncommon" type of AVNRT the echo is initiated at the time of discontinuity in the retrograde AV nodal conduction curve, when conduction shifts from the fast to the slow retrograde AV nodal pathway. The P wave is usually negative in leads II, III, and aV$_F$ and positive or isoelectric in lead I.[63] Variations of the P-QRS relation with or without block occur not infrequently.[64] Conduction through the slow AV nodal pathway retrogradely is supported by the following findings: (1) tachycardia is usually nonsustained; (2) tachycardia cannot be initiated by an atrial premature impulse and does not occur spontaneously during sinus rhythm[65]; and (3) tachycardia cannot be initiated after atropine. From this one can deduce that if tachycardia with a P'R interval shorter than the RP' interval occurs spontaneously, the presence of an accessory pathway with slow retrograde conduction can be assumed to exist.[65]

When reentry involves the bypass tract, there may be evidence of Wolff-Parkinson-White (WPW) syndrome, or the bypass may be concealed. [61,66,67] With AV reentry tachycardia associated with either the WPW syndrome or concealed bypass, retrograde atrial excitation occurs at the end of ventricular depolarization. Therefore the retrograde P wave is seen after the QRS and is not superimposed totally or partially on the QRS, as with the common form of AVNRT, an important distinction between these two common types of supraventricular tachycardia. Also, the presence of ST segment depression >2 mm, T wave inversion, or both during narrow QRS tachycardia is believed to suggest AV reentry.[68] The presence and utilization of an accessory AV pathway in the tachycardia reentrant loop can be excluded if the atria and ventricles are activated simultaneously or when VA conduction is absent. Additionally, persistence of tachycardia during anterograde AV block excludes an accessory AV pathway as a necessary component of the tachycardia circuit (see Figure 16–13). The incidence of 2:1 AV block is about 10 percent, and the site of the block is below the AV node, probably in the His bundle.[69] Another finding that favors utilization of the bypass tract is the initiation of tachycardia by a late-coupled premature ventricular complex.[70] Automatic junctional tachycardia may present similar findings. Their characteristics were discussed earlier.

In the typical form of atrial flutter with 2:1 conduction, negative flutter waves in the inferior leads with the RP interval greater than the PR interval may be mistaken for abnormal P waves associated with low atrial ectopic tachycardia, retrograde P waves from the uncommon type of AVNRT, or the permanent form of junctional reciprocating tachycardia. A special attempt should be made to search for the other flutter wave, which may be mostly or partially masked by the QRS complex. Lead V_1 is often helpful for this purpose.

Vagal stimulation such as carotid sinus massage may be helpful for distinguishing AVNRT from tachycardias due to increased automaticity (Figure 16–23). The maneuver may terminate AV nodal as well as SA nodal and AV reentry tachycardia, or it may have no effect on these rhythms. With ectopic atrial tachycardia and intraatrial reentry tachycardia, vagal stimulation does not terminate the arrhythmia but may cause transient AV block. With sinus tachycardia it may lower the sinus rate slightly, a temporary effect. Vagal stimulation has no effect on atrial flutter but may increase the AV block and reveal the characteristic flutter waves more clearly. Automatic junctional tachycardia and the permanent form of junctional reciprocating tachycardia do not respond to the maneuver. Pacing and various drugs, including adenosine, can be used to terminate tachycardia when intranodal tachycardia is sustained and not terminated by vagal maneuvers. Adenosine administration may be helpful in differentiation between reentrant (atrial, AVNRT, AVRT) tachycardias and focal automatic tachycardias.[71,72]

The AVNRT is usually terminated by a single premature stimulus when the tachycardia rate is slower than 160 beats/min (Figure 16–24). At faster rates, two or more premature atrial stimuli are required to terminate the tachycardia. Cardioversion is not required to terminate this type of tachycardia.

If any of these supraventricular tachycardias are associated with aberrant ventricular conduction, a preexisting intraventricular conduction defect

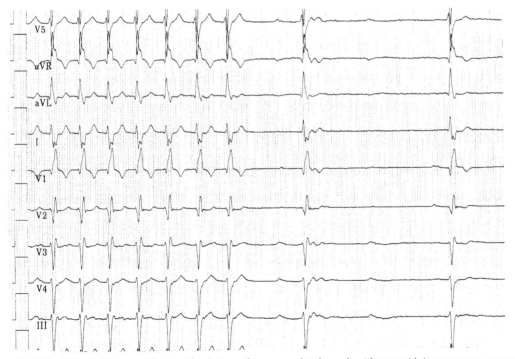

Figure 16–23 ECG of a 77-year-old man with a history of paroxysmal tachycardia. After carotid sinus massage, a complex conducted with a prolonged PR interval is followed by a negative P wave in leads II and III. It suggests that it is a reciprocal atrial complex, and that the wide QRS tachycardia with right bundle branch block and left anterior fascicular block morphology is an atrioventricular nodal reentrant tachycardia.

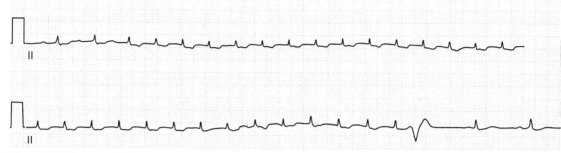

Figure 16–24 Two rhythm strips of lead II recorded on the same day in a 79-year-old man with paroxysmal tachycardia showing the typical onset *(upper strip)* and the typical termination *(lower strip)* of atrioventricular nodal reentrant tachycardia (AVNRT). The onset of AVNRT is preceded by three sinus complexes with progressive lengthening of the P-R interval, and the termination is caused by a premature ventricular complex.

including bundle branch block or ventricular preexcitation of the tachycardia may resemble monomorphic ventricular tachycardia. Their differentiation is discussed in Chapter 17.

Increased QRS voltage has been observed during AVNRT, but the finding is not helpful because it is present also in other reentrant tachycardias.[73–75]

In summary, the common form of AV nodal reentrant tachycardia can be differentiated from the other supraventricular tachycardias if the retrograde P wave is totally or partially superimposed on the QRS complex. Because one cannot always be sure that the former is the case when the P wave cannot be identified, the presence of a retrograde P wave, which is partially seen at the end of the QRS, is practically diagnostic of this arrhythmia. A definitive diagnosis of the uncommon form of AVNRT is difficult without intracardiac electrophysiologic studies because the duration of the RP' interval is similar to that in the AV reentrant tachycardia utilizing concealed A-V bypass. According to Wellens,[76] however, the differentiation can be made on clinical grounds because the uncommon AVNRT is usually paroxysmal, whereas A-V reentry with slow accessory pathway is usually incessant and prone to causing cardiomyopathy. With regard to radiofrequency catheter ablation, in the vast majority of AVNRTs, the slow pathway is ablated in the inferoseptal right atrium, but rare cases of both common and uncommon AVNRTs require ablation in the left atrium or within the coronary sinus.[76a]

Reciprocal Impulses

Reciprocal impulses (echo beats) occur when the impulse activates the chambers (atria or ventricles), returns, and reactivates the same chambers again. The above term is used when the reentry

phenomenon is limited to one or two complexes. If the process continues, reentrant tachycardia develops. The impulses responsible for the appearance of reciprocal complexes may originate from the atrium, AVJ, or ventricle. The fundamental requirement for the genesis of reciprocal complexes is the existence of at least two pathways between the atria and the ventricles. With the exception of WPW syndrome, in which an accessory bundle is present, the two pathways are located in the AVJ. They have refractory periods and speeds of conduction of different lengths, resulting in longitudinal dissociation of the AV junctional tissue.

RECIPROCAL IMPULSES OF JUNCTIONAL ORIGIN

The mechanism responsible for the development of reciprocal impulses originating from the AVJ (Figure 16–25) is analogous to that of AVNRT.

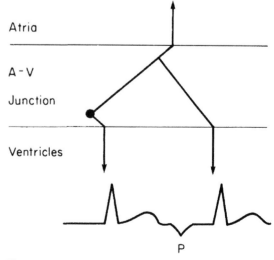

Figure 16–25 Sequence of activation and the QRS-P-QRS pattern in reciprocal junctional complexes.

The junctional impulse is conducted both antegradely and retrogradely. The anterograde conduction results in ventricular depolarization and a QRS complex. The retrograde impulse is blocked in one of the two junctional pathways and is conducted with considerable delay in the other pathway to activate the atria. Subsequently, it enters the previously unused pathway, which by now is able to conduct the impulse anterogradely and activate the ventricles again, producing the reciprocal or echo complex. For the echo impulse to occur, a long anterograde (see Figures 16–8 and 16–18) or a long retrograde conduction time (RP interval) (Figure 16–26) is necessary. This is occasionally precipitated by a retrograde Wenckebach phenomenon with gradual prolongation of the RP interval before the appearance of the reciprocal impulse.

The ECG shows the following:

1. The P wave sandwiched between two closely grouped QRS complexes is inverted in the inferior leads.
2. The RP interval is longer than 0.20 second.
3. The PR interval (from the retrograde P wave to the second QRS) is variable but often prolonged.
4. The first QRS complex is the same as the basic QRS complex of the patient. The second QRS complex may be aberrantly conducted because of the relatively short RR interval.

RECIPROCAL IMPULSES OF ATRIAL ORIGIN

The ECG shows a P-QRS-P pattern. The first P wave is the result of a premature ectopic atrial impulse. The PR interval usually is prolonged. The second P wave, or atrial echo, is a retrograde P wave (see Figure 16–8). A ventricular echo may follow, and reciprocating (reentrant) tachycardia may be initiated (see Figure 16–17).

RECIPROCAL IMPULSES OF VENTRICULAR ORIGIN

The ECG of a reciprocal impulse of ventricular origin (Figure 16–27) reveals a QRS-P-QRS pattern. The first QRS complex is the result of an ectopic ventricular impulse and is therefore wide. The P wave results from retrograde capture of the atria, and the RP interval is prolonged. The second QRS complex, the reciprocal complex (also called *return extrasystole*), is usually normal because the return impulse follows the intraventricular conduction pathways unless there is aberrant ventricular conduction.

An interesting clinical manifestation of dual pathways in the AV node is simultaneous conduction through both pathways by a single impulse, resulting in one P wave followed by two QRS complexes.[77,78] This phenomenon is not common and must be differentiated from the more common "pseudosimultaneous" asynchronous fast and slow pathway conduction, which is present when, after termination of atrial pacing, two ventricular complexes follow one P wave because of sustained, slow conduction through the slow pathway.[79] Double atrial responses to a single ventricular impulse may also occur owing to simultaneous conduction via the two AV nodal retrograde pathway.[80]

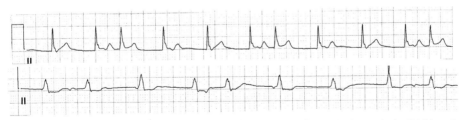

Figure 16–26 Reciprocal impulses following prolongation of the RP interval. *Top,* Atrioventricular (AV) junctional rhythm with short and long RP intervals in a 51-year-old man after a coronary artery bypass graft operation. The longer RP intervals in the second, sixth, and ninth complexes are followed by reciprocal ventricular complexes. *Bottom,* AV junctional rhythm at a rate of 72 beats/min with variable PR and RP intervals in a 78-year-old man with coronary artery disease and previous inferior myocardial infarction. The first, fourth, and eighth complexes with long RP intervals are followed by ventricular reciprocal complexes.

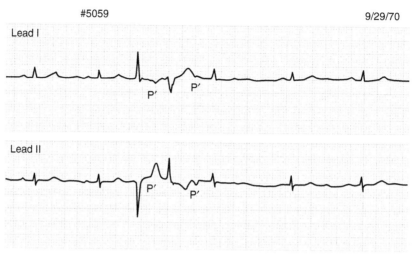

Figure 16–27   Reciprocal complex originating from the ventricle. The simultaneously recorded leads I through III show retrograde capture of the atria by the ectopic ventricular impulse, which returns to reactivate the ventricle. This results in an abnormal QRS complex due to aberrant ventricular conduction. Retrograde capture of the atria occurs again and is followed by another ventricular echo complex with normal morphology.

REFERENCES

1. Truex R, Smythe M: Reconstruction of the human atrioventricular node. Anat Rec 158:11, 1967.
2. McGuire MA, Bourke JP, Robotin MC, et al: High resolution mapping of Koch's triangle using sixty electrodes in humans with atrioventricular junctional ("AV nodal") reentrant tachycardia. Circulation 88:2315, 1993.
3. Langendorf R, Simon AJ, Katz LN: A-V block in A-V nodal rhythm. Am Heart J 27:1, 1944.
4. Lancaster JF, Leonard JJ, Leon DF, et al: The experimental production of coronary sinus rhythm in man. Am Heart J 70:89, 1965.
5. Lau SH, Cohen SI, Stein E: P waves and P loops in coronary sinus and left atrial rhythms. Am Heart J 79:201, 1970.
6. Waldo AL, Vitikainen KJ, Harris PD, et al: The mechanism of synchronization in isorhythmic AV dissociation. Circulation 38:880, 1968.
7. Hwang W, Langendorf R: Auriculoventricular nodal escape in the presence of auricular fibrillation. Circulation 1:930, 1950.
8. Scherlag BJ, Lazzara R, Helfant RH: Differentiation of AV junctional rhythms. Circulation 68:304, 1973.
9. Garson A, Gillette PC: Junctional ectopic tachycardia in children: electrocardiographic, electrophysiologic and pharmacologic response. Am J Cardiol 44:298, 1979.
10. Ruder MA, Davis JS, Eldar M, et al: Clinical and electrophysiologic characterization of automatic junctional tachycardia in adults. Circulation 73:930, 1986.
11. Wu D, Denes P, Amat-y-Leon F, et al: Clinical, electrocardiographic and electrophysiologic observations in patients with paroxysmal supraventricular tachycardia. Am J Cardiol 41:1045, 1978.
12. Cohen SI, Voukydis P: Supraventricular origin of bidirectional tachycardia: report of a case. Circulation 50:634, 1974.
13. Morris SN, Zipes DP: His bundle electrocardiography during bidirectional tachycardia. Circulation 48:32, 1973.
14. Rosenbaum MB, Elizari MV, Lazzari JO: The mechanism of bidirectional tachycardia. Am Heart J 78:4, 1969.
15. Cohen SI, Deisseroth A, Hecht HS: Infra-His bundle origin of bidirectional tachycardia. Circulation 47:1260, 1973.
16. Pick A, Dominguez P: Nonparoxysmal AV nodal tachycardia. Circulation 16:1022, 1957.
17. Konecke LL, Knoebel SB: Nonparoxysmal junctional tachycardia complicating acute myocardial infarction. Circulation 45:367, 1972.
18. Fisch C: Electrocardiography of Arrhythmias. Philadelphia, Lea & Febiger, 1990, pp 264–265.
19. Phibbs B: Interference, dissociation, and semantics: a plea for rational nomenclature. Am Heart J 65:283, 1963.
20. Marriott HJL, Menendez MM: AV dissociation revisited. Prog Cardiovasc Dis 8:522, 1966.
21. Segers M, Lequime J, Denolin H: Synchronization of auricular and ventricular beats during complete heart block. Am Heart J 33:685, 1947.
22. Waldo AL, Vitikainen KJ, Harris PD, et al: The mechanism of synchronization in isorhythmic AV dissociation. Circulation 38:880, 1968.
23. Bigger JT, Goldreyer BN: The mechanism of supraventricular tachycardia. Circulation 62:679, 1971.
24. Goldreyer BN, Damato AN: The essential role of atrioventricular conduction delay in the initiation of paroxysmal supraventricular tachycardia. Circulation 63: 423, 1970.
25. Damato AN, Lau SH, Bobb G: Studies on ventriculoatrial conduction and the reentry phenomenon. Circulation 61:423, 1970.
26. Wellens HJ, Wesdorp JC, Duren DR, et al: Second degree block during reciprocal atrioventricular nodal tachycardia. Circulation 53:595, 1976.
27. Denes P, Wu D, Dhingra RC, et al: Demonstration of dual AV nodal pathways in patients with paroxysmal supraventricular tachycardia. Circulation 68:549, 1973.
28. Wu D, Denes P, Dhingra R, et al: Determinants of fast- and slow-pathway conduction in patients with dual atrioventricular nodal pathways. Circ Res 36:782, 1975.
29. Rosen KM, Bauernfeind RA, Swiryn S, et al: Dual AV nodal pathways and AV nodal reentrant paroxysmal tachycardia. Am Heart J 101:691, 1981.

30. Bauernfeind RA, Swiryn S, Strasberg B, et al: Analysis of anterograde and retrograde fast pathway properties in patients with dual atrioventricualr nodal pathways. Am J Cardiol 49:283, 1982.

31. Wu D, Denes P, Amat-y-Leon F, et al: An unusual variety of atrioventricular nodal reentry due to retrograde dual atrioventricular nodal pathways. Circulation 56:50, 1977.

32. Shen WK, Munger TM, Stanton MS, et al: Effects of slow pathway ablation on fast pathway function in patients with atrioventricular nodal reentrant tachycardia. J Cardiovasc Electrophysiol 8:627, 1997.

33. Sanchez-Quintana D, Davies DW, Ho SH, et al: Architecture of the atrial musculature in and around the triangle of Koch: its potential relevance to atrioventricular nodal reentry. J Cardiovasc Electrophysiol 8:1396, 1997.

34. Olgin JE, Ursell P, Kao AK, et al: Pathological findings following slow pathway ablation for AV nodal reentrant tachycardia. J Cardiovasc Electrophysiol 7:625, 1996.

35. Ward DE, Camm J: Mechanisms of junctional tachycardias in the Lown-Ganong-Levine syndrome. Am Heart J 105:169, 1983.

36. Casta A, Woff GS, Mehta AV, et al: Dual atrioventricular nodal pathways: a benign finding in arrhythmiafree children with heart disease. Am J Cardiol 46:1013, 1980.

37. Boyle NG, Anselme F, Monahan K, et al: Origin of junctional rhythm during radiofrequency ablation of atrioventricular nodal reentrant tachycardia in patients without structural heart disease. Am J Cardiol 80: 575, 1997.

38. Mazgalev TN: The dual AV nodal pathways: are they dual and where they are? J Cardiovasc Electrophysiol 8:1408, 1997.

39. Kuo C-T, Lin K-H, Cheng N-J, et al: Characterization of atrioventricular nodal reentry with continuous atrioventricular node conduction curve by double atrial extrastimulation. Circulation 99:659, 1999.

40. Anselme F, Hook B, Monahan K, et al: Heterogeneity of retrograde fast pathway conduction pattern in patients with atrioventricular nodal reentry tachycardia. Circulation 93:960, 1996.

41. Chen S-A, Tai C-T, Lee S-H, et al: AV nodal reentrant tachycardia with unusual characteristics: lessons from radiofrequency catheter ablation. J Cardiovasc Electrophysiol 9:321, 1998.

42. Lee KL, Chun HM, Liem LB, et al: Multiple atrioventricular nodal pathways in humans: electrophysiogic demonstration and characterization. J Cardiovasc Electrophysiol 9:129, 1998.

42a. Otomo K, Suyama K, Okamura H, et al: Participation of a concealed atriohisian tract in the reentrant circuit of the slow-fast type of atrioventricular nodal reentrant tachycardia. Heart Rhythm 4:703, 2007.

43. Jackman WM, Beckman KJ, McClelland JH, et al: Treatment of supraventricular tachycardia due to atrioventricular nodal reentry by radiofrequency catheter ablation of slow-pathway conduction. N Engl J Med 327:313, 1992.

44. Haissaguerre M, Montserrat P, Warin JF, et al: Closed-chest ablation of retrograde conduction in patients with atrioventricular nodal reentrant tachycardia. N Engl J Med 320:426, 1989.

45. Wu D, Yeh S-J, Wang C-C, et al: A simple technique for selective radiofrequency ablation of the slow pathway in atrioventricular node reentrant tachycardia. J Am Coll Cardiol 21:1612, 1993.

46. Mitrani RD, Klein LS, Hackett FK, et al: Radiofrequency ablation for atrioventricular node reentrant tachycardia: comparison between fast (anterior) and slow (posterior) pathway ablation. J Am Coll Cardiol 21:432, 1993.

47. Akhtar M, Jazayeri MR, Sra J, et al: Atrioventricular nodal reentry: clinical, electrophysiological, and therapeutic considerations. Circulation 88:282, 1993.

48. Josephson ME, Seides SF: Clinical Cardiac Electrophysiology, 2nd ed. Philadelphia, Lea & Febiger, 1993.

49. Josephson ME, Kastor JA: Supraventricular tachycardia: mechanisms and management. Ann Intern Med 87:346, 1977.

50. Zipes DP: Genesis of cardiac arrhythmias: electrophysiological considerations. In: Braunwald E (ed): Heart Disease. Philadelphia, Saunders, 1992.

51. Gaita F, Haissaguerre M, Giustetto C, et al: Catheter ablation of permanent junctional reciprocating tachycardia with radiofrequency current. J Am Coll Cardiol 23:648, 1995.

52. Yagi T, Ito M, Odakura H, et al: Electrophysiologic comparison between incessant and paroxysmal tachycardia in patients with permanent form of junctional reciprocating tachycardia. Am J Cardiol 78:697, 1999.

53. Dorostkar PC, Silka MJ, Morady F, et al: Clinical course of persistent junctional reciprocating tachycardia. J Am Coll Cardiol 33:366, 1999.

54. Brugada P, Bar FW, Vanagt EJ, et al: Observations in patients showing AV junctional echoes with a shorter PR than RP interval. Am J Cardiol 48:611, 1981.

55. Lerman BB, Greenberg M, Overholt ED, et al: Differential electrophysiologic properties of decremental retrograde pathways in long RP′ tachycardia. Circulation 76:21, 1987.

56. Coumel P: Supraventricular tachycardia. In: Krikler DM, Goodwin JF (eds): Cardiac Arrhythmias: The Modern Electrophysiological Approach. Philadelphia, Saunders, 1975.

57. Gomes JA, Hariman RJ, Kang PS, et al: Sustained symptomatic sinus node reentrant tachycardia: incidence, clinical significance, electrophysiologic observations and the effects of antiarrhythmic agents. J Am Coll Cardiol 5:45, 1985.

58. Morady F, Scheinman MM: Paroxysmal supraventricular tachycardia. Part I. Diagnosis. Mod Concepts Cardiovasc Dis 51:107, 1982.

59. Curry PV, Evans TR, Krickler DM: Paroxysmal reciprocating sinus tachycardia. Eur J Cardiol 6:199, 1977.

60. Watanabe Y, Dreifus LS: Sites of impulse formation within the atrioventricular function of the rabbit. Circ Res 22:717, 1968.

61. Wu D, Amat-y-Leon F, Denes P, et al: Demonstration of sustained sinus and atrial reentry as a mechanism of paroxysmal supraventricular tachycardia. Circulation 51:234, 1975.

62. Knight BP, Zivin A, Souza J, et al: A technique for rapid diagnosis of atrial tachycardia in the electrophysiology laboratory. J Am Coll Cardiol 33:775, 1999.

63. Ng K-S, Lauer MR, Young C, et al: Correlation of P-wave polarity with underlying electrophysiologic mechanisms of long RP′ tachycardia. Am J Cardiol 77:1129, 1996.

64. Taniguchi Y, Yeh S-J, Wen M-S, et al: Variation of P-QRS relation during atrioventricular node reentry tachycardia. J Am Coll Cardiol 33:376, 1999.

65. Brugada P, Wellens HJ: Electrophysiology, mechanisms, diagnosis, and treatment of paroxysmal recurrent atrioventricular nodal reentrant tachycardia. In: Surawicz B, Prystowsky EN, Reddy CP (eds): Tachycardias. Boston, Martinus Nijhoff, 1984.

66. Farshidi A, Josephson ME, Horowitz LN: Electrophysiologic characteristics of concealed bypass tracts: clinical and electrocardiographic correlates. Am J Cardiol 41:1052, 1978.

67. Wellens HJ, Durrer D: The role of an accessory pathway in reciprocal tachycardia. Circulation 52:58, 1975.

68. Riva SI, Della Bella P, Fasini G, et al: Value of analysis of ST segment changes during tachycardia in determining type of narrow QRS complex tachycardia. J Am Coll Cardiol 27:1479, 1996.

69. Man KC, Brinkman K, Bogun F, et al: 2:1 Atrioventricular block during atrioventricular node reentrant tachycardia. J Am Coll Cardiol 28:1770, 1996.

70. Anguera I, Roba M, Portiegies M, et al: Narrow QRS complex tachycardia initiated by single spontaneous ventricular premature depolarizations: what is the tachycardia mechanism? J Cardiovasc Electrophysiol 10:1293, 2000.

71. Wakimoto H, Izumida N, Asano Y, et al: Augmentation of QRS wave amplitudes in the precordial leads during narrow QRS tachycardia. J Cardiovasc Electrophysiol 11:52, 2000.

72. Surawicz B: Effect of heart rate on QRS voltage. A simple relation that escaped notice. J Cardiovasc Electrophysiol 11:61, 2000.

73. Oreto G, Luzza F, Badessa F, et al: QRS complex voltage changes associated with supraventricular tachycardia. J Cardiovasc Electrophysiol 12:1358, 2001.

74. Viskin S, Fish R, Glick A, et al: The adenosine triphosphate test: a bedside diagnostic tool for identifying the mechanism of supraventricular tachycardia in patients with palpitations. J Am Coll Cardiol 38:173, 2001.

75. Iwai S, Markovitz SM, Stein KM, et al: Response to adenosine differentiates focal from macroreentrant tachycardia. Validation using three dimensional electroanatomic mapping. Circulation 106:2793, 2002.

76. Wellens HJJ: Twenty-five years of insights into the mechanisms of supraventricular arrhythmias. J Cardiovasc Electrophysiol 14:1020, 2003.

76a. Otomo K, Nagata Y, Uno K, et al: Atypical atrioventricular nodal reentrant tachycardia with eccentric coronary sinus activation: Electrophysiological characteristics and essential effects of left-sided ablation inside the coronary sinus. Heart Rhythm 4:421, 2007.

77. Wu D, Denes P, Dhingra R, et al: New manifestations of dual AV nodal pathways. Eur J Cardiol 2:456, 1975.

78. Sutton FJ, Yu-Chen L: Supraventricular nonreentrant tachycardia due to simultaneous conduction through dual atrioventricular nodal pathways. Am J Cardiol 51:897, 1983.

79. Yeh SJ, Wu Y-C, Lin F-C, et al: Pseudosimultaneous fast and slow pathway conduction: a common electrophysiologic finding in patients with dual atrioventricular nodal pathways. J Am Coll Cardiol 6:927, 1985.

80. Lin FC, Yeh SJ, Wu D: Double atrial responses to a single ventricular impulse due to simultaneous conduction via two retrograde pathways. J Am Coll Cardiol 5:168, 1985.

17 Ventricular Arrhythmias

Ventricular arrhythmias define ectopic activity originating distal to the bifurcation of the His bundle. Excluded is activity originating in the His bundle, even though this structure is situated within the interventricular septum, because the His bundle is part of the atrioventricular (AV) junction. Arrhythmias utilizing the accessory pathway are also excluded from the definition even though ventricular tissue is involved in the circus movement tachycardias.[1]

The ectopic location of the pacemaker in the ventricle alters the sequence of cardiac activation. The excitation no longer follows the normal pathway of the intraventricular conduction network. There is asynchronous activation of the two ventricles. Consequently, the morphology of the QRS complex becomes abnormal, and the duration of the QRS complex is prolonged.

Ventricular arrhythmias may develop as an escape phenomenon because of failure of the sinus or supraventricular impulse to reach the ventricles at the expected time. More commonly, however, ventricular ectopic impulses occur prematurely.

Premature Ventricular Complexes

Premature ventricular complexes (PVCs) are known by several other names, such as ventricular extrasystoles, ventricular premature beats (VPBs), ventricular ectopic complexes (VECs), and ventricular premature depolarizations (VPDs). None of these terms is absolutely satisfactory for this most common of rhythm disorders[2] because prematurity can be recognized only in the presence of regular rhythm, whereas in the presence of atrial fibrillation the prefix "premature," a term that implies an occurrence earlier than expected, may not be valid.[2,3]

ELECTROCARDIOGRAPHIC FINDINGS

1. The ectopic impulses on electrocardiograms (ECGs) are premature in relation to the expected impulse of the basic rhythm.
2. The QRS complex is abnormal in duration and configuration. It is accompanied by secondary ST segment and T wave changes. When the major QRS deflection is upright, the ST segment is depressed and the T wave inverted; and when the major QRS deflection is negative, the ST segment is elevated and the T wave upright. The morphology of the complexes may vary in the same patient.
3. There is usually a full compensatory pause following the PVCs (Figure 17–1).
4. Retrograde capture of the atria may or may not occur.

Coupling Interval

The PVCs with a constant coupling interval usually occur near the end of the T wave (i.e., close to the end of the ventricular refractory period). Early PVCs interrupt the T wave (R-on-T); and late PVCs, called *end-diastolic*, frequently form fusion complexes (Figure 17–2). Most often the coupling interval is considered constant when the variation does not exceed 0.08 second.[4] Occasionally it is influenced by the preceding cycle length.[5]

To determine whether the patterns of PVC coupling hold any clues to the mechanism of PVCs, Surawicz and Macdonald[6] analyzed the coupling interval in 88 subjects who had 10 or more unifocal PVCs in the same lead. In 40 subjects the coupling interval was fixed (varying by less than 120 ms), and in 48 subjects the coupling interval varied by more than 120 ms. Persons without heart disease and three groups of patients with heart disease of varying severity had a similar incidence of fixed and variable coupling intervals. In some cases the coupling interval increased with increasing duration of the RR (and QT) interval, and in some cases the relation was inverse. Most often, however, there was no good correlation between the coupling interval and the preceding RR interval in subjects with varying RR intervals.

Fusion Complexes

Summation or fusion occurs when two pacemakers participate in ventricular activation (Figures 17–3 and 17–4). Ventricular fusion complexes are observed in most cases of ventricular preexcitation where different parts of the ventricles are activated by impulses conducted simultaneously through the AV bypass and the AV node. The presence of fusion complexes is important for the diagnosis of parasystole (Figure 17–5). Fusion complexes are also common when supraventricular complexes coincide with late PVCs or escape impulses. Ventricular fusion complexes can also result from simultaneous stimulation of two ventricular impulses (e.g., fusion of a spontaneous complex and a paced complex or of two competing escape pacemakers) during AV block.[7]

Marriott et al.[8] formulated the following criteria for fusion complexes between supraventricular and ventricular impulses: (1) the contour and duration of fusion complexes are usually intermediate between the contours and durations of two competing pacemakers; (2) the PS (or PJ) interval of the fusion complex cannot be shorter than the PR interval of the supraventricular complex; (3) the PR interval is equal to or shorter than the PR interval of the supraventricular complex; (4) the terminal vector of the fusion complex is always different from that of the complex generated by the supraventricular impulse; and (5) the initial vector may or may not differ from the initial vector of the complex generated by the supraventricular impulse. Exceptions

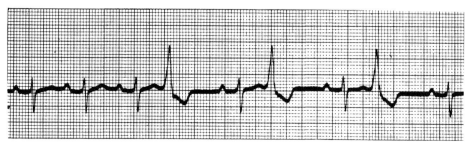

Figure 17–1 Premature ventricular complexes (PVCs). Tracing demonstrates the full compensatory pause after the PVCs. A short run of bigeminal rhythm is present.

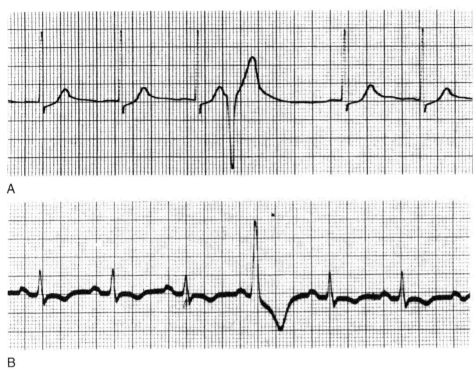

Figure 17–2   **A,** Early premature ventricular complex (PVC) with the R-on-T phenomenon. **B,** Late or end-diastolic PVC.

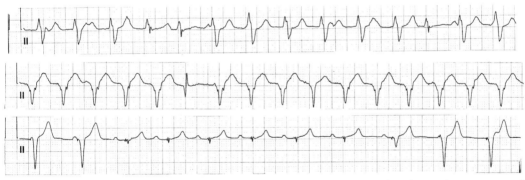

Figure 17–3   ECG strips of lead II. *Top,* Ventricular accelerated rhythm at a rate of 95 beats/min with sinus captures (fifth and twelfth complexes) and fusion complexes (fourth and eighth). *Middle,* Ventricular tachycardia at a rate of 107 beats/min with sinus capture (sixth complex) and fusion (tenth complex). *Bottom,* Intermittent ventricular pacing with a fusion complex (ninth complex).

to these criteria are seen in the presence of bundle branch block, other intraventricular conduction disturbances, and variable AV conduction times during supraventricular rhythm.

Concealed PVC

Concealment of PVC implies the absence of a PVC at the time it was expected to occur. This can be postulated only if there is a regular, predictable arrangement of PVCs. For instance, if a PVC becomes concealed during bigeminal rhythm, there are three sinus complexes, rather than one sinus complex, between two PVCs.

Kinoshita in Japan in 1960[9] and Schamroth and Marriott in the United States in 1961[10] independently observed cases in which there were only odd numbers of sinus complexes between two PVCs (i.e., $2n-1$, where n is any number) and postulated that it is indicative of concealed

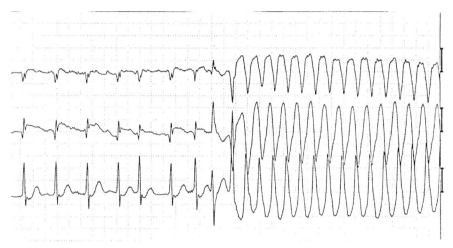

Figure 17–4　Onset of monomorphic ventricular tachycardia (VT) recorded during ambulatory monitoring of a 50-year-old man with coronary artery disease. ECG shows atrial fibrillation with ST segment elevation in the middle (inferior) lead. VT follows abruptly after a fusion complex.

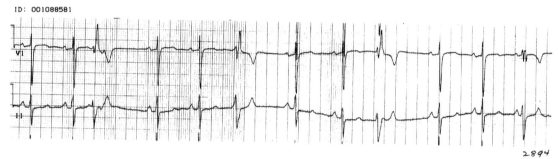

Figure 17–5　Ventricular parasystole. The basic rhythm is sinus with an RR interval of about 800 ms. Parasystolic complexes with right bundle branch block configuration show varying coupling intervals, a fixed interectopic interval of 2600 ms, and fusion in the last complex. (Courtesy of Dr. Charles Fisch.)

bigeminy. They also defined concealed trigeminy as a PVC occurring after two sinus impulses.* In this case concealment was detected by showing that the number of intervening sinus complexes was $3n-1$, where n is any number (e.g., 5, 8, 11, 14). Subsequently, cases of concealed quadrigeminy were found with the number of intervening sinus complexes equal to $4n-1$, and concealed hexageminy with the number of intervening complexes equal to $6n-1$.

---

*This type of trigeminy should be differentiated from a trigeminy where each sinus impulse is followed by two PVCs. Even if the concept of concealed PVCs is plausible, its occurrence does not reveal the mechanism of the PVCs.[9] Schamroth[10] assumed that the concealed PVCs are aborted automatic discharges, whereas Levy et al.[11,12] explained the same phenomenon by varying block in the reentrant circuit and described several additional variants of concealed bigeminy, trigeminy, and a combination of the two.

SITE OF ORIGIN

As a broad general rule, the right ventricular ectopic pacemaker generates a ventricular complex with left bundle branch block (LBBB) pattern, and the left ventricular ectopic pacemaker generates a ventricular complex with right bundle branch block (RBBB) pattern. A superior frontal plane QRS axis under such circumstance suggests a location of the pacemaker in or near the posterior division of the left bundle branch. A rightward QRS axis suggests a location in or near the anterior division of the left bundle branch. A basal location of the pacemaker is associated with dominant anterior QRS forces, with most or all of the precordial leads displaying an upright QRS complex.[13] An apical location generates posteriorly oriented QRS forces and mostly negative QRS complexes in the precordial leads.

The QRS duration of PVCs depends on their site of origin and on the characteristics of tissues activated by the premature impulse in relation to the Purkinje network. It also tends to be wider when the coupling time is short because the impulse conduction is likely to be more aberrant or encounter partially refractory tissue.

It has been shown that in patients with cardiomyopathy the PVCs with notches and shelves of more than 40 ms duration and QRS duration exceeding 160 ms represent markers for a dilated and globally hypokinetic left ventricle.[14] The duration of the QRS complex with ectopic ventricular complexes is usually 0.12 second or longer, but ventricular premature complexes with morphology similar to that of sinus complexes and normal QRS duration can occur. This is seen most commonly in the presence of LBBB on baseline complexes (see Chapter 4). The suggested mechanism explaining the narrow QRS complex of a ventricular ectopic impulse is the origin within the interventricular septum, with equal conduction time to both ventricles below

the region of the block.[15] In the absence of bundle branch block, a septal ectopic impulse conducting with equal delay to both ventricles is expected to simulate an AV junctional complex.

PVCs with different QRS configurations usually indicate a multifocal origin of the ectopic beats (Figure 17–6). Endocardial mapping studies showed, however, that an impulse originating at the same site may produce complexes with distinctly different QRS morphologies because of varying spread of excitation.[16] This means that errors can be made when attempting to localize the site of origin of a PVC on the basis of the morphology of the ventricular complex on the surface ECG, especially in patients with coronary artery disease.[17]

When the ectopic impulses originate from different foci, their coupling intervals are usually different. The changing morphology in the absence of multifocal origin can also occur when the premature complexes are late and cause

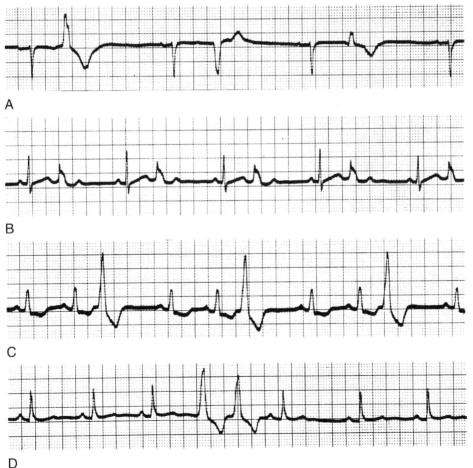

A

B

C

D

Figure 17–6   **A,** Multifocal premature ventricular complexes (PVCs). **B,** PVCs in bigeminy. **C,** PVCs in trigeminy. **D,** PVCs in a couplet.

varying degrees of fusion with the next sinus complex because of the slight change in the sinus rate or changing coupling interval of the premature impulses. Also, in couplets, the morphology of the second QRS complex of the couplet may differ from that of the first complex because of the short RR interval, resulting in additional aberrant conduction caused by relative refractoriness.

In patients with myocardial infarction (MI) and an abnormal Q wave, PVCs may also display a Q wave. Such Q waves may persist when a Q wave is no longer present in the sinus complexes (Figure 17–7).

POSTEXTRASYSTOLIC PAUSE AND VENTRICULOATRIAL CONDUCTION

If the basic rhythm is sinus in origin, a PVC is typically followed by a pause that is fully compensatory. The sum of the RR intervals that precede and follow the ectopic complex (or the RR interval that contains the PVC) equals two RR intervals of the sinus rhythm. The fundamental requirement for the occurrence of a fully compensatory pause is that the sinus rhythmicity is undisturbed by the ectopic impulse. It is observed if one of the following conditions occur: (1) there is ventriculoatrial (VA) block or (2) there is retrograde VA conduction and atrial capture, but the ectopic impulse is either blocked at the sinoatrial (SA) junction, or the sinus impulse is discharged before arrival of the ectopic impulse. The two excitation fronts may meet at the SA junction, in the atria, at the AV junction, or in the ventricles.

Because many patients have sinus arrhythmia, the RR interval that contains the PVC may not be exactly twice the duration of the RR interval of the adjacent sinus complex, even though a fully compensatory pause exists. If the ectopic impulse depolarizes the SA node and resets its rhythmicity, the postextrasystolic pause is no longer fully compensatory. Such depolarization of the SA nodal tissue by an extrinsic impulse may temporarily depress its activity, and a fortuitous "compensatory" pause may be observed.

In most instances the sinus P wave that occurs during the PVC is difficult to recognize within the QRS complex or the T wave (Figure 17–8). The exact state of the VA conduction is therefore often difficult to determine on the surface ECG. With an esophageal lead, retrograde VA conduction was demonstrated in 45 percent of patients with PVCs by Kistin and Landowne.[18] During ventricular pacing the incidence of VA conduction was 89 percent in patients

with normal anterograde AV conduction times and 8 percent in patients with prolonged AV conduction times.

PATTERN OF PRESENTATION

The frequency of the ectopic beats varies widely not only among individuals, but also in the same subject at different periods of observation. Most authors use the adjective *frequent* when there are 5 or more PVCs per minute on the routine ECG or more than 10 to 30 per hour during ambulatory monitoring.

The PVCs may appear in a pattern of bigeminy, trigeminy, or quadrigeminy (see Figure 17–2). The term *complex premature ventricular complexes* usually refers to PVCs that are frequent, are multiform, or show bigeminy, trigeminy, couplets, triplets, or the R-on-T phenomenon.

Lown and Graboys[19] proposed the following grading system for premature ventricular complexes. It was commonly used for prognostic evaluation but today is mainly of historic interest.

0 = No premature ventricular complexes
1 = Occasional (<30 per hour)
2 = Frequent (>30 per hour)
3 = Multiform
4 = Repetitive
        A = Couplets
        B = Salvos of 3
5 = R-on-T

RULE OF BIGEMINY

Langendorf et al.[4] defined the "rule of bigeminy" as a natural consequence of PVCs emerging only after appropriately long diastolic intervals. In such cases a compensatory pause creates conditions for PVC occurrence, and hence bigeminy persisting so long as the compensatory pause remains sufficiently long (see Figures 17–1 and 17–6). According to the rule, bigeminy disappears when the heart rate increases, which is usually the case (Figure 17–9). Even though the rule of bigeminy explains the increased prevalence of PVCs at slow heart rates, it does not explain the mechanism of the PVC because it can represent reentry if propagation through the circuit requires a certain amount of time or an automatic discharge after a long phase 4 depolarization.

INTERPOLATED PVCs

An interpolated PVC is sandwiched between two consecutive sinus complexes without disturbing the sinus rhythm (Figure 17–10). It occurs mostly when the sinus rate is slow and the

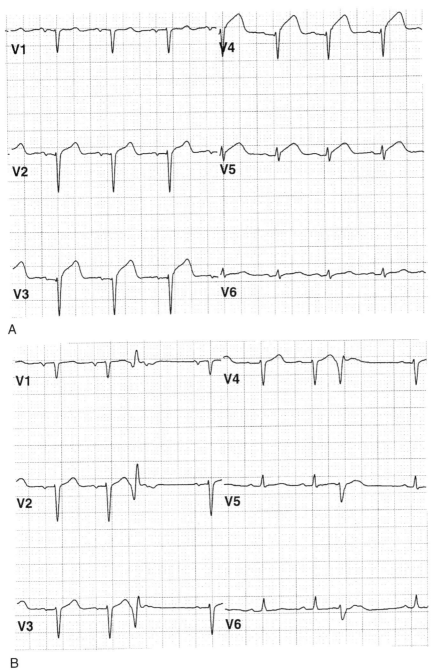

Figure 17–7 **A,** EGC precordial leads from an 86-year-old woman recorded 5 days after an acute anterior myocardial infarction documented by typical ECG evolution and enzyme elevation. Note the abnormal ST segment elevation in leads V_2–V_4 and nearly absent R waves in leads V_1–V_4. **B,** Three months later her pattern is normal except for "poor R wave progression," which is not specific. Another supporting, albeit nonspecific, finding is the morphology of the ventricular premature complex.

premature complex is early. The PR interval of the sinus couples following the PVC is nearly always prolonged because of concealed retrograde conduction of the ectopic ventricular impulse, which renders the AV junction partially refractory to the closely following sinus impulse.

Katz et al.[20] established that disturbances of AV conduction caused by an interpolated PVC affect the conduction not only of the first but also of the second postextrasystolic complex as a result of changing the RP-PR relation. This accounts for a postponed compensatory pause.[21]

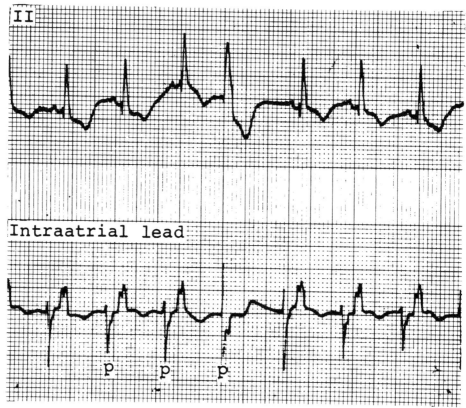

Figure 17–8   Premature ventricular complexes (fourth complete complex) masking the P wave, which is revealed by a simultaneous intraatrial electrogram.

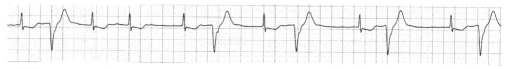

Figure 17–9   ECG strip of lead II illustrating the "rule of bigeminy": preferential occurrence and perpetuation of premature ventricular complexes (PVCs) after long RR intervals. Note the absence of PVCs after a shorter RR interval (fourth cycle). Underlying rhythm is atrial fibrillation.

COUPLETS AND TRIPLETS

Couplets and triplets (two or three PVCs in succession, respectively) (see Figures 17–6 and 17–10) seldom occur in the absence of concomitant single PVCs. Typically the number of PVCs exceeds by several orders of magnitude the number of couplets, whereas the episodes of couplets are usually more frequent than those of triplets and nonsustained ventricular tachycardia (VT). The morphologies of the PVCs of the couplets may differ from each other, but more frequently the morphologies are the same. Triplets (see Figure 17–10) are also called *salvos* and are sometimes considered nonsustained VT.

Kuo and Surawicz[22] have shown that couplets occur significantly more often in patients with proved or suspected ventricular parasystole than in those with fixed coupling intervals of the PVCs. Of several possible mechanisms proposed to explain this association, the most plausible is reentry within the parasystolic focus or its vicinity.[22,23] In such cases the mechanism of the second complex of the couplet is the same as that of a single PVC, which may explain the more frequent occurrence of couplets than of triplets and longer runs of nonsustained VT. This hypothesis is consistent with the observation that repetitive reentry is more difficult to elicit than single reentry during programmed electrical stimulation.

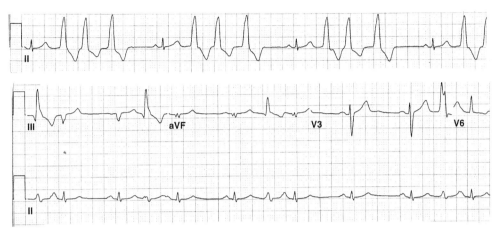

Figure 17–10   *Top*, Three ventricular ectopic complexes in a row, called *triplets, salvos,* or *nonsustained ventricular tachycardia. Bottom,* Interpolated premature ventricular complexes (PVCs). Sinus P wave after the interpolated PVC is superimposed on a T wave, but lengthening of the PR interval can be appreciated.

Surawicz et al.[24] examined the QRS morphology of PVCs in patients with permanent ventricular pacemakers and found that in 20 of 80 patients the QRS morphology of the PVC was similar to that of the preceding paced complex, which suggested that the couplet was caused by reentry in the vicinity of the pacing site (i.e., parasystolic focus). Two PVCs in a row (assumed repeated reentry) were observed in only one patient, and no VT following a paced complex was encountered.

The proposed mechanism of couplets discussed earlier cannot be considered universal. Couplets are frequently associated with sustained and nonsustained VT in the absence of identifiable parasystole. In these patients the coupling interval of the first and second complex of the couplet correlated closely with the first cycle length of the VT, a finding compatible with the hypothesis that the couplet in this setting represents attempted but aborted VT.[25]

Aberrant Intraventricular Conduction

Aberrant intraventricular conduction can be divided arbitrarily into physiologic and pathologic types. The former, but not the latter, can be explained by the cycle length–dependent action potential duration and the retrograde invasion of the anterogradely blocked conduction pathway.

Physiologic Aberration

Physiologic aberration is also known as the Ashman phenomenon.[26] Intraventricular conduction

disturbances occur when the refractoriness in a segment of the conducting system (usually a bundle branch or a fascicle) had insufficient time to complete recovery. The most likely site of delayed recovery is in the segment with the longest intrinsic refractory period, which is usually the right bundle branch.

Physiologic aberration can be produced in nearly all normal subjects by selecting an appropriate combination of a long cycle followed by a short cycle. This is because after a long cycle the time-dependent refractoriness of the AV node tends to shorten, the voltage-dependent refractoriness of the bundle branch becomes longer, and the relatively short voltage-dependent refractoriness of the His bundle does not impede the impulse transmission toward the bundle branches.

In 1967, Cohen et al.[27] produced aberration of the RBBB type in nearly all studied subjects (including six normal persons) and aberration of the LBBB type in two of these subjects. They concluded that aberrant conduction "must be considered a physiological event."

In another pacing study of 52 subjects by Cohen and colleagues,[28] multiple patterns of aberrant conduction were observed in 29 cases. RBBB was induced in 31 cases, RBBB with left anterior fascicular block in 27, left anterior fascicular block in 14, left posterior fascicular block in 6, RBBB with left posterior fascicular block in 7, and LBBB in 6.

In practice, aberration of the supraventricular premature complexes is observed often (Figure 17–11). The most common sites of conduction delay are the right bundle branch and the left anterior fascicle of the left bundle branch (see Figure 17–11). Frequently, in the presence

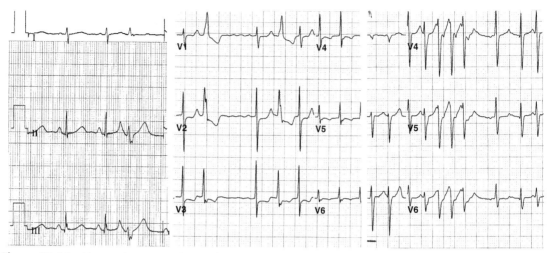

Figure 17–11 Aberrant intraventricular conduction. *Left,* Premature atrial complex conducted with aberration (right bundle branch block [RBBB] morphology). *Middle,* Atrial fibrillation with two complexes conducted after long pauses with aberration (RBBB morphology); the short RR interval after the complex with wide QRS favors the diagnosis of aberration versus premature ventricular complexes. *Right,* Four consecutive complexes conducted with aberration because of the rapid rate during atrial fibrillation; the diagnosis of aberration is supported by polymorphism.

of two or more supraventricular premature complexes, only the first is conducted with aberration. The degree of aberrancy may vary. Different gradations of abnormalities may be seen in the same individual, often related to the degree of prematurity of the supraventricular impulse.

Runs of aberrant PVCs can form a "wide QRS tachycardia" (Figure 17–12), possibly caused by long sequences of cycle lengths shorter than the refractory period of the conducting system, a mechanism postulated by Gouaux and Ashman[29] in 1947 and popularized by Langendorf[30] in 1950. An alternative mechanism of continuing aberration is continuing retrograde invasion from the contralateral bundle branch, a mechanism documented by several investigators during intracardiac extrastimulation.[31,32]

Akthar et al.[33] examined the site of conduction delay during functional bundle branch block in 14 subjects with normal intraventricular conduction. All subjects developed RBBB; 9 of them also developed LBBB and bilateral bundle branch block. During RBBB, the block was proximal to the site of the right bundle potential recording in all but 2 subjects.

Chilson et al.[34] studied the rate-dependent refractoriness of the right and left bundle branches in humans. They found that during long cycles the relative refractory period of the right bundle branch was greater than that of the left bundle branch, but during short cycles the relative refractory period of the left bundle branch was greater than that of the right bundle branch. This explains the occurrence of functional

RBBB and LBBB in the same person. Cohen et al.[35] showed that an aberrant QRS complex was followed by retrograde activation of the His bundle. They suggested that, following anterograde conduction in the left bundle branch, the blocked right bundle branch was invaded retrogradely, causing a His bundle echo. This has been shown to occur in subjects with normal function of the intraventricular conduction system, in whom sustained conduction delay in the right bundle branch could be induced by ventricular pacing because of repeated anterograde concealment by impulses conducted retrogradely via the left bundle branch.[36] This may be the reason why the cycle in which the bundle branch block disappears is nearly always longer than the cycle in which acceleration-dependent bundle branch block develops.

"Pathologic" Aberration

Fisch et al.[37] studied 40 patients with a rate-dependent aberration that differed from the physiologic aberration as follows: (1) the aberration occurred after relatively long cycles (i.e., at slow heart rates) and in some cases without a change in cycle length; (2) the aberration was less dependent on the typical sequence of a short cycle preceded by a long cycle; (3) in most patients the conduction block was in the left bundle branch; and (4) nearly all patients had structural heart disease. In a similar group of 15 patients with organic heart disease and rate-dependent bundle branch block (10 patients with LBBB and 5 with RBBB), Denes et al.[38]

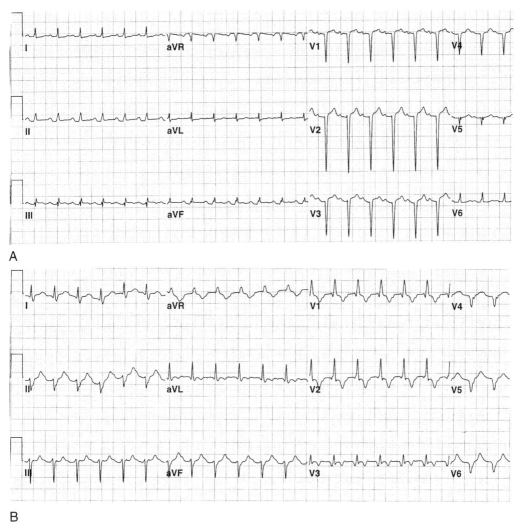

A

B

Figure 17–12   ECG of a 29-year-old man with acute anterior myocardial infarction. **A,** Sinus rhythm at a rate of 152 beats/min; QRS is 70 ms. Note the QS pattern in leads V_1–V_5. **B,** Same day: the sinus rhythm is at a rate of 146 beats/min, and there is aberrant ventricular conduction with a pattern of incomplete right bundle branch block and left anterior fascicular block. QRS is 118 ms, and there is a wide Q wave in lead V_3 and a QS pattern in leads V_4–V_6.

found that the onset of rate-dependent bundle branch block was usually abrupt and caused by loss of the normal decrease in the refractory period of the bundle branch accompanying the decrease in cycle length. It was manifested by an abnormal shape of the relation between the refractory period of the bundle branches and the cycle length in these patients.

Fisch[39] also reported the transient appearance of bundle branch block after termination of VT in three patients with organic heart disease. Although two of these patients had rate-dependent bundle branch block, the posttachycardia bundle branch block could not be explained by a critical increase in cycle length but was assumed to be provoked by VT.

DIFFERENTIATION OF PVCs FROM PREMATURE SUPRAVENTRICULAR COMPLEXES WITH ABERRANT VENTRICULAR CONDUCTION

The differential diagnosis of PVCs versus premature supraventricular complexes with aberrant ventricular conduction is not difficult when the abnormal QRS complex is preceded by a *premature* P wave, indicating that the ectopic beat is supraventricular (atrial or junctional) in origin. The absence of a fully compensatory pause further supports such a diagnosis. If no P wave can be identified, the ectopic focus may be located in the AV junction or ventricle. A fully compensatory pause following the premature complex favors its ventricular origin, but the absence of a fully compensatory pause does not exclude such a possibility, as retrograde depolarization of the SA node may have occurred. A normal sinus P wave may appear after the QRS complex in either a premature junctional or ventricular complex if there is no retrograde atrial capture. If a retrograde P wave is identifiable after the QRS complex and the RP interval is less than 0.11 second, the premature complex is likely to be AV junctional, as the RP interval is too short for VA conduction unless an accessory pathway is present. An RP interval of 0.20 second or longer is suggestive, but not diagnostic, of an ectopic ventricular complex, as the retrograde conduction time of a junctional impulse is less likely to exceed this duration.[40]

The morphology of the QRS complex may be of some assistance in distinguishing aberrant conduction from ventricular ectopy. The abnormal QRS complex is more likely to be aberrant if its initial forces are similar to those of the sinus impulse and if there is an RBBB pattern with an rSR pattern in lead V_1[41] (see Figure 17–11). Conversely, if the QRS complexes in all precordial leads are either all positive or all negative, ventricular ectopic complexes are more likely.[42]

DIAGNOSIS OF PVCs IN THE PRESENCE OF ATRIAL FIBRILLATION

Atrial fibrillation and atrial flutter with variable block create numerous opportunities for aberration. Under these circumstances, the differential diagnosis between aberration and PVCs may be difficult or impossible. The differential diagnosis is discussed in Chapter 15.

Heart Rate Turbulence

The concept of heart rate turbulence (HRT) was introduced by Schmidt et al in 1999.[43] The HRT indicates short-term fluctuation in sinus cycle length (an increase followed by a decrease over a 10- to 15-beat period that follows a PVC. The absence of HRT is considered to be a noninvasive predictor of adverse cardiac events following MI.[44]

Clinical Correlation

PVCs seldom occur in healthy children, but from adolescence on they begin to increase in frequency exponentially with advancing age.[45] The "complexity"—defined as multiformity, bigeminy, couplets, triplets, and runs of nonsustained

VT—also increases with advancing age. The presence of heart disease contributes to the increased frequency and complexity of PVCs even when cardiac function remains normal or minimally impaired. An even greater increase in frequency and complexity tends to accompany impairment of ventricular function and development of congestive heart failure.[45,46]

Apparently Healthy Individuals

The prevalence of PVCs in otherwise healthy adults monitored with 24-hour ambulatory ECGs ranged from 17 to 100 percent but most commonly from 40 to 55 percent.[47–49] Complex PVC forms may be present in 7 to 22 percent of subjects and in as many as 77 percent when older subjects were studied. A considerable variation in the number and complexity of the PVCs occurs from day to day and hour to hour in the same individual in all age groups. In one study of 165 hospital patients, those without organic heart disease had PVCs predominantly of right ventricular origin.[50]

In normal individuals PVCs may increase, decrease, or be totally suppressed by exercise.[51–53] They may be absent at rest but precipitated by exercise. In the studies of McHenry et al.,[54] 6 percent of clinically normal subjects had ventricular arrhythmias when they exercised on the treadmill to increase their heart rate up to 130 beats/min. The incidence of ventricular arrhythmias increased with increasing levels of exercise, and 44 percent of the subjects developed arrhythmias when the heart rate was increased to more than 170 beats/min. The arrhythmias may appear during or immediately after exercise.

No definite relation between PVCs and smoking or coffee, tea, or alcohol intake has been established. Generally, the frequency of PVCs tends to decrease during sleep[52,55] in normal subjects and those with heart disease.

In certain patients, frequent PVCs can cause left ventricular dysfunction which may subside after catheter ablation of the foci of PVC origin.[55a]

Heart Disease

As a rule, the reported incidence of ventricular arrhythmias varies depending on the duration of observation. In patients with chronic coronary artery disease without acute MI, the incidence was about 90 percent when the ECG was recorded for 6 to 24 hours.[52,53]

Patients with coronary artery disease are more prone to develop ventricular arrhythmias with exercise. The incidence of such arrhythmias in these patients is more than four times that of age-matched normal subjects at comparable heart rates.[54] The incidence of complex ventricular arrhythmias also is higher in patients with coronary artery disease. Patients with three-vessel disease and abnormal left ventricular wall motion have a significantly higher incidence of exercise-induced ventricular arrhythmias. Most investigators agree, however, that exercise-induced ventricular arrhythmias are of questionable value as predictors of untoward events in patients with ischemic heart disease.[55–58] In patients with acute MI, the PVCs can be detected in all patients by continuous monitoring.[59]

PVCs also are commonly encountered in patients with other types of organic heart disease, including hypertensive and rheumatic heart disease and cardiomyopathies. In patients with rheumatic or valvular heart disease, ventricular arrhythmias are seen most often when there is cardiac enlargement or congestive heart failure.

PVCs comprise the most common arrhythmia in patients with mitral valve prolapse syndrome. They are seen in about one third of routine ECGs of these patients.[60] Ambulatory ECG monitoring by Winkle and associates[61] revealed an even higher incidence, with 50 percent of the patients showing frequent PVCs (which they defined as more than 425 complexes in 24 hours) and another 25 percent exhibiting occasional PVCs.

Frequent PVCs are the most common arrhythmias in patients with digitalis excess. They account for about half of the arrhythmias induced by the drug[62] and are often multifocal or bigeminal. Antiarrhythmic drugs used to treat arrhythmia can also increase the incidence of PVCs, a phenomenon known as *proarrhythmia*. Among electrolyte imbalances, hypokalemia is frequently associated with the appearance of ventricular arrhythmias.[63]

PROGNOSTIC SIGNIFICANCE

The prognostic significance of PVCs depends mainly on the population involved. Rodstein et al.[64] found no increased mortality among 712 insured persons with extrasystoles on their routine ECGs who were followed for an average 18 years. Their life expectancy was normal if they had no other evidence of cardiac abnormality or hypertension, regardless of whether the subjects had simple or complex PVCs. In the presence of hypertension or other cardiac abnormality, however, PVCs were associated with a mortality rate more than twice that expected.

The prognostic implications of complex ventricular ectopic complexes in patients with coronary artery disease varied among studies. De Soyza et al.[65] found that complex ventricular arrhythmias were not associated with an increased risk of sudden death in patients with chronic stable angina. In three large series of patients with acute MI examined before their hospital discharge and followed for 1 to 3 years, the presence of complex ventricular arrhythmias increased the risk of sudden death by about threefold.[54,66,67] In the Cardiac Arrhythmia Pilot Study, 360 patients who had more than 10 PVCs per hour during the early post-MI period and received no antiarrhythmic agents were followed by 24-hour ambulatory ECGs for 1 year. Patients who had more than 10 PVCs per hour 1 year after MI had a threefold increase in mortality compared with those who had fewer than 3 PVCs per hour.[68] In the GISSI-2 study, 8676 post-MI patients who were treated with thrombolytic agents during the acute phase of the illness were followed for 6 months.[69] The incidence of sudden death (2.1 percent) was significantly higher among patients who had more than 10 PVCs per hour than in those who had fewer than 10 PVCs per hour (0.8 percent).

An increased risk of sudden death also is found for patients who have arrhythmias several months after MI.[70,71] In the Coronary Drug Project,[72] among 2,035 survivors of MI, mortality during a 3-year follow-up was nearly twice as high among those with any PVCs in the resting baseline 12-lead ECG as in those who had no PVCs. In the Danish Verapamil Infarction Trial,[73] the presence of more than 10 PVCs predicted increased mortality 1 week and 1 month after MI but not after 16 months. In the Canadian Assessment of Myocardial Infarction Study, PVCs had no independent predictive value of mortality.[74]

Ventricular Parasystole

Parasystolic rhythms are believed to be automatic. Automaticity is an inherent property of cardiac fibers endowed with the capacity to develop diastolic depolarization (i.e., pacemaker fibers). Normally the heart rate is usurped by pacemakers with the steepest slope of diastolic depolarization located in the SA node. The pacemakers with the slowest intrinsic rate are the ventricular Purkinje fibers with the gentlest slope of diastolic depolarization, whereas the intrinsic rate of subsidiary pacemakers in the atria and the AV junction is intermediate between that of the SA mode and Purkinje fibers.

During normal activity originating in the SA node, the slower diastolic depolarization of all subsidiary pacemaker fibers is constantly suppressed by the activity of the dominant pacemaker and becomes evident only as an escape mechanism when the propagation wave originating in the faster pacemakers fails to reach the subsidiary pacemakers and suppress their activity. Under certain circumstances, however, two rhythms—one originating in the faster, dominant pacemaker and the other in the slower, subsidiary pacemaker—can coexist. This is known as *paraarrhythmia* or, more commonly, *parasystole*.

To explain the presence of parasystole, it is necessary to assume that the slower pacemaker is not disturbed by the spread of excitation from the dominant pacemaker; that is, it enjoys protection. This implies the presence of an entrance block into the site of the ventricular automatic (parasystolic) focus, which thus has an opportunity to continue its diastolic depolarization until it reaches a threshold of excitation and spreads out as an ectopic impulse. The successful propagation of such an impulse can take place when the myocardium ceases to be refractory after propagation of the dominant pacemaker. Propagation of the ectopic pacemaker during the refractory period (most of the QT interval) is not possible, which means that the ectopic pacemaker encounters an exit block.

Because of the usual lack of synchronization between the rates of the dominant pacemaker and the parasystolic pacemaker, the emerging ectopic impulses bear no fixed time relation (although exceptions occur) to the dominant pacemaker, which means that their coupling intervals vary. Variable coupling intervals represent an important characteristic of a parasystolic rhythm.

The inherent rate of a parasystolic pacemaker can be deduced if the dominant rhythm becomes temporarily suppressed (e.g., by vagal stimulation), allowing two or more ectopic impulses to appear in succession. A more practical way to determine the rate of the parasystolic pacemaker is to measure the durations of interectopic intervals, which may contain variable numbers of impulses that were prevented from emerging because of an exit block. The cycle length of the parasystole may be revealed by finding a common divisor. The search for the common divisor is helped by the availability of a long record. The long records often reveal time intervals of absent ectopic impulses that cannot be accounted for by the presence of refractoriness. The occurrence of such intervals free of parasystolic activity is defined as intermittent parasystole.

Even in the absence of intermittence, however, the calculated interectopic intervals are not absolutely constant, which may be explained in part by the autonomic influences and more importantly by the process known as *modulation*. The concept of modulated pacemaker activity originates in the observations of Weidmann,[75] who showed that the course of diastolic depolarization in Purkinje fibers is reset to a steeper or flatter slope following application of subthreshold depolarizing or hyperpolarizing current pulses.

Moe and co-workers[76,77] showed that the stimuli applied during the early and late courses of diastolic depolarization have opposite effects on the course of diastolic depolarization; the earliest stimulus has the maximal effect in one direction and the last stimulus in the opposite direction. This means that each perturbation can produce a phase response curve that typically consists of a period of acceleration followed by a period of retardation. The perturbation assumed to be responsible for modulation of the parasystolic pacemaker is the spread of excitation of the dominant pacemaker, which influences electrotonically the zone of protection without actual invasion of this zone and without abolition of protection. Because the electrotonic modulation takes place variously during different phases of pacemaker activity, one can determine when the dominant pacemaker will accelerate or delay diastolic depolarization and thereby accurately describe the characteristics of the so-called phase response curve that modulates the rhythm of pacemaker activity.

In most subjects, parasystolic rates range between 30 and 66 beats/min[78] but may be as slow as 20 beats/min and as rapid as 400 beats/min. Parasystolic VT is present when the rate is more than 70 beats/min (Figure 17–13). Fusion complexes are frequently found in subjects with parasystole. The morphology is variable depending on the proportion of the ventricle activated by the two impulses. Fusion complexes occur with all types of ventricular arrhythmias but are seen more commonly with ventricular parasystole (see Figure 17–5).

Ventricular parasystole is seen more often than atrial or AV junctional parasystole. In the early literature, it was reported to occur in 1.0 to 1.5 per 1000 ECGs,[78,79] but the examination of short ECG strips probably underestimates the frequency of ventricular parasystole. In the study of Surawicz and Macdonald,[6] examination of extended records revealed that variable coupling intervals occurred more frequently than the fixed coupling intervals. In 32 of 48 persons with a variable coupling interval, a least-common divisor of interectopic intervals was established, permitting the labeling of these

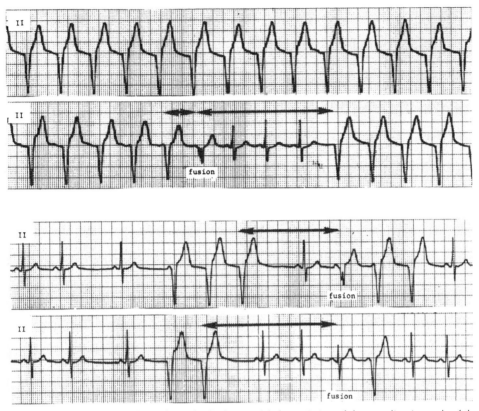

Figure 17–13 Parasystolic ventricular tachycardia (VT). Note (1) the variation of the coupling intervals of the ectopic complexes initiating the various episodes of VT; (2) the mathematic relation between the RR intervals of the ectopic complexes; and (3) the presence of fusion complexes. (Courtesy of Dr. Kenneth Gimbel.)

cases as parasystole, but in the remaining cases a common divisor could not be found because the interectopic intervals were either too long or too erratic.

Parasystole was associated nearly always with an exit block or intermittence. In some cases of parasystole, the interectopic intervals increased progressively in the manner consistent with Wenckebach periodicity; in some cases, shorter and longer interectopic intervals alternated; and in some cases of intermittent parasystole, each new run of parasystolic rhythm was initiated by a PVC with the same coupling interval. The latter observation is consistent with the prevailing notion that the fixed coupling interval need not be attributed to reentry. Conversely, Malinow and Langendorf[7] pointed out that a variable coupling interval does not rule out reentry.

The fixed coupling interval of parasystole was attributed by Langendorf and Pick[80] to one of the following possibilities: (1) mutual protection of the two pacemakers; (2) a fortuitous numeric relation between the two pacemaker rates; (3) discharge only during the supernormal phase; and (4) unilateral protection with discharge of the dominant pacemaker by the parasystolic pacemaker, referred to as "reversed coupling."

Levy et al.[81] showed that a feedback mechanism involving a baroreceptor reflex arc could explain the fixed coupling interval of parasystole. This may explain the observation that the exercise-induced increase in heart rate can reveal parasystolic mechanism when the coupling interval is fixed at rest.[82] Because a fixed-rate electronic pacemaker can be viewed as a parasystolic focus, the interaction between the pacemaker rhythm and the spontaneous sinus rhythm can provide helpful information about "protection."

Steffens[83] showed that the PVC-free intermittent period resulted from discharge of the parasystolic focus by the dominant pacemaker (i.e., loss of protection). Parasystole resumed with the onset of entrance block. This also explained the fixed coupling interval, the duration of which equals the parasystolic cycle length minus the dominant cycle length plus the ventricular conduction time to the parasystolic focus.

Ventricular parasystole is seen in the presence of various heart diseases and in persons without heart disease.[84] It does not appear to have any particular prognostic significance, and there is no evidence that it responds differently to drug therapy than PVCs with a fixed coupling interval.

Monomorphic VT (Paroxysmal VT)

In monomorphic VT there is a rapid succession of three or more ectopic ventricular complexes.[85] The tachycardia is called *sustained* if it lasts longer than 30 seconds or requires intervention for termination. There are two definitions of nonsustained VT: Spontaneous nonsustained VT consists of three or more consecutive PVCs,[86] whereas induced nonsustained arrhythmia consists of six or more impulses lasting less than 29 seconds. Figure 17–14 is the record of a patient who had both sustained and nonsustained VT on two occasions.

VENTRICULAR RATE

The ventricular rate during paroxysmal VT is usually 140 to 200 beats/min, but a rate as slow as 120 beats/min is seen occasionally. An ectopic ventricular rhythm with a rate below 110 beats/min is generally referred to as *accelerated*

ventricular rhythm or *nonparoxysmal ventricular tachycardia* (see Figure 17–3). When the ventricular rate is more than 200 beats/min and the tracing resembles a continuous sine wave, the rhythm is usually called *ventricular flutter*.

REGULARITY

The RR interval during monomorphic VT is constant in more than 90 percent of cases. Some variation of the interval is often seen during the early part of an episode, especially when the rate of the tachycardia is slow.[87] Geibel et al.[88] found that the cycle length at the onset of tachycardia varied from –18 percent to 12 percent of the mean cycle length. During 74 episodes of sustained monomorphic VT induced by pacing, Volosin et al.[87] found that the average difference between the maximum and minimum RR intervals per episode was 127 ± 72 ms. In 45 percent of the episodes, the difference was less than 150 ms, and the maximum observed during one episode was 290 ms (Figure 17–15). The variability of the cycle length decreased as the episode continued, and the cycle length stabilized by 20 beats in about 70 percent of cases.[87] In patients with irregular nonsustained VT, the longest interval during VT is usually the first or the last interectopic interval.

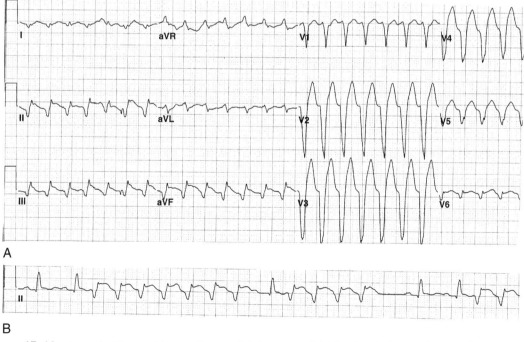

A

B

Figure 17–14   ECGs of a 66-year-old man with acute inferior myocardial infarction. **A,** Sustained ventricular tachycardia (VT) at a rate of 170 beats/min with left bundle branch block morphology. **B,** Episodes of nonsustained VT with the same morphology interrupted by conducted sinus impulses recorded 1 day later.

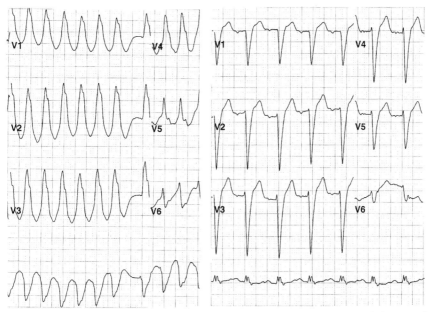

Figure 17-15   ECGs of a 42-year-old woman with idiopathic dilated cardiomyopathy, severe left ventricular dysfunction, pulmonary hypertension, low cardiac output, and normal coronary arteries. On the *left*, the ventricular tachycardia (VT) at a rate of 171 beats/min, QRS duration of 158 ms, and right bundle branch block morphology. Tachycardia is irregular. The diagnosis of VT is supported by the QRS morphology in lead V_1 and positive concordance. Tachycardia with the same morphology was induced by extrastimulation in the laboratory. ECG recorded *(right)* on the preceding day shows the sinus rhythm with left bundle branch block.

ONSET AND TERMINATION

Most VTs are initiated by PVCs (see Figure 17-4), although initiation by supraventricular impulses is known to occur. Qi et al.[25] examined the premature index (PI), defined as the coupling interval/QT interval ratio, during 469 episodes of VT in 122 patients. The PI of the PVC initiating VT was less than 1 (R-on-T) during only 62 (13 percent) VTs in 14 patients, and the PI of the second complex of VT was less than 1 during only 24 episodes of VT. Although the range of PIs was similar for single PVCs not initiating VT and those initiating VT, for individual patients the PI of the PVC initiating VT was longer than the PI of isolated PVCs. The relation was not affected by gender, age, presence of heart disease, or drug therapy. The coupling interval of the first VT complex was longer than the first interectopic interval during VT in 72 percent of patients. Similar findings were observed by other investigators.[88,90] The relatively long coupling interval required for initiation of tachycardia may be explained by the required critical recovery time for completion of reentry.[25,91]

Anderson et al.[92] divided spontaneous sustained monomorphic VTs into two types based on the type of onset. In type 1 VT, the initiating early cycle PVC (possibly triggering) was morphologically distinct;

in type 2 VT, the QRS complex of the initial complex was identical to subsequent complexes. Heart rate and heart rate variability did not change before type 1 VT, but RR interval dynamics changed before type 2, which suggested that with type 2 the short-term changes in neurohumoral activity contributed to VT initiation.

Gomes and associates[89] noted that a short–long cycle sequence often precedes the onset of VT. The short cycle consists of a sinus complex followed by a PVC. The ensuing compensatory pause before the appearance of the next sinus complex represents the long cycle. Such a sequence (sinus–PVC–pause–sinus–VT) is often seen at the onset of polymorphic VT (see Chapter 18).

AV DISSOCIATION

In patients with underlying sinus rhythm, the atria may remain under the control of the sinus impulse. The atrial and ventricular rhythms are independent of each other, and there is no demonstrable relation between the P waves and QRS complexes (Figure 17-16). The P wave during VT may be misdiagnosed, as certain components of the wide QRS complex or the ventricular repolarization may resemble P waves (Figure 17-17). It is recommended, therefore, to support the diagnosis by noting the presence

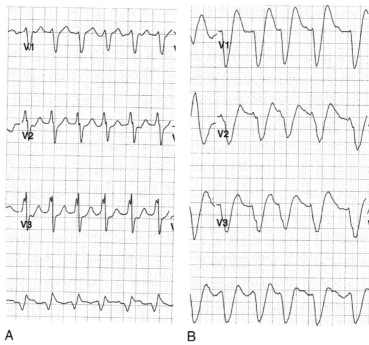

A   B

Figure 17–16 Recognition of sinus P waves during ventricular tachycardia (VT). From top to bottom: leads V_1, V_2, V_3, II. **A,** VT with left bundle branch block morphology at a rate of 135 beats/min. In lead II, sinus P waves can be recognized in the first and fifth complexes; corroborating evidence consists of a corresponding notch during the ST segment in leads V_2 and V_3. **B,** VT at a rate of 120 beats/min. P wave is seen in lead II (at the bottom) during the ST segment and is corroborated by corresponding P waves in lead V_1.

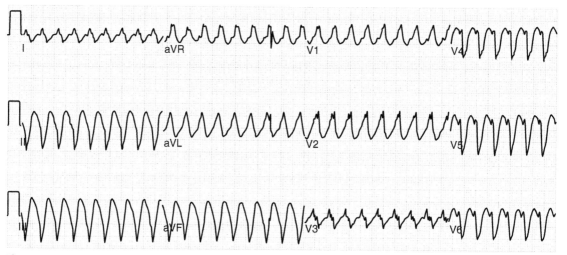

Figure 17–17 ECG of a 63-year old man with severe ischemic cardiomyopathy and documented ventricular tachycardia with a pattern of right bundle branch block and superior axis. The initial deflections in leads V_3–V_6 resemble P waves, but synchronization with lead V_2 shows that these deflections correspond to the QRS complex.

of a synchronous deflection in another lead (see Figures 17–16 and 17–17).

The atrial rate is usually slower than the ventricular rate. However, retrograde impulse conduction to the atria from the ventricular focus often occurs during VT (Figure 17–18). In 21 cases of VT studied by Kistin[93] with esophageal leads, 1:1 VA conduction was demonstrated in 10 cases, VA conduction with variable block in 4, and independent atrial rhythm in 7. The RP interval of the retrograde conducted beats is, as a rule, 0.11 second or longer. Wellens

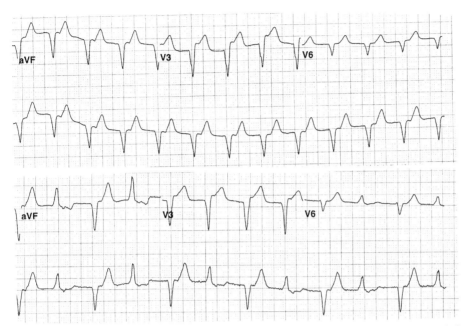

Figure 17–18 ECGs of a 51-year-old woman who developed an accelerated ventricular rhythm after thrombolytic therapy for an acute anterior myocardial infarction. *Top,* Monomorphic accelerated ventricular rhythm at a rate of 97 beats/min with retrograde conduction to the atria. *Bottom,* At 58 minutes later there is a regular bidirectional accelerated ventricular rhythm (89 beats/min) with retrograde conduction to the atria. After cessation of the ectopic rhythm, the QRS complex during sinus rhythm was narrow (not shown).

and Lie[94] found 1:1 VA conduction in 29 (64 percent) of 45 consecutive patients with VT in whom intracavitary atrial recordings were obtained. VA conduction was uncommon when the ventricular rate was rapid, being seen in only one of seven patients with a rate of more than 200 beats/min. Among the 122 cases of VT reported by Akhtar and co-workers,[95] 25 percent had 1:1 VA conduction and another 20 percent had VA conduction with varying degrees of VA block.

VENTRICULAR CAPTURE AND FUSION COMPLEXES

Occasionally, ventricular capture by conducted supraventricular impulse results in QRS complexes with normal or aberrant supraventricular morphology appearing during VT (see Figure 17–3). Their presence is helpful for confirming the ventricular origin of the ectopic tachycardia. Fusion complexes, known as *Dressler beats,* have the same significance.[96] According to Fisch,[97] fusion and captures are present in only 5 percent of patients with VT.

USING THE ECG TO LOCALIZE THE SITE OF ORIGIN OF VT

Demonstrating the exact site of origin of the VT requires exact mapping. The approximate location can be identified on the basis of QRS morphology on the surface ECG. Most often RBBB morphology (VT-RBBB) (see Figures 17–15, 17–17, and 17–19) is associated with a left ventricular origin of VT. The LBBB morphology (VT-LBBB) and inferior axis is usually localized in the right ventricular outflow tract in the absence of heart disease.[98] Left bundle branch morphologies are present in all right VTs, and occasionally from the left ventricular site of the septum. In patients with ischemic or dilated cardiomyopathy, VT-LBBB is also associated more often with left VT (see Figures 17–14 and 17–16). Josephson and associates[99] proposed that the left ventricular site of origin of VT with LBBB configuration may be explained by preferential left-to-right transseptal activation or other alterations of the conduction pathway. VT-LBBB is also seen in patients with arrhythmogenic right ventricular dysplasia[100–102] or Uhl's anomaly,[103] after surgical repair of tetralogy of Fallot, and in patients with no apparent heart disease.[46 98,104,105]

In the presence of myocardial infarction, VT nearly always arises in the left ventricle or intraventricular septum. VTs in the left ventricle have RBBB morphology, and VTs adjacent to the left septum have LBBB morphology. VTs with RBBB morphology arising from the apex usually have a right and superior axis. VTs with LBBB morphology and a right inferior axis arise on

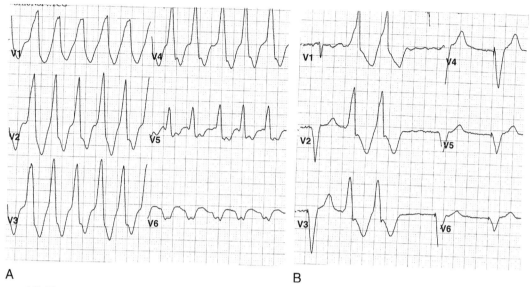

Figure 17–19 **A,** ECG of a 77-year-old man with severe ischemic cardiomyopathy (left ventricular ejection fraction about 20 percent) treated with amiodarone. It shows ventricular tachycardia (VT) at a rate of 141 beats/min and a QRS duration of 216 ms. The pattern in leads V_1 and V_6 is nearly pathognomonic of VT. **B,** Additional proof is obtained by the configuration of premature ventricular complexes in a couplet that follows a paced ventricular complex in a record made on another day.

the upper half of the septum. VTs with RBBB morphology and a right inferior axis may arise on the septum or on the free wall.

Miller et al.[106] correlated the findings in the 12-lead ECG during VT with the endocardial site of origin obtained by mapping in 108 patients with a prior MI. They found that the specific site of origin is more difficult to determine with anterior infarction than with inferior infarction. In tachycardias with an LBBB pattern the sites of origin clustered on or were adjacent to the septum, whereas in those with RBBB morphology the location could be either septal or the free wall of the left ventricle (see the section on Idiopathic VT).

Some features on the ECG can give clues to the underlying substrate, which is most useful in the ablation therapy. The following text is abstracted from a paper by Josephson and Callans.[107] They note that the more rapid the initial forces, the more likely VT is arising from normal myocardium (Figure 17–20). Slurring of the initial force is often seen when the tachycardia arises from the scar or from the epicardium. VTs originating in very diseased myocardium have lower amplitude complexes than those arising in the normal substrate. The presence of notching of the QRS is a sign of scar tissue. The presence of qRr, qr, or QR complexes is highly suggestive of an infarct.

The site of origin of VT affects QRS width. Septal VTs exhibit generally less wide QRS complexes than VTs originating on the free wall. The

QRS axis is related more to the superior/inferior activation of normal muscle. Thus right superior axis VTs arise from apical, septal, or apical lateral regions, whereas inferior axis VTs arise in the basal areas of the heart, right ventricular outflow tract, high left ventricular septum, or high lateral left ventricle. A left inferior axis is more likely to be present in a VT arising from a superior area of the right free wall or from the top of ventricular septum.

Positive concordance is seen only in VTs arising at the base of the heart (left ventricular outflow tract along the mitral or aortic valves, or the basal septum) and negative concordance is seen only in VTs originating near the apical septum, in which case the activation moves away from the chest wall.

QS complexes reflect activation away from the recording site (i.e., the QS complexes in the inferior leads suggest that the activation is originating in the inferior wall, whereas QS complexes recorded in the anterior leads indicate activation moving from the anterior wall).

POLYMORPHISM (OR PLEOMORPHISM) OF VT

These terms signify two or more morphologies of the same sustained VT. Polymorphous VT is similar to torsade de pointes (see Chapter 18), except that the QT interval is not prolonged. It is seen mostly in patients with coronary artery

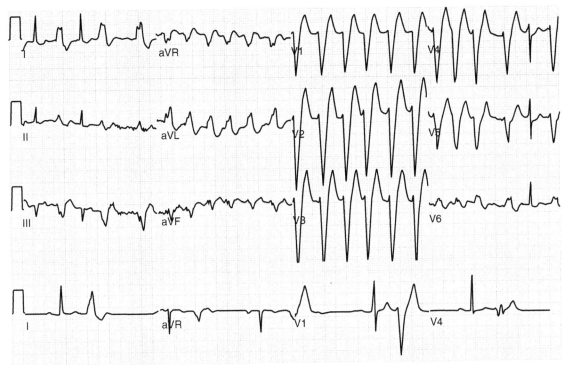

Figure 17–20 ECG of an 86-year-old man with hypertension and normal systolic ventricular function. *Top,* Ventricular tachycardia (VT) with left bundle branch block morphology at the heart rate of 137 beats/min with sinus captures (leads I-III) and fusion complexes (leads V₄–V₆). *Bottom,* ECG made 3 days earlier shows sinus rhythm with premature ventricular complexes (PVCs) exhibiting the same morphology as the VT. Note the rapid initial deflection of the PVCs and during VT .

disease, including those with acute myocardial ischemia and MI.[108] The incidence of this arrhythmia is lower than that of torsade de pointes. Josephson et al.[109] have shown that multiple morphologies (i.e., the presence of VT-RBBB and VT-LBBB) in the same patient usually reflect variable exit sites or a variable ventricular activation pattern. Kimber et al.[110] found that in patients with pleomorphic VT the site of origin of the VT remained relatively constant, whereas the changes in the QRS configuration resulted from changes in the direction of propagation and different patterns of ventricular activation. The uncommon bidirectional VT (see Figure 17–18) is probably generated in such a way in most cases. Buxton et al.[111] showed that conversion of inducible polymorphic VT to uniform VT after procainamide administration occurred almost exclusively in patients with previous MI and abnormal left ventricular function.

FASCICULAR TACHYCARDIA AND NARROW QRS VT

In some but not all fascicular VTs the QRS complex is narrow, and some but not all VTs with a narrow QRS complex are fascicular in origin. A left anterior fascicular origin is suggested by VT-RBBB with an inferior axis (Figure 17–21); and left posterior fascicular VT is suggested by VT-RBBB with a superior axis.[112] In one study,[113] VT with narrow QRS complex (i.e., 110 ms or less) was present in about 5 percent of VTs; the morphology was fascicular in only two of five cases. The diagnosis of VT with fascicular morphology or narrow QRS complex is established by the usual criteria: AV dissociation, fusion complexes, and HV interval shorter than during the sinus rhythm.[114]

Ventricular Escape Complexes and Idioventricular Rhythm

Ventricular escape complexes occur when the rate of supraventricular impulses reaching the ventricles is slower than the inherent rate of the ectopic ventricular pacemaker (Figure 17–22). In most instances, escape complexes associated with bradyarrhythmias originate from the AV junction. Ventricular escape complexes occur when junctional automaticity is impaired or when the block

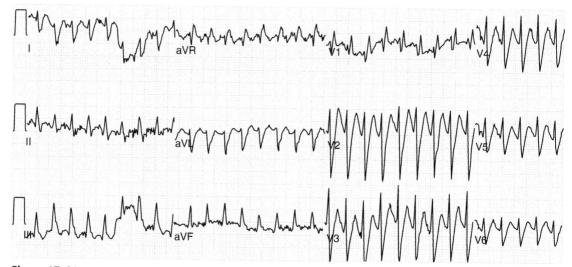

Figure 17–21 ECG of a 65-year-old man with presumably left anterior fascicular tachycardia suggested by right bundle branch block and left posterior fascicular morphology. Earlier ECG on the same day showed sinus tachycardia and normal QRST pattern (not shown).

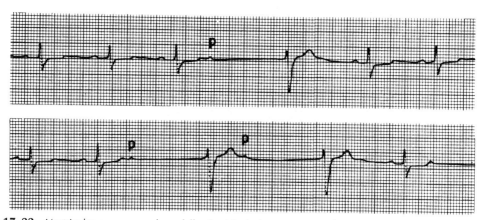

Figure 17–22 Ventricular escape complexes following blocked premature atrial complexes.

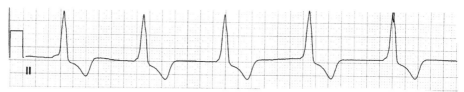

Figure 17–23 ECG lead II from a 56-year-old man following thrombolytic treatment of an acute inferior myocardial infarction. Note the marked sinus bradycardia and ventricular escape rhythm (46 beats/min), configuration of left bundle branch block, and a QRS duration of 170 ms. A P wave is seen at the foot of the first and fifth R waves.

is at a level distal to the His bundle. A sequence of three or more consecutive ventricular escape complexes is called *slow ventricular rhythm.*

The ventricular rate in idioventricular rhythm is usually 30 to 40 beats/min but may be as slow as 20 beats/min or as fast as 50 beats/min (Figure 17–23). The QRS complexes are usually wide, but escape complexes originating in the ventricular septum may have near-normal duration and configuration. Escape complexes from the right bundle branch system generally have LBBB morphology, and escape complexes from the left bundle branch system usually have RBBB morphology. Escape rhythms may arise from the left anterior (Figure 17–24) or left posterior (Figure 17–25) fascicle.

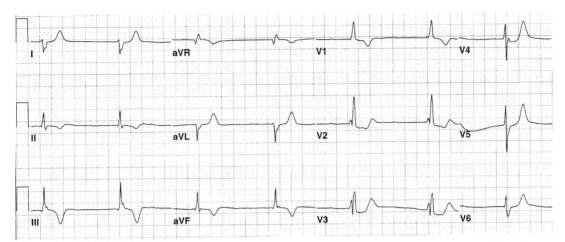

Figure 17–24 Ventricular escape rhythm originating at or near the left anterior fascicle at a rate of 44 beats/min in a 60-year-old man with atrial fibrillation and complete atrioventricular block. Note the right bundle branch block pattern and left posterior fascicular block. QRS is 122 ms. Junctional rhythm with aberrant conduction cannot be ruled out.

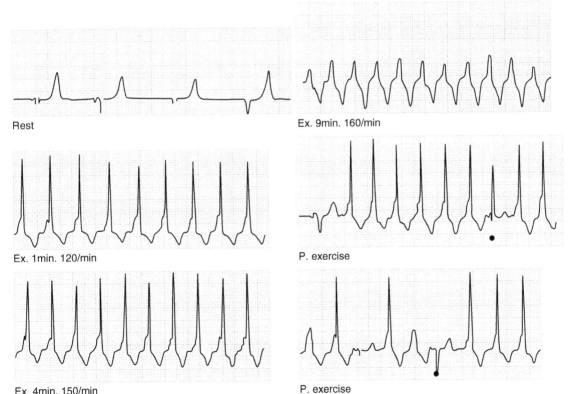

Figure 17–25 Ventricular escape rhythm originating at or near the left posterior fascicle at a rate of 38 beats/min in an 80-year-old woman with marked sinus bradycardia. Note the right bundle branch block pattern and left anterior fascicular block. QRS is 114 ms. Junctional rhythm with aberrant conduction cannot be ruled out.

Slow ventricular rhythm may be simulated by the AV junctional escape rhythm with preexisting intraventricular conduction defect. The differentiation is sometimes impossible based on the body surface ECG. The diagnosis of ventricular rhythm is supported by the presence of capture or fusion complexes.

ACCELERATED VENTRICULAR RHYTHMS

Accelerated ventricular rhythms, termed by Schamroth[115] *idioventricular tachycardia* or *nonparoxysmal VT,*[116] are ectopic ventricular rhythms at rates intermediate between escape rhythms (rate less than about 40 beats/min) and VT at rates above 100 to 120 beats/min (see Figures 17–18 and 17–26). The rhythm is accelerated because it is faster than the inherent rate of ventricular pacemakers, even when it is 100 beats/min or less. The ventricular origin of these rhythms can be demonstrated by the usual ECG criteria (e.g., AV dissociation, fusion, or capture complexes) and recording of His bundle potentials.[117] They are believed to be automatic and are usually readily overdriven by faster supraventricular pacemakers. The slower ectopic ventricular rate also allows more opportunities for complete or partial activation of the ventricles by supraventricular impulses. Therefore ventricular capture or fusion complexes are seen much more commonly with this type of arrhythmia than with the paroxysmal variety. Because the VT rate and the sinus rate are often

similar, an isorhythmic dissociation is a common finding.

Most of the episodes of nonparoxysmal VT are transient, lasting seconds, minutes, or hours (Figure 17–27). In some cases the RR interval of the nonparoxysmal VT was the exact multiple of the RR interval of the rapid VT. This relation suggests that exit block of the rapid ventricular ectopic impulse is responsible for the appearance of nonparoxysmal VT in some instances.

Accelerated idioventricular rhythm was first described as nonparoxysmal VT by Rothfeld and associates in patients with acute MI,[118] in whom the incidence of this arrhythmia was reported to vary between 8 and 36 percent.[118,119] In patients with acute MI[120] this arrhythmia is seen during the first 24 hours after reperfusion in 90 percent of patients, most often during the first few hours. The frequency begins to decrease 8 to 12 hours after reperfusion (see Chapter 7 for additional discussion). Accelerated idioventricular rhythm usually occurs in the presence of sinus bradycardia. The prognosis is not adversely affected, probably because the ventricular rate is in the normal range. Paroxysmal VT often coexists in the same patient, however.

The arrhythmia also is seen in patients with other types of heart disease, such as primary myocardial disease and hypertensive, rheumatic, and congenital heart disease.[121] It also may be caused by digitalis.[116] Occasionally, no evidence of heart disease is found. Such an example is shown in Figure 17–27.

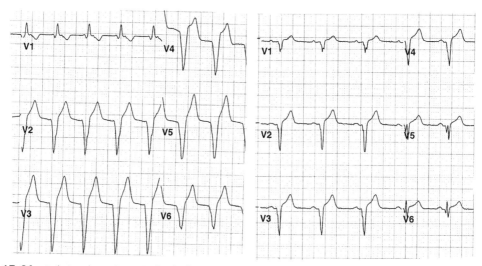

Figure 17–26   *Left,* Accelerated ventricular rhythm at a rate of 105 beats/min after thrombolytic treatment of a 43-year-old man with an acute anterior myocardial infarction caused by occlusion of the left anterior descending coronary artery in its proximal portion. QRS duration is 152 ms. *Right,* Nine hours later, note the sinus rhythm at a rate of 84 beats/min; QRS duration is 94 ms.

G.F.   Hosp. No. 303 8

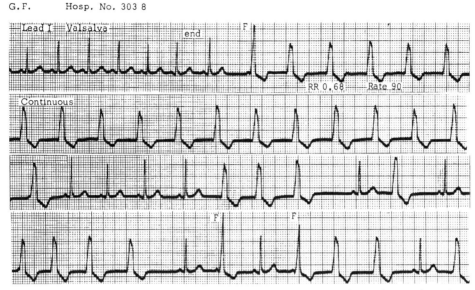

Figure 17–27   Accelerated ventricular rhythm in a 15-year-old girl with no other evidence of organic heart disease. She has no symptoms. The ectopic rhythm is intermittent and occurs when the sinus rhythm is slow. Fusion complexes are present.

PARASYSTOLIC VT

It is believed that VT may originate from a parasystolic focus (see Figure 17–13). The diagnosis is suggested by the VT morphology being the same as that of documented ventricular parasystole. The ventricular rate is usually 70 to 140 beats/min. Most of the patients have organic heart disease, especially coronary artery disease with MI. Parasystolic VT is seen occasionally in young, otherwise healthy individuals.[122]

INCESSANT VT

Ventricular tachycardia is described as incessant if the tachycardia is recurrent and the episodes present during a large part of the day and night, interrupted by only a few sinus complexes. In the 21 infants studied by Garson et al.,[123] VT continued during more than 90 percent of the day and night; the VT rate ranged from 167 to 440 beats/min (average 260 beats/min). Surgical exploration revealed myocardial hamartomas (Purkinje cell tumors) or histiocytoid cardiomyopathy in 13 patients and rhabdomyomas in 2 (i.e., lesions amenable to excision). The incessant VT observed in adults, some of whom can be treated with antiarrhythmic drugs, appear to differ from incessant VTs in infants in terms of substrate.

CATECHOLAMINERGIC POLYMORPHIC VT

Catecholaminergic polymorphic VT, which is often bidirectional, is believed to result from abnormalities in ryanodine receptors that are responsible for release of calcium from sarcoplasmic reticulum following the calcium entry into the cell. The tachycardia is often induced by exercise or stress and may terminate in sudden death. Resting ECG and cardiac structure are normal.[124–126]

Idiopathic VT

The term *idiopathic* implies a structurally normal heart in young and middle-aged subjects and a normal QT interval, although biopsy or magnetic resonance imaging[127,128] may detect microscopic or subtle macroscopic abnormalities. In most cases idiopathic VTs are amenable to ablation. Idiopathic VT comprises about 10 percent of all VTs and can be classified in three ways on the basis of (1) symptoms, (2) site of origin, and (3) response to drugs and interventions.

Classification by Symptoms

Two syndromes merit management considerations: (1) repetitive monomorphic VT and (2) paroxysmal sustained monomorphic VT. *Repetitive monomorphic VT* is characterized by repetitive runs of nonsustained VT interspersed with sinus rhythm. Frequent PVCs usually are present. The arrhythmia is often asymptomatic and found incidentally during studies done for other reasons. The VT may be suppressed with exercise. The QRS morphology is usually LBBB with normal or right axis. Callans et al.[129] reported that repetitive monomorphic VT can arise from the outflow tract of the right or left ventricle. Tachycardias with a precordial R wave transition at or before lead V_2 are consistent with a left ventricular origin. The tachycardia is usually not inducible with programmed ventricular stimulation. Some of these patients show a warm-up phenomenon with gradual acceleration of the rate after tachycardia begins, which suggests an automatic mechanism (see later discussion). The prognosis is usually excellent.

Paroxysmal sustained monomorphic VT is similar to the repetitive monomorphic type, but the episodes of tachycardia tend to be more widely spread out in time. The episodes are often sustained when they occur. This type of VT is more likely to be inducible with programmed ventricular stimulation, and induction is often facilitated by isoproterenol.

Classification by Site of Origin

VTs arising from the anterior septal side of the right ventricular outflow tract, from the right or left coronary cusp passing to the right or left side of the septum, and from the pulmonary artery give rise to LBBB morphologies with right inferior axis. VTs arising in the left ventricle from the mitral annulus adjacent to the aortic valve or from the epicardium at the outflow tract may have RBBB morphology. The major difference between VTs with LBBB morphology arising from the right or left sides of the heart is that early R wave progression is present when VTs originate in the left ventricle or in the aortic cusp. R waves in V_1 and V_2 and a transition by lead V_3 are characteristic of left-side outflow tract VTs, whereas later transitions at V_3 and V_4 characterize VTs arising from the right ventricular outflow tract or pulmonary artery. In posterior septal right ventricular outflow tract VTs, the axis becomes more leftward. Free wall right ventricular outflow tract VTs have lower QRS amplitude, and the QRS is notched in the inferior leads. In addition, the VTs with free wall origins have a later R wave transition in the precordial leads to V_4 and V_5. On the left side, there is not only the early transition, but also persistent dominant R waves across the precordium with small or absent S waves out to the apex. The R wave in V_2 is broad and occupies a greater percentage of the QRS width than in VTs originating on the right side. A broad R wave in the lead V_1 is often present in VTs with LBBB morphology originating from the right coronary cusp.[111]

VTs originating along the mitral annulus superiorly, laterally, and occasionally inferiorly have RBBB morphology with dominant R waves across the precordium, whereas epicardial VTs that follow the anterior coronary vein often show a loss of R wave in V_1 and V_2 with a broad R wave from V_3 to V_6. The VTs arising from the right ventricular outflow tract just above the His bundle have a left inferior axis that is usually about +30 degrees.[111]

Idiopathic right ventricular tachycardia is the most common type, found in about 70 percent of patients. The origin is usually in the right ventricular outflow tract. The ECG morphology is that of LBBB, usually with an inferior or a rightward axis.[130] It is often exercise induced and catecholamine sensitive. The postulated mechanism is cyclic adenosine monophosphate (cAMP)-mediated triggered activity. In a small number of patients, VT originates in the tricuspid annulus; their ECG shows usually R wave amplitude >0.5 mV in lead I and positive QRS polarity in lead aVL.[130a]

Idiopathic left ventricular tachycardia is a less common tachycardia. It is seen predominantly in young patients, who are usually symptomatic and have episodes of sustained VT.[131,132] Lerman et al.[133] subdivided this syndrome into three subgroups. The most prevalent form, verapamil-sensitive intrafascicular tachycardia, originates in the region of the left posterior fascicle of the left bundle. This tachycardia is adenosine insensitive and is thought to be due to reentry. A second type is analogous to adenosine-sensitive right ventriclar outflow tachycardia. It appears to originate from deep within the interventricular septum and exits from the left side of the septum. This form responds to verapamil and is thought to be due to cAMP-mediated triggered activity. A third form is propranolol sensitive. It is not initiated by programmed electrical stimulation, and the drug responses suggest an automatic mechanism.

Classification by Response to Drugs

Verapamil-sensitive tachycardia encompasses a heterogeneous group of tachycardias. Lee et al.[134] found that, of 32 patients, 69 percent had VT with RBBB morphology and 31 percent had VT with LBBB morphology. Verapamil-sensitive VT exhibits properties of both reentrant and triggered arrhythmia and is inconsistently dependent on both exogenous catecholamines for induction and intravenous adenosine for termination.

Catecholamine- or *exercise-sensitive tachycardia* most often has an LBBB-like morphology (Figure 17–28). Gill et al.[135] suggested that there are at least two possible mechanisms of this idiopathic VT. First, VT initiated without cycle length changes

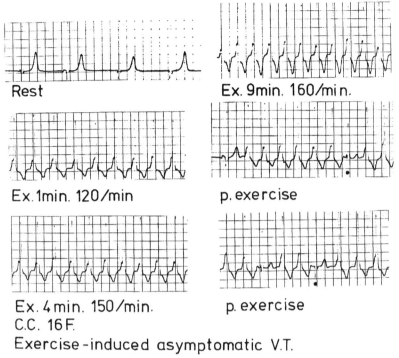

Rest

Ex. 9min. 160/min.

Ex. 1min. 120/min

p. exercise

Ex. 4min. 150/min.
C.C. 16 F.

p. exercise

Exercise-induced asymptomatic V.T.

Figure 17–28   Exercise-induced ventricular tachycardia with left bundle branch block morphology in a 16-year-old girl. ECG strips of lead II are shown at rest, during exercise (Ex.), and after exercise (p. exercise). Dots mark fusion and sinus capture complexes. Note that the rate of tachycardia increases progressively with increasing duration of exercise, which means that the ectopic focus is probably automatic and presumably under sympathetic control. (From Surawicz B: Automaticity. *In:* Fisch C, Surawicz B (eds): Cardiac Electrophysiology and Arrhythmias. New York, Elsevier, 1991.)

is more common and more likely to have an inferior axis, suggesting an outflow tract origin. It is probably related to triggered activity secondary to delayed diastolic depolarizations. Second, VT initiated with a long–short sequence is more often nonsustained. It may have a superior axis and is probably related to early afterdepolarizations. In children, catecholamine-sensitive VT may be a variant of long QT syndrome (see Chapter 24).[136]

Adenosine-sensitive VT is another type. Lerman et al.[137] suggested that termination of VT by adenosine is strongly suggestive of a cAMP-mediated triggered mechanism rather than reentry. Among 14 patients in whom VT was terminated by adenosine, the VT originated in the right ventricular outflow tract in 10, right ventricular apex in 1, and left ventricular septum in 3.[128] Yeh et al.[138] found that adenosine-terminated VT originated from the anterolateral left ventricle in only 4 of 53 consecutive cases.

CLINICAL CORRELATION

As a general rule, the incidence of nonsustained and sustained monomorphic VT mirrors the severity of the structural heart disease. The incidence is low in subjects without heart disease.

The reported incidence of VT in patients with acute MI during continuous ECG monitoring varies between 6 and 40 percent. Among 820 patients monitored by 24-hour Holter recording for 8 to 14 days after acute MI, Bigger and colleagues[139] found nonsustained VT in 11 percent and sustained VT in 2 percent. In a more recent survey of 40,895 patients with ventricular arrhythmias receiving thrombolytic treatment in the GUSTO-I study,[140] 4188 (10.7 percent) had sustained VT, ventricular fibrillation (VF), or both. These arrhythmias had a negative impact on the patients' early outcome and predicted significantly higher mortality 1 year later among the survivors.[141]

In patients with congestive heart failure secondary to ischemic or dilated cardiomyopathy, about half of deaths are caused by arrhythmias, which include VT, VT degenerating into VF, and VF. In seven studies of such patients summarized by Packer,[142] the incidence of VT ranged from 39 to 60 percent. In eight studies reviewed by Surawicz,[45] the incidence of nonsustained VT ranged from 49 to 100 percent (average 65 percent). In many of these studies ventricular arrhythmias were detected during single 24-hour ambulatory monitoring, and thus it is likely that longer monitoring would have revealed an even higher incidence of VT. In the seven studies summarized by Packer,[142] the total mortality averaged 37.4 percent, and sudden cardiac death averaged 14.3 percent per year. In the eight studies reviewed by Surawicz,[45] the average incidence of sudden cardiac death was 21.4 percent during follow-up of 11 to 34 months. The introduction of automatic implantable cardioverter defibrillators drastically reduced the incidence of sudden arrhythmic death among these patients. The prognostic role of nonsustained VT is debatable. In the collaborative study of patients with heart failure treated with vasodilator drugs, nonsustained VT was present in 80 percent of all patients but was not an independent predictor of all-cause mortality or sudden death.[143]

VT and VF are responsible for sudden death in patients with hypertrophic cardiomyopathy, some of whom are young athletes. The association between right VT and arrhythmogenic right ventricular dysplasia was emphasized by Marcus et al.[101] Paroxysmal VT may occur for the first time during pregnancy[144] and is responsible for syncope in some patients with mitral valve prolapse.[145,146] In adult patients late after repair of tetralogy of Fallot, the risk factors for sustained VT included low cardiac index, outflow tract aneurysm, pulmonary regurgitation,[147] and QRS prolongation.[148] Several cases of familial VT have been reported, characteristically with female preponderance.[106]

Digitalis intoxication is a common cause of paroxysmal VT. It was responsible for 25 percent of the cases in one study.[149] The incidence has been much lower in recent years because the digitalis dosage used is generally lower. Many of the class I *antiarrhythmic drugs* can cause VT and VF.[150–154]

Ventricular tachycardia may develop because of nonpenetrating *trauma* to the heart, causing myocardial contusion or electrical injury involving the heart. It also may be the result of cardiac catheterization and cardiac surgery because of mechanical irritation of the ventricles. It has been observed in patients after coronary artery bypass surgery when no such arrhythmia was seen preoperatively.[155] Severe hypokalemia and hyperkalemia can cause VT.[63,156] VT and other types of arrhythmia also have been implicated in substance abuse, including "sudden sniffing death" as a result of inhaling aerosols propelled by fluorinated hydrocarbons.[157,158]

Role of Programmed Electrical Stimulation

Programmed electrical stimulation (PES), introduced in 1972 for diagnostic purposes, evolved into a procedure utilized for clinical management of patients with life-threatening VTs. The results of a typical study are examined in terms of: (1) the presence or absence of inducible arrhythmia; (2) the type of inducible arrhythmia; and (3) suppression or modification of inducible arrhythmia by therapy.

The most commonly practiced stimulation protocol utilizes the right ventricular apex as the single stimulation site, pacing at three basic rates, and applying a maximum of three extrastimuli. It seldom initiates sustained VT in persons without heart disease or a history of ventricular tachyarrhythmia, but it can initiate the clinically occurring sustained monomorphic VT in nearly 100 percent of patients with previous MI, in 75 to 90 percent of patients with idiopathic VT, and in 50 to 60 percent of patients with dilated cardiomyopathy or mitral valve prolapse.[159] Rarely the results are improved by stimulation from an additional right ventricular site, stimulation from the left ventricle, or addition of isoproterenol.

The prognostic significance of nonsustained VT induced by pacing in patients with structural heart disease has been disputed because several studies suggest that the substrate of nonsustained VT is not necessarily the same as that of sustained VT. For instance, the rate of nonsustained VT observed during ambulatory monitoring tends to be considerably slower than the rate of spontaneous or induced sustained VT in the same person. In one study[160] the rate of spontaneous nonsustained VT averaged 150 beats/min compared with 246 beats/min for sustained VT.

Induction of polymorphic VT is considered a nonspecific response because an aggressive stimulation protocol can induce it even in persons without heart disease or a history of spontaneous sustained VT. For the same reason, induction of VF is considered a nonspecific finding, the incidence of which increases with the use of aggressive stimulation protocols.

The usefulness of PES for selecting helpful drugs is limited because drugs that prevent inducibility can be identified in no more than 20 to 25 percent of patients; sometimes drugs are helpful even if they do not suppress inducibility; and therapeutic failures occur even when inducibility is suppressed. Variable results depend on the stimulation protocol.

Mechanisms of Ventricular Arrhythmias

The mechanism of PVCs is not known. It appears that each of the three factors (advancing age, presence of heart disease, impaired ventricular function) not only increases the PVC frequency but also facilitates the formation of repetitive forms. These associations suggest the role of an abnormal matrix that would favor a reentrant mechanism but could equally well enhance normal or abnormal automaticity. It is plausible that, analogous to VTs, more than one mechanism plays a role in the genesis of PVCs. The following mechanisms have been postulated in the genesis of VT: (1) reentry; (2) normal automaticity; (3) abnormal automaticity; (4) triggering by late afterdepolarizations; and (5) triggering by early afterdepolarizations. Whereas it is customary to apply the term *triggering* only to arrhythmias dependent on afterdepolarizations, it must be acknowledged that a trigger must be present at the onset of any arrhythmia. Indeed, the concept of a receptive matrix and an effective trigger is common to each of the postulated mechanisms discussed next.

REENTRY

Reentry is a common mechanism that is believed to play a dominant role in the precipitation and maintenance of life-threatening supraventricular and ventricular tachyarrhythmias. This discussion of clinical reentry is confined to monomorphic VTs. The rules governing maintenance of the circus movement in all models of reentry call for: (1) unidirectional block; (2) slow conduction around the site of block, allowing for reexcitation of the previously blocked site, and continuing propagation along the same path; and (3) physical interruption of the circuit,

which terminates and prevents reinitiation of the circus movement. Figure 17–29 shows a short reentrant circuit involving the junction between a Purkinje fiber and ventricular muscle with a unidirectional block in the Purkinje fiber.

The length of the functional reentry pathway is related to the wavelength of the electrical impulse. The latter is defined by the distance traveled by the depolarization wave during the time the tissue restores excitability to propagate another impulse. The wavelength equals the conduction velocity (in meters per second) multiplied by the duration of the functional refractory period (in seconds). In the anatomically defined circuit, a wavelength shorter than the circuit implies the presence of an excitable gap, defined as the time interval between the recovery of excitability (or the end of the refractory period) and the arrival of the next impulse. The tissue within the gap may be fully excitable or partially refractory. A fully excitable gap is likely to be present in an anatomically defined pathway when the conduction time is longer than the recovery time. A propagated impulse from a premature stimulus arriving at the path of reentry during the excitable gap can interfere with the reentrant arrhythmia by: (1) interrupting it; (2) resetting its cycle; or (3) merging with the reentrant propagation (i.e., entraining it).

Unidirectional block can be continuous or transient. It has been attributed to depressed conduction, prolonged refractoriness, or both. Newer studies have emphasized the role of abnormal anisotropy.[161]

Reentry is suggested by the following findings: (1) VT can be induced and terminated by

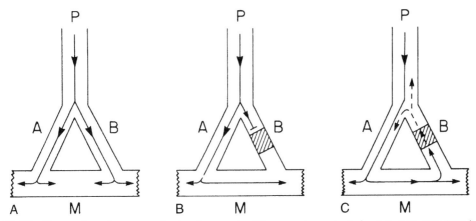

Figure 17–29   Theory of reentry as a mechanism for genesis of the premature ectopic beat. **A,** Activation impulse is conducted normally through the Purkinje fiber (P) and its branches (A and B) to depolarize the myocardium (M). **B,** Area (hatched) of impaired conductivity and excitability in branch B, where the normal antegrade impulse is blocked. **C,** This refractory area has recovered when the impulse arrives later from the retrograde direction. Its activation generates an impulse that propagates (as indicated by the interrupted lines) and causes premature depolarization of the myocardium. Sustained paroxysmal tachycardia occurs if the process is perpetuated.

extrastimuli; (2) there is an inverse relation between the coupling interval of the initiating extrastimulus and the following cycle length that precedes VT; (3) there is continuous diastolic or end-diastolic activity during VT; (4) there are fragmented late potentials during sinus rhythm, a finding suggestive of slow conduction; (5) the characteristic behavior of entrainment and resetting; (6) the possibility of mechanical interruption by incision, cooling, or radiofrequency ablation; and (7) there is mapping out of the reentrant circuit. Pogwizd et al.[162] performed three-dimensional computer-assisted intraoperative mapping of as many as 156 intramural sites in patients with healed MI and refractory VT and defined the mechanism of VT as either intramural reentry or a focal mechanism. In the focal VTs the sites of marked conduction delay were distant from the sites of stimulation. Pogwizd et al.[163] confirmed that spontaneous and induced VTs in patients with end-stage idiopathic cardiomyopathy can arise in the subendocardium or subepicardium. In some cases of post-myocardial monomorphic VT, the Purkinje system appeared to form part of the re-entry circuit.[163a]

A so-called phase 2 reentry has been described in isolated tissues.[164] This arrhythmia appears to be a manifestation of re-excitation rather than reentry and is a result of juxtaposition of myocardial cells at different membrane potential during phase 2 (plateau) of the ventricular transmembrane action potential.[164] This mechanism has been postulated in patients in whom ventricular arrhythmias were precipitated by a sinus complex with an elevated J point and ST segment and T wave changes.[165] Such a mechanism has been suggested to explain arrhythmias in patients wih Brugada syndrome (see Chapter 7).

Reentry Incorporating Bundle Branches

Programmed electrical stimulation showed bundle branch reentry in more than half of the patients studied by Akthar et al.[166] This occurred when an appropriately timed right ventricular premature impulse (V_2) was conducted with delay to the site of the His bundle recording (H) and was followed by a spontaneous impulse with an H_2V_3 longer than the HV interval of the sinus impulses. It was assumed that V_2, which was blocked retrogradely in the right bundle branch (i.e., the site of unidirectional block), was conducted across the septum and returned by way of the left bundle branch and His bundle to the right ventricle through the previously blocked right bundle branch. The reentry

depends on the critical lengthening of the V_2H_2 or V_3H_3 intervals.

Bundle branch reentry can become continuous, giving rise to macroreentrant VT, which has been shown to be the mechanism operating in 6 percent of patients with sustained VT.[167] The QRS morphology is of the LBBB or RBBB type (when the site of unidirectional block is the left bundle branch). The affected patients frequently have intraventricular conduction disturbances and a prolonged HV interval. Most have dilated cardiomyopathy, but it is seen also in one third of patients with VT occurring after valve surgery.[168] The importance of this type of reentry is that it can be managed selectively by ablation of the bundle branch in nearly all cases.[169]

Intramyocardial Reentry

With intramyocardial reentry the reentry pathway is a macrocircuit comprising a tract of surviving tissue traversing the infarct and the remaining healthy tissue.[170] Studies by Josephson et al.[171–173] suggested that many cases of inducible (and thus presumably reentrant) VT in patients with ischemic and dilated cardiomyopathy originate in a small (micro-reentrant) focus that is well protected from invasion during circus movement. Localizing the circuit to a small area in the ventricle was suggested by the finding that large areas of the ventricles could be captured by ventricular extrastimuli (or by sinus capture) without any effect on the tachycardia.

NORMAL AUTOMATICITY

The concept of automaticity was introduced into the discussion of ventricular escape complexes and ventricular parasystole. The automatic Purkinje fibers are depolarized from a membrane potential negative to −70 mV by a sodium entry–dependent mechanism. The automatic tachycardias are not inducible and are not interrupted by extrastimulation. They are believed to originate in small protected foci that are amenable to ablation. The automatic VT is typically catecholamine sensitive; that is, it can be induced by isoproterenol or exercise and suppressed by β-adrenergic drugs (see Figure 17–28). The arrhythmia is also amenable to overdrive suppression.

ABNORMAL AUTOMATICITY

Abnormal automaticity can arise in any depolarized Purkinje fiber or nonautomatic ventricular fiber at membrane potentials positive to about −60 mV when the sodium channel is depressed or inactivated and when the depolarization is mediated by the calcium channel. Abnormal automaticity can be readily elicited in vitro, but its role in human arrhythmias is difficult to document. In support of the mechanism of abnormal automaticity is suppression by verapamil, but such a finding is not specific for abnormal automaticity because depolarized verapamil-sensitive tissue may be incorporated into a reentrant circuit, and arrhythmias triggered by delayed depolarizations are also sensitive to verapamil.

TRIGGERING BY DELAYED AFTERDEPOLARIZATIONS

The discovery of abnormal automaticity demonstrated that reentry is not the only mechanism for arrhythmias initiated by extrastimulation. This property is shared by delayed afterdepolarizations (DADs) that arise in tissues with intracellular calcium overload, which in practice is most often a result of treatment with digitalis. It has been shown that the amplitude and frequency of afterdepolarizations (i.e., depolarizations occurring after the end of the action potential during diastole) are increased by a higher rate of stimulation and higher calcium concentration. Digitalis-induced afterdepolarizations in Purkinje fibers can reach threshold and initiate automatic activity even when normal pacemaker activity is depressed.[174,175] DADs can be also induced by high concentrations of isoproterenol and cAMP. Calcium overload is difficult to document in clinical arrhythmias, but it may be suspected in the presence of digitalis toxicity. Vos et al.[176] found that flunarazine, a blocker of calcium overload, delayed the occurrence of ouabain-induced arrhythmias in animals but had no effect on arrhythmias attributed to normal or abnormal automaticity.

It is generally believed that arrhythmias in which increasing prematurity shortens the interval between the extrastimulus and the first complex of the tachycardia are caused by triggered DADs, rather than by reentry.

TRIGGERING BY EARLY AFTERDEPOLARIZATIONS

Triggering by early afterdepolarizations (EADs) is a mechanism that is easily elicited in vitro but difficult to prove in the clinical setting. EADs arise before the end of repolarization and, unlike DADs, tend to appear after long pauses. When applied to EADs, the term *triggering* denotes that an afterdepolarization that does not elicit ectopic activity triggers another

afterdepolarization, which gives rise to ectopic activity. Such arrhythmias are implicated in the setting of long QT interval and are believed to play a role in the genesis of torsade de pointes.[177]

ECG CLUES TO THE MECHANISM OF VENTRICULAR ARRHYTHMIAS

Reentry may be postulated for PVCs with fixed coupling and for about 90 percent of monomorphic nonsustained and sustained VTs in the presence of structural heart disease. It is also involved in ventricular fibrillation.

Normal automaticity is the postulated mechanism of escape complexes and escape rhythms, parasystolic rhythms, accelerated ventricular rhythms, and certain idiopathic VTs. Arrhythmia triggered by DADs can be suspected when the VT is triggered by a supraventricular tachycardia, as may occur in the presence of digitalis toxicity.

With automatic tachycardias the first interectopic interval tends to be longer, and the rate increases gradually ("warming-up" effect); however, reentrant tachycardias also accelerate.[178,179]

Triggering by EADs is suspected in torsade de pointes and long QT syndrome. This is particularly true when the polymorphic tachycardia is preceded by a sequence of long cycle–short cycle, often causing an R-on-T phenomenon.

REFERENCES

1. Reddy CP, Surawicz B: Terminology of tachycardias: historical background and evolution. PACE 6:1123, 1983.
2. Janse MJ: The premature beat. Cardiovasc Res 26:89, 1992.
3. Scherf D, Schott A: Extrasystoles and Allied Arrhythmias, 2nd ed. London, Heinemann, 1973.
4. Langendorf R, Pick A, Winternitz M: Mechanisms of intermittent ventricular bigeminy. I. Appearance of ectopic beats dependent upon length of cycle, the "rule of bigeminy." Circulation 11:422, 1955.
5. Schamroth L, Dolara A: Paroxysmal ventricular tachycardia with rate-dependent coupling intervals. Circulation 36:255, 1967.
6. Surawicz B, Macdonald MG: Ventricular ectopic beats with fixed and variable coupling: incidence, clinical significance and factors influencing the coupling interval. Am J Cardiol 13:198, 1964.
7. Malinow MR, Langendorf R: Different mechanisms of fusion beats. Am Heart J 35:448, 1948.
8. Marriott HJ, Schwartz NL, Bix HH: Ventricular fusion beats. Circulation 26:880, 1962.
9. Kinoshita S: Concealed ventricular extrasystoles due to interference and due to exit block. Circulation 52:230, 1975.
10. Schamroth L: Genesis and evolution of ectopic ventricular rhythm. Br Heart J 28:244, 1966.
11. Levy MN, Adler DS, Levy JR: Three variants of concealed bigeminy. Circulation 51:646, 1975.

12. Levy MN, Mori I, Kerin N: Two variants of concealed trigeminy. Am Heart J 93:183, 1977.

13. Rosenbaum MB: Classification of ventricular extrasystoles according to form. J Electrocardiol 2:289, 1969.

14. Moulton KP, Medcalf T, Lazzara R: Premature ventricular complex morphology: a marker for left ventricular structure and function. Circulation 81:1245, 1990.

15. Simon AJ, Langendorf R: Intraventricular block with ectopic beats approaching normal QRS duration. Am Heart J 27:340, 1944.

16. Booth DC, Popio KA, Gettes LS: Multiformity of induced unifocal ventricular premature beats in human subjects: electrocardiographic and angiographic correlations. Am J Cardiol 49:1643, 1982.

17. Josephson ME, Horowitz LN, Waxman HL, et al: Sustained ventricular tachycardia: role of the 12-lead electrocardiogram in localizing site of origin. Circulation 64:257, 1981.

18. Kistin AD, Landowne M: Retrograde conduction from premature ventricular contractions: a common occurrence in the human heart. Circulation 3:738, 1951.

19. Lown B, Graboys TB: Management of patients with malignant ventricular arrhythmias. Am J Cardiol 39:910, 1977.

20. Katz LN, Langendorf R, Cole SL: An unusual effect of interpolated ventricular premature systoles. Am Heart J 28:167, 1944.

21. Langendorf R: Ventricular premature systoles with postponed compensatory pause. Am Heart J 46:401, 1953.

22. Kuo CS, Surawicz B: Coexistence of ventricular parasystole and ventricular couplets: mechanism and clinical significance. Am J Cardiol 44:435, 1979.

23. Singer DH, Paramasweran A, Drake FT, et al: Ventricular parasystole and re-entry: clinical electrophysiological correlations. Am Heart J 88:79, 1974.

24. Surawicz B, Kuo CS, Reddy CP: Re-entry near the site of the ventricular parasystolic focus: an ECG study of patients with artificial ventricular pacemakers. J Electrocardiol 13:103, 1980.

25. Qi WH, Fineberg NS, Surawicz B: The timing of ventricular premature complexes initiating chronic ventricular tachycardia. J Electrocardiol 17:377, 1984.

26. Ashman R, Byer E: Aberration in the conduction of premature ventricular impulses. J La State Med Soc 8:62, 1946.

27. Cohen SI, Lau SH, Haft JL, et al: Experimental production of aberrant ventricular conduction in man. Circulation 36:673, 1967.

28. Cohen SI, Lau SH, Stein E, et al: Variations of aberrant ventricular conduction in man: evidence of isolated and combined block within the specialized conduction system. Circulation 38:899, 1968.

29. Gouaux JL, Ashman R: Auricular fibrillation with aberration simulating ventricular paroxysmal tachycardia. Am Heart J 34:366, 1947.

30. Langendorf R: Aberrant ventricular conduction. Am Heart J 41:700, 1951.

31. Spurrell RA, Krikler DM, Sowton E: Retrograde invasion of the bundle branches producing aberration of the QRS complex during supraventricular tachycardia induced by programmed electrical stimulation. Circulation 50:487, 1974.

32. Wellens HJ, Durrer D: Supraventricular tachycardia with left aberrant conduction due to retrograde invasion into the left bundle branch. Circulation 38:474, 1968.

33. Akthar M, Gilbert C, Al-Nouri M, et al: Site of conduction delay during functional block in the His-Purkinje system in man. Circulation 61:1239, 1980.

34. Chilson DA, Zipes DP, Heger JJ, et al: Functional bundle branch block: discordant response of right and left bundle branches to changes in heart rate. Am J Cardiol 54:313, 1984.

35. Cohen SL, Lau SH, Scherlag BJ, et al: Alternate patterns of premature ventricular excitation during induced atrial bigeminy. Circulation 39:819, 1969.

36. Lehmann MH, Denker S, Mahmud R, et al: Functional His-Purkinje system behavior during sudden ventricular rate acceleration in man. Circulation 68:767, 1983.

37. Fisch C, Zipes DP, McHenry PL: Rate dependent aberrancy. Circulation 68:714, 1973.

38. Denes P, Wu D, Rosen KM, et al: Electrophysiological observations in patients with rate dependent bundle branch block. Circulation 51:244, 1973.

39. Fisch C: Bundle branch block after ventricular tachycardia: a manifestation of "fatigue" or "overdrive suppression." J Am Coll Cardiol 3:1562, 1984.

40. Scherf D, Cohen J: The Atrioventricular Node and Selected Cardiac Arrhythmias. Orlando, Grune & Stratton, 1964.

41. Sandler IA, Marriott HJL: The differential morphology of anomalous ventricular complexes of RBBB-type in lead V_1. Circulation 31:551, 1965.

42. Marriott HJL, Thorne DC: Dysrhythmic dilemmas in coronary care. Am J Cardiol 27:327, 1971.

43. Schmidt G, Malik M, Barthel P, et al: Heart-rate turbulence after ventricular premaure beats as a predictor of mortality after acute myocardial infarction. Lancet 353:1390, 1999.

44. Watanabe MA, Schmidt G: Heart rate turbulence: a 5-year review. Heart Rhythm 1:732, 2004.

45. Surawicz B: Prognosis of ventricular arrhythmias in relation to sudden cardiac death: therapeutic implications. J Am Coll Cardiol 10:435, 1987.

46. Surawicz B: Ventricular arrhythmias: why is it so difficult to find a pharmacologic cure? J Am Coll Cardiol 14:1401, 1989.

47. Brodsky M, Wu D, Denes P, et al: Arrhythmias documented by 24 hour continuous electrocardiographic monitoring in 50 male medical students without apparent heart disease. Am J Cardiol 39:390, 1977.

48. Glasser SP, Clark PE, Appelbaum HJ: Occurrence of frequent complex arrhythmias detected by ambulatory monitoring: findings in an apparently healthy asymptomatic elderly population. Chest 75:565, 1979.

49. Kostis JB, Moreyra AE, Amendo MT, et al: The effect of age on heart rate in subjects free of heart disease: studies by ambulatory electrocardiography and maximal exercise stress test. Circulation 65:141, 1982.

50. Lewis S, Kanakis C, Rosen KM, et al: Significance of origin of premature ventricular contractions. Am Heart J 97:159, 1979.

51. Jelinek MV, Lown B: Exercise stress testing for exposure of cardiac arrhythmias. Prog Cardiovasc Dis 16:497, 1974.

52. Kennedy HL, Underhill SJ: Frequent or complex ventricular ectopy in apparently healthy subjects: a clinical study of 25 cases. Am J Cardiol 38:141, 1976.

53. McHenry PL, Fisch C, Jordan JW, et al: Cardiac arrhythmias observed during maximal treadmill exercise testing in clinically normal men. Am J Cardiol 29:331, 1972.

54. McHenry PL, Morris SN, Kavalier M, et al: Comparative study of exercise-induced ventricular arrhythmias in normal subjects and patients with documented coronary artery disease. Am J Cardiol 37:609, 1976.

55. Lown B, Tykocinski M, Garfein A, et al: Sleep and ventricular premature beats. Circulation 48:691, 1973.

55a. Bogun F, Crawford T, Reich S, et al: Radiofrequency ablation of frequent, idiopathic premature ventricular complexes: Comparison with a control group without intervention. Heart Rhythm 4:863, 2007.

56. Bigger JT, Dresdale RJ, Heissenbuttel RH, et al: Ventricular arrhythmias in ischemic heart disease: mechanism, prevalence, significance and management. Prog Cardiovasc Dis 19:255, 1977.

57. Faris JV, McHenry PL, Jordan JW, et al: Prevalence and reproducibility of exercise-induced ventricular arrhythmias during maximal exercise testing in normal man. Am J Cardiol 37:617, 1976.

58. Froelicher VF, Thomas MM, Pillow C, et al: Epidemiologic study of asymptomatic men screened by maximal treadmill testing for latent coronary artery disease. Am J Cardiol 34:770, 1974.

59. Romhilt DW, Bloomfield SS, Chou T, et al: Unreliability of conventional electrocardiographic monitoring for arrhythmia detection in coronary care units. Am J Cardiol 31:457, 1973.

60. Devereux RB, Perloff JK, Reichek N, et al: Mitral valve prolapse. Circulation 54:3, 1976.

61. Winkle RA, Goodman DJ, Popp RL: Simultaneous echocardiographic-phonocardiographic recordings at rest and during amytal nitrate administration in patients with mitral valve prolapse. Circulation 51:522, 1975.

62. Chou TC: Digitalis-induced arrhythmias. In: Fowler NO (ed): Treatment of Cardiac Arrhythmias, 2nd ed. New York, Harper & Row, 1977.

63. Surawicz B: Relationship between electrocardiogram and electrolytes. Am Heart J 73:814, 1967.

64. Rodstein M, Wolloch L, Gubner RS: Mortality study of the significance of extrasystoles in an insured population. Circulation 44:617, 1971.

65. De Soyza N, Bennett FA, Murphy ML, et al: The relationship of paroxysmal ventricular tachycardia complicating the acute phase and ventricular arrhythmia during the late hospital phase of myocardial infarction in long-term survival. Am J Med 64:377, 1978.

66. Kostis JB, McCrone K, Moreyra AE, et al: Premature ventricular complexes in the absence of identifiable heart disease. Circulation 63:1351, 1981.

67. Moss AJ, Davis HT, DeCamilla J, et al: Ventricular ectopic beats and their relation to sudden cardiac death after myocardial infarction. Circulation 60: 998, 1979.

68. Hallstrom AP, Bigger JT, Roden D, et al: Prognostic significance of ventricular premature depolarizations measured 1 year after myocardial infarction in patients with early postinfarction asymptomatic ventricular arrhythmia. J Am Coll Cardiol 20:259, 1992.

69. Maggioni AP, Zuanetti G, Franzosi MG, et al: Prevalence and prognostic significance of ventricular arrhythmias after acute myocardial infarction in the fibrinolytic era: GISSI-2 results. Circulation 87:312, 1993.

70. Kotler MN, Tabatznik B, Mower MM, et al: Prognostic significance of ventricular ectopic beats with respect to sudden death in the late postinfarction period. Circulation 47:959, 1973.

71. Ruberman W, Weinblatt E, Goldberg JD, et al: Ventricular premature complexes and sudden death after myocardial infarction. Circulation 64:297, 1981.

72. Coronary Drug Project Research Group: Prognostic importance of premature beats following myocardial infarction: experience in the Coronary Drug Project. JAMA 223:1116, 1973.

73. Nilsen MV, Rasmussen V, Hansen JF, et al: Prognostic implications of ventricular ectopy one week, one month, and sixteen months after an acute myocardial infarction. Clin Cardiol 21:905, 1998.

74. Rouleau JL, Talajic M, Sussex B, et al: Myocardial infarction patients in the 1990s: their risk factors, stratification and survival in Canada: the Canadian Assessment of Myocardial Infarction (CAMI) study. J Am Coll Cardiol 22:119, 1996.

75. Weidmann S: Effect of current flow on the membrane potential of cardiac muscle. J Physiol (Lond) 115:527, 1951.

76. Jalife J, Hamilton AY, Lamanna VR, et al: Effects of current flow on pacemaker activity of the isolated kitten sinoatrial node. Am J Physiol 238:H307, 1980.

77. Jalife J, Moe GK: Phasic effects of vagal stimulation on pacemaker activity of the isolated sinus node of the young cat. Circ Res 45:595, 1979.

78. Chung EKY: Parasystole. Prog Cardiovasc Dis 11:64, 1968.

79. Cohen H, Langendorf R, Pick A: Intermittent parasystole: mechanism of protection. Circulation 68:761, 1973.

80. Langendorf R, Pick A: Parasystole with fixed coupling. Circulation 35:304, 1967.

81. Levy MN, Lee MH, Zieske H: A feedback mechanism responsible for fixed coupling in parasystole. Circ Res 31:846, 1972.

82. Michelson EL, Morganroth J, Spear JF, et al: Fixed coupling: different mechanisms revealed by exercise-induced changes in cycle length. Circulation 58: 1002, 1978.

83. Steffens TG: Intermittent ventricular parasystole due to entrance block failure. Circulation 64:442, 1971.

84. Myburgh DP, Lewis BS: Ventricular parasystole in healthy hearts. Am Heart J 82:307, 1971.

85. Katz LN, Pick A: Clinical Electrocardiography and the Arrhythmias. Philadelphia, Lea & Febiger, 1956.

86. Wellens JH, Brugada P, Stevenson WG: Programmed electrical stimulation of the heart in patients with life-threatening ventricular arrhythmias: what is the significance of induced arrhythmias and what is the correct stimulation protocol? Circulation 72:1, 1985.

87. Volosin KJ, Beauregard LM, Fabiszewski R, et al: Spontaneous changes in ventricular cycle length. J Am Coll Cardiol 17:409, 1991.

88. Geibel A, Zehender M, Brugada P: Changes in cycle length at the onset of sustained tachycardias: importance of antitachycardiac pacing. Am Heart J 115: 588, 1988.

89. Gomes JA, Alexopoulos D, Winters SL, et al: The role of silent ischemia, the arrhythmic substrate and the short-long sequence in the genesis of sudden cardiac death. J Am Coll Cardiol 14:1618, 1989.

90. Tye KH, Samant A, Desser KB, et al: R on T or R on P phenomenon? Relation to the genesis of ventricular tachycardia. Am J Cardiol 44:632, 1979.

91. Holland OB, Nixon JV, Kuhnert L: Diuretic-induced ventricular ectopic activity. Am J Med 70:762, 1981.

92. Anderson KP, Shusterman V, Aysin B, et al: Distinctive RR dynamics preceding two modes of onset of spontaneous sustained ventricular tachycardia. J Cardiovasc Electrophysiol 10:897, 1999.

93. Kistin AD: Retrograde conduction to the atria in ventricular tachycardia. Circulation 24:236, 1961.

94. Wellens HJJ, Lie KI: Ventricular tachycardia: the value of programmed electrical stimulation. In: Krikler DM, Goodwin JF (eds): Cardiac Arrhythmias: The Modern Electrophysiological Approach. Philadelphia, Saunders, 1975, p 182.

95. Akhtar M, Shenasa M, Jazayeri MR, et al: Wide QRS complex tachycardia. Ann Intern Med 109:905, 1988.

96. Dressler W, Roesler M: The occurrence in paroxysmal ventricular tachycardia of ventricular complexes transitional in shape to sinoauricular beats. Am Heart J 44:485, 1952.

97. Fisch C: Electrocardiography of Arrhythmias. Philadelphia, Lea & Febiger, 1990, p 131.

98. Buxton AE, Waman HL, Marchlinski FE, et al: Right ventricular tachycardia: clinical and electrophysiologic characteristics. Circulation 68:917, 1983.

99. Josephson ME, Horowitz LN, Farshidi A, et al: Recurrent sustained ventricular tachycardia. 2. Endocardial mapping. Circulation 57:440, 1978.

100. Manyari DE, Klein GJ, Gulamhusein S, et al: Arrhythomogenic right ventricular dysplasia: a generalized cardiomyopathy? Circulation 68:251, 1983.

101. Marcus FI, Fontaine GH, Guiraudon G, et al: Right ventricular dysplasia: a report of 24 adult cases. Circulation 65:384, 1982.

102. Nava A, Thiene G, Canciani B, et al: Familial occurrence of right ventricular dysplasia: a study involving nine families. J Am Coll Cardiol 12:1222, 1988.

103. Fontaine G, Guiradon G, Frank R, et al: Modern concepts of ventricular tachycardia. Eur J Cardiol 8:565, 1978.

104. Miller JM, Marchlinski FE, Buxton AE, et al: Relationship between the 12-lead electrocardiogram during ventricular tachycardia and endocardial site of origin in patients with coronary artery disease. Circulation 77:759, 1988.

105. Josephsom ME, Callans DJ: Using the twelve-lead electrocardiogram to localize the site of origin of ventricular tachycardia. Heart Rhythm 2:443, 2004.

106. Wren C, Rowland E, Burn J, et al: Familial ventricular tachycardia: a report of four families. Br Heart J 63:169, 1990.

107. Lemery R, Brugada P, Bella PD, et al: Nonischemic ventricular tachycardia. Clinical course and long-term follow-up in patients without clinically overt heart disease. Circulation 78:990, 1989.

108. Wolfe CL, Nibley C, Bhandari A, et al: Polymorphous ventricular tachycardia associated with acute myocardial infarction. Circulation 84:1543, 1991.

109. Josephson ME, Horowitz LN, Farshidi A: Recurrent sustained ventricular tachycardia: pleomorphism. Circulation 59:459, 1979.

110. Kimber SK, Downar E, Harris L, et al: Mechanisms of spontaneous shift of surface electrocardiographic configuration during ventricular tachycardia. J Am Coll Cardiol 20:1397, 1992.

111. Buxton AE, Josephson ME, Marchlinski FE, et al: Polymorphic ventricular tachycardia induced by programmed stimulation: response to procainamide. J Am Coll Cardiol 21:90, 1993.

112. Cohen HC, Gozo EG, Pick A: Ventricular tachycardia with narrow QRS complexes (left posterior fascicular tachycardia). Circulation 45:1035, 1972.

113. Hayes JJ, Stewart RB, Greene HL, Bardy GH: Narrow QRS ventricular tachycardia. Ann Intern Med 114:460, 1991.

114. Weiss J, Stevenson WG: Narrow QRS ventricular tachycardia. Am Heart J 112:843, 1986.

115. Schamroth L: Idioventricular tachycardia. J Electrocardiol 1:205, 1968.

116. Schamroth L: Genesis and evolution of ectopic ventricular rhythms. Br Heart J 28:244, 1966.

117. Gallagher JJ, Damato AN, Lau SH: Electrophysiologic studies during accelerated idioventricular rhythms. Circulation 64:671, 1971.

118. Rothfeld EL, Zucker IR, Parsonnet V, et al: Idioventricular rhythm in acute myocardial infarction. Circulation 37:203, 1968.

119. Lichstein E, Ribas-Meneelier C, Gupta PK, et al: Incidence and description of accelerated ventricular rhythm complicating acute myocardial infarction. Am J Med 58:192, 1975.

120. Goldberg S, Greenspon AJ, Urban PL, et al: Reperfusion arrhythmia: a marker of restoration of antegrade flow during intracoronary thrombosis for acute myocardial infarction. Am Heart J 105:26, 1983.

121. Massumi RA, Ali N: Accelerated isorhythmic ventricular rhythms. Am J Cardiol 26:170, 1970.

122. Chung EKY, Walsh TJ, Massie E: Ventricular parasystolic tachycardia. Br Heart J 27:392, 1965.

123. Garson AJr, Smith RT, Moak JP, et al: Incessant ventricular tachycardia in infants; myocardial hamartomas and surgical cure. J Am Coll Cardiol 10:619, 1987.

124. Swan H, Piippo K, Heikkila P, et al: Arrhythmic disorder mapped to chromosome 1q42-q43 causes malignant polymorphic ventricular tachycardia in structurally normal hearts. J Am Coll Cardiol 34:2035, 1999.

125. Laitinen P, Brown KM, Swan H, et al: Mutations in the cardiac ryanodine receptor (RyR2) gene in familial polymorphic ventricular tachycardia. Circulation 103:488, 2001.

126. Francis J, Sankar V, Nair VG, et al: Catecholaminergic polymorphic ventricular tachycardia. Heart Rhythm 2:550, 2005.

127. Carlson MD, White RD, Trohman RG, et al: Right ventricular outflow tract ventricular tachycardia: detection of previously unrecognized anatomic abnormalities using cine magnetic resonance imaging. J Am Coll Cardiol 24:720, 1994.

128. Markowitz SM, Litvak BL, Ramirez de Arellano EA, et al: Adenosine-sensitive ventricular tachycardia: right ventricular abnormalities delineated by magnetic resonance imaging. Circulation 96:1192, 1997.

129. Callans DJ, Menz V, Schwartzman D, et al: Repetitive monomorphic tachycardia from the left ventricular outflow tract: electrocardiographic patterns consistent with a left ventricular origin. J Am Coll Cardiol 29:1023, 1997.

130. Gumbrielle TP, Bourke JP, Doig JC, et al: Electrocardiographic features of septal location of right ventricular outflow tract tachycardia. Am J Cardiol 79:213, 1997.

130a.Tada H, Tadokoro K, Ito S, et al: Idiopathic ventricular arrhythmias originating from the tricuspid annulus: Prevalence, electrocardiographic characteristics, and results of radiofrequency catheter ablation. Heart Rhythm 4:7, 2007.

131. Ohe T, Shimomura K, Aihara N, et al: Idiopathic sustained left ventricular tachycardia: clinical and electrophysiologic characteristics. Circulation 77:560, 1988.

132. Zivin A, Goyal R, Daoud E, et al: Idiopathic left ventricular tachycardia with left and right bundle branch block configurations. J Cardiovasc Electrophysiol 8:441, 1997.

133. Lerman BB, Stein KM, Markowitz SM: Mechanisms of idiopathic left ventricular tachycardia. J Cardiovasc Electrophysiol 8:571, 1997.

134. Lee KL, Lauer MR, Young C, et al: Spectrum of electrophysiologic and electropharmacologic characteristics of verapamil-sensitive ventricular tachycardia in patients without structural heart disease. Am J Cardiol 77:967, 1996.

135. Gill JS, Prasad K, Blaszyk K, et al: Initiating sequences in exercise-induced idiopathic ventricular tachycardia of left bundle branch-like morphology. PACE 21:1873, 1998.

136. Leenhardt A, Lucet V, Denjoy I, et al: Catecholaminergic polymorphic ventricular tachycardia in children: a 7-year follow-up of 21 patients. Circulation 91:1512, 1995.

137. Lerman BB, Stein KM, Markowitz SM, et al: Catecholamine facilitated reentrant ventricular tachycardia: uncoupling of adenosine's antiadrenergic effects. J Cardiovasc Electrophysiol 10:17, 1999.

138. Yeh S-J, Wu D-S, Wang C-C, et al: Adenosine-sensitive ventricular tachycardia from the anterobasal left ventricle. J Am Coll Cardiol 30:1339, 1997.

139. Bigger JT, Fleiss JL, Rolnitzky LM, et al: Prevalence, characteristics and significance of ventricular tachycardia detected by 24-hour continuous electrocardiographic recordings in the late hospital phase of acute myocardial infarction. Am J Cardiol 58:1151, 1986.

140. Miller FC, Krucoff MW, Satler LF, et al: Ventricular arrhythmias during reperfusion. Am Heart J 112: 928, 1986.

141. Newby KH, Thompson T, Stebbins A, et al: Sustained ventricular arrhythmias in patients receiving thrombolytic therapy. Circulation 98:2567, 1998.

142. Packer M: Sudden unexpected death in patients with congestive heart failure: a second frontier. Circulation 72:681, 1985.

143. Singh SN, Fisher SG, Carson PE, et al: Prevalence and significance of nonsustained ventricular tachycardia in patients with premature ventricular contractions and heart failure treated with vasodilator therapy. J Am Coll Cardiol 32:942, 1998.

144. Brodsky M, Doria R, Allen B, et al: New-onset ventricular tachycardia during pregnancy. Am Heart J 123:933, 1992.

145. Jeresaty RM: Sudden death in the mitral valve prolapse-click syndrome. Am J Cardiol 37:317, 1976.

146. Shappel SD, Marshall CE, Brown RE, et al: Sudden death and the familial occurrence of the midsystolic click, late systolic murmur syndrome. Circulation 48:1128, 1973.

147. Harrison DA, Harris L, Siu SC, et al: Sustained ventricular tachycardia in adult patients late after repair of tetralogy. J Am Coll Cardiol 30:1368, 1997.

148. Balaji S, Lau YR, Case CL, et al: QRS prolongation is associated with inducible ventricular tachycardia after repair of tetralogy of Fallot. Am J Cardiol 80:160, 1997.

149. Mackenzie GJ, Pascual S: Paroxysmal ventricular tachycardia. Br Heart J 26:441, 1964.

150. Bellet S: Clinical Disorders of the Heart Beat. Philadelphia, Lea & Febiger, 1963.

151. Creamer JE, Nathan AW, Camm AJ: The proarrhythmic effects of antiarrhythmic drugs. Am Heart J 114:397, 1987.

152. Dhein S, Muller A, Gerwin R, et al: Comparative study on the proarrhythmic effects of some antiarrhythmic agents. Circulation 87:617, 1993.

153. Selzer A, Wray HW: Quinidine syncope: paroxysmal ventricular fibrillation occurring during treatment of chronic atrial arrhythmias. Circulation 30:17, 1964.

154. Stanton MS, Prystowsky EN, Fineberg NS, et al: Arrhythmogenic effects of antiarrhythmic drugs: a study of 506 patients treated for ventricular tachycardia or fibrillation. J Am Coll Cardiol 14:209, 1989.

155. Michelson EL, Morganroth J, MacVaugh H: Postoperative arrhythmias after coronary artery and cardiac valvular surgery detected by long-term electrocardiographic monitoring. Am Heart J 97:442, 1979.

156. Surawicz B: Role of electrolytes in etiology and management of cardiac arrhythmias. Prog Cardiovasc Dis 8:364, 1966.

157. Bass M: Sudden sniffing death. JAMA 212:2075, 1970.

158. Flowers NV, Horan LG: Nonanoxic aerosol arrhythmias. JAMA 219:33, 1972.

159. Wellens JJH, Brugada O, Stevenson WG: Programmed electrical stimulation of the heart in patients with life-threatening ventricular arrhythmias: what is the significance of induced arrhythmias and what is the correct stimulation protocol?. Circulation 72:1, 1985.

160. Kim SG, Mercando AD, Fisher JD: Comparison of the characteristics of nonsustained ventricular tachycardia on Holter monitoring and sustained ventricular tachycardia observed spontaneously or induced by programmed stimulation. Am J Cardiol 60:288, 1987.

161. Spach MS: Anisotopic structural complexities in the genesis of ventricular arrhythmias. Circulation 84: 1448, 1991.

162. Pogwizd SM, Hoyt RH, Saffitz JE, et al: Reentrant and focal mechanisms underlying ventricular tachycardia in the human heart. Circulation 86:1872, 1992.

163. Pogwizd SM, McKenzie JP, Cain ME: Mechanisms underlying spontaneous and induced ventricular arrhythmias in patients with idiopathic dilated cardiomyopathy. Circulation 98:2404, 1998.

163a. Bogun F, Good E, Reich S, et al: Role of Purkinje fibers in post-infarction ventricular tachycardia. J Am Coll Cardiol 48:2500, 2006.

164. Lucas A, Antzelevitch C: Phase 2 reentry as a mechanism of initiation of circus movement reentry in canine epicardium exposed to simulated ischemia. Cardiovasc Res 32:593, 1996.

165. Thomsen PEB, Joergensen RM, Kanters JK, et al: Phase 2 reentry in man. Heart Rhythm 2:797, 2005.

166. Akthar M, Damato AN, Batsford WP, et al: Demonstration of reentry within the His Purkinje system in man. Circulation 50:1150, 1974.

167. Caceres J, Jazayeri M, McKinnie J, et al: Sustained bundle branch reentry as a mechanism of clinical tachycardia. Circulation 79:256, 1989.

168. Narasimhan C, Jazayeri MR, Sra J, et al: Ventricular tachycardia in valvular heart disease: facilitation of sustained bundle-branch reentry in valve surgery. Circulation 96:4307, 1997.

169. Tchou P, Jazayeri M, Denker S, et al: Transcatheter electrical ablation of right bundle branch block: a method of treating macroreentrant ventricular tachycardia attributed to bundle branch reentry. Circulation 78:246, 1988.

170. De Bakker JM, van Capelle FJL, Janse MJ, et al: Macroreentry in the infarcted human heart: the mechanism of ventricular tachycardias with a "focal" activation pattern. J Am Coll Cardiol 18:1005, 1991.

171. Waxman HL, Josephson ME: Ventricular tachycardia in man. In: Surawicz B, Reddy CP, Prystowsky EN (eds): Tachycardias. The Hague, Martinus Nijhoff, 1984.

172. Josephson ME, Horowitz LN, Farshidi A: Continuous local electrical activity: a mechanism of recurrent ventricular tachycardia. Circulation 57:659, 1978.

173. Josephson ME, Horowitz LN, Farshidi A, et al: Sustained ventricular tachycardia: evidence for protected localized reentry. Am J Cardiol 422:416, 1978.

174. Ferrier GR, Saunders JH, Mendez C: A cellular mechanism for the generation of ventricular arrhythmias by acetylstrophanthidin. Circ Res 41:600, 1973.

175. Rosen MR, Gelband H, Hoffman BF: Correlation between effects of ouabain on the canine electrocardiogram and transmembrane potentials of isolated Purkinje fibers. Circulation 67:65, 1973.

176. Vos MA, Gorgels APD, Leumissen JDM, et al: Flumarazine allows differentiation between mechanisms of arrhythmias in the intact heart. Circulation 81:342, 1990.

177. Surawicz B: Electrophysiologic Basis of ECG and Cardiac Arrhythmias. Baltimore, Williams & Wilkins, 1995, p 206.

178. Julian DT, Valentine PA, Miller GG: Disturbances of rate, rhythm and conduction in acute myocardial infarction: a prospective study of 100 consecutive unselected patients with the aid of electrocardiographic monitoring. Am J Med 37:915, 1964.

179. Kaltenbrunner W, Cardinal R, Dubuc M, et al: Epicardial and endocardial mapping of ventricular tachycardia in patients with myocardial infarction. Circulation 84:1058, 1991.

18 Torsade de Pointes, Ventricular Fibrillation, and Differential Diagnosis of Wide QRS Tachycardias

Torsade de Pointes
Paroxysm
Clinical Correlation
Most Common Causes of TDP
Mechanism of TDP
Other Polymorphic VTs

Ventricular Flutter and Fibrillation

Commotio Cordis

Differential Diagnosis of Tachycardia with Wide QRS Complex
Mechanism of Regular Wide QRS Tachycardia
AV Dissociation
Differential Diagnosis of VT versus Preexcited Tachycardia

Torsade de Pointes

Torsade de pointes (TDP), a polymorphic ventricular tachycardia (VT) associated with a prolonged QT interval or increased U wave amplitude, is amenable to suppression by an increase in heart rate.[1–3] When defined in this manner, the arrhythmia has been recognized as a syndrome rather than a distinctly different VT or ventricular fibrillation.

To satisfy the description of torsade de pointes, the axis of the QRS complex must change direction after a certain number of complexes as though the complex rotated around the baseline. The phasic variation of the polarity and amplitude of the QRS complexes may be apparent only if several synchronous leads are recorded.[4]

The intervals between complexes vary, and the rate of tachycardia is usually 200 to 250 beats/min but may range from 150 to 300 beats/min. It has been observed that the episodes of fast TDP (heart rate >220 beats/min) are characterized by longer duration, are preceded by faster heart rate, and degenerate more often into ventricular fibrillation.[5] In addition to its characteristic morphologic features, TDP differs from sustained monomorphic VT by the difficulty of arrhythmia induction with programmed electrical stimulation and by the characteristic pattern of onset. In most cases TDP is preceded by a sequence of a long RR interval of the dominant cycle followed by a short extrasystolic interval with premature depolarization interrupting the T wave (R-on-T phenomenon) (Figure 18–1). Kay and associates[6] reported that such a sequence was seen during 41 of the 44 episodes of TDP that occurred in 32 patients. Such a sequence is not pathognomonic for TDP, however, as Gomes et al.[7] also noted it frequently preceding ventricular tachycardia and ventricular fibrillation. The presence of severe bradycardia, as seen with advanced atrioventricular (AV) block or sinoatrial (SA) block, in the basic rhythm before the onset of TDP has been noted on many occasions[8–10] (see Figure 18–1).

PAROXYSM

An episode of TDP consists of two or more cycles. Each cycle begins or ends at the point where the amplitude of the QRS complexes is the smallest and the polarity of the complexes changes. There are usually 5 to 20 complexes in each cycle. Because of the wide QRS complexes and rapid rate, it is often difficult to distinguish the QRS and T waves. In some instances, when multiple simultaneous leads are recorded, the tachycardia appears to be monophasic in one lead but presents the typical TDP in another.[1] Torsade de pointes appears to be less disorganized than ventricular fibrillation; the rhythm is usually self-terminating but may degenerate into ventricular fibrillation. The attack also may end with sinus arrest with slow ventricular escape rhythm before the basal rhythm resumes (Figure 18–2).

J.H.   76 M   8-10-72
Pacemaker failure

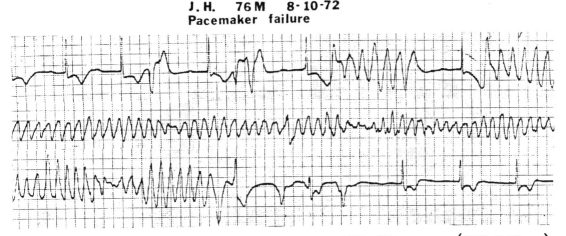

Contin. record. Complete AVB & pacing since 1966. AVJ   escape (QRS: 0.09 sec)

Figure 18–1   Continuous strip of ECG lead II in a 76-year-old man with failure of an electronic pacemaker, implanted 6 years earlier. Ventricular premature complexes (VPC) with varying coupling intervals (CI) in the presence of complete AV block and AV junctional escape rhythm. QT interval is 0.54 second. *Top strip:* The CI of the VPC decreases progressively: 0.56 second (4th complex), 0.52 second (6th complex), 0.50 second (9th complex), and 0.48 second (16th complex). Note the long pauses before the complexes followed by a VPC. The VPC with the shortest CI is followed by ventricular fibrillation and torsade de pointes, continuing through the middle strip and part of the bottom strip.

CLINICAL CORRELATION

TDP is generally seen in conditions associated with QT prolongation.[11] The risk is increased with increasing QTc duration and in the presence of (1) hypokalemia, potassium deficiency, and perhaps hypomagnesemia; (2) impaired ventricular function; (3) severe bradycardia and second- or third-degree AV block; (4) T wave alternans; and (5) R-on-T phenomenon.[12,13] Female gender is also a relative risk factor, as in most series there is female preponderance of this arrhythmia (ratio of female:male is about 3:1). The clinical conditions known to predispose to TDP are as follows:

1. *Congenital long QT syndrome (see Chapter 24).*
2. *Poisoning with organophosphorus compounds.[14]*
3. *Intracranial hemorrhage[15,16] and complications of air encephalography.[17]*
4. *Treatment with antiarrhythmic drugs.* This represents one of the three most common causes of TDP. The largest number of cases has been reported in patients treated with quinidine,[18–20] in whom the incidence of torsade is approximately 1.5 percent per year[21] (Figure 18–3). Arrhythmia tends to occur early, within 1 week of initiating treatment. In one study of 31 patients, approximately two thirds had a prolonged QT while not receiving quinidine.[22] Other aggravating factors include structural heart disease, hypokalemia, and abrupt rate slowing.[21]

TDP has been reported in patients treated with procainamide and its metabolite N-acetylprocainamide[23,24] and in those treated with disopyramide.[25] Other drugs in the class IA category reported to have induced TDP include aprindine and ajmaline.[26,27] There are case reports of TDP attributed to class IB drugs (e.g., mexiletine) and class IC drugs (e.g., propafenone). TDP also occurs during treatment with class III drugs, such as sotalol,[28,29] ibutilide, azimilide, dofetilide, and amiodarone.[6,18,30] In patients in whom ibutilide was administered intravenously for treatment of atrial fibrillation, TDP occurred in 5.6 percent of women and in 3 percent of men during or within 45 minutes of completion of ibutilide infusion.[31] In patients treated with azimilide the incidene of TDP is 1 percent but, unlike other IKr blockers, the TDP events are not concentrated in the first week.[31a] The incidence of TDP appears to be lower in patients treated with amiodarone than with other drugs that prolong the QT interval.[32,33] Other antiarrhythmic drugs that prolong QTc and can induce TDP are the calcium channel–blocking drugs bepridil[34] and prenylamine.[35]

5. *Metabolic disturbances.* TDP associated with significant QT prolongation has been reported in patients with hypothyroidism[36,37]

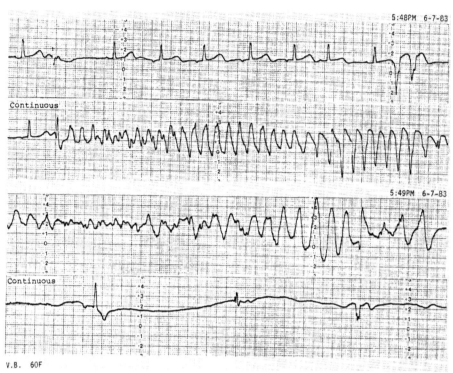

Figure 18–2 Torsade de pointes (TDP) resulting from quinidine administration in a 60-year-old woman who had a previous myocardial infarction and was receiving digoxin and quinidine for the control of supraventricular and ventricular tachyarrhythmias. Because of recurrent dizziness, an ambulatory ECG was obtained. During the recording, she had a syncope episode. The tracing at the time of syncope (5:48 PM) shows TDP followed by ventricular fibrillation and sinus arrest with ventricular escape complexes. Sinus rhythm returned in about 1 minute. Note the prolongation of the QT interval (0.48 second) in the top strip during sinus and ectopic atrial rhythm. There is a ventricular couplet followed by a pause and a supraventricular complex, which in turn is followed by an ectopic ventricular complex that falls on the terminal part of the T wave and initiates a 45-second episode of TDP. Thus a long–short cycle initiating sequence is present (see text discussion). The quinidine and digoxin levels were within therapeutic range. The patient did not have recurrence of syncope after quinidine administration was discontinued.

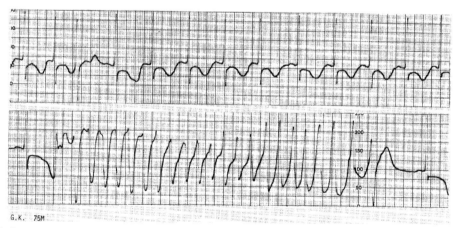

Figure 18–3 Torsade de pointes resulting from quinidine administration in a 75-year-old man who had syncope while receiving quinidine. The *upper strip* shows a basic sinus rhythm. There is marked prolongation of the QT interval, measuring 0.56 second. *Bottom strip:* There is an ectopic ventricular complex falling on the T wave of the preceding sinus complex. The ectopic complex initiates an episode of ventricular tachyarrhythmia. The tachycardia has a rate of about 200 beats/min. The RR interval is irregular. The QRS complexes have negative polarity during the first part of the episode and upright polarity during the second part.

or anorexia nervosa and during treatment with "liquid protein" diets, other fad weight-reducing diets, and therapeutic starvation.[38–40] Hypokalemia is a well-known risk factor for this arrhythmia, either alone or in association with other factors.[13,41,42] Hypocalcemia appears to be a rare cause of TDP[43]; the same is true of hypomagnesemia.

6. *Concomitant use of drugs that compete for or inhibit the hepatic cytochrome P-450 3A4.* This isoenzyme is essential for the metabolism of drugs that prolong the QT interval. The two drug categories that inhibit this enzyme are (1) antifungal drugs such as ketoconazole, itraconazole, miconazole, and fluconazole; and (2) macrolide antibiotics such as erythromycin, clarithromycin, and troleandomycin. The reported arrhythmias in patients treated with terfenadine and cisapride occurred usually during concomitant administration of a drug in these two categories.[44–46]

7. *Other drugs.* Case reports of TDP associated with QT lengthening incriminate a variety of drugs. A partial list includes thioridazine, amantadine, vincamine, ketanserin, astemizole, pentamidine, trimethoprim-sulfamethoxazole, vasopressin, and a mixture of Chinese medical herbs.[47–55] Undoubtedly, more drugs will be added to the list in the future. See also Chapter 21.

8. Transient QT prolongation often occurs during the acute phase of *myocardial infarction* (MI).[56] In a series of 771 consecutive patients with acute MI, TDP was observed in 1.2 percent.[57] Drugs and electrolyte imbalance were not implicated in these patients. TDP also was reported in a few patients with chronic stable coronary artery disease[58] (in some such cases the QT interval is not prolonged) (Figure 18–4), variant angina,[59,60] and myocarditis.[61] Mitral valve prolapse may rarely cause TDP.[58]

9. *Other conditions.* TDP has been reported in several other conditions associated with QT lengthening (e.g., after ionic contrast injections into the coronary artery[62]) and in patients with pheochromocytoma.[63]

MOST COMMON CAUSES OF TDP

In one of the largest series collected over 11 years, Salle et al. found that of 60 cases of TDP, 21 were associated with severe bradycardia, 16 were linked to potassium depletion, and 23 were caused by drugs.[64]

MECHANISM OF TDP

Many experimental studies suggest that TDP is initiated by a process known as *early afterdepolarizations*, which may also contribute to maintenance of the arrhythmia. An alternative hypothesis proposes that essential to the maintenance and perhaps to the initiation of TDP is the presence of dispersion of ventricular repolarization.[65]

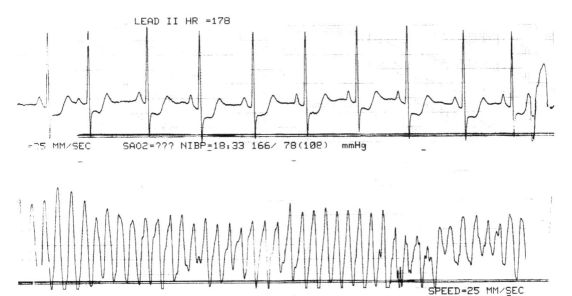

Figure 18–4   ECG recorded during ambulatory monitoring in a patient with angina pectoris (continuous tracing). Early premature ventricular complex interrupts the T wave and initiates torsade de pointes. ST segment depression precedes the event.

OTHER POLYMORPHIC VTs

The definition of TDP does not include polymorphic tachycardias, which are morphologically indistinguishable from TDP but occur in the absence of prolonged ventricular repolarization. Such tachycardias may be present during acute myocardial ischemia, in patients with structural heart disease (e.g., ischemic or dilated cardiomyopathy in which the polymorphic ventricular tachycardias coexist with other types of ventricular tachyarrhythmia), and in the presence of QT lengthening resulting from QRS prolongation without appreciable lengthening of repolarization[66a] (e.g., after treatment with class IC antiarrhythmic or certain antidepressant drugs).

Leenhardt and associates[66] described a "short-coupled variant" of TDP in 14 patients with syncope but no structural heart disease. The episodes of VT had the typical characteristics of TDP except the QT interval was normal. The coupling interval of the first tachycardia complex was unusually short, indicating increased dispersion of repolarization. Of these 14 patients, 5 died suddenly within 7 years.

Ventricular Flutter and Fibrillation

The electrocardiographic (ECG) pattern of ventricular flutter (VFl) shows regular, continuous waves, usually of large amplitude (Figure 18–5). The tracing often resembles a continuous sine wave, with no distinction among the QRS complex, ST segment, and T wave. The rate of the undulations is usually more than 200 per minute. Differentiation between VT and VFl is based mainly on the morphology of the waveforms rather than on the rate. Ventricular flutter is diagnosed when the individual component of the ventricular complex is no longer recognizable.

Ventricular fibrillation (VF) is defined as chaotic asynchronous fractionated activity of the heart. The ECG shows irregular deflections of varying amplitude and contour. No definitive P waves, QRS complexes, or T waves can be recognized. The rate of the undulations varies between 150 and 500 per minute (Figure 18–6). The pattern of disorganized electrical activity

during VF is similar to that in atrial fibrillation (see Chapter 15). Recently, epicardial activity during VF induced by burst pacing in patients undergoing cardiac surgery was sampled with a sock containing 256 unipolar contact electrodes.[66a] It was shown that VF was driven by co-existent multiple complex wavelets and single periodic sources (mother rotors).[66a]

Ambulatory monitoring shows that in patients with coronary artery disease, VF may be preceded by a variety of events such as VT, VF, frequent premature ventricular contractions (PVCs), ST deviation caused by myocardial ischemia, R-on-T phenomenon, long pauses, lengthening of the QT interval, supraventricular arrhythmias, or sinus tachycardia.[67] None of these events is highly sensitive or highly specific. Campbell et al.[68] studied ventricular arrhythmias that occurred within the first 12 hours of acute MI and reported that R-on-T initiated the primary VF in 16 of 17 patients, whereas it initiated VT in only 4 of 265 VT episodes. R-on-T frequently occurs in the absence of arrhythmia and is not a reliable predictor of VF. Adgey et al.[69] found that R-on-T initiated primary VF in 33 of 48 (69 percent) patients, whereas the remaining VF episodes were preceded by VT (19 percent) or late ventricular ectopic complexes (12 percent). Similar results were reported by other investigators. VF was observed in 20 percent of patients with documented MI monitored within 1 hour after the onset of symptoms and in only 1 of 98 patients later than 10 hours after the onset of symptoms.[70] The recurrence rate of VF in patients with initial primary VF occurring within 1 hour after onset of MI was 16 percent; it was higher among the hospitalized survivors who had no acute myocardial infarction.[71] In another study, the incidence of recurrent VF in a large group of hospital patients was 2.4 percent.[72] It has been reported that in patients with acute MI the risk of primary VF is determined by cumulative ST deviation and family history of sudden death.[72a]

Cases of VF in the absence of previously documented organic heart disease or a long QT comprise a small fraction of victims of sudden cardiac death in all published series. These

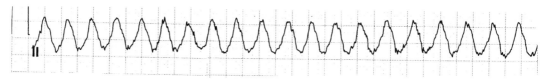

Figure 18–5   Ventricular flutter.

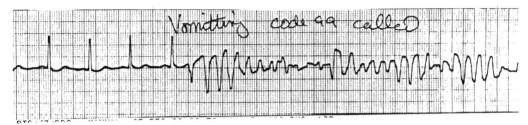

Figure 18–6   Ventricular fibrillation.

arrhythmias predominantly affect men[73] and represent a variety of etiologies and mechanisms (e.g., exercise-induced familial or sporadic, possible "forme fruste" of long QT syndrome, abnormally short ventricular refractory period, or coronary spasm). For a more detailed discussion of VF and its mechanisms, the reader is referred to two review articles[74,75] and the author's textbook.[76]

Commotio Cordis

Commotio cordis is a term applied to sudden death resulting from nonpenetrating chest wall impact in the absence of injury to the ribs, sternum, and heart, thereby differing from cardiac contusion. The common causes include the impact of baseballs, footballs, lacrosse sticks, and hockey pucks. The mean age of affected individuals was 14 years. Among more than 140 cases collected in the registry begun in 1998, the death rate was 84%, presumably caused by ventricular tachyarrhythmia.[77] In terms of mechanism, it is believed to represent a mechanically induced ionic channel dysfunction.[78]

Differential Diagnosis of Tachycardia with Wide QRS Complex

A regular tachycardia with a rate of 120 to 200 beats/min and a QRS duration of 0.12 second or longer may represent one of the following rhythms:

1. Ventricular tachycardia
2. Aberrant ventricular conduction (see Figure 17–11)
3. Preexisting left (LBBB) or right (RBBB) bundle branch block
4. Preexisting nonspecific intraventricular conduction defect
5. Anterograde conduction through the bypass tract in patients with the Wolff-Parkinson-White (WPW) syndrome (see Chapter 20)
6. Anterograde conduction over an atriofascicular or nodoventricular connection (see Chapter 20)

An irregular wide QRS complex tachycardia may represent one of the following rhythms:

1. Atrial fibrillation with aberrant ventricular conduction, bundle branch block, or intraventricular conduction defect.
2. Atrial fibrillation with ventricular preexcitation. In the presence of a short refractory period of the bypass tract, the ventricular rate can be rapid. Indeed, if the ventricular rate in atrial fibrillation is >220 beats/min or the shortest RR interval is <250 ms, the presence of a bypass should be seriously considered because the AV node is not capable of conducting impulses at such rates in adults.
3. Polymorphic VT (e.g., catecholaminergic tachycardia) (see Chapter 17).
4. Torsade de pointes.

MECHANISM OF REGULAR WIDE QRS TACHYCARDIA

Morphology of Premature Complexes during Supraventricular Rhythm

The availability of a previous or subsequent record during sinus rhythm helps to recognize the preexisting intraventricular conduction defect. If PVCs are present and their morphology is identical to those of the tachycardia complexes, the ventricular origin of the ectopic rhythm can be assumed (see Figure 17–18). Conversely, the presence of premature supraventricular complexes with aberrant ventricular conduction and morphology identical to that of the tachycardia complexes supports the diagnosis of supraventricular tachycardia (see Figure 17–11).

Onset of Tachycardias

When the tachycardia is intermittent and its onset is recorded, supraventricular tachycardia can be diagnosed if the episode is initiated by a premature P wave. If the paroxysm begins with a QRS complex, however, the tachycardia may be ventricular or supraventricular. If the first wide QRS complex of the tachycardia is preceded by a sinus P wave with a PR interval shorter than that of the conducted sinus complexes, the tachycardia is usually ventricular.

AV DISSOCIATION

Identification of atrial activity independent of ventricular activity establishes the presence of AV dissociation and offers strong evidence but not absolute proof of VT. AV dissociation also may be seen in AV junctional tachycardias with retrograde second-degree block.[79,80] Conversely, a 1:1 atrial:ventricular relation does not exclude VT because it may represent 1:1 retrograde VA conduction (Figure 18–7). Finding an RP interval of <0.10 second favors junctional tachycardia, as the time interval is too short for VA conduction in the absence of a bypass pathway. However, rapid VA conduction may take place when the PR interval during sinus rhythm is short (Figure 18–8). Similarly, a longer RP interval does not exclude junctional rhythm because retrograde conduction of the junctional impulse may be delayed. Appearance of retrograde P waves may be simulated by portions of the QRS complex. This can be detected by aligning the suspected P wave with the QRS complex in other simultaneously recorded leads (Figure 18–9).

Positive and Negative Concordance

The terms *positive* and *negative concordance* indicate that the QRS complexes in all six precordial leads have the same polarity (i.e., all positive or all negative). The finding of positive or negative concordance favors VT (see Figures 17–14 and 17-15), but exceptions occur (Figure 18–10).

Capture and Fusion Complexes

Although capture and fusion complexes with a normal QRS duration occur in only about 5 percent of VTs, their appearance constitutes some of the strongest evidence for VT. It should be remembered, however, that during supraventricular tachycardia with LBBB, intermittent premature narrow QRS complexes may represent fusion complexes between bundle branch block and an ipsilateral PVC. This is because the PVC from the left ventricle with RBBB morphology, when superimposed on the underlying LBBB complex, results in pseudonormalization of the ventricular complex (see Chapter 4). A short HV interval of such PVCs suggests that their origin is in the fascicles.[81] A narrow QRS complex may appear also during irregular supraventricular tachycardia with LBBB morphology if the LBBB is rate dependent.

Other exceptions are caused by fusion of the supraventricular impulses with the wide QRS complex. This is caused by conduction through an anomalous pathway with sinus complexes that are transmitted through the normal AV pathway.[82]

Vagal Stimulation and Adenosine Administration

In most instances, termination or slowing of wide QRS tachycardia by vagal stimulation or adenosine implies a supraventricular origin,

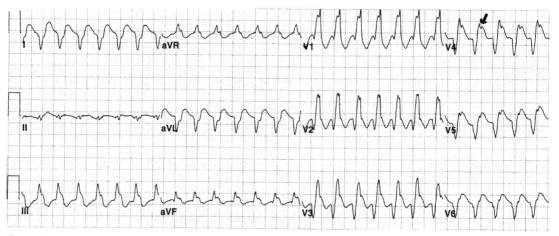

Figure 18–7 Ventricular tachycardia with retrograde ventriculoatrial conduction in a 76-year-old man with ischemic cardiomyopathy. Arrow points at the P wave. The morphology is right bundle branch block, and the QRS duration is 160 ms.

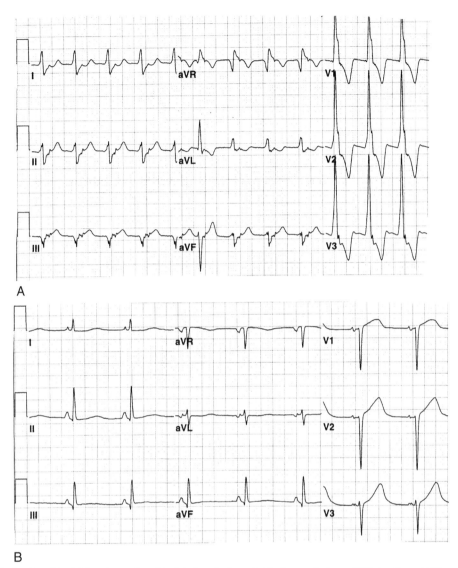

Figure 18–8 **A,** Wide QRS tachycardia with right bundle branch block morphology, QRS duration of 196 ms, and short RP interval in a 68-year-old woman with three-vessel coronary artery disease, previous inferior myocardial infarction, and inducible ventricular tachycardia (VT) with RBBB morphology. **B,** ECG during sinus rhythm shows a relatively short PR interval of 118 ms, suggesting that the short RP during VT is caused by rapid ventriculoatrial transmission.

although exceptions occur. Waxman and Wald[83] reported well-documented episodes of VT that were terminated by carotid sinus massage after pretreatment with edrophonium. The subset of adenosine-sensitive idiopathic VT is discussed in Chapter 17.

Morphology of the QRS Complex

The markers differentiating VT from supraventricular tachycardia with aberrant conduction listed previously are useful but are available for only a small number of the wide QRS tachycardias that may be in need of urgent diagnosis.

Hence the need to analyze the morphology of the QRS complexes must be emphasized. In some patients with bundle branch block or fascicular block, the morphology of the QRS complexes during VT is nearly identical to that of supraventricular complexes.[84] In most cases, however, the morphologies of supraventricular complexes conducted with aberration and ventricular ectopic complexes differ from each other. Therefore VT is frequently suspected when the QRS complexes do not resemble typical bundle branch block complexes. Because an impulse blocked in the bundle branch spreads through the other bundle branch and the

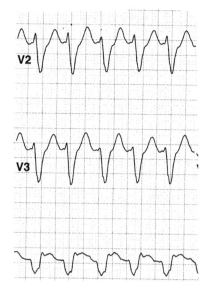

Figure 18–9 Pseudo P waves during ventricular tachycardia (VT) on an ECG of a 69-year-old man with documented VT. Negative deflections after the QRS complex in lead II (at the bottom) resemble retrograde P waves, but they are synchronous with the terminal portion of the QRS complex in other leads.

Purkinje fibers, the onset of the QRS deflection is inscribed relatively rapidly (Figure 18–11). In contrast, the QRS onset of an ectopic ventricular complex is slower. Therefore differences in the speed of inscription of the initial QRS deflection are helpful for the differential diagnosis of the two types of wide QRS tachycardia (Figure 18–12).

Diagnostic mistakes can be made because there may be slow onset of the QRS complex during supraventricular tachycardia with aberration during preexcitation, after MI, during treatment with sodium channel–blocking drugs, or in the presence of hyperkalemia. Figure 18–13A shows supraventricular tachycardia with slow onset of the QRS complex in a patient with bundle branch block and MI (Figure 18–13B). Conversely, rapid onset of the QRS complex can occur during VT if the latter originates in or near the rapidly conducting fascicles (Figure 18–14) and when the initial QRS force is cancelled by two opposing slow wave fronts. Rapid onset of the QRS complex during VT has been attributed also to the origin of VT in a normal ventricular substrate (see Chapter 17 and Figure 17–20).

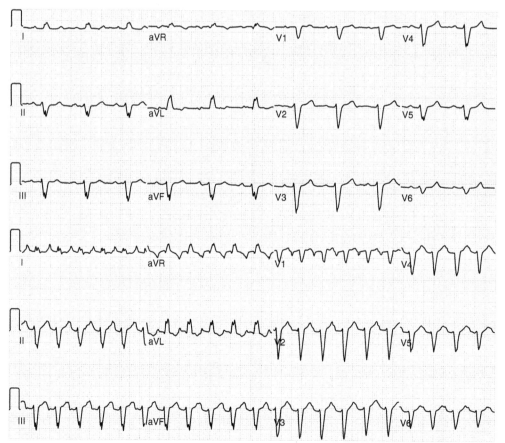

Figure 18–10 ECG of a 69-year-old woman with a concordant pattern of QRS in left bundle branch block (QRS duration 128 ms) during sinus rhythm *(top)* and supravenricular tachycardia *(bottom)* simulating ventricular tachycardia.

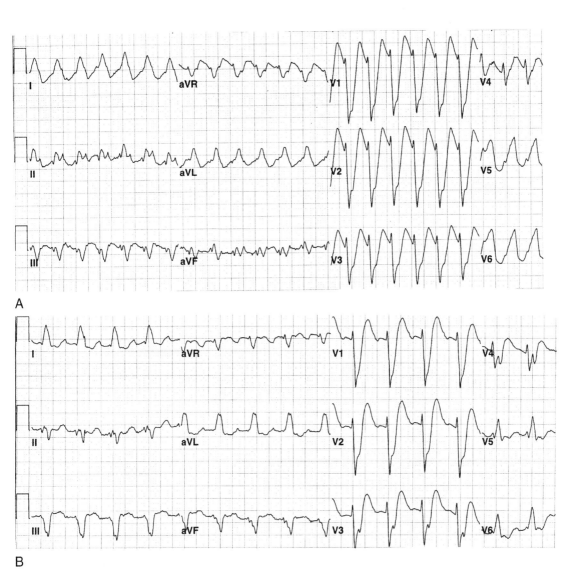

Figure 18–11   **A,** Wide QRS tachycardia (159 beats/min) and a QRS duration of 186 ms in a 65-year-old man with ischemic cardiomyopathy. The rapid onset of the QRS complex suggests that the tachycardia is supraventricular. **B,** ECG recorded during sinus rhythm confirms the diagnosis.

Criteria Based on Correlations with Intracardiac Studies

The mechanism of any wide QRS tachycardia can be established by means of intracardiac recording. In patients with VT, regular activation of the His bundle is either absent or occurs later than during supraventricular tachycardia, and intracardiac ECGs are abnormal in more than 50 percent of the cases[84] (Figure 18–15).

Because most intracardiac studies utilize ECG leads V_1, V_2, and V_6, the proposed criteria for the differential diagnosis between supraventricular tachycardia with aberration and VT refer to the QRS morphology in these three leads. Based on the polarity of the main QRS deflection

in lead V_1, wide QRS tachycardias have been divided into RBBB-like and LBBB-like morphologies. Based on intracardiac recordings, Wellens[85] established the following diagnostic criteria for VT with RBBB-like QRS morphology: (1) in lead V_1 are monophasic R or biphasic qR, QR, RS; (2) in lead V_6 are rS, QS, qR.

For VT with LBBB-like morphology Kindwall et al.[86] established the following diagnostic criteria: (1) R wave in lead V_1 or V_2 >30 ms; (2) any Q wave in V_6; (3) a duration of ≥60 ms from the onset of QRS to the nadir of the S wave in V_1 or V_2; and (4) notching of the downstroke of the S wave in V_1 or V_2. Common to all these criteria for VT is the slow onset of the QRS complex or an abnormal Q wave.

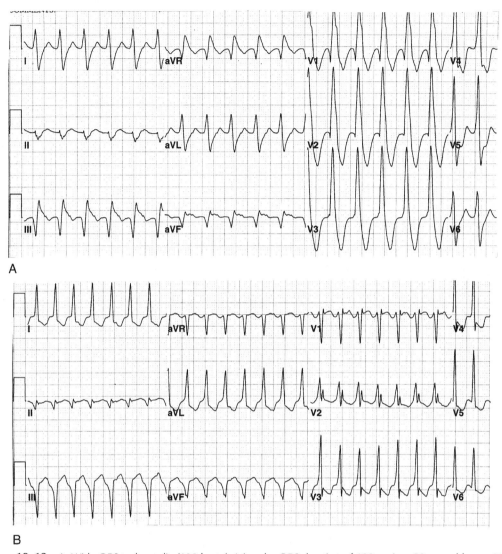

Figure 18–12   **A,** Wide QRS tachycardia (138 beats/min) and a QRS duration of 190 ms in a 58-year-old man. He had ischemic cardiomyopathy, status post coronary artery bypass graft operation, and multiple episodes of inducible nonsustained ventricular tachycardia (VT), but no inducible sustained VT. Onset of QRS is slow. **B,** ECG of the same patient recorded 2 days earlier shows supraventricular tachycardia of uncertain mechanism at a rate of 178 beats/min, QRS duration of 120 ms, and left bundle branch block. Onset of QRS is rapid. During sinus rhythm (not shown) the QRS morphology was the same as during supraventricular tachycardia.

Brugada et al.[87] combined these two sets of criteria for VT and developed a simplified approach to analysis of wide QRS tachycardia of uncertain mechanism, shown in Figure 18–16. It can be seen that VT can be diagnosed if there are no rS complexes in any precordial lead (negative concordance), if the interval from R to S exceeds 100 ms, in the presence of AV dissociation, and if the morphologic criteria for VT proposed by Wellens[85] are present in lead V_1, V_2, or V_6. When these four features were absent, supraventricular tachycardia with aberration can be diagnosed by exclusion.

In a sample of 554 wide QRS tachycardias, the four-step approach to the differential diagnosis shown in Figure 18–16 yielded a sensitivity of 98.7 percent and a specificity of 96.5 percent. In the presence of RBBB-like QRS morphology in lead V_1, qR or the RS complex had a specificity of 98 percent and a sensitivity of 30 percent for VT, and a triphasic QRS complex had a specificity of 91 percent and a sensitivity of 82 percent for supraventricular tachycardia with aberration. In lead V_6, R/S >1 had a specificity of 94 percent and a sensitivity of 41 percent for VT; QS had a specificity of 100 percent and a sensitivity of

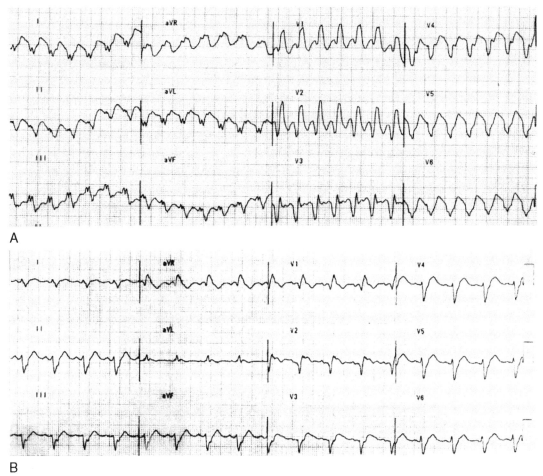

Figure 18–13   **A,** Supraventricular wide QRS tachycardia simulating ventricular tachycardia because of the slow onset of QRS. **B,** ECG of the same patient during sinus rhythm shows nearly the same pattern (minor differences can be attributed to different rate-dependent aberration and perhaps different lead placement) as during tachycardia (i.e., right bundle branch block with anterior myocardial infarction). The latter accounts for the slow onset of the QRS complex.

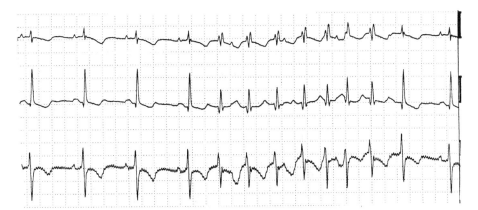

Figure 18–14   Three simultaneous ECG leads during ambulatory monitoring show a seven-beat run of ventricular tachycardia (VT) with a QRS complex of 0.11 second. Note the atrioventricular dissociation and fusion (sixth complex of VT).

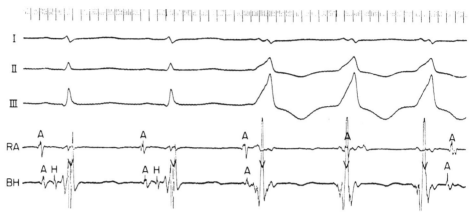

Figure 18–15   His bundle recording from a patient with ventricular tachycardia (VT). Simultaneous leads I, II, and III and bipolar electrograms from the high right atrium (RA) and bundle of His (BH) area are shown. In the two sinus beats (first and second complexes), His bundle potential (H) is present between the atrial (A) and ventricular (V) potentials. With the development of VT, the bundle of His deflection is no longer seen before the ventricular deflection. (Courtesy of Dr. Winston Gaum, Cincinnati, OH.)

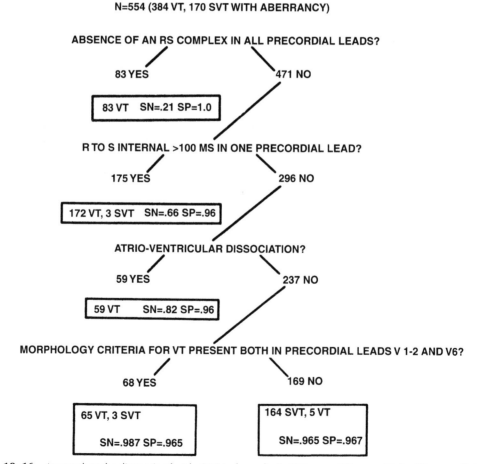

Figure 18–16   Approach to the diagnosis of wide QRS tachycardia in 554 cases. SN = sensitivity; SP = specificity; VT = ventricular tachycardia. (From Brugada P, Brugada J, Mont L, et al: A new approach to the differential diagnosis of a regular tachycardia with a wide QRS complex. Circulation 83:1649, 1991.)

29 percent for VT; and the triphasic QRS complex had a specificity of 64 percent and a sensitivity of 95 percent for supraventricular tachycardia with aberration. In the presence of LBBB-like QRS morphology, the specificity of the criteria proposed by Kindwell et al.[86] for VT was 89 percent and the sensitivity was 100 percent.

Brugada et al.[87] failed to classify correctly only 11 of 554 wide QRS tachycardia. This is remarkably high diagnostic accuracy that may be peculiar to the sample of patients referred for diagnostic studies to the clinical electrophysiology laboratory.

The rate of tachycardia is of no help in the differential diagnosis except for unusually rapid rates of certain supraventricular tachyarrhythmias (e.g., atrial flutter and atrial fibrillation) conducted through an accessory pathway. The QRS duration tends to be wider during VT than during supraventricular tachycardia with aberration. Akthar et al.[88] found that the QRS duration during VT averaged 169 ± 29 ms, 138 ± 14 ms during supraventricular tachycardia with aberration, and 156 ± 24 ms during antidromic conduction through an accessory pathway. The QRS was ≤140 ms in nearly all cases of RBBB aberration and <160 ms in all cases of LBBB aberration. They also reported that positive concordance (QRS upright in all precordial leads) and right superior axis in the frontal plane from -90 to $+180$ degrees had a specificity of 100 percent for VT.

DIFFERENTIAL DIAGNOSIS OF VT VERSUS PREEXCITED TACHYCARDIA

Stierer et al.[89] analyzed the morphologic differences between VT and supraventricular tachycardia with anterograde conduction over an accessory pathway (preexcited tachycardia) with a QRS complex >0.12 second in 149 consecutive VTs and 149 consecutive preexcited regular tachycardia. They found that the following characteristics were specific for VT but were absent with preexcited tachycardia: (1) predominantly negative QRS complexes in leads V_4–V_6; (2) presence of a QR complex in one or more leads V_2–V_6; and (3) more QRS complexes than P waves (when AV dissociation was present during VT). The sensitivity and specificity of these three markers of VT were 75 percent and 100 percent, respectively.

REFERENCES

1. Dessertenne F: La tachycardie ventriculaire a deux foyers opposes variable. Arch Mal Coeur 59:263, 1966.
2. Coumel P, Leclerq JF, Lucet V: Possible mechanisms of the arrhythmias in the long QT syndrome. Eur Heart J 6:115, 1985.
3. Nguyen PT, Scheinman MM, Seger J: Polymorphous ventricular tachycardia: clinical characterization, therapy and QT interval. Circulation 74:340, 1986.
4. Sclarovsky S, Strasberg B, Lewin RF, et al: Polymorphous ventricular tachycardia: clinical features and treatment. Am J Cardiol 44:339, 1979.
5. Kukla P, Slowiak-Lewinska T, Szczuka K, et al: Fast and slow torsade de pointes—electrocardiographic characteristics. Kardiol Pol 60:342, 2004.
6. Kay GN, Plumb VJ, Arciniegas JG, et al: Torsades de pointes: the long–short initiating sequence and other clinical features: observations in 32 patients. J Am Coll Cardiol 2:806, 1983.
7. Gomes JA, Alexopoulos D, Winters SL, et al: The role of silent ischemia, the arrhythmic substrate and the short–long sequence in the genesis of sudden cardiac death. J Am Coll Cardiol 14:1618, 1989.
8. Motte G, Coumel P, Abitbol G, et al: Le syndrome de QT long et syncopes par "torsades de pointes." Arch Mal Coeur 63:831, 1970.
9. Steinbrecher UP, Fitchett DH: Torsade de pointes: a cause of syncope with atrioventricular block. Arch Intern Med 140:1223, 1980.
10. Fontaine G, Frank R, Lascault G, et al: Torsades de pointes initiated by slow ventricular stimulation. Arch Mal Coeur 76:918, 1983.
11. Surawicz B, Knoebel SK: Long QT: good, bad and indifferent. J Am Coll Cardiol 4:398, 1984.
12. Chou TC, Wenzke F: The importance of R on T phenomenon. Am Heart J 96:191, 1978.
13. Surawicz B: R on T phenomenon: dangerous and harmless. J Appl Cardiol 1:39, 1986.
14. Ludomirsky A, Klein HO, Sarelli P, et al: Q-T prolongation and polymorphous ("torsades de pointes") ventricular arrhythmias associated with organophosphorus insecticide poisoning. Am J Cardiol 49:1654, 1982.
15. Di Pasquale G, Pinelli G, Andreoli A, et al: Torsade de pointes and ventricular flutter-fibrillation following spontaneous cerebral subarachnoid hemorrhage. Int J Cardiol 18:163, 1988.
16. Grossman MA: Cardiac arrhythmias in acute central nervous system disease. Successful management with stellate ganglion block. Arch Intern Med 136:203, 1976.
17. Vourc'h G, Tannieres ML: Cardiac arrhythmia induced by pneumoencephalography. Br J Anesth 50:833, 1978.
18. Keren A, Tzivoni D, Gavish D, et al: Etiology, warning signs and therapy of torsades de pointes: a study of 10 patients. Circulation 64:1167, 1981.
19. Koster RW, Wellens HJ: Quinidine-induced ventricular flutter and fibrillation without digitalis therapy. Am J Cardiol 38:519, 1976.
20. Selzer A, Wray HW: Quinidine syncope: paroxysmal ventricular fibrillation occurring during treatment of chronic atrial arrhythmias. Circulation 30:17, 1964.
21. Roden DM, Woosley RL, Primm RK: Incidence and clinical features of the quinidine-associated long QT syndrome: implications for patient care. Am Heart J 11:1088, 1986.
22. Bauman JL, Bauernfeind RA, Hoff JV, et al: Torsade de pointes due to quinidine: observations in 31 patients. Am Heart J 107:425, 1984.

23. Strasberg B, Sclarovsky S, Erdberg A, et al: Procaina-mide-induced polymorphous ventricular tachycardia. Am J Cardiol 47:1309, 1981.
24. Smith WM, Gallagher JJ: "Les torsades de pointes": an unusual ventricular arrhythmia. Ann Intern Med 93:578, 1980.
25. Nicholson WJ, Martin CE, Gracey JG, et al: Disopyramide-induced ventricular fibrillation. Am J Cardiol 43:1053, 1979.
26. Scagliotti D, Strasberg B, Hai HA, et al: Aprindine-induced polymorphous ventricular tachycardia. Am J Cardiol 49:1297, 1982.
27. Kaul U, Mohan JC, Narula J, et al: Ajmaline-induced torsade de pointes. Cardiology 72:140, 1985.
28. Kuck KH, Kunze RP, Roewer N, et al: Sotalol-induced torsade de pointes. Am Heart J 107:179, 1984.
29. Stratmann HG, Kennedy HL: Torsades de pointes associated with drugs and toxins: recognition and management. Am Heart J 113:1470, 1987.
30. Westveer DC, Gadowski GA, Gordon S, et al: Amioadorone-induced ventricular tachycardia. Ann Intern Med 97:561, 1982.
31. Gowda RM, Khan IA, Punikollu G, et al: Female preponderance in ibutilide-induced torsade de pointes. Int J Cardiol 95:219, 2004.
31a. Pratt CM, Al-Khalidi HR, Brum JM, et al: Cumulative experience of azimilide-associated torsades de pointes ventricular tachycardia in the 19 clinical studies comprising the azimilide database. J Am Coll Cardiol 48:471, 2006.
32. Brown MA, Smith WM, Lubbe WF, et al: Amioadorone-induced torsades de pointes. Eur Heart J 7:234, 1986.
33. Moro C, Romero J, Corres Peiretti MA: Amioadorone and hypokalemia: a dangerous combination. Int J Cardiol 13:365, 1986.
34. Manouvrier J, Sagot M, Caron C, et al: Nine cases of torsade de pointes with bepridil administration. Am Heart J 111:1005, 1986.
35. Abinader AG, Shahar J: Possible female preponderance in prenylamine-induced "torsade de pointes" tachycardia. Cardiology 70:37, 1983.
36. Fredlund BO, Olsson SB: Long QT interval and ventricular tachycardia of "torsade de pointe" type in hypothyroidism. Acta Med Scand 213:231, 1983.
37. Pechter RA, Osborn LA: Polymorphic ventricular tachycardia secondary to hypothyroidism. Am J Cardiol 57:882, 1986.
38. Isner JM, Sours HE, Paris AL, et al: Sudden, unexpected death in avid dieters using the liquid-protein-modified-fast diet: observations in 17 patients and the role of the prolonged QT interval. Circulation 60:1401, 1979.
39. Singh BN, Gaarder TD, Kanegae T, et al: Liquid protein diets and torsade de pointes. JAMA 240:115, 1978.
40. Surawicz B, Waller BF: The enigma of sudden cardiac death related to dieting. Can J Cardiol 11:228, 1995.
41. Ruder MA, Flaker GC, Alpert MA, et al: Hypokalemia as a cause of cardiac arrest: results of electrophysiological testing and long-term follow-up. Am Heart J 110:490, 1985.
42. Curry P, Stubbs W, Fitchett D, et al: Ventricular arrhythmias and hypokalemia. Lancet 2:231, 1976.
43. Khan MM, Logan KR, McComb JM, et al: Management of recurrent ventricular tachyarrhythmia associated with QT prolongation. Am J Cardiol 47:1301, 1981.
44. Pratt CM, Hertz RP, Ellis BE, et al: Risk of developing life-threatening ventricular arrhythmia with terfenadine in comparison with over-the-counter antihistamines, ibuprofen, and clemastine. Am J Cardiol 73:346, 1994.

45. Monahan BP, Ferguson CL, Killeavy ES, et al: Torsades de pointes occurring in association with terfenadine use. JAMA 264:2788, 1990.
46. Honig PK, Wortham DC, Zamani K, et al: Terfenadine-ketoconazole interaction: pharmacokinetic and electrocardiographic consequences. JAMA 269:1513, 1993.
47. Giles TD, Modlin RK: Death associated with ventricular arrhythmia and thioridazine hydrochloride. JAMA 205:98, 1968.
48. Sartori M, Pratt CM, Young JB: Torsade de pointes: malignant cardiac arrhythmia induced by amantidine poisoning. Am J Med 77:388, 1984.
49. Dany PF, Liozon F, Goudoud K, et al: Torsades de pointes et arrhythmies ventriculaires graves par administration parenterale de vincamine. Arch Mal Coeur 73:298, 1980.
50. Aldariz AE, Romero H, Baroni M, et al: QT prolongation and torsade de pointes ventricular tachycardia produced by ketanserin. PACE 9:836, 1986.
51. Simons FE, Kesselman MS, Giddins NG, et al: Astemizole-induced torsade de pointes. Lancet 2:624, 1988.
52. Bibler MR, Chou TC, Toltzis RJ, et al: Recurrent ventricular tachycardia due to pentamidine-induced cardiotoxicity. Chest 94:1303, 1988.
53. Lopez JA, Harold JG, Rosenthal MC, et al: QT prolongation and torsades de pointes after administration of trimathoprim-sulfamethoxazole. Am J Cardiol 59:375, 1987.
54. Mauro VF, Bingle JF, Ginn SM, et al: Torsade de pointes in a patient receiving intravenous vasopressin. Crit Care Med 16:200, 1988.
55. Bryer-Ash M, Zehender J, Angelchik P, et al: Torsades de pointes precipitated by a Chinese herbal remedy. Am J Cardiol 60:1185, 1987.
56. Doroghazi RM, Childers R: Time-related changes in the QT interval in acute myocardial infarction. Am J Cardiol 41:684, 1978.
57. Grenadier E, Alpan G, Maor N, et al: Polymorphous ventricular tachycardia in acute myocardial infarction. Am J Cardiol 53:1280, 1984.
58. Horowitz LN, Greenspan AM, Spielman SR, et al: Torsades de pointes: electrophysiologic studies in patients without transient pharmacologic or metabolic abnormalities. Circulation 63:1120, 1981.
59. Chiche P, Haiat R, Steff P: Angina pectoris with syncope due to paroxysmal atrioventricular block: role of ischaemia; report of two cases. Br Heart J 36:577, 1974.
60. Slama R, Motte G, Coumel PH, et al: Le syndrome "alongement de QT et syncopes par torsades de pointes." Laval Med 42:353, 1971.
61. Krikler DM, Curry PVJ: Torsades de pointes: an atypical ventricular tachycardia. Br Heart J 38:117, 1976.
62. Wolf GL, Hirschfeld JW: Changes in QTc interval induced with Renografin-76 and Hypaque-76 during coronary arteriography. J Am Coll Cardiol 1:1489, 1983.
63. Shimizu K, Miura Y, Meguro Y, et al: QT prolongation with torsade de pointes in pheochromocytoma. Am Heart J 124:235, 1992.
64. Salle P, Ray JL, Bernasconi P, et al: Torsade de pointes: a propos of 60 cases. Ann Cardiol Angeiol (Paris) 34:381, 1985.
65. Surawicz B: Electrophysiologic substrate of torsade de pointes: dispersion of repolarization or early afterdepolarization? J Am Coll Cardiol 14:172, 1989.
66. Leenhardt A, Glaser E, Burguera M, et al: Short-coupled variant of torsade de pointes: a new electrocardiographic entity in the spectrum of idiopathic ventricular tachyarrhythmias. Circulation 89:206, 1994.

66a. Nash MP, Mourad A, Clayton RH, et al: Evidence for multiple mechanisms in human ventricular fibrillation. Circulation 114:536, 2006.

67. Bardy GH, Olson WH: Clinical characteristics of spontaneous onset of sustained ventricular tachycardia and ventricular fibrillation in survivors of cardiac arrest. *In:* Zipes DP, Jalife J (eds): Cardiac Electrophysiology from Cell to Bedside. Philadelphia, Saunders, 1990.

68. Campbell RW, Murray A, Julian DG: Ventricular arrhythmias in first 12 hours of acute myocardial infarction. Br Heart J 46:351, 1981.

69. Adgey AA, Develin JE, Webb SW, et al: Initiation of ventricular fibrillation outside hospital in patients with acute ischemic heart disease. Br Heart J 47:55, 1982.

70. O'Doherty M, Tayler DI, Quinn E, et al: Five hundred patients with myocardial infarction monitored within one hour of symptoms. BMJ 286:1405, 1983.

71. Weaver WD, Cobb LA, Hallstrom AP: Ambulatory arrhythmias in resuscitated victims of cardiac arrest. Circulation 66:212, 1982.

72. Lie KI, Liem KL, Schuilenburg RM, et al: Early identification of patients developing late in-hospital ventricular fibrillation after discharge from the coronary care unit. Am J Cardiol 41:674, 1978.

72a. Dekker LRC, Bezzina CR, Henriques JPS, et al: Familial sudden death is an important risk factor for primary ventricular fibrillation. A case-control study in acute myocardial infarction patients. Circulation 114:1140, 2006.

73. Lemery R, Brugada P, Della Bella P, et al: Ventricular fibrillation in six adults without overt heart disease. J Am Coll Cardiol 13:911, 1989.

74. Surawicz B: Ventricular fibrillation. Am J Cardiol 28:268, 1971.

75. Surawicz B: Ventricular fibrillation. II. Progress report since 1971. Clin Prog Pacing Electrophysiol 2:395, 1984.

76. Surawicz B: Electrophysiologic Basis of ECG and Cardiac Arrhythmias. Baltimore, Williams & Wilkins, 1995, pp 353–377.

77. Maron BJ, Poliac LC, Link MS, et al: Blunt impact to the chest leading to sudden death from cardiac arrest during sports activities. N Engl J Med 333:337, 1995.

78. Link MS, Maron BJ, Estes M III: Ventricular fibrillation secondary to nonpenetrating chest wall impact (commotion cordis). *In:* Kohl P, Sachs F, Franz MR (eds): Cardiac Mechano-Electric Feedback and Arrhythmias. Philadelphia, Saunders, 2005, pp 137–144.

79. Di Marco JP, Sellers TD, Bellardinelli L: Paroxysmal supraventricular tachycardia with Wenckebach block: Evidence for reentry within the upper portion of the atrioventricular node. J Am Coll Cardiol 3:1551, 1984.

80. Bauernfeind RA, Wu D, Denes P, et al: Retrograde block during dual pathway atrioventricular nodal reentrant paroxysmal tachycardia. Am J Cardiol 42:499, 1978.

81. Massumi RA, Hilliard G, De Maria A, et al: Paradoxic phenomenon of premature beats with narrow QRS in the presence of bundle-branch block. Circulation 42:543, 1973.

82. Kistin AD: Problems in the differentiation of ventricular arrhythmia from supraventricular arrhythmia with abnormal QRS. Prog Cardiovasc Dis 9:1, 1966.

83. Waxman MB, Wald RW: Termination of ventricular tachycardia by an increase in cardiac vagal drive. Circulation 56:385, 1977.

84. Cassidy DM, Vassallo JA, Miller JM, et al: Endocardial catheter mapping in patients with sinus rhythm: relationship to underlying heart disease and ventricular arrhythmia. Circulation 73:645, 1986.

85. Wellens HJ, Bar FW, Lie KI: The value of the electrocardiogram in the differential diagnosis of a tachycardia with a widened QRS complex. Am J Med 64:27, 1978.

86. Kindwall KE, Brown J, Josephson ME: Electrocardiographic criteria for ventricular tachycardia in wide complex left bundle branch block morphology tachycardia. Am J Cardiol 61:1279, 1988.

87. Brugada P, Brugada J, Mont L, et al: A new approach to the differential diagnosis of a regular tachycardia with a wide QRS complex. Circulation 83:1649, 1991.

88. Akhtar M, Shenasa M, Jazayeri M, et al: Wide QRS complex tachycardia. Ann Intern Med 109:905, 1988.

89. Stierer G, Gursoy S, Frey B, et al: The differential diagnosis on the electrocardiogram between ventricular tachycardia and preexcited tachycardia. Clin Cardiol 17:306, 1994.

19 Atrioventricular Block; Concealed Conduction; Gap Phenomenon

Atrioventricular Block	AV Block with Preserved Retrograde
AV Conduction Defect with Normal	VA Conduction
PR Interval	Multilevel AV Block
First-Degree AV Block	Clinical Correlation of AV Block
Second-Degree AV Block	Vagal Stimulation and Drugs
2:1 AV Block	
High-Grade or Advanced AV Block	**Concealed Conduction**
Differential Diagnosis of Second-Degree	Concealed Conduction in the AV Junction
AV Block	Concealed Conduction in the Bundle
Complete (Third-Degree) AV Block	Branch System
Postextrasystolic Depression of AV	Concealed Conduction of Atrial Impulses
Conduction and Paroxysmal AV Block	into the Bundle Branch during Atrial
Comparison of AV and Ventriculoatrial	Flutter and Atrial Fibrillation
Conduction	
	Gap Phenomenon

Atrioventricular Block

The atrioventricular (AV) conduction defect traditionally is divided into incomplete and complete block. Incomplete AV block includes first-degree, second-degree, and advanced AV block. Complete AV block, also known as third-degree AV block, is often incorrectly called "complete heart block." The block may be located proximal to, in, or distal to the His bundle.[1] When it is proximal to the His bundle, the block may be in the atrium (intraatrial) or AV node (AV nodal). The distal infranodal block includes intrahisian and infrahisian types.[2-4] With intraatrial block there is prolongation of the PA time (normal 25 to 45 ms), which represents the interval between the onset of the P wave in the surface electrocardiogram (ECG) and the deflection A recorded by the intracardiac electrode at the low right atrium (Figure 19–1).

With AV nodal block there is an increase in the AH interval (normal 60 to 140 ms), which is the interval between deflection A from the low right atrium to the onset of the first rapid deflection of the His bundle electrogram (H). With intrahisian block (or block within the His bundle itself), the duration of the His bundle potential, or BH time, exceeds 20 ms (normal

15 to 20 ms). The His bundle potential is "split." With infrahisian block, the conduction defect is at the level of the bundle branches, and there is prolongation of the HV time (normal 35 to 55 ms), which is the interval between the onset of the His bundle potential and the onset of ventricular depolarization recorded on the intracardiac electrogram (V) or any of the surface leads. Although the His bundle recording can offer more accurate assessment of AV conduction than the surface ECG, it is not routinely obtained in clinical practice because it is seldom needed to make a reasonable therapeutic decision.

All degrees of AV block may be intermittent or persistent. The degree of the conduction defect also may vary from time to time. It is not uncommon for a patient to experience a transient episode of complete AV block resulting in syncope in the absence of premonitory first- or second-degree AV block.

AV CONDUCTION DEFECT WITH NORMAL PR INTERVAL

Conduction delay in part of the AV conduction system may not be sufficient to prolong the PR interval above the upper limit of normal, which is 0.20 second in adults. This arbitrary limit has no particular physiologic counterpart,

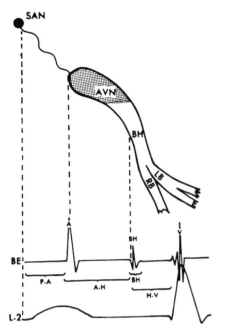

Figure 19–1 Atrioventricular conduction system and the corresponding bipolar intracardiac electrogram (BE) and standard surface ECG (L-2). A = bipolar atrial electrogram; A-H = conduction time through the AVN; AVN = atrioventricular node; BH = bundle of His; H-V = conduction time through the His Purkinje system; RB and LB = right and left bundle branches, respectively; SAN = sinoatrial node; V = bipolar ventricular electrogram recorded from the area of the AV junction. (Adapted from Narula OS, Schlerlag BJ, Samet P, et al: Atrioventricular block: localization and classification by His bundle recordings. Am J Med 50:146, 1971.)

and in some computer programs the upper limit of normal is set at 0.21 second. Often a change in duration of the PR interval, even to a value that is still within normal limits, is more revealing than a stable interval exceeding the normal limit.

A normal PR interval does not rule out disturbed AV conduction. Thus of 96 patients with a normal PR interval and an abnormally wide QRS complex studied by Puech, more than half had a prolonged HV interval (>55 ms).[4] The

HV prolongation was more common in patients with left bundle branch block (LBBB) or right bundle branch block (RBBB) with left fascicular block.[4,5] Bilateral bundle branch block is suspected when HV prolongation is attributed to a conduction delay in the unblocked fascicle.

FIRST-DEGREE AV BLOCK

With first-degree AV block (Figure 19–2) the range of PR prolongation is usually 0.21 to 0.40 second. Occasionally, the interval is as long or longer than 0.60 second. When prolongation is marked, the P wave may be superimposed on the preceding T wave, or it may simulate a U wave. This is more likely to occur at rapid heart rates (Figure 19–3).

The degree of prolongation may change even in the same individual. The interval may shorten when the heart rate increases and lengthen when the vagal tone is increased. Occasionally one observes a phenomenon of two markedly different PR intervals in the same subject, presumably due to conduction through two different AV nodal pathways (i.e., fast and slow) (Figure 19–4; see also Chapter 16).

Fisch et al.[6] reported findings in 21 patients with sinus rhythm and PR intervals consistent with dual AV nodal physiology. Eighteen patients exhibited an abrupt, persistent PR interval change. In two patients the PR interval alternated between the slow and fast pathways, and in one the ECG suggested simultaneous conduction along both pathways in response to a single stimulus. A similar phenomenon is probably responsible for the presence of two RP intervals (Figure 19–5).

In patients with first-degree AV block and a narrow QRS complex, the conduction is most commonly delayed in the AV node with prolongation of the AH time.[7] Less common is prolongation of the PA or BH time, and least common is prolongation of the HV interval.[3] PR prolongation caused by interatrial block is

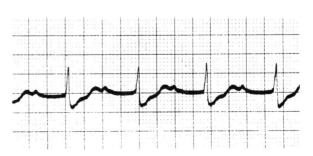

Figure 19–2 First-degree atrioventricular block. PR 0.36

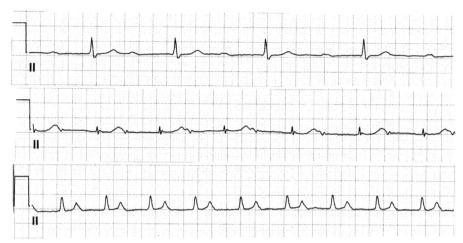

Figure 19–3 Marked PR prolongation at various heart rates. *Top,* PR interval of 580 ms duration in the presence of a heart rate of 45 beats/min. *Middle,* PR interval is about 560 ms. The P wave is partly merged with the T wave in the presence of a heart rate of 65 beats/min. *Bottom,* PR interval is about 480 ms. The P wave is superimposed on the T wave in the presence of a heart rate of 94 beats/min.

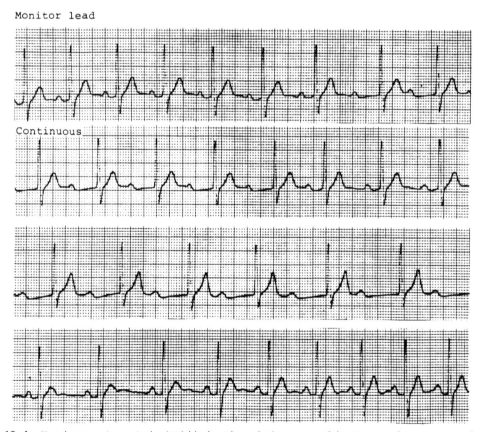

Figure 19–4 First-degree atrioventricular (AV) block with marked variation of the PR interval in an apparently healthy individual, probably caused by dual AV conduction. The PR interval varies from 0.18 to 0.66 second. The shorter PR interval is associated mostly with a more rapid heart rate.

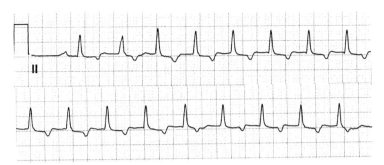

Figure 19–5 Continuous tracing of ECG lead II shows the onset of apparent reciprocating atrioventricular (AV) nodal tachycardia after the sinus complex with a PR interval of 280 ms. After the first two complexes, the RR intervals vary by <40 ms. The first RP interval is 260 ms; the next RP interval is 200 ms; the subsequent 10 RP intervals are 240 to 260 ms, and the 12th and 16th RP interval are 180 and 100 ms, respectively. Variations in the RP interval at a nearly constant ventricular rate may be explained by dual AV nodal pathways.

seen in patients with an endocardial cushion defect.[8]

In patients with first-degree AV block and bundle branch block, the HV interval is often prolonged, particularly in those with LBBB. However, the conduction delay may occur at other sites and at more than one site.

SECOND-DEGREE AV BLOCK

With second-degree AV block, there is intermittent failure of the supraventricular impulse to be conducted to the ventricles. Some of the P waves are not followed by a QRS complex. The conduction ratio (P/QRS ratio) may be set at 2:1, 3:1, 3:2, 4:3, and so forth; or it may vary from time to time in a haphazard fashion. When describing the conduction sequence, it is important to specify whether the ratio refers to conduction or block. For example, if only every third P wave is followed by a QRS complex, there is 3:1 conduction or 3:2 block. Interchangeable use of the terms *conduction* and *block* can create misunderstandings.

There are two types of second-degree AV block: I and II. Type I also is called *Wenckebach phenomenon* or *Mobitz type I* and represents the more common type. Type II is also called *Mobitz type II* and is less common.

Type I Second-Degree AV Block: Wenckebach Phenomenon

ECG Findings

The ECG findings with type I second-degree AV block are as follows:

1. Progressive lengthening of the PR interval until a P wave is blocked.
2. Progressive shortening of the RR interval until a P wave is blocked.
3. RR interval containing the blocked P wave is shorter than the sum of two PP intervals.

In the so-called typical case of type I second-degree AV block, the greatest increment of PR prolongation takes place in the second conducted impulse after the pause (Figure 19–6). In the subsequent impulses the PR interval continues to increase, but the degree of the

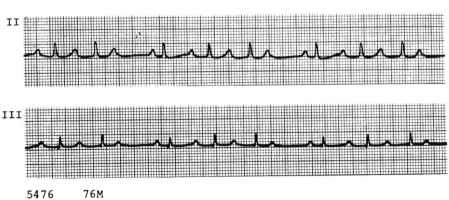

5476   76M

Figure 19–6 Type I second-degree atrioventricular block with typical Wenckebach phenomenon.

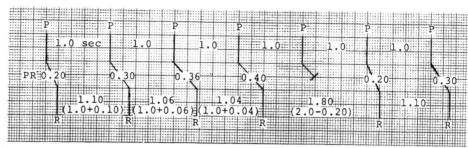

Figure 19–7   Progressive shortening of the RR interval during a typical Wenckebach period. Although there is progressive prolongation of the PR interval, the increment of increase decreases.

increment decreases. Progressive shortening of the RR interval until a blocked P wave occurs is the result of the decrease in the increment of PR prolongation, as shown in Figure 19–7. Assuming the PP interval is 1.0 second, the PR interval increases stepwise from 0.20 to 0.30 to 0.36 to 0.40 second, following which the P wave is blocked. Therefore 5:4 conduction is present. The increments of the PR interval of the conducted beats are 0.10, 0.06, and 0.04 second, respectively. The RR intervals are 1.0±0.10 (1.10), 1.0±0.06 (1.06), and 1.0±0.04 second (1.04), respectively. The same diagram shows that marked shortening of the PR interval after the pause results in an earlier appearance of the QRS complex, which explains why the RR interval that contains the blocked P wave is shorter than the two PP intervals. The sequence between one pause and the next is referred to as a "Wenckebach period."

Because of the periodic pauses, the rhythm has a character of "group beating," a finding that is an important clue to the diagnosis of Wenckebach phenomenon. Paradoxically, the typical Wenckebach phenomenon is not the most common

pattern of type I second-degree AV block, as the exceptions exceed the rule. Prolongation of the PR interval may not be progressive (Figure 19–8). The largest increment of the PR interval is sometimes seen just before block occurs (see Figure 19–8). When the Wenckebach period is long, many successive cycles may not show any measurable change in the PR interval (see Figure 19–8). In most clinical studies the atypical periodicity occurs more frequently than the typical periodicity. This is because under most circumstances the PP intervals are not absolutely regular, the PR/RP relations do not remain constant, and there are changes in autonomic tone, all of which can affect AV nodal conductivity and modify the typical pattern of Wenckebach periodicity.[9]

AV nodal Wenckebach periodicity can be induced in nearly all subjects when atrial refractoriness permits achievement of the critical rate required to elicit this phenomenon. During electrophysiologic studies, the point at which progressive shortening of the coupling of atrial premature stimuli induces Wenckebach period is a useful marker of refractoriness. It has been

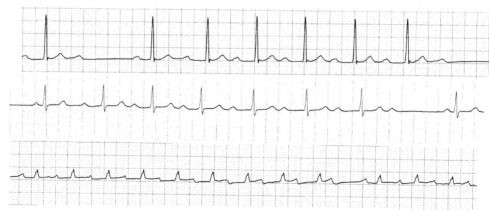

Figure 19–8   Atypical Wenckebach periodicity. *Top,* 7:6 atrioventricular (AV) conduction with lengthening of the RR interval before the block. *Middle,* 8:7 AV conduction with shortening of the first two RR intervals and subsequent lengthening of RR intervals. *Bottom,* 10:9 AV conduction with shortening of the first two RR intervals and subsequent constant RR intervals until the appearance of the block.

shown that the Wenckebach block point remains stable during long-term follow-up in patients with intact AV conduction.[10]

Electrophysiologic Correlation

In patients with type I block and narrow QRS complexes, the block is usually located in the AV node[4,11] and the progressive PR lengthening is associated with progressive prolongation of the AH interval until the P wave is blocked with an absent His bundle potential. Occasionally, the block is in the His bundle, which can be recognized by progressive prolongation of the interval between the split His potentials and absence of the second part of the split His potential after the blocked P wave.

Often intrahisian block can be distinguished from intranodal block on the body surface ECG, because with infrahisian block the AV conduction ratio worsens after atropine administration (which increases the sinus rate) and improves with carotid sinus massage (which decreases the sinus rate), whereas opposite effects are observed if the block is intranodal.[12] When type I second-degree AV block is associated with bundle branch block, the site of the block may be the AV node, the His bundle, or the contralateral bundle branch. In about 75 percent of cases the block is in the AV node; in the other 25 percent it is infranodal.[4,11]

Mechanism of Wenckebach Periodicity

Wenckebach periodicity appears most commonly in slowly conducting tissue when propagation depends on a depressed sodium channel or calcium channel. Of the two structures with predominantly calcium channel–dependent conduction, Wenckebach periodicity is seen much more frequently in the AV node than in the sinus node, perhaps because AV transmission manifests on the surface ECG but sinoatrial conduction does not. Experimental studies suggest that the progressive slowing of conduction in the AV node is related to a progressive, time-dependent decline of excitability.[13,14] Wenckebach periodicity may occur also in any cardiac tissue in which the conduction is

normally fast, such as the ventricular conduction system (see Figure 4–6) or myocardium.

Type II Second-Degree AV Block: Mobitz Type II

ECG Findings

Type II second-degree AV block exhibits the following ECG signs: (1) there are intermittent blocked P waves and (2) during the conducted impulses the PR intervals may be normal or prolonged, but they remain constant. Slight shortening may occur, however, in the first impulse after the blocked cycle as a result of improved conduction following block. In some cases the shorter interval from P to QRS is due to an escape complex.[15] Some investigators require the presence of a constant PR interval in all complexes as a strict diagnostic criterion for Mobitz type II block.[16]

Electrophysiologic Correlation

Most patients with type II second-degree AV block have associated bundle branch block (Figures 19–9 to 19–11). In these patients the block is usually located distal to the His bundle (see Figure 19–11).[17] In about 27 to 35 percent of patients with Mobitz type II block, the lesion is in the His bundle[4,11] and the QRS complex is narrow[11] (Figure 19–12). Rarely, the site is the AV node.[18]

2:1 AV BLOCK

When the AV conduction ratio is 2:1, it is often impossible to determine whether the second-degree AV block is type I or II. A long rhythm strip may help by recording an episode of changing conduction ratio and observing the behavior of the PR interval (Figure 19–13). The wide QRS complex in the conducted impulses favors the diagnosis of type II (see Figure 19–13). When the atrial rate is increased by exercise or atropine, the AV block in type I tends to decrease and that in type II tends to increase.[12,15] In the absence of such additional information, however, it is advisable to be noncommittal as to the type of Mobitz block when dealing with 2:1 AV block.

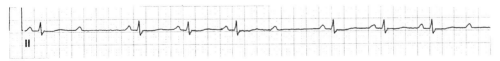

Figure 19–9 Mobitz type II atrioventricular block. ECG strip of lead II from a 78-year-old man with regular sinus rhythm at a rate of 56 beats/min, incomplete right bundle branch block, constant PR interval of 188 ms, and nonconducted P waves.

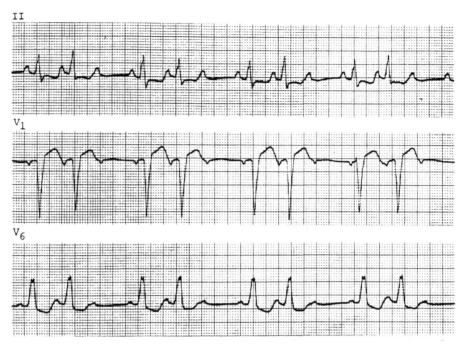

Figure 19–10 Mobitz type II second-degree atrioventricular block. There is 3:2 conduction. The QRS complex has left bundle branch block morphology.

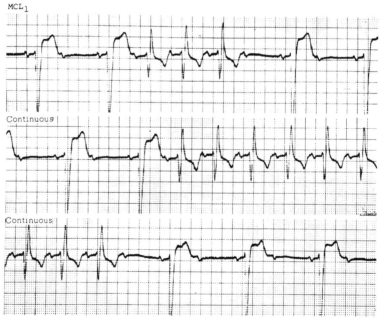

Figure 19–11 Mobitz type II second-degree atrioventricular block resulting from bilateral bundle branch block. The monitor lead shows changing left and right bundle branch block patterns. A His bundle recording demonstrated that the block was distal to the His bundle (not shown).

HIGH-GRADE OR ADVANCED AV BLOCK

When the AV conduction ratio is 3:1 or higher, the rhythm is called *advanced AV block*. In some

cases only occasional ventricular captures are observed, and the dominant rhythm is maintained by a subsidiary pacemaker. Identifying the type of second-degree block in such instances is also difficult. A comparison of the

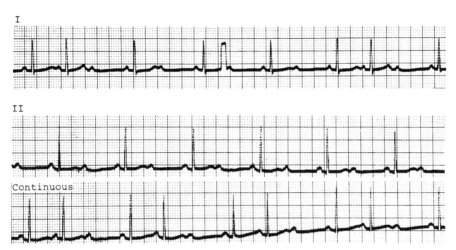

I

II

Continuous

Figure 19–12   Mobitz type II second-degree atrioventricular block with narrow QRS complex. The patient had recurrent episodes of syncope. Because of the narrow QRS complex, the block is probably at the level of the His bundle.

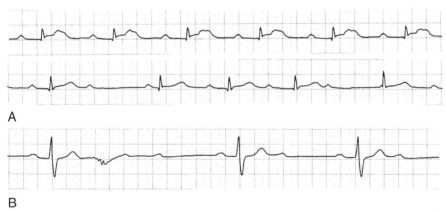

A

B

Figure 19–13   Two examples of 2:1 atrioventricular (AV) block. **A,** ECG lead II of a 59-year-old man with inferior myocardial infarction, 2:1 AV block, and a PR interval of 316 ms. QRS duration is 92 ms, and there is fusion of the P and T waves. *Bottom:* ECG recorded the next day shows Wenckebach periods (Mobitz type I block) with an AV junctional escape complex and blocked P wave. **B,** ECG lead II from a 78-year-old man with predominant 2:1 AV block, PR interval of 256 ms, and left bundle branch block (QRS is 130 ms). The presence of a nonconducted P wave following the premature ventricular complex at the beginning of the strip in conjunction with the constant PR interval confirm that the 2:1 AV block represents a Mobitz type II block.

PR intervals of the occasional captured complexes may provide a clue. If the PR interval varies and its duration is inversely related to the interval between the P wave and its preceding R wave (RP), type I block is likely. A constant PR interval in all captured complexes suggests type II block.[15]

Not infrequently the advanced AV block occurs in patients in whom the PR interval is normal or only slightly prolonged. The failure of AV conduction in such cases is caused by a functional block that is most often localized in the AV node. The block is caused by concealed conduction of the atrial impulses that fail to reach the ventricles but prolong the refractoriness of the

AV node. Figure 19–14 shows three cases of advanced AV block. In the first case the success or failure of conduction depends on the duration of the preceding RP interval (see Figure 19–14). In the second case, high-degree AV block with a normal PR interval in the conducted impulses may be related to repeated concealed conduction associated with sinus tachycardia. In the third case sinus tachycardia is also present, but the AV conduction appears impaired, as the PR interval of the conducted impulse is 600 ms. In this case the appearance of occasional conduction is difficult to explain unless one postulates dissipation of concealment before the conducted impulse.

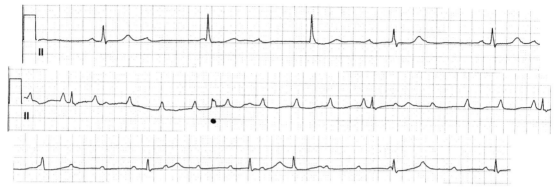

Figure 19–14 Advanced atrioventricular block. *Top,* The first and second RR intervals are escape intervals at a rate of about 1800 ms. The first sinus complex is conducted with a PR interval of 220 ms; the subsequent four P waves at a rate of 60 beats/min are not conducted to the ventricles; the sixth P wave is conducted with a PR interval of 450 ms and is preceded by an RP interval of 960 ms; the seventh P wave is blocked, but the eighth P wave is conducted with a PR interval of 200 ms, being preceded by an RP interval of 1500 ms. The RP intervals preceding nonconducted P waves are shorter (740 and 860 ms) than the RP intervals preceding the conducted P waves. *Middle,* Sinus tachycardia at a rate of 100 beats/min. Three sinus complexes with right bundle branch block pattern appear to be conducted because the PR interval is constant (although coincidence cannot be ruled out). The block is attributed to repeated concealed conduction. The dot marks an artifact. *Bottom,* Sinus rhythm at a rate of about 110 beats/min. The first, second, fourth, and fifth RR intervals are regular escape intervals of about 1660 ms duration. The P wave after the third QRS complex appears to be conducted with a PR interval of 600 ms. It is possible that the conduction took place because of dissipated concealment.

DIFFERENTIAL DIAGNOSIS OF SECOND-DEGREE AV BLOCK

Second-degree AV block may be simulated by blocked premature atrial impulses (see Chapter 14). This occurs especially when the coupling interval of the premature atrial impulse is relatively long. Careful measurement of the PP cycle length and examination of the P wave morphology can clarify the diagnosis. Conversely, ventriculophasic sinus arrhythmias are present with some second-degree AV blocks. The PP intervals that contain the QRS complexes are shorter than those that do not. The blocked P waves may be mistaken for blocked premature atrial complexes.

An AV conduction ratio of 2:1 may simulate sinus bradycardia when the nonconducted P waves fall on the preceding T waves and escape recognition (see Figure 19–13) or are mistaken for U waves. Conversely, the U waves in patients with sinus bradycardia may be mistaken for blocked P waves, causing an erroneous diagnosis of second-degree AV block.

COMPLETE (THIRD-DEGREE) AV BLOCK

With third-degree AV block there is complete failure of the supraventricular impulses to reach the ventricles. The atrial and ventricular activities are independent of each other. The ventricular excitation is initiated by a subsidiary pacemaker distal to the site of the block, which may be in the AV junction, His bundle, or bundle branches. If the block is in the main bundle branches, it is called *bilateral bundle branch block*. If it involves the right bundle branch and two divisions of the left bundle branch, it is called *trifascicular block*.

ECG Findings

In patients with sinus rhythm and complete AV block, the PP and RR intervals are regular, but the P waves bear no constant relation to the QRS complexes (Figure 19–15). The PR interval varies, and the PP intervals may be slightly irregular because of sinus arrhythmia. Ventriculophasic sinus arrhythmias can be demonstrated in about 30 to 40 percent of patients with complete AV block.[19]

In the presence of atrial fibrillation, complete AV block is recognized by the regularity of the ventricular rhythm (see Figures 15–19 and 15–20). The same applies to atrial flutter or ectopic atrial tachycardia, but as an additional requirement the flutter or ectopic P waves should have no demonstrable relation to the QRS complexes (see Figure 15–1).

The morphology of the QRS complexes depends mainly on the location of the block. The escape pacemaker usually originates from a site just distal to the region of the block. If the block is proximal to the bifurcation of the His bundle, the escape pacemaker is likely to be within the AV junction, and the QRS complexes are narrow (Figure 19–16) unless bundle

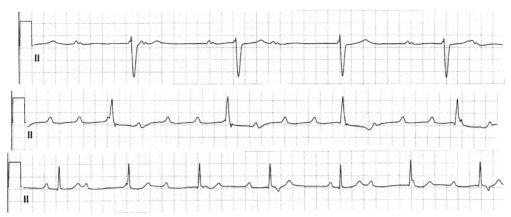

Figure 19–15 Complete atrioventricular (AV) block. ECG strips of lead II. *Top*, Escape rhythm at a rate of 34 beats/min, QRS duration of 156 ms, and a pattern indicating right bundle branch block (RBBB) and left anterior fascicular block. The presumed site of the escape pacemaker is at or near the left posterior fascicle. *Middle*, Escape rhythm at a rate of 30 beats/min, QRS duration of 144 ms, and RBBB pattern. The presumed site of the escape pacemaker is the Purkinje fiber in the left ventricle. *Bottom*, Escape rhythm is at a rate of 50 beats/min, and the QRS duration is 84 ms. The presumed site of the escape pacemaker is the AV junction. Note that retrograde conduction is preserved in the presence of anterograde AV block.

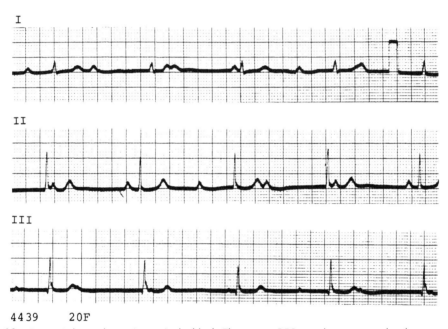

4439   20F

Figure 19–16 Congenital complete atrioventricular block. The narrow QRS complexes suggest that the escape pacemaker is junctional in origin. No other associated congenital defects were found.

branch block coexists. If the block is below the bifurcation of the His bundle, the escape rhythm is of ventricular origin and the QRS complexes are wide (see Figure 19–15). Therefore in the presence of complete AV block, narrow QRS complexes indicate an AV junctional location of the block, but wide QRS complexes may be the result of bilateral bundle branch block, trifascicular block, or AV junctional block with unilateral bundle branch block. This relation

between the duration of the QRS complexes and the location of the block was confirmed by histologic studies of the conduction system in a limited number of patients in whom His bundle records were available.[20]

The ventricular rate associated with complete AV block usually depends on the origin of the escape pacemaker. The rate of AV junctional escape rhythm is usually 40 to 60 beats/min. The rate of the ventricular pacemaker is usually

II

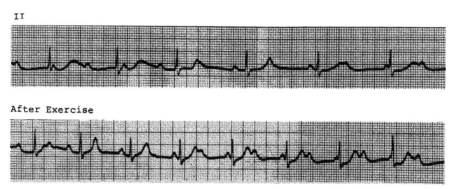

After Exercise

Figure 19–17   Effect of exercise on the ventricular rate in a patient with congenital complete atrioventricular (AV) block. The QRS complexes are narrow, and the ventricular rate increases after exercise. The escape pacemaker probably is located in the proximal part of the AV junction.

30 to 40 beats/min, but it may be as low as 20 beats/min or as high as 50 beats/min. If the pacemaker is high in the AV junction, the ventricular rate may be increased by exercise or vagolytic agents[21] (Figure 19–17). An escape rhythm from the ventricle or low AV junction is generally not affected by such maneuvers.

Electrophysiologic Correlation

His bundle recordings indicate that the site of block in patients with complete AV block may be proximal to, within, or distal to the His bundle. With chronic, acquired, complete AV block the site of the block is distal to the His bundle in about 50 to 60 percent of cases, and the QRS complexes are wide.[1,4] When the block is proximal to or within the His bundle, the QRS complexes are more often narrow than wide. In the presence of acute AV block resulting from inferior myocardial infarction (MI), infections, or drugs, the block is usually proximal to the His bundle. A complete AV block associated with acute anterior MI is usually distal to the His bundle.

POSTEXTRASYSTOLIC DEPRESSION OF AV CONDUCTION AND PAROXYSMAL AV BLOCK

The postextrasystolic AV block associated with delayed escape intervention is usually of short duration.[22] In some cases, however, the absence of AV conduction persists for several seconds and leads to syncope. Two examples of such a block, also known as *paroxysmal AV block*, are shown in Figure 19–18. The mechanism is unclear, but concealed discharge of escape pacemakers may be suspected. Study of Brignole et al.,[23] which utilized the implantable event recorders, showed that in patients with bundle branch block, syncope, and a negative

conventional workup, including electrophysiological study, the syncope was often caused by a paroxysmal AV block. In only a minority of their cases, however, was the block preceded by a premature complex.

COMPARISON OF AV AND VENTRICULOATRIAL CONDUCTION

Akhtar et al.[24] compared the facility to conduct impulses in the anterograde and retrograde directions in 50 patients using incremental atrial and ventricular pacing and the extrastimulation technique. Ventriculoatrial (VA) conduction was absent in 11 patients. In an additional 25 patients, AV conduction was "better" than VA conduction because the onset of Wenckebach periodicity in the AV node occurred at a faster pacing rate. In 8 patients the VA and AV conductions were equal, and in 6 the onset of Wenckebach periodicity occurred at a faster rate during VA conduction. The authors concluded that in most patients anterograde conduction is better than retrograde conduction. The region of maximum refractoriness (i.e., atrium, AV node, His-Purkinje systems, ventricular myocardium) varied among patients and was usually not the same during anterograde as during retrograde conduction in the same patient. Figure 19–20 shows an example of AV conduction that is considerably longer than VA conduction.

AV BLOCK WITH PRESERVED RETROGRADE VA CONDUCTION

AV block with preserved VA conduction is not rare (see Figure 19–15). The first comprehensive review of this phenomenon, by Winternitz and Langendorf,[25] appeared in 1944. The pathologic lesions in the autopsied cases were near the bifurcation of the His bundle.

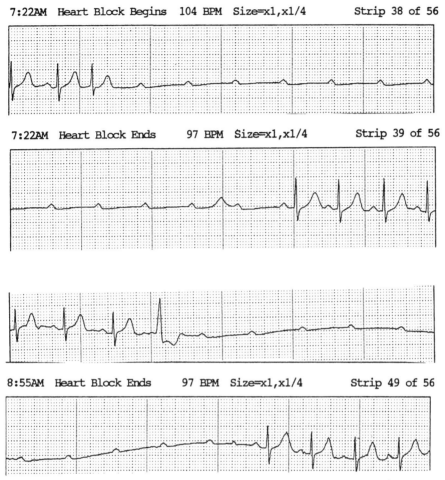

Figure 19-18 ECG strips recorded during ambulatory monitoring show prolonged depression of atrioventricular conduction after an atrial premature complex (*top*) and after a ventricular premature complex (*bottom*).

MULTILEVEL AV BLOCK

The presence of AV block at two levels can be detected by the occurrence of Wenckebach periods at alternate complexes. Alternating Wenckebach periodicity has been demonstrated both below and above the His bundle.[26,27] Most episodes are attributed to multilevel block.[28] The phenomenon is not uncommon, particularly during atrial flutter.

Kosowsky et al.[29] classified ECGs of patients with multilevel AV block into two groups based on the nature of the conduction defect at their uppermost level of block. Of their 36 patients, 24 had an integral conduction response (2:1 in all cases) at the uppermost level of the block and Wenckebach periods at the lower level of the block; 12 patients had a nonintegral conduction ratio (e.g., 5:4, 4:3) at the upper level with either integral or nonintegral block at the lower level. Complex patterns of conduction can be produced by pacing in patients with bilevel block.[30]

CLINICAL CORRELATION OF AV BLOCK

Normal Subjects

A PR interval longer than 0.2 second occasionally is seen in apparently healthy individuals. It was found in 0.52 percent of 67,375 asymptomatic male pilots examined by Johnson and associates.[31] The PR interval ranged from 0.21 to 0.39 second but rarely exceeded 0.28 second. The incidence of first-degree AV block in normal subjects is higher when a 24-hour ambulatory ECG is obtained,[32,33] which in some instances reflects the presence of dual AV nodal conduction. Second-degree AV block with Wenckebach phenomenon also may be seen in young individuals mostly during sleep,[32,33] and it has been reported on routine ECGs of trained athletes.[34] None of 16 subjects with prolonged PR intervals among 1000 healthy young aviators had clinical evidence of heart disease during 10 years of follow-up.[35]

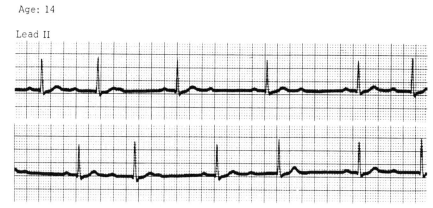

Figure 19–19   Type I second-degree atrioventricular block due to digitalis intoxication.

Mymin et al.[36] examined the long-term prognosis of first-degree AV block in a 30-year longitudinal study of 3983 healthy men. First-degree AV block was present in 52 patients on entry into the study, and in 124 the PR interval became prolonged during follow-up. Two thirds had a PR interval of 0.22 to 0.23 second. The study showed that first-degree AV block with moderate PR prolongation was a benign finding. Mortality was not increased, and the AV block progressed to higher grades in only two cases.[36]

VAGAL STIMULATION AND DRUGS

Transient AV block may be produced by vagal stimulation, such as carotid sinus massage, Valsalva maneuver, or hiccups.[37] It may be the mechanism responsible for syncope in patients with hypersensitive carotid sinus reflex.[38]

Digitalis (due to its vagal action) (see Figure 19–19), β-adrenergic blocking drugs, verapamil, and diltiazem can produce varying degrees of AV block, particularly when used in combination or in subjects with a diseased conduction system. Other offending drugs include class IA and IC sodium channel blockers and amiodarone.

Coronary Artery Disease

AV block in patients with coronary artery disease may be acute or chronic, transient or permanent. With acute MI, varying degrees of AV conduction defect occur in about 16 to 21 percent of patients: first-degree AV block in 8 to 13 percent, second-degree block in 3.5 to 10.0 percent, and complete AV block in 2.5 to 8.0 percent.[39,40] The MILIS Study Group[41] found complete AV block in 38 of 698 patients during acute MI.[32,33] The occurrence was more frequent among patients with preceding major abnormalities of AV or intraventricular conduction. Another study suggested that the incidence of complete AV block during acute MI has declined since the advent of thrombolytic therapy.[42]

The ECG manifestations are closely related to the location of the infarct. AV block is more common in patients with inferior MI (Figure 19–21) caused by occlusion of the right coronary artery proximal to the takeoff of the

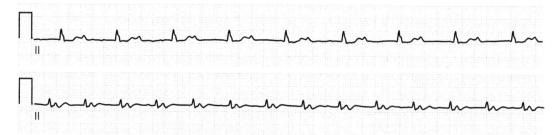

Figure 19–20   Strips of selected ECG leads of a 80-year-old man made on 2 consecutive days. ECG is normal except for rhythm and conduction disturbances. *Top,* Sinus rhythm with PR interval of 540 ms at a heart rate of 65 beats/min. *Bottom,* Probably an atrioventricular junctional rhythm at a rate of 101 beats/min with negative (retrograde) P waves within the T wave.

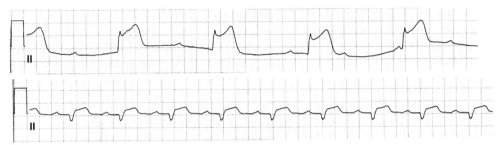

Figure 19–21   Strips of ECG lead II of a 64-year-old man. *Top,* Complete atrioventricular (AV) block with an AV junctional escape rhythm at a rate of 38 beats/min. *Bottom,* At 26 hours later there is a sinus rhythm with 1:1 AV conduction and a PR interval of 260 ms.

artery supplying the AV node (see Chapter 8). The block is proximal to the His bundle.[4] If the block is high grade or complete, the escape rhythm is usually junctional in origin. First-degree or type I second-degree AV block often precedes the complete AV block. As a rule, the AV block is transient, and normal conduction resumes within less than 1 week after the acute episode.[40,43] Structural damage of the AV node is usually absent.[44,45]

Some degree of AV block may be seen in up to 21 percent of patients with acute anterior MI[46] (Figure 19–22). The reported incidence of second- and third-degree AV block is 5 and 7 percent, respectively.[40,43]

The block is the result of extensive damage to the interventricular septum, caused usually by occlusion of the left anterior descending coronary artery proximal to the takeoff of the septal perforators. RBBB alone, RBBB with left anterior or left posterior fascicular block, or LBBB alone often precedes the development of bilateral or trifascicular AV block.[45,46] The PR interval is usually normal or minimally prolonged before the sudden onset of second- or third-degree AV block. Although the initial episode of the AV block is mostly transient, there is a relatively high incidence of recurrence of the high-degree AV block after the acute event.[47] In the Danish TRACE study, the presence of a complete AV block was associated with a fourfold increase in mortality (i.e., to 60% in patients with anterior MI and from 10% to 25% of patients with inferior MI).[48]

In the past, infarction and ischemia of the septum caused by coronary artery disease were thought to be the most important causes of chronic complete AV block, but more recent pathologic studies have shown that this is not the case (Table 19–1).[49] Only 15 of 100 chronic complete AV blocks examined by Davies were caused by coronary artery disease.[49]

Degenerative Diseases of the Conducting System

Table 19–1 shows that among the 100 autopsied cases of chronic complete AV block examined by

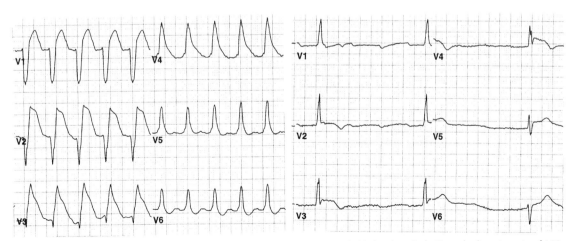

Figure 19–22   ECG from a 79-year-old man with acute anterior myocardial infarction. *Left,* Sinus rhythm at a rate of 122 beats/min and acute injury pattern. *Right,* At 17 hours later there is complete atrioventricular block with an escape rhythm at a rate of 30 beats/min.

TABLE 19-1	Cause of Chronic AV Block (100 Autopsied Cases)

Cause	No. of Cases
Idiopathic bilateral bundle branch fibrosis	46
Ischemic coronary artery disease	
Destruction of both bundle branches	14
Destruction of AV node	1
Cardiomyopathy	13
Calcific valve disease	8
Myocarditis	4
Connective tissue disorder	3
Amyloidosis	3
Transfusion siderosis (only AV node affected)	2
Congenital heart block (only main bundle affected)	3
Gumma of interventricular septum	3
Total	100

Adapted from Davies MJ: Pathology of Conducting Tissue of the Heart. New York, Appleton-Century-Crofts, 1971.
AV, Atrioventricular.

Davies, the most common cause (46 percent of cases) was idiopathic bilateral bundle branch fibrosis. Lenègre is credited with establishing the link between the sclerodegenerative lesions of the bundle branches and chronic complete AV block.[50] The pathologic process described by Lenègre is also called *idiopathic bilateral bundle branch fibrosis*, and the AV block is called *primary heart block*.

Lev described similar degenerative lesions, which he referred to as *sclerosis of the left side of the cardiac skeleton*.[51] There is progressive fibrosis and calcification of the mitral annulus, central fibrous body, pars membranacea, base of the aorta, and summit of the muscular ventricular septum. Various portions of the His bundle or the bundle branches may be involved, resulting in AV block. The difference between so-called Lenègre disease and Lev disease[52] consists probably in the prevalence of valve calcifications in the latter versus pure fibrosis of the summit of the ventricular septum in the former. Cardiac calcifications associated with complete AV block have been found also in Paget's disease.[53] The chronic AV block seen in patients with hypertension is thought to be due to coronary arteriosclerosis or sclerosis of the left side of the cardiac skeleton exacerbated by hypertension.[54]

Myocardial Diseases

Atrioventricular conduction defects are seen in idiopathic and secondary cardiomyopathies, particularly the former (see Table 19–1). Varying degrees of AV block are observed in about 15 percent of patients with dilated idiopathic cardiomyopathy but in only about 3 percent of those with the hypertrophic variety.[55] Among secondary cardiomyopathies, myocardial sarcoidosis is well known for its frequent association with AV block. Other causes are infiltrative diseases such as amyloidosis and hemachromatosis, neuromuscular diseases such as progressive muscular dystrophy, and connective tissue diseases such as systemic lupus erythematosus, dermatomyositis, scleroderma, Reiter's disease, and Marfan syndrome.[56] AV block also has been described in association with rheumatoid heart disease,[57] but it is more commonly seen with ankylosing spondylitis.[58] Tumors, primary or metastatic, may involve the AV node, His bundle, or bundle branches to produce AV block.

AV block may occur with all types of acute myocarditis. Prolongation of the PR interval is a common finding in patients with acute rheumatic fever, with the incidence ranging from 25 to 95 percent in various reported series. Type I second-degree AV block also may occur, but complete AV block is uncommon.[59]

The AV block seen with acute rheumatic fever is not included in the diagnostic criteria for rheumatic carditis. In 508 patients with acute rheumatic fever reviewed by Clarke and Keith,[59] no significant difference in the PR interval was found between patients with or without carditis. The transient appearance of incomplete AV block is not uncommon with other forms of myocarditis of viral or bacterial origin. Among bacterial infections, diphtheria was once a well-known cause of complete AV block. The parasitic Chagas heart disease is known to be associated with both acute and chronic AV block.

Valvular Heart Diseases

In patients with calcific aortic stenosis, a chronic partial or complete AV block may occur when extended calcifications involve the main bundle or its bifurcation, resulting in degeneration and necrosis of the conduction tissue.[49] Occasionally, massive calcification of the mitral annulus causes AV block.[60] In patients with bacterial endocarditis, especially on the aortic valve, AV block may be caused by extension of the infectious process to the adjacent conduction tissue.

Congenital Heart Disease

Congenital complete AV block occurs most commonly in the absence of other evidence of organic heart disease. The site of the block is most commonly the AV node and less often the bundle of His.[61] In patients with congenital complete AV block, abnormally wide QRS complexes occur less frequently and have been considered more ominous than QRS complexes of normal duration.[61] In a study conducted by Engle, abnormally wide QRS complexes were present in 18 of 128 patients with congenital complete AV block without associated congenital malformations.[61] In children with complete AV block, the ventricular rate is usually >40 beats/min. In one study, a persistent heart rate at rest of <50 beats/min significantly correlated with the incidence of syncope.[62]

A congenital AV block may be hereditary[63,64] and may occur in infants born to mothers with systemic lupus erythematosus.[65] Among patients who have other congenital cardiac defects, AV block is frequently seen in those with corrected transposition of the great vessels. In adult patients with congenital heart disease, AV block (usually incomplete) is seen more commonly in association with atrial septal defect and Ebstein anomaly.

Trauma

AV block may be induced during open heart surgery in the area of the AV conduction tissue. It is seen in patients operated on to correct a ventricular septal defect, tetralogy of Fallot, or left ventricular outflow tract obstruction. The conduction defect may be the result of edema, transient ischemia, or disruption of the conduction tissue. Complete AV block following surgery for congenital heart disease resolves in two thirds of patients, usually by the ninth postoperative day.[66]

In some cases, complete AV block is created purposefully by interrupting the His bundle when all other measures fail to slow the ventricular rate in patients with atrial fibrillation. Complete AV block also has been reported in patients who sustained nonpenetrating or penetrating trauma of the chest.[67] Also, after alcohol septal ablation for the treatment of obstructive hypertrophic cardiomyopathy, the occurrence of complete AV block requiring a pacemaker is not uncommon.[68,69]

▌ Concealed Conduction

Concealed conduction, mentioned earlier, is a common manifestation applicable to the surface ECG. It defines a nonrecordable event that modifies the expected behavior of the recorded event. The concealment is most frequently localized in the AV node during anterograde (atrial) or retrograde (ventricular) propagation of an impulse that, upon reaching the AV node and modifying its refractoriness, fails to complete its passage across the AV junction. The concealed presence of such an impulse can be deduced from the unexpected changes in conduction, refractoriness, excitability, or automaticity of the subsequent impulse. It has been shown that 1-ms change in the timing of the atrial premature response could determine whether a block occurred that resulted in concealment or conduction in the AV node.[70]

The concept of concealed conduction antedates electrocardiography.[71] Of note are the experimental studies of Scherf and Shookhoff[70] and the analysis of human ECGs by Langendorf.[72] Langendorf's simplest example of this phenomenon was lengthening of the PR interval after an interpolated premature ventricular or AV junctional complex (Figure 19–23). Other examples are disturbances of AV junctional automaticity by anterograde or retrograde concealment of supraventricular or ventricular impulses reaching the AV node. Concealment can be uncovered by direct recording from the sites of concealment, such as recording AV nodal action potentials of impulses propagated from the atria and not reaching the ventricles or impulses propagated from the ventricles and not reaching the atria.[73]

Various types of single or multiple concealment of cardiac impulses are discussed in textbooks dedicated to complex arrhythmias.[71,74] Here only a few representative examples of this phenomenon are outlined. An interested reader encountering an observation that may include concealed conduction should be guided by the following principles formulated by Fisch:[71]

Any manifestation of concealed conduction can be accurately defined in the context of the following descriptors: the site of origin of the concealed impulse and, when possible, the mechanism responsible for the impulse formation (i.e., concealed reciprocation or concealed His bundle discharge), the anatomic site of concealment (i.e., AV node), and the effect of the concealed impulse on the behavior of the subsequent impulse. The latter may take form of delayed conduction, conduction block, displacement of pacemaker, enhancement of conduction, or a combination of the above.

CONCEALED CONDUCTION IN THE AV JUNCTION

In Figure 19–23, the retrogradely conducted interpolated ectopic impulse reaches the AV junction and prolongs its refractoriness, remaining concealed and failing to complete its passage to the atria. Conduction of the postextrasystolic sinus impulse in the invaded and incompletely recovered AV junction is slowed, resulting in prolongation of the PR interval. A similar explanation is suggested for the occurrence of an alternating PR interval and resulting bigeminal rhythm in Figure 19–24.

In some cases concealed conduction restores failed conduction in the AV junction, possibly due to retrograde concealed conduction of the premature ventricular impulse entering the AV junction. Early depolarization of the AV junction by the premature impulse results in its

earlier recovery, shifting the refractoriness of the AV junction "leftward" to allow conduction of the next supraventricular impulse at a time when such impulse was previously blocked. The same effect can cause paradoxical shortening of the PR interval. This phenomenon is often called "peeling," or peeling back of the refractory period.[71]

The effect of anterograde concealed conduction on impulse conduction may be observed during atrial fibrillation. The irregular ventricular response during atrial fibrillation is probably the result of the varying depth and frequency of the concealed conduction into the AV junction.[75] A long RR interval after repeated concealments is usually followed by an AV junctional escape pacemaker. If the RR is longer than the expected junctional escape interval, however, a concealed discharge of the junctional pacemaker may be suspected (Figure 19–25).

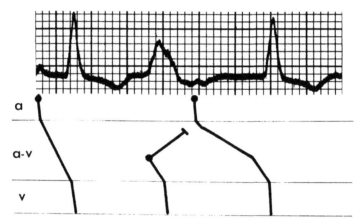

Figure 19–23   Interpolated premature complex, presumably from the atrioventricular junction conducted with aberration to the ventricles and causing prolongation of the PR interval. a = atrium; a-v = atrioventricular junction; v = ventricle. (From Schamroth L, Surawicz B: Concealed interpolated AV junctional extrasystoles and AV junctional parasystole. Am J Cardiol 27:703, 1971.)

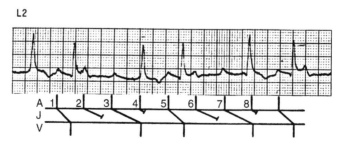

Figure 19–24   Sinus rhythm with 2:1 atrioventricular block and alternation of the PR interval. P_1 with an RP interval of 400 ms conducts with a PR interval of 200 ms. P_2 is blocked. P_3 with an RP interval of 680 ms conducts with a P_3R interval of 440 ms. P_4 with an RP interval of 0 ms is blocked. The rhythm is bigeminal because of alternation of the PR interval. Unexpected prolongation of P_3R and P_7R is attributed to concealed conduction of P_2 and P_6, respectively. In the Lewis diagram: A = atria; J = junction; V = ventricle. (From Knoebel S, Fisch C: Concealed conduction. In Fisch C [ed]: Complex Electrocardiography. Philadelphia, FA Davis, 1973, p 22.)

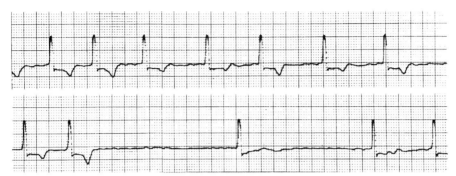

Figure 19–25   Concealed conduction in atrial fibrillation. The unexpected marked prolongation of the RR interval on the bottom strip can best be explained by repeated concealed conduction in the atrioventricular junction and concealed discharge of the junctional pacemaker. The RR intervals are longer than the expected junctional escape interval.

Pseudo AV block due to concealed His extrasystole is another example of the effect of concealed depolarization on AV conduction.[76] If premature His extrasystole occurs soon after the preceding sinus impulse, it is completely concealed because it fails to propagate either anterogradely or retrogradely.[77] No QRS or P can be detected on the surface ECG, but when the next sinus impulse arrives at the His bundle the latter is still refractory and fails to conduct. A blocked sinus P wave is seen unexpectedly, accounting for the phenomenon of pseudo AV block. In Figure 19–26, His extrasystoles are (1) conducted anterogradely and retrogradely; (2) conducted only anterogradely or retrogradely; and (3) not conducted in either direction. The latter is implied by the presence of an unexpected nonconducted sinus P wave. Figure 19–27 shows a concealed His discharge that blocks propagation of the following atrial impulse into the ventricles, resulting in a so-called pseudo AV block. Figure 19–28 shows a transient 2:1 AV block attributed to concealed conduction in the presence of AV junctional parasystolic rhythm, which is slightly faster than the sinus rhythm.

Concealed conduction may play a role in the phenomenon of tachycardia-induced AV block, a cause of syncope that is usually associated with impaired conduction in the distal part of the AV junction (Figure 19–29).[78] This phenomenon falls also into the category of the previously discussed paroxysmal AV block.[71] Concealed conduction is probably responsible for a concomitant increase in R-R and P-R interval after short runs of atrial tachycardia or atrial flutter shown in Figure 19–30.

CONCEALED CONDUCTION IN THE BUNDLE BRANCH SYSTEM

Concealed conduction of impulses in the bundle branch may account for the following manifestations of transient appearance and disappearance of bundle branch block.

Perpetuation of aberrant ventricular conduction (functional bundle branch block) is initiated by a sudden increase in the ventricular rate. The aberrancy persists even though the ventricular rate returns to its previous level. Such a phenomenon can be explained by transseptal concealed conduction. The supraventricular impulse, which is conducted through the bundle branch that is not refractory, traverses the interventricular septum to depolarize the blocked bundle branch. When the next impulse arrives, the previously refractory bundle continues to remain refractory because it was depolarized late via transseptal conduction of the impulse from the contralateral bundle branch. This process is believed to perpetuate aberrancy. An example is shown in Figure 19–31. In bradycardia- or deceleration-dependent bundle branch block, the conduction defect is attributed to spontaneous diastolic depolarization (phase 4 depolarization) of the bundle branch. At slower heart rates, diastolic depolarization may reach a takeoff potential at which impulse propagation fails and conduction block occurs. With an increase in heart rate, the block dissipates. Concealed conduction from a premature impulse can accelerate or depress the course of diastolic depolarization and alter the cycle length at which bundle branch block is present or absent. A similar mechanism is responsible for modulated ventricular parasystole (see Chapter 17). Examples of bradycardia-dependent LBBB are shown in Figures 4–16 and 4–17.

CONCEALED CONDUCTION OF ATRIAL IMPULSES INTO THE BUNDLE BRANCH DURING ATRIAL FLUTTER AND ATRIAL FIBRILLATION

The ability of an atrial impulse to get past the AV junction into the bundle branch system has been demonstrated in humans by electrophysiologic studies.[79] Figure 19–32 shows an ECG of a patient with atrial fibrillation, complete AV

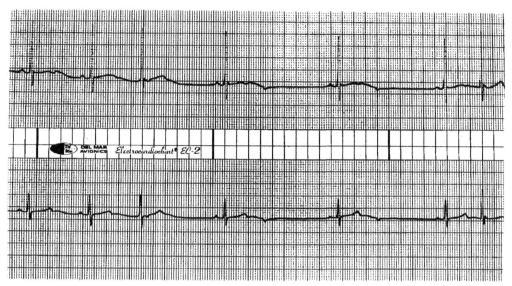

I.C. 18M

A

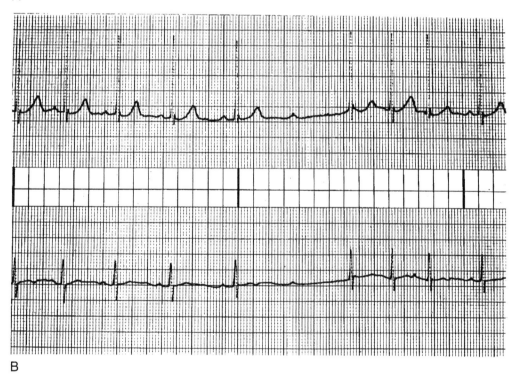

B

Figure 19–26 Pseudo atrioventricular (AV) block due to concealed His extrasystole. The tracings were recorded with a two-channel Holter monitor. **A,** There is sinus rhythm with premature junctional complexes. The third complex is a premature junctional complex with retrograde atrial capture. The negative P waves after the third and fourth sinus complexes are retrograde P waves from premature junctional complexes with anterograde block resulting in an absence of QRS complexes. The last complex is premature junctional without retrograde P wave. **B,** The sinus P wave, which is not followed by QRS, is most likely due to refractoriness of the His bundle caused by premature His depolarization with both anterograde and retrograde block occurring before the blocked sinus P wave. The blocked P wave is followed by two more junctional complexes. The patient is an 18-year-old man with mitral valve prolapse. During his 24-hour Holter monitor numerous junctional extrasystoles are seen, but there is no evidence of an AV conduction defect other than the nonconducted sinus P wave shown in the tracing.

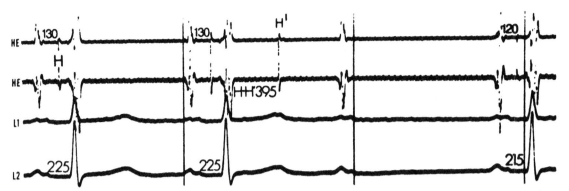

Figure 19–27   Pseudo type II atrioventricular block following the third P wave caused by a concealed premature His bundle discharge (H'). The intracardiac recordings are from the His bundle (HL) and ECG leads I and II (L1, L2). H = His bundle deflection; H-H = interval between two His bundle deflections. (From Fisch C, Zipes DP, McHenry PL: Electrocardiographic manifestations of concealed junctional ectopic impulses. Circulation 53:217, 1976.)

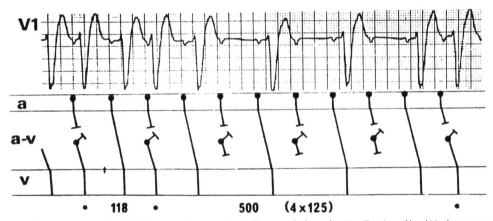

Figure 19–28   Atrioventricular (AV) junctional parasystole with concealed conduction. Tracing of lead V_1 shows pseudo second-degree AV block. Dots at the bottom indicate manifest parasystolic impulses. Interectopic intervals are expressed in 0.01 second. a = atrium; a-v = atrioventricular junction; v = ventricle. (From Lindsay AL, Schamroth L: Atrioventricular junctional parasystole with concealed conduction simulating second degree atrioventricular block. Am J Cardiol 31:397, 1973.)

block, and marked slowing of the presumed fascicular escape rhythm, possibly caused by concealed conduction, although other interpretations of this phenomenon are possible.

Gap Phenomenon

The term "gap" of conduction defines a zone within the cardiac cycle during which premature impulses fail to propagate, whereas premature responses outside that zone (i.e. earlier or later) evoke propagated responses. The existence of gaps depends on the presence of nonhomogeneous refractoriness in different parts of the conducting system. In 1981, Reddy et al. reported that six types of gap had been described for anterograde conduction and three types for retrograde conduction.[80] The common mechanism of all types of gap involves a proximal delay, allowing more time for distal recovery.

The two most commonly cited anterograde gaps are type I (a gap in AV conduction) and type II (a gap in the bundle branch).[81] With both types there is prolongation of the P'R interval of the conducted premature complex. With type I gap, the resumption of AV conduction with an early premature complex is due to a delay in the conduction of the impulse in the AV node. The delay allows sufficient time for the His-Purkinje system to recover and conduct. With type II gap, the delay of the premature impulse is within the proximal His-Purkinje system, allowing impulse propagation to the affected bundle branch after its recovery from refractoriness.[82]

The sequence of AV conduction in type I gap is illustrated in Figure 19–33A. Among the three premature atrial complexes (P'), those with the longest and shortest RP' interval (0.40 and 0.20 second, respectively) are conducted, but the one with the intermediate RP' interval (0.30 second) is blocked. The P' with the

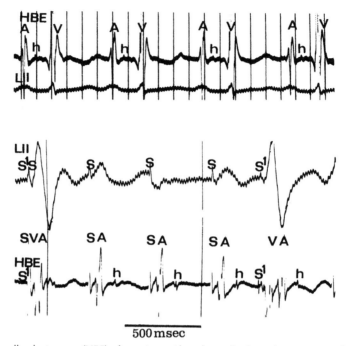

Figure 19–29 His bundle electrogram (HBE) of a patient with tachycardia-dependent paroxysmal atrioventricular block. *Top,* Normal AH (100 ms) and prolonged HV (65 ms) intervals during 1:1 conduction. *Bottom,* Effect of rapid atrial pacing at a rate of 150 beats/min. Atrial depolarizations (A) follow atrial pacing stimulus artifacts (S). His bundle spikes are present after each atrial depolarization (AH interval is = 125 ms). The absence of a ventricular complex (V) after h indicates a block below the level of recording of the His bundle spike. S¹ = ventricular pacing spike. (From Aravindakshan V, Surawicz B, Daoud FS: Depression of escape pacemakers associated with rapid supraventricular rate in patients with atrioventricular block. Circulation 50:255, 1974.)

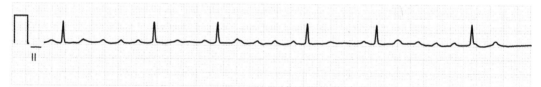

Figure 19–30 ECG strip of a 71-year-old man. ECG is normal except for short runs of atrial tachycardia or atrial flutter. The non-conducted atrial impulses cause lengthening of the R-R interval and of the P-R interval, probably due to concealed conduction within the atrioventricular junction.

shortest RP′ interval is conducted because of the longer delay in the AV node. The P′R interval of the conducted P′ is longer, and consequently the RR interval containing the shortest RP′ is equal to or longer than the RR interval containing the longest RP′.

Figure 19–33B illustrates a type II gap. Aberrant ventricular conduction with RBBB morphology occurs when the premature atrial complex is early but normal ventricular conduction resumes upon further shortening of the coupling interval.

The gap is not the only mechanism that explains the unexpected conduction of an early premature impulse. Another mechanism invoked to explain such phenomena is called supernormality,[71,73] a favorite hypothesis offered when other explanations fail. Supernormal excitability and supernormal conduction are sound physiologic concepts,[73] but a discussion of this subject is beyond the scope of this textbook. In 1962 Pick et al.[83] stated, "The application of the concept of supernormal conduction in conjunction with that of concealed conduction and of unidirectional block permits a satisfactory interpretation of some otherwise inexplicable features of AV block in clinical electrocardiography." This statement has not lost its validity, but speculations may cease to be necessary when technical means are available to examine various properties of the conducting system critically during intracardiac electrophysiologic studies.

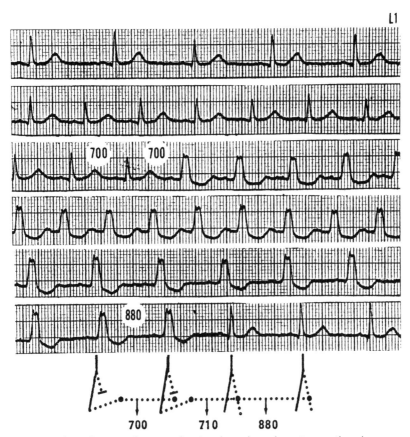

Figure 19–31 Unexpected persistence of an acceleration-dependent aberration attributed to concealed transseptal conduction from the right bundle branch (RBB) to the left bundle branch (LBB). The basic rhythm is sinus with gradual acceleration of the heart rate. When the RR interval shortens to 700 ms, left bundle branch block (LBBB) appears and persists at longer RR intervals up to 880 ms. Persistence of the LBBB at cycles longer than the critical RR cycle for initiation of LBBB is explained by the concealed transseptal conduction from the RBB to the LBB, which is believed to shorten the LBB-to-LBB interval to 700 ms, resulting in LBBB. This implies that the LBB-to-LBB interval, shown in the diagram below the figure, rather than the manifest QRS-to-QRS interval, determines whether conduction is normal or aberrant. The authors of this report also considered other explanations for this phenomenon. (From Fisch C, Zipes DP, McHenry PL: Rate-dependent aberrancy. Circulation 48:714, 1973.)

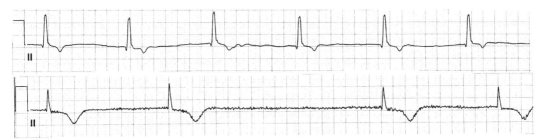

Figure 19–32 ECG strips of lead II from a 90-year-old man with atrial fibrillation and complete atrioventricular block. *Top,* Escape pacemaker at a rate of 41 beats/min with right bundle branch block and left posterior fascicular block QRS morphology, presumably from or near the site of the left anterior fascicle. *Bottom,* The same escape pacemaker at a slower rate. The second RR interval is approximately twice as long as the first and third RR intervals, which suggests the possibility of an exit block.

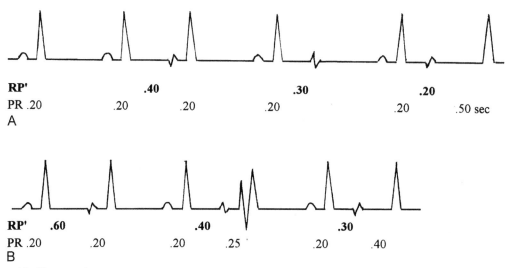

Figure 19–33 Gap phenomenon. **A,** Gap in atrioventricular (AV) conduction is shown. Relatively late premature complex with an RP′ interval of 0.40 second is conducted. As the premature complex appears earlier (RP′ = 0.30 second), it is blocked. However, when the premature complex occurs even earlier (RP′ = 0.20 second) it is conducted with a prolonged PR interval (0.50 second). An AV conduction gap is therefore present. **B,** Bundle branch conduction gap. As the RP′ interval of the premature complex decreases from 0.60 to 0.40 to 0.30 second, the QRS complex changes from normal to right bundle branch block morphology and back to normal when the ectopic atrial complex is most premature (RP′ = 0.30 second). The latter is associated with a long PR′ interval (0.40 second). See text for explanation.

REFERENCES

1. Rosen KM, Dhingra RC, Loeb HS, et al: Chronic heart block in adults: clinical and electrophysiological observations. Arch Intern Med 131:663, 1973.
2. Kastor JA, Josephson ME: Treatment of atrioventricular block. In Fowler NO (ed): Cardiac Arrhythmias, Diagnosis and Treatment, 2nd ed. New York, Harper & Row, 1977, p 188.
3. Narula OS, Scherlag BJ, Samet P, et al: Atrioventricular block: localization and classification by His bundle recordings. Am J Med 50:146, 1971.
4. Puech P: Atrioventricular block; the value of intracardiac recordings. In Krikler DM, Goodwin JF (eds): Cardiac Arrhythmias: The Modern Electrophysiological Approach. Philadelphia, Saunders, 1975, p 81.
5. Dhingra RC: His bundle recording in acquired conduction disease. Arch Intern Med 135:397, 1975.
6. Fisch C, Mandrola JM, Rardon DP: Electrocardiographic manifestations of dual atrioventricular node conduction during sinus rhythm. J Am Coll Cardiol 29:1015, 1997.
7. Damato AN, Lau SH, Helfant R, et al: A study of heart block in man using His bundle recordings. Circulation 39:297, 1969.
8. Waldo AL, Kaiser GA, Bowman FO Jr, et al: Etiology of the P-R interval in patients with an endocardial cushion defect. Circulation 48:19, 1973.
9. Kupfer JM, Kligfield P: A generalized description of Wenckebach behavior with analysis of determinants of ventricular cycle-length variation during ambulatory electrocardiography. Am J Cardiol 67:981, 1991.
10. Andersen HR, Nielsen JC, Thomsen PEB, et al: Atrioventricular conduction during long-term follow up of patients with sick sinus syndrome. Circulation 98: 1315, 1998.
11. Narula OS, Samet P: Wenckebach and Mobitz type II AV block due to block within the His bundle and bundle branches. Circulation 41:947, 1970.
12. Mangiardi LM, Bonamini R, Conte M, et al: Bedside evaluation of atrioventricular block with narrow QRS complexes: usefulness of carotid sinus massage and atropine administration. Am J Cardiol 49:1136, 1982.
13. Delmar M, Michaels DC, Jalife J: Slow recovery of excitability and the Wenckebach phenomenon in the single guinea pig ventricular myocyte. Circ Res 65:761, 1989.
14. Hoshino K, Anumonwo J, Delmar M, et al: Wenckebach periodicity in single atrioventricular nodal cells from the rabbit heart. Circulation 82:2201, 1990.
15. Langendorf R, Cohen H, Gozo EG: Observations on second degree atrioventricular block, including new criteria for the differential diagnosis between type I and type II block. Am J Cardiol 29:111, 1972.
16. Barold SS, Friedberg HD: Second degree atrioventricular block: a matter of definition. Am J Cardiol 33:311, 1974.
17. Zipes DP: Second-degree atrioventricular block. Circulation 60:465, 1979.
18. Rosen KM, Loeb HS, Gunnar RM, et al: Mobitz type II block without bundle branch block. Circulation 44:1111, 1971.
19. Schamroth L: Ventriculophasic atrial extrasystoles associated with complete atrioventricular block. Am J Cardiol 21:593, 1968.
20. Ohkawa S, Sugiura M, Itoh Y, et al: Electrophysiologic and histologic correlations in chronic complete atrioventricular block. Circulation 64:215, 1981.
21. Scherlag BJ, Lazzara R, Helfant RH: Differentiation of "A-V junctional rhythms." Circulation 48:304, 1973.
22. Pick A, Langendorf R, Katz LN: Depression of cardiac pacemakers by premature impulses. Am Heart J 41:49, 1951.
23. Brignole M, Menozzi C, Moya A, et al: Mechanism of syncope in patients with bundle branch block and negative electrophysiological test. Circulation 104:2045, 2001.
24. Akhtar M, Damato AN, Batsford WP, et al: A comparative analysis of antegrade and retrograde conduction patterns in man. Circulation 52:766, 1975.

25. Winternitz M, Langendorf R: Auriculoventricular block with ventriculoauricular response. Am Heart J 27:301, 1944.

26. Halpern MS, Nau GJ, Levi RJ, et al: Wenckebach periods of alternate beats: clinical and experimental observation. Circulation 48:41, 1973.

27. Amat-y-Leon F, Chuquimia R, Wu D, et al: Alternating Wenckebach periodicity: a common electrophysiologic response. Am J Cardiol 36:757, 1975.

28. Castellanos A, Interian A, Cox MM, et al: Alternating Wenckebach periods and allied arrhythmias. PACE 16:2285, 1993.

29. Kosowsky BD, Latif P, Radoff AM: Multilevel atrioventricular block. Circulation 54:914, 1976.

30. Castellanos A, Cox MM, Fernandez PR, et al: Mechanisms and dynamics of episodes of progression of 2:1 atrioventricular block in patients with documented two-level conduction disturbances. Am J Cardiol 70:193, 1992.

31. Johnson RL, Averill KH, Lamb LE: Electrocardiographic findings in 67,375 asymptomatic subjects. VII. Atrioventricular block. Am J Cardiol 6:153, 1960.

32. Brodsky M, Wu D, Denes P, et al: Arrhythmia documented by 24 hour continuous electrocardiographic monitoring in 50 male medical students without apparent heart disease. Am J Cardiol 39:390, 1977.

33. Sobotka RA, Mayer JH, Bauernfeind RA, et al: Arrhythmias documented by 24-hour continuous ambulatory electrocardiographic monitoring in young women without apparent heart disease. Am Heart J 101:753, 1981.

34. Zeppilli P, Fenici R, Sassara M, et al: Wenckebach second-degree A-V block in top-ranking athletes: an old problem revisited. Am Heart J 100:281, 1980.

35. Packard JM, Graettinger JS, Graybiel A: Analysis of the electrocardiograms obtained from 1000 young healthy aviators: ten year follow-up. Circulation 10:384, 1954.

36. Mymin D, Matheson FAL, Tate RB, et al: The natural history of primary first-degree atrioventricular heart block. N Engl J Med 315:1183, 1986.

37. Harrington JT, De Sanctis RW: Hiccup-induced atrioventricular block. Ann Intern Med 72:105, 1969.

38. Hutchinson EC, Stock JTT: Carotid sinus syndrome. Lancet 2:445, 1960.

39. Meltzer LE, Kitchell JB: The incidence of arrhythmias associated with acute myocardial infarction. Prog Cardiovasc Dis 9:50, 1966.

40. Stock RJ, Macken DL: Observations on heart block during continuous electrocardiographic monitoring in myocardial infarction. Circulation 38:993, 1968.

41. Lamas GA, Muller JE, Turi ZG, et al: A simplified method to predict occurrence of complete heart block during acute myocardial infarction. Am J Cardiol 57:1213, 1986.

42. Harpaz D, Behar S, Gottlieb S, et al: Complete atrioventricular block complicating acute myocardial infarction in the thrombolytic era. J Am Coll Cardiol 34:1721, 1999.

43. Norris RM: Heart block in posterior and anterior myocardial infarction. Br Heart J 31:352, 1969.

44. Lev M, Kinare SG, Pick A: The pathogenesis of atrioventricular block in coronary disease. Circulation 42:409, 1970.

45. Sutton R, Davies M: The conduction system in acute myocardial infarction complicated by heart block. Circulation 38:987, 1968.

46. Rotman W, Wagner GS, Wallace AG: Bradyarrhythmias in acute myocardial infarction. Circulation 45:703, 1972.

47. Hindman MC, Wagner GS, JaRo M, et al: The clinical significance of bundle branch block complicating acute myocardial infarction. 2. Indications of temporary and permanent pacemaker insertion. Circulation 58:689, 1978.

48. Aplin M, Engstrom T, Vejlstrup NG, et al on behalf of the TRACE Study Group: Prognostic importance of complete atrioventricular block complicating acute myocardial infarction. Am J Cardiol 92:853, 2003.

49. Davies MJ: Pathology of Conducting Tissue of the Heart. New York, Appleton-Century-Crofts, 1971.

50. Langendorf R, Pick A: Concealed intraventricular conduction in the human heart. Adv Cardiol 14:40, 1975.

51. Lev M: Anatomical basis for atrioventricular block. Am J Med 37:742, 1964.

52. Rosenbaum MB, Elizari MV, Lazzari JO, et al: The Hemiblocks. Oldsmar, FL, Tampa Tracings, 1970.

53. King M, Huang J-M, Glassman E: Paget's disease with cardiac calcification and complete heart block. Am J Med 46:302, 1969.

54. Lev M, Bharati S: Atrioventricular and intraventricular conduction disease. Arch Intern Med 135:405, 1975.

55. Flowers NV, Horan LG: Electrocardiographic and vectorcardiographic features of myocardial disease. In Fowler NO (ed): Myocardial Diseases. Orlando, Grune & Stratton, 1973.

56. Bear ES, Tung MY, Bordiuk J: Marfan's syndrome with complete heart block and junctional rhythm. JAMA 217:335, 1971.

57. Hoffman FG, Leight L: Complete atrioventricular block associated with rheumatoid disease. Am J Cardiol 16:585, 1965.

58. Weed CL, Kurlander BG, Mazzarella JA: Heart block in ankylosing spondylitis. Arch Intern Med 117:800, 1966.

59. Clarke M, Keith JD: Atrioventricular conduction in acute rheumatic fever. Br Heart J 34:472, 1972.

60. Rytand DA, Lipsitch LS: Clinical aspects of calcification of mitral annulus fibrosis. Arch Intern Med 78:544, 1946.

61. Lev M, Cuadris H, Paul MH: Interruption of the atrioventricular bundle with congenital atrioventricular block. Circulation 43:703, 1971.

62. Karpawich PP, Gillette PC, Garson A, et al: Congenital complete atrioventricular block: clinical and electrophysiologic predictors of need for pacemaker insertion. Am J Cardiol 48:1098, 1981.

63. Lynch HT, Mohuddin S, Moran J, et al: Hereditary progressive atrioventricular conduction defect. Am J Cardiol 36:297, 1975.

64. Waxman MB, Catching JD, Felderhof CH, et al: Familial atrioventricular heart block. an autosomal dominant trait. Circulation 51:226, 1975.

65. Goble MM, Dick MII, McCune WJ, et al: Atrioventricular conduction in children of women with systemic lupus erythematosus. Am J Cardiol 71:94, 1993.

66. Weindling SN, Saul P, Gamble WJ, et al: Duration of complete atrioventricular block after congenital heart surgery. Am J Cardiol 82:525, 1998.

67. Lev M: The pathology of atrioventricular block. Cardiovasc Clin 4:159, 1972.

68. Reinhard W, Ten Cate FJ, Scholten M, et al: Permanent pacing for complete atrioventricular block after nonsurgical (alcohol) septal reduction in patients with obstructive hypertrophic cardiomyopathy. Am J Cardiol 93:1064, 2004.

69. Chen AA, Palacios IF, Mela T, et al: Acute predictors of subacute complete heart block after alcohol ablation for obstructive hypertrophic cardiomyopathy. Am J Cardiol 97:264, 2006.

70. Scherf D, Shookhoff C: Reizleitungsstoerungen im Buendel. I. Wien Arch Inn Med 10:97, 1925.

71. Fisch C: Electrocardiography of Arrhythmias. Philadelphia, Lea & Febiger, 1990.

72. Langendorf R: Concealed AV conduction: the effect of block impulses on the formation and conduction of succeeding impulses. Am Heart J 35:542, 1948.

73. Surawicz B: Electrophysiologic Basis of ECG and Cardiac Arrhythmias. Baltimore, Williams & Wilkins, 1995.

74. Pick A, Langendorf R: Interpretation of Complex Arrhythmias. Philadelphia, Lea & Febiger, 1979.

75. Moore EN, Knoebel SB, Spear JF: Concealed conduction. Am J Cardiol 28:406, 1971.

76. Rosen KM, Rahimtoola SH, Gunnar RM: Pseudo AV block secondary to premature non-propagated His bundle depolarizations: documentation by His bundle electrocardiography. Circulation 42:367, 1970.

77. Langendorf R, Mehlman JS: Blocked (nonconducted) A-V nodal premature systoles imitating first and second degree A-V block. Am Heart J 34:500, 1947.

78. Aravindakshan V, Surawicz B, Daoud FS: Depression of escape pacemakers associated with rapid supraventricular rate in patients with atrioventricular block. Circulation 50:255, 1974.

79. Berkowitz WD, Lau SH, Patton RD, et al: The use of His bundle recordings in the analysis of unilateral and bilateral bundle branch block. Am Heart J 81:340, 1971.

80. Reddy CP, Damato AN, Akhthar M: Intra His Purkinje gap phenomenon during retrograde conduction in man. J Electrocardiol 14:1, 1981.

81. Gallagher JJ, Damato AN, Caracta AR, et al: Gap in AV conduction in man: types I and II. Am Heart J 85:78, 1973.

82. Aghe AS, Castellanos A, Wells D, et al: Type I, type II, and type III gaps in bundle-branch conduction. Circulation 47:325, 1973.

83. Pick A, Langendorf R, Katz LN: The supernormal phase of atrioventricular conduction. Circulation 26:388, 1962.

20 Ventricular Preexcitation (Wolff-Parkinson-White Syndrome and Its Variants)

The syndrome of short PR interval with an abnormal QRS complex and paroxysmal tachycardia was first described by Wolff, Parkinson, and White[1] in 1930. It also is called the *ventricular preexcitation syndrome*. The term *Wolff-Parkinson-White (WPW) pattern* defines the ventricular preexcitation seen in the absence of the preexcitation-dependent tachycardia.[2]

Figure 20–1 shows the four preexcitation pathways: atrioventricular (Kent bundle) and three types of Mahaim fibers (i.e., atriofascicular, sometimes called the *Brechenmacher tract*; nodoventricular; fasciculoventricular). The atrioventricular (AV) bypass is the most common type of preexcitation, generating the typical pattern of short PR interval, delta wave, wide QRS complex, and T wave vector directed opposite to the delta vector.

In patients with AV bypass tracts the impulse may be conducted only through the AV node, only through the bypass tract (full preexcitation), and simultaneously through the AV node and the AV bypass tract, giving rise to a wide range of fusion complexes. With an increasing contribution of conduction through the AV bypass tract, the QRS complex widens and the HV interval shortens.[3] Conversely, with an increasing contribution of conduction through the AV node (e.g., during exercise), the PR and HV intervals lengthen and the QRS complex shortens.

Progressive shortening of the PR interval with corresponding widening of the QRS complex, and vice versa, without change in the duration of the P-end QRS interval is called the *concertina effect* (Figure 20–2). In about half of patients with the WPW pattern, the characteristic electrocardiographic (ECG) changes appear only intermittently.[4,5] In some cases the change from the preexcitation pattern to normal AV conduction (and vice versa) occurs in the same tracing (Figure 20–3). The capacity for preexcitation to go in the anterograde direction may become lost with time. In a longitudinal electrophysiologic study of 29 patients with the WPW pattern but without symptoms, Klein and Gulamhusein[6] found that 9 subjects lost this capacity when they were reexamined after 36 months.

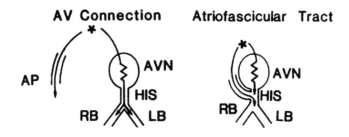

Figure 20–1   Classification of preexcitation syndromes. AP = accessory pathway; AVN = atrioventricular node; RB and LB = right and left bundle branch. See text discussion. (From Prystowsky EN, Miles WM, Heger JJ, et al: Preexcitation syndromes: mechanisms and management. Med Clin North Am 68:831, 1984, by permission.)

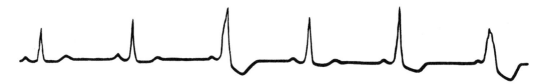

Lead II of a patient with intermittent WPW pattern.

Figure 20–2   ECG lead II of a patient with intermittent preexcitation demonstrates a "concertina" effect in which increasing preexcitation shortens the PR interval and lengthens the QRS complex, with the interval from P to the end of QRS remaining constant. This tracing also is an example of secondary T wave changes, with the T wave becoming more negative as the QRS duration increases. Of the six consecutive complexes, the first is conducted through the atrioventricular (AV) node alone and the sixth presumably through the accessory pathway (AP) alone (fully preexcited), whereas the second, fourth, fifth, and third complexes show increasing degrees of fusion between the AV nodal and AP conduction.

Wolff-Parkinson-White ECG Pattern

The WPW ECG pattern with full preexcitation contains the following elements:

1. A PR interval of less than 0.12 second, with a normal P wave
2. Abnormally wide QRS complex with a duration of 0.11 second or more
3. The presence of initial slurring of the QRS complex, the delta wave
4. Secondary ST segment and T wave changes

PR INTERVAL

The duration of the PR interval is affected by the degree of preexcitation. In fully preexcited

complexes, the duration of the PR intervals equals the duration of the P wave or its initial portion. In most instances it is 0.06–0.11 second. In about 12 percent of cases, PR is longer than 0.12 second; a duration of up to 0.20 second has been reported,[7,8] predominantly in variant forms of the preexcitation associated with Mahaim bypass fibers. If the baseline PR interval is relatively long, the interval may shorten considerably, but the duration remains in the normal range. In such cases the diagnosis of preexcitation may be confirmed if the tracing during normal AV conduction is available for comparison.

In the absence of coexisting atrial pathology, the P wave morphology is normal. The WPW pattern cannot be diagnosed with certainty if there is a short PR interval without a delta wave.

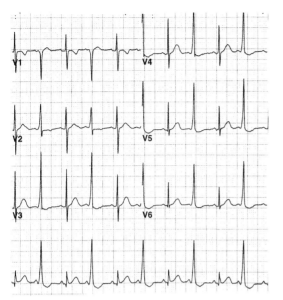

Figure 20–3   ECG precordial leads and the strip of lead II (at the bottom) show alternating normal and preexcited complexes in a 3-year-old girl with Wolff-Parkinson-White syndrome.

A short PR interval with an inverted P wave in the standard limb leads may be caused by an ectopic atrial or AV junctional pacemaker.

QRS COMPLEX

When the ventricles are depolarized entirely by the impulse conducted through the accessory pathway (AP), the QRS duration is increased, usually to 0.11 to 0.16 second. In some series,[7,9] however, the QRS duration was less than 0.10 second in almost one third of the cases, presumably due to fusion between preexcited and normally conducted complexes. The sum of the PR and QRS intervals usually remains within the normal range.

A normal "septal" q wave is seldom found in the preexcited complexes. Its presence in lead V_6 is believed to exclude preexcitation.[10]

Complete normalization of the WPW pattern was attributed by Massumi and Vera[11] to the following mechanisms: (1) the bypass tract failed to conduct at rapid atrial rates or with early atrial premature complexes; (2) the AP became refractory after long pauses and at slow rates, presumably because of phase 4 depolarization; (3) the origin of the ventricular impulse was situated in the His bundle; and (4) conduction through the AV node was faster than through the AV bypass tract.

DELTA WAVE

The delta wave is the most important finding in the WPW pattern. It depicts slow conduction through the bypass tract and ventricular myocardium between the site of bypass tract insertion and the site at which ventricular activation proceeds via the rapidly conducting Purkinje system. The duration of the delta wave varies between 0.02 and 0.07 second. Theoretically, the delta wave should be present in all leads, but it may become isoelectric and be easily overlooked in the leads with the lead axis, which is nearly perpendicular to the initial QRS forces.

When the delta wave is negative, the downward deflection may resemble the abnormal Q wave associated with myocardial infarction. Such a pseudoinfarction pattern may be seen in up to 70 percent of patients with the WPW pattern. Anterior myocardial infarction (MI) may be simulated by the negative delta waves in the right precordial leads, lateral MI by a negative delta wave in lead aV_L (Figure 20–4), and inferior MI by a negative delta wave in leads II, III, aV_F (Figures 20–5 and 20–6). The large upright delta wave in lead V_1 may simulate true posterior MI (Figure 20–7A) or right bundle branch block.

ST SEGMENT AND T WAVE CHANGES

The altered sequence of ventricular activation in patients with the WPW pattern results in secondary repolarization abnormalities. Most commonly, the direction of the ST segment displacement and the T wave polarity are opposite to the direction of the delta wave and the major deflection of the QRS complex. The changes are similar to those of ventricular hypertrophy or bundle branch block. In some cases, however, no apparent ST segment and T wave abnormalities are seen (Figure 20–8). Attention has been called to different types of T wave abnormality that persist after ablation of the APs, resulting in cessation of preexcitation. These abnormalities have been sometimes called "T wave memory" to indicate that they completely regress within several weeks after ablation[12] (Figure 20–9). The origin of these T wave abnormalities has been attributed to the lengthening of ventricular action potentials at the preexcited site, induced by preexcitation and slowly subsiding after ablation.[13]

Clinical Significance

It has been estimated that the WPW pattern is present in 0.15 to 0.20 percent of the general population.[7] The incidence may be higher if concealed forms (see later discussion) are

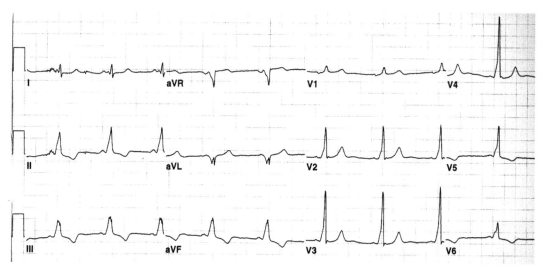

Figure 20–4   ECG of a 44-year-old man with left lateral bypass tract. The negative delta wave in lead aV$_L$ simulates basal or lateral myocardial infarction.

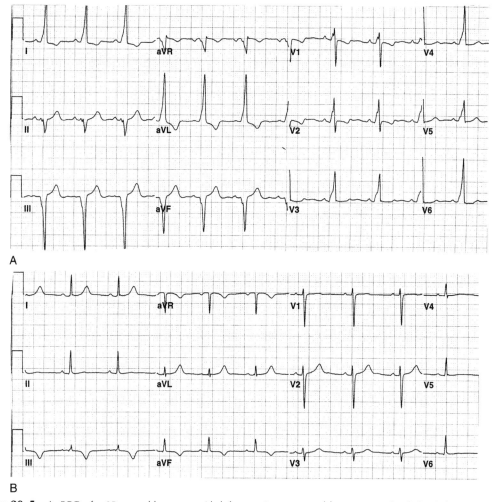

Figure 20–5   **A,** ECG of a 25-year-old woman with left posterior paraseptal bypass tract simulating inferior myocardial infarction. **B,** Normal atrioventricular conduction after ablation of the bypass tract. The deeply inverted symmetric T wave in leads III and aV$_F$ represents a transient postablation abnormality also known as the "memory" T wave.

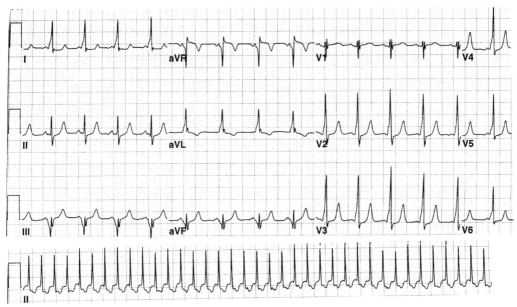

Figure 20–6   *Top,* ECG of a 7-year-old girl with the Wolff-Parkinson-White pattern (probably right anterior accessory pathway). *Bottom,* Lead II recorded on another day shows narrow QRS tachycardia at a rate of 278 beats/min with negative P waves inscribed during the ST segment, which is typical of atrioventricular reentrant tachycardia.

counted.[3] The incidence of other clinically recognizable types of bypass tract is much lower. The WPW pattern occurs more often in males than females. Most subjects (about two thirds) with the WPW pattern have no associated organic heart disease.[7,14,15] In the presence of coronary, hypertensive, or rheumatic heart disease, the WPW pattern is usually an unrelated finding. There is a higher incidence of this pattern in patients with dilated and obstructive types of cardiomyopathy. With the latter type (see Figure 20–23), the reported incidence is 4 percent.[16] With the congestive type of primary myocardial disease, the WPW pattern is more often seen with the familial variety.[17] Patients with hyperthyroidism are said to have a high incidence of the WPW pattern.[18] In one series of patients with the WPW pattern, hyperthyroidism was present in 6 percent of the subjects. The WPW syndrome may become apparent during pregnancy owing to the observed sensitivity of women with preexcitation to supraventricular arrhythmias in this condition.[19]

Of the 163 patients reported by Gallagher and associates,[20] 12 had mitral valve prolapse syndrome. All but one had left-sided bypass. WPW syndrome has been reported also in association with AV block, sick sinus syndrome, tuberous sclerosis, and cardiac tumors.[21] It has been hypothesized that tumor tissue (e.g., rhabdomyoma) becomes an AP that functions like a Kent bundle.[22] In a reported case of mesothelioma of the AV node the WPW syndrome appeared to be coincidental.[21]

Among patients with congenital heart disease, the WPW pattern is seen most commonly in patients with Ebstein's anomaly (Figure 20–10). Schiebler and co-workers[23] reported that this anomaly was present in 24 of 83 patients with congenital heart disease and the WPW pattern. About 5 to 10 percent of patients with Ebstein's anomaly have the WPW pattern,[24] nearly always with a right-sided AP.[25,26] Other associated congenital heart diseases include atrial septal defect (Figure 20–11), tricuspid atresia, corrected transposition of the great vessels, ventricular septal defect, tetralogy of Fallot, and coarctation of the aorta.[27,28]

Tachyarrhythmias

Paroxysmal tachycardias are the most important clinical manifestations in patients with WPW syndrome. They were recorded in 13 to 80 percent of patients with the WPW pattern. The incidence is closely related to the population sampled: It was low (13 percent) when the WPW pattern was diagnosed from routine ECGs among a clinically healthy population.[29] In hospitalized or cardiac clinic patients with this pattern, paroxysmal tachycardias occurred in 40 to 80 percent.[7,12] In many cases the tachyarrhythmia is the first clue to the diagnosis of preexcitation syndrome.

Paroxysmal supraventricular tachycardia is responsible for 75 to 80 percent of all paroxysmal tachycardias in patients with WPW syndrome.[18,30] If the tachycardia is a reciprocating

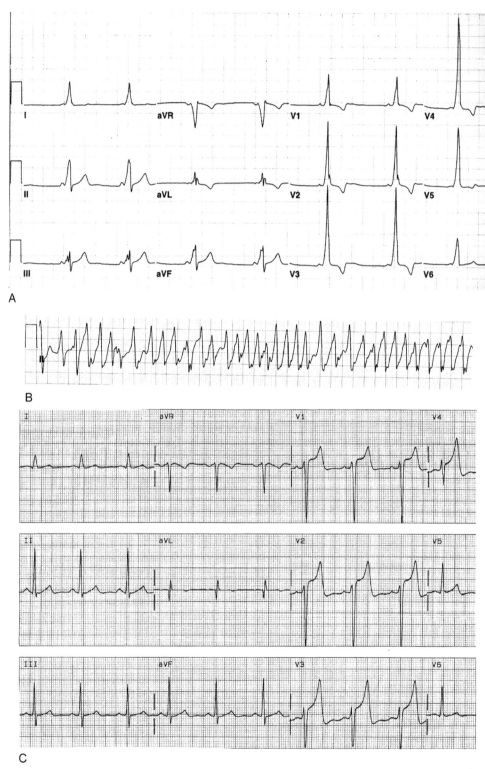

Figure 20–7   ECG of a 28-year-old man with Wolff-Parkinson-White (WPW) syndrome. **A**, WPW pattern suggestive of left anterior paraseptal bypass tract and simulating posterior myocardial infarction. **B**, Strip of lead II during atrial fibrillation with a ventricular rate of 249 beats/min. **C**, Normal atrioventricular conduction after ablation of the bypass tract.

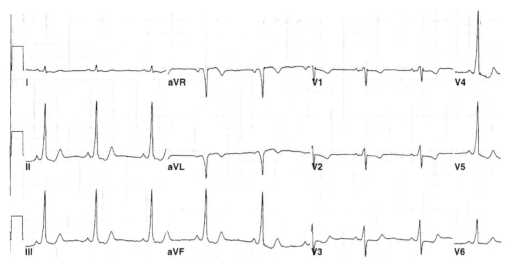

Figure 20–8   ECG of a 76-year-old woman with an asymptomatic Wolff-Parkson-White pattern suggestive of a left anterior bypass tract. The T waves are upright in several leads in which the delta wave is upright.

or reentrant type, it is called *AV reentrant tachycardia*. The tachycardia loop in such cases is formed by the atrium, AV node, His-Purkinje system, and ventricular myocardium in the anterograde direction, returning to the atrium via AP in the retrograde direction. A circus movement is therefore established (Figure 20–12).

In such patients the delta wave is not observed during the tachycardia, and the duration of the QRS complex is normal (narrow). This tachycardia is called *orthodromic AV reentrant tachycardia* (see Figures 20–6 and 20–13C). The heart rate is usually 140 to 250 beats/min, which is generally faster than the rate of tachycardia due to reentry in the AV node.[20] The cycle length of tachycardia depends on the total conduction time in all elements but most importantly in the AV node. Therefore the rate of tachycardia is enhanced by rapid conduction through the AV node, which may manifest as a short PR interval.[31,32] Tachycardia is often initiated by premature atrial or ventricular complexes (Figure 20–14). It can also be induced by a premature atrial or ventricular stimulus, due either to anterograde block in the accessory pathway when pacing the atrium or to unidirectional retrograde block in the His-Purkinje system when pacing the ventricle.[33]

Diagnostic criteria on the surface ECG and in the intracardiac electrogram during tachycardia include the following[3,34]: (1) the P wave is negative in lead I; (2) PR is longer than RP when the retrograde pathway is fast (most common pattern) and shorter than RP when the retrograde pathway is slow; (3) the P wave is inscribed after, not during, the QRS complex; and (4) the

tachycardia cycle length is prolonged in the presence of functional ipsilateral bundle branch block (BBB). The difference between the cycle length without and with ipsilateral BBB equals the conduction time from the nonblocked bundle branch across the septum to the terminals of the blocked bundle branch. Wellens and Durrer[35] reported that this interval ranged from 20 to 50 ms. However, Kerr et al.[36] found that in the presence of ipsilateral BBB the minimum VA interval increased by an average of 61 ms, whereas no change in cycle length occurred in the presence of contralateral BBB. It should be added that the increase in tachycardia cycle length in the presence of ipsilateral BBB is too small to be detected when the accessory pathway is located in the septum (septal pathway) or when an increase in AV conduction time counteracts the delay caused by the BBB.

Coumel and Attuel[37] described a phenomenon called the "paradoxical capture." They showed that if BBB was present during tachycardia, a premature impulse elicited in the ventricle of the blocked bundle branch could be followed by a VA interval shorter than the VA interval of the tachycardia complexes because there is no delay caused by conduction around the blocked bundle branch.

Criterion (5) is an occasional occurrence of electrical alternans during tachycardia. This is probably not a peculiarity of the circuit but rather the consequence of rapid rates during AV reentrant tachycardia, which are frequently faster than AV node reentrant tachycardia.[38]

Criterion (6) is the sequence of the atrial excitation. The earliest excitation of the impulse

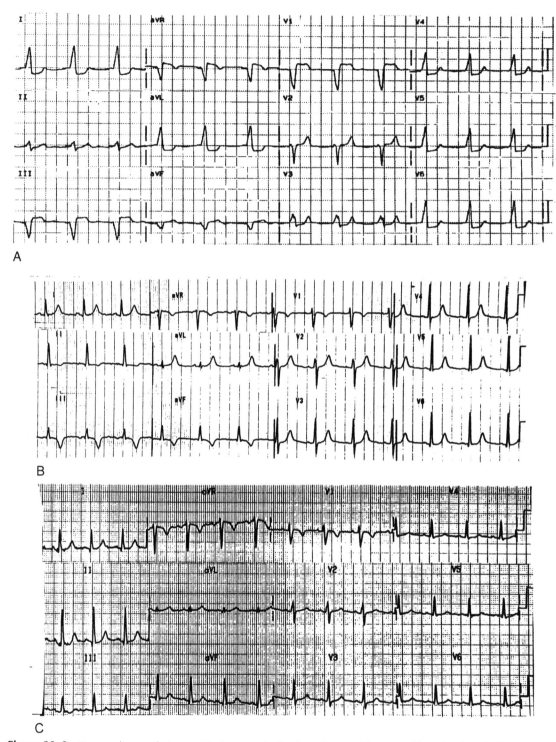

Figure 20–9 T wave changes during ventricular preexcitation in a 45-year-old woman (**A**) on the day of ablation of the right posterior accessory pathway (**B**) and 40 days later (**C**). See text discussion. (From Surawicz B: Transient T wave abnormalities after cessation of ventricular preexcitation: memory of what? J Cardiovasc Electrophysiol 7:51, 1996.)

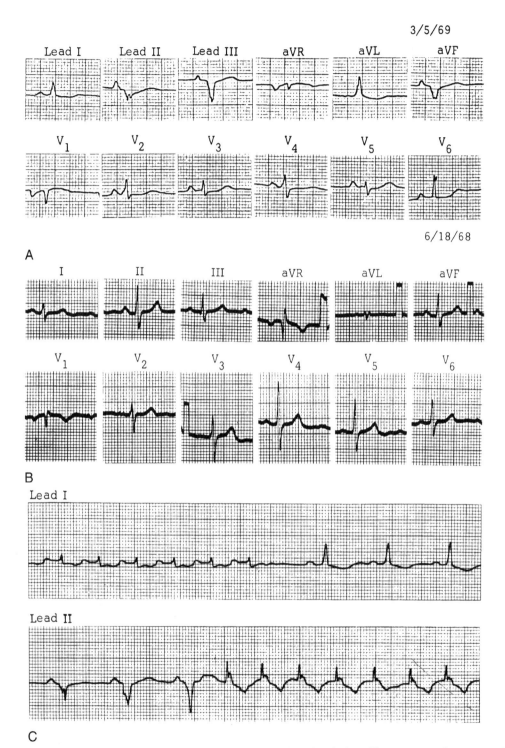

Figure 20–10   ECG of a 35-year-old woman with Ebstein's anomaly with right lateral bypass tract and recurrent episodes of orthodromic atrioventricular (AV) reentrant tachycardia. **A,** Abnormal P waves. The QRS morphology is consistent with ventricular preexcitation. The PR interval is within normal limits (0.14 second). **B,** Tracing recorded during normal AV conduction. The PR interval is longer. There is borderline abnormal right axis deviation. Lead V_1 shows a QR pattern. **C,** Tracing demonstrating intermittent AV reentrant tachycardia with a retrograde P wave following the QRS. Note the change in morphology of the QRS complexes during tachycardia. Epicardial mapping during sinus rhythm with the Wolff-Parkinson-White pattern revealed early ventricular excitation at the lateral border of the right ventricle near the AV groove. During orthodromic AV reentrant tachycardia, the same area was the latest among the mapping sites to be activated. The findings suggest a right lateral location of the bypass.

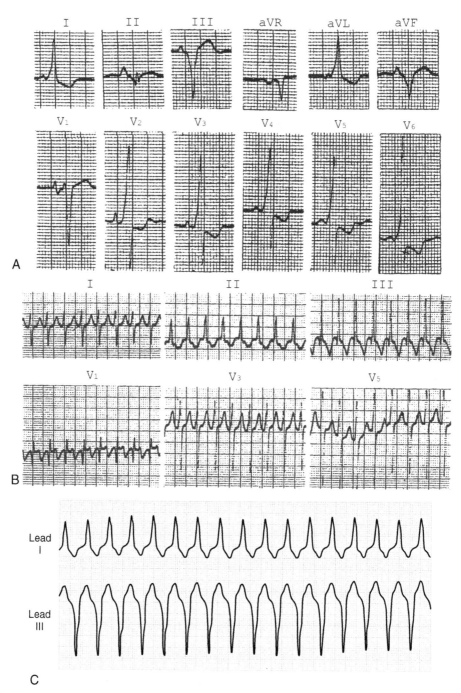

Figure 20–11   Wolff-Parkinson-White (WPW) syndrome in a 28-year-old man with ostium secondum type atrial septal defect. **A,** During sinus rhythm there is a WPW pattern, with a pseudoinfarction pattern in the inferior leads. **B,** During atrio-ventricular (AV) reentrant tachycardia the QRS complex is narrow and the delta wave is no longer present, suggesting normal anterograde AV conduction (orthodromic tachycardia). The morphology of the QRS complexes is consistent with right ventricular hypertrophy. **C,** On another occasion the patient developed tachycardia with wide QRS complexes similar to those during sinus rhythm, suggesting anomalous anterograde AV conduction through the bypass (antidromic tachycardia). The rhythm was later proved to be atrial flutter with 2:1 conduction.

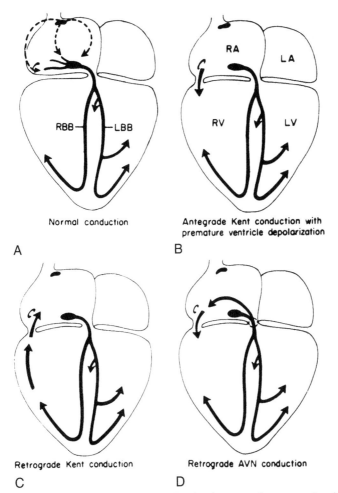

Normal conduction

A

Antegrade Kent conduction with
premature ventricle depolarization

B

Retrograde Kent conduction

C

Retrograde AVN conduction

D

Figure 20–12   Most common mechanism responsible for the development of paroxysmal tachycardia associated with Wolff-Parkinson-White syndrome. **A,** Normal conduction pathways of atria and ventricles. **B,** Anterograde Kent conduction with premature ventricular depolarization. **C,** Excitation impulse conducts anterogradely through the normal atrioventricular (AV) conduction system and returns to the atrium retrogradely through the accessory pathway. A circus movement is therefore established, resulting in orthodromic AV reentrant tachycardia. **D,** The impulse is conducted anterogradely through the Kent bundle and retrogradely through the AV node (AVN). The reentrant supraventricular tachycardia has wide QRS complexes simulating ventricular tachycardia and is called *antidromic AV reentrant tachycardia.* (From Dreifus LS, Nichols H, Morse D, et al: Control of recurrent tachycardia of Wolff-Parkinson-White syndrome by surgical ligature of the A-V bundle. Circulation 38:1030, 1968, by permission of the American Heart Association.)

conducted retrogradely via the AV node takes place near the atrial septum. Evidence of retrograde conduction through the AV bypass tract is established when the earliest excitation site is remote from the septum. Atrial excitation becomes eccentric to the His bundle, and the earliest atrial activation site is recorded, depending on the location of the bypass tract, at sites surrounding the circumference of the mitral and tricuspid valves using multiple endocardial electrodes in the coronary sinus and right atrium.[3,36,39] The site of earliest atrial excitation helps locate the site of the bypass tract when it is situated at a distance from the AV node and the His bundle. However, intermediate septal

bypass tracts located in close proximity to the AV node and His bundle cannot be detected in this manner.

Some bypass sites are in close proximity to each other (e.g., posterior septal and left posterior bypass tracts), and the location of the site of the earliest atrial activation is not as helpful as directional conduction times established by multiple electrode catheters[40] or differences between the time of activation of the His bundle and atria.[41] Also, anteroseptal, midseptal, and right anterior free wall pathways may be best distinguished using programmed stimulation of the summit of the right ventricular septum and especially with changes in the VA interval when

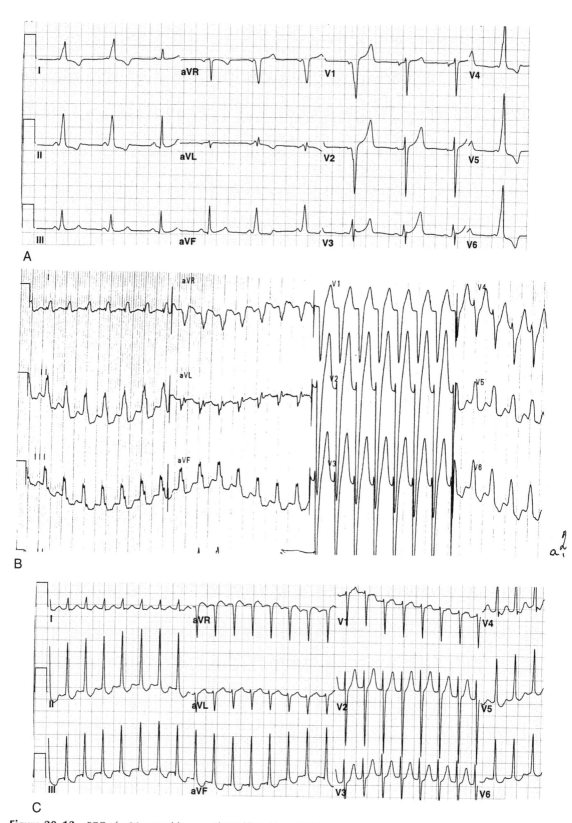

Figure 20–13   ECG of a 36-year-old man with Wolff-Parkinson-White syndrome. **A,** Intermittent preexcitation with a pattern suggestive of right anteroseptal bypass tract. **B,** Antidromic tachycardia at a rate of 175 beats/min. **C,** Orthodromic atrioventricular reentrant tachycardia at a rate of 185 beats/min with P wave inscribed during the ST segment.

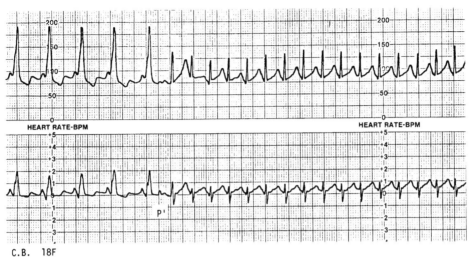

C.B.   18F

Figure 20–14   Orthodromic atrioventricular (AV) reentrant tachycardia initiated by a premature atrial complex. The first five complexes of the simultaneously recorded leads show sinus rhythm with ventricular preexcitation. A premature atrial complex (P′) initiates the narrow QRS complex tachycardia (orthodromic AV reentrant tachycardia) at a rate of 186 beats/min. During the tachycardia the retrograde P waves can be seen after the QRS complexes, most distinctly in the bottom strip.

right bundle branch block (RBBB) develops during orthodromic reentrant tachycardia.[42]

Criterion (7) is the demonstration that the impulse is conducted from the ventricle to the atria at the time when the His bundle is refractory. Conversely, the presence of AV block during continuing tachycardia (see Figure 16–13) rules out the tachycardia utilizing the AV bypass tract.

The effect of drugs is criterion (8). The effective refractory period of the AV node and of the AP is lengthened by different categories of drugs (i.e., adenosine, β-adrenergic blockers, calcium channel blockers, and digitalis for the AV node and class 1A sodium channel blockers for the AP). Therefore the response to a drug may be helpful occasionally in the differential diagnosis between AV node reentrant and AV reentrant tachycardia. These criteria, however, are not reliable in the presence of atypical electrophysiologic properties of the AV node or the AP.

AP WITH DECREMENTAL CONDUCTION

In some cases of AV reentrant tachycardia, the AP conducts the impulse as slowly as or slower than the normally conducting AV node. Such decremental conduction was found in 7.6 percent of APs in 653 patients.[43] Most of these atypical APs are located in the posteroseptal region,[44] and the associated tachycardia is called the *permanent form of junctional reciprocating tachycardia,* as was first described by Coumel et al.[45] (see Chapter 16). Patients with AP located in the left

or right free wall also have been reported.[44,46,47] The tachycardia tends to be "incessant." It is usually initiated by lengthening of the PR interval or a premature complex and can be produced or aggravated by antiarrhythmia drugs.[48]

ATRIAL FIBRILLATION AND ATRIAL FLUTTER

Atrial fibrillation was mentioned in the original description of the syndrome by Wolff, Parkinson, and White in 1930. In 1952, Langendorf et al.[49] pointed out that preexcitation should be suspected if the ventricular rate during atrial fibrillation with a wide QRS complex is unusually rapid.

Castellanos et al.[50] have shown that the rapid ventricular rate is associated with a short, effective refractory period of the AP. This association was confirmed by Wellens and Durrer[51] during atrial fibrillation induced in patients with WPW syndrome.

Atrial fibrillation and flutter (see Figures 20–7B and 20–15) are less common than AV reentrant tachycardia in the WPW syndrome. The reported incidence of atrial fibrillation was 20 to 35 percent[18,20,30,44,52] and that of atrial flutter was 7 percent[44] among patients with tachyarrhythmias. In most cases the atrial impulses during atrial fibrillation and atrial flutter are conducted to the ventricles through the AP. Therefore the preexcited QRS complexes are wide with an additional increase in duration caused by aberrant ventricular conduction. The latter is often present because the ventricular rate may be as rapid as 220 to 360 beats/min

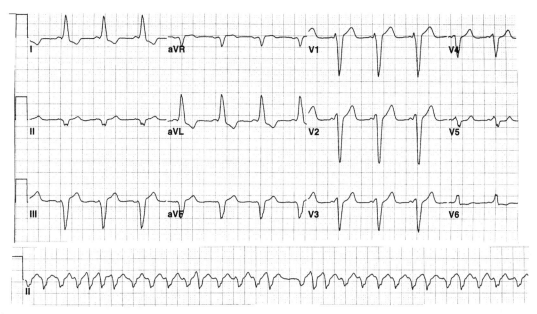

Figure 20–15 *Top*, ECG of a 46-year-old woman with Wolff-Parkinson-White syndrome and a pattern suggestive of right posterior paraseptal bypass tract. The pattern simulates left bundle branch block. *Bottom*, Strip of lead II shows atrial fibrillation with a ventricular rate of 197 beats/min.

(see Figure 20–7B). Such a rapid rate is possible in the presence of a short, effective refractory period of the accessory bundle.

Because of the rapid ventricular response during atrial fibrillation, patients with the WPW syndrome may develop ventricular fibrillation that results in sudden death.[25,53] Klein and co-workers[5] found that a short, effective refractory period (i.e., 250 ms or less) increases the risk of ventricular fibrillation in the presence of atrial fibrillation, atrial flutter, or other rapid atrial tachycardia. The presence of multiple APs also renders the patient more susceptible to the development of this potentially lethal arrhythmia.[54]

The occurrence of atrial fibrillation appears to be facilitated by the presence of reentrant tachycardia. This is suggested by the low recurrence rate of atrial fibrillation after surgical[55] and catheter[56] ablation. The probable mechanism of atrial fibrillation is stimulation during the atrial vulnerable period by the impulse returning to the atria (see Chapter 15).

With atrial flutter, the regular rhythm with wide QRS complexes is often mistaken for paroxysmal ventricular tachycardia (see Figure 20–11). The AV conduction ratio may be 2:1 or 1:1. Indeed, atrial flutter with 1:1 conduction is rare in the absence of the WPW syndrome unless the atrial rate is relatively slow owing to treatment with sodium channel–blocking drugs.

With atrial fibrillation, the erroneous diagnosis of ventricular tachycardia can often be avoided because of the gross irregularity of the ventricular response (see Figures 20–7B and 20–15). The presence of the WPW syndrome is often suspected from the rhythm strip alone if the ventricular rate during atrial fibrillation exceeds about 200 beats/min. Such a rapid ventricular response would be unusual if the impulses were conducted via the normal AV conduction system. Although ventricular tachycardia can occur in subjects with WPW syndrome, it is unrelated to the syndrome unless tachycardia originates in the bypass tissue.

ABORTED SUDDEN DEATH WITH THE WPW SYNDROME

Among 690 patients with the WPW syndrome referred to the Academic Hospital in Maastricht, the Netherlands,[57] aborted sudden death outside the hospital setting occurred in 15 (2.2 percent). Ventricular fibrillation was the first manifestation of the WPW syndrome in 8 patients; the remaining patients had atrial fibrillation, circus movement tachycardia, or both. The location of the AP was septal in 11 patients, left lateral in 4, and right lateral in 1.

ELECTROPHYSIOLOGIC PROPERTIES OF THE APs

Anterograde refractoriness of the AP is studied by delivering atrial premature stimuli (A_1A_2); retrograde refractoriness is studied by delivering ventricular premature stimuli (V_1V_2). The anterograde effective refractory period is the longest A_1A_2 interval recorded nearest the AP at which A_2 conducts to ventricles without preexcitation. The retrograde effective refractory period is the longest V_1V_2 interval recorded nearest the AP with the activation sequence compatible with retrograde conduction through the accessory bypass tract.

Unlike the AV node, conduction time through the AV bypass tract is not dependent on the cycle length, and this is helpful for evaluating AP function. However, atypical patterns of conduction can occur through both the AP and the AV node. This means that conduction through the AP becomes time dependent; conversely, the AV nodal transmission becomes virtually time independent.

CONCEALED AP: CONCEALED WPW SYNDROME

An accessory AV pathway may be capable only of retrograde conduction. Anterograde block in the AP with preserved retrograde conduction results in an absence of the WPW pattern on the surface ECG (i.e., concealment of the bypass tract). However, the bypass tract can be utilized in the retrograde direction as a link in the AV reentrant circuit.[58-60]

The pathway is called *concealed accessory pathway* or *bypass*. Its existence can be documented only by intracardiac studies.[58,60-63] When a reentrant tachycardia occurs in association with such a concealed bypass, the condition is called *concealed WPW syndrome*. It is the most common variant form of WPW syndrome and occurs in about 20 to 30 percent of patients with APs.[64,65]

Patients with this syndrome have AV reentrant tachycardia when a sinus or an atrial impulse is conducted to the ventricle through the normal AV conduction system. From the ventricle the impulse is conducted retrogradely through the concealed bypass to reactivate the atrium and initiate a reciprocating tachycardia. Such a mechanism may be responsible for many reentrant tachycardias that were formerly attributed to AV nodal reentry. Paroxysms of atrial flutter or fibrillation may develop in such patients if the retrograde activation of the atrium occurs during its vulnerable period.

In most of the reported cases of concealed WPW syndrome, the AP is located on the left side of the cardiac chambers.[60,61] In a few cases the location is right sided or septal. The site of the anterograde conduction block appears to be located almost always near the AP–ventricular interface.[66]

Farshidi and associates[34] considered the following findings during tachycardia to be suggestive of a concealed bypass tract: (1) negative P wave in lead I (because of left-sided bypass and early left atrial depolarization), (2) P wave during the ST segment, and (3) increased cycle length if functional left bundle branch block (LBBB) develops.

Atrioventricular reentrant tachycardia due to the presence of a concealed AP is shown in Figure 20–16. A less common type of unidirectional block is a retrograde unidirectional block in the AP. This can be detected by means of ventricular stimulation in 5 percent of patients with single APs. In such cases the accessory bypass tract can cause antidromic reentrant tachycardia or "preexcited" atrial tachyarrhythmias, or it can serve as an "innocent bystander" in patients with AV nodal reentrant tachycardia.

Anatomic Findings: Localization of the AP by Routine ECG

Ventricular preexcitation was once believed to be the result of congenital clefts in the fibrous AV ring that are occupied by muscular bridges serving as APs. Later, anatomic studies at autopsy and during surgery showed that the APs (Kent bundles) skirt but do not perforate the fibrous annulus.[67,68] They may be found in the right (tricuspid) or left (mitral) side of the AV ring as well as in the interventricular septal area.[69]

With the advent of ablation treatment of refractory tachyarrhythmias in patients with WPW syndrome, precise localization of the site of the AP became important. The extensive surgical experience from Duke University indicated that the routine ECG was useful for localizing an approximate site of the AP in most cases.[20,25,70] Figure 20–17 shows a schematic drawing of the cross section of AV ring depicting 10 sites of preexcitation, and Figure 20–18 shows the polarity of the delta wave at these sites in the 12-lead ECG.

Rodriguez et al.[71] found it helpful to distinguish the major AP locations by the differences in the frontal plane QRS axis combined with differences in locations of the frontal plane delta wave axis. Arruda et al.[72] developed an ECG algorithm for identifying AP ablation sites based on correlations of a 12-lead ECG with the successful radiofrequency ablation site in 135 patients with a single anterogradely conducting AP. This algorithm correctly identified the AP location in 87 percent of patients and was subsequently successfully tested prospectively in 121 patients. AP locations were

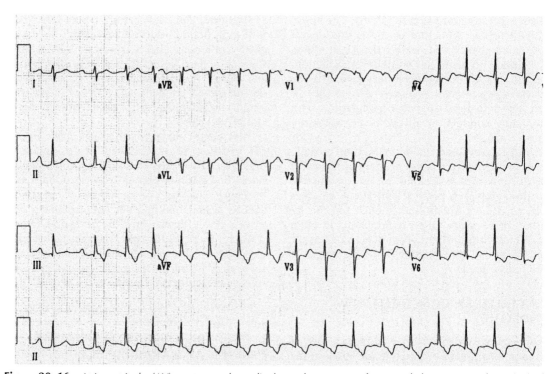

Figure 20–16 Atrioventricular (AV) reentrant tachycardia due to the presence of a concealed accessory pathway (AP). The ECG shows first-degree AV block. The first complex is sinus in origin. The second complex is followed by an atrial echo, which initiates AV reentrant tachycardia. The fact that the QRS complex in the first complex is normal without a delta wave indicates that the AP is concealed. The presence of a left-sided concealed AP was documented during electrophysiologic studies. The patient also has a standby dual AV nodal pathway manifested by two different PR intervals on different ECGs (not shown).

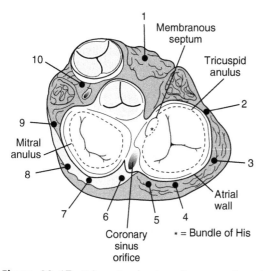

Figure 20–17 Schematic drawing of cross-section of atrioventricular ring depicting 10 sites of epicardial preexcitation. 1 = right anterior paraseptal; 2 = right anterior; 3 = right lateral; 4 = right posterior; 5 = right posterior paraseptal; 6 = left posterior paraseptal; 7 = left posterior; 8 = left lateral; 9 = left anterior; 10 = left anterior paraseptal. (Reprinted with permission from Gallagher JJ, Pritchett ELC, Sealy WC, et al: The preexcitation syndromes. Prog Cardiovasc Dis 20: 285, 1978.)

divided into three main regions, which were further subdivided as shown in Figure 20–19.

The *septal APs* were subdivided into five regions, as follows:

1. Anteroseptal tricuspid annulus and right anterior paraseptal (AS/RAPS), which includes APs located up to 10 mm anterior to the His bundle, in which both the AP and a His potential can be recorded from the same bipolar electrode

2. Midseptal tricuspid annulus (MSTA), which includes APs located at the septal section of the tricuspid annulus between the posteroseptal and anteroseptal regions

3. Posteroseptal tricuspid annulus (PSTA), including APs located near the coronary sinus (CSOs)

4. Posteroseptal mitral annulus (PSMA)

5. Subepicardial posteroseptal APs, which consist of APs that required ablation from within the subepicardial venous system (occasionally at the left posterior region), including the middle cardiac vein and other coronary veins or in anomalies of

DELTA WAVE POLARITY

	I	II	III	AVR	AVL	AVF	V$_1$	V$_2$	V$_3$	V$_4$	V$_5$	V$_6$
(1)	+	+	+(±)	−	±(+)	+	±	±	+(±)	+	+	+
(2)	+	+	−(±)	−	+(±)	±(−)	±	+(±)	+(±)	+	+	+
(3)	+	±(−)	−	−	+	−(±)	±	±	±	+	+	+
(4)	+	−	−	−	+	−	±(+)	±	+	+	+	+
(5)	+	−	−	−(+)	+	−	±	+	+	+	+	+
(6)	+	−	−	−	+	−	+	+	+	+	+	+
(7)	+	−	−	±(+)	+	−	+	+	+	+	+	−(±)
(8)	−(±)	±	±	±(+)	−(±)	±	+	+	+	+	−(±)	−(±)
(9)	−(±)	+	+	−	−(±)	+	+	+	+	+	+	+
(10)	+	+	+(±)	−	±	+	±(+)	+	+	+	+	+

Figure 20–18 Expected polarity at 10 sites of ventricular insertion of accessory atrioventricular connections for each of 12 standard ECG leads, based on analysis of initial activation at 40 ms of ventricular depolarization in documented cases of single accessory pathways with no associated anomalies. ± = isoelectric; + = positive; − = negative. (Reprinted with permission from Gallagher JJ, Pritchett ELC, Sealy WC, et al: The preexcitation syndromes. Prog Cardiovasc Dis 20: 285, 1978.)

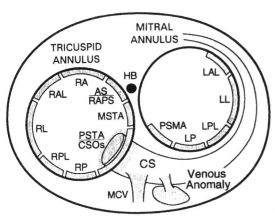

Figure 20–19 The heart as viewed in the left anterior oblique projection. Nomenclature used to describe accessory pathway locations. AS = anteroseptal; CS = coronary sinus venous anomaly (coronary sinus diverticulum); CSOs = coronary sinus ostium; HB = His bundle; LAL = left anterolateral; LL = left lateral; LP = left posterior; LPL = left posterolateral; MCV = middle cardiac vein (coronary vein); MSTA = mid-septal tricuspid annulus; PSMA = posteroseptal mitral annulus; PSTA = posteroseptal tricuspid annulus; RA = right anterior; RAL = right anterolateral; RAPS = right anterior paraseptal; RL = right lateral; RP = right posterior; RPL = right posterolateral. (From Arruda MS, McClelland JH, Wang X, et al: Development and validation of an ECG algorithm for identifying accessory pathway ablation site in Wolff-Parkinson-White syndrome. J Cardiovasc Electrophysiol 9:2, 1998, by permission.)

the coronary sinus such as a diverticulum (subepicardial)

The *right free-wall APs* were subdivided into five regions, as follows:

1. Right anterior (RA)
2. Right anterolateral (RAL)
3. Right lateral (RL)
4. Right posterolateral (RPL)
5. Right posterior (RP)

The *left free-wall APs* were subdivided into four regions, as follows:

1. Left anterolateral (LAL)
2. Left lateral (LL)
3. Left posterolateral (LPL)
4. Left posterior (LP)

The polarity of the delta wave was measured during the initial 20 ms of the preexcitation and was classified as positive (+), negative (−), or isoelectric (+−). The algorithm is shown in Figure 20–20 and is described as follows:

Step 1: If the delta wave in lead I is (−) or (±) or the R/S in lead V$_1$ is >1, a left free-wall AP is present. If this criterion is fulfilled, lead aV$_F$ is examined. If the delta wave in lead aV$_F$ is (+), an LL/LAL AP is identified. If a delta wave in lead aV$_F$ is (±) or (−), the AP is located at the LP/LPL region. If the criteria in leads I and V$_1$ are not fulfilled, a septal or right-free wall AP pathway is identified. Proceed to step 2.

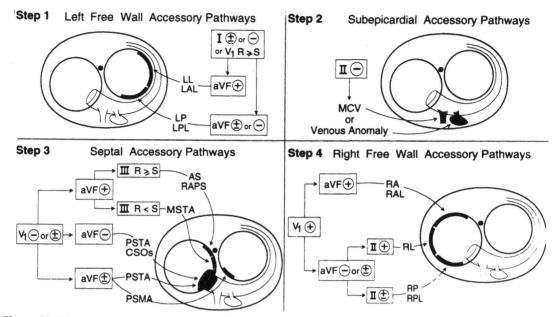

Figure 20–20   Stepwise ECG algorithm for predicting accessory pathway location. Abbreviations as in Figure 20–19. See text for explanation. (From Arruda MS, McClelland JH, Wang X, et al: Development and validation of an ECG algorithm for identifying accessory pathway ablation site in Wolff-Parkinson-White syndrome. J Cardiovasc Electrophysiol 9:2, 1998, with permission.)

Step 2: Lead II is examined. A (−) delta wave in lead II identifies the subepicardial posteroseptal AP. If the delta wave in lead II is (±) or (+), proceed to step 3.

Step 3: Lead V_1 is examined. A (−) or (±) delta wave identifies a septal AP. If this criterion is fulfilled, lead aV_F is examined. If the delta wave in lead aV_F is (−), an AP is identified that is located at the PSTA/CSOs. If the delta wave is (+−) in lead aV_F, the AP may be located close to either PSTA or the PSMA. A (+) delta wave in aV_F identifies the AS/RAPS or MS regions. These two regions are differentiated by examining the R/S ratio in lead III: R >S identifies AS/RAPS AP, and R <S identifies an AP located along MSTA. If the delta wave in lead V_1 is (+) (after having excluded patients with a left free-wall APs, in step 1), a right free-wall AP is identified. Proceed to step 4.

Step 4: In patients with right free-wall APs, examine lead aV_F. A (+) delta wave in lead aV_F identifies RA/RAL. If the delta wave in aV_F is (±) or (−), examine lead II. A (+) delta wave in lead II identifies RP/RPL.

Earlier, Chiang et al.[73] suggested a similar algorithm based on comprehensive analysis of the delta wave in the limb leads and an R/S ratio in leads V_1 and V_2 in 369 patients who underwent successful radiofrequency ablation.

CORRELATION OF THE LOCATION OF AN AP AND ELECTROPHYSIOLOGIC PROPERTIES

In four series of patients in which a total of 906 APs were successfully ablated by catheter or surgery, 560 (61.8 percent) pathways were located in the free wall of the left ventricle.[44,65,66,74] The remaining 115 pathways (38.2 percent) were in the free wall of the right ventricle, 61 were in the anteroseptal area, 158 were in the posteroseptal area, and 12 were in the midseptal area. About 21 to 30 percent of the pathways were concealed.

In a study of 817 patients who underwent ablation of APs, Haissaguerre and co-workers[75] reported the following breakdown: About 50 percent of pathways were left lateral, about 25 percent were posteroseptal, about 15 percent were right lateral, about 5 percent were Mahaim fibers, and about 5 percent were APs with retrograde decremental conduction properties giving rise to permanent junctional reciprocating tachycardia. Location of APs in close proximity to the His bundle (parahisian) was identified in 8 of 582 consecutive patients who underwent radiofrequency ablation of APs.[76]

Among the 384 symptomatic patients with a single AP studied by de Chillou and associates,[44] the concealed AP was more common in the left free wall or in a posteroseptal location. The researchers also found that the decremental conduction property in the AP was related to the location of the pathway. Anterograde decremental conduction property was associated only with right free pathways, and retrograde decremental conduction was found only in patients with a posteroseptal or left free wall pathway.

MULTIPLE APs

The presence of more than one AP is not unexpected if one accepts the premise that such pathways result from an imperfect separation between the atria and the ventricles during cardiac development. In addition to offering diagnostic and therapeutic challenges, multiple pathways increase the probability of multiple reentrant circuits. For example, in a case reported by Portillo et al.,[77] three APs and two internodal pathways produced three types of reciprocal tachycardia.

The incidence of multiple pathways in patients with WPW syndrome studied electrophysiologically ranges from 5 to 15 percent. Of 388 patients with APs studied at Duke University, 52 (13 percent) had multiple APs.[78] The following criteria were proposed to recognize the presence of multiple pathways[78]: (1) two or more patterns of preexcitation during sinus rhythm, atrial pacing, atrial fibrillation, or antidromic circus movement; (2) two or more pathways of atrial activation during orthodromic circus movement or ventricular pacing; and (3) an antidromic tachycardia using another AP as the retrograde limb of the tachycardia or vice versa. The incidence of multiple pathways is increased in patients with Ebstein's anomaly and those with atrial fibrillation or ventricular fibrillation.[79]

ANTIDROMIC REENTRANT TACHYCARDIA

Antidromic reentrant tachycardia is a wide QRS tachycardia with the morphology of a fully preexcited ventricular complex. The conduction proceeds in the anterograde direction through the bypass tract and returns via the His bundle and AV node (see Figure 20–13B). This is the least common cause of wide QRS tachycardia. It occurs in about 10 percent of patients with WPW syndrome undergoing electrophysiologic evaluation[80]; and one third of these patients harbor multiple APs. There is also a relatively high incidence of atrial fibrillation and ventricular fibrillation. The diagnosis is established by the following criteria: (1) QRS morphology identical to that of the fully preexcited complex; (2)

establishment of circus movement; and (3) documented participation of both ventricles and atria in the reentrant circuit.

Conditions favorable for development of antidromic tachycardia include: (1) short, effective refractory period of the entire retrograde VA conduction system; (2) short anterograde effective refractory period of the AP; and (3) location of the bypass tract farther from the AV node.[81] In a study of 30 patients with antidromic AV reentrant tachycardia, Parker and associates[81] found that the pathways in these patients were located at least 5 cm away from the AV node, and no patient with a posteroseptal AP had this form of tachycardia.

Reentrant Tachycardia Associated with a Short PR Interval and Lown-Ganong-Levine Syndrome

In the early literature, the short PR interval was attributed to the presence of paranodal fibers described by James.[82] The sinus impulse is conducted through these fibers and bypasses most or all of the AV node, thereby avoiding the normal delay at the AV node. The QRS complex is normal in duration and morphology. Other explanations for the short PR interval include a small, underdeveloped AV node,[83,84] a preferential fast pathway, or unusually rapid conduction in an anatomically normal AV node.[20,85-87]

The ECG findings of Lown-Ganong-Levine (LGL) syndrome[88] include the following:

1. PR interval less than 0.12 second (in adults), with normal P wave
2. Normal QRS duration
3. Paroxysmal tachycardia

The mechanisms, and even the mere existence, of such a syndrome have been disputed; even if the term remains in use, it should not be applied to the ECG findings of short PR interval and normal QRS, with no history of paroxysmal tachycardia. In such cases, when the history of tachycardia is unknown, the term *accelerated AV conduction* is appropriate. The early literature suggested that this syndrome may be caused by the atriofascicular bypass tract.[89] Indeed, an infant with short PR, supraventricular tachycardia, and atriofascicular connection was described.[90] However, such cases are rare, and, as discussed in Chapter 16, most cases of enhanced AV conduction manifested by an AH interval of 60 ms or short PR interval during sinus rhythm are believed to represent but one of a continuous spectrum of normal AV nodal physiology.[91] The mechanism of tachycardia in such cases is either AV nodal reentry[29] or AV reentry via a concealed bypass tract.[92] Another cause of short PR may be excessive sympathetic stimulation. In one case, short PR in a patient with pheochromocytoma disappeared when the tumor was resected.[93]

Atrial fibrillation and atrial flutter are occasionally observed in patients with a short PR interval, and the ventricular response may be rapid. Ventricular rates as fast as 300 beats/min have been reported.[94] Ventricular tachycardia also has been described.[29,95,96]

Mahaim-Type Preexcitation

In 1941 Mahaim and Winston[97] described muscular bridges connecting the AV node and ventricular myocardium, as well as discrete connections between the fascicles to the ventricles. Almost all Mahaim fibers are right sided. Depending on the origin of the fibers, these bypass tracts may be called *atriofascicular, nodoventricular* (or *nodofascicular*), or *fasciculoventricular* connections[98,99] (see Figure 20–1). A sinus impulse may therefore travel to the right atrium and upper part of the AV node with the normal delay, but it is followed by premature excitation of the basal part of the ventricular myocardium, resulting in the inscription of a delta wave. This variant form of preexcitation with a normal PR interval and delta wave cannot be differentiated from the occasional cases of ventricular preexcitation via the bundle of Kent with a normal PR interval caused by a long intraatrial conduction time or slow conduction in the bypass tract[60]

(Figure 20–21). Furthermore, many patients with Mahaim fibers show no delta wave on their ECG during sinus rhythm (Figure 20–22). Preexcitation, not manifested during sinus rhythm, may be shown by rapid atrial pacing when the delay in the AV node occurs and the His bundle deflection is displaced into the QRS complex.

Reentrant tachycardia in patients with the nodoventricular- or atriofascicular-type Mahaim fibers typically has LBBB morphology with a superior axis. The excitation proceeds over a macroreentry circuit, with the Mahaim fibers serving as the anterograde limb and the His-Purkinje system as the retrograde limb.[68,100,101] Bardy and colleagues[100] suggested that the following findings during tachycardia with LBBB morphology were predictive of the presence of nodoventricular (nodofascicular) fibers: ventricular rate of 134 to 270 beats/min; QRS axis of 0 to −75 degrees; QRS duration of 0.15 second or less; R wave in lead I; rS wave in lead V_1; and precordial transition from a negative to a positive QRS complex after lead V_4. These findings were present in 12 of the 13 patients in their study. Nodoventricular tachycardia is illustrated in Figure 20–22.

It has been suggested that the "nodoventricular pathway" is a variant of the AV bypass tract (i.e., an anomalous connection between the right atrium and the right bundle branch[102,103] or the right ventricular myocardium).[103] The absence of preexcitation and delta waves during sinus rhythm is explained by slow conduction and decremental properties of the pathway. The reentrant circuit involves anterograde conduction

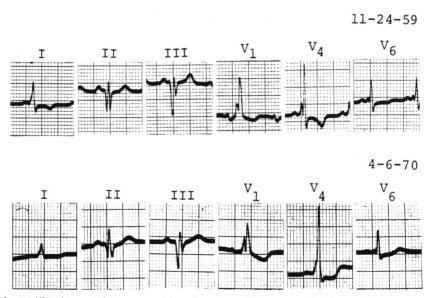

Figure 20–21 Wolff-Parkinson-White pattern with prolongation of the PR interval with age. The PR interval in the tracing in 1959 is 0.11 second. It increases to 0.16 second in 1970. The QRS morphology is essentially unchanged.

over the accessory pathway and retrograde conduction over the bundle branches. Nevertheless, the existence of nodofascicular (or nodoventricular) pathways cannot be dismissed.[104] Nodofascicular tachycardia should be suspected if: (1) intermittent anterograde preexcitation is recorded; (2) the tachycardia can be initiated with a single atrial premature stimulus producing two ventricular complexes; and (3) a single ventricular extrastimulus initiates supraventricular tachycardia without a retrograde His deflection.[105]

In the absence of reentrant tachycardia, Mahaim fibers can be suspected when two different morphologies of the ventricular complex appear within a short time interval without any intervening clinical events (see Figure 27–10).

ATRIOFASCICULAR TRACTS

Evidence from electrophysiologic studies, catheter ablation, and surgery has definitely established that right atriofascicular fibers crossing the tricuspid annulus serve as the basis for

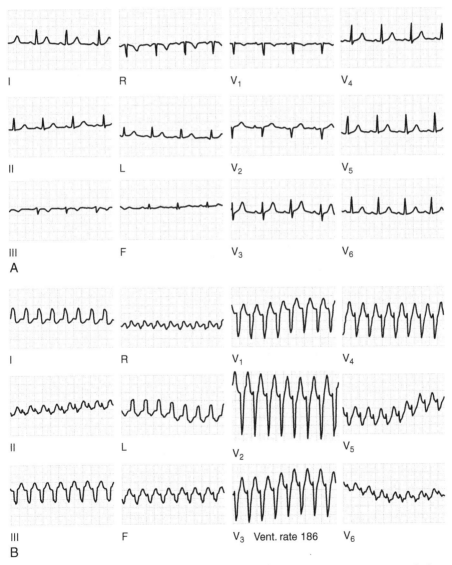

Figure 20–22 Nodoventricular tachycardia in a 14-year-old girl with recurrent episodes of tachycardia but no other evidence of organic heart disease. **A,** The resting 12-lead ECG is within normal limits, but the absence of Q waves in leads I, V_5, and V_6 and the small R waves in leads V_1 and V_2 are uncommon at this age. **B,** During tachycardia the QRS complexes have a left bundle branch block appearance. The heart rate is 186 beats/min. The other findings are similar to those described by Bardy and colleagues.[100] Electrophysiological studies supported the diagnosis of nodoventricular tachycardia. During sinus rhythm, the AH and HV intervals and the QRS duration are normal (not shown). With atrial pacing at increasing rates (shorter S_1S_1 interval) there was progressive lengthening of the AH interval, but the HV interval was progressively shortened. The QRS duration gradually increased, but 1:1 AV conduction was maintained.

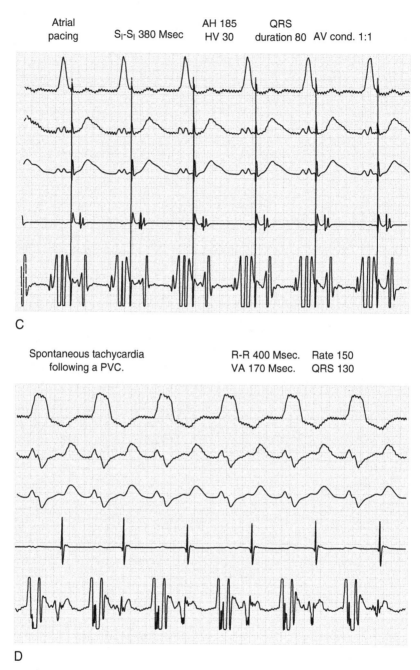

Figure 20–22 cont'd   **C,** Various measurements when the pacing interval (S_1S_1) was 380 ms; AH interval, 185 ms; HV interval, 30 ms; QRS duration, 80 ms; AV conduction, 1:1. These findings suggest the presence of an accessory pathway (Mahaim fibers) that bypasses the His bundle. **D,** During the study an episode of tachycardia developed spontaneously following a premature ventricular complex. The morphology of the QRS complexes is identical to that in **B.** The His bundle potential is not seen. There is retrograde atrial activation. (Courtesy of Dr. Winston Gaum, Cincinnati, OH.)

typical Mahaim conduction in most if not all of these patients.[106] A case of atriofascicular pathway inserting into the left bundle branch has been reported.[107] The physiologic properties of these fiber tracts were found to be similar to those in the AV node.[108]

FASCICULOVENTRICULAR FIBERS

Fasciculoventricular Mahaim fibers arise from the His bundle or bundle branches and enter the ventricles. The PR interval is normal, the HV interval is shortened, and there is slight ventricular preexcitation manifested by slurring of the initial QRS portion. No specific arrhythmias have been associated with this condition,[3] but the AV bypass tracts often coexist with the fasciculoventricular fiber tracts.[109]

AUTOMATICITY IN THE AP

Impulse formation within the AP was postulated by Pick and Katz in 1955.[110] Cases reported by Lerman and Josephson[111] and by Deam et al.[112] support the existence of such a phenomenon, even though the bypass tract is usually composed of ordinary myocardial fibers. Automaticity was found in 5 of 40 patients with Mahaim fibers, a finding suggestive of the presence of AV nodal–like structures in these fibers.[113]

LONGITUDINAL DISSOCIATION IN THE AP

Similar to the AV node, a fast and a slow pathway (with decremental conduction) are known to coexist in some accessory pathways. The resulting longitudinal dissociation can be diagnosed during orthodromic or antidromic tachycardia by sudden changes in cycle length, AV or VA intervals without changes in AV nodal conduction, pattern of preexcitation, and sequence of activation.[114]

Ventricular Hypertrophy, BBB, and MI in the Presence of the WPW Pattern

Because of the altered sequence of ventricular activation, the usual diagnostic criteria for left (LVH) and right (RVH) ventricular hypertrophy cannot be applied in patients with the WPW pattern. In patients with LVH the voltage is increased (Figure 20–23), but the voltage can be increased in the absence of hypertrophy. The evidence of LBBB may be masked, but the presence of RBBB associated with the preexcitation pattern is often recognized when there is a typical slow, anteriorly and rightward-directed terminal QRS portion. When the WPW pattern with a right-sided AP pattern and RBBB coexist, the findings are highly suggestive of Ebstein's anomaly[115] (Figure 20–24).

The frequent occurrence of the pseudoinfarction pattern in the WPW syndrome has been emphasized. In addition, preexcitation usually obscures the abnormal Q waves of true MI (Figure 20–25). An interesting example may be seen in Figure 20–26, in which the appearance of the WPW pattern obscures the presence of an old anterior MI but creates a pseudoinfarction pattern in the inferior leads. In patients with the WPW pattern and acute MI, ST segment elevation suggestive of myocardial injury may be seen

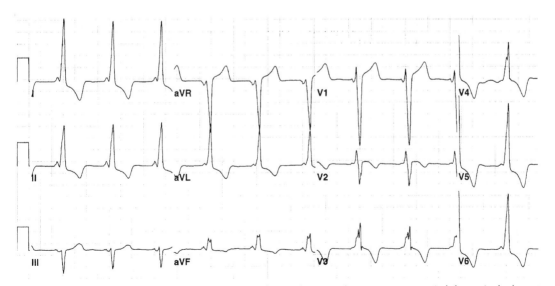

Figure 20–23   ECG of a 58-year-old man with hypertrophic cardiomyopathy, severe asymmetric left ventricular hypertrophy, and asymptomatic ventricular preexcitation. Patient also had significant stenosis of the left anterior descending coronary artery, treated with angioplasty.

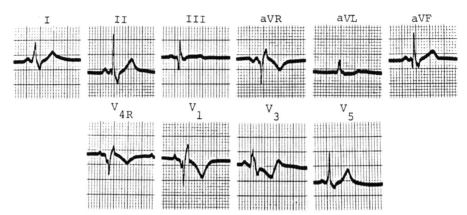

Figure 20–24   Ebstein's anomaly with Wolff-Parkinson-White (WPW) pattern. The presence of both a WPW pattern and a right bundle branch block pattern is highly suggestive of Ebstein's anomaly. (Courtesy of Dr. Samuel Kaplan, Cincinnati, OH.)

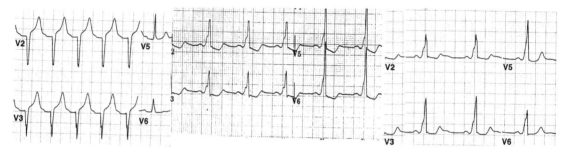

Figure 20–25   Four ECG precordial leads of a 71-year-old man with previous anterior myocardial infarction (MI). *Left,* Sinus tachycardia with normal atrioventricular conduction. *Middle,* Wolff-Parkinson-White pattern, suggestive of left posterior paraseptal bypass tract; there is ST segment depression in leads V_2–V_5 during an angina pectoris attack. *Right,* Ten hours later, after treatment with intravenous nitroglycerin, there is regression of the ST segment depression. The pattern of anterior MI is obscured by preexcitation.

in leads that normally would display isoelectric or depressed ST segments (Figure 20–27). Also, an abnormal ST segment depression suggestive of myocardial ischemia can be recognized in the presence of the WPW pattern (see Figure 20–25).

Effects of Drugs

The greatest threat to life from ventricular pre-excitation is a rapid ventricular rate during atrial fibrillation and other atrial tachyarrhythmias. The rapid rate is facilitated by a short, effective refractory period of the AP. A shortened effective refractory period may be caused also by digitalis and vagal stimulation. Digitalis, β-adrenergic drugs, and calcium channel blockers such as verapamil and diltiazem suppress transmission through the AV node and thereby facilitate transmission through the AP. Being composed of ventricular muscle fibers,

the AP responds in the same way as other ventricular myocardium to the action of drugs and neurotransmitters. Accordingly, conduction is slowed by sodium channel–blocking drugs, whereas refractoriness is prolonged by class IA and class III antiarrhythmia drugs.

Radiofrequency Ablation of APs

Current techniques make APs amenable to successful radiofrequency catheter ablation at all locations.[75,76] Some posteroseptal APs can be successfully ablated only from inside the coronary sinus or its branches.[116] They were reported to have a characteristic ECG pattern with a positive steep delta wave in lead aV_R and a deep S wave in lead V_6.[116] Radiofrequency current applied to the tricuspid annulus can safely eliminate tachycardia in patients with Mahaim fibers.[106]

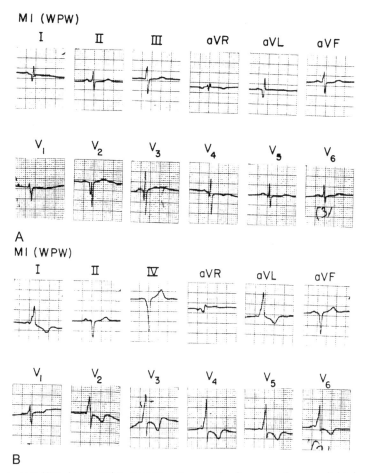

Figure 20–26 Effect of Wolff-Parkinson-White (WPW) pattern on the diagnosis of myocardial infarction (MI). **A,** During normal conduction through the atrioventricular node, the ECG shows a previous anterior and high lateral MI pattern. **B,** In the presence of a WPW pattern there is a pseudoinfarction pattern in the inferior leads, but the anterior and lateral infarction are no longer recognizable.

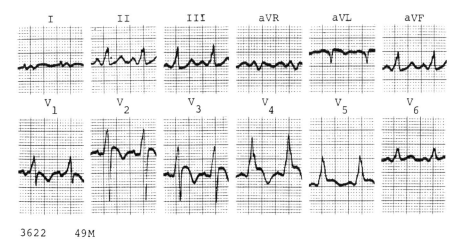

Figure 20–27 Acute myocardial infarction (MI) in the presence of a Wolff-Parkinson-White (WPW) pattern in a 49-year-old man with the typical symptoms and enzyme changes of acute MI. The tracing shows a WPW pattern. The presence of acute injury is indicated by the ST segment elevation in leads V_3–V_5. In uncomplicated cases of WPW pattern, the ST segment is either isoelectric or depressed in leads with an essentially upright QRS complex.

REFERENCES

1. Wolff L, Parkinson J, White PD: Bundle branch block with short P-R interval in healthy young people prone to paroxysmal tachycardia. Am Heart J 5:685, 1930.
2. Willems JL, DeMedina EO, Bernard R, et al: Criteria for intraventricular conduction disturbances and preexcitation. J Am Coll Cardiol 5:1261, 1985.
3. Prystowsky EN, Miles WM, Heger JJ, et al: Preexcitation syndromes: mechanisms and management. Med Clin North Am 68:831, 1984.
4. Berkman NL, Lamb LE: The Wolff-Parkinson-White electrocardiogram. N Engl J Med 278:492, 1968.
5. Klein GJ, Bashore TM, Sellers TD, et al: Ventricular fibrillation in the Wolff-Parkinson-White syndrome. N Engl J Med 301:1080, 1979.
6. Klein GJ, Gulamhusein SS: Intermittent preexcitation in the Wolff-Parkinson-White syndrome. Am J Cardiol 52:292, 1983.
7. Chung KY, Walsh TJ, Massie E: Wolff-Parkinson-White syndrome. Am Heart J 69:116, 1965.
8. Wolff L: Anomalous atrioventricular excitation (Wolff-Parkinson-White syndrome). Circulation 19: 14, 1959.
9. Grant RB, Tomlison FB, Van Buren JK: Ventricular activation in the pre-excitation syndrome (Wolff-Parkinson-White). Circulation 18:355, 1958.
10. Bogun F, Kalusche D, Li Y-G, et al: Septal Q waves in surface electrocardiographic lead V_6 exclude minimal ventricular preexcitation. Am J Cardiol 84:101, 1999.
11. Massumi RA, Vera Z: Patterns and mechanisms of QRS normalization in patients with Wolff-Parkinson-White syndrome. Am J Cardiol 28:541, 1971.
12. Surawicz B: Transient T wave abnormalities after cessation of ventricular preexcitation: Memory of what? J Cardiovasc Electrophysiol 7:51, 1996.
13. Inden Y, Hirai M, Takada Y, et al: Prolongation of activation-recovery interval over a preexcited region before and after catheter ablation in patients with Wolff-Parkinson-White syndrome. J Cardiovasc Electrophysiol 12:939, 2001.
14. Hejtmancik MT, Herrmann GR: The electrocardiographic syndrome of short P-R interval and broad QRS complexes: a clinical study of 80 cases. Am Heart J 54:708, 1957.
15. Willus FA, Carryer HM: Electrocardiograms displaying short P-R intervals with prolonged QRS complexes: an analysis of sixty-five cases. Proc Staff Meet Mayo Clin 21:438, 1946.
16. Frank S, Braunwald E: Idiopathic hypertrophic subaortic stenosis: clinical analysis of 126 patients with emphasis on the natural history. Circulation 37:759, 1968.
17. Flowers NV, Horan LG: Electrocardiographic and vectorcardiographic features of myocardial disease. In Fowler NO (ed): Myocardial Diseases. Orlando, Grune & Stratton, 1973.
18. Chung EK: Tachyarrhythmias in Wolff-Parkinson-White syndrome. JAMA 237:376, 1977.
19. Kounis NG, Zavras GM, Papadaki PJ, et al: Pregnancy-induced increase of supraventricular arrhythmia in Wolff-Parkinson-White syndrome. Clin Cardiol 18:137, 1995.
20. Gallagher JJ, Pritchett ELC, Sealy WC, et al: The preexcitation syndromes. Prog Cardiovasc Dis 20: 285, 1978.
21. Bharati S, Bauernfeind R, Josephson M: Intermittent preexcitation and mesothelioma of the atrioventricular node: a hitherto undescribed entity. J Cardiovasc Electrophysiol 6:823, 1995.
22. Van Hare GF, Phoon CK, Munkebeck F, et al: Electrophysiologic study and radiofrequency ablation in patients with intracardiac tumors and accessory pathways: is the tumor the pathway? J Cardiovasc Electrophysiol 7:1204, 1996.
23. Schiebler GL, Adams P, Anderson RC, et al: The Wolff-Parkinson-White syndrome in infants and children. Pediatrics 24:585, 1959.
24. Lev M, Gibson S, Miller RA: Ebstein's disease with Wolff-Parkinson-White syndrome. Am Heart J 49:724, 1955.
25. Gallagher JJ, Gilbert M, Svenson RH, et al: Wolff-Parkinson-White syndrome: the problem, evaluation, and surgical correction. Circulation 51:767, 1975.
26. Schiebler GL, Adams P, Anderson RC, et al: Clinical study of twenty-three cases of Ebstein's anomaly of the tricuspid valve. Circulation 19:165, 1959.
27. Giardina ACV, Ehlers KH, Engle ME: Wolff-Parkinson-White syndrome in infants and children. a long-term follow-up study. Br Heart J 34:839, 1972.
28. Swiderski J, Lees MH, Nadas AS: The Wolff-Parkinson-White syndrome in infancy and childhood. Br Heart J 24:561, 1962.
29. Benditt DG, Pritchett ELC, Smith WH, et al: Characteristics of atrioventricular conduction and the spectrum of arrhythmias in Lown-Ganong-Levine syndrome. Circulation 57:454, 1978.
30. Wellens HJ: Wolff-Parkinson-White syndrome. I. Diagnosis, arrhythmias and identification of the high risk patient. Mod Concepts Cardiovasc Dis 52:53, 1983.
31. Denes P, Wu D, Amat-y-Leon F, et al: Determinants of atrioventricular reentrant paroxysmal tachycardia in patients with Wolff-Parkinson-White syndrome. Circulation 58:415, 1978.
32. Holmes DR, Hartzler GO, Maloney JD: Concealed retrograde bypass tracts and enhanced atrioventricular nodal conduction. Am J Cardiol 45:1053, 1980.
33. Akhtar M, Lehmann MH, Denker ST, et al: Electrophysiologic mechanisms of orthodromic tachycardia initiation during ventricular pacing in the Wolff-Parkinson-White syndrome. J Am Coll Cardiol 9:89, 1987.
34. Farshidi A, Josephson ME, Horowitz LN: Electrophysiologic characteristics of concealed bypass tracts: clinical and electrocardiographic correlates. Am J Cardiol 41:1052, 1978.
35. Wellens HJ, Durrer D: The role of an accessory atrioventricular pathway in reciprocal tachycardia. Circulation 52:58, 1975.
36. Kerr CR, Gallagher JJ, German LD: Changes in ventriculoatrial intervals with bundle branch block aberration during reciprocating tachycardia in patients with accessory atrioventricular pathways. Circulation 66:196, 1982.
37. Coumel P, Attuel P: Reciprocating tachycardia in overt and latent preexcitation. Eur J Cardiol 14:423, 1974.
38. Kay GN, Pressley JC, Packer DL, et al: Value of the 12-lead electrocardiogram in discriminating atrioventricular nodal reciprocating tachycardia from circus movement atrioventricular tachycardia utilizing a retrograde accessory pathway. Am J Cardiol 59:296, 1987.
39. Gallagher JJ, Pritchett ELC, Benditt DG, et al: New catheter techniques for analysis of the sequence of retrograde atrial activation in man. Eur J Cardiol 6:1, 1977.
40. Hood MA, Cox JL, Lindsay BD, et al: Improved detection of accessory pathways that bridge posterior septal and left posterior regions in the Wolff-Parkinson-White syndrome. Am J Cardiol 70:205, 1992.
41. Miller JM, Rosenthal ME, Gottlieb CD, et al: Usefulness of the HA interval to accurately distinguish atrioventricular nodal reentry from orthodromic septal bypass tract tachycardias. Am J Cardiol 68:1037, 1991.

42. Scheinman MM, Wang Y-S, Van Hare GF, et al: Electrocardiographic and electrophysiologic characteristics of anterior, midseptal and right anterior free wall accessory pathways. J Am Coll Cardiol 20:1220, 1992.
43. Murdock CJ, Leitch JW, Teo WS, et al: Characteristics of accessory pathways exhibiting decremental conduction. Am J Cardiol 67:506, 1991.
44. De Chillou C, Rodriguez LM, Schlapfer J, et al: Clinical characteristics and electrophysiological properties of atrioventricular accessory pathways: importance of the accessory pathway location. J Am Coll Cardiol 20:666, 1992.
45. Coumel P, Cabrol C, Fabiato A, et al: Tachycardie permanente par rythm reciproque. Arch Mal Coeur 60:1830, 1967.
46. Farre D, Ross D, Weiner I, et al: Reciprocal tachycardias using accessory pathways with long conduction times. Am J Cardiol 44:1099, 1979.
47. Okumura K, Henthorn RW, Epstein AE, et al: "Incessant" atrioventricular reciprocating tachycardia utilizing left lateral AV bypass pathway with a long retrograde conduction time. PACE 9:332, 1986.
48. Krikler D, Curry P, Attuel P, et al: "Incessant" tachycardias in Wolff-Parkinson-White syndrome. Br Heart J 38:885, 1976.
49. Langendorf R, Lev M, Pick R: Auricular fibrillation with anomalous AV excitation (WPW syndrome) imitating ventricular paroxysmal tachycardia. Acta Cardiol (Brux) 2:241, 1952.
50. Castellanos A, Myerburg RJ, Craparo K, et al: Factors regulating ventricular rates during atrial flutter and fibrillation in preexcitation (Wolff-Parkinson-White) syndrome. Br Heart J 35:811, 1973.
51. Wellens HJ, Durrer D: Wolff-Parkinson-White syndrome and atrial fibrillation. Am J Cardiol 34:777, 1974.
52. Campbell RWF, Smith RA, Gallagher JJ, et al: Atrial fibrillation in the preexcitation syndrome. Am J Cardiol 40:514, 1977.
53. Dreifus LS, Haiat R, Watanabe Y: Ventricular fibrillation: a possible mechanism of sudden death in patients with Wolff-Parkinson-White syndrome. Circulation 43:520, 1971.
54. Iesaka Y, Yamane T, Takahashi A, et al: Retrograde multiple and multifiber accessory pathways in the Wolff-Parkinson-White syndrome: potential precipitating factor of atrial fibrillation. J Cardiovasc Electrophysiol 9:141, 1998.
55. Sharma AD, Klein GJ, Guiraudon GM, Milstein S: Atrial fibrillation in patients with Wolff-Parkinson-White syndrome: incidence after surgical ablation of the accessory pathway. Circulation 72:161, 1985.
56. Haissaguerre M, Fischer B, Labbé T, et al: Frequency of recurrent atrial fibrillation after catheter ablation of overt accessory pathways. Am J Cardiol 69:493, 1992.
57. Timmermans C, Smeets JLRM, Rodriguez L-M, et al: Aborted sudden death in the Wolff-Parkinson-White syndrome. Am J Cardiol 76:492, 1995.
58. Wellens HJ, Durrer D: Patterns of ventriculo-atrial conduction in the Wolff-Parkinson-White syndrome. Circulation 69:22, 1974.
59. Zipes DP, DeJoseph RL, Rothbaum DA: Unusual properties of accessory pathways. Circulation 69:1200, 1974.
60. Sung RJ, Tamer DM, Castellanos A, et al: Clinical and electrophysiologic observations in patients with concealed accessory atrioventricular bypass tracts. Am J Cardiol 40:839, 1977.
61. Gillette PC: Concealed anomalous cardiac conduction pathways: a frequent cause of supraventricular tachycardia. Am J Cardiol 40:848, 1977.

62. Narula OS: Retrograde pre-excitation: comparison of antegrade and retrograde conduction intervals in man. Circulation 50:1129, 1974.
63. Neuss H, Schlepper M, Thormann J: Analysis of reentry mechanisms in three patients with concealed Wolff-Parkinson-White syndrome. Circulation 51:75, 1975.
64. Fitzpatrick AP, Gonzales RP, Lesh MD, et al: New algorithm for the localization of accessory atrioventricular connections using a baseline electrocardiogram. J Am Coll Cardiol 23:107, 1994.
65. Jackman WM, Wang X, Friday KJ, et al: Catheter ablation of accessory atrioventricular pathways (Wolff-Parkinson-White syndrome) by radiofrequency current. N Engl J Med 324:1605, 1991.
66. Kuck KH, Friday KJ, Kunze KP, et al: Sites of conduction block in accessory atrioventricular pathways: basis for concealed accessory pathways. Circulation 82: 407, 1990.
67. Becker AE, Anderson RH, Durrer D, et al: The anatomic substrates of Wolff-Parkinson-White syndrome. Circulation 57:870, 1978.
68. Gallagher JJ, Smith WM, Kasell HJ, et al: Role of Mahaim fibers in cardiac arrhythmias in man. Circulation 64:176, 1981.
69. Ferrer MI: Pre-Excitation, Including the Wolff-Parkinson-White and Other Related Syndromes. Mount Kisco, NY, Futura, 1976.
70. Tonkin AM, Wagner GS, Gallagher JJ, et al: Initial forces of ventricular depolarization in the Wolff-Parkinson-White syndrome. Circulation 52:1030, 1975.
71. Rodriguez L-M, Smeets JLMR, de Chillou C, et al: The 12-lead electrocardiogram in midseptal, anteroseptal, posteroseptal and right free wall accessory pathways. Am J Cardiol 72:1274, 1993.
72. Arruda MS, McClelland JM, Wang X, et al: Development and validation of an ECG algorithm identifying accessory pathway ablation site in Wolff-Parkinson-White syndrome. J Cardiovasc Electrophysiol 9:2, 1998.
73. Chiang C-E, Chen S-A, Teo WS, et al: An accurate stepwise electrocardiographic algorithm for localization of accessory pathways in patients with Wolff-Parkinson-White syndrome from a comprehensive analysis of delta waves and R/S ratio during sinus rhythm. Am J Cardiol 76:40, 1995.
74. Calkins H, Langberg J, Sousa J, et al: Radiofrequency catheter ablation of accessory atrioventricular connections in 250 patients. Circulation 85:1337, 1992.
75. Haissaguerre M, Gaita F, Marcus FI, et al: Radiofrequency catheter ablation of accessory pathways; a contemporary review. J Cardiovasc Electrophysiol 5:532, 1994.
76. Haissaguerre M, Marcus FI, Poquet F, et al: Electrocardiographic characteristics and catheter ablation of parahissian accessory pathways. Circulation 90:1124, 1994.
77. Portillo B, Portillo-Leon N, Zaman L, et al: Quintuple pathways participating in three distinct types of atrioventricular reciprocating tachycardia in a patient with Wolff-Parkinson-White syndrome. Am J Cardiol 50:347, 1982.
78. Colavita PG, Packer DL, Pressley JC, et al: Frequency, diagnosis and clinical characteristics of patients with multiple accessory atrioventricular pathways. Am J Cardiol 59:601, 1987.
79. Teo WS, Klein GJ, Guiraudon GM, et al: Multiple accessory pathways in the Wolff-Parkinson-White syndrome as a risk factor for ventricular fibrillation. Am J Cardiol 67:889, 1991.
80. Atie J: New observations on the role of accessory pathways in tachycardias in man [thesis]. Thesis. Maastricht University, 1990, Chapter 6.

81. Packer DL, Gallagher JJ, Prystowsky EN: Physiologic substrate for antidromic reciprocating tachycardia. Circulation 85:574, 1992.

82. James TN: Morphology of the human atrioventricular node, with remarks pertinent to its electrophysiology. Am Heart J 62:756, 1961.

83. Caracta AR, Damato AN, Gallagher JJ, et al: Electrophysiologic studies in the syndrome of short P-R interval, normal QRS complex. Am J Cardiol 31:245, 1973.

84. Childers R: The AV node: normal and abnormal physiology. Prog Cardiovasc Dis 19:361, 1977.

85. Denes P, Wu D, Rosen KM: Demonstration of dual AV pathways in a patient with Lown-Ganong-Levine syndrome. Chest 65:343, 1974.

86. Holmes DR, Hartzler GO, Merideth J: The clinical and electrophysiologic characteristics of patients with accelerated atrioventricular nodal conduction. Mayo Clin Proc 57:339, 1982.

87. Wiener I: Syndromes of Lown-Ganong-Levine and enhanced atrioventricular nodal conduction. Am J Cardiol 52:637, 1983.

88. Lown B, Ganong WF, Levine SA: The syndrome of short P-R interval, normal QRS complex and paroxysmal rapid heart action. Circulation 5:693, 1952.

89. Moller P: Criteria for the LGL syndrome. Am Heart J 91:539, 1976.

90. Brechenmacher C, Coumel P, Fauchier JP, et al: Syndrome de Wolff-Parkinson-White par association de fibres atriohissiennes et de fibres de Mahaim. Arch Mal Coeur 69:1275, 1976.

91. Jackman WM, Prystowsky EN, Naccarelli GV, et al: Reevaluation of enhanced atrioventricular nodal conduction: evidence to suggest a continuum of normal atrioventricular nodal physiology. Circulation 67:441, 1983.

92. Ward DE, Camm J: Mechanisms of junctional tachycardias in the Lown-Ganong-Levine syndrome. Am Heart J 105:169, 1983.

93. Huang SK, Rosenberg MJ, Denes P: Short PR interval and narrow QRS complex associated with pheochromocytoma: electrophysiologic observations. J Am Coll Cardiol 3:872, 1984.

94. Moleiro F, Mendoza I, Medina-Ravell V, et al: One to one atrioventricular conduction during atrial pacing at rates of 300/minute in absence of Wolff-Parkinson-White syndrome. Am J Cardiol 48:789, 1981.

95. Castellanos A, Castillo CA, Agha AS, et al: His bundle electrograms in patients with short P-R intervals, narrow QRS complexes and paroxysmal tachycardias. Circulation 43:667, 1971.

96. Myerburg RJ, Sung RJ, Castellanos A: Ventricular tachycardia and ventricular fibrillation in patients with short P-R intervals and narrow QRS complexes. PACE 2:568, 1979.

97. Mahaim I, Winston MR: Recherches d'anatomie comparee et de pathologie experimentale sur les connexions hautes de faisceau de His-Tawara. Cardiologia 5:189, 1941.

98. Anderson RH, Becker AE, Brechenmacher C, et al: Ventricular preexcitation: a proposed nomenclature for its substrates. Eur J Cardiol 3:27, 1975.

99. Klein GJ, Yee R, Sharma AD: Longitudinal electrophysiologic assessment of asymptomatic patients with the Wolff-Parkinson-White electrocardiographic pattern. N Engl J Med 19:1229, 1989.

100. Bardy GH, Fedor JM, German LD, et al: Surface electrocardiographic clues suggesting presence of a nodofascicular Mahaim fiber. J Am Coll Cardiol 3:1161, 1984.

101. Klein LS, Hackett, Zipes DP, et al: Radiofrequency catheter ablation of Mahaim fibers at the tricuspid annulus. Circulation 87:738, 1993.

102. Tchou P, Lehmann MH, Jazayeri M, et al: Atriofascicular connection or a nodoventricular Mahaim fiber? Electrophysiologic elucidation of the pathway and associated reentrant circuit. Circulation 77:837, 1988.

103. Murdock CJ, Leitch JW, Klein GJ, et al: Epicardial mapping in patients with "nodoventricular" accessory pathways. Am J Cardiol 68:208, 1991.

104. Scheinman M: Nodoventricular Mahaim pathway concept. Circulation 91:910, 1995.

105. Hamdan MH, Kalman JM, Lesh MD, et al: Narrow complex tachycardia with VA block: diagnostic and therapeutic implications. PACE 21:1196, 1998.

106. Grogin HR, Lee RJ, Kwasman M, et al: Radiofrequency catheter ablation of atriofascicular and nodoventricular Mahaim traces. Circulation 90:272, 1994.

107. Mecca A, Telfer A, Lanzarotti C, et al: Symptomatic atrioventricular block in atriofascicular pathway inserting into the left bundle branch without apparent atrioventricular node function. J Cardiovasc Electrophysiol 8:922, 1997.

108. Lee P-C, Kanter R, Gomez-Marin O, et al: Quantitative assessment of the recovery property of atriofascicular/atrioventricular-type Mahaim fibers. J Cardiovasc Electrophysiol 13:535, 2002.

109. Sternick EB, Gerken LM, Vrandecic MO, et al: Fasciculoventricular pathways: clinical and electrophysiologic characteristics of a variant of preexcitation. J Cardiovasc Electrophysiol 14:1057, 2003.

110. Pick A, Katz LN: Disturbances of impulse formation and conduction in the pre-excitation (WPW) syndrome: their bearing on its mechanism. Am J Med 19:759, 1955.

111. Lerman BB, Josephson ME: Automaticity of the Kent bundle: confirmation by phase 3 and phase 4 block. J Am Coll Cardiol 5:996, 1985.

112. Deam AG, Burton ME, Walter PF, et al: Wide complex tachycardia due to automaticity in an accessory pathway. PACE 18:2106, 1995.

113. Sternick EB, Sosa EA, Timmermans C, et al: Automaticity in Mahaim fibers. J Cardiovasc Electrophysiol 15:738, 2004.

114. Atie J, Brugada P, Brugada J, et al: Longitudinal dissociation of atrioventricular accessory pathways. J Am Coll Cardiol 17:161, 1991.

115. Robertson PGC, Emslie-Smith D, Lowe KG, et al: The association of type B ventricular pre-excitation and right bundle branch block. Br Heart J 25:755, 1963.

116. Takahashi A, Shah DC, Jais P, et al: Specific electrocardiographic features of manifest coronary vein posteroseptal accessory pathway. J Cardiovasc Electrophysiol 9:1015, 1998.

21 Effect of Drugs on the Electrocardiogram

Antiarrhythmia Drugs
Classification
Clinical Application
Proarrhythmic Effects of Antiarrhythmia
  Drugs
Individual Drugs

Digitalis
Digitalis Intoxication
The More Common Arrhythmias

Correlation of Digitalis Toxicity with
  Serum Glycoside Levels

Miscellaneous Drugs
Epinephrine, Norepinephrine,
  Isoproterenol
Vagolytic Drugs
Anesthetic and Analgesic Agents
Antiparasitic Drugs
Arsenic

Drugs can affect the electrocardiogram (ECG) indirectly or directly. Examples of indirect action include hypokalemia or hyperkalemia caused by a diuretic drug, cessation of fever-induced tachycardia by an antibiotic, or regression of a left ventricular hypertrophy pattern by an antihypertensive drug. The pertinent indirect effects are discussed in the appropriate chapters.

The direct effects on the ECG result from specific electropharmacologic actions, which can be separated into several categories. When a new drug becomes available for clinical use, it is important to learn about its assignment to a specific category. This is because the fundamental electrophysiologic properties of a drug in a given category can predictably determine its effect on the ECG. The ability to deduce the possible ECG changes based on knowledge of the drug's fundamental properties is useful because it obviates the need to commit to memory the details of each drug's action on each ECG component. The following general principles may be helpful.

The *specific actions* of drugs are as follows:
1. Vagal action slows the activity of the pacemakers and prolongs atrioventricular (AV) conduction.
2. Sympathetic action has an opposite effect.
3. β-adrenergic block has an effect similar to the vagal effect.
4. Anticholinergic agents have an effect similar (but not identical) to sympathetic action.
5. Sodium channel–blocking effect slows conduction in all cardiac fibers except the sinoatrial (SA) node and the AV node. In the latter structures, conduction depends mainly on the calcium channel.

6. Sodium channel–enhancing effect plays no role in current pharmacotherapy, but future development of drugs with such properties is possible. The depression of conduction by sodium channel–blocking drugs can be overcome by an increase in extracellular sodium concentration and to a degree by increased sympathetic stimulation (e.g., isoproterenol).
7. Potassium channel–blocking drugs prolong repolarization (i.e., the duration of cardiac action potential) and thereby prolong the duration of the effective refractory period.
8. Potassium channel–opening drugs have an opposite effect. They have not been used for this purpose in practice at the time of this writing.
9. The two calcium channel–blocking drugs verapamil and diltiazem slow automaticity and conduction in the SA and AV nodes but not in other cardiac tissues. The dihydropyridine class of calcium channel–blocking drugs, which shares the negative inotropic and vascular effects with the above two drugs, is devoid of significant action on the SA and AV nodes at therapeutic concentrations.
10. Block of the sodium-potassium pump by digitalis glycosides shortens the duration and alters the repolarization slope of the ventricular action potential because of altered sodium, potassium, and calcium transmembrane gradients.
11. *Use-dependent* (or rate-dependent) *effect* describes an increase in the sodium channel

block (i.e., increased slowing of conduction) associated with increased heart rates.

12. *Reverse use-dependent effect* applies to potassium channel–blocking drugs and means that the degree of block increases with decreasing heart rate; that is, the action potential duration (and refractoriness) deviates toward longer values from the predicted RR-dependent duration more at slow heart rates than at fast heart rates.

The above 12 actions may affect the ECG in the following manner:

1. Sinus rate is increased by sympathetic stimulation and anticholinergic action.
2. Sinus rate is decreased by vagal stimulation and β-adrenergic blocking action.
3. P wave duration may be expected to increase by both sodium channel– and potassium channel–blocking drugs.
4. PR (AH) interval is increased by vagal stimulation and β-adrenergic blocking action as well as by calcium channel blocking action and adenosine or adenosine triphosphate (ATP).
5. HV interval is prolonged by sodium channel–blocking drugs.

6. QRS duration is prolonged by sodium channel–blocking drugs.
7. Accessory pathway conduction is slowed by sodium channel–blocking drugs.
8. QT intervals (and JT intervals) are shortened by digitalis and prolonged by potassium channel–blocking drugs. The same applies to the refractoriness of the accessory pathway.
9. Use-dependent effect is manifested by increased QT duration at fast heart rates (Figure 21–1).
10. Reverse use dependence is manifested by excessive QT lengthening at slow heart rates (Figure 21–2).

Antiarrhythmia Drugs

CLASSIFICATION

The purpose of classifying antiarrhythmia drugs is to categorize their action and to fit new drugs with similar action into established categories. The most successful and widely accepted classification is that first proposed by Vaughan

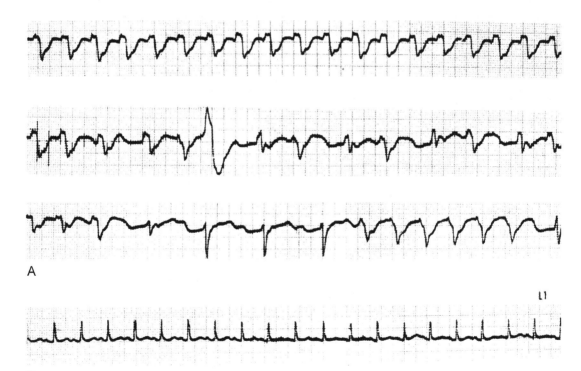

A

B

Figure 21–1 **A,** Rate-dependent effects of quinidine on the ECG of a patient treated with quinidine sulfate. The QRS complex is wider when the rate is rapid; it is also wider in the premature complexes with shorter coupling intervals than in those with longer coupling intervals. **B,** Control tracing in the same lead in the absence of quinidine. (Courtesy of Dr. Charles Fisch, M.D., Indianapolis, IN.)

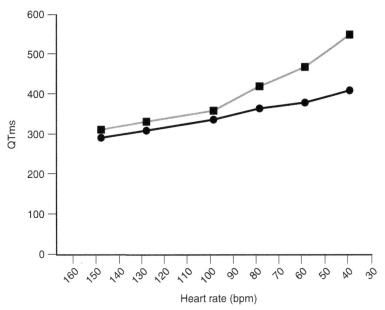

Figure 21–2 Reverse use dependence is a process caused by blocking the repolarizing potassium current (iKr) by class III drugs such as sotalol or dofetilide. It is manifested on the ECG by disproportionately more lengthening of the QT interval at slow heart rates than at fast heart rates *(top curve)* compared to that of the control with no drug *(bottom curve).*

Williams in 1970 and 1975 and subsequently modified by others.[1] The classification is useful for practical purposes, even though the inherent weakness of this or any other classification is that most of the arrhythmia drugs have more than one action.

Class I Action

The class I drugs are divided into three categories: A, B, and C. The differences between these categories reflect the differences in the kinetics of the interaction between the drug and the sodium channel entry into the cell interior during depolarization and to some extent the differences in the interaction with other channels. The detailed description of these differences is beyond the scope of this textbook, and the interested reader is referred to textbooks of pharmacology and basic electrophysiology[1] and review articles.[2]

Class IA drugs include quinidine, procainamide, disopyramide, and ajmaline. These drugs block not only the sodium channel but also one or more of the potassium channels and to a degree the calcium channel. On the ECG these drugs are seen to prolong the P wave (may be difficult to recognize), the QRS duration, and the JT component of the QT interval. Characteristically, the QRS duration is more prolonged at rapid rates (see Figure 21–1).

Class IB drugs include lidocaine, tocainide, mexiletine, and phenytoin. These drugs block the sodium current predominantly at rapid heart rates and in depolarized (e.g., acutely ischemic) tissue. For practical purposes the effects of these drugs on the ECG are not recognizable.

Class IC drugs include encainide, flecainide, propafenone, moricizine, and tricyclic antidepressants (e.g., imipramine and amitriptyline). These drugs block sodium entry into the myocyte more tenaciously at therapeutic doses and have a strong use-dependent effect. On the ECG the drugs prolong the QRS duration and QT interval (but not JT), particularly at rapid heart rates and in the early premature complexes. Because of QRS widening at rapid heart rates, supraventricular tachycardias can mimic ventricular tachycardias.[3]

Class II Action

Antiarrhythmic drugs in class II (i.e., β-adrenergic blockers) depress automaticity of the SA node and prolong conduction time through the AV node (AH interval). They may suppress the effects of β-adrenergic stimulation on automaticity and ameliorate the adverse balance between the energy supply and demand in the heart. On the ECG these drugs decrease the sinus rate, prolong the PR interval, may produce SA and AV conduction block, and depress both the escape and accelerated automatic rhythms.

Class III Action

Class III action prolongs repolarization, most often by blocking one of the potassium channels, but it may be produced also by other mechanisms, such as increased inward sodium current. Some of the potassium channel–blocking drugs in this category are sotalol, amiodarone, bretylium, dofetilide,[4] ibutilide,[5] sematilide,[6] and almokalant.[7] On the ECG these drugs prolong the QT intval (and JT interval) without QRS prolongation (with the exception of amiodarone) and exhibit the property of reverse use dependence.

Class IV Action

Class IV action inhibits the calcium inward current, which can have a direct effect on slow channel–dependent (e.g., SA and AV nodes) automaticity, conduction, and refractoriness, and an indirect effect on processes involving the intracellular calcium concentration (e.g., myocardial ischemia). On the ECG, verapamil and diltiazem decrease the sinus rate and prolong AV conduction (AH interval).

Class V Action

Class V action refers to "specific bradycardia agents" acting on the SA node. At the time of this writing, these drugs have not been approved for clinical use.

CLINICAL APPLICATION

Antiarrhythmia drugs can depress normal automaticity, abnormal automaticity, and triggered activity caused by delayed or early afterdepolarizations. They can stop or prevent reentry by improving or depressing conduction.[1] Improved conduction can eliminate the unidirectional block or accelerate the returning wavefront by engaging the still-refractory tissue. Depressed conduction can prevent or terminate reentry by transforming a unidirectional block into a bidirectional block. Drugs that prolong repolarization and refractoriness also can terminate or prevent reentry by blocking propagation of the reentering impulse. The effects of antiarrhythmic drugs on conduction and refractoriness in human hearts are consistent with the drug effects on determinants of conduction and refractoriness in single cardiac fibers in vitro.[1]

PROARRHYTHMIC EFFECTS OF ANTIARRHYTHMIA DRUGS

The administration of antiarrhythmia agents may, paradoxically, aggravate the arrhythmias that are being treated or cause new rhythm disorders. Such effect, which is often called *proarrhythmia*, usually occurs when the dosage of the drugs does not exceed the therapeutic range. Characteristically, the arrhythmogenic effect usually appears within a few hours or a few days after initiation of treatment.[8]

The reported incidence of proarrhythmia ranges from 3.4 to 16.4 percent, depending to a large extent on the antiarrhythmia agents used and the type of proarrhythmia included in the study.[8–10] The arrhythmogenic effect is seldom caused by drugs with class II and IV action or by class IB drugs. Proarrhythmia is predominantly associated with slow use-dependent conduction (e.g., incessant ventricular tachycardia) during treatment with class IC drugs or a reverse use-dependent effect on refractoriness (e.g., torsade de pointes during treatment with class IA drugs or drugs with pure class III action).[8,10–14] Proarrhythmia is described as *primary* when it is unrelated to any identifiable arrhythmogenic factor other than the underlying arrhythmia or heart disease. It is called *secondary* when its occurrence requires the presence of an adjunctive factor, such as high plasma concentration of the antiarrhythmic drug, concomitant medications, electrolyte disturbances, or myocardial ischemia.[12]

Ventricular proarrhythmia has received the most attention because of its potentially serious consequences. Aggravation of preexisting ventricular ectopic activity is often difficult to recognize because of the marked variation in the number and complexity of premature ventricular complexes (PVCs) in the absence of any antiarrhythmic drugs. Velebit and associates[8] suggested the following changes as evidence of drug-induced aggravation of arrhythmia:

1. A fourfold increase in the hourly frequency of PVCs compared with the control period
2. A tenfold increase in the hourly frequency of couplets or ventricular tachycardia compared with the control period
3. The first occurrence of sustained ventricular tachycardia not present during control studies

Refinement of these criteria has been proposed because some investigators question the accuracy of the criteria when the ectopic PVCs are infrequent during the control period.[9] In patients who are treated for ventricular tachycardia, 10 percent shortening of the tachycardia cycle length also is considered evidence of aggravation of the arrhythmia.[14]

Figures 18–2 and 18–3 are examples of quinidine-induced torsade de pointes, which is probably the most generally recognized form of drug-induced ventricular tachyarrhythmia.

INDIVIDUAL DRUGS

Quinidine

Quinidine is discussed in greater detail as a prototype of an antiarrhythmia drug that slows conduction and prolongs refractoriness. Therapeutic doses of quinidine have little effect on the sinus rate even though it directly decreases the automaticity of the pacemaker fibers in the SA node. At the AV junction, the conduction time is often decreased because the direct depressing action of the drug is counteracted by the vagolytic effect. Automaticity is depressed in the Purkinje system. Quinidine slows conduction and prolongs refractoriness in the His-Purkinje system, atria, and ventricles.

With high or toxic doses of the drug, the automaticity of the SA node may be depressed, resulting in sinus bradycardia or sinus arrest, or it may be increased, resulting in sinus tachycardia. SA and AV conduction may be impaired, and the intraventricular conduction time may be markedly prolonged.

The ECG findings consist of the following:

1. Decreased amplitude of the T wave or T wave inversion
2. ST segment depression
3. Prominent U waves
4. Prolongation of the QTc interval
5. Notching and widening of the P waves
6. Increased QRS duration

Toxic effects include marked widening of the QRS complex, various degrees of AV block, ventricular arrhythmias, syncope, and sudden death (usually associated with torsade de pointes); less often there is marked sinus bradycardia, sinus arrest, or SA block. In the meta-analysis of randomized control trials for maintenance of sinus rhythm after cardioversion from chronic atrial fibrillation, the odds of death in the quinidine-treated group were approximately threefold that of the control group.[15]

Prolongation of the QTc interval is related to the increased duration of the action potential of the ventricular muscle fibers. The degree of prolongation may give some indication of the intensity of the quinidine effect, but it cannot be used as a reliable sign to guide therapy. Because the U wave is often prominent and merged with the T wave, accurate determination of the QT interval is difficult. Figure 21–3 illustrates prolongation of the QT interval as a result of quinidine, but the exact measurement of the interval is difficult because of the T wave merger with U waves. The ST segment, T wave, and U wave changes caused by quinidine often closely mimic those seen in patients with hypokalemia.

Notching and widening of the P waves may occur in patients with sinus rhythm. Although these changes may be seen with therapeutic doses of the drug, they are observed most often when the plasma level is in the toxic range. In patients with coarse atrial fibrillation or atrial flutter, widening of the fibrillatory or flutter waves may be seen with a decrease in the atrial rate. This may occur even when the plasma level of the drug is as low as 1.7 to 2.7 mg/L.[16]

With large doses and a high blood concentration of quinidine, the QRS complex may widen progressively. The widening is diffuse, affecting the entire QRS complex. Although this is generally considered a late change, careful measurements by Heissenbuttel and Bigger in 20 patients receiving quinidine revealed an increased QRS duration in every patient.[17] The mean increase was 12 ms at a plasma drug concentration of 2 to 5 mg/L. Prolongation of the duration above 25 percent of the control value, however, usually is considered a toxic sign. Higher quinidine concentrations can cause ventricular tachycardia (Figure 21–4).

Prolongation of the PR interval represents a late toxic change and occurs only when the serum concentration of quinidine reaches a high level, usually above 10 mg/L. Therapeutic concentrations (mean value 4.6 mg/L), however, as shown by Josephson and associates who recorded His bundle electrograms, tended to shorten the AV nodal conduction time.[18]

Considerable ECG variability is present at similar plasma quinidine concentrations among individuals. Patients with advanced heart disease may be particularly sensitive to the drug. Both the quinidine plasma level and the ECG should be used to guide therapy. It is of note that quinine has the same electrophysiologic properties as quinidine.[19]

Procainamide

The electrophysiologic effects of procainamide are similar to those of quinidine except that the drug it is not anticholinergic.[20,21] The ECG changes that result from therapeutic doses of procainamide are usually less pronounced than those from quinidine. The sinus rate is not affected in a predictable way. The P wave may be slightly widened and the PR interval slightly prolonged. The QRS duration is increased generally in proportion to the plasma level of the drug but usually does not exceed the normal range.

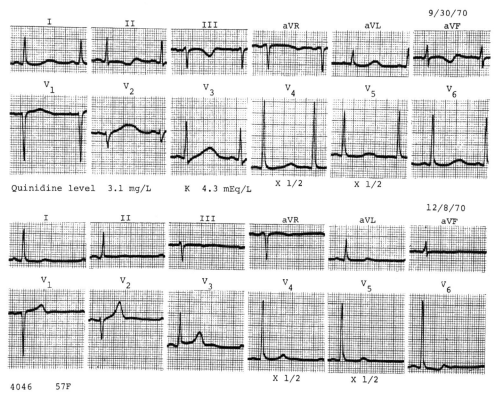

Figure 21–3 QT interval prolongation, T wave changes, and T wave merger with U wave as a result of quinidine. This 57-year-old woman with hypertensive disease was given quinidine (300 mg q6h) to control frequent premature ventricular complexes (a treatment currently considered inappropriate). The tracing from 9/30/70 shows prolongation of the QT interval, even though the exact measurement is difficult because of the prominent U waves. There is T wave inversion in leads II, III, and aV_F. ECG also suggests left ventricular hypertrophy. The tracing of 12/8/70 was recorded 4 days after quinidine was discontinued. The QT interval has shortened, the U waves are separated from T waves, and the T waves in the inferior leads have become essentially isoelectric.

The QTc interval is prolonged but usually less than the prolongation caused by quinidine. The T waves are lower in amplitude or notched, and the U waves become more prominent.[22]

High or toxic procainamide doses may cause high-degree AV block, marked widening of the QRS duration (Figure 21–5), ventricular premature complexes, ventricular tachycardia, torsade de pointes, ventricular fibrillation, or asystole.[23–25] These manifestations are seen more frequently with intravenous than with oral administration of the drug.

Disopyramide Phosphate

The effects of disopyramide on the ECG are similar to those of quinidine,[26–28] but the QRS widening and QTc prolongation are less conspicuous with the usual therapeutic doses of the drug.[29] However, marked depression of sinus node function may occur in patients with sinus node disease.[30] Preexisting AV block or an intraventricular conduction defect also may

be aggravated by disopyramide.[31] Ventricular tachycardia, ventricular fibrillation, and torsade de pointes have been reported in patients receiving the drugs, especially in those with QTc interval prolongation[31,32] (Figure 21–6). Slowing of conduction may be manifested by slower rates of ventricular tachycardia and atrial flutter.

Lidocaine, Mexiletine, Tocainide, Phenytoin

Clinically, lidocaine, mexiletine, tocainide, and phenytoin cause no noticeable changes of the P wave, PR interval, QRS complex, QT interval, or T wave.[33–35] Although in vitro lidocaine depresses the current involved in phase 4 depolarization in Purkinje fibers,[36] the clinical relevance of this change is uncertain, as therapeutic lidocaine concentrations have little effect on the automaticity of the escape pacemakers both proximal and distal to the His bundle.[37,38] An unusual case of sinus arrest after administration of an average customary dose of lidocaine is shown in Figure 21–7.

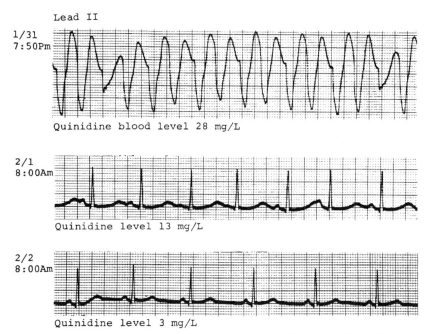

Figure 21–4   Quinidine intoxication in a 20-year-old woman who ingested 4 g of quinidine sulfate in a suicide attempt. The first rhythm strip (7:50 PM, 1/31/68) was recorded about 3 hours after the ingestion and shortly after she had a syncopal episode. The rhythm is paroxysmal ventricular tachycardia. The third and fifteenth QRS complexes are probably sinus captures. The plasma quinidine level at that time was 28 mg/L. At 8 AM the following day the quinidine level had decreased to 13 mg/L. The rhythm is sinus with a PR interval of 0.18 second. The QRS duration is normal. There is prolongation of the QT interval with prominent U waves. A premature atrial complex is present. The tracing recorded at 8 AM on 2/2/68 is within normal limits, and the quinidine plasma level was 3 mg/L.

Propafenone, Flecainide, Encainide, Moricizine

The sinus rate on the ECG is unaffected by propafenone, flecainide, encainide, or moricizine; the PR interval and QRS duration are prolonged (especially in the case of encainide); and the QT interval may or may not be appreciably increased.[39–41] Propafenone differs from the other class IC agents in that it also has β-adrenergic properties[42] and may cause sinus node slowing. The QTc lengthens to the extent that the QRS duration increases.[42–44] Slowing of conduction results in slower rate of atrial flutter (Figure 21–8). Similar to other class IC agents, propafenone increases the refractory period of the accessory pathway in patients with Wolff-Parkinson-White (WPW) syndrome.

β-Adrenergic Blocking Agents

Many β-adrenergic blocking agents are available for clinical use. Their electrophysiologic actions are similar, but propranolol in high doses also has a direct quinidine-like effect on conduction. The drugs depress the automaticity of the SA node and Purkinje fibers; they prolong the AV conduction time and the effective refractory period of the AV node.[45]

Therapeutic doses of β-adrenergic blocking drugs administered orally slow the sinus rate and may prolong the PR interval, but they have no significant effect on the P, QRS, T, or U wave.[46] The QTc interval is sometimes shortened. In the presence of atrial tachyarrhythmias, especially atrial fibrillation and atrial flutter, these agents decrease the ventricular rate[47] and may cause various degrees of AV block in patients with preexisting disease of the AV conduction system or in those receiving digitalis and either verapamil or diltiazem.

Intravenous administration of propranolol was reported to produce AV block, SA block, shortening of the QTc interval, and occasionally slight peaking and increased amplitude of the T wave.[48,49] No significant ECG effects, except for slowing the ventricular rate due to the action on the AV node, have been seen in patients treated with the ultrashort-acting β-adrenergic blocking agent esmolol.[50]

Amiodarone and Dronedarone

Amiodarone has multiple effects on cardiac ionic channels. It depresses sodium and calcium inward currents and at least two components of potassium repolarizing currents, interacts with the α-adrenergic and muscarinic receptors, alters

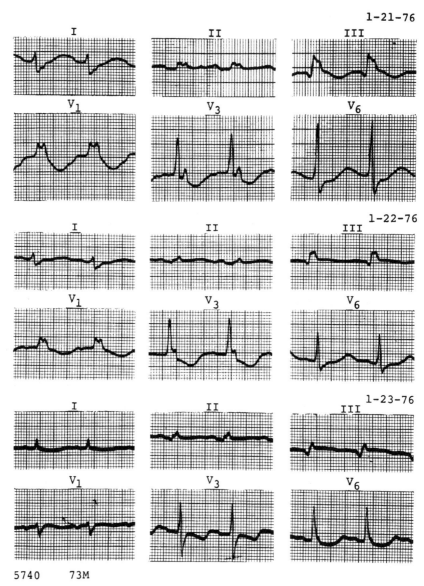

Figure 21-5 Procainamide intoxication in a 73-year-old man who was given procainamide (6 mg/min IV) on 1/21/76. The tracing recorded on that date reveals first-degree atrioventricular block and marked prolongation of the QRS complex, with a duration of 0.20 second. The morphology of the QRS complexes resembles that of right bundle branch block. Additional primary ST and T wave changes are present. On 1/22/76, after procainamide was discontinued, the PR interval and QRS duration have shortened. There are fewer ST and T wave changes. The QT interval, which now can be measured more accurately, is prolonged. On the next day (1/23/76) the PR interval is within normal limits, and the QRS duration has decreased to 0.12 second. ST and T wave abnormalities are still present, especially in the precordial leads.

sodium/potassium pump activity, and affects thyroid function.[1] It is listed as a class III drug because the potassium channel–blocking effects prolong the QT interval. This effect, however, is rarely seen after intravenous amiodarone administration.

Amiodarone is probably the most potent antiarrhythmia drug and is frequently effective in the treatment of supraventricular and ventricular ectopic rhythms resistant to other drugs.

By slowing the ventricular rate, amiodarone may transform a poorly tolerated ventricular tachycardia into a tolerable one (Figure 21-9).

Amiodarone is slowly accumulated in and dissipated from the body. Use of the drug appears to be associated with a low incidence of proarrhythmic effects and less than a 1.0 percent incidence of torsade de pointes.[51] The undesirable effects on other organs, however, result in a high incidence of intolerance.

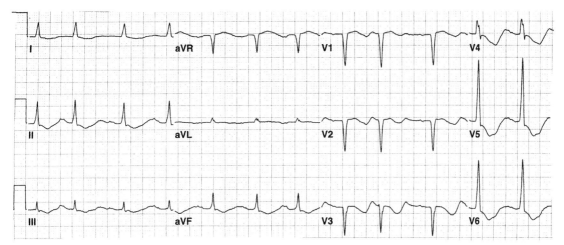

Figure 21–6   ECG of a 68-year-old woman treated with disopyramide for atrial tachyarrhythmias shows sinus rhythm with premature atrial complexes, notched P wave, QRS duration of 96 ms, and QTc of 526 ms. Torsade de pointes occurred on the same day this ECG was recorded.

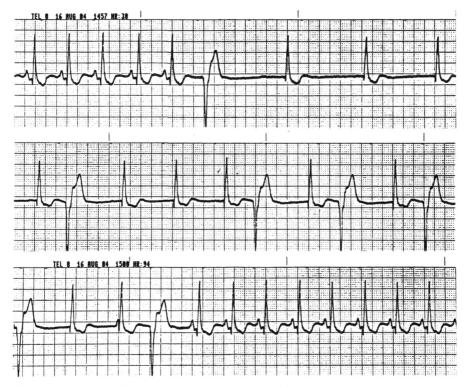

Figure 21–7   Sinus arrest due to lidocaine. The patient is a 56-year-old man who underwent aortocoronary artery bypass surgery. Lidocaine (100 mg) was administered intravenously as a bolus postoperatively for treatment of ventricular arrhythmias. The tracing was recorded 2 minutes after the injection. Note the normal sinus rhythm followed by the appearance of sinus arrest with junctional escape rhythm and premature ventricular complexes. Normal sinus rhythm resumed after about 3 minutes.

The electrophysiologic effects of amiodarone consist of depression of sinus node automaticity and prolonged conduction and refractory periods of the atrium, AV node, His-Purkinje system, and ventricle.[31,52] In patients with WPW syndrome, administration of amiodarone prolongs the refractory period of the accessory pathway, reportedly more consistently in the anterograde direction than in the retrograde direction.[14,53] The drug is particularly effective for treating arrhythmias associated with WPW syndrome because amiodarone affects conduction and refractoriness in all components of the long reentrant pathway.

Sinus bradycardia is commonly seen on the ECGs of patients receiving amiodarone, and occasional cases of SA block and sinus arrest have been described.[54–57] The PR interval may be prolonged[52,53] and the QRS duration increased.[52] The QTc interval is usually lengthened[52,56,58] (Figure 21–10). The T waves may become wider and notched with prominent U waves. The interval between the peak and the end of T wave is prolonged.[59] The repolarization changes usually begin to appear after the fourth day of loading treatment, become pronounced after 7 to 10 days, and persist 15 to 21 days after the drug is discontinued.[59] Mitchell and co-workers[60] showed that the effect of amiodarone on sinus node automaticity and atrial and AV nodal conduction reached their maximum within 2 weeks, whereas the effect on ventricular repolarization (and therefore on the QTc interval) did not reach maximum until 10 weeks after oral administration of the drug was begun. Dronedarone is a benzofuran derivative with electropharmacologic profiles closely resembling that of amiodarone, but with structural differences intended to eliminate the effects of amiodarone

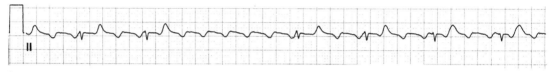

Figure 21–8 ECG rhythm strip of lead II shows atrial flutter at a rate of 180 beats/min with 4:1 ventricular response in a patient treated with propafenone. Before propafenone the rate of atrial flutter was 244 beats/min.

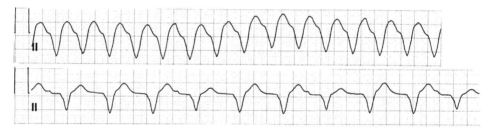

Figure 21–9 ECG rhythm strips of lead II from a 43-year-old man with ventricular tachycardia. *Top,* Before treatment with amiodarone the ventricular rate is 147 beats/min and the QRS duration 196 ms. *Bottom,* After treatment with oral amiodarone the ventricular rate is 92 beats/min and the QRS duration 200 ms.

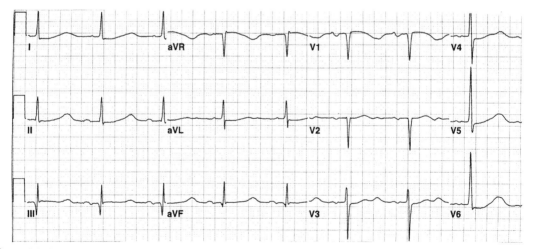

Figure 21–10 ECG of a 72-year-old woman treated with oral amiodarone following electrocardioversion of atrial fibrillation to sinus rhythm. The wide P wave suggests left atrial enlargement. The PR interval is 190 ms and the QRS duration 104 ms. The QT interval appears prolonged but is difficult to measure because of fusion of the T wave with the U wave. In lead aV$_L$ the U wave amplitude is low, and there is a notch between the end of the T wave and the onset of the U wave. The QT interval in lead aV$_L$ is 520 ms. The duration of the QT+U interval is 716 ms.

on thyroid and pulmonary function, resulting in fewer side effects. The elimination half-life of dronaderone is 1 to 2 days compared with 30-55 days for amioadorone.[60a]

Bretylium Tosylate

After intravenous administration of bretylium, there is a brief initial sympathomimetic phase of action followed by adrenergic neuronal blockade. Bretylium causes an initial transient increase in the heart rate followed by a later decrease. The drug lengthens the duration of the action potential and refractory periods of the atrial, ventricular, and Purkinje fibers; but in the doses used, the QRS duration and QTc interval are unchanged.[61] Bretylium has a reputation for effectively suppressing life-threatening ventricular tachyarrhythmias that are refractory to treatment with other antiarrhythmia drugs, but the alleged antifibrillatory action of the drug could not have been predicted from its pharmacologic and electrophysiologic properties.[62]

Sotalol

Sotalol[63] is a class III antiarrhythmic agent that also has a β-adrenergic blocking effect. On the ECG sotalol is shown to decrease the heart rate and increase the PR interval. There are no significant changes in the QRS duration. The most significant change is prolongation of the QTc interval, usually by 40 to 110 ms[63–65] (Figure 21–11). Consistent with the reverse use-dependent effect, prolongation of the QT interval is more pronounced at a slow heart rate and may not be apparent during tachycardia.[63,66,67] To achieve greater prolongation of refractoriness, low-dose sotalol has been

combined with a class IA drug, but the reverse use dependence has not been eliminated.[68,69] Like other antiarrhythmic agents that prolong the QTc interval, the drug may cause torsade de pointes.[70]

Calcium Channel–Blocking Agents: Verapamil and Diltiazem

In patients with normal sinus node function, the calcium channel blockers cause no significant heart rate slowing.[71] In patients with sinus node disease, however, verapamil and diltiazem may cause severe sinus bradycardia and occasionally sinus arrest.[72,73] The calcium channel–blocking agents have no effect on the HV interval or the effective refractory period of the atria, ventricles, or His-Purkinje system.[74] The effects of these drugs on the accessory pathway in patients with WPW syndrome are variable.[75] In some patients, verapamil shortens the anterograde effective refractory period of the accessory pathway.[76] Prolongation of conduction via the AV node may facilitate conduction through the accessory pathway and accelerate conduction via the AV bypass tract during atrial tachyarrhythmias in patients with WPW syndrome. This can lead to ventricular fibrillation and cardiac arrest.[77]

The effect of calcium channel blockers on the sinus rate on the 12-lead ECG varies depending on the balance between the direct action of the drugs and the antagonistic sympathetic reflex secondary to their hypotensive action. The PR interval is lengthened by verapamil and diltiazem, but second- and third-degree AV blocks rarely develop. The calcium channel–blocking agents have no effect on the QRS duration or QTc interval.[74]

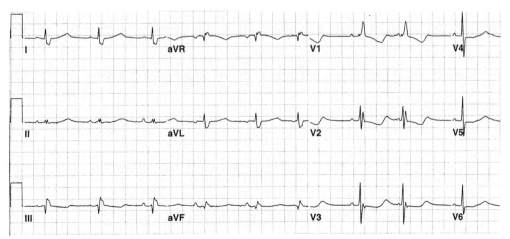

Figure 21–11   ECG of a 77-year-old woman treated with sotalol after electrocardioversion of atrial fibrillation to sinus rhythm shows right bundle branch block. The QT interval is difficult to measure accurately, but it measures 480 ms in lead aV$_L$, in which the U wave is absent, and 610 ms in leads V$_2$–V$_4$, in which the T wave has merged with the U wave.

Adenosine and ATP

Both adenosine and ATP depress the automaticity of the sinus node and AV nodal conduction.[78,79] The AV conduction delay is caused by prolongation of the AH interval without any demonstrable effect on the HV conduction time. After rapid bolus injection of the drugs, AV block of varying degree usually occurs within 20 seconds and lasts for about 10 to 20 seconds.[78,79] The mechanism by which the AV conduction is delayed differs from the β-adrenergic blocking and vagal actions.[78,79]

Adenosine and ATP have been used to terminate AV nodal reentrant tachycardia and orthodromic AV reentrant tachycardia[80,81] (Figure 21–12). The incidence of transient second-degree AV block and various supraventricular and ventricular arrhythmias after termination of the reentrant tachycardia is high.[80]

Psychotropic Drugs (Phenothiazines, Tricyclic Antidepressants, Lithium)

The electrophysiologic effects of the phenothiazines on ventricular repolarization are similar to those of quinidine, but the QRS duration usually remains normal. The most common ECG changes caused by the phenothiazines are widening, flattening, notching, or inversion of the T wave; prolongation of the QTc interval; and prominence of the U wave (Figure 21–13).[19,82,83] These repolarization abnormalities are seen more frequently in patients receiving thioridazine (Mellaril) than in those receiving chlorpromazine (Thorazine) or, even less, trifluoperazine (Stelazine).[83] The changes are dose related.

With thioridazine, repolarization abnormalities are usually not seen when the dosage is less than 100 mg/day. T wave abnormalities are present in about half of patients when the dosage

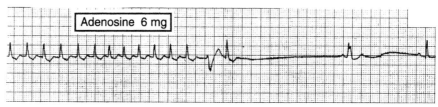

Figure 21–12   Effect of intravenous administration of adenosine on atrioventricular reentrant tachycardia. The negative P wave is recognizable within the ST segment during tachycardia. The first complex after the pause appears to show ventricular preexcitation.

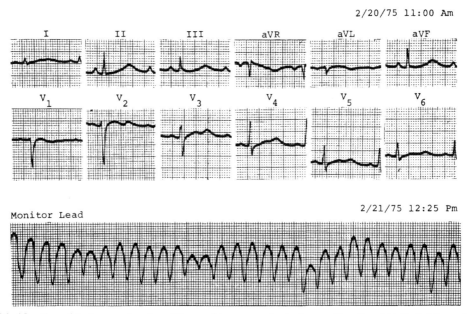

Figure 21–13   Phenothiazine overdose in a 40-year-old woman who took more than 2 g of Mellaril 3 hours before the 12-lead ECG was recorded. The tracing shows prominent U waves. The QT interval is prolonged, but exact measurement is difficult because of the superimposed U wave. The patient developed multiple episodes of ventricular tachycardia during the next 2 days. One of the episodes is shown here.

level is 100 to 300 mg/day and in about three fourths of patients when the dosage is >300 mg/day[82] (see Figure 21–13). The effects usually appear within 1 to 2 days after starting therapy and reach their maximum in 4 to 5 days. They are seen more often in women than in men.[82] High doses of the drug may cause supraventricular and ventricular tachyarrhythmias. Ventricular tachycardia and fibrillation were responsible for sudden death in some of these patients.[84,85]

The ventricular repolarization changes produced by the tricyclic antidepressants are similar to those caused by the phenothiazines but are usually less pronounced.[86–88] In contrast, the slowing of conduction manifested by increased QRS duration is more marked, particularly at rapid heart rates (use-dependent effect) (Figure 21–14). Niemann and associates[89] found that the presence of sinus tachycardia, prolonged QRS duration, prolonged QTc interval, and rightward shift of the terminal 40-ms QRS vector are useful ECG signs of tricyclic antidepressant cardiotoxicity. Their absence practically rules out overdose of the drug.

The most common ECG changes associated with therapeutic doses of lithium carbonate are T wave abnormalities.[90,91] Flattening or occasional inversion of the T wave is seen in 20 to 30 percent of lithium-treated patients.[90] The QT interval is not prolonged, and the T wave changes are reversible within 2 weeks after the drug is discontinued. In a number of case

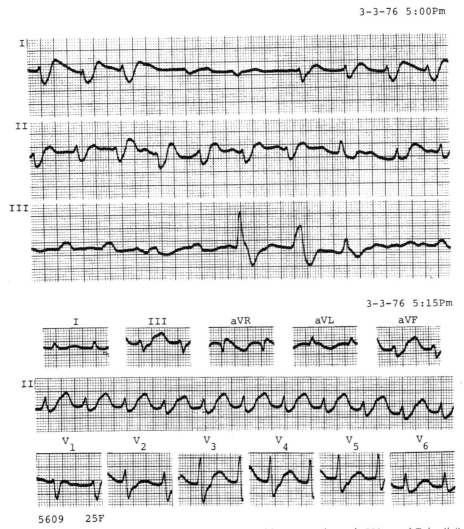

Figure 21–14 Tricyclic antidepressant overdose in a 25-year-old woman who took 500 mg of Tofranil (imipramine) 4 hours before the 5 PM tracing was recorded. The three standard limb leads show wide QRS complexes of varying morphology. The exact rhythm cannot be determined. She was severely hypotensive at this time. Fifteen minutes later the tracing shows probable supraventricular rhythm with intraventricular conduction defect.

reports, lithium caused sinus node dysfunction, including marked sinus bradycardia, sinus pauses, and sinoatrial (SA) block.[90–95] Such effects, however, are uncommon relative to the number of population taking the drug.

Of 97 consecutive patients receiving lithium and examined by Hagman and colleagues,[92] only 2 had sinus node depression possibly caused by lithium. In one report,[93] sinus node dysfunction induced by lithium was associated with hypothyroidism. Isolated cases of lithium toxicity causing supraventricular and ventricular tachyarrhythmias, AV and intraventricular conduction defects, and QT prolongation have been described.[90] Occasional premature ventricular complexes and first-degree AV block have been attributed to the drug, but many such case reports are not well documented.

Digitalis

Digitalis is used clinically because it exerts a positive inotropic effect and because it slows transmission in the AV node in patients with supraventricular tachyarrhythmias. The positive inotropic effect is due to inhibition of the sodium/potassium pump at the outer cell membrane. The action of digitalis on the AV node is primarily vagal and can be counteracted by atropine (Figure 21–15). Digitalis also has an antiadrenergic and a slight direct action, both of which augment the vagal effect of the drug on conduction in the AV node.

Digitalis has two potentially proarrhythmia effects: (1) shortening of the refractory period in the atria, ventricles, His-Purkinje system,

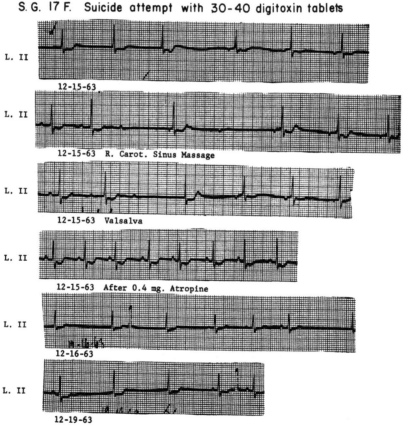

Figure 21–15 ECG of a 17-year-old woman after she attempted suicide by ingesting 3.0 to 4.0 mg (30 to 40 tablets) of digitoxin. Top three strips, recorded on the day of ingestion, show depression of sinoatrial (SA) node activity, supraventricular escape complexes, and slowing of the ventricular rate after carotid (R. Carot.) sinus massage and after the Valsalva maneuver. The fourth strip, recorded on the same day, shows regular sinus rhythm at a rate of 90 beats/min and a normal PR interval after intravenous administration of 0.4 mg atropine sulfate. The lower strips, recorded 1 and 4 days after digitoxin ingestion, show persistent depression of SA node activity and supraventricular escape complexes. (From Surawicz B, Mortelmans S: Factors affecting individual tolerance to digitalis. *In:* Fisch C, Surawicz B [eds]: Digitalis. Orlando, Grune & Stratton 1969.)

and accessory pathways; and (2) a narrow margin between therapeutic and toxic action on the sodium/potassium pump regulating intracellular calcium concentration.

Administration of therapeutic doses of digitalis decreases the automaticity of the SA node. At the AV junction the drug slows conduction but enhances automaticity.[96] The increase in the PR interval is due to prolongation of the AH interval, but the HV interval is unchanged. Digitalis may cause an increase in the automaticity of the His-Purkinje system by increasing the slope of diastolic depolarization in the Purkinje fibers. This action is responsible for the production of digitalis-induced AV junctional and ventricular tachyarrhythmias. The effects of digitalis on ventricular repolarization are responsible for the characteristic ST segment and T wave changes associated with administration of the drug. The QT interval is shortened. Application of suction electrodes during cardiac catheterization in humans showed that the monophasic action potential recorded from the endocardial surface of the ventricles had a steeper repolarization slope and shortened total duration.[97] The most common digitalis effects on the ECG are as follows:

1. Prolonged PR interval
2. ST segment depression
3. Decreased amplitude of the T wave, which may become diphasic (negative-positive) or negative
4. Shortened QT interval
5. Increased U wave amplitude

After administration of digitalis, the earliest ECG changes usually consist of decreased amplitude of the T wave and shortening of the QT interval. The more typical finding, however, is sagging of the ST segment, with the first part of the T wave "dragged down" by the depressed ST segment (Figure 21–16). Therefore the T wave becomes diphasic, with the initial portion being negative and the terminal portion positive. As the ST segment depression becomes more pronounced, the entire T wave may become inverted.[19]

Sometimes digitalis-induced T wave changes are atypical (i.e., pointed, inverted) and resemble those seen with myocardial ischemia or pericarditis.[19] The QT interval is shortened by digitalis, however, and it is usually normal with pericarditis and prolonged with myocardial ischemia. In about 10 percent of patients receiving digitalis, there is peaking of the terminal portion of the T wave.[98]

The U wave may become more prominent with digitalis therapy. The increased amplitude usually is best seen in the mid-precordial leads and may simulate QT lengthening (Figure 21–17). The degree of the increase is usually less than that resulting from hypokalemia or quinidine or amiodarone administration.

The characteristic ST and T wave changes caused by digitalis are not always present. Furthermore, the degree of change has no consistent relation to the amount of digitalis administered or the serum level of the glycoside. Toxic systemic manifestations of the drug or arrhythmias may occur in the absence of any significant

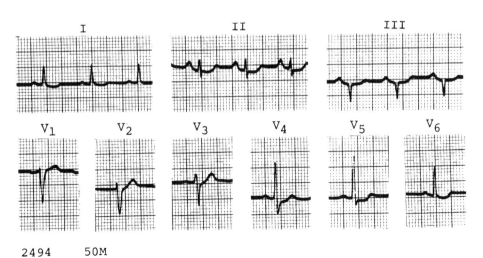

2494   50M

Figure 21–16 Digitalis effect in a 50-year-old man with no evidence of heart disease who took about 5 mg of digoxin in a suicide attempt 1 day before the tracing was recorded. The plasma digoxin level at the time of the recording was 4.1 ng/mL. Note the sagging of the ST segment, especially in leads I, II, and V_4–V_6. The T waves in leads II and V_5 are biphasic. No arrhythmia was observed.

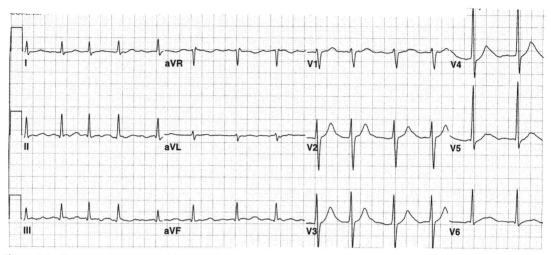

Figure 21–17 ECG of a 55-year-old man with atrial fibrillation treated with digoxin. Prolongation of the QT interval is simulated by fusion of the T wave with the U wave, best seen in leads V_2–V_4. The amplitude of the U wave is increased. Normally at this heart rate the U wave amplitude is too low to be recognizable.

ST segment or T wave changes. Conversely, marked repolarization abnormalities may be present when the doses are therapeutic or subtherapeutic. These changes also are more likely to be pronounced during tachycardia. Digitalis is one of the common causes of a false-positive ECG response during exercise testing to detect ischemia. Such a false-positive response was reported in 50 percent of normal subjects.[99]

The secondary ST segment and T wave changes in patients with ventricular hypertrophy or bundle branch block may simulate or mask the repolarization abnormalities associated with digitalis. The digitalis effect may be recognized, however, if there is definite "sagging" of the ST segment with an upward concavity. The duration of the QT interval is also sometimes helpful. With left ventricular hypertrophy or left bundle branch block, the QT interval is usually prolonged, whereas a digitalis effect may be suspected if the interval is normal or shortened.

DIGITALIS INTOXICATION

The diversity of actions affecting normal and abnormal automaticity, excitability and conduction, and the ability to elicit delayed afterdepolarizations (see Chapter 17) explains the diversity and complexity of cardiac arrhythmias and conduction disturbances caused by digitalis toxicity. A marked decline in complex arrhythmias has occurred concomitant with blood concentration–guided use of the drug, resulting in both lower blood and (presumably) myocardial drug concentration.[1] Reversal of digitalis toxicity now can be accomplished rapidly using highly specific antibodies.[100]

Although gastrointestinal symptoms are common and neurologic manifestations may occur, cardiac complications are the most serious toxic effect of digitalis. The drug is known to produce almost all types of cardiac arrhythmia, resulting from either disturbed impulse formation or impaired conduction. The only exceptions are atrial flutter and bundle branch block, which are rarely caused by digitalis. Different arrhythmias are often seen in the same patient within a relatively short time. Digitalis toxicity should be suspected especially when evidence of increased automaticity and impaired conduction are present at the same time. Although some of the arrhythmias are characteristic of digitalis toxicity, none is pathognomonic.

THE MORE COMMON ARRHYTHMIAS

Ventricular ectopic complexes are the most common arrhythmias and often represent the earliest manifestation of digitalis intoxication. They account for almost half of the arrhythmias caused by digitalis. They may be unifocal or multifocal. Bigeminal and trigeminal rhythms are particularly characteristic. When PVCs due to digitalis are not recognized and the drug administration is continued, more serious ventricular arrhythmias, such as ventricular tachycardia and ventricular fibrillation, may develop. The latter, however, may occur in the absence of the warning premature complexes. Digitalis also may cause a more benign accelerated idioventricular rhythm.

AV block of varying degree is the next most common arrhythmia induced by digitalis. In patients with sinus rhythm, slight prolongation of the PR interval is generally considered to be a therapeutic effect; more marked prolongation of the PR interval should be considered a warning sign of toxicity. Second- and third-degree AV block, when caused by digitalis, can be viewed as definitive evidence of intoxication.

Digitalis-induced second-degree AV block is usually of the Wenckebach type. Mobitz type II second-degree AV block is rare. Complete AV block caused by digitalis, as a rule, is associated with narrow QRS complexes unless an intraventricular conduction defect preexists. In patients with atrial fibrillation, advanced-degree AV block manifests as excessive slowing of the ventricular rate. A regular ventricular rhythm in the presence of atrial fibrillation suggests complete AV block (Figure 21–18).

Digitalis may cause abnormal enhancement of impulse formation at the AV junction, resulting in accelerated junctional rhythm. The rate of the junctional discharge is usually 70 to 130 beats/min, and the rhythm is regular. If the junctional pacemaker fails to capture the atria, AV dissociation occurs.[101] The atrial and ventricular rhythms are independent, and the ventricular rate is generally faster than the atrial rate.

Digitalis used to be the most frequent cause of a form of bidirectional tachycardia[102,103] (Figure 21–19). This rare arrhythmia may be AV junctional in origin, with regular alteration of two types of QRS complex, but well-documented cases of bidirectional ventricular tachycardia originating in the ventricle also have been reported.

Lown and associates[104] stressed the importance of digitalis in the genesis of ectopic atrial tachycardia with block, an arrhythmia known as paroxysmal atrial tachycardia (PAT) with block. Loss of potassium is responsible for precipitation of PAT with block in many digitalized patients. It was estimated that, among hospitalized patients, about 73 percent of those with this arrhythmia had the arrhythmia induced by digitalis.[104] Both the incidence of arrhythmia and its precipitation by digitalis have decreased in recent years.

The atrial rate in PAT with block is usually 150 to 200 beats/min. The degree of AV block varies (Figure 21–20), with second-degree block and the Wenckebach phenomenon being most common. Occasionally there is 1:1 conduction with a normal PR interval, and the AV block is demonstrated only during carotid sinus massage.

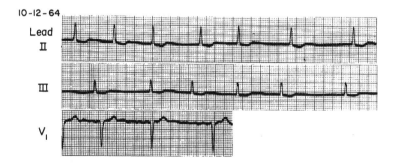

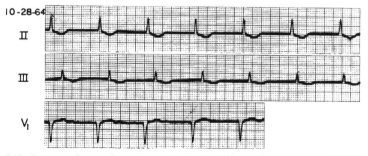

Figure 21–18   Atrial fibrillation with complete atrioventricular (AV) block. The tracing on 10/12/64 shows atrial fibrillation with controlled ventricular response. The ST and T wave changes are consistent with a digitalis effect. The regular RR interval in the tracing of 10/28/64 suggests a complete AV block with junctional escape rhythm. Digitalis toxicity is strongly suspected. (From Chou TC: Digitalis-induced arrhythmias. *In:* Fowler NO [ed]: Cardiac Arrhythmias: Diagnosis and Treatment. New York, Harper & Row, 1977.)

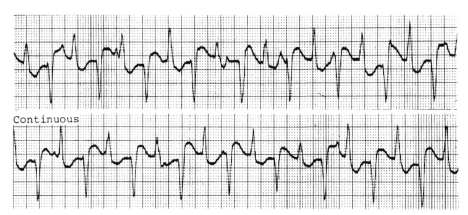

Figure 21-19 Bidirectional tachycardia caused by digitalis in a 54-year-old man with cardiomyopathy. The rhythm strip shows an atrial rate of 72 beats/min and a ventricular rate of 168 beats/min. There is atrioventricular dissociation. The alternate QRS complexes have opposite directions. The 12-lead ECG (not illustrated) showed a right bundle branch block pattern in all complexes.

Shortening of atrial refractory period can facilitate induction of atrial fibrillation, which is reported to account for about 10 percent of the arrhythmias induced by digitalis. The role of the drug in such an event is often difficult to document. Only if sinus rhythm returns after the drug is discontinued can the cause–effect relation be assumed.

The bradyarrhythmias are caused by the vagal effect of digitalis (see Chapter 13; Figure 21–15).

CORRELATION OF DIGITALIS TOXICITY WITH SERUM GLYCOSIDE LEVELS

The serum glycoside level is of considerable value for confirming the diagnosis of digitalis-induced arrhythmias. A digoxin level >2 ng/mL is generally considered indicative of digitalis overdosage. Considerable overlap of the serum glycoside concentration is found, however, among patients with and without toxicity. Toxic manifestations are seen in some patients with serum levels <2.0 ng/mL, but toxicity is absent in others with levels of 3.0 ng/mL.[105] Treatment with digitalis requires understanding the factors that modify sensitivity and tolerance to the drug.[106]

❚ Miscellaneous Drugs

EPINEPHRINE, NOREPINEPHRINE, ISOPROTERENOL

Epinephrine administered subcutaneously produces tachycardia and occasional PVCs. Rapid intravenous administration of 0.25 mg epinephrine has also caused various repolarization abnormalities, including ST segment elevation simulating acute myocardial ischemia.[107]

The effect of intravenous epinephrine infusion in different types of congenital long QT syndrome is described in Chapter 24.

Intravenous infusions of norepinephrine and isoproterenol at customary rates are associated with increased P wave amplitude, depressed PR segment, slightly shortened PR and QRS intervals, and variable T wave changes. Biberman et al.[108] studied the sequence of ECG changes during infusion of isoproterenol administered at a rate of 3 to 6 μg/min for 4 to 6 minutes in 11 healthy subjects with normal ECGs. During the early phase of infusion the T wave amplitude decreased in all subjects, and previously upright T waves became negative in one or more of leads I, II, and V$_3$–V$_6$. These changes were accompanied by an increase in heart rate without change in the QT interval (i.e., lengthening of the QTc interval). The maximal T wave inversion occurred usually within 30 to 40 seconds after starting the infusion and was always associated with hysteresis of the QT interval. Subsequently, the T wave became gradually more upright and the U wave amplitude increased. After an average of 2 minutes, the T wave and QTc interval were not significantly different from those in the control. After about 4 minutes, the amplitude of the upright T wave frequently exceeded that of the control (Figure 21–21). The change from negative to normal upright T waves during the second phase of isoproterenol action is similar to the often-observed effect of exercise in subjects with nonspecific T wave inversions at rest becoming upright during exercise-induced tachycardia.

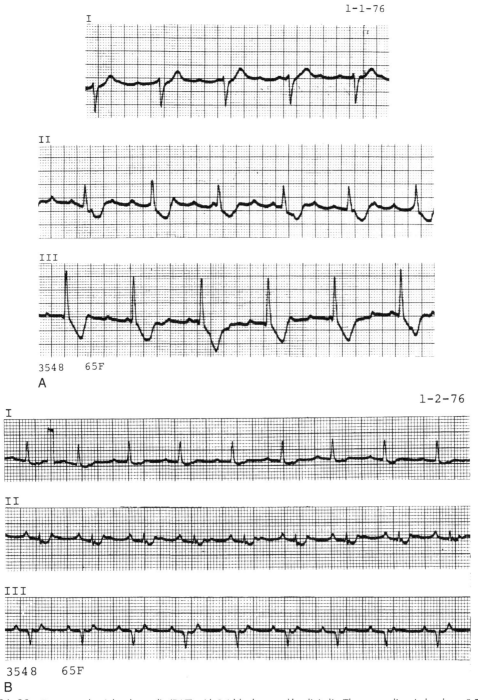

Figure 21–20   Paroxysmal atrial tachycardia (PAT) with 2:1 block caused by digitalis. The serum digoxin level was 3.7 ng/mL.

VAGOLYTIC DRUGS

Administration of vagolytic drugs (e.g., atropine) produces an effect resembling spontaneous tachycardia (i.e., increased P wave amplitude, shortened PR interval, and decreased T wave amplitude).[19]

ANESTHETIC AND ANALGESIC AGENTS

Transient prolongation of the PR interval, deviation of the ST segment, T wave abnormalities, and various rhythm disturbances may occur

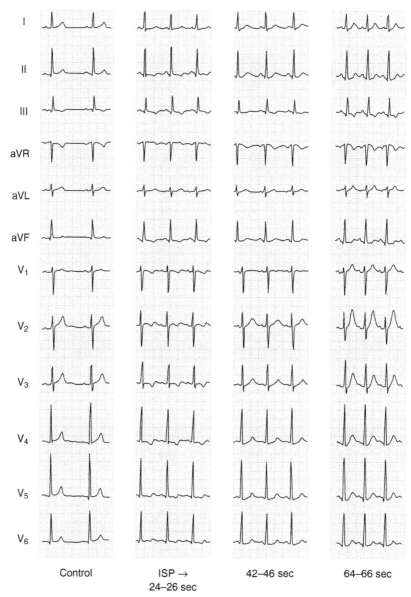

Figure 21–21   Sequence of T wave changes during intravenous isoproterenol infusion at a rate best seen in leads V_2–V_4. See text discussion. (From Biberman L, Sarma RN, Surawicz B: T wave abnormalities during hyperventilation and isoproterenol infusion. Am Heart J 81:166, 1971.)

during anesthesia with all commonly employed agents.[19]

In normal subjects, doses of succinylcholine used for endotracheal intubation (1 mg/kg) have no apparent effect on the plasma potassium concentration or the ECG; but in patients with soft tissue injuries, hyperkalemia associated with typical ECG manifestations was observed.[109] Curare and gallamine have no apparent effect on the ECG and do not cause hyperkalemia in subjects with soft tissue injuries.

ANTIPARASITIC DRUGS

Administration of emetine for treatment of amebiasis or alcoholism has caused T wave abnormalities, lengthening of the QTc interval, and occasional deviation of the ST segment.[19] Similar ECG abnormalities may occur after administration of chloroquine, plasmaquin, and atabrine. Treatment of schistosomiasis with various antimony compounds produced progressive T wave abnormalities associated with an increased QTc interval in nearly all patients.[19]

ARSENIC

Chronic arsenic intoxication produced QRS widening of 0.10 to 0.16 second, depression of the ST segment, QT prolongation, and T wave lowering in 56 percent of patients.[19] Episodes of ventricular tachycardia[110] and ventricular fibrillation[111] have been reported. A case of complete AV block was attributed to arsenic trioxide used to treat leukemia.[112]

REFERENCES

1. Surawicz B: Electropharmacology of antiarrhythmic drugs and digitalis. In: Electrophysiologic Basis of ECG and Cardiac Arrhythmias. Baltimore, Williams & Wilkins, 1995, pp 454–490.
2. Task Force of the Working Group on Arrhythmias of the European Society of Cardiology: The Sicilian gambit. Circulation 84:1831, 1991.
3. Crijns HJ, van Gelder IC, Lie KI: Supraventricular tachycardia mimicking ventricular tachycardia during flecainide treatment. Am J Cardiol 52:1303, 1988.
4. Rasmussen HS, Allen MJ, Blackburn KJ, et al: Dofetilide, a novel class III antiarrhythmic agent. J Cardiovasc Pharmacol 20:S96, 1992.
5. Di Marco JP: The ibutilide for atrial arrhythmias study group cardioversion of atrial flutter by intravenous ibutilide, a new class III antiarrhythmic agent. J Am Coll Cardiol 17:324A, 1991.
6. Wong W, Pavlou HN, Birgersdotter UM, et al: Pharmacology of the class III antiarrhythmic agent sematilide in patients with arrhythmias. Am J Cardiol 69:206, 1992.
7. Carmeliet E: Use-dependent block and use-dependent unblock of the delayed rectifier K⁺ current by almokalant in rabbit ventricular myocytes. Circ Res 73:857, 1993.
8. Velebit V, Podrid P, Lown B, et al: Aggravation and provocation of ventricular arrhythmias by antiarrhythmic drugs. Circulation 65:886, 1982.
9. Morganroth J: Risk factors for the development of proarrhythmic events. Am J Cardiol 59:32E, 1987.
10. Stanton MS, Prystowsky EN, Fineberg NS, et al: Arrhythmogenic effects of antiarrhythmic drugs: a study of 506 patients treated for ventricular tachycardia or fibrillation. J Am Coll Cardiol 14:209, 1989.
11. Horowitz LN: Drugs and proarrhythmia. In: Zipes DP, Rowlands DJ (eds): Progress in Cardiology. Philadelphia, Lea & Febiger, 1988, p 109.
12. Horowitz LN, Zipes DP, Bigger JT, et al: Proarrhythmia, arrhythmogenesis or aggravation of arrhythmia: a status report, 1987. Am J Cardiol 59:54E, 1987.
13. Mason JW: A comparison of seven antiarrhythmic drugs in patients with ventricular tachyarrhythmias. N Engl J Med 329:452, 1993.
14. Zipes DP: Proarrhythmic effects of antiarrhythmic drugs. Am J Cardiol 59:26E, 1987.
15. Coplen SE, Antman EM, Berlin JA, et al: Efficacy and safety of quinidine therapy for maintenance of sinus rhythm after cardioversion. a meta-analysis of randomized control trials. Circulation 82:1106, 1990.
16. Wegria R, Boyle MN: Correlation between effects of quinidine sulfate on heart and its concentration in blood plasma. Am J Med 4:373, 1948.
17. Heissenbuttel RH, Bigger JT: The effect of oral quinidine on intraventricular conduction in man: correlation of plasma quinidine with changes in QRS duration. Am Heart J 80:453, 1970.
18. Josephson M, Seides S, Batsford W, et al: The electrophysiological effects of intramuscular quinidine on the atrioventricular conducting system in man. Am Heart J 87:55, 1974.
19. Surawicz B, Lasseter KC: Effect of drugs on the electrocardiogram. Prog Cardiovasc Dis 13:26, 1970.
20. Hoffman BF, Rosen MR, Wit AL: Electrophysiology and pharmacology of cardiac arrhythmias. VII. Cardiac effects of quinidine and procaine amide. Am Heart J 89:804, 1975.
21. Vaughan Williams EM: A classification of antiarrhythmic actions reassessed after a decade of new drugs. J Clin Pharmacol 24:129, 1984.
22. Kayden HT, Brodie BB, Steele JM: Procaine amide: a review. Circulation 15:118, 1957.
23. Castellanos A, Salhanick L: Electrocardiographic patterns of procainide amide toxicity. Am J Med Sci 253:52, 1967.
24. Stearns NS, Callahan EJ, Ellis LB: Value and hazards of IV procaine amide therapy. JAMA 148:360, 1952.
25. Strasberg S, Sclarovsky S, Erdberg A, et al: Procainamide-induced polymorphous ventricular tachycardia. Am J Cardiol 47:1309, 1981.
26. Bleifer B, Castellanos A, Wells DE, et al: Electrophysiologic effect of the antiarrhythmic agent disopyramide phosphate. Am J Cardiol 35:282, 1975.
27. Danilo P, Rosen MR: Cardiac effects of disopyramide. Am Heart J 92:532, 1976.
28. Josephson MD, Caracta AR, Jau SH, et al: Electrophysiological evaluation of disopyramide in man. Am Heart J 86:721, 1973.
29. Koch-Weser J: Drug therapy: disopyramide. N Engl J Med 300:957, 1979.
30. LaBarre A, Strauss HC, Scheinman MM, et al: Electrophysiologic effects of disopyramide phosphate on sinus node function in patients with sinus node dysfunction. Circulation 59:226, 1979.
31. Singh BH, Collett JT, Chew CYC: New perspectives in the pharmacologic therapy of cardiac arrhythmias. Prog Cardiovasc Dis 22:243, 1980.
32. Morady F, Scheinman MM, Desai J: Disopyramide. Ann Intern Med 96:337, 1982.
33. Anderson JL, Manson JW, Winkle RA, et al: Clinical electrophysiologic effects of tocainide. Circulation 57:685, 1978.
34. Helfant RH, Schlerlag BJ, Damato AN: The electrophysiological properties of diphenylhydantoin sodium as compared to procaine amide in the normal and digitalis intoxicated heart. Circulation 36:108, 1967.
35. Grossman JI, Cooper JA, Frieden J: Cardiovascular effects of infusion of lidocaine on patients with heart disease. Am J Cardiol 24:191, 1969.
36. Coraboeuf E, Deroubaix S, Second D, et al: Comparative effects of three class I antiarrhythmic drugs on plateau and pacemaker currents of sheep cardiac Purkinje fibres. Cardiovasc Res 22:375, 1988.
37. Aravindakshan V, Kuo CS, Gettes LS: Effect of lidocaine on escape rate in patients with complete atrioventricular block. Am J Cardiol 40:177, 1977.
38. Kuo CS, Reddy CP: Effect of lidocaine on escape rate in patients with complete atrioventricular block. B. Proximal His bundle block. Am J Cardiol 47:1315, 1981.
39. Barbey JT, Thompson KA, Echt DS, et al: Antiarrhythmic activity, electrocardiographic effects and pharmacokinetics of the encainide metabolites O-desmethyl encainide and 3-methoxy-O-desmethyl encainide in man. Circulation 77:380, 1988.
40. Jackman WM, Zipes DP, Naccarelli GV, et al: Electrophysiology of oral encainide. Am J Cardiol 49:1270, 1982.
41. Mason JW: Basic and clinical cardiac electrophysiology of encainide. Am J Cardiol 58:18C, 1986.
42. Somberg JC, Tepper D, Landau S: Propafenone: a new antiarrhythmic agent. Am Heart J 115:1274, 1988.
43. Chilson DA, Heger JJ, Zipes DP, et al: Electrophysiologic effects and clinical efficacy of oral propafenone therapy in patients with ventricular tachycardia. J Am Coll Cardiol 5:1407, 1985.

44. Funck-Brentano C, Kroemer HK, Lee JT, et al: Propafenone. N Engl J Med 322:518, 1990.
45. Berkowitz WD, Wit AL, Lau SH, et al: Effects of propranolol on cardiac conduction. Circulation 40:855, 1969.
46. Gettes LS, Surawicz B: Long-term prevention of paroxysmal arrhythmias with propranolol therapy. Am J Med Sci 254:257, 1967.
47. Epstein SE, Braunwald E: Beta-adrenergic receptor blocking drugs: mechanism of action and clinical applications. N Engl J Med 275:1175, 1966.
48. Schamroth L: Immediate effects of intravenous propranolol on various cardiac arrhythmias. Am J Cardiol 18:438, 1966.
49. Stern S, Eisenberg S: The effect of propranolol (Inderal) on the electrocardiogram of normal subjects. Am Heart J 77:192, 1969.
50. Gray RJ, Bateman TM, Czer LS, et al: Esmolol: a new ultrashort-acting beta-adrenergic blocking agent for rapid control of heart rate in postoperative supraventricular tachyarrhythmias. J Am Coll Cardiol 5:1451, 1985.
51. Hohnloser SH, Klingenheben T, Singh BN: Amioadorone-associated proarrhythmic effects: a review with special reference to torsade de pointes tachycardia. Ann Intern Med 121:529, 1994.
52. Saksena S, Rothbart ST, Shah Y, et al: Clinical efficacy and electropharmacology of continuous intravenous amiodarone infusion and chronic oral amiodarone in refractory ventricular tachycardia. Am J Cardiol 54:347, 1984.
53. Wellens HJJ, Lie KI, Bar FW, et al: Effect of amiodarone in the Wolff-Parkinson-White syndrome. Am J Cardiol 38:189, 1976.
54. Heger JJ, Prystowsky EN, Jackman WM, et al: Amiodarone: clinical efficacy and electrophysiology during long-term therapy for recurrent ventricular tachycardia or ventricular fibrillation. N Engl J Med 305:539, 1981.
55. Minardo JD, Heger JJ, Miles WM, et al: Clinical characteristics of patients with ventricular fibrillation during antiarrhythmic drug therapy. N Engl J Med 319:257, 1988.
56. Rosenbaum MB, Chiale PA, Halpern MS, et al: Clinical efficacy of amiodarone as an antiarrhythmic agent. Am J Cardiol 38:934, 1976.
57. Touboul P, Atallah G, Gressard A, et al: Effects of amiodarone on sinus node in man. Br Heart J 42:573, 1979.
58. Harris L, McKenna WJ, Rowland E, et al: Side effects of long-term amiodarone therapy. Circulation 67:45, 1983.
59. Smetana P, Pueyo E, Hnatjova K, et al: Effect of amiodarone on the descending limb of the T wave. Am J Cardiol 92:742, 2003.
60. Mitchell LB, Wyse G, Gillis AM, et al: Electropharmacology of amiodarone therapy initiation: time courses of onset of electrophysiologic and antiarrhythmic effects. Circulation 80:34, 1989.
60a. Singh BN, Connolly SJ, Crijns HJGM, et al: Dronedarone for maintenance of sinus rhythm in atrial fibrillation or flutter. N Engl J Med 337:987, 1987.
61. Duff HJ, Roden DM, Yacobi A, et al: Bretylium: relations between plasma concentrations and pharmacologic actions in high-frequency ventricular arrhythmias. Am J Cardiol 55:395, 1985.
62. Koch-Weser J: Drug therapy. Bretylium. N Engl J Med 300:473, 1979.
63. Hohnloser SH, Woosley R: Sotalol. N Engl J Med 331:31, 1994.
64. Nademanee K, Feld G, Hendrickson J, et al: Electrophysiologic and antiarrhythmic effects of sotalol in patients with life-threatening ventricular tachyarrhythmias. Circulation 72:555, 1985.
65. Ruder MA, Ellis T, Lebsack C, et al: Clinical experience with sotalol in patient with drug-refractory ventricular arrhythmias. J Am Coll Cardiol 13:145, 1989.
66. Okada Y, Ogawa S, Sadanaga T, et al: Assessment of reverse use-dependent blocking actions of class III antiarrhythmic drugs by 24-hour Holter electrocardiography. J Am Coll Cardiol 27:84, 1996.
67. Funck-Brentano C, Kiblur Y, Le Cox F, et al: Rate dependence of sotalol-induced prolongation of ventricular repolarization during exercise in humans. Circulation 83:536, 1991.
68. Dorian P, Newman D, Berman N, et al: Sotalol and type-I in combination prevent recurrence of sustained ventricular tachycardia. J Am Coll Cardiol 22:106, 1993.
69. Lee SD, Newman D, Ham M, et al: Electrophysiologic mechanisms of antiarrhythmic efficacy of a sotalol and class Ia drug combination; elimination of reverse-use dependence. J Am Coll Cardiol 29:100, 1997.
70. Jackman WM, Friday KJ, Anderson JL, et al: The long QT syndrome: a critical review, new clinical observations and unifying hypothesis. Prog Cardiovasc Dis 31:115, 1988.
71. Mitchell LB, Schroeder JS, Mason JW: Comparative clinical electrophysiologic effects of diltiazem, verapamil and nifedipine: a review. Am J Cardiol 49:629, 1982.
72. Breithardt G, Seipel L, Wiebringhaus E, et al: Effects of verapamil on sinus node function in man. Eur J Cardiol 8:379, 1978.
73. Carrasco HA, Fuenmayor A, Barboza JS, et al: Effect of verapamil on normal sino-atrial node function and on sick sinus syndrome. Am Heart J 96:760, 1978.
74. Singh BH, Hecht HS, Nademanee K, et al: Electrophysiologic and hemodynamic effects of slow-channel blocking drugs. Prog Cardiovasc Dis 25:103, 1982.
75. Spurrell RAJ, Krikler DM, Sowton E: Effects of verapamil on electrophysiological properties of anomalous atrioventricular connection in Wolff-Parkinson-White syndrome. Br Heart J 36:256, 1974.
76. Gulamhusein S, Ko P, Carruthers SG, et al: Acceleration of the ventricular response during atrial fibrillation in the Wolff-Parkinson-White syndrome after verapamil. Circulation 65:348, 1982.
77. McGovern B, Garan H, Ruskin JN: Precipitation of cardiac arrest by verapamil in patients with Wolff-Parkinson-White syndrome. Ann Intern Med 104:791, 1986.
78. DiMarco JP, Sellers D, Berne RM, et al: Adenosine: electrophysiologic effects and therapeutic use for terminating paroxysmal supraventricular tachycardia. Circulation 68:1254, 1983.
79. Favale S, DiBiase M, Rizzo U, et al: Effect of adenosine and adenosine-5'-triphosphate on atrioventricular conduction in patients. J Am Coll Cardiol 5:1212, 1985.
80. Belhassen B, Glick A, Laniado S: Comparative clinical and electrophysiologic effects of adenosine triphosphate and verapamil on paroxysmal reciprocating junctional tachycardia. Circulation 77:795, 1988.
81. Sharma AD, Klein GJ: Comparative quantitative electrophysiologic effects of adenosine triphosphate on the sinus node and atrioventricular node. Am J Cardiol 61:330, 1988.
82. Huston JR, Bell GE: The effect of thioridazine hydrochloride and chlorpromazine on the electrocardiogram. JAMA 198:134, 1966.
83. Banta TA, St. Jean A: The effect of phenothiazines on the electrocardiogram. Can Med Assoc J 91:537, 1964.
84. Alexander CS, Nini A: Cardiovascular complications in young patients taking psychotropic drugs. Am Heart J 78:757, 1969.
85. Hollister LE, Kosek JC: Sudden death during treatment with phenothiazine derivatives. JAMA 192:93, 1965.
86. Burckhardt D, Raeder E, Muller V, et al: Cardiovascular effects of tricyclic and tetracyclic antidepressants. JAMA 239:213, 1978.

87. Giardina E, Bigger JT, Glassman AH, et al: The electro-cardiographic and antiarrhythmic effects of imipramine hydrochloride at therapeutic plasma concentrations. Circulation 60:1045, 1979.

88. Marshall JB, Forker AD: Cardiovascular effects of tricyclic antidepressant drugs: therapeutic usage, overdose, and management of complications. Am Heart J 103:401, 1982.

89. Niemann JT, Bessen HA, Rothstein RJ, et al: Electrocardiographic criteria for tricyclic antidepressant cardiotoxicity. Am J Cardiol 57:1154, 1986.

90. Mitchell JE, MacKenzie TB: Cardiac effects of lithium therapy in man: a review. J Clin Psychiatry 43:47, 1982.

91. Tilkian AG, Schroeder JS, Kao JJ, et al: The cardiovascular effects of lithium in man. Am J Med 661:665, 1976.

92. Hagman A, Arnman K, Ryden L: Syncope caused by lithium treatment: report of two cases and a prospective investigation of the prevalence of lithium-induced sinus node dysfunction. Acta Med Scand 208:467, 1979.

93. Numata T, Abe H, Terao T, et al: Possible involvement of hypothyroidism as a cause of lithium-induced sinus node dysfunction. PACE 22:954, 1999.

94. Wellens HJJ, Cats VM, Duren DR: Sympatomatic sinus node abnormalities following lithium carbonate therapy. Am J Med 59:285, 1975.

95. Wilson JR, Kraus ES, Bailas MM, et al: Reversible sinus-node abnormalities due to lithium carbonate therapy. N Engl J Med 294:1223, 1976.

96. Hoffman BF: Effects of digitalis on electrical activity of cardiac fibers. In: Fisch C, Surawicz B (eds): Digitalis. Orlando, Grune & Stratton, 1969.

97. Shabetai R, Surawicz B, Hammill W: Monophasic action potentials in man. Circulation 38:341, 1968.

98. Levine HD, Angelakos ET: Late peaking of the T wave as a digitalis effect. Am Heart J 68:320, 1964.

99. Kawai C, Hultgren HN: The effect of digitalis upon the exercise electrocardiogram. Am Heart J 68:409, 1964.

100. Haber E: Antibodies and digitalis: the modern revolution in the use of an ancient drug. J Am Coll Cardiol 5:111A, 1985.

101. Pick A, Dominguez P: Nonparoxysmal A-V nodal tachycardia. Circulation 16:1022, 1957.

102. Rosenbaum MB, Elizari MV, Lazzari JO: Mechanism of bidirectional tachycardia. Am Heart J 78:4, 1969.

103. Morris SN, Zipes DP: His bundle electrocardiography during bidirectional tachycardia. Circulation 48:32, 1973.

104. Lown B, Wyatt NF, Levine HD: Paroxysmal atrial tachycardia with block. Circulation 21:129, 1960.

105. Smith TW, Haber E: Digoxin intoxication: the relationship of clinical presentation to serum digoxin concentration. J Clin Invest 49:2377, 1970.

106. Surawicz B: Factors affecting tolerance to digitalis. J Am Coll Cardiol 5:69A, 1985.

107. Nordenfeldt O: Ueber funktionelle Veraenderungen der P und T Zacken in Electrokardiogramm. Acta Med Scand Suppl 119:1, 1941.

108. Biberman L, Sarma RN, Surawicz B: T wave abnormalities during hyperventilation and isoproterenol infusion. Am Heart J 81:166, 1971.

109. Mazze RL, Esene HM, Houston JB: Hyperkalemia and cardiovascular collapse during administration of succinylcholine to the traumatized patient. Anesthesiology 31:540, 1969.

110. Goldsmith S, From AHL: Arsenic-induced atypical ventricular tachycardia. N Engl J Med 303:1096, 1980.

111. St Petery J, Gross C, Victorica BA, et al: Ventricular fibrillation caused by arsenic poisoning. Am J Dis Child 120:367, 1970.

112. Huang C-H, Chen W-J, Wu C-C, et al: Complete atrioventricular block after arsenic trioxide treatment in acute promyelocytic leukemic patient. PACE 22:965, 1999.

Electrolytes, Temperature, Central Nervous System Diseases, and Miscellaneous Effects

Electrolytes	Hypothermia
Potassium	Hyperthermia
Calcium	
Sodium	**Miscellaneous Compounds**
Magnesium	
pH	**Central Nervous System Diseases**
Temperature	

Electrolytes

The specific electrocardiographic (ECG) changes caused by electrolyte imbalance are attributed to the effect of the altered concentration of ions on the transmembrane potentials of cardiac cells. Such changes are usually reversible, and their development and regression follow a predictable course. They can be modified, however, by a number of variables, the most important of which are (1) variation in the basic ECG pattern upon which the abnormalities caused by electrolyte imbalance are superimposed; (2) nonspecific effects owing to changes in the rate or rhythm caused by abnormal electrolyte concentrations; (3) repolarization changes secondary to intraventricular conduction disturbances caused by the abnormal electrolyte concentration; and (4) modifications introduced by the effect of one electrolyte on the concentration and activity of other electrolytes.

Another variable assumed to be responsible for the commonly encountered inaccuracy of the ECG in predicting the concentration is the effect of intracellular concentrations of electrolytes, but this factor is not likely to play an important role.[1] There is ample evidence that all patterns of electrolyte imbalance can be produced or corrected by rapidly altering the extracellular concentration of electrolytes.[1]

The accuracy of the ECG diagnosis improves when the interpreter is alert to the possibility of an electrolyte imbalance, when control tracings are available for comparison, and when the patient is followed with serial tracings. Monitoring the ECG during intravenous administration of potassium and calcium salts or of agents that lower the concentrations of these ions contributes to the effectiveness and safety of such therapy.

POTASSIUM

ECG Manifestations of Hyperkalemia

When the plasma K concentration exceeds approximately 5.5 mM, the T waves become tall and peaked; and when the plasma K concentration exceeds 6.5 mM, QRS changes are usually present (Figure 22–1). Hyperkalemia cannot be diagnosed with certainty on the basis of T wave changes alone. Braun et al.[2] found that the characteristic tall, steep, narrow, and pointed T waves were present in only 22 percent of patients with hyperkalemia, whereas in the remainder the tall T wave could not be distinguished from similar T waves of other etiology.

A correct ECG diagnosis of hyperkalemia can usually be made when plasma K concentrations exceed 6.7 mM.[1] Characteristically, the uniformly wide QRS complex due to hyperkalemia differs from the ECG pattern of bundle branch block or preexcitation because widening affects both the initial and terminal portions of the QRS complex (Figures 22–2 and 22–3). The

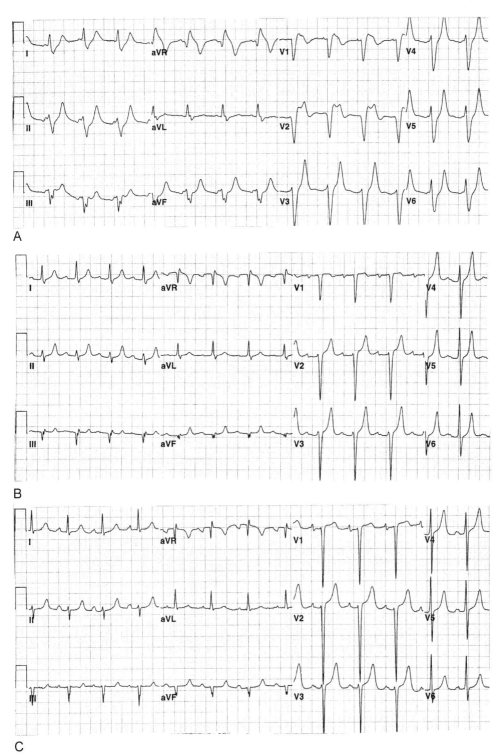

Figure 22–1   ECGs of a 46-year-old woman with chronic renal insufficiency. **A,** Plasma K concentration (Kp) is 8.0 mEq/L. There is a regular rhythm at a rate of 87 beats/min. P waves are not recognizable. The slow onset of QRS simulates P waves; the QRS duration is about 220 ms. T waves are tall, narrow, and sharply peaked. **B,** Three hours later, after treatment, the Kp is 6.0 mEq/L. Note the sinus rhythm at a rate of 90 beats/min. The PR interval is 240 ms, and the QRS duration is 116 ms. T waves are tall, narrow, and sharply peaked. **C,** Kp is now 4.2 mEq/L. Sinus rhythm is present at a rate of 87 beats/min. The PR interval is 180 ms, and the QRS duration is 96 ms. T waves are lower and wider than in **B**.

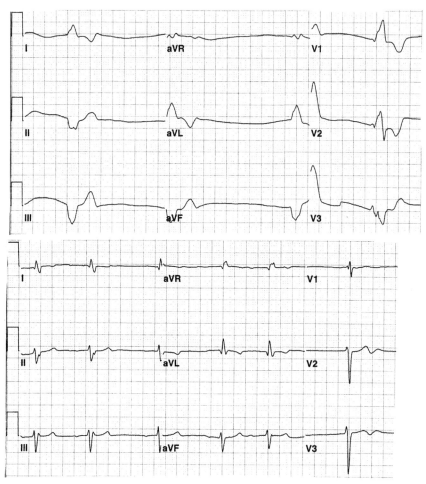

Figure 22–2   ECGs of a 76-year-old man with chronic renal failure and atrial fibrillation. *Top,* Kp is 8.1 mEq/L. There is irregular rhythm at a rate of 36 beats/min. The QRS duration is about 360 ms. Secondary T waves are not as tall, narrow, or sharply peaked as with less severe hyperkalemia and a lesser degree of intraventricular conduction disturbance. *Bottom,* After treatment the Kp is 3.9 mEq/L. Atrial fibrillation is present with a ventricular rate of 54 beats/min. Note the right bundle branch block and left axis deviation. The QRS duration is 130 ms.

wide S wave in the left precordial leads sometimes helps differentiate the pattern of hyperkalemia from that of typical left bundle branch block (LBBB), whereas the wide initial portion of the QRS complex may help differentiate the pattern of hyperkalemia from that of typical right bundle branch block (RBBB).

In some patients with hyperkalemia, however, the wide QRS complex resembles the typical pattern of LBBB or RBBB (see Figure 22–3). The QRS axis may shift superiorly (see Figure 22–3) or sometimes inferiorly, suggesting a nonuniform delay of conduction in the major divisions of the left bundle branch. Slow intraventricular conduction is associated with prolongation of the HV interval, which parallels the increase in the QRS duration.[3] The QRS duration increases progressively with an increasing plasma K concentration, and there is a rough correlation between the duration of the QRS complex and the plasma K concentration. Rarely, initial QRS portion is inscribed rapidly. Figure 22–4 shows pattern of advanced hyperkalemia with a rapid initial QRS deflection that simulates a pacemaker spike. Cases of yet inadequately explained normal ECG in patients with plasma K concentrations of 6.5 to 9.0 mEq/L have been observed and reported, but they lacked firm verification.

The pattern of advanced hyperkalemia is nearly identical to that recorded from dying hearts. Sometimes in patients with advanced hyperkalemia the ST segment deviates appreciably from baseline and simulates the "acute injury" pattern, which resembles the pattern of acute myocardial ischemia (Figure 22–5). Such ST deviation disappears rapidly when hyperkalemia regresses during treatment with hemodialysis.[4] The "injury current"

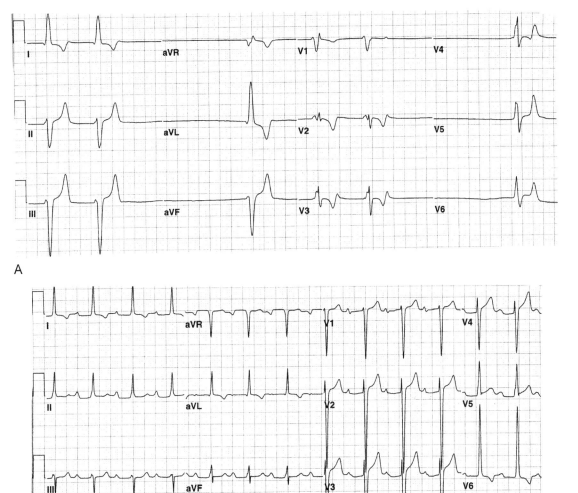

Figure 22–3 ECGs of a 36-year-old man with hypertension, diabetes mellitus, and end-stage renal disease. **A,** The Kp is 8.4 mEq/L. The rhythm is irregular at a rate of 36 beats/min. P waves are absent; the slow onset of QRS simulates P waves; the QRS duration is 182 ms; and the T waves are tall and narrow. **B,** After treatment of hyperkalemia, 53 minutes later, there is a sinus rhythm at a rate of 86 beats/min. The PR interval is 298 ms, and the QRS duration is 104 ms. The pattern of left ventricular hypertrophy is now recognizable.

responsible for the ST segment deviation is probably caused by nonhomogeneous depolarization in different portions of the myocardium. Deviation of the ST segment or a monophasic pattern can be readily produced by topical application of K on the ventricular surface or an intracoronary KCl injection.[5]

When the plasma K concentration exceeds 7.0 mM, the P wave amplitude usually decreases, and the duration of the P wave increases because of the slower conduction in the atria. The PR interval is frequently prolonged, but most of the prolongation tends to result from an increase

in P wave duration. When the plasma K concentration exceeds about 8.0 mM, the P wave frequently becomes invisible (see Figures 22–1 and 22–3). In the presence of a wide QRS complex, a low or absent P wave helps differentiate the pattern of hyperkalemia from that of intraventricular conduction disturbances of other origin.

A regular rhythm in the absence of P waves has been attributed to sinoventricular conduction via atrionodal tracts in the presence of sinoatrial (SA) block. This concept is supported by the observations that when the P wave disappeared

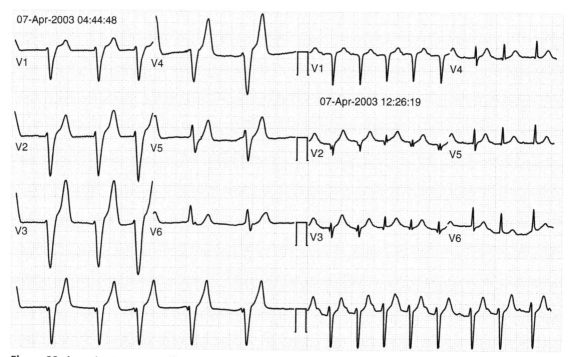

Figure 22–4 *Left,* ECG pattern of hyperkalemia in a 74-year-old woman with renal insufficiency (Ks = 7.8 mEq/L). Note the rapid onset of QRS duration, which in lead II (at the bottom of the tracing) simulates a pacemaker spike. QRS duration is 204 ms. P waves are absent. *Right,* Nearly 8 hours later after treatment. Note the sinus tachycardia (116 beats/min). QRS duration is 108 ms.

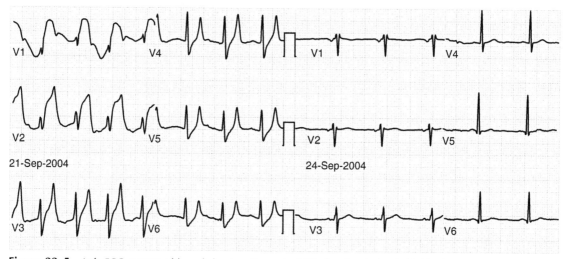

Figure 22–5 *Left,* ECG pattern of hyperkalemia with marked ST elevation in leads V_1–V_3. Acute injury pattern in a 36-year-old man with acute renal insufficiency (Ks = 7.3 mEq/L). Also of note: QRS duration is 138 ms; tall, narrow, peaked T waves in leads V_4–V_6; P waves are still present. *Right,* After treatment: sinus rhythm; incomplete right bundle branch block; QRS = 88 ms; low T amplitude.

during hyperkalemia in dogs, the electrical activity was recorded from the SA node, crista terminalis,[6] and atrionodal tracts,[7] and each QRS complex was preceded by a His bundle electrogram.

A regular rhythm in the absence of P waves can be caused by displacement of the pacemaker into the atrioventricular (AV) junction or the Purkinje fibers, but precise localization of the pacemaker in patients with absent P waves is usually not possible. When the plasma K concentration exceeds about 10 mM, the ventricular rhythm may become irregular owing to the simultaneous activity of several escape pacemakers in the depressed myocardium. The combination of an irregular rhythm and an absent P wave may simulate atrial fibrillation (see Figure 22–3). In patients with preexisting atrial fibrillation and hyperkalemia, the ventricular rate is usually slow (see Figure 22–2).

An increase in the plasma K concentration to above 12 to 14 mM causes ventricular asystole or ventricular fibrillation. The latter may or may not be preceded by acceleration of the ventricular rate.[8] When the heart rate is rapid, the ECG simulates ventricular tachycardia (Figure 22–6). The ECG pattern of hyperkalemia can be made more normal by increasing the concentrations of plasma calcium and sodium[9] and more abnormal by decreasing the concentration of plasma calcium and possibly that of sodium.

Understanding the above-described ECG changes produced by hyperkalemia may be facilitated by correlating these changes with concomitant changes in the atrial and ventricular transmembrane action potential. This is shown in Figure 22–7, which is based on experimental work

in isolated perfused rabbit hearts.[10] Figure 22–7A shows that the action potential duration in atrial fibers is shorter than in ventricular fibers. Figure 22–7B shows the more rapid repolarization that is responsible for the narrow and peaked T wave when the K concentration is increased to 6.0 mM. Figure 22–7, parts C to E, demonstrate that a progressive increase in the K concentration produces a progressive decrease in resting membrane potential, which decreases the maximum velocity of depolarization (V_{max}). This in turn slows intraatrial and intraventricular conduction, resulting in an increased duration of the P wave and the QRS complex.[11] At a K concentration of 12.0 mM ventricular depolarization is exceedingly slow, portions of the ventricular myocardium undergo repolarization before depolarization is completed, and determining the end of the QRS complex may be difficult to impossible (see Figure 22–7E). Figures 22–7C,D show that the atrial fiber is more depolarized than the ventricular fiber. In Figure 22–7C the P wave is wide and of low amplitude, and in Figure 22–7D the P wave is barely discernible. In Figure 22–7E the P wave is absent because the low-amplitude atrial depolarization does not reach the threshold to produce a propagated response.

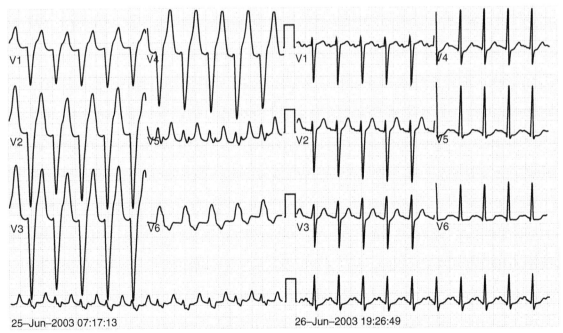

25–Jun–2003 07:17:13   26–Jun–2003 19:26:49

Figure 22–6   *Left* (June 25), ECG pattern of hyperkalemia simulating ventricular tachycardia with left bundle branch block morphology in a 50-year-old man with renal insufficiency. Ks = 8.0 mEq/L; QRS duration is 164 ms; P waves are absent; T waves are tall and peaked. *Right* (June 26), After treatment, the ECG is normal except for sinus tachycardia (136 beats/min). QRS is 98 ms.

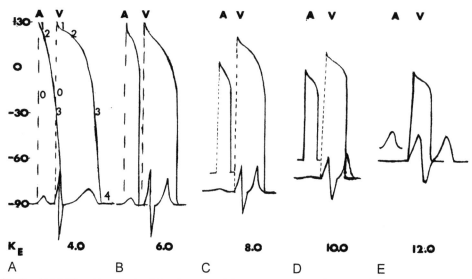

Figure 22–7 Atrial (A) and ventricular (V) action potentials superimposed on the ECG. The numbers on the left designate the transmembrane potential in millivolts, and the numbers at the bottom represent the extracellular K concentration in milliequivalents per liter. See text discussion. (From Surawicz B: Relation between electrocardiogram and electrolytes. Am Heart J 73:814, 1967.)

Antiarrhythmic and Arrhythmogenic Effects of Potassium

In the study of Bettinger et al.,[12] intravenous administration of potassium chloride solution suppressed supraventricular and ventricular ectopic complexes (with the exception of atrial fibrillation and flutter) in about 80 percent of patients. The incidence of suppression was not influenced by the presence or absence of heart disease, plasma K concentration, or treatment with digitalis. The margin between the therapeutic and toxic doses of K was rather narrow, and the antiarrhythmic effect usually occurred when the plasma K concentration increased by 0.5 to 1.0 mM to a level of 5.0 to 6.5 mM. Such an increase in plasma K concentration usually had no effect on the sinus rate. The therapeutic effect of K administration is usually transient.

Administration of K salts with glucose at a slow rate may precipitate serious arrhythmias (including ventricular tachycardia and ventricular fibrillation) in patients with hypokalemia, severe K depletion, or digitalis toxicity.[13] In these patients K is apparently avidly taken up by the cells, and the plasma K concentration falls when K in glucose solution is administered slowly.

Lethal hyperkalemia results predominantly from renal failure and occasionally from an error in the amount of K administered intravenously. The effect of intravenously administered K depends on the rate of administration rather than the absolute amount of potassium given. Large amounts of potassium can be administered at a slow rate, which

allows K to be excreted through the kidneys or transferred into the cells. At rapid administration rates, however, even small amounts of K can be lethal.

ECG Manifestations of Hypokalemia

Understanding the ECG changes due to hypokalemia may be facilitated by correlating these changes with concomitant changes in the ventricular action potential, as shown in Figure 22–8. It can be seen that progressive changes in repolarization are reflected on the ECG as progressive depression of the ST segment, a decrease in T wave amplitude, and an increase in U wave amplitude in the standard limb and precordial leads. So long as the T and U waves are separated by a notch, the duration of the QT interval is unchanged. With more advanced stages of hypokalemia, the T and U waves are fused, and an accurate measurement of the QT interval is not possible.[1] Because the duration of mechanical systole does not change during hypokalemia, one can best describe the pattern of hypokalemia as a gradual shift of the major repolarization wave from systole into diastole. The maximum amplitude of the repolarization wave is inscribed during systole in Figure 22–8A. Repolarization waves during systole and diastole are of equal amplitude in Figure 22–8B, whereas in Figure 22–8C,D the amplitude of the repolarization wave inscribed during diastole is greater than that inscribed during systole. The latter two ECG patterns seen with hypokalemia are most frequently encountered when the plasma K concentration is

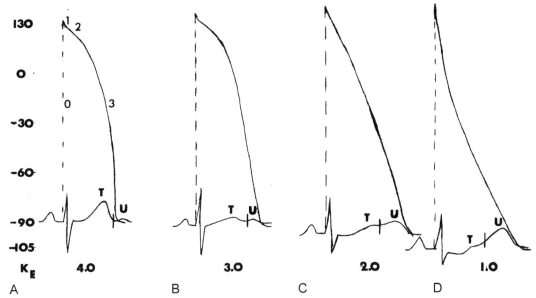

Figure 22–8   Ventricular action potential (on the left) superimposed on the ECG for extracellular K (Ks) 4.0 to 1.0 mEq/L. The numbers on the left designate the transmembrane potential in millivolts. See text discussion. (From Surawicz B: Relation between electrocardiogram and electrolytes. Am Heart J 73:814, 1967.)

<2.7 mM.[1] Previously, Surawicz and Lepeschkin assumed that the second heart sound marked the point of the TU junction and that the apex of a large deflection expected at the time of the occurrence of the normal U wave apex represents either a U wave of large amplitude or a normal U wave elevated by underlying prolonged ventricular repolarization. It is equally possible that the U wave amplitude remains unchanged, however, and that analogous to congenital or acquired long QT syndromes the abnormal repolarization during hypokalemia is caused by fusion of a prolonged T wave with a normal U wave, which means a prolonged QT interval with an unrecognizable U wave.[14]

The ECG diagnosis of hypokalemia is usually based on abnormalities of the ST segment, T wave, and U wave. In an attempt to evaluate the pattern of hypokalemia quantitatively, Surawicz et al.[15] considered the following three ECG features: (1) depression of the ST segment of ≥0.5 mm; (2) U wave amplitude >1 mm; and (3) U wave amplitude greater than the T wave amplitude in the same lead. The limb lead and the precordial lead, each with the tallest U wave, were analyzed on each of the ECGs.

The ECG was considered to be "typical" of hypokalemia if three or more of these features were present in the two leads; it was considered "compatible" with hypokalemia if two of these features or one related to the U wave were present. When the plasma K concentration was <2.7 mEq/L, the ECG was "typical" in 78 percent and "compatible" in 11 percent of all patients. When the plasma K concentration was 2.7 to 3.0 mEq/L, the ECG was "typical" in 35 percent and "compatible" with hypokalemia in 35 percent of patients. Other investigators obtained full agreement of the ECG and laboratory findings in patients whose plasma K concentration was <2.3 mEq/L[16] or <3.0 mEq/L.[17] Typical patterns of hypokalemia are shown in Figures 22–9 to 22–11.

When the ECG was monitored during administration of K in patients with hypokalemia, changes in the amplitude of the T and U waves reflected fairly accurately the changes in the plasma K concentration.[13]

Recognizing hypokalemia is frequently difficult in the presence of tachycardia, which decreases the amplitude of the T and U waves and often causes ST segment depression. Moreover, during tachycardia the U wave usually merges with the terminal portion of the T wave and with the P wave. The only indication that a U wave is present may be prolonged descent of an apparently normal T wave. In such cases the P wave is usually superimposed on the U wave. When this occurs, the P wave is tilted because its onset is situated farther from the baseline than its end[15] (see Figure 22–9). P wave tilting, however, is not always caused by an underlying U wave. When the rate is rapid or when the PR or QT interval is prolonged, the P wave may be superimposed on the descent of the T wave.

In the presence of a left ventricular hypertrophy (LVH) pattern, the U wave amplitude is frequently

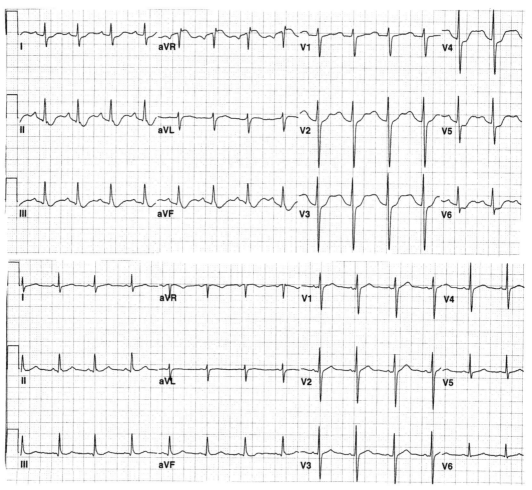

Figure 22–9   ECGs of a 43-year-old man with distal renal tubular acidosis and muscular weakness. *Top,* Kp is 1.5 mEq/L. Sinus rhythm is present at a rate of 97 beats/min. The PR is 220 ms, and the QRS is 110 ms. This is a typical pattern of hypokalemia with ST segment depression and U wave amplitude exceeding the T wave amplitude in several leads. In some leads the P wave is tilted because it is superimposed on the U wave. *Bottom,* After correction of hypokalemia, there is sinus rhythm at a rate of 90 beats/min. ECG is normal. The PR is 116 ms, and the QRS is 82 ms. The ST segment is no longer depressed, and the T wave amplitude exceeds that of the U wave.

increased (as part of the overall amplitude increases) even in the absence of hypokalemia. The latter may be suspected when the ST segment is depressed in the right precordial leads because in the presence of an uncomplicated LVH pattern the ST segment in these leads is usually elevated. Digitalis often causes ST segment and T wave changes similar to those caused by hypokalemia, but it does not increase the U wave amplitude to the same degree as hypokalemia does.

Digitalis usually causes a more distinct separation of the T wave from the U wave than hypokalemia because digitalis shortens the QT interval (see Figure 21–16). Concomitant administration of digitalis with quinidine and other drugs that prolong QT results in a pattern indistinguishable from that of hypokalemia.[1]

The U wave amplitude is also increased during bradycardia, particularly in the presence of complete AV block and in some patients with a "cerebrovascular accident (CVA) pattern" (see later discussion). In these patients the T wave amplitude is also frequently increased, and the T/U wave amplitude ratio is usually not altered.

When hypokalemia is advanced, both the amplitude and duration of the QRS interval are increased. The QRS complex is widened diffusely (but seldom by more than 0.02 second in adults). The QRS widening may be more pronounced in children.[18] The increased duration of the QRS is the result of widening without a change in shape, which suggests that it is caused by slower intraventricular conduction without changes in the depolarization sequence. The amplitude and duration

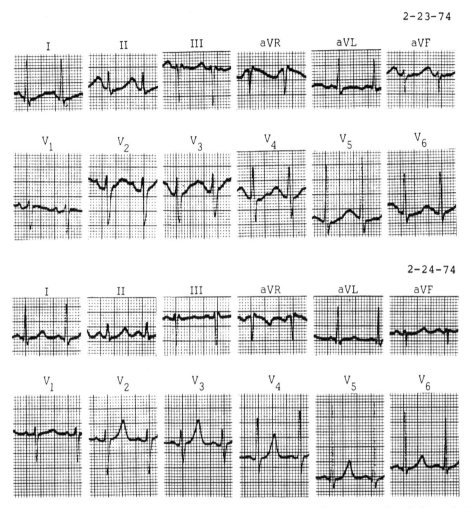

Figure 22–10 Hypokalemia associated with periodic paralysis in a 33-year-old woman with periodic paralysis. The top tracing (2/23/74) was recorded when the serum potassium level was 2.4 mEq/L. ST segment depression and low amplitude of the T wave are seen in leads I, II, aV$_F$, and V$_4$–V$_6$. Prominent U waves are best seen in leads II, III, aV$_F$, and V$_3$–V$_6$. The bottom tracing was recorded the next day, after the serum potassium level was restored to normal.

of the P wave in hypokalemia are usually increased, and the PR interval is often slightly or moderately prolonged (see Figure 22–9).

Arrhythmogenic Effects

Hypokalemia promotes the appearance of supraventricular and ventricular ectopic complexes (see Figures 22–11 and 22–12). In a study of 81 patients not treated with digitalis whose plasma K concentration was ≤3.2 mEq/L, the incidence of ventricular ectopic complexes was 28 percent; that of supraventricular ectopic complexes, 22 percent; and that of AV conduction disturbances, 12 percent. The incidence of ectopic complexes was three times higher and the incidence of AV conduction disturbances

two times higher than the corresponding incidences in the control hospital population.[19]

Arrhythmias appearing in patients with severe hypokalemia are of the same type as in patients with digitalis toxicity; that is, nonparoxysmal atrial tachycardia with block (see Figure 22–12) and various types of AV dissociation. These arrhythmias are attributed to a combination of increased automaticity of ectopic pacemakers and at least some degree of AV conduction disturbance. Similar to digitalis, hypokalemia increases sensitivity to vagal stimulation.

In patients with severe hypokalemia, serious ventricular tachyarrhythmias, including ventricular tachycardia, torsade de pointes, and ventricular fibrillation, have been reported in the absence of heart disease or digitalis therapy.[13,15,19–21]

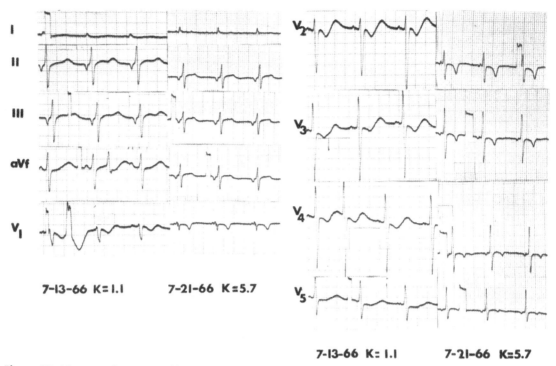

Figure 22–11   ECG of a 65-year-old woman with chronic pyelonephritis and vomiting in the presence of hypokalemia (7/13) and after K repletion (7/21). There was a typical pattern of hypokalemia on 7/13 and ventricular ectopic complexes with a short coupling interval in leads aV_F and V_2. The plasma K concentration is shown in milliequivalents per liter. During hypokalemia the T and U waves are fused. After treatment the Kp was 5.7 mEq/L. The U wave is not discernible. (From Surawicz B: Relation between electrocardiogram and electrolytes. Am Heart J 73:814, 1967.)

Hypokalemia is frequently present in patients with acute myocardial infarction[22,23] or after resuscitation from out-of-hospital ventricular fibrillation[24] possibly due to treatment with thiazide diuretics[20,22,24] or administration of sodium bicarbonate during resuscitation.[24] Hypokalemia may be precipitated by intense sympathetic stimulation that shifts K into the skeletal muscle and the liver,[25] an effect attributed to β_2-receptor stimulation by the circulating epinephrine.[26]

Modification of Potassium Effects by Other Electrolytes

Hypocalcemia frequently accompanies hyperkalemia in patients with renal insufficiency (see Figure 12–27). Its presence may be expected to aggravate AV and intraventricular conduction disturbances and facilitate the appearance of ventricular fibrillation.

Hypercalcemia is also present in some patients with renal insufficiency and hyperkalemia because of secondary hyperparathyroidism or overzealous therapy with calcium. Hypercalcemia may be expected to counteract the effect of hyperkalemia on the AV and intraventricular

conduction disturbances and to prevent ventricular fibrillation.

Abnormal sodium concentrations may also modify the ECG pattern of hyperkalemia. Hypernatremia may be expected to counteract, and hyponatremia to augment, the effects of increased K concentration on AV and intraventricular conduction disturbances. In hypokalemic patients with hypocalcemia, the ST segment is prolonged (Figure 22–13). Arrhythmias in hypokalemic patients with hypocalcemia were as common as in those without hypocalcemia.[19] Similarly, the incidence of arrhythmias was the same in hypokalemic patients with and without acidosis.[19]

CALCIUM

Changes in extracellular calcium concentration have a profound effect on the duration of the plateau (phase 2) of the action potential. The duration of the plateau increases at low extracellular calcium concentrations and shortens at high calcium concentrations. Because the plateau duration of the ventricular action potential determines the duration of the ST segment, the changes in calcium concentration

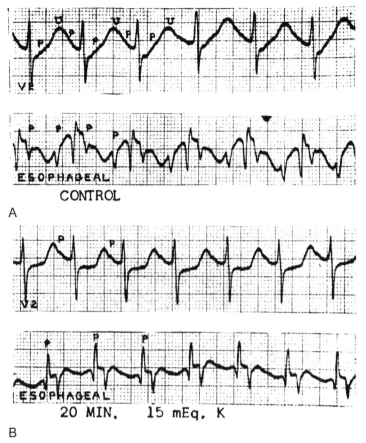

Figure 22–12 ECG lead V_2 (at the top of each panel) and esophageal lead (at the bottom of each panel) of a 34-year-old woman with a plasma K level of 1.0 mEq/L caused by vomiting. Top panel shows hypokalemia pattern and indistinct P waves in lead V_2. The P waves and the 2:1 atrioventricular block are seen clearly in the esophageal lead. After intravenous administration of 15 mEq K (two lower strips), ectopic atrial tachycardia and 2:1 block are no longer present. (From Bettinger JC, Surawicz B, Crum WB, et al: The effect of intravenous administration of potassium chloride on ectopic rhythms, ectopic beats, and disturbances in AV conduction. Am J Med 21:521, 1956.)

predominantly affect the duration of the ST segment and thereby the duration of the QT interval.

Hypercalcemia

The ST segment is short or absent in the presence of hypercalcemia and the duration of the QTc interval is decreased[1] (Figure 22–14; see also Figure 12–25). Bronsky et al.[27] found that the QTc interval was inversely proportional to the serum calcium level up to 16 mg/dL. The interval between the onset of QRS and the onset of the T wave (Q-oT) became shorter at higher calcium levels, although the T wave was prolonged and the QT interval became more normal. Nierenberg and Ransil[28] found that the interval from the onset of QRS to the apex of the T wave (Q-aT) correlated more closely than the QTc or Q-oTc with the serum calcium levels.

Q-aTc interval of 0.27 second or less was associated with hypercalcemia in more than 90 percent of the cases. Lind and Ljunghall[29] examined ECG changes of 139 patients with primary hyperparathyroidism (and hypercalcemia). A decrease in the ST segment and the Q-oT interval correlated significantly with increasing serum calcium concentration, but the QRS and PR durations did not. In other studies hypercalcemia was associated with slight prolongation of the QRS duration.[1]

Hypercalcemia usually does not alter the morphology of the P waves and T waves, but a slight, statistically significant increase in T wave duration was reported.[29] The U wave amplitude is either normal or increased.[1] In the presence of hypercalcemia associated with hypokalemia, a short QT interval with increased U wave amplitude results in a distinct pattern, most often seen in patients with multiple myeloma (Figure 22–15).

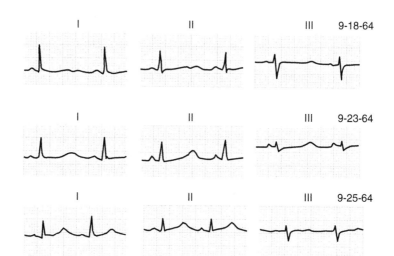

Figure 22–13   Hypocalcemia and hypokalemia in a 31-year-old man with chronic renal failure. The tracing on 9/18/64 shows prolongation of the QT interval, especially the ST segment. The U waves are prominent. The serum calcium level was 5.8 mg/dL, and the potassium level was 3.3 mEq/L. On 9/23/64 the serum potassium level was 2.8 mEq/L. The U waves become more prominent, and in most of the leads they are superimposed on the T waves. The ST segment remains prolonged. On 9/25/64 the serum calcium level was increased to 6.5 mg/dL, and the potassium level was increased to 3.5 mEq/L. The tracing shows definite shortening of the ST segment, and the U waves are less prominent.

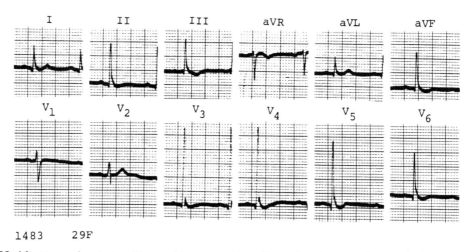

Figure 22–14   Hypercalcemia in a 29-year-old woman with malignant lymphoma involving multiple organs, including bone. The serum calcium level was 17.4 mg/dL. She was not receiving digitalis. The heart was found to be normal at autopsy. Note the short QT interval. The ST segment is almost absent. The flat T waves may or may not be related to hypercalcemia.

Cardiac arrhythmias are uncommon in patients with hypercalcemia. It has been postulated, however, that sudden death of patients during hyperparathyroid crisis and other conditions associated with severe hypercalcemia may be caused by ventricular fibrillation.[30] Second- or third-degree AV blocks have been reported in patients with severe hypercalcemia.[30,31]

Hypocalcemia

In the presence of hypocalcemia, the ST segment and the QTc interval are prolonged (Figure 22–16; see also Figure 12–24). The duration of the ST segment is inversely related to the plasma calcium concentration.[1] Usually lengthening of the ST segment, Q-aT, and the QT interval are the only ECG abnormalities; but the QTc interval seldom exceeds 140 percent of normal. Therefore a QTc interval of more than 140 percent usually suggests that the U wave is incorporated into the T wave and that QU is being measured.[32] Hypocalcemia usually can be recognized on the ECG because, with the possible exception of hypothermia, there are no other agents or metabolic abnormalities that prolong the duration of the ST segment without

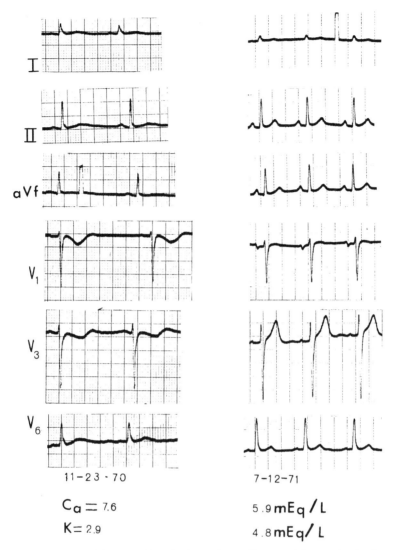

Figure 22–15 ECG of a 41-year-old man with multiple myeloma. Plasma calcium and potassium concentrations (in mEq/L) are shown at the bottom. On the left, hypercalcemia is manifested by near-absence of the ST segment, and hypokalemia is reflected in the increased U wave amplitude, best seen in lead V_3. On the right, the pattern is normal at normal plasma Ca and K concentrations.

changing the duration of the T wave (a possible exception to this statement may be LQT3 pattern; see Chapter 24). Measurements of the ST segment duration, however, may be difficult when it is depressed or elevated or when the T wave is diphasic.[1] In patients with a prolonged QT interval due to hypocalcemia, the U wave is usually absent or not recognizable. The heart rate, P wave configuration, and duration of the PR interval and the QRS complex are usually normal, and no significant rhythm disturbances are noted. The results of correlation between serum calcium and the QTc are variable.[16,33] A good correlation between the duration of the ST segment and the plasma calcium concentration was found in patients with hypocalcemia induced by administration of the calcium-

binding agent ethylenediaminetetraacetic acid (EDTA).[34] In these patients the ECG pattern was not obscured by the effects of other electrolyte abnormalities. Because the ECG is affected by the concentration of ionized calcium rather than total calcium, it apparently correlates better with the calcium concentration in the protein-free cerebrovascular fluid than with the calcium concentration in the blood.[35] In the presence of hypocalcemia, the polarity of the T wave may remain unchanged. Sometimes, however, the T wave becomes low, flat, or sharply inverted in leads with an upright QRS complex.[36] The change in T wave polarity suggests a change in the sequence of repolarization, presumably due to unequal lengthening of ventricular action potentials in different regions of the

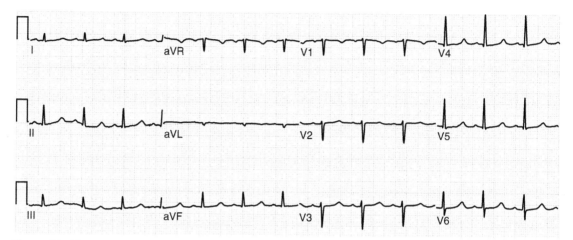

Figure 22–16   Prolonged QTc (532 ms) caused by hypocalcemia (Ca_s = 6.0 mg/L) in a 44-year-old woman. Note the prolonged ST segment with normal duration and morphology of the T wave.

myocardium. Figure 12–24 shows that intravenous calcium administration shortens the QT interval and restores normal T wave polarity in a patient with hypocalcemia.

Prolongation of the QTc interval is associated with an increased duration of the ventricular refractory period. This effect per se, in the absence of a concomitant increase in dispersion of refractoriness or changes in conduction, may be expected to be antiarrhythmic, perhaps similar to the class III action of the antiarrhythmic drugs. Moderate hypocalcemia induced by administration of Na_2 EDTA suppressed supraventricular and ventricular ectopic complexes in about 50 percent of patients.[37] The ectopic complexes suppressed by hypocalcemia reappeared after calcium administration.[37]

SODIUM

High sodium levels prolong the duration of the cardiac action potential, but the clinical significance of this change is uncertain. A prolonged QT interval caused by delayed inactivation of the sodium current in patients with congenital long QT syndrome (type 3) is described in Chapter 24. The effect of high or low sodium levels on the ECG, cardiac rhythm, and conduction is probably negligible within the limits of the plasma sodium concentration compatible with life. However, in the presence of intraventricular conduction disturbances caused by hyperkalemia, the duration of the QRS complex is shortened by hypernatremia and prolonged by hyponatremia.

MAGNESIUM

Magnesium concentrations within the range encountered in clinical situations have no important effect on the action potential, at least at normal potassium and calcium concentrations.[38] Studies of isolated perfused rabbit hearts suggested that hypomagnesemia may augment the QT lengthening induced by hypocalcemia, but clinical studies produced no supporting evidence for such a phenomenon,[1] probably because the effect of magnesium deficiency that modulates the effect of calcium deficiency on the plateau of the action potential in vitro does not manifest in vivo until the concentrations of these two ions fall to levels that are not compatible with life.[39]

Hypomagnesemia and hypermagnesemia do not produce specific ECG patterns in animals and humans. Personal experience suggests that neither hyper- nor hypomagnesemia has a detectable effect on the QT interval in humans. In fact, in children with tetany the lack of QT prolongation would favor deficiency of magnesium rather than of calcium.

Evidence that hypomagnesemia is responsible for cardiac arrhythmias is limited to case reports. In some cases, other associated causes could be suspected because of QT prolongation[40,41] or the presence of hypokalemia on admission[42,43] (Figure 22–17).

Magnesium sulfate solution administered intravenously has been used empirically for several decades[44,45] to suppress a variety of supraventricular and ventricular arrhythmias in the absence and presence of digitalis therapy.[46] The precise mechanism of antiarrhythmic action of acute magnesium administration has not been elucidated. Magnesium blocks the calcium channel, modifies the effect of hyperkalemia, and exerts modulating effects on several potassium currents.[5]

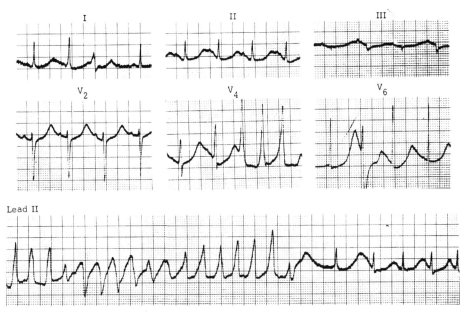

Figure 22–17   Ventricular tachycardia and torsade de pointes, probably caused by electrolyte imbalance, in a 63-year-old woman with diagnosis of hypertension, diabetes mellitus, and chronic alcoholism. The tracing shows prolongation of the QT interval, with probable prominent U waves and an episode of ventricular tachycardia in lead V_4. Long lead II shows an episode of torsade de pointes. The serum potassium level was 2.9 mEq/L, and the calcium level was 7.9 mg/dL. Serum magnesium level determined 2 days later was 0.7 mg/dL. It is likely that the hypokalemia and hypomagnesemia are responsible for the ventricular arrhythmias.

Hypermagnesemia depresses AV and intraventricular conduction. In animal experiments, AV conduction may be depressed when the magnesium concentration reaches 3 to 5 mM. The latter concentrations are higher than those that can cause respiratory arrest. In humans, infusion of magnesium salts lengthens the sinus node recovery time, AV conduction time, and QRS duration during ventricular pacing.[47] A number of these actions can influence cardiac arrhythmias and conduction disturbances. It appears plausible that the antiarrhythmic effect of magnesium is caused by improved conduction in depolarized myocardium.[5]

pH

Acidosis and alkalosis usually are associated with an altered concentration of potassium and ionized calcium. It is difficult to determine whether modification of the extracellular pH per se causes specific ECG changes.

Temperature

A low temperature slows and a high temperature accelerates the ion fluxes and various metabolic processes that determine the electrophysiologic properties of the heart.

HYPOTHERMIA

A lowered temperature is associated with gradual action potential duration lengthening, predominantly caused by lengthening of the plateau of the action potential. The velocity of depolarization decreases both secondary to depolarization and independent of depolarization. Decreased velocity of depolarization causes slowing of conduction, and the prolonged action potential duration is associated with lengthening of the refractory period. In humans profound hypothermia affects both depolarization and repolarization, but moderate hypothermia causes T wave abnormalities without appreciable QRS changes (Figure 22–18). Homogeneous cooling of the entire heart causes an increase in T wave duration without a change in polarity, a pattern observed during accidental hypothermia.[48] Cooling the posterior wall of the heart by drinking ice water usually produces deviation of the T wave vector anteriorly and superiorly, causing T wave inversion in leads II and III.[35]

Hypothermia is frequently associated with the appearance of a J wave (also called an *Osborne wave*), which is a slow upright deflection between the end of the QRS complex and the early portion of the ST segment (see Figures 22–18 and 22–19). They are most commonly observed in leads II, III, aV_F, V_5, and V_6. The J wave increases in amplitude

CASE V.F. LEAD 1

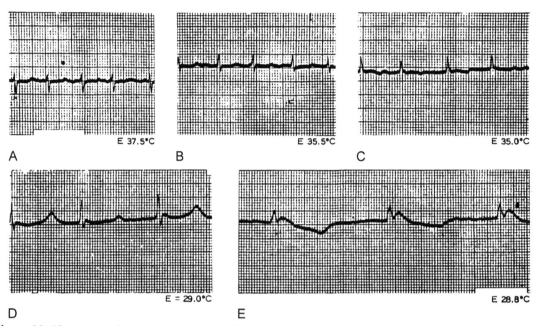

Figure 22–18 Sequential ECG changes during induction of hypothermia. **A,** Control. The temperature is 37.5°C, and there is atrial fibrillation. The QRS is 0.06 second, and the T wave is upright. **B,** Temperature is 35.5°C. An RS complex is present, and the ventricular rate is slower. **C,** Temperature is 35°C. The S wave has disappeared. The QRS is 0.07 second, and the T wave is inverted. **D,** Temperature is 29°C. There is marked slowing of the ventricular rate. The QRS is 0.12 second. The S wave has reappeared, and there is elevation of the J junction and marked QT prolongation. **E,** Temperature is 28.8°C a few seconds before the development of ventricular fibrillation. QRS is 0.13 second, and there is a prominent elevated J wave. (From Schwab RH, Lewis DW, Killough JH, et al: Electrocardiographic changes occurring in rapidly induced deep hypothermia. Am J Med Sci 248:290, 1964.)

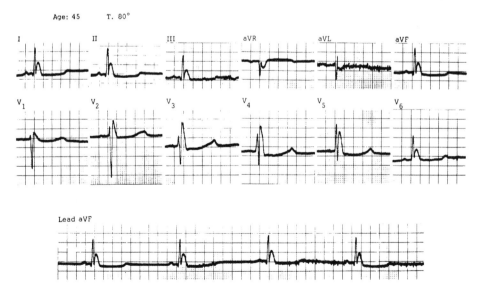

Figure 22–19 Hypothermia. The body temperature was 80°F. Note the J waves in all leads, with prolonged QT interval and low T waves. Intermittent baseline oscillation is present as a result of somatic muscle tremors. The heart rate is 32 beats/min.

as the body temperature falls. The genesis of this deflection has been difficult to explain. The timing is compatible with atrial repolarization, but the large amplitude of the J wave and its appearance in the absence of P waves makes this explanation unlikely. Yan and Antzelevitch[49] postulated that the J wave could be caused by the transmural potential gradient at the onset of ventricular repolarization, which has been observed in vitro. This gradient is attributed to the presence of a prominent notch during early repolarization in the epicardium and not in the endocardium, presumably reflecting differences in reactivation of the transient outward current (i_{to}), which participates in repolarization during the early portion of the action potential. It is of note that the occurrence of J waves is not limited to hypothermia. They may also be present during extreme hypercalcemia, with various disorders of the central and peripheral nervous system,[50] with vasospastic angina[51] and with other miscellaneous conditions.[52] A deflection similar to the J wave is present also in patients with Brugada syndrome (see Chapter 7). During rapid induction of deep hypothermia in patients prepared for surgery, atrial fibrillation appeared at temperatures ranging from 32.0°C to 22.5°C (average 27.2°C).

Among 12 studied patients, ventricular fibrillation occurred in 10 and cardiac standstill in 2. Ventricular fibrillation was preceded by widening of the QRS complex and the appearance of a J wave (see Figure 22–16). The temperature at which the J wave appeared was 1°C to 9°C warmer than the temperature at the onset of ventricular fibrillation (15°C to 30°C).[53] Okada[54] studied 60 patients with accidental hypothermia (body temperature 34°C or lower). At about 25°C, 32 patients had sinus rhythm with P wave of low amplitude, 23 had atrial fibrillation, and the remaining had AV junctional rhythm. In most cases, in this and other studies, atrial fibrillation developed at a temperature below 32°C, and it usually subsided during rewarming.

HYPERTHERMIA

Immersion of lightly anesthetized dogs and monkeys into 45°C water resulted in cardiac arrest from ventricular fibrillation or asystole within about 2 to 5 hours.[55] In humans, fever is associated with tachycardia, but the effect of increased temperature is difficult to discern from that of increased sympathetic stimulation. Persons susceptible to malignant hyperthermia are at risk of ventricular tachycardia or ventricular fibrillation, particularly during anesthesia.[56]

Miscellaneous Compounds

In humans, alcohol, coffee, and tobacco produce no detectable specific ECG abnormalities. The longitudinal Normative Aging Study revealed that an increase in bone lead level was associated with increased QRS duration and increased risk of intraventricular and AV conduction disturbances.[57]

Central Nervous System Diseases

In 1954, Burch et al.[58] identified a specific ECG pattern peculiar to certain patients with cerebrovascular accident (CVA). This pattern occurs most frequently in patients with intracranial hemorrhage, but it has been found also in those with other intracranial lesions. The typical ECG pattern is characterized by a conspicuous increase in T wave amplitude, prolonged QT interval (by 20 ms or more) (Figure 22–20), and an occasional increase in U wave amplitude. In one series,[59] ECG changes were seen in 71.5 percent of patients with subarachnoid hemorrhage and in 57.1 percent of those with cerebral hemorrhage. The abnormally wide T waves of increased amplitude are more often negative than positive, resembling other "giant T waves" (see Chapter 23). Surawicz[60] found this pattern in 29 percent of 89 patients with intracranial hemorrhage, 10 percent of patients with primary intracranial aneurysm, and 7 percent of patients with acute cerebrovascular thrombosis and increased intracranial pressure. The pattern was found in only 1 of 30 patients with hypertensive encephalopathy and 1 of 32 patients with brain metastases.[60] Similar percentages have been found by other investigators. In one study of 186 patients with cerebrovascular hemorrhage, the QT interval was prolonged only in patients with frontal lobe damage.[61] In another study of 89 patients with subarachnoid hemorrhage, the QT interval exceeded 115 percent of normal in 19 percent of patients.[62] In yet another study, the QT was prolonged in 11 of 20 patients.[63]

The observation that the CVA pattern appeared in several patients after cryohypophysectomy associated with diabetes insipidus, as shown in Figure 22–21, suggested that the pattern could result from injury of the hypothalamus.[64] This would explain the association of the pattern with subarachnoid hemorrhage, because hypothalamic lesions occur frequently after rupture of aneurysms of the anterior and posterior communicating arteries.[65]

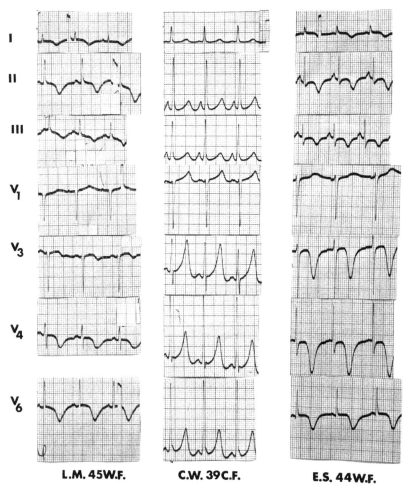

Figure 22-20 Typical ECG pattern after cerebrovascular accidents in three women who were 45, 39, and 44 years old, respectively. All had subarachnoid hemorrhage, a prolonged QT interval, and an increased amplitude of an upright or inverted T wave. (From Surawicz B, Knoebel SK: Long QT: good, bad, or indifferent. J Am Coll Cardiol 4:398, 1984.)

On rare occasions, an ECG pattern identical to that in patients with cerebral lesions appears after extracranial manipulation of the autonomic nervous system (e.g., after transabdominal truncal vagotomy for treatment of peptic ulcer disease, after presumed destruction of the sympathetic nerve fibers during radical lymph node dissection of the right side of the neck,[66,67] or with a neck hematoma).[68] Global T wave inversion was reported also in association with nonconvulsive status epilepticus, and in one case report preceded the stroke.[69,69a] The typical CVA pattern is usually a transient phenomenon lasting only a few days and can be reversed by intravenous administration of isoproterenol.[70]

In a study of Kuo and Surawicz,[71] the pattern most similar to that of CVA in patients appeared in an experimental animal with combined left stellate ganglion transection and right stellate stimulation. It has been reported that some patients with cerebrovascular disease develop less typical T wave changes, consisting of a lowered T wave amplitude or T wave notching.[72]

Elevation or depression of the ST segment may occur. The former may simulate the injury pattern of acute ischemia.[73] Occasionally the ST elevation is diffuse, mimicking acute pericarditis (Figure 22-22). Regional wall motion abnormalities were observed in a group of patients with subarachnoid hemorrhage associated with ST segment elevation in at least two consecutive leads.[74] In some cases abnormal Q waves develop, and the erroneous diagnosis of acute myocardial infarction may be made.[74-76] Appearance of a J wave has been reported.[76] Tall P waves were frequently encountered in one series.[77]

Rhythm disturbances may occur in patients with central nervous system disease. They include sinus bradycardia, sinus tachycardia,

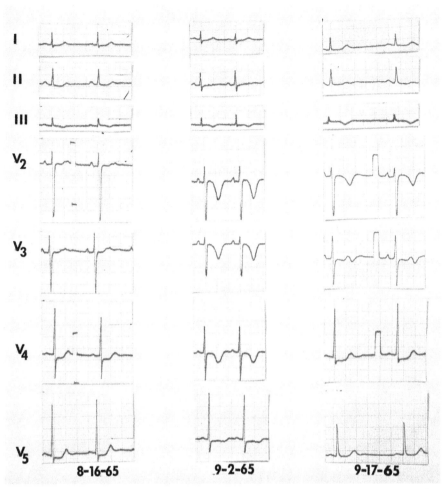

Figure 22–21 ECG of a 52-year-old woman treated with a 0.25-mg daily maintenance dose of digoxin before *(left)*, 3 days after *(middle)*, and 18 days after *(right)* cryohypophysectomy. The deeply inverted symmetric T waves with a prolonged QT interval are similar to changes induced by subarachnoid hemorrhage. (From Surawicz B: The pathogenesis and clinical significance of primary T wave abnormalities. *In:* Schalant RC, Hurst JW [eds]: Advances in Electrocardiography. Orlando, Grune & Stratton, 1972.)

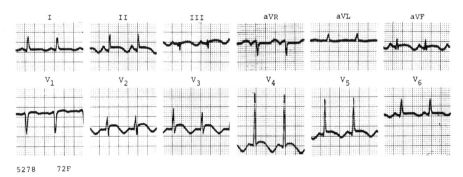

Figure 22–22 Cerebral thrombosis in a 72-year-old woman who was comatose on admission when this ECG was obtained. There is diffuse ST segment elevation involving all leads except leads aV_R and aV_L. There also is T wave inversion in most of the leads, with prolongation of the QT interval. The pattern suggests the possibility of acute pericarditis, but prolongation of the QT interval is evidence against the diagnosis. At autopsy there was extensive cerebral atherosclerosis, with scattered large infarcts in the cerebral and cerebellar hemispheres and pons. Although there also was generalized atherosclerosis of the coronary arteries, there was no evidence of pericarditis or myocardial infarction.

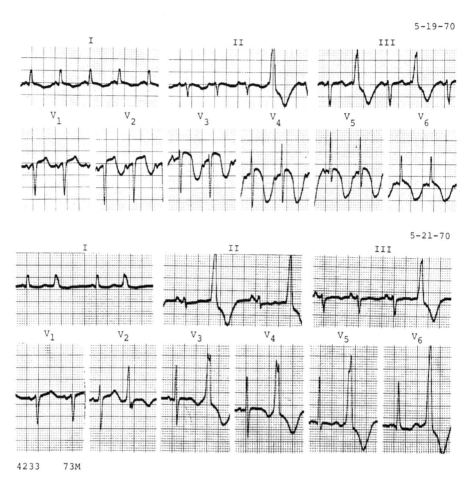

Figure 22–23 Head injury in a 73-year-old man with fracture of the skull. The tracings were recorded after the patient underwent craniotomy with evacuation of epidural, subdural, and left temporal lobe hematoma. There are frequent premature ventricular complexes, with periods of bigeminal rhythm. The tracing on 5/19/70 shows sinus tachycardia and left anterior fascicular block. There are QS complexes in leads V_1 and V_2. ST segment elevation and wide and inverted T waves are present in all the precordial leads except lead V_1, which shows an upright T wave. It was uncertain whether these abnormalities were due to the original head injury or the intracranial surgical procedure. The tracing on 5/21/70 shows the appearance of R waves in leads V_1 and V_2, and the ST and T wave changes have much improved. At autopsy the heart showed left ventricular hypertrophy, with 60 percent narrowing of the left circumflex coronary artery. No evidence of myocardial infarction was found.

AV junctional rhythm, premature ventricular complexes (Figure 22–23), and ventricular tachycardia.[78] Chou[79] observed the development of atrial fibrillation after head injury in a few young persons.

REFERENCES

1. Surawicz B: Relation between electrocardiogram and electrolytes. Am Heart J 73:814, 1967.
2. Braun HA, Surawicz B, Bellet S: T waves in hyperpotassemia. Am J Med Sci 230:147, 1955.
3. Ettinger PO, Regan TJ, Oldewurtel HA: Hyperkalemia, cardiac conduction and the electrocardiogram: a review. Am Heart J 88:360, 1974.
4. Levine HD, Wanzer SH, Merrill JP: Dialyzable currents of injury in potassium intoxication resembling acute myocardial infarction or pericarditis. Circulation 13:29, 1956.
5. Surawicz B: Electrophysiologic Basis of ECG and Cardiac Arrhythmias. Baltimore, Williams & Wilkins, 1995, pp 426–453.
6. Hariman RJ, Chen Chia M: Effects of hyperkalemia on sinus nodal function in dog: sino-ventricular conduction. Cardiovasc Res 17:509, 1983.
7. Racker DK: Sinoventricular transmission in 10 mM K^+ by canine atrioventricular nodal inputs. Circulation 83:1738, 1991.
8. Surawicz B: Methods of production of ventricular fibrillation. In: Surawicz B, Pellegrino E (eds): Sudden Cardiac Death. Orlando, Grune & Stratton, 1964, p 64.
9. Garcia-Palmieri MR: Reversal of hyperkalemic cardiotoxicity with hypertonic saline. Am Heart J 64:483, 1962.
10. Surawicz B, Lepeschkin E, Herrlich HC, et al: Effect of potassium and calcium deficiency on the monophasic action potential, electrocardiogram and contractility of isolated rabbit hearts. Am J Physiol 196:1302, 1959.

11. Gettes LS, Surawicz B, Shiue JC: Effect of high K, low K, and quinidine on QRS duration and ventricular action potential. Am J Physiol 203:1135, 1962.
12. Bettinger JC, Surawicz B, Bryfogle JW, et al: The effect of intravenous administration of potassium chloride on ectopic rhythms, ectopic beats and disturbances in AV conduction. Am J Med 21:521, 1956.
13. Kunin AS, Surawicz B, Sims EA: Decrease in serum potassium concentration and appearance of cardiac arrhythmias during infusion of potassium with glucose in potassium-depleted patients. N Engl J Med 266:228, 1962.
14. Surawicz B: U wave: facts, hypotheses, misconceptions, and misnomers. J Cardiovasc Electrophysiol 9:1117, 1998.
15. Surawicz B, Braun AH, Crum WB, et al: Quantitative analysis of the electrocardiographic pattern of hypopotassemia. Circulation 16:750, 1957.
16. Dreifus LS, Pick A: A clinical correlative study of the electrocardiogram in electrolyte imbalance. Circulation 14:815, 1956.
17. Bickel G, Plattner H, Fabre J: Les repercussions cardiaques des alterations du metabolism du potassium. Arch Mal Coeur 47:203,1954.
18. Cherry JC, Surawicz B: Unusual effects of potassium deficiency on the heart of a child with cystinosis. Pediatrics 30:414, 1962.
19. Davidson S, Surawicz B: Ectopic beats and atrioventricular conduction disturbances in patients with hypopotassemia. Arch Intern Med 20:280, 1967.
20. Redleaf PD, Lerner IJ: Thiazide-induced hypokalemia with associated major ventricular arrhythmia. JAMA 206:1302, 1968.
21. Salvador M, Thomas C, Mazeng M, et al: Troubles du rhythme directment induits ou favorises par les depletions potassiques. Arch Mal Coeur 63:230, 1970.
22. Beck OA, Hochrein H: Initial serum potassium level in relation to cardiac arrhythmias in acute myocardial infarction. Z Kardiol 66:187, 1977.
23. Hulting J: In-hospital ventricular fibrillation and its relation to serum potassium. Acta Med Scand Suppl 647:109, 1981.
24. Thompson RG, Cobb LA: Hypokalemia after resuscitation from out-of-hospital ventricular fibrillation. JAMA 248:2860, 1982.
25. Vick RL, Todd EP, Luedke DW: Epinephrine-induced hypokalemia: relation to liver and skeletal muscle. J Pharmacol Exp Ther 181:139, 1972.
26. Brown MJ, Brown DC, Murphy MB: Hypokalemia from beta2-receptor stimulation by circulating epinephrine. N Engl J Med 309:1414, 1983.
27. Bronsky D, Dubin A, Waldstein SS, et al: Calcium and the electrocardiogram II. The electrocardiographic manifestations of hyperparathyroidism and of marked hypercalcemia from various other etiologies. Am J Cardiol 7:833, 1961.
28. Nierenberg DW, Ransil BJ: Q-aTc interval as a clinical indicator of hypercalcemia. Am J Cardiol 44:243, 1979.
29. Lind L, Ljunghall S: Serum calcium and the ECG in patients with primary hyperparathyroidism. J Electrocardiol 27:99, 1994.
30. Voss DM, Drake EH: Cardiac manifestations of hyperparathyroidism, with presentation of a previously unreported arrhythmia. Am Heart J 73:235, 1967.
31. Crum WD, Till HJ: Hyperparathyroidism with Wenckebach's phenomenon. Am J Cardiol 6:836, 1960.
32. Surawicz B, Lepeschkin E: Electrocardiographic pattern of hypopotassemia with and without hypocalcemia. Circulation 8:801, 1953.
33. Yu PNG: Electrocardiographic changes associated with hypocalcemia and hypercalcemia. Am J Med Sci 224:413, 1952.
34. Surawicz B, MacDonald MG, Kaljot V, et al: Treatment of cardiac arrhythmias with salts of ethylendiamine tetraacetic acid (EDTA). Am Heart J 58:493, 1959.
35. Lepeschkin E: Modern Electrocardiography, vol 1. Baltimore, Williams & Wilkins, 1951.
36. Surawicz B, Gettes LS: Effects of electrolytes on the action potential. In: Dreifus LS, Likoff W(eds): Mechanisms and Therapy of Cardiac Arrhythmias. Orlando, Grune & Stratton, 1965.
37. Surawicz B: Use of the chelating agent, EDTA, in digitalis intoxication and cardiac arrhythmias. Prog Cardiovasc Dis 2:432, 1959.
38. Surawicz B, Lepeschkin E, Herrlich HC: Low and high magnesium concentrations at various calcium levels: effect on the monophasic action potential, electrocardiogram, and contractility of isolated rabbit hearts. Circ Res 9:811, 1961.
39. Surawicz B: Is hypomagnesemia or magnesium deficiency arrhythmogenic? J Am Coll Cardiol 14:1093, 1989.
40. Loeb HS, Petras RJ, Gunnar RM, et al: Paroxysmal ventricular fibrillation in two patients with hypomagnesemia. Circulation 37:210, 1968.
41. Ramee SR, White CJ, Svinarich JT, et al: Torsades de pointes and magnesium deficiency. Am Heart J 110:164, 1985.
42. Chadda KD, Gupta PK, Lichstein E: Magnesium in cardiac arrhythmia. N Engl J Med 287:1102, 1972.
43. Dyckner T, Wester PO: Magnesium deficiency contributing to ventricular tachycardia. Acta Med Scand 212:89, 1982.
44. Boyd LJ, Scherf D: Magnesium sulphate in paroxysmal tachycardia. Am J Med Sci 206:43, 1943.
45. Szekely P, Wynne NA: The effects of magnesium on cardiac arrhythmias caused by digitalis. Clin Sci 10:241, 1951.
46. Iseri LT, Fairshter RD, Hardemann JL, et al: Magnesium and potassium therapy in multifocal atrial tachycardia. Am Heart J 110:789, 1985.
47. DiCarlo LA, Morady F, de Buitleir M, et al: Effects of magnesium sulfate on cardiac conduction and refractoriness in humans. J Am Coll Cardiol 7:1356, 1986.
48. Trevino A, Raze B, Beller BM: The characteristic electrocardiogram of accidental hypothermia. Arch Intern Med 127:470, 1971.
49. Yan G-X, Antzelevitch C: Cellular basis for the electrocardiographic J wave. Circulation 93:372, 1996.
50. Gussak I, Bjerregaard P, Egan TM, et al: ECG phenomenon called the J wave. J Electrocardiol 28:49, 1995.
51. Maruyama M, Atarashi H, Ino T, et al: Osborn waves associated with ventricular fibrillation in a patient with vasospastic angina. J Cardiovasc Electrophysiol 13:486, 2002.
52. Patel A, Getsos JP, Moussa G, et al: The Osborn wave of hypothermia in normothermic patients. Clin Cardiol 17:273, 1994.
53. Schwab RH, Lewis DW, Killough JH, et al: Electrocardiographic changes occurring in rapidly induced deep hypothermia. Am J Med Sci 248:290, 1964.
54. Okada M: The cardiac rhythm in accidental hypothermia. J Electrocardiol 17:123, 1984.
55. Eshel G, Safar P, Sassano J, et al: Hyperthermia-induced cardiac arrest in dogs and monkeys. Resuscitation 20:129, 1990.
56. Huckell VF, Staniloff HM, Britt BA, et al: Cardiac manifestations of malignant hyperthermia susceptibility. Circulation 58:916, 1978.

57. Cheng Y, Schwartz J, Vokonas PS, et al: Electrocardiographic conduction disturbances in association with low-level lead exposure (the Normative Aging Study). Am J Cardiol 82:594, 1998.

58. Burch GE, Meyers R, Abildskov JA: A new electrocardiographic pattern observed in cerebrovascular accidents. Circulation 9:719, 1954.

59. Kreus KE, Kemila SJ, Takata JK: Electrocardiographic changes in cerebrovascular accidents. Acta Med Scand 185:327, 1969.

60. Surawicz B: The pathogenesis and clinical significance of primary T wave abnormalities. *In:* Schlant RC, Hurst JW (eds): Advances in Electrocardiography. Orlando, Grune & Stratton, 1972.

61. Yamour BJ, Svidharan MR, Rice JR, et al: Electrocardiographic changes in cerebrovascular hemorrhage. Am Heart J 99:294, 1980.

62. Stober T, Kunze K: Electrocardiographic alterations in subarachnoid hemorrhage. J Neurol 227:99, 1982.

63. Eisalo A, Peresalo J, Halonen PJ: Electrocardiographic abnormalities and some laboratory findings in patients with subarachnoid hemorrhage. Br Heart J 34:217, 1970.

64. Surawicz B: Electrocardiographic pattern of cerebrovascular accident. JAMA 197:213, 1966.

65. Jenkins JS, Buekell M, Carter AB, et al: Hypothalamic pituitary-adrenal function after subarachnoid hemorrhage. BMJ 4:707, 1969.

66. Gallivan GJ, Levane H, Canzonetti AJ: Ischemic electrocardiographic changes after truncal vagotomy. JAMA 211:798, 1970.

67. Hugenholtz PG: Electrocardiographic changes typical for central nervous system disease after right radical neck dissection. Am Heart J 74:438, 1967.

68. Chou TM, Sweeney JP, Massie BM: Marked T wave inversion after internal jugular cannulation complicated by neck hematoma. Am Heart J 128:1038, 1994.

69. Spencer RGS, Cox TS: Global T-wave inversion associated with status epilepticus. Ann Intern Med 129:163, 1998.

69a. Lindberg DM, Jauch EC: Neurogenic T waves preceding acute ischemic stroke. Circulation 114:369, 2006.

70. Daoud FS, Surawicz B, Gettes LS: Effect of isoproterenol on T wave abnormalities. Am J Cardiol 30: 810, 1972.

71. Kuo CS, Surawicz B: Ventricular monophasic action potential changes associated with neurogenic T wave abnormalities and isoproterenol administration in dogs. Am J Cardiol 38:170, 1976.

72. Abildskov JA, Millar K, Burgess MJ, et al: The electrocardiogram and the central nervous system. Prog Cardiovasc Dis 13:210, 1970.

73. Cropp GJ, Manning GW: Electrocardiographic changes simulating myocardial ischemia and infarction associated with spontaneous intracranial hemorrhage. Circulation 22:25, 1960.

74. Kono T, Morita H, Kuroiwa T, et al: Left ventricular wall motion abnormalities in patients with subarachnoid hemorrhage: neurogenic stunned myocardium. J Am Coll Cardiol 24:636, 1994.

75. Chou TC, Susilavorn B: Electrocardiographic changes in intracranial hemorrhage. J Electrocardiol 2:193, 1969.

76. Abbott JA, Cheitlin MD: The nonspecific camel-hump sign. JAMA 235:413, 1976.

77. Hersch C: Electrocardiographic changes in subarachnoid hemorrhage, meningitis, and intracranial space occupying lesions. Br Heart J 26:785, 1964.

78. Grossman MA: Cardiac arrhythmias in acute central nervous system disease. Arch Intern Med 136:203, 1976.

79. Chou T-C: Electrocardiography in Clinical Practice: Adult and Pediatric, 4th ed. Philadelphia, Saunders, 1996, p 547.

23 | T Wave Abnormalities

Secondary T Wave Abnormalities	Fear, Anxiety, and Nervous Tension
	Hyperventilation
Primary T Wave Abnormalities	Orthostatic Abnormalities
Uniform Changes in the Shape or	Miscellaneous Primary T Wave
Duration of Ventricular APs	Abnormalities
Asynchronous Repolarization	Rapidly Reversible T Wave
Ischemic and Postischemic T Wave	Abnormalities
Abnormalities	
Pericarditis	**Concomitant ST-T Abnormalities**
Myocardial Disease Processes	
Mitral Valve Prolapse Syndrome and	**Nonspecific ST and T Abnormalities**
Floppy Mitral Valve	
Diffuse ("Global") T Wave Inversion	**Computerized Analysis of T Wave**
Isolated T Wave Inversion in Adults	**Morphology and Spatial Orientation**
Apparent Dysfunction of the Autonomic	**of the T Wave**
Nervous System	

Of all the components of the electrocardiogram (ECG), the T wave has the greatest potential for misinterpretation because the line dividing normal from abnormal is not sharp, and structural and functional disturbances can cause similar patterns of abnormal repolarization.

Cellular electrophysiology has contributed to the understanding of normal and abnormal ventricular repolarization.[1] The shape of the normal T wave is largely determined by the asynchrony of phase 3 of the ventricular action potentials (see Figure 1–1). Consistent with the smooth course of the ventricular actional potential (AP), the T wave is smooth and rounded, and it contains little frequency content in excess of 10 cycles per second. The characteristic form of the T wave helps differentiate between the T wave and the P wave, which usually displays notches that are indicative of higher-frequency components. When the T wave is notched in the precordial leads, however, a second summit may be as pointed as a P wave component.

The T wave abnormalities are classified as primary and secondary (Table 23–1). The concept of a ventricular gradient (see Chapter 1) allows one to define the primary and secondary T wave abnormalities according to their independence of or dependence on changes in the QRS complex.[2,3] The area of the primary T wave is equal to the ventricular gradient, and the primary T wave describes variations of the ventricular gradient as a function of time.[4]

A secondary T wave is a deflection that would follow a given QRS complex if ventricular recovery properties were uniform. In theory, secondary T wave abnormalities can be recognized by measuring the ventricular gradient planimetrically.

Secondary T Wave Abnormalities

Secondary T wave abnormalities can be expected under any conditions of an altered depolarization sequence. An instructive example of secondary T wave changes is shown in Figure 20–2. In practice, the recognition of secondary T wave abnormalities is not difficult when the T wave vector deviates opposite to that of the main QRS vector in the presence of ventricular hypertrophy or left bundle branch block (LBBB) patterns, opposite the slow terminal QRS component in the presence of right bundle branch block (RBBB), and opposite the delta wave in the presence of the ventricular preexcitation pattern (see Figure 20–2). However, recognition of the secondary T wave abnormalities may be difficult in the presence of conditions that generate both primary and secondary T wave abnormalities. The secondary T wave abnormalities caused by left ventricular hypertrophy reflect an abnormally wide QRS/T angle in both the frontal and horizontal planes in the presence of an unchanged ventricular gradient. During typical evolution of the left ventricular "strain" pattern, the phase of T wave lowering precedes the stage of inversion (see Chapter 3). Differences between the shape of the secondary and primary T wave changes in the same patient

TABLE 23–1	Classification of T Wave Abnormalities		
Sequence of Depolarization	Shape and Duration of Ventricular APs	Sequence of Repolarization	Type of Abnormality
Abnormal	Normal	Abnormal	Secondary
Normal	Uniformly abnormal	Normal	Primary
Normal	Nonuniformly abnormal	Abnormal	Primary

From Surawicz B: The pathogenesis and clinical significance of primary T wave abnormalities. *In:* Schlant R, Hurst JW (eds): Advances in Electroradiology. Orlando, Grune & Stratton, 1972.
APs = action potentials.

are shown in Figure 23–1. In the typical pattern of right ventricular hypertrophy, the QRS/T angle is wide and the T wave is upright in the leads in which the QRS area is negative (i.e., lead I) and the left precordial leads. In patients with chronic lung disease and deep S waves in the standard limb and left precordial leads, the T wave tends to be directed opposite to the main QRS axis.

In the presence of RBBB, the T wave vector is directed opposite to the vector of the terminal wide QRS component. The constancy of the QRS-T area in many cases of intermittent RBBB or during progression from incomplete to complete RBBB has generally validated the concept of a ventricular gradient under such circumstances.

In the presence of LBBB, the T wave is usually directed opposite to the main QRS axis. Therefore the negative T waves in the leads with a deep S wave suggest the presence of additional primary T wave abnormalities (Figure 23–2). The persistence of an upright T wave in leads with a tall R wave (e.g., lead I or V_6) does not require the same interpretation, as it may result from lowering of a T wave that had been taller in the absence of LBBB or from differences between the location of the transition zone for the T wave and the QRS complex. Secondary T wave inversion in the presence of LBBB is usually initiated by a depressed downsloping ST segment followed by a steeper ascent to the baseline (see Figures 4–1, 4–2, 4–4, and 4–5).

Primary T Wave Abnormalities

Table 23–1 shows that the primary T wave abnormalities may be caused by uniform alteration in the shape and/or duration of all ventricular APs, without a change in the sequence of repolarization; or they may be due to nonuniform changes in the shape and/or duration of the ventricular APs resulting in an altered sequence of repolarization. Abnormal T waves may also be caused by various combinations of primary and secondary mechanisms.

UNIFORM CHANGES IN THE SHAPE OR DURATION OF VENTRICULAR APs

Uniform changes in the shape or duration of ventricular APs are caused predominantly by electrolyte imbalance or drugs, and they are reversible. They are discussed in Chapters 21 and 22. The effect of temperature change also belongs in this category (see Chapter 22).

ASYNCHRONOUS REPOLARIZATION

The T wave abnormalities caused by asynchronous repolarization account for the largest number of organic and functional disturbances of ventricular repolarization. Numerous studies have shown that local changes in the duration of recovery can alter the duration, amplitude, and polarity of the T wave without changes in the QRS complex. Calculations based on experimental data have shown that small alterations in the local form of the AP may cause large-percentile changes in the configuration of the T wave.[5] This means that the ventricular gradient is highly sensitive to local differences in the duration of repolarization and that the T wave may be considered "some special detector for differences in repolarization of the various parts of the ventricle."[5]

Characteristically, these primary T wave abnormalities do not alter the course or duration of the ST segment. However, they are often associated with prolonged QTc interval and an increased duration of the aTeT interval. The lengthening of these intervals suggests that the T wave abnormalities are caused by regional prolongation of the ventricular APs.

ISCHEMIC AND POSTISCHEMIC T WAVE ABNORMALITIES

Primary T wave abnormalities associated with myocardial ischemia and myocardial infarction are of greatest practical importance. The T wave

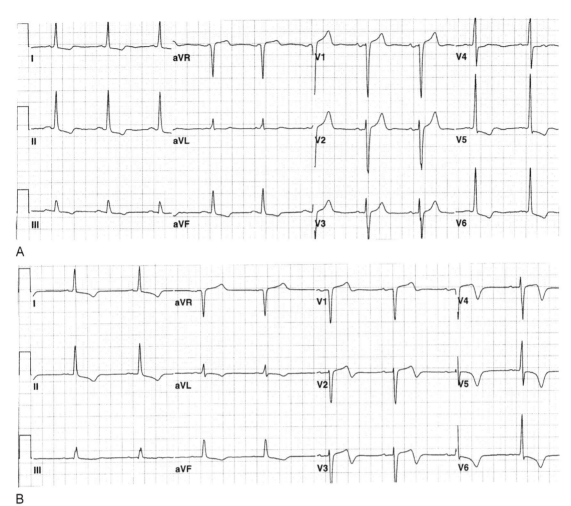

Figure 23–1 Differences between the shape of the secondary and primary T wave changes on the ECG of a 70-year-old man with hypertensive and coronary artery disease. **A**, Typical secondary ST segment and T wave changes in the presence of a left ventricular hypertrophy pattern. The ST segment is upsloping and slightly elevated in the right precordial leads and downsloping in the left precordial leads. The T wave is upright in leads V_1–V_3, notched in transitional lead V_4, and inverted in leads V_5 and V_6. U wave polarity is concordant with the T wave polarity. **B**, ECG recorded the next day after an episode of chest pain associated with cardiac enzyme elevation. The QRS complex is practically unchanged, but the T wave is inverted in all precordial leads. Typical of the primary T wave changes caused by myocardial ischemia, the ST segment remains nearly flat, and is followed by a terminal T wave inversion. The QTc interval increased from 404 ms in **A** to 466 ms in **B**.

pattern that is prevalent in patients with ischemic heart disease is sometimes referred to as a "coronary T wave." Typically, the ST segment is not displaced, the T wave vector is abnormal, the angle between the ascent and the descent is more acute (pointed configuration), and the QTc interval is prolonged. (See also Chapters 7 to 9.)

PERICARDITIS

The primary T wave changes seen with pericarditis are discussed in Chapter 11.

MYOCARDIAL DISEASE PROCESSES

The T wave abnormalities in patients with non-ischemic cardiomyopathies are usually secondary to QRS abnormalities produced by ventricular hypertrophy. Sometimes, however, primary T wave abnormalities precede changes in the QRS complex.[6] Coltart and Meldrum[7] found that the ventricular AP from a muscle band excised from the heart of a patient with hypertrophic obstructive cardiomyopathy had a slow slope of phase 3 and 498-ms duration compared with an average 308-ms duration of the ventricular action

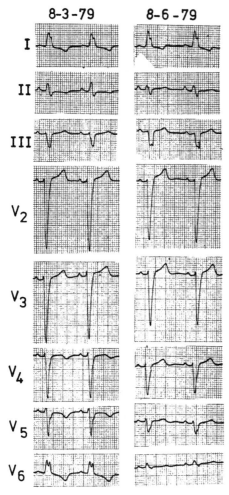

8-3-79   **8-6-79**

I

II

III

V₂

V₃

V₄

V₅

V₆

Figure 23–2 Differences between secondary (8/6/79) and primary T wave changes (8/3/79) on the ECG of a patient with left bundle branch block and myocardial infarction. The differences are similar to those described for Figure 23–1 and are best seen in leads II, V₄, and V₅. (From Surawicz B: ST-T abnormalities. *In:* MacFarlane PW, Lawrie TD [eds]: Comprehensive Electrocardiology. New York, Pergamon, 1989.)

potential in eight control human subjects. This observation explains the primary T wave abnormalities and prolonged QTc in patients with obstructive cardiomyopathy.

Several conditions associated with primary T wave changes in patients with myocardial damage are discussed in Chapter 9.

MITRAL VALVE PROLAPSE SYNDROME AND FLOPPY MITRAL VALVE

The most typical ECG abnormalities in patients with mitral valve prolapse are flattening or inversion of T waves in leads II, III, and aV_F with or without ST segment depression. They occur in

15 to 42 percent of patients in the larger reported series[8–10] and often resemble T waves caused by myocardial ischemia. In some patients, similar changes are present in the left precordial leads (Figure 23–3). T wave changes in the right precordial leads were reported to be associated with prolapse of both leaflets.[9] Diffuse T wave inversion (see later discussion) has also been described but is uncommon. Spontaneous variations of the T wave may occur, and normalization by exercise is not uncommon.[8,10] Exercise may precipitate a horizontal ST segment depression in patients with normal coronary arteriograms.[8,11] A false-positive response to exercise was found in 53 percent of patients with the syndrome and chest pain.[12]

The genesis of the T wave abnormalities is unclear. It is conceivable that they are caused by prolonged repolarization in the abnormal left ventricular ridge described for this syndrome.[13] Primary T wave abnormalities frequently occur also in patients with mitral insufficiency caused by a floppy mitral valve in Marfan syndrome.[14]

DIFFUSE ("GLOBAL") T WAVE INVERSION

The term "diffuse inversion" is applied when the T wave is inverted (and often symmetric) in all standard leads except aV_R, although leads V₁, III, and aV_L are occasionally spared (Figure 23–4). The term "global" was used by Walder and Spodick,[15] who found such a pattern in 100 cases among the approximately 30,000 consecutive routine ECGs they interpreted. Among these patients, 82 were women and 18 were men. The QTc interval was prolonged. The most common causes were myocardial ischemia and central nervous system disorders. Other conditions included pericarditis, myocarditis, apical hypertrophic cardiomyopathy, cardiac metastases, carotid endarterectomy, cocaine abuse, and pheochromocytoma. In some cases, no associated condition was apparent. After following these cases for up to 11 years, Walder and Spodick[16] concluded that the long-term prognosis depended on the underlying or associated disease and that the striking diffuse T wave changes per se do not imply a poor prognosis. Brscic et al.[17] reported a series of 17 patients (all women) with global T wave inversion with "ischemic" chest pain, normal coronary arteriograms, and intact left ventricular function. In another series of nine patients (seven women), the pattern was associated with acute cardiogenic but nonischemic pulmonary edema.[18] The ECG changes gradually resolved within 1 week and had no immediate prognostic implications.

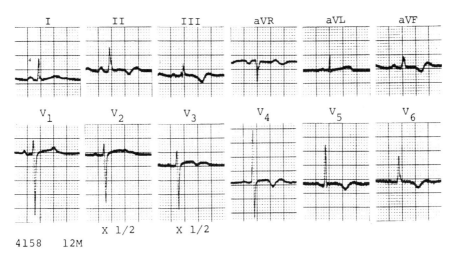

Figure 23–3 Mitral valve prolapse syndrome in a 12-year-old asymptomatic boy. A mid-systolic click and a late systolic murmur were heard in the mitral area. Rhythm strips showed frequent premature supraventricular complexes. The 12-lead ECG shows T wave inversion in the inferior leads and leads V_3–V_6 and prominent U waves.

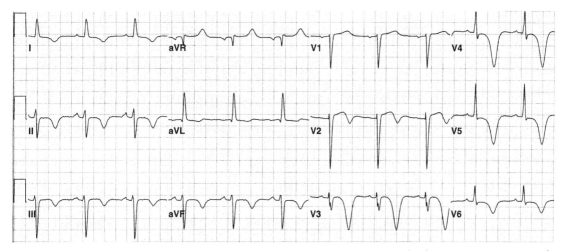

Figure 23–4 ECG of a 78-year-old woman admitted to the hospital with dyspnea and pulmonary congestion. Note the typical pattern of "global" T wave inversion with prolonged QTc (527 ms). Myocardial infarction was ruled out by the absence of cardiac enzyme elevation. Echocardiography and left heart catheterization revealed normal dimensions of cardiac chambers and no wall motion abnormalities; coronary angiography showed no obstructive disease.

The pattern of global T wave inversion does not differ substantially from the pattern of the giant negative T waves seen most often with myocardial ischemia, subarachnoid hemorrhage, and apical cardiomyopathy with a spade-like configuration of the ventricle (see Chapter 12). It has been reported that the characteristic giant T wave pattern may appear at an early stage of the disease, before the appearance of the spade-like configuration.[19] Another cause of global T wave inversion is the presence of a 2:1 advanced or complete atrioventricular (AV) block (Figure 23–5).

ISOLATED T WAVE INVERSION IN ADULTS

Another rare variant is an isolated negative T wave in the mid-precordial leads V_3 and V_4. In such cases the T wave tends to be diphasic rather than frankly negative. This pattern sometimes occurs in the absence of heart disease. Under these circumstances the region in which the T wave is abnormal over the precordium is small, and small downward electrode shifting usually reveals an upright T wave.

In a series of 86 consecutive patients with isolated T wave inversion reported by Okada

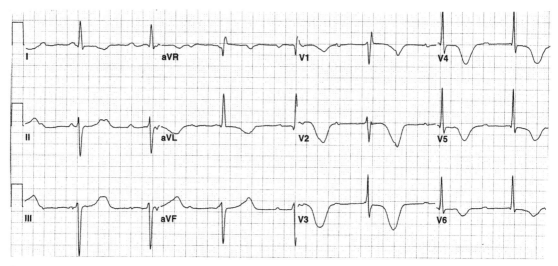

Figure 23–5 Marked T wave inversion and QTc prolongation (604 ms) in an asymptomatic 88-year-old man with complete atrioventricular block.

et al.,[20] 23 had no symptoms and represented a normal variant. The remaining 63 patients had chest pain. Among the latter, 19 were considered to represent a normal variant, whereas most of the others had coronary artery disease. The presence or absence of structural heart disease could be differentiated by recording additional precordial leads. In the absence of heart disease, the area of negative T waves extended rightward and downward and in patients with heart disease leftward and upward.[20]

APPARENT DYSFUNCTION OF THE AUTONOMIC NERVOUS SYSTEM

The ECG pattern associated with cerebrovascular accidents is discussed in Chapter 22. Other T wave abnormalities in patients with various dysfunctions of the autonomic nervous system are probably caused by the effects of nonhomogeneous sympathetic stimulation on ventricular repolarization.[21] Such a mechanism may explain T wave abnormalities preceding hypertensive crises in patients with pheochromocytoma or abnormalities from adrenal or pituitary insufficiency[21] (see Chapter 12), as well as diffuse T wave abnormalities occurring occasionally after electroconvulsive therapy.[22]

Visceral reflexes are believed to be responsible for the rapidly reversible T wave changes present in some patients with acute abdominal processes (cholecystitis, peritonitis, appendicitis, pancreatic necrosis, and ileus).[3] These ECG abnormalities may simulate myocardial ischemia in patients with pathologic conditions of the heart and coronary vessels.[23,24] T wave abnormalities in patients with acute and subacute pancreatitis

are caused in some cases by pericarditis or myocardial necrosis induced by circulating enzymes from the damaged pancreas.[6]

FEAR, ANXIETY, AND NERVOUS TENSION

Fear (especially fear of operation), anxiety, worry, longing suggested by hypnosis, and other emotional factors may produce T wave abnormalities in persons without heart disease.[6] It has been shown that T wave abnormalities in anxious subjects may disappear after reassurance and rest, even without a change in the heart rate.

Several studies have reported T wave abnormalities in a vaguely defined syndrome of neurocirculatory asthenia (NCA) characterized by tachycardia, hyperventilation, labile blood pressure, and low effort tolerance (i.e., characteristics of many subjects with mitral valve prolapse syndrome). However, it has been shown conclusively that NCA is not associated with a characteristic ECG pattern.[6]

HYPERVENTILATION

The effect of hyperventilation on the ECG has been studied predominantly in subjects with normal ECGs at rest before a stress test is done to detect myocardial ischemia. Hyperventilation causes predominantly transient T wave inversion in leads with an upright T wave and sometimes ST segment depression. The incidence of T wave abnormalities varies depending on the duration and vigor of the hyperventilation and the number of recorded leads.[25]

Biberman et al.[26] found that T wave inversion was present in all normal volunteers studied during the early stage of vigorous hyperventilation, but not during the late stage of rapid hyperventilation or during prolonged slow hyperventilation (Figure 23–6). Biberman et al.[26] showed that the T wave abnormalities produced by hyperventilation could not be attributed to alkalosis; changes in the plasma sodium, potassium, or magnesium concentrations; or changes in heart position. The T wave abnormalities produced by hyperventilation were always accompanied by tachycardia but could not be attributed solely to a critical increase in heart rate. This conclusion is in agreement with previous studies in which the T wave became inverted after hyperventilation but remained upright when tachycardia was induced by exercise,[27,28] intravenous administration of propantheline, or breathing air containing 5 percent CO_2.[29,30]

Transient T wave inversion during hyperventilation is similar to the transient T wave abnormalities during isoproterenol infusion[26] and can be explained by an asynchronous shortening of ventricular repolarization during the early phase of sympathetic stimulation. In keeping with this hypothesis are the observations that T wave abnormalities produced by hyperventilation can be prevented by pretreatment with propranolol[31,32] while maintaining the heart rate at which hyperventilation caused T wave abnormalities.[31]

Unlike the T wave inversion that may be considered a physiologic finding, the ST segment depression observed occasionally during short- or long-lasting hyperventilation may be associated with myocardial ischemia, although it appears also in subjects without coronary artery disease. Therefore it should be evaluated in the same manner as the exercise-induced or postexercise-induced ST segment depression.[33–35]

ORTHOSTATIC ABNORMALITIES

In the upright position the ventricular gradient decreases, the QRS/T angle widens,[36] and T wave changes occur in most young individuals.[37] However, the incidence of unequivocal orthostatic T wave abnormalities varies among patient groups. Lepeschkin and Surawicz[38] found an abnormal orthostatic ECG in only 3 percent of individuals with a negative exercise test but in 30 percent of subjects with junctional ST segment depression and in 23 percent of patients with ischemic heart disease and a positive exercise test. In patients with NCA, orthostatic T wave

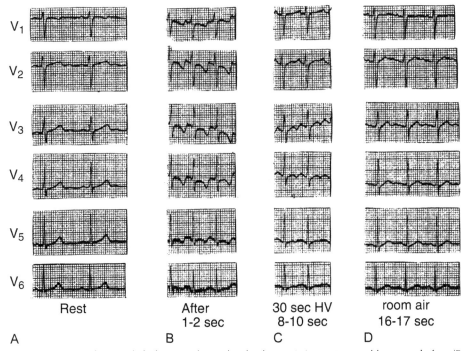

Figure 23–6 Simultaneously recorded electrocardiographic leads V_1–V_6 in a 21-year-old woman before (Rest) and at various intervals after 30 seconds (sec) of vigorous hyperventilation (HV). The T wave is inverted early but becomes upright 16 to 17 seconds after HV. (From Biberman L, Sarma RN, Surawicz B: T wave abnormalities during hyperventilation and isoproterenol infusion. Am Heart J 81:166, 1971.)

abnormalities occurred in 43 percent of women and 30 percent of men.[39]

Transient orthostatic T wave abnormalities have been attributed to increased sympathetic activity.[40] Intravenous administration of propranolol prevents orthostatic T wave abnormalities.[6] Suppression of the orthostatic changes by β-adrenergic blocking drugs does not result solely from the decrease in heart rate.[32]

MISCELLANEOUS PRIMARY T WAVE ABNORMALITIES

Postprandial Abnormalities

A decrease in T wave amplitude or T wave inversion in leads I, II, and V_2–V_4 occurs frequently within 30 minutes after a meal of about 1200 calories.[41] Postprandial T wave abnormalities occurred in 3.9 percent of 2000 young, healthy airmen.[42] These abnormalities may arise from lowering of the plasma potassium concentration, tachycardia, and possibly sympathetic stimulation. It has been shown that various nonspecific T wave abnormalities may disappear when the ECG is recorded after fasting.[43]

Injection of Ionic Contrast Material into Coronary Arteries

Injection of ionic contrast material into coronary arteries produces transient prolongation of the QTc interval and changes in T wave morphology. These T wave changes are sometimes associated with prolongation of the QRS complex, but in most cases they are primary. As a rule, the

T wave vector is directed away from the area perfused by the contrast material.[44] These T wave changes have been attributed to the regional prolongation of repolarization caused by the high sodium concentration in the contrast medium[44] or the medium's calcium-binding properties. Shabetai et al.[45] showed that transient T wave abnormalities that occur during injection of contrast into the right coronary artery were associated with prolongation of the ventricular monophasic action potential (MAP) in the right ventricle without changes in MAP in the left ventricle.[45]

Postextrasystolic Abnormalities

The cause of occasional primary T wave changes in the first and sometimes also the second or third postextrasystolic complex is not known (Figure 23–7). The association of postextrasystolic T wave inversion with prolongation of the QT interval[46] suggests asynchronous repolarization during adjustment to a new cycle length. The postextrasystolic T wave changes apparently occur more frequently in patients with heart disease than in those without it,[46–48] but the reason for this association is not obvious.

Posttachycardia Abnormalities

In about 20 percent of patients with paroxysmal tachycardia, the normal upright T wave becomes inverted for hours or days after termination of the episode[3] or interruption of tachycardia by ablation.[49] This may occur after ventricular or supraventricular tachycardia and is unrelated to the age of the patient or to the presence or

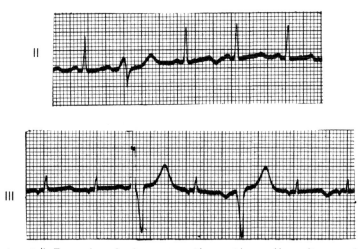

Figure 23–7 Postextrasystolic T wave inversion in a person with no evidence of heart disease and a normal ECG except for premature ventricular complexes. (From Surawicz B: ST-T abnormalities. *In:* MacFarlane PW, Lawrie TD [eds]: Comprehensive Electrocardiology. New York, Pergamon, 1989.)

absence of heart disease.[6] The abnormalities often persist longer than would be expected on the basis of physiologic adjustment to the new cycle. The mechanism is probably similar to that of the postpacing, post-LBBB, and post-preexcitation abnormalities (see following discussion).

Right Ventricular Pacing

Ventricular pacing frequently produces T wave inversion in the nonpaced sinus complexes (Figures 23–8 and 23–9). These T wave changes occur without any change in the QRS duration. The T wave abnormalities increase with increased

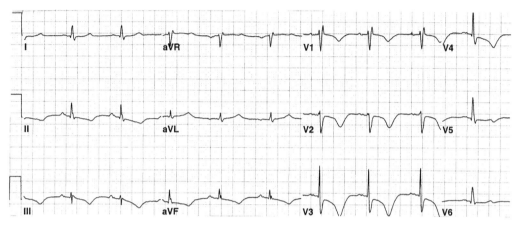

Figure 23–8 Assumed postpacing T wave abnormalities in a 85-year-old man after 1.5 years of intermittent ventricular pacing. The presently inverted T waves were upright before pacemaker implantation, and there were no intervening cardiac events.

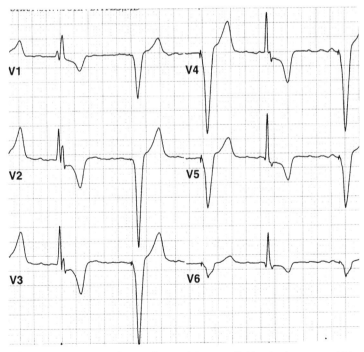

Figure 23–9 Assumed postpacing T wave abnormalities. ECG precordial leads of a 69-year-old man with an implanted ventricular pacemaker show atrial fibrillation with both paced and nonpaced ventricular complexes and right bundle branch block. In the nonpaced complexes, the T waves are deeply inverted. Before pacemaker implantation, the T waves were upright in the left precordial leads.

duration of pacing and the amount of energy applied during pacing. The site of stimulation determines the vector of the T wave. After pacing the endocardial surface of the right ventricle, or the epicardial surface and apex of the left ventricle, abnormal T waves appear predominantly in leads II, III, and V_3–V_5; but after pacing the right ventricular outflow tract, the T wave inversions occur mainly in leads V_1 and V_2.[50] In some cases, T wave abnormalities persisted for 1 to 2 years after termination of the pacing. T wave changes do not appear after atrial pacing or after ventricular pacing during the ventricular refractory period.[50] Thus the T wave abnormalities appear to be related to the presence of abnormal depolarization in the stimulated area. Goyal et al.[51] noted that changes in T wave morphology correlated with changes in the monophasic AP morphology at the right ventricular septum and that the lingering effects on the repolarization process were evident after pacing episodes as brief as 1 minute.[51]

Shvilkin et al.[52] found that the combination of a positive T wave in lead aV_L, positive or isoelectric T wave in lead I, and maximal precordial T wave inversion greater than T wave inversion in lead III had a 92% sensitivity and 100% specificity for T wave abnormalities following pacing right ventricle at the apex, presumably because such distribution of T wave abnormalities is not likely to be caused by myocardial ischemia or myocardial infarction.

LBBB and Ventricular Preexcitation

Transient T wave abnormalities have been observed for variable periods of time after the disappearance of LBBB[53] or ventricular preexcitation.[54] In patients with preexcitation, T wave abnormalities persisted for days, weeks, and sometimes up to 3 months (see Figure 20–9). The incidence of transient T wave abnormalities and the magnitude of the T wave abnormalities increase with increasing degree of preexcitation (i.e., the duration of the preexcited QRS complex).[55,56] No T wave abnormalities occurred in patients with concealed AV bypass conducting only in the retrograde direction. The pattern of primary T wave changes produced by ventricular preexcitation depends on the location of the accessory pathway connections. The septal and posterior connections are associated with more prominent anteriorly directed T wave deflections (i.e., increased amplitude of the T wave in the right and mid-precordial leads) and deviation of the T wave vector superiorly (i.e., negative T waves in leads II, III, and aV_F). The left lateral connections are associated with rightward deviation of the T wave in the frontal plane (i.e.,

T wave inversion or flattening in the left "lateral" leads).[57] The distribution of body surface potentials studied before and 1 day and 1 week after ablation of accessory pathways strongly suggests that the transient T wave abnormalities after cessation of preexcitation are caused by AP prolongation over the preexcited area[58] and that substantial recovery of action potential duration takes place within 1 week after the ablation.[58]

The gradual disappearance of primary T wave abnormalities following normalization of intraventricular conduction has been considered a possible manifestation of repolarization "memory." This implies that the abnormal sequence of activation is "remembered" for some time after return to a normal activation pattern.[53] Another term applied to describe such a phenomenon is "electrical remodeling." It is of interest that similar abnormalities have not been recorded in patients with intermittent RBBB.

Normal Variants and Unexplained T Wave Abnormalities

Abnormalities of the T wave have been found in 0.5 to 2.0 percent of normal persons in various population groups.[6] In a study of 122,043 men without heart disease, aged 16 to 50 years, Hiss and Lamb[59] found a 1.15 percent overall incidence of T wave abnormalities, with the highest incidence in the youngest and the oldest age groups. T wave abnormalites occurred most frequently in the lateral precordial leads. Fisch[60] found no ST or T wave abnormalities in 776 normal individuals younger than age 25 years, whereas 15.7 percent of normal persons older than 65 years had abnormal T waves.

RAPIDLY REVERSIBLE T WAVE ABNORMALITIES

"Rapidly reversible T wave abnormalities" characterizes a category of primary T wave abnormalities that disappear spontaneously with a change in posture or heart rate or within minutes after administering potassium or catecholamines. Such changes may be present only at a slow heart rate or only at a rapid heart rate, or they may be independent of the heart rate.

T Wave Abnormalities Reversed by an Increase in Heart Rate

In certain subjects without heart disease, primary T wave abnormalities appear only at normal or slow heart rates and disappear after a certain critical increase in heart rate with exercise, hyperventilation, pacing, or administration of atropine

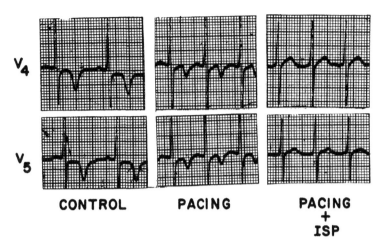

Figure 23–10   ECG leads V_4 and V_5 of a 55-year-old man with diabetes mellitus, increased left ventricular end-diastolic pressure, and a normal coronary arteriogram recorded before (control) and during atrial pacing and during pacing and isoproterenol (ISP) infusion. The normalization of T waves after ISP cannot be attributed to the increase in heart rate. The QT interval during pacing without ISP is 320 ms and that during pacing with ISP is 340 ms. (From Daoud F, Surawicz B, Gettes LS: Effect of isoproterenol on the abnormal T wave. Am J Cardiol 30:810, 1972.)

or isoproterenol. This type of purely rate-dependent T wave abnormality can be identified most conclusively with atrial pacing because the rate-dependent effects of exercise, hyperventilation, and isoproterenol may be attributed to the sympathetic stimulation. The suppression of T wave abnormalities by atropine more likely results from a nonspecific increase in heart rate than from the vagolytic action of the drug because, in persons with normal T waves, atropine tends to decrease the T wave amplitude.

T Wave Abnormalities Reversed by a Decrease in Heart Rate

Various nonspecific T wave abnormalities are often associated with tachycardia and disappear when the heart rate slows.[6] It has been reported that intravenous administration of 10 to 20 mg propranolol abolishes ST segment and T wave abnormalities and prevents orthostatic and exercise-induced changes in patients with T wave abnormalities arising from myocardial ischemia or myocarditis.[61]

Rapidly Reversible Rate-Independent T Wave Abnormalities

A moderate increase in the potassium concentration can change an abnormally low or negative T wave to an upright T wave without a change in heart rate. During the 1950s a diagnostic test consisting of administration of about 10 g of potassium salts orally was employed to differentiate between the irreversible T wave abnormalities produced by structural heart disease and

the reversible T wave changes attributed to functional and nonspecific T wave abnormalities. The test proved to be unsafe.

A safer but more cumbersome test that can be used for the same purpose consists of intravenous administration of isoproterenol. In the study of Daoud et al.,[62] isoproterenol was administered at a rate of 2 to 6 μg/min for 30 to 90 seconds to 80 patients with various T wave abnormalities. The isoproterenol infusion increased the heart rate by 27 to 55 (average 37) beats/min. In patients with secondary T wave abnormalities arising from hypertrophy and bundle branch block and in patients with primary T wave abnormalities after myocardial infarction or pericarditis, administration of isoproterenol altered only the amplitude, not the polarity, of the T wave. In patients (with or without heart disease) with various primary T wave abnormalities and a normal QRS complex, isoproterenol transiently shifted the abnormal T wave vector to the left and anteriorly by 60 to 180 degrees and "normalized" the ECG (see Figure 12-26). These changes did not result from an increase in heart rate because they did not occur after a similar increase in heart rate by atropine or pacing (Figure 23–10).[63] The results of this study help us understand the fairly common occurrence of T wave normalization during exercise-induced tachycardia.

Concomitant ST-T Abnormalities

As a result of the differences in the underlying mechanisms at the cellular level, the behavior of the ST segment and the T wave differ from each other in a variety of conditions discussed earlier. An example is myocardial ischemia, which frequently produces both ST segment and T wave changes, although the ST segment changes may occur without T wave changes and vice versa.

Despite the fundamental differences in the genesis of the ST segment and the T wave, electrocardiographers frequently use the expression "ST-T changes" to describe the patterns associated with the alterations of one or both of these two repolarization components. One reason for applying this term may be the lack of a distinct point of demarcation between the end of the ST segment and the onset of the T wave. Another reason is that the ST segment and the T wave abnormalities commonly coexist in the presence of secondary repolarization abnormalities (e.g., left ventricular hypertrophy or LBBB) or when primary repolarization abnormalities affect both the plateau and phase 3 of repolarization (e.g., effect of digitalis and type IA antiarrhythmia drugs). Nevertheless, in a variety of other situations the ECG diagnosis gains in precision when the ST segment, T wave, and U wave are analyzed as separate components rather than as a single complex of "repolarization."

Nonspecific ST and T Abnormalities

Ventricular repolarization changes are probably the most common ECG abnormalities. Their diagnostic usefulness, however, is often curtailed owing to the perceived notion of low specificity reflected in the commonly used terms "nonspecific repolarization abnormalities" and "nonspecific ST, T, or ST-T changes." These terms are appropriate when the interpreter is unable to render an opinion because it carries a risk of being incorrect, but they deprive the clinician of useful information when a specific cause can be suggested with a high degree of probability. The interpretation of abnormal ventricular repolarization can be facilitated by using available clinical information and by noting the following suggestions:

1. Define whether the abnormalities affect only the ST segment, only the T wave, or both.
2. Assess the abnormality as slight, moderate, or marked.
3. Based on the analysis of the QRS complex and the contour of the ST segment and T wave changes, determine whether the changes are likely to be secondary to

hypertrophy and an intraventricular conduction disturbance.

4. Assume that terminal T wave inversion without deviation of the ST segment from the baseline is probably a primary abnormality that often indicates acute or chronic myocardial ischemia.
5. Consider that the probability of myocardial ischemia is increased when: (1) a pattern of progression or regression can be detected in serial tracings; (2) a constellation of leads suggests possible localization of the ischemic region; (3) the QTc interval is considerably prolonged; and (4) the U wave is inverted.
6. Consider that secondary and primary T wave changes can coexist.
7. Consider that tachycardia alone can precipitate both ST segment depression and T wave abnormalities.
8. Remember that a negative T wave may represent a normal finding in leads III, aV_L, and V_1. Moreover, a negative T wave in lead V_2 may represent a normal "juvenile" pattern in young adults.
9. Consider that marked QT lengthening associated with ST segment depression and fusion of the T and U waves may reflect a drug effect or hypokalemia.

When no clues are available to suggest a specific diagnosis or a cause of the abnormality, it is appropriate to characterize the undiagnosed abnormalities as nonspecific. When such abnormalities are minimal or slight, it is appropriate to acknowledge this in the report. In the United States and other countries with a high prevalence of ischemic heart disease, the presence of moderate or marked primary T wave abnormalities in the adult population should be considered probable manifestations of ischemic heart disease. In my opinion, the diagnostic usefulness of the ST segment and T wave abnormalities improves when the interpretations are couched in terms of probable specificity, rather than placing the emphasis on the absence of specific findings.

Computerized Analysis of T Wave Morphology and Spatial Orientation of the T Wave

The widely perceived failure of QT dispersion in the 12-lead ECG as a prognostic marker of cardiac events in clinical practice spawned studies testing alternative ways to characterize the nonhomogeneity of ventricular repolarization. Several approaches aided by computer-based methodology have been undertaken to characterize the morphology and the spatial orientation of abnormal T waves. The details of methods analyzing various descriptors of T wave morphology,[64,65] T wave complexity derived from principal component analysis,[66] T wave axis deviation,[67] and the shape of the T wave loop[68] are beyond the scope of this textbook inasmuch as the practical usefulness of this information must await the passage of time.

REFERENCES

1. Surawicz B, Saito S: Exercise testing for detection of myocardial ischemia in patients with abnormal electrocardiogram at rest. Am J Cardiol 41:943, 1978.
2. Wilson FN, MacLeod AG, Barker PS: The T deflection of the electrocardiogram. Trans Assoc Am Physicians 46:29, 1931.
3. Lepeschkin E: Modern Electrocardiography. Baltimore, Williams & Wilkins, 1951.
4. Abildskov JA, Burgess MJ, Lux RL, et al: The expression of normal ventricular repolarization in the body surface distribution of T potentials. Circulation 54:901, 1976.
5. Schaefer H, Haas HG: Electrocardiography. In: Hamilton WF, Dow P (eds): Handbook of Physiology, vol I, sect 2: Circulation. Washington, DC, American Physiological Society, 1962.
6. Surawicz B: ST-T abnormalities. In: MacFarlane PW, Lawrie TD (eds): Comprehensive Electrocardiology. New York, Pergamon, 1989.
7. Coltart DJ, Meldrum SJ: Hypertrophic cardiomyopathy: an electrophysiological study. BMJ 4:217, 1970.
8. Barlow JB, Pocock WA: The problem of non-ejection systolic clicks and associated mitral systolic murmurs: emphasis on the billowing mitral leaflet syndrome. Am Heart J 90:636, 1975.
9. Jeresaty RM: Mitral valve prolapse-click syndrome. Prog Cardiovasc Dis 15:623, 1973.
10. Procacci PM, Savran SV, Schreiter SL, et al: Prevalence of clinical mitral valve prolapse in 1169 young women. N Engl J Med 294:1086, 1976.
11. Massie B, Botvinick EH, Shames D, et al: Myocardial perfusion scintigraphy in patients with mitral valve prolapse. Circulation 57:19, 1978.
12. Engel PJ, Alpert BL, Triebwasser JH, et al: Exercise testing in mitral valve prolapse. Am J Cardiol 41:430, 1978.
13. Ehlers KH, Engle MA, Levin AR, et al: Left ventricular abnormality with late mitral insufficiency and abnormal electrocardiogram. Am J Cardiol 26:333, 1970.
14. Bowers D: An electrocardiographic pattern associated with mitral valve deformity in Marfan's syndrome. Circulation 23:30, 1961.
15. Walder LA, Spodick DH: Global T wave inversion. J Am Coll Cardiol 17:1479, 1991.
16. Walder LA, Spodick DH: Global T wave inversion: long-term follow-up. J Am Coll Cardiol 21:1652, 1993.
17. Brscic E, Brusca A, Presbitero P, et al: Ischemic chest pain and global T-wave inversion in women with normal coronary arteriograms. Am J Cardiol 80:245, 1997.
18. Littmann L: Large T wave inversion and QT prolongation associated with pulmonary edema: a report of nine cases. J Am Coll Cardiol 34:1106, 1999.
19. Suzuki J-I, Shimamoto R, Nishikawa J-I, et al: Morphological onset and early diagnosis in apical hypertrophic cardiomyopathy: a long term analysis with nuclear magnetic resonance imaging. J Am Coll Cardiol 33:146, 1999.
20. Okada M, Yotsukura M, Shimada T, et al: Clinical implications of isolated T wave inversion in adults: electrocardiographic differentiation of the underlying causes of this phenomenon. J Am Coll Cardiol 24:739, 1994.
21. Surawicz B: The pathogenesis and clinical significance of primary T-wave abnormalities. In: Schlant RC, Hurst JW (eds): Advances in Electrocardiography. Orlando, Grune & Stratton, 1972.
22. O'Brien KE, Pastis N, Conii JB: Diffuse T-wave inversions associated with electroconvulsive therapy. Am J Cardiol 93:1573, 2004.
23. Averbuck SH: Acute generalized postoperative peritonitis simulating coronary artery occlusion. J Mt Sinai Hosp 8:335, 1942.
24. Fulton MC, Marriott HJ: Acute pancreatitis simulating myocardial infarction in the electrocardiogram. Ann Intern Med 59:730, 1963.
25. Kemp GL, Ellestad MH: The significance of hyperventilation and orthostatic T-wave changes on the electrocardiogram. Arch Intern Med 121:518, 1968.
26. Biberman L, Sarma RN, Surawicz B: T-wave abnormalities during hyperventilation and isoproterenol infusion. Am Heart J 81:166, 1971.
27. Salvetti A, Cella PL, Arrigoni P, et al: Comportamento della fase di ripolarizzazione ventricolare dopo sforzo e dopo iperventilazione volontaria in giovani sani. Cuore Circ 48:192, 1964.
28. Yu PN, Yim BJ, Stanfield CA: Hyperventilation syndrome. Arch Intern Med 103:902, 1959.
29. Christensen BC: Studies on hyperventilation. II. Electrocardiographic changes in normal man during voluntary hyperventilation. J Clin Invest 25:880, 1946.
30. Christensen BC: Variations in the carbon dioxide tension in the arterial blood and the electrocardiogram in man. Acta Physiol Scand 12:389, 1946.
31. Furberg C, Tengblad CF: Adrenergic beta receptor blockade and the effect of hyperventilation on the electrocardiogram. Scand J Clin Lab Invest 18:467, 1966.
32. Pentimone F, Pesola A, L' Abbaate A, et al: Effetto del propranolol sulle modificazioni elettocardiographiche secondaria alla prova da iperventillazione volontaria ed alla prova ortostatica. Cuore Circ 51:79, 1967.
33. McHenry PL, Cogan OJ, Elliott WC, et al: False positive ECG response to exercise secondary to hyperventilation: cineangiographic correlation. Am Heart J 79: 683, 1970.
34. Lary D, Goldschlager N: Electrocardiographic changes during hyperventilation resembling myocardial ischemia in patients with normal coronary arteriogram. Am Heart J 87:383, 1974.
35. Ardissino D, De Servi S, Barberis P, et al: Significance of hyperventilation-induced ST segment depression in patients with coronary artery disease. J Am Coll Cardiol 13:804, 1989.
36. Schweitzer P, Hildebrand T, Kivanova H, et al: Der Einfluss der adrenergen Blockade auf die orthostatischen Veraenderungen der Integralvektoren von QRS. Z Kreislaufforsch 56:316, 1967.
37. Hiss RG, Smith GB, Lamb LE: Pitfalls in interpreting electrocardiographic changes occurring while monitoring stress procedures. Aerospace Med 31:9, 1960.
38. Lepeschkin E, Surawicz B: Characteristics of true-positive and false-positive results of electrocardiographic Master two-step exercise test. N Engl J Med 258:511, 1958.
39. Levander Lindgren M: Studies in neurocirculatory asthenia (Da Costa's syndrome). I. Variations with regard to

symptoms and some pathophysiological signs. Acta Med Scand 172:665, 1962.

40. Wendkos MH, Logue RB: Unstable T waves in leads II and III in persons with neurocirculatory asthenia. Am Heart J 31:711, 1946.

41. Simonson E, McKinlay CA: The meal test in clinical electrocardiography. Circulation 1:1006, 1950.

42. Sears GA, Manning GW: Routine electrocardiography: postprandial T wave changes. Am Heart J 56:591, 1958.

43. Sleeper JC, Orgain ES: Differentiation of benign from pathologic T waves in the electrocardiogram. Am J Cardiol 11:338, 1963.

44. MacAlpin RN, Weidner WA, Kattus AA, et al: Electrocardiographic changes during selective coronary cineangiography. Circulation 34:627, 1966.

45. Shabetai R, Surawicz B, Hamill W: Monophasic action potentials in man. Circulation 38:341, 1968.

46. Mann RH, Burchell HB: The significance of T wave inversion in sinus beats following ventricular extrasystoles. Am Heart J 47:504, 1954.

47. Levine HD, Lown B, Streeper RB: The clinical significance of postextrasystolic T wave changes. Circulation 6:538, 1952.

48. Meyer P, Schmidt C: Troubles postextrasystoliques de la repolarisation. Arch Mal Coeur Vaiss 42:1175, 1949.

49. Paparella N, Ouyang F, Fuca G, et al: Significance of newly acquired negative T waves after interruption of paroxysmal reentrant supraventricular tachycardia with narrow QRS complex. Am J Cardiol 85:261, 2000.

50. Chatterjee K, Harris A, Davies G, et al: Electrocardiographic changes subsequent to artificial depolarization. Br Heart J 31:770, 1969.

51. Goyal R, Syed ZA, Mukhopadhyay S, et al: Changes in cardiac repolarization following short periods of pacing. J Cardiovasc Electrophysiol 9:269, 1998.

52. Shvilin A, Ho KKL, Rosen MR, et al: T-vector direction differentiates postpacing from ischemic T-wave inversion in precordial leads. Circulation 111:969, 2005.

53. Rosenbaum MB, Blanco HH, Elizari MV, et al: Electrotonic modulation of the T wave and cardiac memory. Am J Cardiol 50:213, 1982.

54. Nicolai P, Medvedovsky JL, Delaage M, et al: Wolff-Parkinson-White syndrome: T wave abnormalities during normal pathway conduction. J Electrocardiol 14:295, 1981.

55. Hirai M, Tsuboi N, Hayashi H, et al: Body surface distribution of abnormally low QRST areas in patients with Wolff-Parkinson-White syndrome: evidence for

56. Kalbfleisch SL, Sousa J, El-Atassi R, et al: Repolarization abnormalities after catheter ablation of accessory atrioventricular connections with radiofrequency current. J Am Coll Cardiol 18:1761, 1991.

57. Surawicz B: Transient T wave abnormalities after cessation of ventricular preexcitation: memory of what? J Cardiovasc Electrophysiol 7:51, 1996.

58. Akahoshi M, Hirai M, Inden Y, et al: Body-surface distribution of changes in activation-recovery intervals before and after catheter ablation in patients with Wolff-Parkinson-White syndrome: clinical evidence for "electrical remodeling" with prolongation of action-potential duration over a preexcited area. Circulation 96:1566, 1997.

59. Hiss RG, Lamb LE: Electrocardiographic findings in 122,043 individuals. Circulation 25:947, 1962.

60. Fisch C: The electrocardiogram in the aged. In: Noble RJ, Rothbaum D (eds): Geriatric Cardiology. Philadelphia, FA Davis, 1981.

61. Furberg C: Adrenergic beta blockade and electrocardiographic ST-T changes. Acta Med Scand 181:21, 1967.

62. Daoud FS, Surawicz B, Gettes LS: Effect of isoproterenol on the abnormal T wave. Am J Cardiol 30:810, 1972.

63. Wasserburger RH, Corliss RJ: Value of oral potassium salts in differentiation of functional and organic T wave changes. Am J Cardiol 10:673, 1962.

64. Zabel M, Malik M, Hnatkova K, et al: Analysis of T-wave morphology from the 12-lead electrocardiogram for prediction of long-term prognosis in male US veterans. Circulation 105:1066, 2002.

65. Oikarinen L, Vaananen H, Dabek J, et al: Relation of twelve-lead electrocardiographic T-wave morphology description to left ventricular mass. Am J Cardiol 90:1032, 2002.

66. Okin PM, Devereux RB, Fabsitz RR, et al: Principal component analysis of the T wave and prediction of cardiovascular mortality in American Indians. The Strong Heart Study. Circulation 105:714, 2002.

67. Rautaharju PM, Nelson JC, Kronmal RA, et al: Usefulness of T-axis deviation as an independent risk indicator for incident cardiac events in older men and women free from coronary heart disease (The Cardiovascular Health Study). Am J Cardiol 88:118, 2001.

68. Perkiomaki JS, Hyytinen-Oinas M, Karsikas M, et al: Usefulness of T-wave loop and QRS complex loop to predict mortality after acute myocardial infarction. Am J Cardiol 97:353, 2006.

continuation of repolarization abnormalities before and after catheter ablation. Circulation 88:2674, 1993.

24 QT Interval, U Wave Abnormalities, and Cardiac Alternans

QT Interval

The normal QT interval is discussed in Chapter 1. A recently published distribution of QTc values in apparently healthy persons is shown in Figure 24–1. Abnormal shortening of the QTc interval results from a shortened or absent ST segment. Shortening of the QTc is seldom recognized and, except for a hypercalcemia and digitalis effect, has not played a role in clinical practice. Recently, however, a syndrome of short QT associated with sudden death became recognized as a distinct channelopathy (see later discussion).

Lengthening of the QT interval, however, is a common finding of undiminished theoretic and practical interest. Such lengthening may be caused in part or exclusively by increased QRS duration, but the subsequent text deals only with the conditions associated with predominant or exclusive lengthening of repolarization.

PROLONGED QT INTERVAL

Clinical manifestations of a prolonged QT interval can be divided into those that result in: (1) marked QTc prolongation (i.e., >125 percent of the average normal value) (Table 24–1); and (2) moderate QT prolongation (i.e., approximately 115 to 125 percent of the average normal value) (Table 24–2). Several reported causes of minor and inconsistent QTc prolongation are considered separately. Subdivision into these categories is based exclusively on personal experience and is not categoric. Each of the conditions that can cause marked QT prolongation may also cause less or no QT prolongation. The conditions listed as causing moderate QT prolongation in Table 24–2 seldom cause QT prolongation as marked as do the conditions in Table 24–1. Thus the conditions listed in Tables 24–1 and 24–2 may be used as guidelines for the differential diagnosis when confronted with marked or moderate QTc prolongation of uncertain origin.

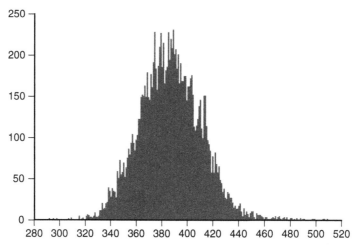

Figure 24–1 QTc values in 12,012 healthy persons. (With permission of authors and publishers in Gallagher MM, Magliano G, Yap YG, et al: Distribution and prognostic significance of QT intervals in the lowest half centile in 12,012 apparently healthy persons. Am J Cardiol 98:933, 2006.)

TABLE 24-1	Causes of Marked QT Lengthening* (>125%)

Congenital
Neurogenic, including organophosphorus
Severe hypothermia
Hypokalemia
Severe hypocalcemia
Fad diets
Contrast injections into coronary artery
Antiarrhythmic drugs classes IA and III
Severe bradycardia, atrioventricular block (see
　Figure 24–5), myocardial ischemia,
　postresuscitation, unexplained (occasionally)**

*Excluding that secondary to QRS widening.
**Probably predominantly neurogenic.

TABLE 24-2	Causes of Moderate QT Prolongation* (115–125%)

Postischemic, transmural, and nontransmural
　myocardial infarction
Various cardiomyopathies and after cardiac
　surgical trauma
Moderate hypokalemia and hypocalcemia
Class IA and III antiarrhythmic agents,
　tranquilizers
Hypothyroidism and pituitary insufficiency
Neurogenic or unexplained (occasionally)

*Excluding that secondary to QRS widening.

CONGENITAL LONG QT SYNDROME

Familial prolongation of the QT interval associated with congenital deafness and sudden cardiac death due to ventricular arrhythmia was first reported by Jervell and Lange-Nielsen of Norway.[1] This condition is autosomal recessive and is less common and more severe[2] than the subsequently described autosomal-dominant congenital long QT syndrome associated with sudden death and normal hearing reported in families in Ireland[3] and Italy[4,5] (Romano-Ward syndrome).

The natural history of the disorder is extremely variable, the appearance of symptoms is sporadic and unpredictable, and the duration of the QT interval undergoes marked spontaneous variations (Figure 24–2). Numerous clinical observations of ventricular arrhythmia have shown that syncope and sudden death are provoked by increased sympathetic stimulation and emotional stress, such as fright[1,6] or startling noises (Figure 24–3). In some cases, continuous recordings are available[7–9] that show prolongation of the QT interval precipitated by noxious psychic stimuli and the concomitant appearance of ventricular premature complexes and ventricular tachycardia degenerating into ventricular fibrillation. Evidence for autonomic dysfunction in patients with long QT syndrome include a reported inability to increase the heart rate appropriately with exercise[10–12] or after administration of atropine[13] and inappropriate adjustment of the QT interval to tachycardia induced by exercise or during the Valsalva maneuver.[14–17] Such dysfunction does not occur uniformly in all patients.

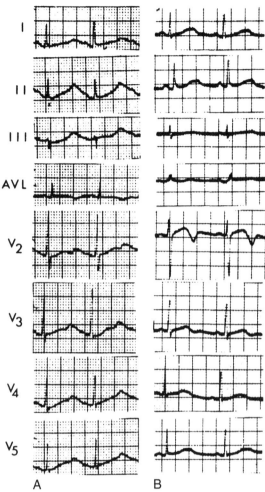

I

II

III

AVL

V₂

V₃

V₄

V₅

A   B

Figure 24–2 ECGs on different days from a 15-year-old girl with congenital long QT syndrome. The QT lengthening is much greater in **A** than in **B,** although the heart rates are similar. (From Surawicz B, Knoebel SK: Long QT, good, bad, and indifferent. J Am Coll Cardiol 4:398, 1984.)

Syncope and sudden cardiac death are caused usually by the characteristic polymorphous ventricular tachycardia (torsade de pointes) or ventricular fibrillation. These arrhythmias occur in the setting of large dispersion of ventricular repolarization[18,19] and are precipitated usually by a ventricular premature complex interrupting the T wave.[4,13,20–23]

It has been suspected for some time that congenital long QT syndrome (LQTS) was an abnormality of ion channel proteins that control the duration of the ventricular action potential; that is, potassium channel block or prolonged inactivation of the sodium channel (i.e., a leaky sodium channel).

During the early 1990s a linkage was identified between the LQTS phenotype and abnormalities

at several chromosomal locations. Keating et al.[24] analyzed the DNA of members of multiple families from the international registry of congenital LQTS and found mutations in two genes in some affected families. Both genes encoded cardiac channels in families linked to chromosomes 3 and 7. This established congenital LQTS as primarily a disease of cardiac ion channels (channelopathy) with marked genetic heterogeneity. Since then, the horizons of genetic molecular biology have expanded in many directions. The defective genes have been mapped to five chromosomes and identified in various types of LQTS. The Jervell and Lange-Nielsen syndrome is caused by two genes that encode the slowly activating delayed rectifier potassium channel (KCNQ1) and KCNEI, whereas the Romano-Ward syndrome is caused by mutations in eight different genes. These include: KCNQI (LQTI), KCNH2(LQT2), SCN5A (sodium channel-LQT3), ANKB (protein ankyrin involved in anchoring calcium and sodium channel to the cellular membrane (LQT4), KCNEI (mink, LQT5), KCNE 2 (LQT6), KCNJ2(LQT7, Andersen's syndrome), and CACNAIC (LQT8, Timothy syndrome). This means that of the eight genes, six encode for cardiac potassium channel, one for the sodium channel, and one for the protein ankyrin (ankyrin-B syndrome).[25,26,26a] It is believed that the ECG differences in repolarization patterns in congenital LQTS can identify LQTI, LQT2, and possibly LQT3 genotypes.[27] The long QT in LQTI and LQT2 is caused mostly by T wave lengthening, but the T waves in LQT2 are lower and more notched than in LQTI,[28] whereas in patients with LQT3 lengthening of QT is due predominantly to an increased duration of the ST segment.[29] The epinephrine test is another way to expose the differences between the three most common channelopathies.[30,31] Low-dose epinephrine infusion shortens the QT interval in control subjects and those with LQT2 and LQT3 but paradoxically lengthens it in subjects with LQTI.[30,31] Sinus bradycardia may be present in LQT3 patients as a result of sodium channel mutations.[32] Also, certain types of the T and U abnormalities, such as prolonged terminal portion of T wave downslope and wide T-U junction, have been reported as distinct anomalies in Andersen-Tawil syndrome (LQT7).[33] It has also been reported that different types of LQTS require application of different preventive and therapeutic measures.[34,35] A more detailed survey of the growing literature about various aspects of LQTS is beyond the scope of this textbook.

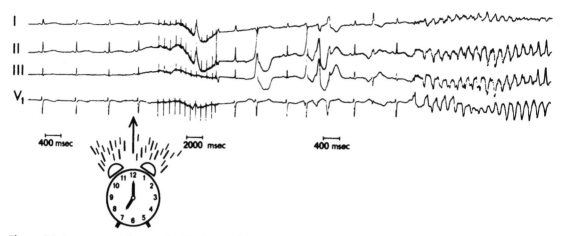

Figure 24–3 Initiation of ventricular fibrillation after an auditory stimulus (alarm clock) in a 14-year-old girl with congenital long QT syndrome. QT interval lengthening is followed by ventricular premature complexes, torsade de pointes, and ventricular fibrillation. The middle of the tracing is recorded at a slower speed than the beginning and the end. (From Wellens HJ, Vermeulen A, Durrer D: Ventricular fibrillation occurring upon arousal from sleep by auditory stimuli. Circulation 46:661, 1972.)

ACQUIRED BRADYARRHYTHMIAS

The marked QT lengthening in patients with bradycardia in the presence of complete A-V block (Figure 24–5) may cause torsade de pointes, particularly when morphology of the T waves is like in LQT2 syndrome.[35a]

CEREBROVASCULAR ACCIDENT

See Chapter 22.

ANTIARRHYTHMIC AND PSYCHOTROPIC DRUGS

See Chapter 21.

POISONING WITH ORGANOPHOSPHOROUS COMPOUNDS

The organophosphorous compounds inhibit cholinesterase and produce intense vagal stimulation. The mechanism of QT lengthening in this condition is poorly understood, but the electrocardiographic (ECG) patterns and the arrhythmias (i.e., torsade de pointes) are similar to those in patients with congenital LQTS.[36]

METABOLIC DISTURBANCES

See Chapter 22.

OBESITY, WEIGHT LOSS, DIETING

Frank et al.[37] studied the ECGs of 1029 obese persons, of whom 85 percent were women. The QTc tended to increase slightly with an increase in weight, but a QTc >0.44 second was found in only 7.8 percent of the subjects and a QTc >0.47 second in 12 persons. These values appear to be within the range of QT distribution in the general population. In contrast, El-Gamal et al.[38] found that the duration of the QTc interval is significantly associated with obesity and that obesity may be one of the most common causes of prolonged QTc interval. Conventional dieting appears to result in shortening rather than lengthening of the QTc,[39] whereas QTc lengthening has been reported in persons using a liquid protein diet.

Isner et al. reviewed 17 cases of unexplained sudden death in the users of liquid protein diet for weight reduction.[40] The ECG was recorded before death in nine women and one man, and their QTc intervals ranged from 0.46 to 0.70 second. Similar findings were reported by others,[41,42] although some of the cases appear in multiple reviews. In their review article, Surawicz and Waller[43] concluded that sudden cardiac death during use of liquid protein products remains an enigma, but other methods of properly supervised diets are not associated with a prolonged QT interval and appear to be safe.

Lengthening of the QTc has been reported in some patients with anorexia nervosa.[36] Isner et al.[44] speculated about the possibility of neurogenic QT lengthening caused by hypothalamic-pituitary disturbances believed to be associated frequently with anorexia nervosa. Prolonged starvation is associated with low voltage, which makes it difficult to measure the QT interval accurately. This may account for conflicting reports about the effects of starvation on the QTc interval. Simonson et al.[45] found no evidence of QTc lengthening after 3 months of semistarvation, resulting in

24 percent weight loss, but Hellerstein and Santiago-Stevenson[46] and Burch et al.[47] reported that the QTc was occasionally prolonged in cases of cardiac cachexia and atrophy.

PROLONGED QTc AND MYOCARDIAL DAMAGE

In many patients with rheumatic, congenital, or hypertensive heart disease and various cardiomyopathies, the QT interval is slightly to moderately prolonged. This is frequently due, at least in part, to prolongation of the QRS complex; however, asynchronous repolarization unrelated to the abnormal sequence of activation may also be important. Moderate or occasionally marked QTc lengthening occurs transiently in most patients after open heart

operations (see Chapter 11). Early after operation, this may be a lingering effect of hypothermia. Prolonged QT is seen often after cardiac resuscitation even in cases when the QT interval is not known to be prolonged before the arrest (Figure 24–4).

PREDICTIVE VALUE OF QT INTERVAL IN HEART DISEASE

There are at least two rationales for QTc lengthening being predictive of an adverse prognosis for survivors of myocardial infarction. One could assume that a longer QTc interval is associated with a more extensive mass of scarred or poorly functioning myocardium. However, it is not known whether the magnitude of the QTc lengthening bears a relation to the age, location, and extent of

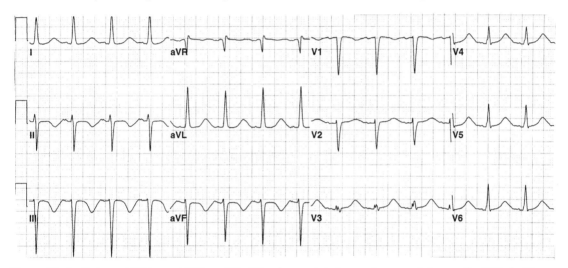

Figure 24–4   Prolonged QT interval (500 ms; QTc 602 ms), recorded after cardiac resuscitation, on the ECG of a 68-year-old hypertensive, diabetic, morbidly obese woman who had not been treated with any drugs. In addition to long QT, note the left axis deviation and increased voltage in the lead aV$_L$ suggestive of left ventricular hypertrophy.

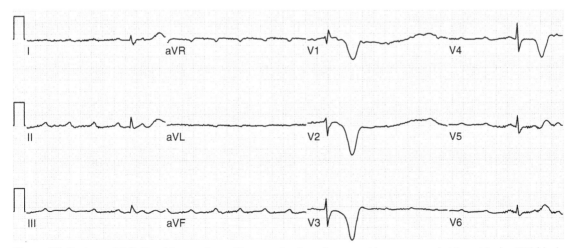

Figure 24–5   Long QT (640 ms) in a patient with severe bradycardia, caused by paroxysmal atrioventricular (AV) block with an escape rhythm at 17 beats/min. On the same day when the AV block dissipated with return of regular sinus rhythm, QTc was normal (not shown).

the infarction. In addition, if the QT lengthening is secondary to a more extensive mass of affected myocardium, the prolonged QTc would not be expected to represent an independent prognostic marker. Alternatively, one could assume that the lengthening of QTc reflects an increased dispersion of ventricular repolarization, a marker of a potentially arrhythmogenic electrophysiologic substrate.

The baseline QTc in a healthy population entering the Framingham Heart Study was not predictive of cardiac mortality or sudden cardiac death.[48] However, in a cohort of Dutch civil servants and their spouses, QTc lengthening (>440 ms) was predictive of increased cardiovascular-related mortality.[49] Similarly, in a population of healthy older adults, QTc interval >450 ms in men and >470 ms in women was reported to be an independent risk factor for sudden cardiac death.[50]

In some studies of patients with heart disease, QTc lengthening was not an independent risk factor for sudden death due to cardiac arrest[51] or death after acute myocardial infarction.[52,53] In other studies, QTc lengthening was a predictor of sudden cardiac death in patients with unstable angina pectoris,[54] with chronic ischemic heart disease,[55] and at 1 year after myocardial infarction.[56]

See also Chapters 7, 8, and 9.

MITRAL VALVE PROLAPSE

The possible role of prolonged QTc as a contributor to arrhythmias in patients with mitral valve prolapse has received increasing attention. In two studies,[57,58] QTc prolongation (>0.43 second) was found in 29 of 40 patients[57] and in 44 of 94 patients, respectively.[58] In another report[59] the average QTc of 56 patients with mitral valve

prolapse was 0.48 second compared with 0.38 second in 62 normal volunteers. In contrast to these reports are the results of the Framingham study[60] in which a QTc >0.44 second was present in 5 percent of 208 subjects with mitral valve prolapse and in 7 percent of 2727 subjects without it. Similarly, Cowan and Fye[61] found no significant difference in the distribution of QTc between patients with mitral valve prolapse and controls.

MISCELLANEOUS CONDITIONS

Lesser degrees of QTc prolongation (usually <115 percent) have been reported in a variety of conditions, including diabetes mellitus, chronic alcoholism, alcoholic liver disease,[62] depression, and induction and maintenance of anesthesia.[63,64] In most of these reports the QTc values are not abnormal but are significantly longer than in the respective matched control groups. Variable QTc prolongation can also be caused by accidental or induced hypothermia and several drugs outside the antiarrhythmic and psychotropic categories, such as quinine, probucol, atabrine, emetine, calcium channel blocker prenylamine, ketanserin (a selective blocker of 5-hydroxytryptamine-2 receptors), vincamine, chloralhydrate, methadone, pimozide, ziprasidone, haloperidol, tamoxifen, arsenic preparations, doxepin, pentamidine, and certain antibiotic and antiinfective agents (e.g., erythromycin, ampicillin, sparfloxacin, moxifloxacin, trimethoprim sulfa). Some of these and other drugs have been withdrawn because of QT prolongation associated with the risk of torsade de pointes.[65] The list has been growing with an increasing number of case reports. Figure 24–6 shows QT prolongation attributed to use of the drug orlaan.

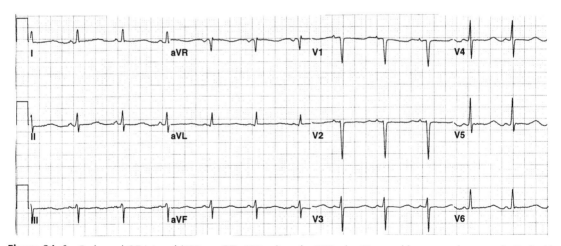

Figure 24–6 Prolonged QT interval (532 ms; QTc 602 ms) on the ECG of a 43-year-old woman who was admitted with torsade de pointes. The QT prolongation was attributed to treatment with the drug orlaan used to manage her narcotic addiction. The patient had no history of heart disease and no abnormal cardiac findings, but the QT interval had not returned to normal after orlaan was eliminated from the body.

SHORT QT SYNDROME (SQTS)

Association of short QT interval with sudden death was mentioned in 1993 by Algra et al.,[66] reported as a short-coupled variant of torsade de pointes by Leenhardt et al.,[67] and introduced as a clinical syndrome by Gussak et al.[68] The QT is considered short when it is <330 ms. However, QTc <320 ms was found in 0.1% in a cohort of 10,282 middle-aged subjects[68a] whereas not a single case of QTc <300 ms was recorded in a sample of 479,120 ECGs from 106,432 patients.[68b] In the study of families with history of sudden cardiac death by Gaita et al.[69] the QTc did not exceed 280 ms. In addition to the short QT, the T waves are often tall and peaked. The syndrome has been linked to to gain-of-function mutations in several potassium channels controlling ventricular repolarization and causing stronger than normal K currents, or loss of function mutations in the cardiac calcium channel.[26,70,70a]

█ Abnormal U Wave

NEGATIVE U WAVE

The negative U wave in the standard ECG leads other than aV_R (and occasionally III and aV_F) seldom occurs in the absence of heart disease or other ECG abnormalities. Holzmann and Zurukzoglu[71] found that 197 of 200 patients with a negative U wave had heart disease. Of the 100 patients reported by Ameur-Hendrich et al.,[72] 99 had heart disease; and in the study of Kishida et al.[73] only 25 of 488 patients (5.1 percent) with a negative U wave had no other ECG abnormalities.

Inversion of the U wave has been reported during attacks of variant angina pectoris.[74] During exercise testing, U wave inversion was found to be a specific (specificity 93 percent) but not a sensitive (sensitivity 21 percent) marker for stenosis of the left anterior descending coronary artery[75] (Figure 24–7). In the study of Kishida et al.,[73] the largest subgroup of patients with a negative U wave had systemic hypertension. In most cases of hypertensive, ischemic, or left-sided valvular heart disease the U wave is inverted in the left precordial leads; but in patients with right ventricular hypertrophy the U wave is usually inverted in the right precordial leads (Figure 24–8).

Kishida et al.[73] reviewed the records of 130 patients in whom the U wave changed polarity, from negative to positive or vice versa, in the same lead within less than 1 year. In 107 patients, the change from a negative to a positive U wave occurred during medical treatment and in 23 patients after a surgical procedure

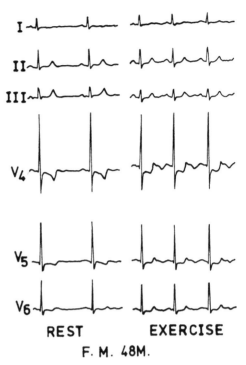

Figure 24–7 U wave inversion associated with ST segment depression in a patient with an akinetic segment of the anterior left ventricular wall caused by previous myocardial infarction.

(e.g., kidney transplantation, aortic valve replacement, coronary artery bypass graft). Changes in the polarity of the U wave were not accompanied by any consistent change in the T wave or ST segment, which suggests that changes in U wave polarity are independent of the electrophysiologic processes that control ventricular repolarization.

Tamura et al.[76] found negative U waves in 31 of 141 patients with acute anterior myocardial infarction. Patients with a negative U wave had smaller infarcts, less ST segment elevation, better collateral circulation, and a larger amount of stunned but viable myocardium.[77] Figure 24–9 shows an ECG from a patient in whom the appearance of negative U waves preceded the occurrence of myocardial infarction.

INCREASED AMPLITUDE OF UPRIGHT U WAVE

Positive inotropic interventions (e.g., catecholamines, calcium, digitalis, or postextrasystolic potentiation) tend to increase the U wave amplitude. Digitalis and hypercalcemia do not appreciably change the temporal relation between the T wave and the U wave (i.e., the U wave begins from the baseline after the end of the T wave). After intravenous administration of

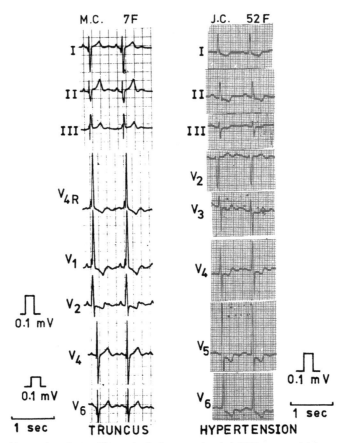

Figure 24–8   Negative U wave in patients with ventricular hypertrophy. *Left,* ECG pattern of right ventricular hypertrophy with negative U waves in leads V_{4R}, V_1, and V_2. *Right,* Pattern of left ventricular hypertrophy with negative U waves in leads V_4–V_6.

epinephrine or isoproterenol, however, the U wave appears earlier, resulting in its fusion with the terminal T wave portion.[78] U wave amplitude is also increased during bradycardia.

The amplitude of a positive U wave in patients with myocardial ischemia has not been studied systematically. Kataoka et al.[79] suggested that in some patients with myocardial ischemia a positive U wave of increased amplitude in the precordial leads represents the reciprocal polarity of a negative U wave associated with inferoposterior myocardial ischemia.

T WAVE AND U WAVE FUSION IN THE PRESENCE OF A PROLONGED QT INTERVAL

Lengthening of the QT interval (without a change in QTc) results most often from a decrease in the heart rate, which is associated with increased ventricular filling and a longer ejection period. Under these conditions the relation between the QT interval and the onset of the U wave remains unchanged; that is, the U wave begins from the baseline synchronously with

the second heart sound. If the increased diastolic interval occurs abruptly, however (e.g., during atrial fibrillation or after a premature impulse[80]), fusion between the T wave and the U wave may occur.

The nonphysiologic types of QT interval lengthening caused by global or regional increases in the ventricular action potential duration result in fusion of the T wave and the U wave. So long as the QT interval is prolonged by less than about 90 to 110 ms and the timing of the U wave does not change, the U wave apex remains recognizable. With progressively increased duration of the QT interval, the point of the TU junction deviates progressively from baseline. More than about 100 ms of QT lengthening results in complete obfuscation of a normally timed U wave. The difficulty of measuring the QT in such cases is illustrated in Figures 24–9 and 24–10.

In the absence of T wave notching or QT prolongation, distinguishing the T wave from the U wave and accurately measuring the QT interval present no difficulties. When the T wave is notched, however, the distant peak can be mistaken for the U wave. This is seldom a problem

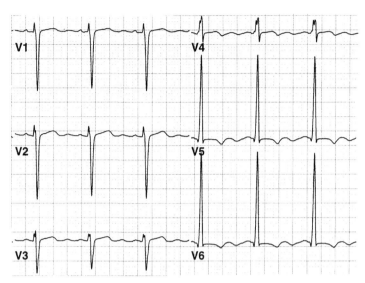

Figure 24–9   Negative U waves in leads V_4–V_6 on the ECG of a 32-year-old hypertensive woman with angina pectoris 1 day before the occurrence of acute anterior wall myocardial infarction. The pattern suggests left ventricular hypertrophy, which could have been responsible or co-responsible for the U wave inversion.

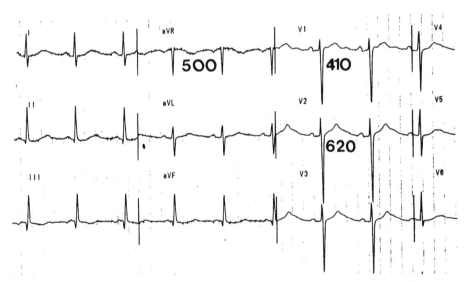

Figure 24–10   This ECG exemplifies the difficulty of measuring the QT interval when the T wave is fused with the U wave. The true QT is assumed to measure 500 ms in lead aV_R, in which the U wave is not detectable, allowing the end of the T wave to be defined. In lead V_2, the QT+U interval measures 620 ms; and in lead V_1, where the T wave is notched, the QT measured to the nadir of the notch is 410 ms.

because the T wave is seldom notched in all 12 leads, and the end of the T wave can be determined in one of the leads with a monophasic contour. The interval between notches is usually shorter than the aT-aU interval (i.e., <170 to 220 ms). The notches are usually situated >0.2 mV above the baseline, whereas T-U fusion occurs usually <0.2 mV above the baseline. One can also take advantage of the absence or near-absence of the U wave in leads I, aV_L, and aV_R (see Figures 24–10 and 24–11), which allows accurate QT measurement in these leads. When the QT interval is prolonged by <100 ms at heart rates of 50 to 100 beats/min, the end of the T wave can be measured at the intersection of these two deflections.[81]

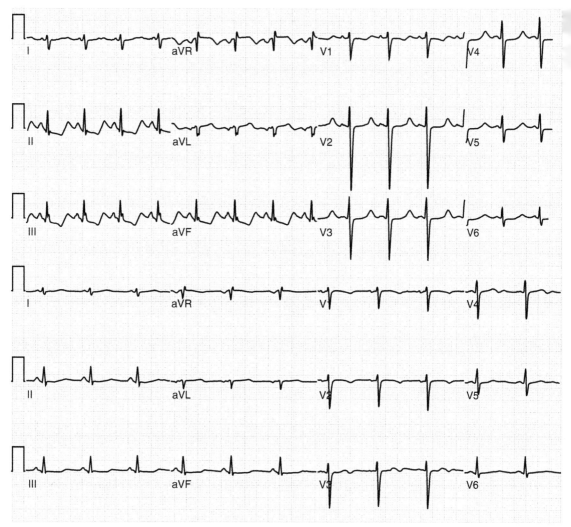

Figure 24–11 Upper tracing shows an example of difficulty measuring the QT interval in the presence of fusion of T wave and U wave caused by hypokalemia (Ks = 2.3 mEq/L). In the precordial leads the QT+U complex measures 510 ms, whereas in lead aV$_L$, in which the U amplitude is low and the T wave end is discernible (end of T wave marked by a vertical line), the QT interval measures 400 ms. The notch between T and U apex can be discerned in lead I. In the lower tracing, in the ECG recorded next day after correction of hypokalemia, the QT interval measures 434 ms and the U wave of low amplitude is separated from the T wave more distinctly.

NOMENCLATURE FOR PROLONGED QT INTERVAL IN THE PRESENCE OF SUSPECTED T WAVE AND U WAVE FUSION

When the QT interval is prolonged by more than about 100 ms at heart rates within the range of 50 to 100 beats/min, the T wave occupies the territory of the U wave and masks it. Under such circumstances it is proper to designate the interval from the beginning of QRS to the end of the T wave as the QT interval or acknowledge the fusion by using the terms *QT + U interval* or *Q(T+U) interval* (see Figures 24–10 and 24–11).

The term "QT(U)" is inappropriate because it does not describe the fusion of two waves but suggests that the terms QT and QU can be used interchangeably. Even more inappropriate than the term "QT(U) interval" is the designation "QU prolongation," a term implying that the given interval is longer than the normal rate-dependent QU interval, usually without comparing it with the available normal rate-dependent QU values.[82]

Electrical Alternans

Electrical and mechanical alternans may be concurrent or dissociated from each other. At the cellular level, mechanical alternans in the ventricular myocardium is usually accompanied by an alternating shape of the ventricular action potential.[83,84]

ALTERNANS OF T WAVE, U WAVE, AND QT INTERVAL

In clinical electrocardiography, ventricular repolarization alternans is most frequently associated with abrupt rate changes[85] or a prolonged QT interval.[84] Alternans of the T wave is the consequence of an alternating duration or shape of the ventricular action potential (or both). It may be expected to occur when the diastolic interval becomes sufficiently brief to produce measurable shortening of the following action potential, which in turn lengthens the subsequent diastolic interval and perpetuates continuation of alternation. The longer the QT interval, the longer is the shortest cycle length at which alternans can occur. When the QT interval is prolonged, the T wave tends to encroach on the U wave, resulting in fusion between the two waves. Under such circumstances, alternans has been described as U alternans or QU alternans.

A prolonged QT interval not only predisposes to T wave alternans but also frequently reflects the presence of an electrophysiologic substrate generating torsade de pointes.[86] Therefore it is not surprising that T wave alternans has been implicated as a precursor of torsade de pointes. This association may be only a fortuitous result of a common electrophysiologic abnormality.

Alternans of the T wave that is dependent on critical shortening of the diastolic interval frequently manifests when the duration of the ventricular action potential approaches or exceeds the cycle length. Therefore a QT interval occupying nearly the entire cycle length can be seen in many cases of repolarization alternans associated with a long QT interval (Figure 24–12). T wave alternans associated with a long QT has been reported in some of the following conditions: congenital LQTS,[87–89] hypocalcemia,[90,92] treatment with quinidine,[92] hypokalemia,[93] hypokalemia with hypocalcemia and hypomagnesemia, and cardiomyopathy associated with hypomagnesemia[94–96] after defibrillation.[97] It may also be unexplained.[98]

In addition to the manifest alternans on the clinical ECG, subtle alternans forms may become detectable by digital processing techniques. It has been shown that these subtle forms of alternans are associated with increased susceptibility to inducible ventricular tachycardia and ventricular fibrillation in patients with coronary artery disease or cardiomyopathy and therefore may represent a noninvasive marker of electrical instability.

ALTERNANS OF CONDUCTION

On the surface ECG, alternans of conduction may manifest as: (1) alternating duration, morphology, or both of the P wave, the QRS complex, or both; (2) alternans of the PR or RP

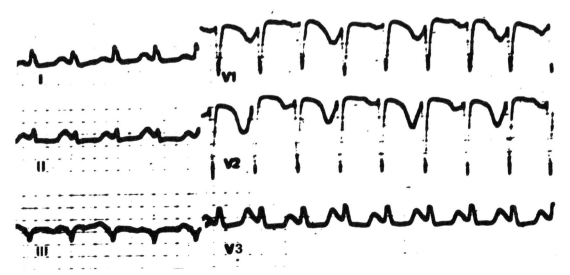

Figure 24–12   T wave alternans in a patient with hypokalemia (K level 2.2 mEq/L) and hypocalcemia (Ca level 3.0 mEq/L). (From Navarro-Lopez F, Chinca J, Sanz G, et al: Isolated T wave alternans. Am Heart J 95:369, 1978.)

interval; (3) alternans of the cycle length; and (4) various combinations of (1) to (3).

The diagnosis of alternans manifested by an alternating cycle length requires documentation of regular impulse formation at a fixed site of origin. Table 24–3 lists structures that may be involved in conduction alternans.

ATRIA

Rapid atrial pacing may result in alternans of atrial electrograms,[99] but P wave alternans is rarely recorded in humans.[100] When present, it is usually accompanied by alternans of the QRS, ST segment, and T wave: so-called total alternans.[101] Alternans of atrial flutter waves and of the PP interval during rapid rates, such as atrial tachycardia, have been recorded.[99,100]

ATRIOVENTRICULAR JUNCTION

Alternation of atrioventricular (AV) conduction in anterograde and retrograde directions has been recorded at normal and rapid heart rates, frequently with rapid pacing.[101] The alternans of AV or ventriculoatrial (VA) conduction can be accompanied by QRS alternans or cycle length alternans. In some cases there is alternation of conduction between two functionally separate AV nodal pathways.[102,103]

BUNDLE BRANCHES AND DISTAL CONDUCTION SYSTEM

Alternation of right (RBBB) or left (LBBB) bundle branch block with normal conduction, known as *2:1 bundle branch block*,[101] may be

tachycardia or bradycardia dependent.[104] The most common type of alternans is between the left bundle branch pattern and either a normal or left ventricular hypertrophy pattern (Figure 24–13). Next in frequency is probably alternans between RBBB and normal conduction or incomplete RBBB, or between two types of intraventricular conduction disturbance (see Figure 24–14).

Alternation of complete RBBB and LBBB conduction during normal sinus rhythm is rare. Alternating conduction along the left anterior and posterior fascicle is most often accompanied by an incomplete or complete RBBB and represents one type of bidirectional ventricular tachycardia.

Subtle changes in QRS duration or amplitude (or both) without definitive changes in the QRS axis or morphology have been observed frequently in the presence of ectopic supraventricular tachycardia with normal QRS duration. In a study of a large number of patients with spontaneous or induced supraventricular tachycardia with a narrow QRS complex, QRS alternans was observed in 22 percent; and of these patients, more than 90 percent were associated with an AV reciprocating tachycardia with retrograde conduction along an accessory pathway[105] (Figure 24–15). Other studies tended to support these findings.[105,106] However, Morady et al.[107] have shown that during rapid pacing alternans is primarily determined by the cycle length of the tachycardia, independent of the mechanism.

TABLE 24-3	Anatomic Structures Involved in Conduction Alternans

Atria
AV junction
Bundle branches
  Single
  Both
Fascicles
Distal Purkinje fibers
Ventricular myocardium
Accessory AV pathway
  Alone
  With AV junction
Various combinations of the above

AV, atrioventricular.

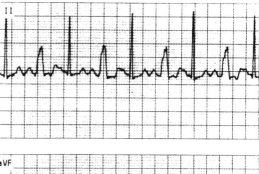
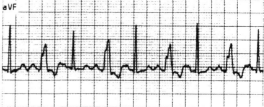

Figure 24–13 Alternans of left bundle branch block and normal ECG complex.

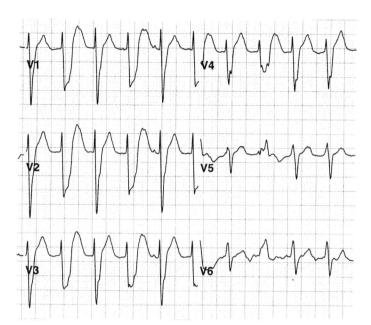

Figure 24–14   Alternans of nonspecific intraventricular conduction complexes with different QRS duration.

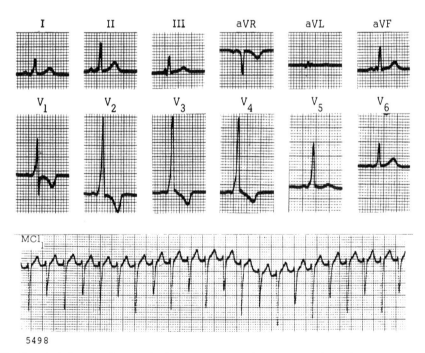

Figure 24–15   Electrical alternans during orthodromic atrioventricular reentrant tachycardia in a 23-year-old woman with Wolff-Parkinson-White syndrome without evidence of organic heart disease.

AV ACCESSORY PATHWAYS

Alternans of conduction has been recorded between an accessory pathway and an AV nodal pathway (see Figure 20–3), between two separate accessory pathways, or within a single accessory pathway.[101]

ALTERNANS ASSOCIATED WITH MYOCARDIAL ISCHEMIA

In patients with ischemic heart disease, ST alternans usually consists of alternating levels of ST elevation in the standard or anterior precordial leads displaying an acute injury pattern with an

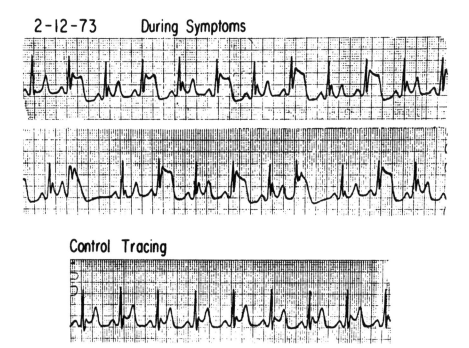

Figure 24–16   Alternans of the ST segment and T wave in a patient with vasospastic angina pectoris. (From Williams RR, Wagner GS, Peter RH: ST-segment alternans in Prinzmetal's angina. A report of two cases. Ann Intern Med 81:51, 1974.)

anteriorly or inferiorly directed ST vector. ST alternans is characteristically associated with vasospastic angina pectoris[108–111] (Figure 24–16) but has been reported during acute myocardial infarction,[112] in the presence of nonvasospastic angina pectoris,[113] during exercise tests,[114–116] and after subarachnoid hemorrhage.[117]

ECG ALTERNANS IN ASSOCIATION WITH CARDIAC MOTION

See Chapter 11.

CLINICAL SIGNIFICANCE OF ELECTRICAL ALTERNANS

Certain forms of electrical alternans can be considered physiologic manifestations of normal electrical adjustment to the new cycle length. Such physiologic forms of alternans may be caused by sudden increases in the heart rate or premature stimuli and are manifested by alterations of refractoriness or repolarization (or both). This form of physiologic alternans is usually nonsustained.

The type of alternans that presents may provide useful diagnostic clues to specific clinical conditions. Electrical alternans in a patient with pericardial effusion, for example, suggests a large effusion with the threat of cardiac tamponade; QRS alternans during narrow QRS tachycardia suggests AV reentry through a manifest or concealed accessory pathway; alternating PR intervals may reveal dual AV nodal conduction pathways; and alternans of the ST segment elevation suggests coronary spasm. T wave alternans in association with a long QT interval conveys a threat of torsade de pointes.

REFERENCES

1. Jervell A, Lange-Nielsen F: Congenital deaf-mutism, functional heart disease with prolongation of QT interval and sudden death. Am Heart J 54:59, 1957.
2. Schwartz PJ, Spazzolini C, Crotti L, et al: The Jervell and Lange-Nielsen syndrome. Natural history, molecular basis and clinical outcome. Circulation 113:783, 2006.
3. Ward O: The electrocardiographic abnormality in familial cardiac arrhythmia. Ir J Med Sci 6:533, 1966.
4. Romano C, Gemme G, Pongiglione R: Aritmie cardiache rare dell'eta pediatrica. Clin Paediatr 45:656, 1963.
5. Garza LA, Vick RL, Nora JJ, et al: Heritable QT prolongation without deafness. Circulation 41:39, 1970.
6. Levine SA, Woodworth CR: Congenital deaf-mutism, prolonged QT interval, syncopal attacks and sudden death. N Engl J Med 259:412, 1958.
7. Wellens HJ, Vermeulen A, Durrer D: Ventricular fibrillation occurring on arousal from sleep by auditory stimuli. Circulation 46:661, 1972.
8. McVay MR, Natarajan G, Reddy CP, et al: Idiopathic long QT syndrome: association of ventricular tachycardia with alternating left and right bundle branch block. J Electrocardiol 15:189, 1982.
9. Tye KH, Desser KB, Benchimol A: Survival following spontaneous ventricular flutter-fibrillation associated with QT syndrome. Arch Intern Med 140:255, 1980.

10. Schwartz PJ, Penti M, Malliani A: The long QT syndrome. Am Heart J 89:378, 1975.
11. Weintraub RG, Gow RM, Wilkinson JL: The congenital long QT syndromes in childhood. J Am Coll Cardiol 16:674, 1990.
12. Vincent GM, Jaiswal D, Timothy KW: Effects of exercise on heart rate, QT, QTc and QT/QS2 in the Romano-Ward inherited long QT syndrome. Am J Cardiol 68:498, 1991.
13. Curtiss EL, Heibel RH, Shaver A: Autonomic maneuvers in hereditary QT interval prolongation (Romano-Ward syndrome). Am Heart J 95:420, 1978.
14. Mitsutaka A, Takeshita A, Kuroiwa A, et al: Usefulness of the Valsalva maneuver in management of the long QT syndrome. Circulation 63:1029, 1981.
15. Tobe TJ, de Langen CDJ, Bink-Boelkens MTE, et al: Late potentials in a bradycardia-dependent long QT syndrome associated with sudden death during sleep. J Am Coll Cardiol 19:541, 1992.
16. Kurita T, Ohe T, Marni N, et al: Bradycardia-induced abnormal QT prolongation in patients with complete atrioventricular block with torsades de pointes. Am J Cardiol 69:628, 1992.
17. Merri M, Moss AJ, Benhorin J, et al: Relation between ventricular repolarization duration and cardiac cycle length during 24-hour Holter recordings: findings in normal patients and patients with long QT syndrome. Circulation 85:1816, 1992.
18. Priori SG, Napolitano C, Diehl L, et al: Dispersion of the QT interval: a marker of therapeutic efficacy in the idiopathic long QT syndrome. Circulation 89:1681, 1995.
19. Surawicz B: Will QT dispersion play a role in clinical decision making? J Cardiovasc Electrophysiol 7:777, 1996.
20. Theisen K, Haider M, Jahrmarker H: Untersuchungen ueber ventrikulaere Tachykardien durch Re-entry bei inhomogener Repolarisation. Dtsch Med Wochenschr 100:1099, 1975.
21. Jervell A, Sivertssen E: Surdo-cardialt syndrom. Nord Med 78:1443, 1967.
22. Mathews EC, Blount AW, Townsend JL: QT prolongation and ventricular arrhythmias, with and without deafness, in the same family. Am J Cardiol 29:702, 1972.
23. Roy PR, Emanuel R, Ismail SA, et al: Hereditary prolongation of the QT interval: genetic observations and management in three families with twelve affected members. Am J Cardiol 37:347, 1967.
24. Keating M, Atkinson D, Dunn C, et al: Linkage of a cardiac arrhythmia, the long QT syndrome, and the Harvey-ras-1 gene. Science 252:704, 1991.
25. Li H, Chen Q, Moss AJ, et al: New mutations in the KVLQT1 potassium channel that cause long-QT syndrome. Circulation 97:1264, 1998.
26. Maron BJ, Towbin JA, Thiene G, et al: Contemporary definitions and classification of the cardiomyopathies. An American Heart Association Scientific Statement from the Council of Clinical Cardiology. Circulation 113:1807, 2006.
26a. Mohler PJ, Scouarnee SL, Denjoy I, et al: Defining the cellular phenotype of "ankyrin-B syndrome" variants: human ANK2 variants associated with clinical phenotypes display a spectrum of activities in cardiomyocytes. Circulation 115:432, 2007.
27. Zhang L, Timothy KW, Vincent GM, et al: Spectrum of ST-T wave patterns and repolarization parameters in congenital long–QT syndrome. ECG findings identify genotypes. Circulation 102:2849, 2000.
28. Kanters JK, Fanoe S, Larsen LA, et al: T wave morphology analysis distinguishes between KvLQT1 and HERG mutations in long QT syndrome. Heart Rhythm 3:285, 2004.
29. Moss AJ, Zareba W, Benhorin J, et al: ECG T-wave patterns in genetically distinct forms of the hereditary long QT syndrome. Circulation 92:2929, 1995.
30. Shimizu W, Noda T, Takaki H, et al: Diagnostic value of epinephrine test for genotyping LQT1, LQT2, and LQT3 forms of congenital long QT syndrome. Heart Rhythm 3:276, 2004.
31. Vyas H, Hejlik J, Ackerman MJ: Epinephrine QT stress testing in the evaluation of congenital long QT-syndrome. Circulation 113:1385, 2006.
32. Veldkamp MW, Wilders R, Baartscher A, et al: Contribution of sodium channel mutations to bradycardia and sinus node dysfunction in LQT3 families. Circ Res 92:976, 2003.
33. Zhang L, Benson W, Tristani-Firouzi M, et al: Electrocardiographic features in Andersen-Tawil syndrome patients with KCNJ2 mutations. Characteristic T-U-wave patterns predict the KCNJ2 genotype. Circulation 111:2720, 2005.
34. Schwartz PJ, Priori SG, Locati EH, et al: Long QT syndrome patients with mutations of the SCN5A and HERG genes have differential responses to Na$^+$ channel blockade and to increases in heart rate: implications for gene-specific therapy. Circulation 92:3381, 1995.
35. Priori SG, Schwartz PJ, Napolitano C, et al: Risk stratification in the long QT syndrome. N Engl J Med 348:1866, 2003.
35a. Topilski I, Rogowski O, Rosso R, et al: The morphology of the QT interval predicts torsade de pointes during acquired bradyarrhythmias. J Am Coll Cardiol 49:320, 2007.
36. Ludomirsky A, Klein HO, Sarelli P, et al: QT prolongation and polymorphous (torsade de pointes): ventricular arrhythmias associated with organophosphorus insecticide poisoning. Am J Cardiol 49:1654, 1981.
37. Frank S, Colliver JA, Frank A: The electrocardiogram in obesity: statistical analysis of 1029 patients. J Am Coll Cardiol 7:295, 1986.
38. El-Gamal A, Gallagher D, Nawras A, et al: Effects of obesity on QT, RR, and QTc intervals. Am J Cardiol 75:956, 1995.
39. Wadden TA, Van Itallie TB, Blackburn GL: Responsible and irresponsible use of very low calorie diets in the treatment of obesity. JAMA 263:83, 1990.
40. Isner JM, Sours HE, Paris AL, et al: Sudden unexpected death in avid dieters using the liquid protein modified fast diet. Circulation 60:1401, 1979.
41. Singh BN, Gaarder TD, Kanagae T, et al: Liquid protein diets and torsade de pointes. JAMA 240:115, 1978.
42. Sours HE, Frattali VP, Brand CD, et al: Sudden death associated with very low calorie weight reduction regimens. Am J Clin Nutr 34:453, 1981.
43. Surawicz B, Waller BF: The enigma of sudden cardiac death related to dieting. Can J Cardiol 11:228, 1995.
44. Isner JM, Roberts WC, Heymsfield SB, et al: Anorexia nervosa and sudden death. Ann Intern Med 102:49, 1985.
45. Simonson E, Henschel A, Keys A: The electrocardiogram of man in semistarvation and subsequent rehabilitation. Am Heart J 35:584, 1948.
46. Hellerstein HK, Santiago-Stevenson D: Atrophy of the heart: a correlative study of eighty-five proved cases. Circulation 1:93, 1950.
47. Burch GE, Phillips JH, Ansari A: The cachectic heart: a clinico-pathologic electrocardiographic and roentgenographic entity. Dis Chest 54:403, 1968.
48. Goldberg RJ, Bengson J, Chen Z, et al: Duration of the QT interval and total and cardiovascular mortality in healthy persons (the Framingham heart study experience). Am J Cardiol 67:55, 1991.

49. Schouten EG, Dekker JM, Mappelink P, et al: QT interval prolongation predicts cardiovascular mortality in an apparently healthy population. Circulation 84:1516, 1991.

50. Straus SMJM, Kors JA, De Bruin ML: Prolonged QTc interval and risk of sudden cardiac death in a population of older adults. J Am Coll Cardiol 47:362, 2006.

51. Algra A, Tijssen JGP, Roelandt JRTC, et al: QTc prolongation measured by standard 12-lead electrocardiography is an independent risk factor for sudden death due to cardiac arrest. Circulation 83:1888, 1991.

52. Pohjola-Sintonen S, Siltanen P, Haapakoski J: Usefulness of QTc interval on the discharge electrocardiogram for predicting survival after acute myocardial infarction. Am J Cardiol 57:1066, 1986.

53. Wheelan K, Mukharji J, Rude RE, et al: Sudden death and its relation to QT interval prolongation after acute myocardial infarction: two year follow-up. Am J Cardiol 57:745, 1986.

54. Gadaleta FL, Llois SC, Lapuente AR, et al: Prognostic value of corrected QT-interval prolongation in patients with unstable angina pectoris. Am J Cardiol 92:203, 2003.

55. Puddu PE, Bourassa MG: Prediction of sudden death from QTc interval prolongation in patients with chronic ischemic heart disease. J Electrocardiol 19:203, 1986.

56. Ahnve S, Gilpin E, Madsen EB, et al: Prognostic importance of QTc interval at discharge after acute myocardial infarction: a multicenter study of 865 patients. Am Heart J 108:395, 1984.

57. Hancock EW, Cohn K: The syndrome associated with mid-systolic click and late systolic murmur. Am J Med 41:183, 1966.

58. Swartz MH, Teichholz LE, Donoso E: Mitral valve prolapse. Am J Med 62:377, 1972.

59. Bekheit SG, Ali AA, Deglin SM, et al: Analysis of QT interval in patients with idiopathic mitral valve prolapse. Chest 61:8205, 1982.

60. Savage DD, Devereux RB, Garrison RJ, et al: Mitral valve prolapse in the general population: clinical features; the Framingham study. Am Heart J 106:577, 1983.

61. Cowan MD, Fye WB: Prevalence of QTc prolongation in women with mitral valve prolapse. Am J Cardiol 63:133, 1989.

62. Day CP, James OFW, Butler TJ, et al: QT prolongation and sudden death in patients with alcoholic liver disease. Lancet 341:1423, 1993.

63. Zehender M, Hohnloser S, Just H: QT-interval prolonging drugs: mechanisms and clinical relevance of their arrhythmogenic hazards. Cardiovasc Drugs Ther 5:515, 1991.

64. Surawicz B, Knoebel SK: Long QT: good, bad or indifferent? J Am Coll Cardiol 4:398, 1984.

65. Roden DM: Drug-induced prolongation of the QT interval. N Engl J Med 350:1013, 2004.

66. Algra A, Tijssen JGP, Roelandt JRTC, et al: QT interval variables from 24 hour electrocardiography and the two year risk of sudden death. Br Heart J 70:43, 1993.

67. Leenhardt A, Glaser B, Burguera M, et al: Short-coupled variant of torsade de pointes: a new electrocardiographic entity in the spectrum of idiopathic ventricular tachyarrhythmias. Circulation 206:89, 1994.

68. Gussak I, Brugada P, Brugada J, et al: Idiopathic short QT interval: a new clinical syndrome? Cardiology 94:99, 2000.

68a. Anttonen O, Juntilla MJ, Rissanen H, et al: Prevalence and prognostic significance of short QT interval in a middle-aged Finnish population. Circulation 116:714, 2007.

68b. Reinig MG, Engel TR: The shortage of short QT intervals. Chest 132:246, 2007.

69. Gaita F, Giustetto C, Bianchi F, et al: Short QT syndrome. A familial cause of sudden death. Circulation 108:965, 2003.

70. Brugada R, Hong K, Dumaine R, et al: Sudden death associated with short-QT syndrome linked to mutations in HERG. Circulation 109:30, 2004.

70a. Antzelevitch C, Pollevick GD, Cordeiro GM, et al: Loss-of-function mutations in the cardiac calcium channel underlie a new clinical entity characterized by ST-segment elevation, short QT intervals, and sudden cardiac death. Circulation 115:442, 2007.

71. Holzmann M, Zurukzoglu W: Die klinische Bedeutung der negativen und diphasischen U-Wellen in menschlichen EKG. Cardiologia 27:202, 1955.

72. Ameur-Hendrich C, Courdier G, Hessel F, et al: Onde U negative a valeur diagnostique et prognostique: a propos de 100 cas. Ann Cardiol Angeiol 25:103, 1976.

73. Kishida H, Cole JS, Surawicz B: Negative U wave: a highly specific but poorly understood sign of heart disease. Am J Cardiol 49:2030, 1982.

74. Miwa K, Murakami T, Kamabara H, et al: U wave inversion during attacks of variant angina. Br Heart J 50:378, 1983.

75. Gerson MC, Phillips F, Morris SN, et al: Exercise-induced U-wave inversion as a marker of stenosis of the left anterior descending coronary artery. Circulation 60:1014, 1979.

76. Tamura A, Watanabe T, Nagase K, et al: Significance of negative U waves in the precordial leads during anterior wall acute myocardial infarction. Am J Cardiol 79:897, 1997.

77. Tamura A, Nagase K, Mikuriya Y, et al: Relation between negative U waves in precordial leads on the admission electrocardiogram and time course of left ventricular wall motion in anterior wall acute myocardial infarction. Am J Cardiol 84:332, 1999.

78. Daoud FS, Surawicz B, Gettes LS: Effect of isoproterenol on the abnormal T wave. Am J Cardiol 30:810, 1972.

79. Kataoka H, Yano S, Tamura A, et al: How epicardial U-wave changes are reflected in body surface precordial electrocardiograms in anterior or inferoposterior myocardial ischemia during coronary angioplasty. Heart 76:397, 1996.

80. Viskin S, Heller K, Barron HV, et al: Postextrasystolic U wave augmentation, a new marker of increased arrhythmic risk in patients without the long QT syndrome. J Am Coll Cardiol 28:1746, 1996.

81. Lepeschkin E, Surawicz B: The measurement of the QT interval of the electrocardiogram. Circulation 4:378, 1953.

82. Surawicz B: U wave: facts, hypotheses, misconceptions, and misnomers. J Cardiovasc Electrophysiol 8:1117, 1998.

83. Saitoh H, Bailey JC, Surawicz B: Alternans of action potential after abrupt shortening of cycle length: differences between dog Purkinje and ventricular muscle fibers. Circ Res 62:1027, 1988.

84. Surawicz B, Fisch C: Cardiac alternans: diverse mechanisms and clinical manifestations. J Am Coll Cardiol 20:483, 1992.

85. Fisch C, Edmands RE, Greenspan K: T wave alternans: an association with abrupt rate change. Am Heart J 81:817, 1971.

86. Surawicz B: Electrophysiologic substrate of torsade de pointes: dispersion of repolarization or early afterdepolarizations? J Am Coll Cardiol 14:172, 1989.

87. Schwartz PJ, Malliani A: Electrical alternation of the T-wave: clinical and experimental evidence of its relationship with the sympathetic nervous system and with the long Q-T syndrome. Am Heart J 89:45, 1975.

88. Bonatti V, Finardi A, Botti G: Recording of monophasic action potentials of the right ventricle in a case of long QT and isolated alternation of the U wave. Arch Mal Coeur 72:1180, 1979.

89. Sharma S, Nair KG, Gadekar HA: Romano-Ward prolonged QT syndrome with intermittent T wave alternans and atrioventricular block. Am Heart J 101:500, 1981.

90. Kimura E, Yoshida K: A case showing electrical alternans of the T wave without change in the QRS complex. Am Heart J 65:391, 1963.

91. Navarro-Lopez F, Chinca J, Sanz G, et al: Isolated T wave alternans. Am Heart J 95:369, 1978.

92. Luca C: Right ventricular monophasic action potential during quinidine induced marked T and U waves abnormalities. Acta Cardiol 32:305, 1977.

93. Ishikawa K, Tateno M: Alternans of the repolarization wave in a case of hypochloremic alkalosis with hypopotassemia. J Electrocardiol 9:75, 1976.

94. Luomanmaki K, Keikkila J, Hartikainen M: T wave alternans associated with heart failure and hypomagnesemia in alcoholic cardiomyopathy. Eur J Cardiol 4:l67, 1975.

95. Ricketts HH, Denison EK, Haywood LJ: Unusual T-wave abnormality: repolarization alternans associated with hypomagnesemia, acute alcoholism and cardiomyopathy. JAMA 217:365, 1969.

96. Reddy CVR, Kiok JP, Khan RG, et al: Repolarization alternans associated with alcoholism and hypomagnesemia. Am J Cardiol 53:390, 1984.

97. Rowland V, Lipschultz T, Benchimol A, et al: Isolated T wave alternans progressing to QRS-T alternation after ventricular defibrillation. Angiology 28:58, 1977.

98. Dolara A, Pozzi L: Electrical alternation of T wave without change in QRS complex. Br Heart J 33:161, 1971.

99. Plumb VJ, Karp RB, James TN, et al: Atrial excitability and conduction during rapid atrial pacing. Circulation 63:1140, 1981.

100. Donato A, Oreto G, Schamroth L: P wave alternans. Am Heart J 116:875, 1988.

101. Fisch C: Electrocardiography of Arrhythmias. Philadelphia, Lea & Febiger, 1990.

102. Moe GK: Reflections on reciprocation. In: Zipes DP, Jalife J (eds): Cardiac Electrophysiology and Arrhythmias. Orlando, Grune & Stratton, 1984.

103. Moe GK, Preston JB, Burlington H: Physiologic evidence for a dual AV transmission system. Circ Res 4:357, 1956.

104. Cohen HC, D'Cruz I, Pick A, et al: Tachycardia and bradycardia-dependent bundle branch block alternans: clinical observations. Circulation 55:242, 1977.

105. Green M, Heddle B, Dassen W, et al: Value of QRS alternation in determining the site of origin of narrow QRS supraventricular tachycardia. Circulation 68:368, 1983.

106. Kremers MS, Wheelan KR, Solodyna M: Role of cycle length, cycle length alternans, and electrocardiographic lead in electrical alternans with rapid atrial pacing. Am J Cardiol 60:613, 1987.

107. Morady F, Di Carlo L, Baerman JM, et al: Determinants of QRS alternans during narrow QRS tachycardia. J Am Coll Cardiol 9:489, 1987.

108. Kleinfeld MJ, Rozanski JJ: Alternans in Prinzmetal's angina. Circulation 55:574, 1977.

109. Rozanski JJ, Kleinfeld MJ: Alternans of the ST segment of T wave: a sign of electrical instability in Prinzmetal's angina. PACE 5:359, 1982.

110. Cheng TC: Electrical alternans: an association with coronary artery spasm. Arch Intern Med 143:1052, 1983.

111. Bekheit S, Turitto G, Fontaine J, et al: Initiation of ventricular fibrillation by supraventricular beats in patients with acute myocardial infarction. Br Heart J 59:190, 1988.

112. Puletti M, Curione M, Righetti G, et al: Alternans of the ST segment and T-wave in acute myocardial infarction. J Electrocardiol 13:297, 1980.

113. Demidowich G, Werres R, Rothfeld D, et al: Electrical alternans of the ST segment in non-Prinzmetal's angina. PACE 3:733, 1980.

114. Rozanski JJ, Kleinfeld M: Occurrence of ST segment electrical alternans during exercise test. PACE 3:339, 1981.

115. Ring ME, Fenster PE: Exercise-induced ST segment alternans. Am Heart J 111:1009, 1986.

116. Wayne VS, Bishop RL, Spodick DH: Exercise induced ST segment alternans. Chest 83:824, 1983.

117. Nakamura Y, Kaseno K, Kubo T: Transient ST-segment elevation in subarachnoid hemorrhage. J Electrocardiol 22:133, 1989.

25 Misplacement of Leads and Electrocardiographic Artifacts

An electrocardiographic (ECG) lead consists of two components: the electrode, which is attached to the patient, and the cable, which connects the electrode to the ECG recorder. Incorrect lead placement may involve applying the electrode in a wrong location, connecting the cable to the wrong electrode, or both. Such errors occur occasionally even when the ECG is recorded by a well-trained, experienced technician. Some mistakes can be identified easily by the ECG interpreter, but others are more difficult or even impossible to recognize, especially if a previous tracing from the same patient is not available for comparison.

Misplacement of the Limb Lead

Because the limb lead electrodes are seldom misplaced, the following discussion is confined to errors in connecting the cables to the electrodes. To distinguish leads recorded with correct cable connections from those with incorrect connections, the latter are cited in quotation marks.

REVERSAL OF LEFT AND RIGHT ARM CABLES

When the left and right arm leads are reversed, a comparison of the resulting ECG (Figure 25–1) from that recorded with correct cable connections (Figure 25–2) reveals the following changes:

1. "Lead I" is upside down because the polarity of the lead is reversed.
2. "Lead II" is actually lead III and vice versa.

3. "Lead aV_R" is actually lead aV_L and vice versa.

The morphology of the complexes in the limb leads therefore resembles that of the patients with mirror-image dextrocardia. However, the precordial leads show normal transition with tall R waves in leads V_5 and V_6, whereas in true mirror-image dextrocardia the QRS complex becomes smaller and displays mostly QS or rS deflections in leads V_3–V_6.

Reversal of the arm leads is the most common lead placement error and is the easiest to recognize because of a negative P wave in lead I in patients with sinus rhythm, which is unusual even in the presence of heart disease. In patients with atrial fibrillation or unidentifiable P waves, the morphology of the ventricular complexes in leads I, V_5, and V_6 should be similar, as the lead axes of all these leads are directed essentially leftward. If the polarity of the QRS complex in lead I is opposite that in the left precordial leads, arm lead reversal is suspected.

REVERSAL OF LEFT ARM AND LEFT LEG CABLES

The following changes are observed if the left arm cable is attached to the left leg and vice versa (Figure 25–3):

1. "Lead I" is actually lead II.
2. "Lead II" is actually lead I.
3. "Lead III" is upside down relative to the actual lead III.
4. "Lead aV_R" is unchanged, but "leads aV_L and aV_F" are reversed.

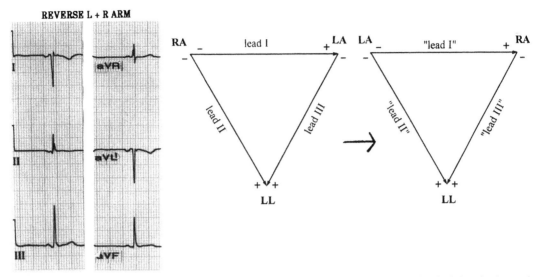

Figure 25–1 Changes in the ECG limb leads from those in the control tracing (Figure 25–2) after the left and right arm lead cables were intentionally reversed. The accompanying diagram depicts the changes in the components of the leads as a result of the cable switch. In this and subsequent diagrams, as well as in the text, leads recorded with placement errors are cited in quotation marks.

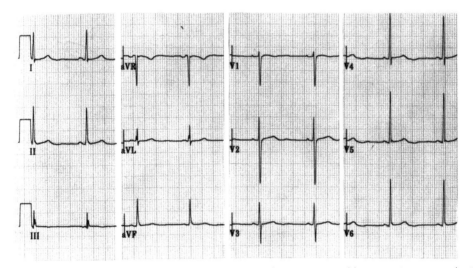

Figure 25–2 Normal ECG recorded with correct lead placement from a 27-year-old woman. It serves as the "control" tracing to be compared with Figures 25–1, 25–3, 25–7 through 25–10, and 25–13, which were recorded with intentional lead misplacements.

Reversal of the left arm and left leg cables is difficult and sometimes impossible to detect if a previously correctly recorded tracing is not available for comparison. Lead misplacement would not have been realized or suspected in Figure 25–3 if the ECG had not been compared with the baseline tracing (see Figure 25–2). One of the exceptions is illustrated in Figure 25–4, in which the sawtooth appearance of the flutter waves is seen in "leads I, III, and aV_L" but not in "lead II." Such a finding

is not seen with atrial flutter, and limb lead reversal is suspected. Because the QRS morphology in "lead aV_R" is what one normally would have expected, reversal of the left arm and left leg cables can be safely assumed.

Difficulty recognizing left arm and left leg lead reversal may result in an erroneous ECG diagnosis even though the clinician gave the interpretation correctly based on the tracing presented. Figure 25–5B is an example of T wave

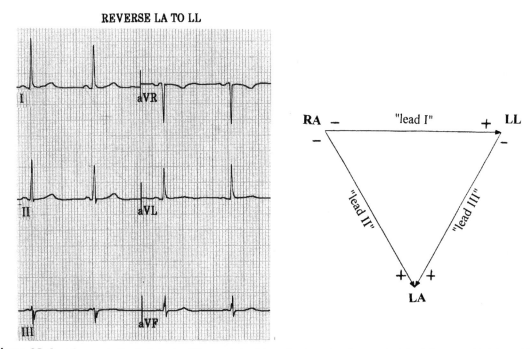

Figure 25–3 Changes in the limb leads of the control subject after intentional reversal of the left arm and left leg cables. "Lead I" is actually lead II, "lead II" is lead I, and "lead III" is upside down. Without the control tracing, the errors in lead placement would not be suspected.

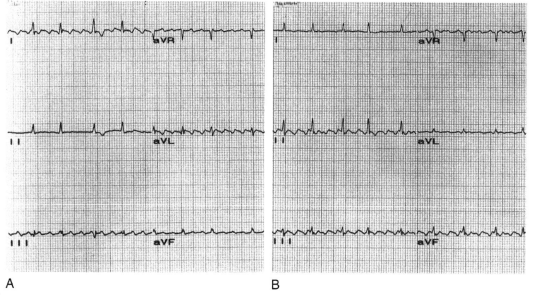

Figure 25–4 Recognition of left arm and left leg cable reversal based on the morphology of the flutter waves. **A,** Limb leads with cable reversal. Note the unusual isoelectric flutter waves in "lead II." **B,** Limb leads with correct lead placement showing the typical sawtooth appearance of the flutter waves in the inferior leads. (Courtesy of Dr. Noble O. Fowler.)

inversion in "leads III and aV_F," suggestive of inferior myocardial ischemia in a healthy 35-year-old man with atypical chest pain, although the tracing recorded with proper lead placement is normal (Figure 25–5A).

REVERSAL OF RIGHT ARM AND RIGHT LEG CABLES

If the cables for the right arm and right leg are switched, the changes in the ECG patterns in the various leads are more pronounced. Because

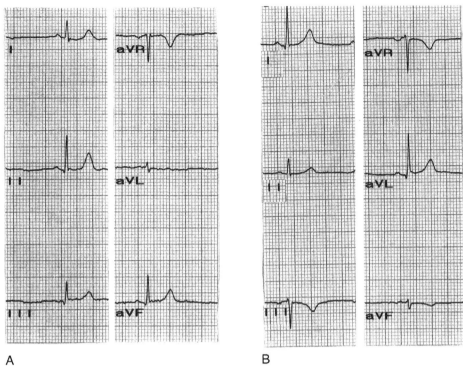

A   B

Figure 25–5   "Abnormal T waves" resulting from left arm and left leg cable reversal. **A,** Recorded from a healthy 35-year-old man with atypical chest pain. The tracing is normal. **B,** Recorded when the left arm and left leg cables were switched by mistake. T wave inversion suggestive of myocardial ischemia appears in leads III and aV$_F$. The "abnormal" pattern due to technical error would not have been recognized if tracing **A** were not available for comparison.

the right leg lead normally serves as a ground, its misplacement on the other limb alters not only the morphology of the complexes but also their amplitude in most of the leads. The potential of the central terminals no longer represent the sum of the potentials from the left arm (VL), right arm (VR), and left leg (VF), as the potentials at both legs are assumed to be equal, and it is no longer zero. Similarly, and usually to a greater degree, the unipolar limb leads are affected. It is now the sum of potentials from the left arm and the left and right legs (or VL + VF + VF). The changes in the amplitude and polarity in each lead varies in the individual cases depending on the potential in each lead when it is attached to the correct limb. They are illustrated in the following list (Figure 25–6) using Figure 25–2 as the control:

1. "Lead I" is actually upside-down lead III. It represents the difference between the right leg and left arm potentials, with the left arm lead designated the positive end.
2. "Lead II" appears as a practically straight line, as it represents the potential difference between the two legs, which have almost equal potentials.
3. "Lead III" is not affected.

4. "Lead aV$_R$" is morphologically similar to the correctly recorded lead aV$_F$ but has a different amplitude with or without a change in polarity.
5. "Leads aV$_L$ and aV$_F$" are morphologically similar to their corresponding leads recorded with correct cable connections but have different amplitudes with or without changes in polarity.

To illustrate the changes in voltage expected in the augmented unipolar limb leads when the right leg (ground) cable is switched with the right arm cable, one may begin with a review of the derivation of these leads.

$$\text{Lead } aV_R = VR - (VL + VF)/2$$
$$\text{Lead } aV_L = VL - (VR + VF)/2$$
$$\text{Lead } aV_F = VF - (VR + VL)/2$$
$$aV_R = VR \times 1.5; aV_L = VL \times 1.5;$$
$$aV_F = VF \times 1.5$$

If the right arm and right leg cables are reversed, the recorded "lead aV$_R$" actually comes from the right leg, which has almost the same potential as the left leg. Therefore,

$$\text{"Lead } aV_R\text{"} = VF - (VL + VF)/2$$

REVERSE RA TO RL

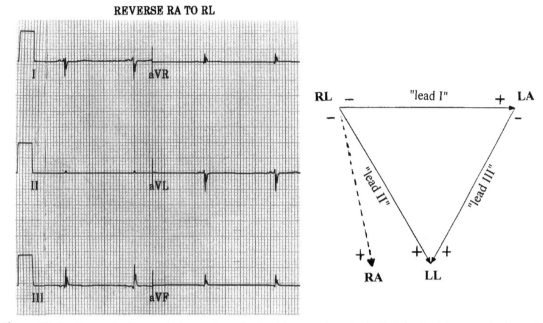

Figure 25–6 Changes in the morphology and amplitude of the complexes in the limb leads of the control subject after intentional reversal of the right arm and right leg cable compared with those in Figure 25–2. See text for a discussion of the changes. An almost straight line in "lead II" should lead one to suspect that the right leg cable has been switched with the right arm cable.

$$\text{"Lead } aV_L\text{"} = VL - (VF + VF)/2$$
$$\text{"Lead } aV_F\text{"} = VF - (VF + VL)/2$$

For example, in Figure 25–1, in which the leads are connected properly:

$$VR = aV_R \times 2/3 = 1.2\text{mV} \times 2/3 = 0.8\text{mV}$$
$$VL = aV_L \times 2/3 = 0.5\text{mV} \times 2/3 = 0.33\text{mV}$$
$$VF = aV_F \times 2/3 = 1.1\text{mV} \times 2/3 = 0.73\text{mV}$$

When the right arm and right leg cables are reversed, the expected potential recorded by:

$$\text{"Lead } aV_R\text{"} = 0.8 - (0.33 + 0.73)/2 = 0.27\text{mV}$$

$$\text{"Lead } aV_L\text{"} = 0.33 - (0.73 + 0.73)/2 = -0.4\text{mV}$$

$$\text{"Lead } aV_F\text{"} = 0.73 - (0.73 + 0.33)/2 = 0.2\text{mV}$$

These values approximate those actually recorded in Figure 25–6. They are not exactly the same, as the calculation is based on the assumption that leads I, II, and III form an equilateral triangle. In reality, these three leads form a scalene triangle.

REVERSAL OF RIGHT ARM AND LEFT LEG CABLES

Misplacement of the right arm and left leg leads results in the following changes, which are illustrated in Figure 25–7:

1. "Lead I" is actually upside-down lead III.
2. "Lead II" becomes upside down.
3. "Lead III" is actually upside-down lead I.
4. "Leads aV_R and aV_F" are reversed, and "lead aV_L" is unchanged.

REVERSAL OF LEFT LEG AND RIGHT LEG CABLES

With reversal of left leg and right leg cables, the ECG is unchanged from that recorded with the cables attached correctly because the potentials at the left and right legs are practically the same.

REVERSAL OF LEFT ARM AND RIGHT LEG CABLES

The changes in the ECG when the left arm and right leg cables are switched are illustrated in Figure 25–8. They include the following:

1. "Lead I" is actually lead II.
2. "Lead II" is unchanged.
3. "Lead III" is a straight line, as it now records the difference in potentials between two legs, which are practically the same.

As in the case of reversal of the right leg and right arm cables, the augmented unipolar limb leads are altered not only in their morphology but also in amplitude because of the associated changes in the potentials of the central terminals.

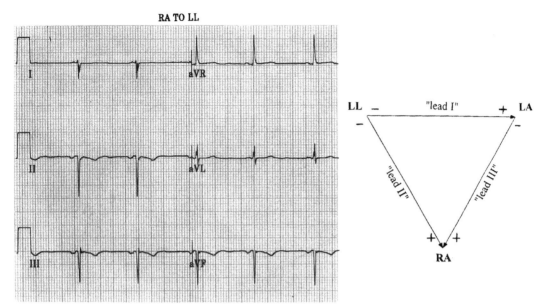

Figure 25–7   Changes in the limb leads of the control subject after intentional reversal of the right arm and left leg cables. Note that the P, QRS, and T waves in lead aV_R are all upright, suggesting that the right arm cable was misplaced. Because all the complexes in the inferior leads appear to be upside down, it may be concluded that the left leg cable is also misplaced. As indicated by the accompanying diagram, "lead I" is actually upside-down lead III, "lead II" becomes upside down, and "lead III" is upside-down lead I. Only lead aV_L is not affected.

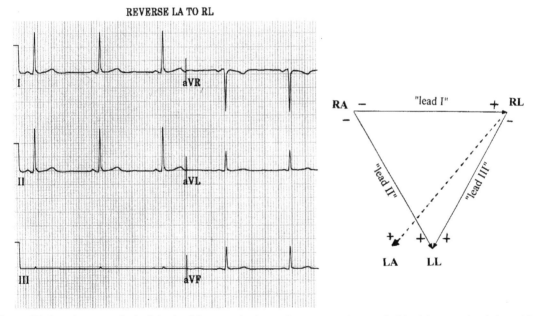

Figure 25–8   Changes in the limb leads of the control subject after intentional reversal of the left arm and right leg cables. "Lead I" is actually lead II. "Lead II" is unchanged. "Lead III" is practically a straight line as it records the difference in potentials between the two legs.

REVERSAL OF BOTH ARM CABLES WITH THEIR CORRESPONDING LEG CABLES

As illustrated in Figure 25–9, switching both arm cables with their corresponding leg cables results in the following changes on the ECG:

1. "Lead I" appears as almost a straight line, as it now records the potential difference of the two legs.
2. "Lead II" is actually upside-down lead III, as it records the potential difference of the left arm and right leg with the left arm serving

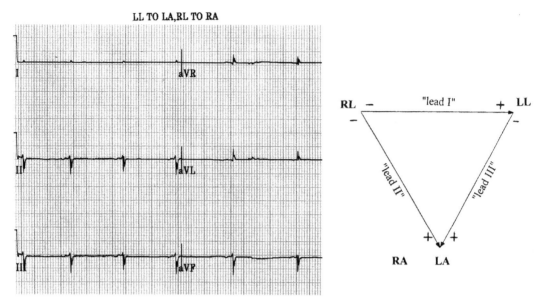

Figure 25–9 Changes in the limb leads of the control subject after intentional reversal of both arm cables with their corresponding leg cables. "Lead I" appears as a practically straight line. "Lead II" is upside-down lead III. "Lead III" becomes upside down.

as the positive instead of the negative electrode as in the case of normal lead placement. As mentioned previously, left and right leg potentials may be assumed to be equal.

3. "Lead III" appears as its own mirror image, as the polarity of its two components is reversed.

4. The amplitude and polarity of "lead aV_R" and "lead aV_L" are the same, as both leads are derived by comparing the potentials at each leg (VF) (which are the same) with the central terminal, which also has the same value for both leads.

MISPLACEMENT OF PRECORDIAL LEAD ELECTRODES

The electrodes may be misplaced simply owing to carelessness, or acting in a hurry. The locations of the electrodes may be too high or too low, as the correct intercostal spaces may not be accurately identified. They also may be more medial or lateral than they should be. This is especially true for leads V_3–V_6. The bony landmarks may be difficult to find in obese subjects.

Misplacement of the electrodes may be difficult to detect unless there are unexpected changes in the ECG in a stable patient whose previous tracings are available for comparison. Even when there is a previous tracing, it is often difficult to decide which one was recorded with proper electrode placement.

Placement of the precordial electrodes at a higher or lower intercostal space may or

may not affect the interpretation of the ECG significantly depending on the individual ECG abnormalities. It is beyond the scope of this text to discuss the potential effects of incorrect electrode placement under each circumstance. Figure 25–10 is an example of the ECG findings that may alert the clinician to the possibility of inaccurate electrode placement.

Figure 25–10A was obtained from a surgical patient with atrial fibrillation. ECGs recorded on the following 2 days showed no significant changes. The tracing recorded 5 days later (Figure 25–10B) showed QS deflections in leads V_1 and V_2, suggestive of anteroseptal infarction. Because the patient's clinical status remained stable, it was suspected that misplacement of the electrodes to a level higher than the standard was responsible for the changes. A repeat tracing (Figure 25–10C) on the same day showed findings similar to those recorded on previous days, supporting the suspicion that the pseudoinfarction pattern in Figure 25–10B was due to a technical error.

MISCONNECTION OF PRECORDIAL LEAD CABLES

In general, misconnection of the cables to properly placed precordial lead electrodes is easier to recognize than misplacement of the electrodes. An abrupt change in the P, QRS, and T wave morphology from the adjacent lead (e.g., V_2–V_3), followed by reversal to some degree in the next lead (e.g., V_4) suggests the possibility of

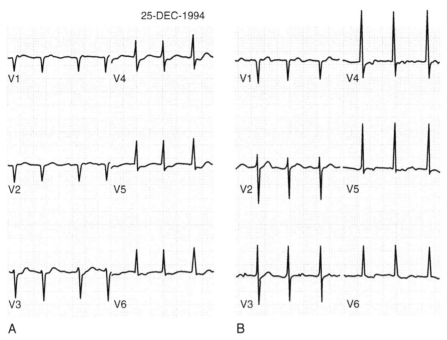

Figure 25–10   Pseudoinfarction pattern due to misplacement of the precordial lead electrodes. **A,** On 12/25/94 there are QS deflections in leads V₁ and V₂ with a decrease in R wave amplitude in lead V₃, suggesting anteroseptal infarction. As the patient's clinical status remained unchanged, technical errors were suspected. **B,** A repeat ECG was recorded on the same day. The QS deflection in lead V₂ is no longer present, and the R wave amplitude in lead V₃ returns to what was seen on the previous days. Apparently, tracing **B** was recorded with the precordial lead electrodes placed at higher than normal levels.

erroneous switching of the adjacent cables (V₂ and V₃). Because the P wave changes are usually independent of those of the QRS-T in most of clinical circumstances, its progression from lead V₁ through V₆ may be helpful for determining whether the QRS changes are real or due to technical error. Figure 25–11 is an example in which the cables for leads V₁ and V₂ were reversed purposefully after the control tracing (Figure 25–2) was recorded. Loss of the R wave amplitude from V₁ to V₂ with T wave inversion in lead V₂ raises the possibility of an anterior infarction. However, these changes occur only in one isolated lead. In addition, the P wave in lead V₂ is biphasic, whereas the P waves in leads V₁ and V₃ are upright, a highly improbable if not impossible presentation.

Recognition of Lead Misplacement: Summary

The following findings are helpful for recognizing errors in lead cable connections or electrode placement and for determining which leads are probably involved:

1. If the complex in lead I (including the P wave) appears to be upside down, the left and right arm cable connections were reversed, provided the precordial leads are not suggestive of mirror-image dextrocardia.

2. If one of the standard limb leads is almost a straight line, the right leg cable was switched with one of the other limb lead cables.

3. In the augmented unipolar limb leads, the lead showing all negative deflections (including the P wave) indicates whether the right arm cable is involved. If such a complex is seen in lead aV_R, the right arm is not involved. If it is seen in lead aV_L, the right arm cable has been switched with the left arm; if it is seen in lead aV_F, it was switched with the left leg cable.

4. Reversal of the left arm and left leg cables is difficult or impossible to recognize without having a previous ECG available for comparison.

5. Misconnection of the precordial lead cables may be suspected if the transition of the complexes including the P waves is not explainable.

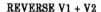

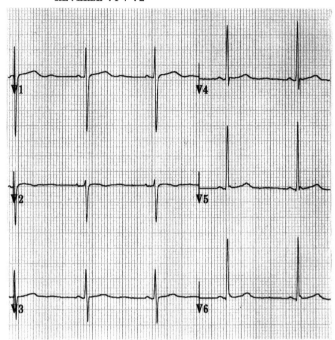

Figure 25–11 Possible anterior infarction pattern resulting from intentional reversal of the cables for leads V_1 and V_2 in the control subject. The tracing shows a decrease in the R wave amplitude from "lead V_1" to "lead V_2," with T wave inversion in "lead V_2." Lead reversal should be suspected because the P wave is upright in "V_1," biphasic in "V_2," and upright again in lead "V_3," which is highly unusual.

6. Misplacement of the precordial electrodes is difficult or impossible to recognize without having a previous tracing available for comparison.
7. If the rhythm is not sinus, recognition of lead misplacement is, with occasional exception, more difficult.

Artifacts

ECG artifacts have two potentially undesirable effects: (1) they may make it difficult to interpret the ECG; or (2) they may cause incorrect interpretation of the ECG.[1,2] Some of the common errors of recording observed in the past have been nearly eliminated by advances in the manufacturing of the equipment. Faulty recorders with poor frequency response (damping), broken stylus, uneven paper transport, incorrect standardization, and excess paste on the skin of the chest are not likely to cause any problems with the present technology. Faulty placement of precordial electrodes (discussed previously) and incorrect identification of the patient can still occur owing to lack of experience or lack of attention by the recording person.

The most common artifacts are caused by skeletal muscle tremor, electrical interference from the network or appliances, and electrode movements. An artifact can be readily recognized if it affects one electrode predominantly (e.g., muscle tremor, jerky movements of one extremity, pulsation of the radial artery under the electrode on one hand). Under such circumstances the leads not connected to the electrode affected by the source of the disturbance are either free of distortion or much less affected by the distortion than the leads connected to the electrode affected by the disturbance. For instance, in Figure 25–12 the artifact affects the electrode on the left arm, and therefore lead II is much less affected than the other limb leads. In Figure 25–13 the artifact affects the right arm, and therefore lead III is much less affected than the other limb leads. Figure 25–14 shows an artifact simulating a long QT interval, which apparently was precipitated by movement of the electrode on the left leg. Similar motion artifacts in the precordial leads can be recognized when they affect few adjacent chest leads. They are usually caused by cardiac pulsations. An example is shown in Figure 25–15. Figure 25–16 shows an intermittently appearing

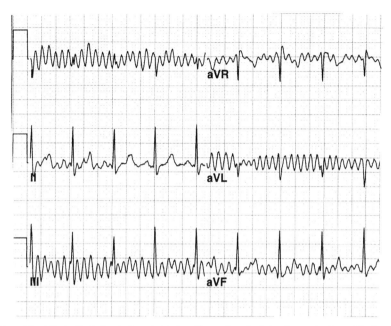

Figure 25–12   An artifact that affects leads II and aV_R less than other limb leads can be traced to the left arm electrode.

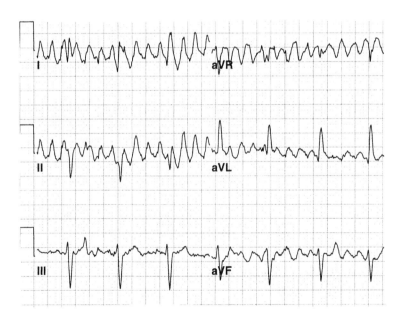

Figure 25–13   An artifact that affects lead III less than other limb leads can be traced to the right arm electrode.

artifact caused by an electric gastric stimulation. Similar artifacts were shown to be caused by an axial blood flow pump after implanting a permanent Jarvik 2000 Heart.[5]

Knight et al.[3] reported 12 artifacts simulating monomorphic or polymorphic ventricular tachycardia. In each of these cases the patient underwent at least one unnecessary intervention. In most such cases the artifacts are superimposed on the regular sinus rhythm, which can be detected by careful inspection. Figure 25–17 shows that portions of the QRS complex of the underlying sinus rhythm are visible within the artifact. Littmann and Monroe[4] pointed out that the intersection of the native complex with the artifact creates visible notches, and that the notch-to-notch intervals can be compared with the RR intervals of the underlying rhythm.

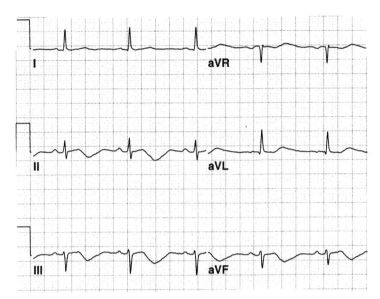

Figure 25–14   An artifact that spares lead I and affects predominantly leads II, III, and aV$_F$ can be traced to the left leg electrode.

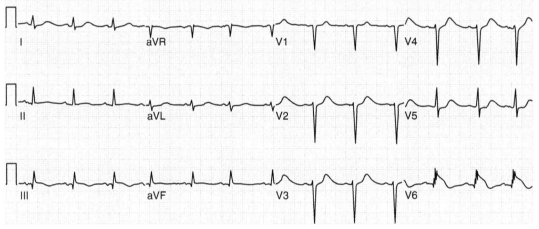

Figure 25–15   An artifact that distorts the terminal T wave portion and simulates ST segment elevation and a negative U wave in lead V$_6$ and a prolonged QT in V$_2$–V$_5$.

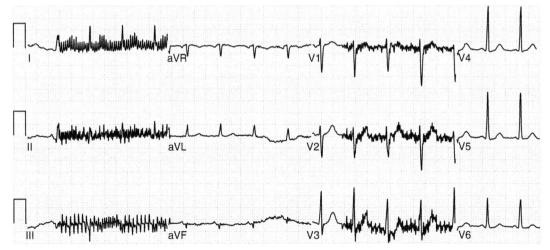

Figure 25–16   An artifact attributed to an electric gastric pump.

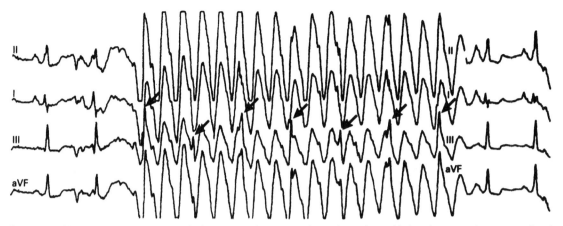

Figure 25–17 ECG artifact that mimicked monomorphic ventricular tachycardia and led to the patient being treated with lidocaine. Arrows point to the native sinus QRS complexes. (From Knight BP, Pelosi F, Michaud GF, et al: Clinical consequences of electrocardiographic artifact mimicking ventricular tachycardia. N Engl J Med 341:1270, 1999.)

REFERENCES

1. Surawicz B: Abnormal electrocardiogram in the absence of heart disease. Assoc Life Insurance Med Directors Ame 60:84, 1976.
2. Surawicz B: Assessing abnormal ECG patterns in the absence of heart disease. Cardiovasc Med 2:629, 1977.
3. Knight BP, Pelosi F, Michaud GF, et al: Clinical consequences of electrocardiographic artifact mimicking ventricular tachycardia. N Engl J Med 341:1270, 1999.
4. Littmann L, Monroe MH: Electrocardiographic artifact [letter]. N Engl J Med 342:590, 2000.
5. Jin XY, Westaby S, Robson D, et al: Unique ECG finding in a patient with an axial blood flow pump. Circulation 104:970, 2001.

26 Electrocardiography of Artificial Electronic Pacemakers

BORYS SURAWICZ • LAWRENCE E. GERING

The electrical pacing of the human heart was initiated in the early 1950s as a resuscitative procedure[1] and has continued to expand since that time, responding to the demands of clinical cardiologists whose challenges have been met sequentially by the ingenuity of electronic technology. The implanted pacemakers became prophylactic with the advent of synchronization made possible by the ability to sense, inhibit, and trigger the intrinsic electrical activity. The next step was to control the heart rate and the atrioventricuular (AV) delay by dual-chamber pacing with the ability to modulate the rate responsiveness. In 2002, dual-chamber pacemakers represented 82.8 percent of all new pacemaker implantations in this country.[2]

More recent advances have been directed at improving the hemodynamics by reducing the recognized adverse effects of asynchronous right ventricular pacing and by the increasing application of the synchronized biventricular pacing. Major preventive action is provided by the implantable cardioverter defibrillators (ICDs) and to some extent by atrial pacing to prevent recurrences of atrial fibrillation.

As indicated by its title, the emphasis of this chapter is electrocardiography. Beyond the scope of this textbook is the detailed coverage of related, but not strictly electrocardiographic (ECG) problems, such as the indications for pacing, selection of appropriate pacing modes, outcomes of therapy, and technical aspects of programming and control of pacemaker function.

Pacemakers Components

An electronic pacemaker system has two major components: the pulse generator and the lead or leads. The pulse generator consists of several components: a power source, which in permanent pacemakers is a sealed battery, most commonly lithium iodide; voltage multipliers that increase the available stimulation amplitude; amplifier circuits that increase the amplitude of sensed cardiac signals; microelectronic circuits that regulate timing of the device and control the action of the pacemaker; a radiofrequency receiver to receive programming information; and a transmitter to provide information from the pacemaker. Most modern pulse generators also include a sensor to modulate the pacing rate; an internal clock may also be included to allow for alteration of the pacing rate based on circadian rhythms. In a permanent pacemaker these components are contained in a hermetically sealed container made of titanium, which is insulated on one side to prevent electrical stimulation of adjacent skeletal muscle. The leads may be unipolar (a single wire extending from the pacemaker to the stimulating electrode) or bipolar (two wires extending to two stimulating electrodes at and near the tip of the lead).

Pacemaker Nomenclature

The pacemaker nomenclature established by the North American Society of Pacing and Electrophysiology (NASPE) and the British Pacing and Electrophysiology Group (BPEG) is designated as NBG code for pacing nomenclature[3] (Table 26–1). The code has five positions. The first position designates the chamber in which stimulation takes place: A = atrium, V = ventricle, and D = dual

chamber, or both A and V. The second position designates the chamber where sensing occurs, and the letters are the same as for the first position sensed. The third position refers to the mode of response. An *I* indicates that a sensed event inhibits the output pulse and causes the pacemaker to recycle for one more timing cycle; *T* indicates that an input pulse is triggered in response to sensed event, and *D* means that both T and I can occur.

For example, the code for the ventricular inhibited pacemaker is VVI. The pacemaker paces the ventricle (V), senses the ventricle (V), and is inhibited (I) by a sensed signal. The D designation is restricted to dual-chamber pacemakers.

The fourth position of the code shows both programmability and rate response. An *R* in the fourth position indicates that the pacemaker incorporates a sensor to modulate the rate idependently of intrinsic cardiac activity. Other functions in the fourth position and the functions in the fifth position are primarily used by manufacturers to describe functions that are beyond the scope of this chapter.

Pacemaker Stimulus Artifact

The pacemaker impulse is recognized on the ECG as a sharp, narrow spike (Figure 26–1). Its duration is generally less than 2 ms,[4] and it appears as a vertical line on the routine ECG. When the pacing spike is large, it is often followed by an exponential voltage decay curve that may distort or even mask the depolarization waveform induced by the pacemaker (Figure 26–2).

TABLE 26–1	NASPE/BPEG Generic (NBG) Pacemaker Codes				
Parameter	Position I	Position II	Position III	Position IV	Position V
Category	Chamber(s) paced	Chamber(s) sensed	Response to sensing	Programmability, rate modulation	Antitachyarrhythmia function(s)
	O = none	O = none	O = none	O = none	O = none
	A = atrium	A = atrium	T = triggered	P = simple programmable	P = pacing (antitachyarrhythmia)
	V = ventricle	V = ventricle	I = inhibited	M = multiprogrammable	S = shock
	D = dual (A + V)	D = dual (A + V)	D = dual (D + I)	C = communicating	D = dual (P + S)
				R = rate modulation	
Manufacturer's designation only	S = single (A or V)	S = single (A or V)		Comma optional here	

Note: Positions I through III are used exclusively for antibradyarrhythmia function.
BPEG = British Pacing and Electrophysiology Group; NASPE = North American Society of Pacing and Electrophysiology.

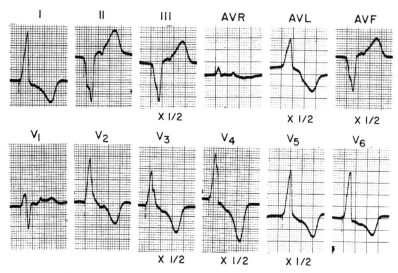

Figure 26–1 Transvenous right ventricular pacemaker with bipolar electrode. The tip of the electrode is located at the apex of the right ventricle. The pacemaker spikes are narrow and of relatively small amplitude. The QRS-T morphology resembles that of complete left bundle branch block. Retrograde capture of the atria is present.

All types of cardiac electrical stimulation require a complete electrical circuit with a cathode (negative) electrode and an anode (positive) electrode. For "bipolar" pacing, the cathode usually is located at the tip of the catheter, and the anode is approximately 1 cm proximal to the tip. The electric current completes the circuit by traversing a relatively small distance from the negative to the positive electrode. For "unipolar" pacing, the cathode is located at the tip of the catheter, and the anode is the exposed metal portion of the pulse generator. The electrical current flows from the tip of the electrode catheter to the pacing device through the body tissue and fluid.

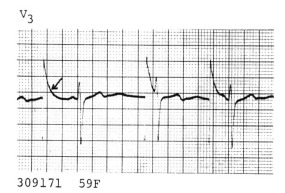

309171   59F

Figure 26–2 Pacemaker spike decay curve. The tracing was recorded from a patient with a malfunctioning unipolar ventricular demand (VVI) pacemaker. There is constant failure to capture and intermittent failure of sensing. The gradual downward inscriptions following the spikes represent the spike decay curves, one of which is indicated by an arrow.

As a rule, pacemakers in the seldom-used unipolar pacing mode cause much larger pacing spikes than those produced by bipolar pacing (see Figures 26–1 and 26–2). Bipolar epicardial-myocardial leads elicit even smaller spikes than the bipolar endocardial leads (Figure 26–3).

Inadvertent stimulation of skeletal muscle occurs more frequently in patients with unipolar pacing, and the longer distance between the electrodes renders the pacemaker more vulnerable to electromagnetic interference and sensing of myopotentials from skeletal muscles (see later discussion).

Regardless of the pacemaker type, placement, or pacing mode, the voltage and polarity of the pacing impulse differ in the various leads of the ECG because both the amplitude and polarity of the spike in a given lead depend on the relation between the axis of the lead and the spatial orientation of the spike vector. For example, with a transvenous bipolar electrode located at the apex of the right ventricle, the vector of the pacing impulse is directed toward the negative side of lead II (because the negative electrode is at the tip of the catheter, and the positive electrode is proximal to it). Therefore lead II usually records a large negative spike and lead aV_R a large positive spike, whereas the leads that are perpendicular to the spike vector record a small deflection. With a unipolar electrode, the vector of the pacer impulse has an orientation parallel to a line joining the tip of the catheter to the pulse generator, the latter having the positive polarity. The direction of the vector

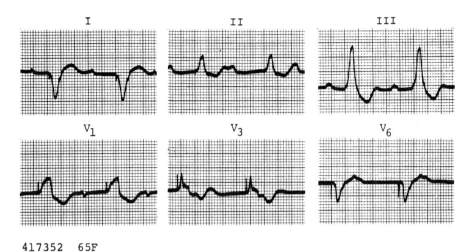

417352 65F

Figure 26–3   Left ventricular epicardial pacing with a bipolar lead. Note the small amplitude of the pacemaker spikes. The QRS complexes show right axis deviation and a right bundle branch block–like pattern. The underlying rhythm is sinus with complete atrioventricular block.

therefore depends on the location of the pulse generator as well as on the pacing site.

Tracings recorded with digital electrocardiography may display unusual pacemaker spikes if they are artificially simulated. Recording devices that enhance pacemaker spikes do so based on sensing high frequency electrical activity. Occasionally, patients with relatively high frequency of spontaneous ventricular activity meet the criteria for enhancement, and an apparent pacemaker spike appears when no pacing has occurred. Pacemaker spikes that are artificially enhanced obviously do not have the same implications for identifying unipolar or bipolar pacing modes. If pacing spikes are not simulated in a digital ECG recording system, the displayed spike amplitude may be highly variable (see Figure 26–3) owing to the short duration of the stimulus (usually <1 ms) and the sampling rate of the recorder (frequently >1 ms). Even experienced electrocardiographers can be led to errors when the spikes are not readily detectable. Standard analog electrocardiography is therefore preferable for detecting pacemaker and lead abnormalities.[5]

Morphology of ECG Complexes

Most pacemakers can be programmed noninvasively through a radiofrequency or an electromagnetic signal to the mode of cardiac pacing best suited to the needs of the individual patient. A single-chamber pacemaker has more limited programmable options than a dual-chamber

pacemaker, such as DDD. The ECG interpretation is easier when one knows the type of pacemaker and programmed parameters, but this information frequently is not available to the reader of the ECG. Although it may be possible to determine the programmed mode by careful analysis of multiple tracings,[6] the findings in a single tracing may be consistent with multiple modes.[7] The ECG characteristics of each mode are described here and must be considered when interpreting "unknown" clinical tracings.

ATRIAL PACING

Sinus node dysfunction is the most common indication for permanent pacemaker implantation, accounting for more than 50 percent of implants.[8,9] Several studies have suggested that atrial-based pacing offers advantages over ventricular pacing in patients with this disorder.[10–12] Single-chamber atrial pacing is an acceptable approach in selected patients,[12] but dual-chamber pacemakers are frequently used because of concern about subsequent development of AV block.

With atrial pacing, the pacer artifacts are followed by ectopic P waves whose waveform depends on the site of stimulation. P wave morphology resembles that of sinus complexes if the site of stimulation is near the sinus node (Figures 26–4 and 26–5). The most common site for implantation of a permanent endocardial atrial pacing lead is the right atrial appendage. If a transvenous catheter is implanted in the coronary sinus, the P wave axis is directed superiorly, and inverted P waves are recorded in the

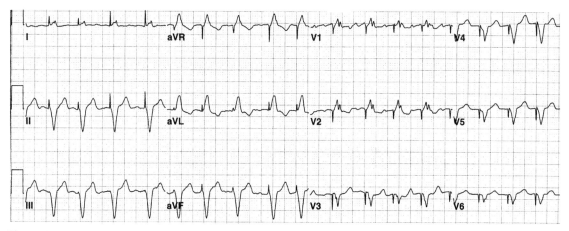

Figure 26–4 Atrial synchronous ventricular pacing with ventricular stimulation from the right ventricular septum. Right bundle branch block with a superior frontal-plane QRS axis is noted. QRS transition occurs to the right of lead V_3. Digital recording results in variable stimulus artifact amplitude.

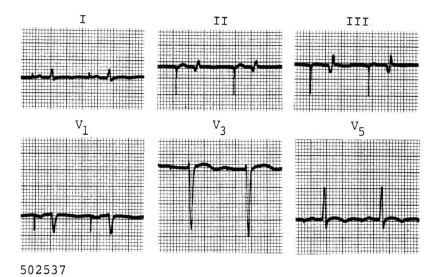

502537

Figure 26–5 Bipolar atrial pacing. The lead was implanted, through a thoracotomy, in the region of the sinoatrial node. The morphology of the P waves resembles that of normal sinus rhythm.

inferior leads (Figure 26–6). Pacing may also be done from more than one atrial site.[13]

Pacing Modes

The modes of atrial pacing can be atrial asynchronous (AOO) or atrial demand, the latter of which may be atrial inhibited (AAI) or atrial triggered (AAT).

The atrial asynchronous (AOO) mode is also called *fixed-rate atrial pacing*. It has no sensing function. Normal ventricular activation depends on an intact AV conduction system. The lead is connected to the atrium, which is paced at a preset rate independent of the patient's own heart

rate or rhythm (Figure 26–7A). This pacing mode is rarely used today.

Atrial demand mode, either atrial inhibited or atrial triggered, paces the atrium and senses the atrial impulse. In the case of AAI pacing, in the presence of spontaneous atrial activity with a rate greater (or the PP interval shorter) than a predetermined level, no stimulus would be delivered (Figure 26–7B). AAI pacing is appropriate for patients with sinus node dysfunction and normal AV conduction. Sensing of the far-field QRS complexes by an AAI pacemaker will cause slowing of the pacing rate because the sensed event from the ventricle resets the lower rate interval. Another problem is that ventricular

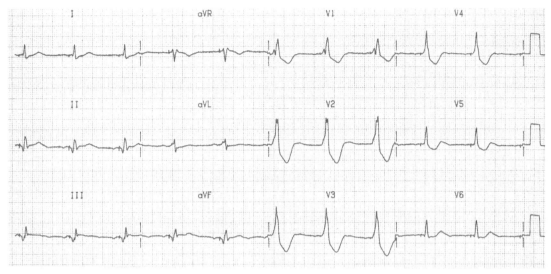

Figure 26–6   Left ventricular pacing via the coronary sinus. Morphology of QRS complexes is a right bundle branch block–like pattern and normal axis. There is no transition in the precordial leads due to pacing from the base of the left ventricle. The atrial lead was positioned in a low posterior right atrial location, resulting in a superiorly directed P wave axis.

AOO

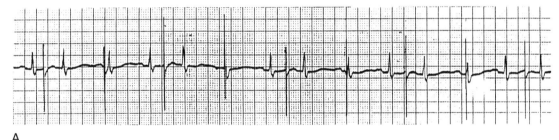

A

AAI

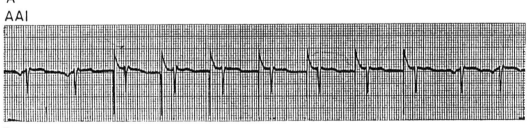

B

Figure 26–7   A, Atrial asynchronous (AOO) pacing. The underlying rhythm is sinus. Competitive fixed-rate atrial pacing occurs with no atrial sensing. Atrial capture does not occur when the atrium is refractory. **B,** Atrial inhibited (AAI) pacing. The underlying rhythm is sinus with intact AV conduction. The pacemaker is inhibited until the intrinsic rate decreases below the programmed pacing rate, at which time pacing begins. Inhibition of the pacemaker again occurs when the intrinsic rate increases above the programmed pacing rate.

premature complexes are often not sensed by the AAI mode because the far-field QRS signal is too weak.

With AAT, the pacer senses the atrial impulse and stimulates the atrium when the atrial rate falls below the programmed rate, but it also delivers stimuli when it senses native P waves. The AAT mode is rarely used as a permanently programmed mode but frequently is helpful as a temporarily programmed mode to assess atrial sensing.

ATRIAL SYNCHRONOUS VENTRICULAR INHIBITED PACING (VDD)

These pacemakers pace only in the ventricle, sense in both chambers, and respond both by inhibition of ventricular input due to intrinsic ventricular activity and by ventricular tracking of P waves.[14] In the VDD mode, sensed atrial events initiate the AV interval (AVI). If an intrinsic ventricular event occurs before the termination of the AVI, ventricular output is inhibited and the lower rate timing cycle is reset. The addition of ventricular sensing prevents bradycardia. This mode of pacing can perform atrial synchronous ventricular inhibited pacing (VDD) with a single lead. The lead is introduced transvenously and has electrodes for ventricular pacing and sensing at the distal tip. Electrodes are also located on the lead in a more proximal position at a point where the lead passes through the atrium. This system is less expensive and easier to implant than a DDD system, but it cannot provide AV synchrony at slow intrinsic atrial rates. This mode of pacing is most appropriate for patients with AV block and intact sinus node function.

VENTRICULAR PACING

With ventricular pacing, the pacer impulse is followed by an abnormal QRS complex, the characteristics of which usually give a fairly good indication of the location of the stimulating electrode. Right ventricular pacing results in QRS complexes similar to those of complete left bundle branch block (LBBB) (see Figure 26–1). In most cases of transvenous ventricular pacing, the tip of the electrode is located at the apex of the right ventricle. The induced sequence of ventricular activation is from right to left and from apex to base. The apex-to-base sequence of depolarization results in a superior orientation

of the QRS vector and superior axis deviation in the frontal plane with negative QRS complexes in leads II, III, and aV$_F$. In many patients, with a typical complete LBBB pattern in the limb leads and right precordial leads there is a predominant negative deflection in leads V$_5$ and V$_6$ (Figure 26–8). This finding is due to the direction of the lead axis of V$_5$ and V$_6$, which is not only leftward but also slightly downward. When the QRS forces are oriented superiorly, they may project on the negative side of the lead axis of the above leads. If the site of stimulation is at the inflow or outflow tract of the right ventricle, the frontal plane QRS axis is usually normal. If the site is located immediately below the pulmonary valve, the QRS axis becomes vertical or even rightward[15] (Figure 26–9).

The QR and qR complexes during right ventricular pacing are abnormal in the absence of fusion complexes except for a qR complex in leads I and aV$_L$, which may be present normally, without indicating myocardial infarction (MI), during stimulation of the right ventricular outflow tract or during biventricular pacing.[16]

The pattern similar to right bundle branch block (RBBB) in the right precordial leads raises concern about possible septal perforation by the pacing electrode, resulting in left ventricular (LV) pacing. In most cases, however, the RBBB-like pattern occurs during right ventricular (RV) pacing in the absence of perforation. This can be recognized by defining the location of the transition zone of the QRS polarity in the precordial leads. When the transition zone is to the right of lead V$_3$ (see Figure 26–4), the pacing is still from the right ventricle, whereas transition at lead V$_3$ or to the left of lead V$_3$ suggests LV pacing.[17]

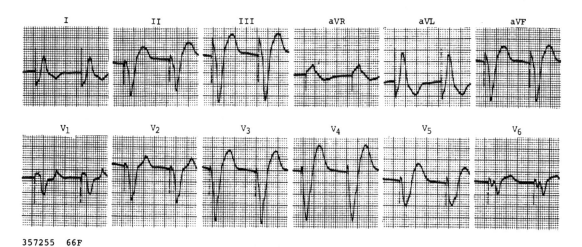

357255   66F

Figure 26–8   Transvenous right ventricular pacing. The left bundle branch block–like QRS complex is predominantly negative in all precordial leads, including V$_5$ and V$_6$.

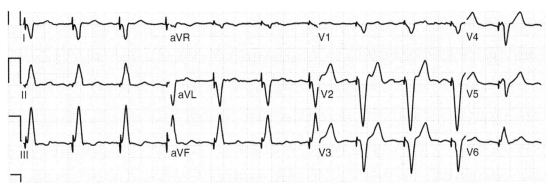

Figure 26–9   Twelve lead ECG during DDD pacing from right ventricular outflow tract shows left bundle branch block pattern with right axis deviation in the frontal plane. (Courtesy of S.S. Barold, MD.)

With LV epicardial-myocardial pacing, the 12-lead ECG displays a complete RBBB pattern. LV pacing from the coronary sinus can also result in an RBBB pattern (see Figure 26–6). The frontal plane axis cannot differentiate precisely an endocardial LV site from the site in the coronary vein system.[16] When the electrode is implanted in the mid to high lateral portions of the left ventricle, there is right axis deviation with negative QRS deflection in leads I and V_6 and an R wave in lead V_1 (see Figures 26–3 and 26–10). When the stimulation site is near the LV apex, an $S_1S_2S_3$ pattern is seen as the activation front advances rightward and superiorly. Occasionally, LV pacing near the apex produces a negative QRS deflection in lead V_1. In that case, it may be impossible to determine from the ECG whether the left or right ventricle is being paced[18] and whether the placement of the LV electrode is correct.[16]

Pacing Modes

The various pacing modes are as follows: ventricular asynchronous (VOO) and ventricular demand, the latter of which may be ventricular inhibited (VVI) or ventricular triggered (VVT).

VOO Pacing

The VOO pacing mode is also called *fixed-rate ventricular pacing*. The pacer delivers stimuli at a

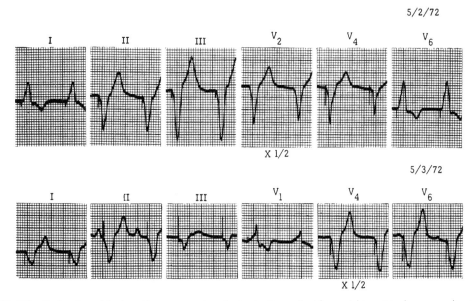

Figure 26–10   Perforation of the heart by a pacemaker electrode. The patient has a right ventricular pacemaker implanted for treatment of complete atrioventricular block. On 5/2/72, the tracing shows functioning right ventricular pacing with QRS-T morphology similar to that of complete left bundle branch block (LBBB). The following day, the electrocardiogram reveals a change from LBBB pattern to right bundle branch block pattern as a result of ventricular perforation, with the tip of the electrode resting on the epicardial surface of the left ventricle.

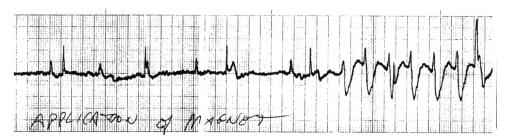

Figure 26–11   Asynchronous ventricular pacing during application of a magnet. Many of the pacemaker stimuli are ineffective, falling on various portions of the spontaneous QRS complexes. The third complex is a fusion complex. The fourth pacing stimulus occurs during the vulnerable period and initiates ventricular tachycardia. Continued asynchronous pacing is noted during ventricular tachycardia.

constant rate independent of the patient's own heart rate or rhythm. The resulting rhythm is a ventricular parasystole. The fixed-rate mode was the only mode available during the early era of pacemakers for treatment of complete AV block[19–21] but is rarely used now, in part because of the risk that the artificial stimulus may fall within the vulnerable period and result in ventricular tachycardia or fibrillation (Figure 26–11). Admittedly, this risk is low in most patients, but it may increase in the presence of myocardial ischemia, electrolyte imbalance, or drug toxicity.[21]

During the follow-up of patients with ventricular demand pacing, an ECG is often obtained while a magnet is applied to the pulse generator. The magnet converts most pacemakers from the demand mode to a fixed-rate mode. It is mostly under this condition that ventricular asynchronous pacing, as well as pacemaker-induced ventricular arrhythmia, is observed clinically.

VVI Pacing

The VVI pacing is the most common type of demand pacing. The VVI pacemaker functions like the AAI pacemaker and generates impulses whenever the patient's ventricular rate falls below the programmed rate (Figures 26–12 and 26–13). The features of the VVI pacing are displayed in Figure 26–13. The QRS marked 1 is sensed by the

pacemaker; complexes 2 and 3 are paced; the ventricular extrasystole (complex 4) and a normal QRS (complex 5) are sensed; and complexes 6 and 7 are paced. The pacemaker refractory period is 300 ms. Inhibition of the pacemaker occurs when the intrinsic rate increases above the programmed lower rate. Therefore the ability to sense ventricular activity is an important function of this type of ventricular pacemaker.

The ECGs of patients with properly functioning ventricular inhibited pacing may present the following findings:

1. All ECG complexes are spontaneous, and the existence of an artificial pacemaker cannot be detected. This occurs when the spontaneous ventricular rate is faster than the pacemaker's pacing rate and all the spontaneous RR intervals are shorter than the pacing interval. The presence of pacing function can be demonstrated by applying an external magnet to the pulse generator to inactivate its sensing circuit and convert it to the fixed-rate mode (see Figure 26–11). Depending on the specific pacemaker, the pacing rate during magnet application may or may not be the same as the pacing rate during its demand mode.

2. All the ventricular complexes are the result of pacemaker stimulation (see Figure 26–6). The spike-to-spike interval (pace interval,

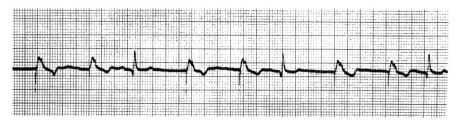

Figure 26–12   Ventricular inhibited pacing (VVI). The third, sixth, and last complexes are sinus complexes that suppress the pacemaker. The interval between spikes is 840 ms.

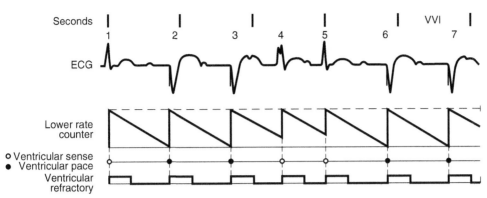

Figure 26–13 Diagram displaying the features of ventricular inhibited pacing (rate = 80 beats/min). The QRS marked 1 is sensed by the pacemaker. Complexes 2 and 3 are a paced ventricular extrasystole (4) and a normal QRS (5) that are then sensed. The sixth and seventh complexes are paced. The pacemaker's refractory period (300 ms) is shown as a rectangle. Complexes 4 and 5 reset and restart the lower rate counter before completion of the ventricular escape interval (equal to automatic interval). (Reproduced with permission from Lindemans PW: Diagrammatic representation of pacemaker function. *In:* Barold SS [ed]: Modern Cardiac Pacing. Mount Kisco, NY, Futura, 1985, pp 323–353.)

automatic interval) remains constant. In adults the pacing rate is commonly set at 60 to 70 beats/min. When a demand pacemaker is pacing uninterruptedly, the ECG is indistinguishable from that seen with a fixed-rate pacing mode.

3. Both spontaneous and paced complexes are present (see Figure 26–12). The spontaneous complexes may be sinus or ectopic supraventricular or ventricular impulses. If a spontaneous complex is followed by a paced complex, the interval from the onset of the spontaneous QRS complex to the pacemaker spike is called the *escape interval*. Depending on the origin of the spontaneous impulse, its potential may not be sensed by the electrode until the later part of the depolarization process. The pacemaker is therefore not reset until part of the QRS complex in the surface ECG is already inscribed. With certain pacemakers the escape interval is deliberately set longer than the pacing interval, a feature called *hysteresis* (see later discussion).

4. Fusion complexes and pseudofusion complexes are seen when the ventricles are simultaneously depolarized by two activation fronts, one from the pacing impulse and one from the spontaneous focus. The morphology of the fusion complexes varies, depending on the portion of the ventricles depolarized by each of the activation fronts, but the QRS duration of the fusion complexes is usually shorter than that of pure paced impulses (see Figures 26–11, 26–14, and 26–15). The QRS complex of a fusion complex may be isoelectric in a single lead, and the diagnosis of fusion relies on

seeing the T wave. Fusion complexes may simulate MI,[22] as shown in Figure 26–15.

Pseudofusion complexes occur when an ineffective pacing impulse is superimposed on a spontaneous complex (Figure 26–16). The pacemaker impulse does not induce ventricular depolarization, and the morphology of the QRS complex with the superimposed spike is the same as that of the nonpaced complex. Pseudofusion complexes occur when the pacemaker discharges during the absolute refractory period before sufficient intracardiac voltage has been generated at the site of the pacing lead to activate its sensing circuit. The pacemaker spike falls within the spontaneous QRS complex generated independently of the electrical changes recorded from the pacing catheter.[23]

Pseudofusion complexes are more likely to be seen in patients with an intraventricular conduction defect or ectopic ventricular complexes.[24] In patients with complete RBBB and an RV artificial pacemaker, there is a delay in the arrival of the activation front of the spontaneous beats at the site of the electrode. The pacemaker may discharge its stimulus at its preset interval in the initial part of the QRS complex because it has not yet sensed the event in progress in the left ventricle. The same phenomenon may be seen in patients with complete LBBB and an LV artificial pacemaker. Pseudofusion complexes may be seen in patients with LV premature ventricular complexes and an RV pacemaker (see Figure 26–16) or with RV premature complexes and an LV pacemaker by a similar

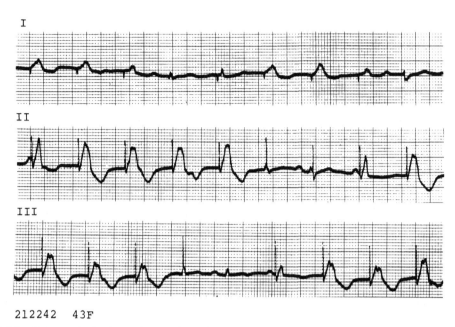

212242   43F

Figure 26–14 Right ventricular demand pacing (VVI) shows fusion complexes. Depending on the proportion of spontaneous and pacer-induced ventricular activation, the morphology of the QRS-T complex varies. The pacemaker rate is 92 beats/min.

mechanism. Pseudofusion complexes do not indicate malfunction of the sensing circuit of the pacemaker and are normal manifestations of a demand pacemaker.

An atrial stimulus also can fall within the QRS complex before the intracardiac ventricular electrogram is sensed. In this situation when an atrial stimulus deforms the QRS complex, the term *pseudopseudofusion* has been applied to indicate that the distortion involves two chambers instead of one, as in the case of pseudofusion complexes (Figure 26–17).[25]

5. Occasionally, certain ventricular ectopic complexes are not sensed by an otherwise properly functioning VVI pacemaker because the abnormal depolarization impulse does not generate adequate signal at the site of the intracardiac electrode. Alternatively, the local electrical voltage may be too low, or the ventricular depolarization vector is perpendicular to the sensing electrodes. Also, the rate of voltage change (dV/dT) may be too slow to be sensed by the pacemaker.

VVI Pacing in the Magnet Mode

Some manufacturers of pacemakers incorporate a "threshold margin test" during the initial part of the magnet mode. The application of a magnet

to such VVI pacemakers initiates asynchronous pacing pulses with the pulse width or amplitude of one of the stimuli having a fixed reduction in output (Figure 26–18). The purpose of this reduction is to ensure that the pacemaker's output is providing a sufficient safety margin to capture the ventricle.

In many pacemakers, the pacing rate in the magnet mode is the same as that during automatic pacing. In some pacemakers, however, the rates are different. In either case, changes in the pacing rate during magnet application may reflect a reduction in the pacemaker's battery voltage. Depending on the particular pacemaker, the degree of change in the pacing rate with magnet application will indicate whether the pacemaker may be electively replaced or the replacement is urgent.

VVT Pacing

The VVT mode of demand pacing functions similarly to the inhibited mode (VVI) by delivering a stimulus at a preset interval when no spontaneous ventricular depolarization is detected. It differs from the VVI mode by additionally delivering a stimulus immediately after a sensed spontaneous QRS. This results in R wave synchronous pacing. On the ECG, each QRS complex is accompanied by a pacing spike. When there is a spontaneous ventricular complex, the

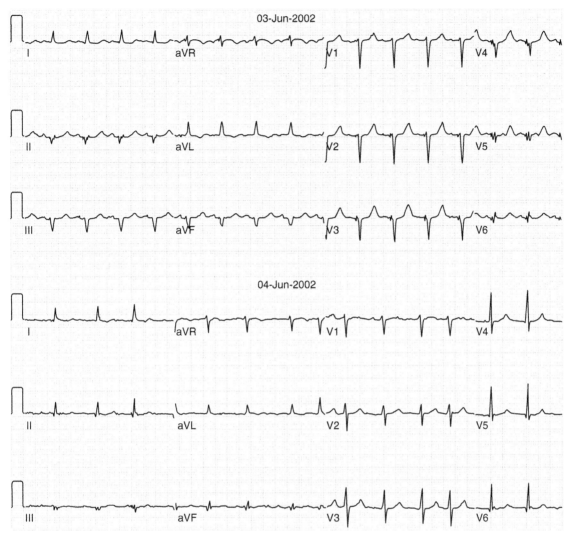

Figure 26–15   Myocardial infarction (MI) simulatd by fusion complexes. ECG of a 58-year-old man admitted for noncardiac surgery. Upper tracing shows sinus complexes and paced fusion complexes; the QRS pattern simulates an extensive anterior MI, of which there was no evidence or history. Lower ECG, recorded 1 day later, shows atrial fibrillation, no pacng, and no evidence of MI.

pacing spike appears shortly after the onset of the QRS during the absolute refractory period of the ventricle and produces a pseudofusion complex. If there is no spontaneous ventricular activation, the pacemaker spike appears at the end of the escape or pacing interval and initiates the QRS complex (Figure 26–19).

Ventricular-triggered pacemakers were originally designed to avoid the potential problem of pacemaker inhibition by extracardiac electrical signals such as those that originated from skeletal muscle or radio transmitters, especially when unipolar leads were used. Modern pacemaker circuitry and an increase in the use of bipolar leads have reduced the likelihood of such interference. Because of the additional power drain and the distortion of the native QRS complexes by the pacing spikes, the triggered mode of pacing is used infrequently as a permanent pacing mode. As in the case of the atrial-triggered mode, the ventricular-triggered mode may be useful as a temporarily programmed mode to assess ventricular sensing problems, particularly an oversensing.

Dual-Chamber Pacing

Dual-chamber pacing may be AV sequential or AV universal (DDD).

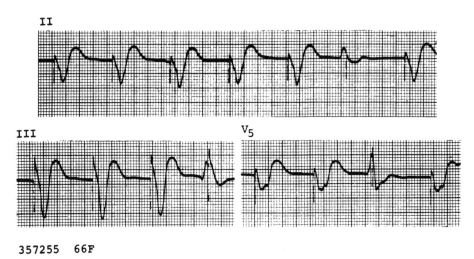

357255   66F

Figure 26–16   Pseudofusion complexes. There is an ineffective pacemaker stimulus falling on the premature complex in each of the three leads.

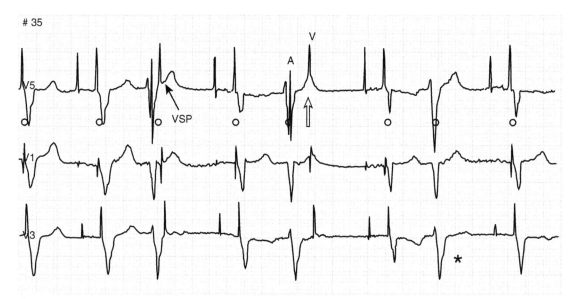

Figure 26–17   Cross talk and pseudopseudofusion. Holter record of DDD pacemaker showing the effect of cross-talk timing cycle during normal pacemaker function. Three leads are recorded simultaneously. The fifth complex is a ventricular premature complex (V) deformed by an atrial stimulus (A). The delivery of atrial stimulus within a QRS complex (capable of being sensed) is called a *pseudopseudofusion complex.* The effective ventricular electrogram of the premature ventricular complex (PVC) (of adequate amplitude to be sensed) occurs within the postarial ventricular blanking period initiated by the atrial stimulus (open arrow). The PVC is therefore unsensed by the ventricular channel of the pacemaker. The subsequent ventricular extrasystole, marked by an asterisk, is sensed normally by the ventricular channel. The third ventricular complex is also deformed by atrial stimulus, but the atrial stimulus occurs earlier, allowing the pacemaker to sense the effective ventricular electrogram beyond the ventricular blanking period but still within ventricular safety period (VSP). Ventricular complexes marked by open circles. (Courtesy of S.S. Barold, MD.)

AV SEQUENTIAL PACING

The AV sequential pacing mode is a dual-chamber pacing mode that paces both the atrium and the ventricle but senses only the ventricle (DVI), or it senses both atrium and ventricle but is capable only of inhibiting pacing but not triggering it (DDI).[26] If ventricular or conducted supraventricular complexes occur at a rate above the programmed rate with DVI pacing, all activities of the pacemaker are suppressed. If no ventricular potential is sensed by the ventricular

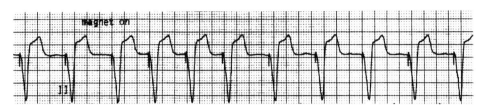

Figure 26–18   Ventricular inhibited pacing (VVI) in the magnet mode, demonstrating the "threshold margin test." With application of a magnet, this pacemaker (manufactured by Medtronic) generates the first three stimuli at a rate of 100 times per minute. The pulse width of the third stimulus is reduced by 25 percent, but this measurement cannot be made on the routine ECG because of the slow paper speed. The pacing rate after the first three stimuli is identical to that during automatic pacing.

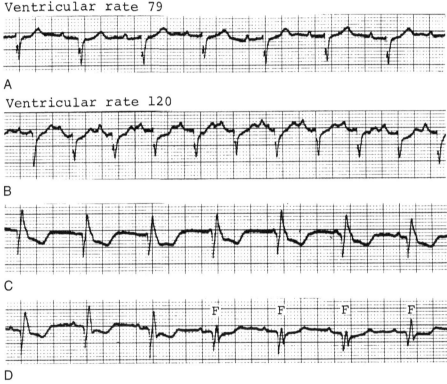

Figure 26–19   Ventricular triggered pacing (VVT). **A,** Recorded during normal sinus rhythm. The pacemaker senses the R waves of the spontaneous complexes and generates stimuli that are superimposed on the initial part of the QRS complexes. **B,** The same phenomenon occurs when the heart rate increases during walking. **C,** The spontaneous ventricular rate falls below 76 beats/min. The pacemaker operates in its demand mode with a rate of 76 beats/min. All ventricular complexes are paced complexes. **D,** Fusion complexes (F) are present and are the result of ventricular depolarization by impulses coming from both the pacemaker and conducted spontaneous impulses. The spontaneous ventricular rate and the pacemaker rate in its demand mode are nearly the same.

electrode at a predetermined interval, atrial pacing occurs. Because the pacemaker does not sense the atrium and the pacing interval is reset by ventricular depolarization, the atrial stimulus is competitive with the native atrial impulse. Atrial fibrillation may develop if the atrial stimulus is delivered during the vulnerable period.

The DDI pacing mode senses native atrial activity and inhibits atrial pacing where appropriate.

This mode, especially when coupled with rate modulation, may be useful in patients with intermittent atrial tachyarrhythmias and AV block. Its use has largely replaced the older DVI mode. AV synchrony is maintained during periods of slow atrial rates, but rapid ventricular pacing in response to atrial tachycardia is not seen owing to inability of the device to trigger ventricular pacing from atrial sensing.

DUAL-CHAMBER PACING AND SENSING WITH INHIBITION AND TRACKING: AV UNIVERSAL PACING (DDD)

DDD pacing mode is most appropriate for patients with normal sinus rhythm and AV block. It is also considered as a mode of choice in neurocardiogenic syndromes with sympathetic cardioinhibition.[27] DDD pacing does not restore rate response in the chronotropically incompetent patient and has limitations in the patients with sinus node dysfunction. Also, in patients with chronic atrial fibrillation, atrial pacing is not possible.

The AV universal mode is the most commonly used dual-chamber pacing mode[27] (Figures 26–20 to 26–22). It senses and paces both the atrium and the ventricle. From the sensed events, it may be inhibited or triggered to pace the atrium,

the ventricle, or both according to the programmed rate limits and AV interval. The operations of the two channels of a DDD pacemaker are intimately linked, and an event detected by one channel generally influences the function of the other. Four different rhythms can occur with normal DDD function: (1) normal sinus rhythm, (2) atrial pacing, (3) AV sequential pacing, and (4) P-synchronous pacing.

Because of the many possible modes of presentation, the ECGs of patients with an AV universal pacemaker are often difficult to interpret without understanding the *timing cycles* of the dual-chamber pacemaker. The traditional dual-chamber pacemakers are designed with ventricular-based or "V-V" lower rate timing (see Figure 26–20). In this system the atrial escape interval (AEI) (the interval from a paced or sensed ventricular complex to the next paced atrial event) is preeminent and controls the paced rate (see Figure 26–20).

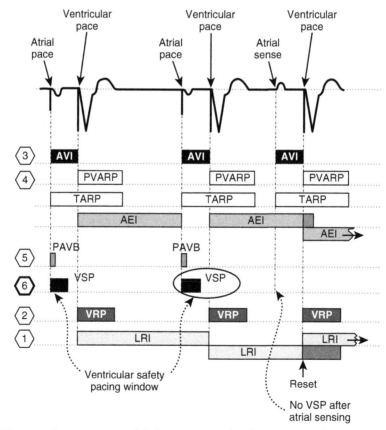

Figure 26–20   Diagrammatic representation of the basic timing cycles of a DDD pacemaker with the addition of the cross-talk intervals: postatrial ventricular blanking period (PAVB) and ventricular safety period (VSP). AEI = atrial escape interval; AVI = AV interval; LRI = lower rate interval (ventricular based); PVAPRP = postventricular atrial refractory period; TARP = total atrial refractory period; VRP = ventricular refractory period. Neither PAVB nor VSP is initiated by atrial sensing. *Reset* refers to the termination and reinitiation by the timing cycle before it has timed out to its completion according to its program duration. See text discussion. (Reproduced with permission from Barold SS, Stroobandt RX, Sinnaeve AF: Cardiac Pacemakers Step by Step. An Illustrated Guide. Malden MA, Blackwell-Futura, 2004.)

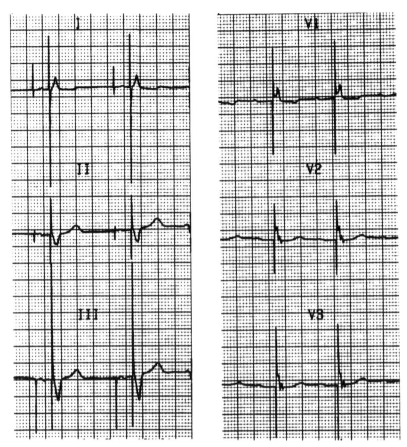

Figure 26–21 Atrioventricular (AV) universal pacemaker (DDD). Leads I, II, and III depict atrial and ventricular pacing at a rate of 60 beats/min (lower limit) with an AV interval of 200 ms. Leads V_1 through V_3 depict sinus rhythm with a rate of 78 beats/min. Atrial pacing is inhibited. Ventricular pacing still occurs because of the delayed spontaneous AV conduction beyond 200 ms.

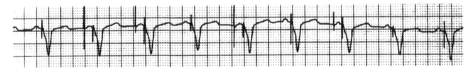

Figure 26–22 Atrioventricular universal (DDD) pacemaker. The tracing shows consistent ventricular pacing. Atrial stimulation is seen intermittently depending on whether the native P wave appeared before the programmed VA interval, which is 700 ms.

Despite its preeminence, the AEI is not a programmed interval but rather is calculated from the programmed lower rate interval (60,000 ms − programmed lower rate interval in ms) minus the programmed AV delay. The paced AV delay is usually 20 to 50 ms longer than the sensed AV delay to allow for the difference in interatrial conduction between intrinsic and paced atrial events.

If AV conduction occurs with an interval shorter than the programmed AV delay, the pacemaker senses the ventricular activity and initiates a new AEI. This results in atrial pacing at a rate faster than the programmed lower rate.

The difference in rate is more pronounced at faster programmed lower rate limits and when there is a more pronounced difference between the programmed AV delay and the native AV conduction interval.

With the development of rate-modulated dual-chamber pacemakers, it is more common to have faster programmed lower rate limits, as the rate modulation may increase the lower rate limit to >100 beats/min during physical activity. As physical activity may also be associated with enhanced AV conduction, shorter native AV conduction intervals may be seen; this may significantly increase the atrial pace rate if "V-V" lower-rate timing is utilized. To avoid this problem, some dual-chamber pacemakers, especially those with rate modulation, use atrial-based, or "A-A" lower rate timing. With this approach the lower rate interval is based on the atrial sensed or paced event without consideration of ventricular events. The AEI is thus lengthened if sensed ventricular activity occurs before the programmed AV delay and there is no increase in the atrial paced rate above the lower rate limit.

The sensing circuits of the atrial and ventricular channels must be enabled and disabled throughout the pacemaker cycle to allow the device to function properly. Sensing in the atrial channel must be controlled to avoid inappropriate sensing of nonatrial events. The atrial channel is refractory during the period beginning with an atrial paced or sensed event and throughout the AV interval (see Figures 26–21 and 26–22). The atrial channel is likewise insensitive for a period of time beginning immediately after sensed or paced ventricular activity (the postventricular atrial refractory period, or PVARP) (see Figure 26–20). Thus the total atrial refractory period is the AV interval plus the PVARP. For many devices the programmable atrial refractory period is the PVARP. The importance of PVARP lies not only in avoiding atrial sensing of ventricular activity but also in avoiding sensing of atrial activity caused by retrograde conduction from a ventricular event. Such retrograde conduction frequently begins with a spontaneous premature ventricular complex and may initiate a acemaker-mediated tachycardia (PMT) or endless-loop tachycardia (see later discussion).

Sensing of the ventricular channel must be completely disabled for a short period during and shortly after the atrial pacing spike. This interval is termed the *postatrial ventricular blanking period* (PAVB in Figure 26–20), during which the device is insensitive to all signals. If it were not for this period, the atrial spike could be sensed as ventricular activity and inhibit ventricular pacing, resulting in so-called cross-talk inhibition (see later discussion). It should be noted that ventricular blanking occurs only with atrial paced and not atrial sensed events.

Following a ventricular paced or sensed event, the ventricular channel is insensitive, the so-called ventricular refractory period. This avoids sensing T waves, which might inhibit subsequent ventricular pacing and would reset the AEI in a device with "V-V" lower rate timing.

The upper tracking limit can be defined either by the duration of the TARP or by a separate timing circuit controlling the ventricular channel.

The upper tracking limit of the dual-chamber pacemaker limits the rate at which ventricular pacing may occur following atrial activity. If atrial activity is sensed and initiates an AV interval that would place a ventricular stimulus earlier than the programmed upper rate limit, the AV interval is extended and the ventricular pulse is delayed until the upper rate limit has been satisfied.

The specifics of the pacemaker features vary among manufacturers and are often programmable. It is essential that such information is known to the ECG interpreter. Without this information, an incorrect diagnosis of pacemaker malfunction may be made. Most DDD pacemakers can be programmed to function in other pacing modes, and adaptive timing cycles can modulate the AV delay and the PVARP. For more details of the DDD pacemaker function, the reader is referred to other texts.[4,27]

MAGNET MODE

As discussed for VVI pacemakers, the application of a magnet against the skin over the implanted pacemaker site serves to reveal the programmed pacing mode, verify capture, and evaluate the status of the pacemaker's power source. The magnet mode also may be helpful for identifying the specific pulse generator, as pacemakers from different manufacturers respond differently to magnet application. Conversely, the specific response to magnet application must be known for each pacemaker to determine whether the response is normal. Otherwise, interpretation of the findings is often erroneous.

Application of a magnet to an AV universal (DDD) pacemaker usually results in asynchronous pacing in both the atrial and ventricular chambers (DOO mode). In some models, magnet application results in asynchronous atrial pacing but ventricular sensing is retained.[28–30] In most devices, however, the atrial and ventricular pacing spikes appear at a specific interval regardless of whether spontaneous complexes are present. The pacing rate and AV interval vary depending on the model and the manufacturer of the pacemaker. A significant decrease from the expected rate usually indicates battery depletion.

Atrial and ventricular capture should occur consistently if there are no spontaneous complexes. They occur intermittently if spontaneous complexes are present and the chambers are stimulated during their refractory periods. Certain DDD pacemakers respond to magnet application with two pacing rates. During the initial part of the magnet mode several complexes are paced at a faster rate, the last being stimulated with

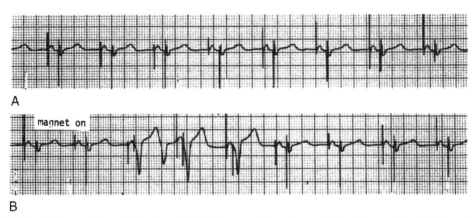

Figure 26–23 Atrioventricular (AV) universal (DDD) pacemaker with and without magnet application. **A,** Tracing recorded without the magnet. The pacing rate is 71 times/min, and the AV interval is 180 ms. There is consistent atrial capture. The ventricular pacing spikes, however, occur at the same time as when spontaneous ventricular depolarization begins, resulting in pseudofusion complexes. **B,** Tracing was obtained while a magnet was applied. There are three pairs of AV stimuli occurring at a rate of 78 times/min with an AV interval of 100 ms (threshold margin test). There is both atrial and ventricular capture. After these three complexes, the pacing rate and AV interval return to the same values seen before the magnet was applied.

reduced pulse width. The AV interval during this period is shortened to avoid competitive depolarization from spontaneous AV conduction (Figure 26–23).

Rate-Responsive Pacing

Rate-responsive pacing is designed to increase the pacing rate and thus the cardiac output in response to increased physical activity.[31–33] A sensor works independently of intrinsic atrial activity. Several types of sensors are available. Those most widely used are vibration- or motion-sensing devices, either a piezoelectric crystal activity sensor fixed to the inside of the pacemaker case or an accelerometer. The crystal detects vibration generated by body motion, and the accelerometer senses motion directly. Circuitry inside the pacemaker then converts these detected vibrations or motion into an increased pacing rate in response to the level of activity being performed.[31–33] Figure 26–24 shows an example of this type of pacemaker.

Other rate-responsive pacemakers have used the right ventricular blood temperature, minute ventilation, the QT interval, mixed venous oxygen saturation, and other physiologic parameters as variables to modulate the pacing rate.[34] Multiple apparent pacing spikes may be recorded from a patient with a pacemaker that senses minute ventilation (Figure 26–25). Some pacemakers use dual sensors (e.g., motion and minute ventilation) in an attempt to provide a more physiologic rate response.

Dual-chamber rate adaptive (DDDR) pacemakers are capable of all modes described for DDD pacemakers. In addition to using P-synchronous pacing as a method for increasing the heart rate, the sensor incorporated in the pacemaker may also drive the increase in heart rate. The resulting rhythm may be sinus driven (alternatively called "P-synchronous") or sensor driven. The relation between the sensor-driven upper rate and the atrial-driven rate can be expressed in three ways: (1) sensor-driven upper rate <atrial-driven upper rate (i.e., a non-useful response); (2) sensor-driven upper rate = atrial-driven upper rate; and (3) sensor-driven upper rate >atrial-driven upper rate, a useful arrangement to avoid tracking of fast atrial rates in patients with bradycardia-tachycardia syndrome and chrontropic incompetence.[4] The ideal patient for DDDR pacing is one with combined sinus and AV node dysfunction, because this mode allows restoration of rate responsiveness and AV synchrony.[27]

DDD PACEMAKER-RELATED ARRHYTHMIAS

Because of the characteristics of the DDD pacemaker, certain tachycardias and irregular rhythms may be seen even though the pacemaker is functioning normally.

Wenckebach Pacemaker Response

The Wenckebach pacemaker response[35,36] is observed when the spontaneous PP interval

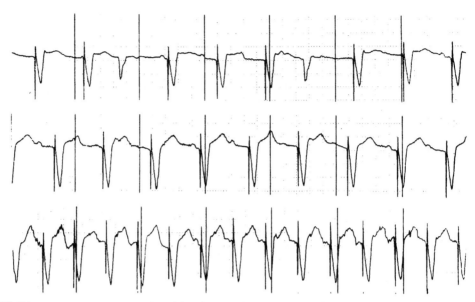

Figure 26–24 Rate-responsive ventricular inhibited pacing (VVI + activity). The tracing was obtained with Holter monitoring. The upper and middle strips show a ventricular pacing rate of 80 times/min. The pacemaker senses and captures properly. The bottom strip was recorded during exercise, and the pacing rate was increased to 124 times/min.

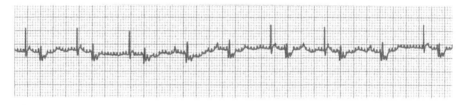

Figure 26–25 Multiple apparent pacing spikes recorded from a patient with a pacemaker that uses a minute ventilation sensor. The pacemaker emits small electrical impulses to measure chest wall impedance. These impulses may be recorded as pseudo-pacing spikes.

(atrial rate) is shorter than the programmed DDD pacemaker upper rate limit, but longer than the TARP. The atrial impulses are sensed (unless they occur during the pacemaker's atrial refractory period), and atrial pacing is inhibited. Ventricular pacing does not occur at the preset AV interval but is delayed until the upper rate limit (the shortest VV interval) is reached (Figure 26–26). Therefore the P-to-V interval is prolonged by an interval that is inversely proportional to the preceding VP interval. This shortening of the VP interval and lengthening of the PV interval is progressive until the P wave falls within the postventricular portion of the atrial refractory period, during which the P wave is not sensed. The unsensed P wave is not followed by a ventricular stimulus. The succeeding P wave, however, is sensed and is followed by ventricular pacing at the programmed AV interval. A long VV interval is observed. The

progressive lengthening of the PV interval until a P wave is no longer followed by a paced QRS complex superficially resembles the Wenckebach type of second-degree AV block.

Pacemaker Circus Movement Tachycardia

The reentry tachycardia occasionally seen in patients with normally functioning DDD, DDR, or VDD pacemakers is sometimes also called *endless-loop tachycardia* (ELT).[37–39] The underlying cause of this pacemaker-induced tachycardia is the presence of retrograde P waves (Figures 26–27 and 26–28). Approximately two thirds of patients with sick sinus syndrome and 20 to 35% of patients with AV block exhibit retrograde VA conduction.[40] The duration of VA conduction ranges from 100 to 300 ms (rarely longer) and is influenced by autonomic tone and drugs.[40a] Only about 5 percent of patients with absent VA

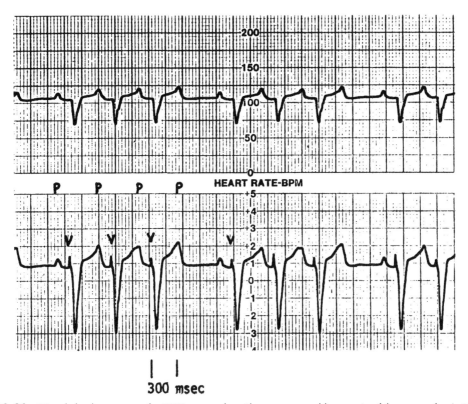

300 msec

Figure 26–26   Wenckebach response of a DDD pacemaker. The programmed lower rate of the pacemaker is 60 and the upper rate 120 pulses/min. The atrioventricular interval is 150 ms, and the postventricular atrial refractory period is 325 ms. The two-channel Holter recording shows that the patient's spontaneous atrial rate is 128 beats/min (PP interval 470 ms). Ventricular pacing occurs at the upper rate limit of 120 pulses/min (VV interval 480 ms) for three beats followed by a pause. There is progressive lengthening of the PV interval and shortening of the VP interval until the pause occurs. The last VP interval before the pause measures 300 ms. The P wave preceding the pause therefore falls within the postventricular atrial refractory period and is not sensed. Ventricular pacing is not triggered until the next P wave appears and the same sequence is repeated.

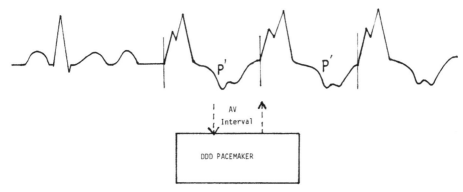

Figure 26–27   Genesis of pacemaker-induced reentry tachycardia. The retrograde P wave (P′) of a paced beat is sensed by the DDD pacemaker and induces delivery of a ventricular stimulus at the end of the programmed atrioventricular interval. The pacemaker serves as a bypass to initiate and perpetuate a reentry tachycardia.

conduction before implantantion acquire VA conduction after pacemaker implantation.[41] Retrograde atrial depolarization is sensed by the atrial component of the pacemaker, which in turn triggers programmed delivery of a ventricular stimulus, resulting in a paced QRS complex with retrograde atrial capture. The same reentrant event repeats itself, resulting in ELT in patients with persistent VA conduction. The rate of the tachycardia cannot exceed the upper rate limit

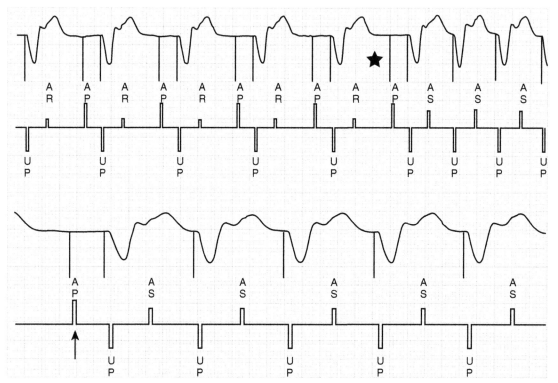

Figure 26–28 DDD pacing and endless-loop tachycardia induced by loss of atrial capture. ECG and marker channel. Lower rate interval = 857 ms; atrioventricular (AV) delay = 200 ms after atrial pacing and 150 ms after atrial sensing; post-ventricular atrial refractory period (PVARP) = 300 ms; upper rate interval = 500 ms. Subthreshold atrial stimulation (AP). Ventricular pacing causes retrograde VA conduction. *Left,* The retrograde P waves fall within the PVARP and are depicted as AR by the marker channel. AR events cannot initiate an AV delay. The PVARP was shortened to 200 ms at the asterisk. The pacemaker then senses the retrograde P wave (AS) and initiates endless-loop tachycardia. (Reproduced with permission from Barold SS, Zipes PD: Cardiac pacemakers and antiarrhythmic devices. *In:* Braunwald E [ed]: Heart Diseases. A Textbook of Cardiovascular Medicine, 5th ed. Philadelphia, Saunders, 1997, pp 705–741.)

programmed for the pacemaker. Lengthening of the atrial refractory period of the pacemaker may decrease the incidence of this complication. Most devices are capable of extending the PVARP after a sensed ventricular event (a premature ventricular complex) to prevent sensing a retrograde P wave. Shortening of AV delay is also useful. Additionally, termination of the tachycardia may occur with a programming feature that allows the device to block sensing of atrial activity periodically when the atrial rate exceeds a preset limit. This feature terminates the endless-loop tachycardia; but if it is sinus tachycardia, only a single ventricular stimulus is omitted, an event not likely to be noted by the patient. Endless-loop tachycardia can also be terminated by applying a magnet over the pacemaker.

Repetitive VA synchrony can also occur in the DDD or DDR mode when the retrograde P wave is unsensed, but the pacemaker continually delivers an ineffectual atrial stimulus that causes an additional ventricular paced complex following each paced ventricular complex. This arrhythmia is often labeled as *non-reentrant.*[41]

OTHER CAUSES OF TACHYCARDIA

Different types of supraventricular tachycardia may induce a variety of pacemaker responses when automatic switching mode is not programmed. A rapid and irregular ventricular rate suggests atrial fibrillation or atrial flutter, provided a defective atrial lead can be ruled out.

Pacemaker tachycardia triggered by myopotentials sensed by the atrial channel of a unipolar DDD pacemaker can be regular or irregular. Sensor-driven tachycardia is rare with accelerometers used in contemporary pacemakers.

OVERDRIVE SUPPRESSION

Overdrive suppression (see Chapter 13) can occur after cessation of pacing.

VENTRICULAR RESYNCHRONIZATION (BIVENTRICULAR PACING)

Ventricular resynchronization with biventricular pacing has become an established therapy for patients with LV dysfunction of various etiology, in particular in the presence of established ventricular asynchrony due to intraventricular conduction disturbances.[42,43,43a] To interpret the ECG during the follow-up of the biventricular pacing, it has been suggested to record four 12-lead ECGs at the time of implantation: (1) intrinsic rhythm, (2) RV paced rhythm, (3) LV paced rhythm, and (4) biventricular paced rhythm.[16]

Biventricular devices permit programming of interventricular interval, usually in steps from +80 ms (LV first) to −80 ms (RV first) in order to optimize hemodynamic function. In the absence of anodal stimulation, increasing the VV interval gradually to +80 ms will progressively widen the QRS complex and alter its morphology by increasing the R wave amplitude in lead V_1. As pointed out by Barold,[44] the varying configuration of QRS in lead V_1 cannot be correlated with the hemodynamic response, and the degree of QRS narrowing is a poor predictor of the mechanical cardiac synchronization.[16]

Evaluation of the ECG pattern of biventricular pacing focuses on simultaneous RV and LV stimulation. The paced QRS complex is often less wide than the QRS complex caused by single-chamber pacing. Loss of capture in one ventricle will cause a change in the morphology of ventricular paced complexes in the 12-lead ECG by displaying ventricular complexes generated by either single-chamber RV or single-chamber LV pacing (see earlier discussion). Also, a shift in the frontal plane axis may be useful in corroborating the loss of capture in one of the ventricles.

During biventricular pacing the QRS complex is often positive in lead V_1 when the RV is paced from the apex. A negative QRS complex in the V_1 position may be caused by lack of LV capture, LV lead displacement, increased latency, or changes in ventricular substrate (e.g., ischemia, scar).

MINIMIZING RV PACING

The recently discovered harmful effects of chronic RV pacing prompted a search for procedures aimed at minimizing its impact. Programmed AV delays and automatic mode switching from DDDR to AAIR represent some of these attempts (Figure 26–29). The reader is referred to other texts for more details.[45,46,46a] In some patients, His bundle stimulation can be satisfactorily performed to synchronize the ventricular contraction.[47]

Adaptive AV Delay, Rate Hysteresis, Fallback Response, Rate Smoothing, Rate-Responsive AV Delay, Mode Switching, Autocapture

Adaptive AV delay is a feature included in some of the DDD pacemakers. With this feature the pacemaker shortens the sensed AV intervals with increasing atrial rate within a programmable range of rates, thereby mimicking the physiologic response of the PR intervals. The purpose of this feature is to provide equivalent AV hemodynamic intervals for spontaneous or paced atrial contractions. It is assumed that the atrial electrode senses the intrinsic atrial impulse after atrial contraction has already begun. Therefore a shorter sensed AV interval provides the same mechanical time sequence generated by a paced atrial beat with a longer paced AV interval.

Adaptive dynamic PVARP with atrial sensing is another provision for adaptation to different atrial rates (see earlier discussion).

Rate hysteresis is present when the pacemaker's escape interval is longer than the pacing interval (Figure 26–30). This feature is provided to allow the patient's own sinus rhythm, which is more physiologic, to be maintained at a lower rate than the pacing rate. In contemporary pacemakers, hysteresis is coupled with a search function that looks for intrinsic activity by periodically extending one or more pacing cycles to the hysteresis interval. If the device then detects intrinsic activity, it will be inhibited and will begin to function at the hysteresis rate. If no intrinsic activity is sensed, pacing will resume at the programmed rate.

In certain pacemakers a *fallback response* is included to limit the time during which the ventricular rate remains at the programmed upper rate.[48] This option is designed to be used in patients who cannot tolerate a sustained upper rate. The response is activated by detection of an atrial rate faster than the programmed upper rate. The fallback mechanism then gradually returns the ventricular rate to more tolerable levels. AV synchrony may or may not be maintained during the fallback response.

Rate smoothing is a programmable option available in some DDD pacemakers. It is designed to eliminate pronounced variations in the ventricular pacing cycle length while tracking atrial activity. It is intended for patients who cannot tolerate marked fluctuations of paced rate. The maximum change in the pacing rate from cycle to cycle is limited to some percentage of the previous RR interval.

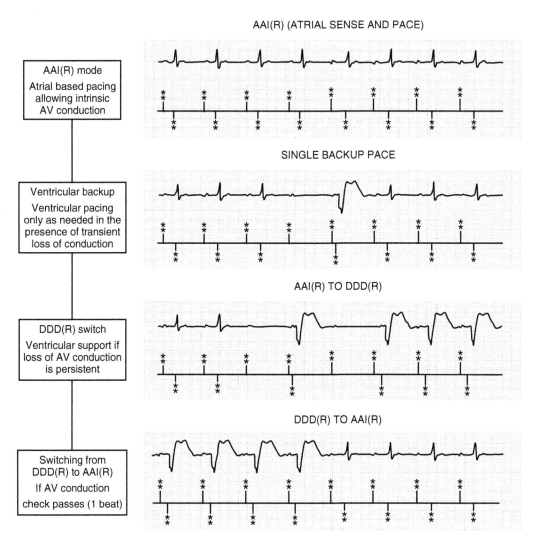

Figure 26–29 ECGs showing the function of Managed Ventricular Pacing (Medtronic) to minimize the impact of right ventricular pacing. AP = atrial paced event; AS = atrial sensed event; V = ventricular paced event; VS = ventricular sensed event. (Courtesy of Medtronic, Inc.)

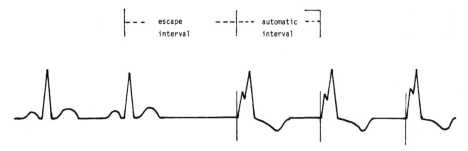

Figure 26–30 Hysteresis. Note the longer escape interval after the spontaneous complexes. Once pacing begins, the rate returns to the programmed automatic rate.

Rate-responsive AV delay allows shortening of the AV interval at faster tracked or paced atrial rates. This allows for more physiologic AV synchrony and higher programmable upper rate limits without shortening the postventricular atrial refractory period.

Mode switching during DDD pacing is also available in many devices. The device can be programmed to behave as a typical AV universal pacemaker until atrial rates exceed those expected for sinus rhythm. Under this condition, the device switches to VVI or DDI mode, usually with rate modulation. This avoids rapid ventricular pacing during atrial arrhythmias.

Autocapture allows the pacemaker to adjust stimulation output according to continuously monitored capture thresholds,[48] decreasing overall current consumption and prolonging the pacemaker's service life. The pacemaker confirms capture while decreasing the amplitude of the pacing stimulus. When capture is not confirmed, the pacemaker delivers a higher-amplitude output pulse shortly after the ineffective pulse. This results in two pacing artifacts preceding the QRS complex on the ECG.

Pacing Failure

Pacing failure (output failure or failure to capture) cannot be recognized if the patient's rhythm is spontaneous with a ventricular rate faster than the pacemaker's preset pacing rate. A magnet may be applied to convert the pacemaker to the fixed-rate mode, and pacing can be examined. In some patients, slowing of the intrinsic heart rate may be accomplished by carotid sinus stimulation to allow the pacemaker to escape. Such a procedure, however, is associated with the potential risk of ventricular asystole if pacing malfunction does exist.

With most pacemakers, a change in the pacing rate due to battery depletion appears earlier in the magnet mode than during automatic pacing. This is frequently a planned indication for pacemaker replacement. Slowing of the automatic pacing rate may be due to malfunction from further battery depletion (Figure 26–31) and in most pacemakers is an indication for urgent pulse generator replacement. With modern pacemakers, a marked increase in the pacing rate (runaway pacemaker) is seldom seen as a sign of battery depletion.

Pacing malfunction also may manifest as failure of the pacemaker impulse to depolarize the ventricles. The failure may be permanent or intermittent and may be caused by inadequate voltage output from the pulse generator, wire fracture, electrode displacement, or an increase in the stimulation threshold at the site of the electrode. Functional failure to capture may also be seen if the pacemaker impulse occurs during the myocardial refractory period (see Figure 26–11).

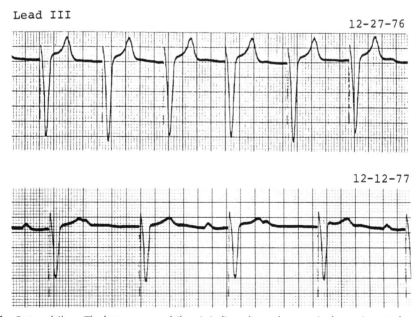

Figure 26–31 Battery failure. The battery power failure is indicated as a decrease in the pacing rate from 70 to 47 beats/min.

Myocardial perforation occasionally is res pon-sible for pacing failure and occurs most frequently during the first few weeks after implantation. An RV endocardial lead may perforate the interventricular septum or, more commonly, the free wall of the right ventricle. The electrode may migrate and rest on the epicardial surface of the left ventricle. On the ECG the morphology of paced complexes may change from an LBBB pattern to an RBBB-like pattern. Indeed, if such morphologic changes occur spontaneously in a patient with an RV transvenous electrode, the diagnosis of myocardial perforation should be suspected (see Figure 26–10).

ECG Signs of Malfunction of Ventricular Pacing

Although other procedures may be employed to evaluate the functions of ventricular pace-makers, only findings detectable by routine ECG are discussed here. Pacemaker malfunction may involve abnormalities of sensing, capture, or heart rate.[49] Loss of sensing ability usually occurs before loss of pacing ability.[50] The source of malfunction may be in the pulse generator, in the lead, at the junction of the cardiac tissue with the electrode, or at the junction of the lead with the pulse generator. The VVI pacing mode is discussed here.

UNDERSENSING

When a ventricular pacemaker in the demand (VVI) mode has completely lost its ability to sense, it performs like a fixed-rate asynchronous pacemaker (Figure 26–32). Such dysfunction cannot be detected if the patient has consistent bradycardia and spontaneous ventricular complexes are absent. In some patients, exercise or drug use accelerate the heart rate, expose spontaneous QRS complexes, and allow one to determine the sensing ability of the pacemaker. In some instances the undersensing is intermittent and may or may not be associated with pacing failure.

The most common cause of undersensing is a low-amplitude electrogram (Figure 26–33). With newly implanted pacing leads, the electrical potential to be sensed may be too low because of underlying myocardial scar, inadequate myocardial or endocardial contact, poor orientation of a bipolar electrode, or inappropriate programming of amplifier sensitivity.[20] Injury current resulting from lead placement, especially seen with active fixation leads, may disturb the rate of discharge (dV/dT) and interfere with sensing.

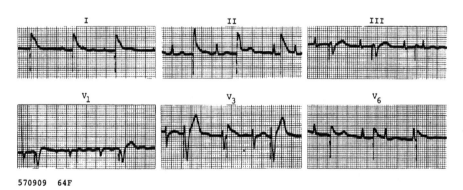

570909   64F

Figure 26–32 Ventricular demand pacemaker (VVI) with sensing malfunction. The pacemaker operates like a fixed-rate pacemaker. The spontaneous ventricular complexes are not sensed. The spontaneous rhythm is atrial fibrillation.

INSPIRATION

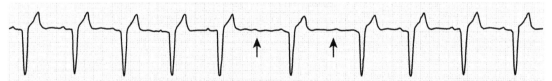

Figure 26–33 Loss of atrial sensing (arrows) during deep inspiration caused by decreased P wave amplitude. (Reproduced with permission from Barold SS, Falkoff MD, Ong TS, et al: Electrocardiography of contemporary DDD pacemakers. In Barold SS, Mugica J [eds]: New Perspectives of Cardiac Pacing. Mount Kisco, NY, Futura, 1988.)

Later loss of signal potential may be the result of acute MI, formation of an insulating fibrous capsule around the electrode, or myocardial perforation with the electrode having migrated to a poor signal area.[24] Hyperkalemia, slow conduction caused by certain types of antiarrhythmic drugs, and cardioversion-defibrillation can also cause transient undersensing.[51] Broken leads or wire insulation tears with current leakage have become less common with the improved quality of the lead wire and insulation.

Findings that may be mistaken for undersensing have been discussed previously, including fusion, pseudofusion, and certain unsensed ventricular ectopic complexes. Artifact caused by recorders that simulate the pacing spike can also be mistaken for undersensing. Functional atrial undersensing with a normally functioning pacemaker is quite common when it occurs during long or extended PVARP.

OVERSENSING

Oversensing of physiologic intracardiac voltage may occur when tall P or T waves may be mistaken for R waves and thereby cause inappropriate triggering with resetting of the pacemaker[23]

(Figure 26–34). Mistaken doubling of the heart rate may occur in the presence of tall, peaked T waves, such as in hyperkalemia. Another cause of oversensing is the myopotential (see next discussion).

MYOPOTENTIAL SENSING

Myopotentials represent electrical activity originating in skeletal muscle. Oversensing of myopotentials occurs almost invariably with unipolar pulse generators. Most myopotential interference originates from the deltopectoral region at the site of a unipolar pacemaker.[52–56] A unipolar ventricular pacemaker may sense such myopotentials and can inhibit ventricular pacing for variable time periods. In a DDD channel myopotential interference is more common in the atrial channel, resulting in a rhythm disturbance. An example is shown in Figure 26–35. Myopotential inhibition in a bipolar pacing system suggests faulty lead insulation.

ABNORMAL LATENCY

The delay from a pacing stimulus to the evoked potential is called *latency*, which is normally <40 ms. Increased latency can be simulated by

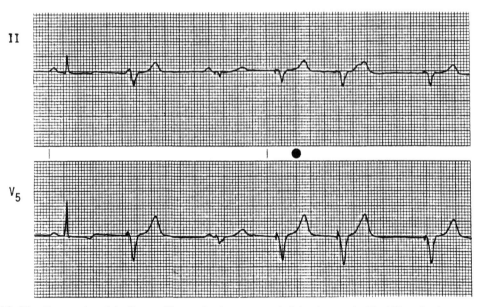

Figure 26–34   Oversensing of the T wave. The two leads were recorded simultaneously. The VVI pacing is programmed to have a pacing rate of 70 beats/min. The first QRS complex is spontaneously conducted. The second, fourth, fifth, and sixth QRS complexes are paced. The third QRS complex is a fusion complex. The spike-to-spike interval of the fourth and fifth complexes is 860 ms, which is the equivalent of the programmed pacing rate. The spike-to-spike interval of the fifth and sixth complexes is much longer. However, the interval between the last pacing spike and the apex of the preceding T wave is 860 ms. The delay of the last pacing spike is therefore most likely the result of sensing of the preceding T wave. The long spike-to-spike interval that involves the second and third complexes can be explained on the same basis.

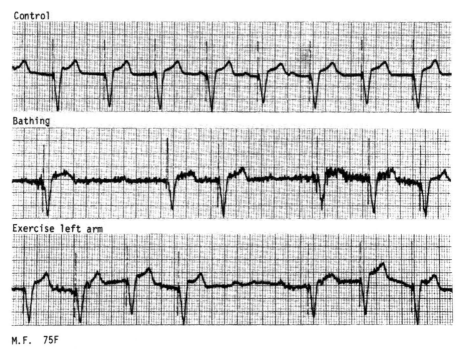

Control

Bathing

Exercise left arm

M.F.   75F

Figure 26–35   Myopotential inhibition of ventricular demand pacing (VVI). The ECG was obtained during telemetry monitoring. In the control tracing obtained while the patient was inactive, the pacemaker is pacing regularly at a rate of 73 beats/min. Intermittent inhibition of the pacemaker occurred while the patient was taking a shower and during left arm exercise. Baseline artifacts due to skeletal muscle potential are present. The pulse generator was implanted overlying the pectoralis muscle, and the lead was unipolar.

an isoelectric onset of the QRS complex in one or more leads. Consequently diagnosis of abnormal latency requires a 12-lead ECG. Abnormalities of latency are caused either by structural myocardial changes (e.g., myocardial ischemia or scar) or by functional reversible abnormalities (e.g., hyperkalemia, antiarrhythmic drugs).

Increased atrial latency is caused usually by atrial disease. The delayed P wave onset results in the delayed mechanical response and suboptimal mechanical AV synchrony.

ELECTROMAGNETIC INTERFERENCE

Electromagnetic interference causing oversensing may come from nonphysiologic sources such as radar, television, and radio transmitters. Electrocautery may inhibit the pacemaker output if it is used within a few inches of the pulse generator. Microwave ovens and weapon detector equipment no longer cause potential problems for proper function of modern pacemakers. Reports have indicated that handheld cellular telephones used in the proximity of permanent pacemakers may interfere with their function.[57,58] Although their effects are not restricted to the sensing

function, it is pertinent to mention that therapeutic irradiation and direct-current countershock applied externally or from a co-implanted cardioverter/defibrillator may damage or reset the pulse generator.[59]

ECG Signs of Malfunction of the AV Universal (DDD) Pacemakers

As in the case of VVI pacemakers, malfunction of DDD pacemakers may be manifested by undersensing or oversensing, an absence of pacing stimuli when expected, a slowed or increased pacing rate, or failure to capture. Those problems that involve only the ventricular channel (see above) and are common to both modes of pacing are not repeated here.

The ECG diagnosis of DDD pacemaker malfunction is usually more difficult because the characteristics of the pulse generators vary with the manufacturer and the different models from the same manufacturer. Misinterpretation of pacemaker malfunction often occurs when the specifics of these characteristics are not known to the electrocardiographer. It also occurs if the interpreter is not informed about the parameters (e.g., pacing rate, pacing mode) that have been reprogrammed since the previous tracing.

Atrial undersensing is one of the most common problems with DDD pacing.[60] It may be due to poor electrode location, lead dislodgement, inadequate P wave amplitude, or problems that involve the lead itself and the pulse generator.

Myopotential interference occurs frequently with unipolar DDD pacemakers, as discussed earlier.[61–63]

CROSS TALK

Unique to the DDD (and DVI) pacemakers is the phenomenon of cross talk, or self-inhibition.[64,65] Cross talk is the inappropriate sensing by one channel of electrical events generated in the other channel (see Figures 26–17 and 26–20). This is seen more commonly as detection of atrial activity or atrial stimulus by the ventricular lead. Sensing of the ventricular stimulus by the atrial lead is obviated by inactivation of atrial sensing after ventricular pacing, but sensing of spontaneous ventricular activity in the atrial lead is another example of cross talk. Depending on the system, cross talk can cause shortening of the paced AV delay and increase the pacing rate. Alternatively it can prolong the interval between the atrial stimulus and the succeeding conducted QRS complex to a value greater than the programmed AV delay.[65]

Most contemporary DDD pacemakers minimize the possibility of cross talk by including the previously described ventricular blanking period after the atrial stimulus. During the ventricular blanking period (usually 10 to 60 ms after the atrial stimulus), no signal can be detected. The ventricular channel then "opens" after this short blanking period so that ventricular sensing can occur during the remainder of the AV delay. Another protective mechanism, known as *ventricular safety pacing*, complements the blanking period but does not prevent cross talk. It merely offsets its consequences. Any event sensed by the ventricular lead during this time triggers ventricular pacing at the end of the triggering period. If this sensed event was "cross talk" from the atrium, ventricular pacing ensures the presence of ventricular activity. If, on the other hand, the sensed event was truly ventricular activity, the ventricular pacing spike falls shortly afterward and probably during ventricular depolarization rather than at the end of the programmed AV delay, avoiding the vulnerable period of the ventricle (Figure 26–36).

▌ Pacemaker Syndrome

According to Barold,[66] the pacemaker syndrome is a clinical problem caused by improper timing of atrial and ventricular contractions precipitating reduced cardiac output and hypotension. The resulting symptoms may be present in about 10 to 20 percent of patients with VVI pacemakers, often in association with retrograde VA conduction. The obvious clinical manifestations

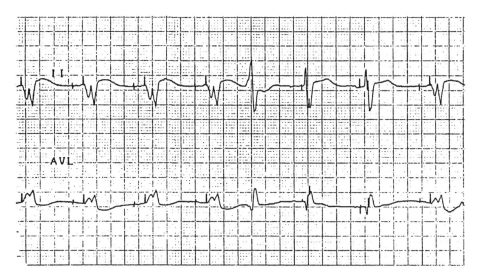

Figure 26–36 Safety pacing. The fifth and sixth QRS complexes are sensed during the early portion of the atrioventricular (AV) interval, and the pacemaker delivers a ventricular stimulus at the conclusion of a shortened AV interval. This stimulus falls during the ventricular refractory period and before the vulnerable period.

include signs and symptoms of heart failure, but there are often subtle manifestations that can be missed. The treatment of pacemaker syndrome is restoration of appropriate AV synchrony and optimizing the AV delay in patients with DDD pacemakers. The MOST study investigators reported severe pacemaker syndrome in nearly 20 percent of VVIR-paced patients who improved with reprogramming to the dual-chamber pacing, and suggested that atrial-based pacemakers be implanted in all patients.[67] However, the meta-analysis of randomized trials showed that, compared with ventricular pacing, the use of atrial-based pacing did not improve survival and cardiac morbidity except for modest reduction of the incidence of atrial fibrillation.[68] For further information the reader is referred to other pertinent studies.[69,70]

Ambulatory Monitoring in Patients with Pacemakers

In general, Holter or event monitoring in pacemaker patients is more useful in the investigation of unexplained symptoms, such as syncope or palpitations[71,72] than in the evaluation of pacemaker function after an unrevealing thorough evaluation in the pacemaker clinic. Asymptomatic lead malfunction, however, may be demonstrated more reliably by Holter monitoring than in the clinic.[73] In routine Holter recordings, the most common abnormalities consist of atrial undersensing and myopotential interference in unipolar systems. The reliable interpretation of recordings from DDD pacemakers may be difficult.

A system that enhances the pacemaker stimulus (and displays it on a separate channel) may be useful. Presently, the pacemaker itself can function as an implantable Holter system.[74,75] The development of electrogram storage and retrieval by pacemakers has added a new dimension to the diagnosis of arrhythmias in patients with pacemakers. The system enables the storage of electrograms with separate channels for atrial and ventricular activity as well as the recording of the onsets and the offsets of the events of interest, which have included detection of tonic-clonic seizures.[76] Also, recent developments have allowed for wireless transmission of pacemaker and lead data. It is anticipated that the memory function will help to facilitate the programming of increasingly complex devices.

POSTPACING T WAVE CHANGES

In patients with artificial ventricular pacemakers, postpacing T wave inversions in the spontaneous complexes may simulate myocardial ischemia. These changes are discussed in Chapters 4 and 23 (see Figures 23–8 and 23–9).

DIAGNOSIS OF MI DURING VENTRICULAR PACING

The QRS complexes generated by right ventricular pacing resemble LBBB, except for the initial forces. Therefore the ST segment and T wave criteria for diagnosis of myocardial ischemia described in Chapter 4 are applicable to the paced RV complexes.[77–79] Thus Sgarbossa et al.[78] proposed the following criteria for the diagnosis of acute injury pattern in the paced ventricular complex: (1) ST elevation ≥5 mm discordant with the QRS complex; (2) ST elevation >1 mm concordant with the QRS complex; and (3) ST depression >1 mm in lead V_1, V_2, or V_3 (Figures 26–37 and 26–38). These findings are associated with a sensitivity of 18 to 53 percent and specificity of 88 to 94 percent.

Pacing from a location at or near to the RV apex can produce a qR pattern in leads I and aV_L, where q wave duration is usually ≤3 ms. The left precordial leads, however, display R, Rs, rS, or QS complexes, and an initial q wave in these leads suggests the presence of a prior

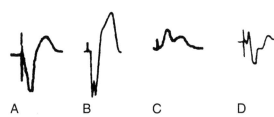

Figure 26–37 Characteristic ECG changes associated with acute myocardial infarction according to Sgarbossa et al.[28] **A,** Normal, expected QRS complex/ST-T wave discordance. **B,** Discordant ST elevation >5 mm. **C,** Concordant ST elevation >1 mm. **D,** ST depression >1 mm in leads V_1, V_2, or V_3. (From Kozlowski FH, Brady WJ, Aufderheide TP, et al: The electrocardiographic diagnosis of acute myocardial infarction in patients with ventricularly paced rhythms. Acad Emerg Med 5:52, 1998.)

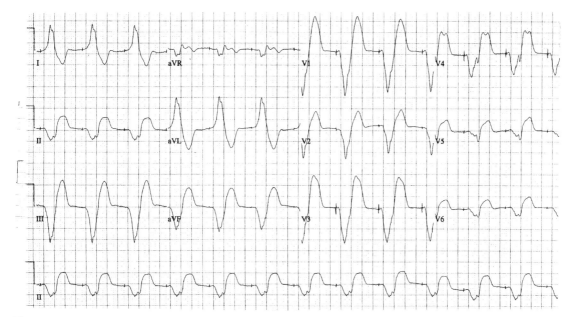

Figure 26–38 Ventricular pacing in a patient with extensive anterior myocardial infarction. There is marked ST segment elevation and absent R waves in leads V_1–V_6. Notching of the upstroke of the QRS complex (Cabrera's sign) is noted in V_4.

anterior MI. The St-qR pattern (*St* refers to the pacing stimulus) in the lateral precordial leads has a specificity approaching 100 percent for anterior MI.[79] Late notching of the ascending limb of the QRS complex in the left precordial leads (Cabrera's sign) (see Figure 26–38) is also highly specific for prior anterior MI.[80]

Inferior MI is more difficult to detect than anterior MI because the QS pattern in the inferior leads is normally recorded during RV apical pacing. A QR or Qr pattern in the inferior leads,

however, does not occur during normal RV pacing and is highly specific for MI (Figure 26–39). An rS pattern in lead aV_R may also be seen with inferior MI but is not specific.[79]

ABNORMALLY WIDE QRS COMPLEX

The very long (e.g., >160 ms) QRS duration of the paced ventricular complex is associated with increased incidence of heart failure and increased mortality.[81,82] It has been found that the risk

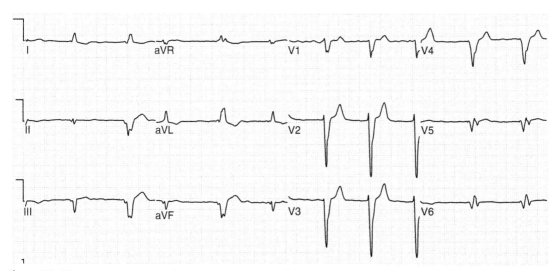

Figure 26–39 Intermittent ventricular pacing in a patient with history of previous inferior and lateral myocardial infarction (MI) caused by occlusion of the dominant left circumflex artery. MI can be recognized in paced complexes by wide Q waves in leads V_5–V_6 and a QS pattern in leads II, III, and aV_F.

increases progressively for each 10-ms increase in the QRS duration of the paced complex.[81]

Reversible widening of QRS complex occurs during treatment with certain antiarrhythmic drugs (see Chapter 22) and during hyperkalemia, which can be suspected in the presence of tall and sometimes peaked T waves and low-amplitude or absent P waves.

REFERENCES

1. Zoll PM: Resuscitation of the heart in ventricular standstill by external electric stimulation. N Engl J Med 247:768, 1952.
2. Birnie D, Williams K, Guo A, et al: Reasons for escalating pacemaker implants. Am J Cardiol 98:93, 2006.
3. Bernstein AD, Fletcher DJC, Hayes DL, et al: The revised NASPE/BPEG generic code for antibradycardia, adaptive-rate, and multisite pacing. North American Society for Pacing and Electrophysiology Group. Pacing Clin Electrophysiol 25:260, 2002.
4. Barold SS: Timing cycles and operatonal characteristics of pacemakers. In: Ellenbogen KA, Kay GN, Wilkoff BL (eds): Clinical Cardiac Pacing and Defibrillation, 2nd ed. Philadelphia, Saunders, 2000, pp 727–825.
5. Fontaine JM, Ursell S, El-Sherif N: Electrocardiography of single-chamber pacemakers. In: El-Sherif N, Samet P (eds): Cardiac Pacing and Electrophysiology. Philadelphia, Saunders, 1991, pp 568–598.
6. Garson A: Stepwise approach to the unknown pacemaker ECG. Am Heart J 119:924, 1990.
7. Hayes DL: Pacemaker electrocardiography. In: Furman S, Hayes DL, Holmes DR (eds): A Practice of Cardiac Pacing. Mount Kisco NY, Futura, 1993, pp 309–359.
8. Kusumoto FM, Goldschlager N: Cardiac pacing. N Engl J Med 334:89, 1996.
9. Anderson HR, Nielsen JC, Thomsen PEB, et al: Long-term follow up of patients from a randomised trial of atrial versus ventricular pacing in sick-sinus syndrome. Lancet 350:1210, 1997.
10. Connolly SJ, Kerr C, Gent M, et al: Dual-chamber versus ventricular pacing: critical appraisal of current data. Circulation 94:578, 1996.
11. Hayes DL, Levine PA: Pacemaker timing cycles. In: Ellenbogen KA, Wood MA (eds): Cardiac Pacing and ICDs, 4th ed. Malden, MA, Blackwell, 2005, pp 265–321.
12. Gregoratos G, Cheitlin MD, Freedman RA, et al: ACC/AHA Guidelines for implantation of cardiac pacemakers and antiarrhythmia devices. J Am Coll Cardiol 31:1175, 1998.
13. Saksena S, Prakash A, Hill M, et al: Prevention of recurrent atrial fibrillation with chronic dual-site right atrial pacing. J Am Coll Cardiol 28:687, 1996.
14. Kruse I, Ryden L, Duffin EL: Clinical evaluation of atrial synchronous ventricular inhibited pacemakers. PACE 3:641, 1980.
15. Castellanos A, Ortiz JM, Pastis N, et al: The electrocardiogram in patients with pacemakers. Prog Cardiovasc Dis 13:190, 1970.
16. Barold SS, Giudici MC, Herweg B, et al: Diagnostic value of the 12-lead electrocardiogram during conventional and biventricular pacing for cardiac resynchronization. Cardiol Clin 24:471, 2006.
17. Coman JA, Trohman RG: Incidence and electrocardiographic localization of safe right bundle branch block configurations during permanent ventricular pacing. Am J Cardiol 76:781, 1995.
18. Buckingham TA: Right ventricular outflow tract pacing. PACE 20:1237, 1997.
19. Chardack WM, Gage AA, Greatbatch W: A transistorized self-contained implantable pacemaker for the long-term correction of complete heart block. Surgery 48:663, 1960.
20. Zoll PM, Linenthal AJ: Long-term electrical pacemakers for Stokes-Adams disease. Circulation 22:341, 1960.
21. Escher DJW: Types of pacemakers and their complications. Circulation 47:1119, 1973.
22. Gould L, Venkataraman K, Goswami MK, et al: Pacemaker-induced electrocardiographic changes simulating myocardial infarction. Chest 63:829, 1973.
23. Barold SS, Gaidula JJ: Evaluation of normal and abnormal sensing functions of demand pacemakers. Am J Cardiol 28:201, 1971.
24. Vera Z, Mason DT, Awan NA, et al: Lack of sensing by demand pacemakers due to intraventricular conduction defects. Circulation 51:815, 1975.
25. Barold SS, Falkoff MD, Ong LS, et al: Characterization of pacemaker arrhythmia due to normally functioning AV demand (DVI) pulse generators. Pacing Clin Electrophysiol 3:712, 1980.
26. Hauser RG: The electrocardiography of AV universal DDD pacemakers. PACE 6:399, 1983.
27. Hayes DL, Zipes DP: Cardiac pacemakers and cardioverter-defibrillators In: Braunwald E, Zipes DP, Libby P (eds): Heart Diseases. Textbook of Cardiovascular Medicine. Philadelphia, Saunders, 2001, pp 775–817.
28. Barold SS, Falkoff MD, Ong LS, et al: Timing cycles of DDD pacemakers. In: Barold SS, Mugica J (eds): New Perspectives in Cardiac Pacing. Mount Kisco, NY, Futura, 1988, pp 69–119.
29. Stokes KB, Kay GN: Artificial electrical stimulation. In: Ellenbogen KA, Kay GN, Wilkoff BL (eds): Clinical Cardiac Pacing and Defibrillation, 2nd ed. Philadelphia, Saunders, 2000, pp 17–52.
30. Hayes DL, Higano ST, Eisinger G: Electrocardiographic manifestations of a dual-chamber, rate-modulated (DDDR) pacemaker. PACE 12:555, 1989.
31. Benditt DG, Mianulli M, Fetter J, et al: Single-chamber cardiac pacing with activity-initiated chronotropic response: evaluation by cardiopulmonary exercise testing. Circulation 75:184, 1987.
32. Dulk KD, Bouwels L, Lindemans F, et al: The activitrax rate responsive pacemaker system. Am J Cardiol 61:107, 1988.
33. Dumen DP, Kostuk WJ, Klein GJ: Activity-sensing, rate-responsive pacing: improvement in myocardial performance with exercise. PACE 8:52, 1985.
34. Fearnot NE, Smith HJ, Geddes LA: A review of pacemakers that physiologically increase rate: the DDD and rate-responsive pacemakers. Prog Cardiovasc Dis 29:145, 1986.
35. Barold SS, Falkoff MD, Ong LS, et al: Basic concepts, upper rate response, retrograde ventriculoatrial conduction, and differential diagnosis of pacemaker tachycardias. In: Saksena S, Goldschlager N (eds): Electrical Therapy for Cardiac Pacing. Philadelphia, Saunders, 1990, p 215.
36. Sutton R, Perrins EJ, Duffin E: Interpretation of dual chamber pacemaker electrocardiograms. PACE 8:6, 1985.
37. Furman S: Newer modes of cardiac pacing. Mod Concepts Cardiovasc Dis 52:1, 1983.
38. Furman S, Fisher JD: Endless loop tachycardia in an AV universal (DDD) pacemaker. PACE 5:486, 1982.
39. Rubin JW, Frank MJ, Boineau JP, et al: Current physiologic pacemakers: a serious problem with a new device. Am J Cardiol 52:88, 1983.

40. Hayes DL, Furman S: Atrio-ventricular and ventriculo-atrial conduction times in patients undergoing pacemaker implantation. Pacing Clin Electrophysiol 6:38, 1983.

40a. Hariman RJ, Pasquariello JL, Gomes JA, et al: Autonomic dependence of ventriculoatrial conduction. Am J Cardiol 56:285, 1985.

41. Barold SS, Levine PA: Pacemaker repetitive nonreentrant ventriculoatrial synchronous rhythm. A review. Interv Card Electrophysiol 5:45, 2001.

42. Daubert JC, Ritter P, LeBreton H, et al: Permanent left ventricular pacing with transvenous leads inserted into the coronary sinus. PACE 21:239, 1998.

43. Jais P, Douard H, Shah DC, et al: Endocardial biventricular pacing. PACE 21:2128, 1998.

43a. Bleeker GB, Mollema SA, Holman ER, et al: Left ventricular resynchronization is mandatory for response to cardiac resynchronization therapy. Circulation 116:1440, 2007.

44. Barold SS: Adverse effects of ventricular desynchronization induced by long-term right ventricular pacing. J Am Coll Cardiol 42:624, 2003.

45. Melzer C, Sowelam S, Sheldon TJ, et al: Reduction of right ventricular pacing in patients with sinus node dysfunction using an enhanced search AV algorithm. Pacing Clin Electrophysiol 28:521, 2005.

46. Sweeney MO, Prinzen FW: A new paradigm for physiologic ventricular pacing. J Am Coll Cardiol 47:282, 2006.

46a. Sweeney MO, Bank AJ, Nsah E, et al: Minimizing ventricular pacing to reduce atrial fibrillation in sinus node disease. N Engl J Med 357:1000, 2007.

47. Orchetta A, Bortnik M, Magnani A, et al: Prevention of ventricular desynchronization by permanent para-Hisian pacing after atrioventricular node ablation in chronic atrial fibrillation. J Am Coll Cardiol 47:1938, 2006.

48. Clarke M, Liu B, Schuller H, et al: Automatic adjustment of pacemaker stimulation output correlated with continuously monitored capture thresholds: a multicenter study. PACE 21:1567, 1998.

49. Hayes DL, Vlietstra RE: Pacemaker malfunction. Ann Intern Med 119:828, 1993.

50. Parsonnet V, Myers GH, Gilbert L, et al: Prediction of impending pacemaker failure in a pacemaker clinic. Am J Cardiol 25:311, 1970.

51. Barold SS, McVenes R, Stokes K: Effect of drugs on pacing threshold in man and canines: old and new facts. In: Barold SS, Mugica J (eds): New Perspectives in Cardiac Pacing. Mount Kisco, NY, Futura, 1993 pp 57–83.

52. Breivik K, Ohm OJ: Myopotential inhibition of unipolar QRS-inhibited (VVI) pacemakers, assessed by ambulatory Holter monitoring of the electrocardiogram. PACE 3:470, 1980.

53. Furman S: Electromagnetic interference. PACE 5:1, 1982.

54. Secemsky SI, Hauser RG, Denes P, et al: Unipolar sensing abnormalities: incidence and clinical significance of skeletal muscle interference and undersensing in 228 patients. PACE 5:10, 1982.

55. Barold SS, Ong LS, Falkoff M, et al: Differential diagnosis of pacemaker pauses. In: Barold SS (ed): Modern Cardiac Pacing. Mount Kisco, NY, Futura, 1985, pp 587–613.

56. Exner DV, Rothscild JM, Heal S, et al: Unipolar sensing in contemporary pacemakers using myopotential testing to define optimal sensitivity settings. J Interv Card Electrophysiol 2:33, 1998.

57. Naegeli B, Osswald S, Deola M, et al: Intermittent pacemaker dysfunction caused by digital mobile telephones. J Am Coll Cardiol 27:1471, 1996.

58. Barbero V, Bartolini P, Donato A, et al: Do European GSM mobile cellular phones pose a potential risk to pacemaker patients? PACE 18:1218, 1995.

59. Katzenberg CA, Marcus FI, Heusinkveld RS, et al: Pacemaker failure due to radiation therapy. PACE 5:156, 1982.

60. Van Mechelen R, Hart C, DeBoer H: Failure to sense P waves during DDD pacing. PACE 9:498, 1986.

61. Halperin JL, Camunas JL, Stern EH, et al: Myopotential interference with DDD pacemakers: endocardial electrographic telemetry in the diagnosis of pacemaker-related arrhythmias. Am J Cardiol 54:97, 1984.

62. Rozanski J, Blankstein RL, Lister JW: Pacer arrhythmias: myopotential triggering of pacemaker-mediated tachycardia. PACE 6:795, 1983.

63. Zimmern SH, Clark MF, Austin WK: Characteristics and clinical effects of myopotential signals in a unipolar DDD pacemaker population. PACE 9:1019, 1986.

64. Barold SS, Ong LC, Falkoff MD, et al: Crosstalk or self-inhibition in dual chamber pacemakers. In: Barold SS (ed): Modern Cardiac Pacing. Mount Kisco, NY, Futura, 1985, pp 615–623.

65. Combs WJ, Reynolds DW, Sharma AD, et al: Cross-talk in bipolar pacemakers. Pacing Clin Electrophysiol 12:1613, 1989.

66. Barold SS: Pacemaker syndrome during atrial-based pacing. In: Aubert AE, Ector H, Stroobandt R (eds): Cardiac Pacing and Electrophysiology. A Bridge to the 21st Century. Dordrecht, The Netherlands, Kluwer, 1994, pp 251–267.

67. Link MS, Hellkamp AS, Estes MA, et al: High incidence of pacemaker syndrome in patients with sinus node dysfunction treated with ventricular-based pacing in the mode selection trial (MOST). J Am Coll Cardiol 43:2066, 2004.

68. Healey JS, Toff WD, Lamas GA, et al: Cardiovascular outcomes with atrial-based pacing compared with ventricular pacing. Meta-analysis of randomized trials, using individual patient data. Circulation 114:11, 2006.

69. Heldman D, Mulvihill D, Nguyen H, et al: True incidence of pacemaker syndrome. Pacing Clin Electrophysiol 13:1742, 1990.

70. Ellenbogen KA, Stambler BS, Orav EJ, et al: Clinical characteristics of patients intolerant to VVIR pacing. Am J Cardiol 86:59, 2000.

71. Barold SS: Usefulness of Holter recordings during cardiac pacing. Standard techniques and intracardiac recordings. Ann Noninvasive Electrocardiol 4:345, 1998.

72. Crawford MH, Bernstein SJ, Deedwania PC, et al: ACC/AHA guidelines for ambulatory electrocardiography: executive summary and recommendations. Circulation 100:886, 1999.

73. Gillis AM, Hiller KR, Rothschild M, et al: Ambulatory electrocardiography for the detection of pacemaker lead failure. PACE 20:1247, 1997.

74. Israel CW, Barold SS: Pacemaker systems as implantable cardiac rhythm monitors. Am J Cardiol 88:442, 2001.

75. Wiegand UK, Bonnemeier H, Eberhardt F, et al: Continuous Holter telemetry of atrial electrograms and marker annotations using a common Holter recording system: impact on Holter electrocardiogram interpretation in patients with dual chamber pacemakers. Pacing Clin Electrophysiol 25:1724, 2000.

76. Ho RT, Wicks T, Wyeth D, et al: Generalized tonic-clonic seizures detected by implantable loop recorder devices: diagnosing more than cardiac arrhyhmias. Heart Rhythm 3:857, 2006.

77. Rosner MH, Brady WJ: The electrocardiographic diagnosis of acute myocardial infarction in patients with ventricular paced rhythms. Am J Emerg Med 17:182, 1999.

78. Sgarbossa EB, Pinski SL, Gates KB, et al: Early electrocardiographic diagnosis of acute myocardial infarction in the presence of ventricular paced rhythm. Am J Cardiol 77:423, 1996.

79. Barold SS, Falkoff MD, Ong LS, et al: Electrocardiographic diagnosis of myocardial infarction during ventricular pacing. Cardiol Clin 5:403, 1987.

80. Castellanos A, Zoble R, Procacci PM, et al: St-qR pattern: new sign of diagnosis of anterior myocardial infarction during right ventricular pacing. Br Heart J 35:1161, 1973.

81. Sweeney MO, Hellkamp AS, Lee KL, et al: Mode selection trial (MOST) Investigators. Association of prolonged QRS duration with death in a clinical trial of pacemaker therapy for sinus node dysfunction. Circulation 111:2418, 2005.

82. Miyoshi F, Kobayashi Y, Itou H, et al: Prolonged paced QRS duration as a predictor for congestive heart failure in patients with right ventricular apical pacing. Pacing Clin Electrophysiol 28:1182, 2005.

27 Ambulatory Electrocardiography

Ambulatory electrocardiographic (ECG) monitoring is a method of recording an ECG for long durations (generally 24 to 48 hours). In honor of Norman J. Holter,[1] an engineer from Helena, Montana, who invented ambulatory ECG monitoring in 1961, the procedure is often called *Holter monitoring*. The methodology has undergone considerable evolution since its introduction into the practice of cardiology.

Modern Holter monitors are cassette recorders or digital recorders that usually record 2 or 3 ECG leads, with some models recording up to 12 leads. The leads generally used are modified bipolar leads V_1 and V_5 and, in the case of three-channel recording, an additional modified lead aV_F. For two-channel recordings, two negative electrodes are placed in the area of the upper sternum and two positive electrodes at the conventional lead V_1 and V_5 positions, respectively. A ground electrode is placed over the right side of the chest. For three-channel recordings, another negative electrode is placed at the left infraclavicular fossa, and the electrode at the conventional lead V_5 position is used as the positive electrode for the modified lead aV_F.

Newer models conform to accepted ECG standards and thus eliminate distortions of low-frequency signals. This allows accurate assessment of ST segment deviations and QT measurement.

Almost all current recorders are equipped with an event marker button that the patient presses to mark the time of a particular symptom. Pressing the button leads to an electronic marker on the tape, so when the tape is analyzed, the symptom noted in a patient's diary can be correlated with the recording. The patient's diary during the monitoring period is an essential part of the information.

Current ambulatory ECG monitoring is undergoing significant renovation with the advent of personal computer technology. In addition to providing a 24-hour (or longer) ECG recording, almost all systems can also provide information regarding hourly heart rates and counts, hourly rhythm disturbances, hourly and day/night ST segment deviation trends, and hourly rates of both supraventricular and ventricular ectopic activity. Most systems also provide information regarding heart rate variability.[2]

All units have time identification whenever the ECG is printed out by an automated program or at the discretion of the operator. A 24-hour trend sheet or digital printout is provided to display the heart rate and ST segment changes in relation to the time of the day as well as the number and characteristics of ventricular and supraventricular ectopic complexes on an hourly basis. Certain playback systems print out the

ECG from the entire Holter tape in a condensed form (Figure 27–1). A printout of the distribution of the frequency of premature complexes, as shown in Figure 27–2, is readily available. Some portions of the tracing may be selected for enlargement and detailed examination.

Even with the most automated scanning system, the computer interpretation is not always reliable. Quantitation of ventricular premature complexes have an average error of 24 percent,[3] and the computer readout often needs editing. Because of the large amount of data recorded

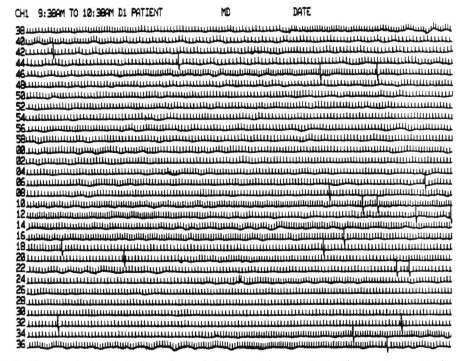

Figure 27–1   Condensed printout of 1 hour of an ambulatory ECG from a patient with premature ventricular complexes.

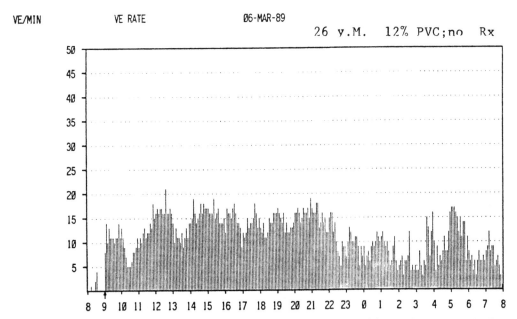

Figure 27–2   Hourly distribution of premature ventricular complexes in a 26-year-old man who is aware of palpitations.

on the tape, the technician should be able to select the pertinent parts of the tape and prepare a printout for the physician's scrutiny. The technician should therefore be experienced in ECG interpretation and know the clinical significance of the common cardiac arrhythmias.

The utilization of personal computer hardware and software has led to more rapid and accurate analysis of Holter monitor tapes. Operator intervention has been reduced considerably, as has the error associated with the analysis. The more advanced systems give the operator considerable leeway for determining whether the complexes are normal or abnormal. This is particularly important in the event of baseline artifact on a recording that may lead to incorrect determinations of ectopic rhythms. Reanalysis may also be performed within minutes using different algorithms, providing more accurate data for patient management.[2]

Event Recorders

Holter monitoring is performed generally for 24 hours. McClellan et al.[3] found that extending the monitoring for an additional day was not cost effective. Transient event recorders have been developed as an alternative to Holter monitoring. These devices are suitable for patients with infrequent symptoms, but are not suitable for patients with syncope or for those who are functionally impaired and therefore unable to activate the recorder. Event recorders should be considered when the suspected symptom may require prompt interpretation or intervention, as analysis of the regular Holter monitoring and the accompanying diary is likely to be performed within 1 to 2 days after occurrence of the recorded symptoms.

The event recorders are roughly the size of a pager and are worn by the patient for 30 days. During this time digital recording can be made at the time of symptomatic episodes and transmitted to a receiving station over the telephone by the patient. These loop recorders record continuously, but only a small window of time is present in memory at any time; the current window is frozen while the device continues to record for 30 to 60 seconds. Some of the loop recorders store up to 30 seconds of ECG before the patient activates the recording.

Event recorders are generally very effective in documenting infrequent events. More recently autotriggered memory loop recorders (AT-MLR) programmed for a variety of arrhythmic events have become available, making it possible to record and analyze the asymptomatic events. The study of Reiffel et al.[4] in a large group of patients showed that standard MLR provided more information than Holter monitors, but the benefit was enhanced even more by the use of AT-MLR.

For patients with very infrequent episodes suggestive of arrhythmia, a period of 30 days may be insufficient. In such cases, small devices implanted under the skin can be activated by a special magnet waved over the implanted device upon the occurrence of the perceived arrhythmia event. The implantable recorder has been useful in determining the cause of syncope in 18 of 21 patients over a mean 5-month period after inserting the implant.[5]

Networking and Databases

Modern ambulatory ECG monitoring systems permit networking and thus allow connections via telephone lines or digital links to outlying locations. The acquisition of data at remote locations may be transmitted over a wide area network to a central location for analysis and interpretation. The final report may be transmitted back to the original source for patient management. This type of networking arrangement may permit greater use of ambulatory ECG monitoring in locations that have no access to such technology. [2,6] The computer operating systems allow digital storage of the ECG strips and final Holter reports. This permits construction of databases containing the data from many patients as well as multiple studies on the same patient.[2]

For more detailed treatment of the technical aspects of ambulatory monitoring, the reader is referred to the guidelines for ambulatory electrocardiography by a task force of the American College of Cardiology and the American Heart Association[7] and review articles.[8,9]

Ambulatory Recording in Normal Subjects

HEART RATE

In young and middle-aged adults, the normal heart rate varies widely during a 24-hour period, day and night. In subjects who do not participate in a regular exercise program, the heart rate over a 24-hour period may range from 35 to 190 beats/min, with an overall average rate of about 80 beats/min.[10] There is distinct diurnal variation. The maximum heart rate usually occurs during late morning and the minimum heart rate at 3 to 5 AM. With increasing age, the maximum heart rate decreases significantly during both day and night. The average heart rate for the 24-hour period, however, is essentially unaffected.[10] The decrease in fluctuation of the heart rate is particularly evident in the elderly. In a group of 98 active subjects 75 years of age or older, only 15 had heart rates that exceeded 100 beats/min intermittently during a 24-hour period.[11] In more than one third of the subjects the heart rate did not vary by more than 10 beats/min during the 24-hour period.

Women generally have faster heart rates than men.[12,13] In 50 healthy young men and 50 healthy young women between the ages of 22 and 28 years studied by the same institution, the average waking and sleeping heart rates were faster in women by about 10 beats/min. The gender-related difference in heart rate persists to a certain degree with advancing age.[13]

The heart rate in normal subjects increases not only with physical exercise but also with mental stress. In a group of house officers presenting cases at medical grand rounds, the average heart rate increased from 73 to 154 beats/min.[14] The fastest heart rate was recorded either during the minutes before or the first few minutes of actual presentation, occasionally reaching 187 beats/min.

It is well known that the heart rate of trained athletes is slower than that of the general population. In one study that compared long-distance runners with untrained young adults, the average heart rates during normal activities during a 24-hour period were 61 and 73 beats/min, respectively.[15] The heart rate of endurance athletes during sleeping hours may be as slow as 24 beats/min.[16]

ECTOPIC COMPLEXES

Isolated asymptomatic supraventricular ectopic complexes may be observed in up to 64 percent of healthy young subjects.[12] In two groups of young adults studied, fewer than 2 percent had more than 100 supraventricular ectopic complexes over a 24-hour period. The frequency of premature complexes is higher in the older population.[15] It was 100 percent in a group of healthy men and women older than 80 years.[17]

The prevalence of ventricular ectopic complexes in otherwise healthy adults monitored with 24-hour ambulatory ECGs ranged from 17 to 100 percent but most commonly was 40 to 55 percent.[7,12,13,18] They are rare in newborns and young children.[19,20] As a rule, the total number of ventricular ectopic complexes in healthy young adults is small: fewer than 100 during a 24-hour period in 96 percent of cases.[10,12] Similar to supraventricular ectopic complexes, the highest incidence of ventricular ectopic complexes was encountered in individuals 60 years of age or older.[16,17] An increase in the duration of monitoring revealed a higher incidence of ventricular ectopic complexes.[13]

Complex ventricular ectopic complexes—defined as >30 beats/hr, multiforms, bigeminy, couplets, or R-on-T phenomenon—are present in 7 to 22 percent of subjects and as many as 77 percent in an older population. Ventricular ectopic complexes may appear or increase in healthy individuals with physical or nonphysical stress,[21,22] but a relation has not been established between premature ventricular complexes (PVCs) and smoking or coffee, tea, or alcohol intake.[7]

TACHYARRHYTHMIAS

Short episodes of atrial tachycardia, usually lasting not more than a few seconds, are occasionally seen on the ambulatory ECGs of otherwise healthy persons. A prevalence of 2 to 5 percent was reported in young adults, but the tachycardia was more frequent in the older population.[12,13] It is thought to be the most common ectopic tachycardia seen on the ambulatory ECG. It occurs in patients of all ages with or without heart disease. The heart rate is generally 100 to 150 beats/min. The rhythm is often slightly irregular, with a gradual increase in rate (warming-up phenomenon), suggesting that the tachycardia is probably automatic. The latter has been referred to as *benign slow paroxysmal atrial tachycardia* or *ectopic atrial tachycardia* (Figure 27–3). The term suggested by Chou[8] is *accelerated atrial rhythm*. With rare exception it is asymptomatic.

Nonsustained ventricular tachycardia (VT) is encountered in apparently healthy young adults but is uncommon.[12] It is usually asymptomatic. Kim et al.[23] used Holter monitoring to examine whether the rate of nonsustained VT was predictive of the rate of sustained VT in the same subject. They found that in 50 patients with nonsustained VT the mean rate was 150 beats/min, which was significantly slower than the rate of spontaneous or induced VT (mean 246 beats/min) in these patients. In a study of 400 patients who underwent coronary angioplasty within 12 hours after onset of acute myocardial infarction (MI), Holter monitoring performed within 10 to 30 days after index MI revealed nonsustained ventricular tachycardia in 10 percent of patients. This finding was associated with increased arrhythmia morbidity.[24]

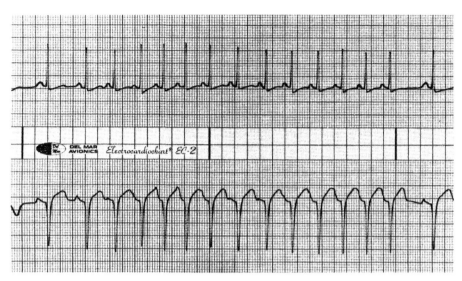

Figure 27–3   Short episode of accelerated atrial rhythm (ectopic atrial tachycardia) in a healthy young man. (From Chou TC, Ceaser JH: Ambulatory electrocardiogram: clinical applications. Cardiovasc Clin 13:321, 1983.)

BRADYARRHYTHMIAS AND CONDUCTION DISTURBANCES

Marked sinus bradycardia is common on the ambulatory ECGs of healthy adults, particularly during sleeping hours. The bradycardia is often associated with transient atrioventricular (AV) junctional escape rhythm, which is observed in 4 to 22 percent of healthy subjects.[12,13] Brief periods of sinus pauses or sinoatrial (SA) block are seen in 28 to 34 percent. First- and second-degree AV blocks with Wenckebach phenomenon have been reported in 1 to 12 percent and 3 to 6 percent of normal subjects, respectively (Figure 27–4). They are seen mostly in young individuals and during sleep. The various bradyarrhythmias are more common in trained athletes.[14]

Correlation with Symptoms of Palpitations, Dizziness, and Syncope

The ambulatory ECG provides a unique opportunity to record cardiac rhythms during normal daily activities and to identify circumstances associated with symptoms. Useful information can be easily obtained if the symptoms occur frequently, but prolonged periods of recording or event monitoring may be needed if the symptoms occur seldom. An example of symptomatic ventricular arrhythmia detected during Holter monitoring is shown in Figure 27–5.

There is a remarkably poor correlation between the presence or absence of cardiac

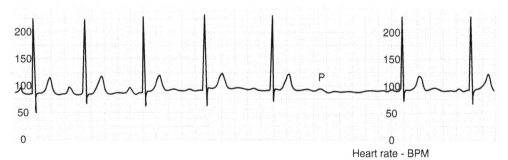

Heart rate - BPM

Figure 27–4   Second-degree atrioventricular block with Wenckebach phenomenon in a healthy young man. P = nonconducted P wave.

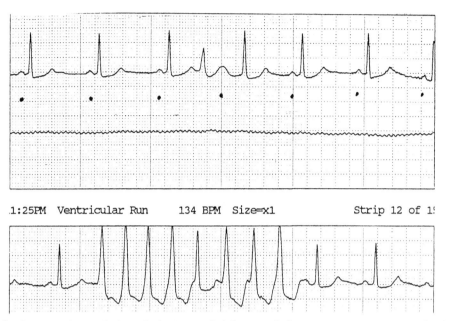

.1:25PM   Ventricular Run   134 BPM Size=x1   Strip 12 of 1!

Figure 27-5   Symptomatic ventricular arrhythmia recorded during ambulatory monitoring. *Top,* Interpolated premature ventricular complex (PVC) with prolonged PR interval after the PVC, a manifestation of concealed conduction. Dots mark P waves. *Bottom,* Nonsustained ventricular tachycardia. The fifth complex during tachycardia is a fusion complex.

arrhythmias and symptoms such as palpitations, fluttering in the chest, and irregular heartbeats. Even sustained paroxysmal tachycardias often go unnoticed. The same patient may have palpitations during some episodes but no symptoms during others (Figure 27–6). Conversely, typical complaints suggestive of arrhythmias often correlate with regular sinus rhythm.

The reported ability of the 24-hour ambulatory ECG to correlate a symptomatic episode with cardiac arrhythmia ranges from 10 to 64 percent.[25] Valuable information also is obtained if rhythm disturbances are absent during the symptomatic periods. It may be that in patients

with dizziness and similar complaints the ambulatory ECG is more often helpful for excluding cardiac arrhythmias as the cause of the symptom than for detecting the cause of a complaint.

Surawicz and Pinto[26] compared symptoms reported during ambulatory ECG recording in 306 hospitalized patients and 278 outpatients who had 20 or more PVCs during waking hours. Complaints compatible with arrhythmia were reported in 6.3 percent of hospital patients and 55 percent of outpatients. The complaints correlated with the presence of ventricular arrhythmias in 19 of 20 (95 percent) hospitalized patients and 67 of 154 (43.5 percent) outpatients. There were

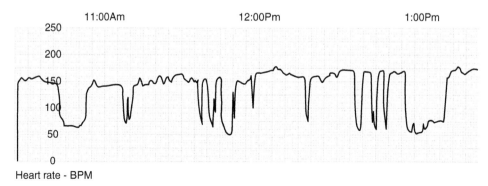

Heart rate - BPM

Figure 27–6   Heart rate trend chart of a 28-year-old woman with Wolff-Parkinson-White syndrome and frequent episodes of orthodromic atrioventricular reentrant tachycardia. Of the many episodes of tachycardia, the patient experienced palpitation only briefly during one episode. (From Chou TC, Ceaser JH: Ambulatory electrocardiogram: clinical applications. Cardiovasc Clin 13:321, 1983.)

no significant age or gender differences among the noncomplainers, appropriate complainers, and inappropriate complainers (symptoms in the absence of arrhythmia) for the outpatients. In a later study, Surawicz (unpublished observations, 1992–1996) correlated symptoms with episodes of supraventricular or ventricular tachycardia (3 to 640 beats in a row) in 601 consecutive patients (inpatients and outpatients) undergoing 24-hour ambulatory ECG monitoring. In this cohort 464 patients had no symptoms, 107 had inappropriate symptoms (i.e., not during the tachycardia episode), and 30 patients (5 percent) had appropriate symptoms.

Arrhythmias capable of producing cardiogenic syncope include bradycardia of <40 beats/min, tachycardia of >150 beats/min, and asystole longer than 3 to 5 seconds, depending on the patient's body position and activity at the time of the arrhythmia.[27] Patients with impaired cardiac function are more likely to have symptoms during tachyarrhythmia or bradyarrhythmia than those without heart disease.

Because of the abnormal sequence of ventricular activation and contraction, ventricular tachycardia can often cause cerebral symptoms at a rate as low as 120 beats/min,[28] whereas patients with supraventricular tachycardia can tolerate faster rates. Focal neurologic abnormalities are rarely due to decreased cerebral flow from cardiac arrhythmias alone, and the ambulatory ECG is unlikely to be helpful in resolving these problems.[29]

Chest Pain

The ambulatory ECG is used to monitor patients in whom chest pain occurs at rest or at night or is associated with stresses other than exercise. It is particularly useful in patients who have chest pain suggestive of Prinzmetal's or vasospastic angina. Occasionally, the continuous recording reveals arrhythmias responsible for the onset of angina.

When the ambulatory ECG is used to evaluate chest pain, it is important to be aware of the limitations inherent in the interpretation of the ST segment changes. As during the graded exercise test, horizontal or downsloping ST segment depression may be a falsely positive finding on the ambulatory ECG.[3] Body position, hyperventilation, cardiac medications, and other factors may contribute to the appearance of ST segment depression resembling that of ischemia.[30] In 50 patients studied by Stern and associates[31] the ambulatory ECG had a sensitivity of

91 percent and a specificity of 78 percent for diagnosing significant coronary artery disease documented by angiography. Patients with abnormal resting ECGs, however, were included in this study, and T wave inversion also was considered a positive sign for myocardial ischemia. In 70 patients studied by Crawford and associates,[32] the sensitivity of the ischemic-type ST segment depression on the ambulatory ECG for detecting significant coronary artery disease was 62 percent (24 of 39 patients), and the specificity was 61 percent. Armstrong and associates[33] studied 50 middle-aged normal men with 24-hour Holter monitoring. Transient horizontal or downsloping ST segment depression of 1 mm or more was recorded in 15 (30 percent) of the subjects. The abnormal ST segment depression lasted 30 seconds to 2 hours, and the magnitude of the depression varied from 1 to 4 mm. These men had no symptoms during an average 36-month follow-up period. This study also demonstrated that isolated T wave inversion on the ambulatory ECG is a nonspecific finding, as 36 percent of the normal subjects had such a finding intermittently. In contrast, it is generally agreed that transient ST segment elevation of 1 mm or more on the ambulatory ECG is a highly specific sign for myocardial ischemia, as it seldom occurs in normal persons without symptoms.[33]

To minimize the incidence of a false-positive diagnosis of myocardial ischemia, a set of control tracings should be obtained at the beginning of the Holter recording with the patient in the supine, sitting, and standing positions and during hyperventilation.

Clues to the Arrhythmia Mechanism

Ambulatory monitoring may provide clues to the mechanism of arrhythmias. This is illustrated in the following four examples.

Figure 27–7 shows the onset of atrial tachycardia, preceded by atrial premature complexes conducted with aberration. The RR interval gradually shortens, indicating a "warming-up" phenomenon, which suggests an automatic mechanism of the tachycardia. Figure 27–8 shows spontaneous termination of torsade de pointes followed by a sinus rhythm with apparent QT prolongation in a patient with frequent presyncopal episodes. Figure 27–9 shows a rhythm strip from a patient with a history of presyncopal episodes. A long period of AV block is explained by the rare phenomenon of depressed AV conduction following an atrial premature complex. Figure 27–10 shows

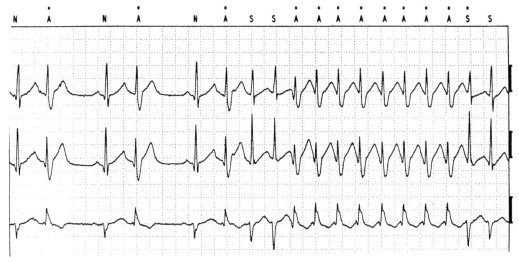

Figure 27–7   Onset of atrial tachycardia preceded by single premature atrial complexes conducted with aberration. The cycle length decreases gradually. Aberrant conduction is present in the first complex of tachycardia because of the Ashman phenomenon and in the fourth through eleventh complexes because of a critically short cycle. Aberration ceases without change in cycle length because the refractory period has adjusted to the new short cycle length.

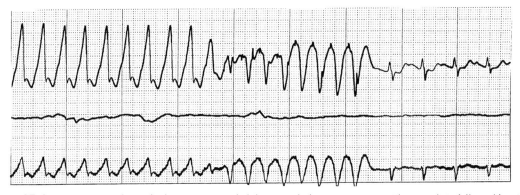

Figure 27–8   Termination of torsade de pointes recorded during ambulatory monitoring. The torsade is followed by sinus complexes with a depressed ST segment and apparent prolongation of the QT interval suggested by the "tilted P waves." These repolarization changes suggest hypokalemia.

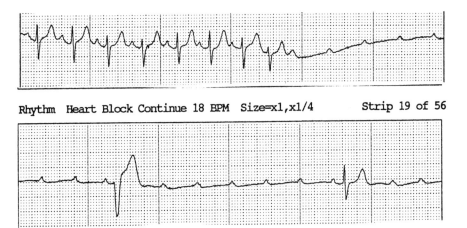

Figure 27–9   Continuous record during ambulatory monitoring shows depression of atrioventricular (AV) conduction after an atrial premature complex, a ventricular escape complex, and resumption of AV conduction with a normal PR interval after 15 nonconducted P waves.

11:39PM AXIS SHIFT   60 BPM Size=x1/2,x1/4

1:21AM PAC   59 BPM Size=x1/2,x1/4

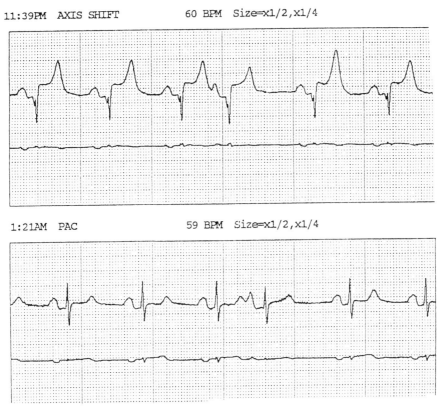

Figure 27-10 ECG strips recorded during ambulatory monitoring show a change in the QRS axis without a change in heart rate or PR interval. The change is apparent also in the atrial premature complex. A subsequent study showed that the pattern in the lower strip at 1:21 AM represents normal conduction, and the pattern in the upper strip at 11:39 PM represents conduction through a nodoventricular bypass tract.

an "axis shift" without a change in the heart rate or the PR interval. This was explained in a subsequent study by a nodoventricular bypass tract.

Patients with Specific Problems

EVALUATION OF ISCHEMIC EPISODES

Holter monitoring has been used to examine patients with unstable or vasospastic angina, detect silent myocardial ischemia, and evaluate antianginal therapy. Figueras and associates[34] studied 23 patients with coronary artery disease and resting or nocturnal angina with continuous hemodynamic and ECG recording. In 11 patients, recurrent episodes of pain were always preceded by an average of 8 minutes of ischemic ECG changes and hemodynamic signs of left ventricular dysfunction. Two patients had transient ischemic ECG and hemodynamic changes without pain.

Among 116 patients with unstable angina, Johnson and co-workers[35] found that the appearance of transient ischemic ST segment displacement or ventricular tachycardia on the Holter recording is an indicator of severe left main or triple-vessel coronary artery disease, variant angina, or impaired prognosis over the subsequent 3 months. Examples of ventricular tachycardia and ventricular fibrillation, believed to be precipitated by myocardial ischemia, are shown in Figures 17-5 and 18-4, respectively.

Continuous ECG monitoring in patients with variant angina reveals serious cardiac arrhythmias in about 50 percent of cases. These arrhythmias include ventricular tachycardia, ventricular fibrillation, complex ventricular ectopic rhythms, second- and third-degree AV block, and asystole.[36-38] They are seen mostly in patients with marked ST segment elevation (4 mm or more).[36-38] Serious ventricular arrhythmias are usually associated with ST segment elevation in the anterior leads, whereas bradyarrhythmias are usually associated with ST elevation in the inferior leads.[36,39] The ventricular arrhythmias may develop during the period of maximal ST segment elevation or during resolution of the ST segment changes.

Previtali and associates[38] suggested that the arrhythmias seen during ST segment elevation represent occlusion arrhythmias, and that those seen during resolution represent reperfusion arrhythmias. The latter occurred more often when the duration of myocardial ischemia was longer.

Patients with variant angina and serious arrhythmias also have been shown to be at a much higher risk for sudden death. Among 114 patients with variant angina followed for a mean period of 26 months by Miller and associates,[37] sudden death occurred in 42 percent of the patients with serious arrhythmias during their anginal episodes compared with 6 percent of those without such arrhythmias.

Asymptomatic episodes of ischemic types of ST segment change are often observed on the ambulatory ECGs of patients with coronary artery disease.[40–44] Such episodes are also seen in patients with exertional or rest angina. The duration and degree of the ST changes tend to be less with the asymptomatic than the symptomatic episodes, but the available evidence suggests that these episodes represent usually silent myocardial ischemia.[41] In 93 patients with silent ischemic episodes on ambulatory ECGs, Mody and co-workers[43] found that the patients who had longer cumulative duration (more than 60 minutes per 24 hours) of ischemia were more likely to have three-vessel and proximal coronary artery disease.

Among patients with anginal chest pain and normal coronary arteries, episodes of ST depression during Holter monitoring were recorded in 17 of 28 (61 percent) patients who had significant ST segment depression during exercise testing and in 5 of 10 (50 percent) patients without ST segment depression during exercise testing.[45] The findings were explained by differences in the response of the coronary microvascular tone to exercise testing and to stimuli operating during daily life.[45]

SICK SINUS SYNDROME

One of the common manifestations of the sick sinus syndrome is a prolonged sinus pause without an escape rhythm during the symptomatic episode. Repeated 24-hour monitoring is often needed to establish a temporal relation between the patient's symptoms and the ECG findings. In some instances, sinus pauses are seen but the patient exhibits no symptoms during the period of monitoring. SA node dysfunction may be suspected, but it is possible that the cause of the patient's symptoms is noncardiac. Brief sinus pauses (up to 2 seconds) may occur in normal subjects, especially during sleep.

In patients with sick sinus syndrome and bradytachyarrhythmias, tachyarrhythmia may be the presenting abnormality. Sinus arrest or cessation of AV transmission often follows an episode of supraventricular tachyarrhythmia, causing dizziness or syncope (Figure 27–11).

CONDUCTION ABNORMALITIES

The ambulatory ECG may be used to detect intermittent conduction abnormalities including

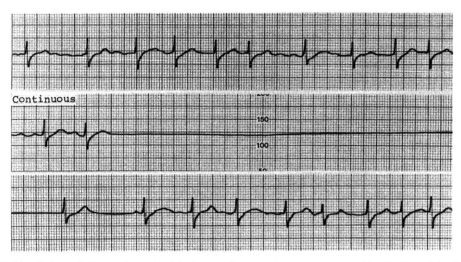

Figure 27–11   Tachycardia in a patient with sick sinus syndrome and recurrent syncope. Ventricular activity during atrial fibrillation stops abruptly and resumes after about 6 seconds. (From Chou TC, Ceaser JH: Ambulatory electrocardiogram: clinical applications. Cardiovasc Clin 13:321, 1983.)

combinations of fascicular block and various degrees of AV block if symptoms suggestive of transient cerebral ischemia appear. A patient with a normal PR interval on the routine ECG may be found by Holter monitoring to have transient high-degree AV block and marked bradycardia. Patients with bifascicular blocks may have transient episodes of second- or high-degree AV block long before the development of permanent complete AV block.[46]

PACEMAKER EVALUATION

Patients with implanted cardiac pacemakers are periodically evaluated with ECGs recorded in the routine manner or by transtelephonic transmission. The ambulatory ECG may be helpful when evaluating patients with pacemakers that appear to function properly on routine evaluation but who have symptoms suggestive of pacemaker malfunction (see Chapter 26).

MITRAL VALVE PROLAPSE

Cardiac arrhythmias, both ventricular and supraventricular, are common in patients with mitral valve prolapse, and sudden death occurs occasionally.[47,48] Many patients with the mitral valve prolapse syndrome are troubled by symptoms of palpitations, lightheadedness, and atypical chest pain. In one study only 27 percent of symptomatic patients were found to have arrhythmias associated with their symptoms.[48] In most cases the negative correlation between symptoms and arrhythmias serves to reassure patients of the benign nature of their symptoms.

PREEXCITATION SYNDROME

In patients with documented Wolff-Parkinson-White (WPW) pattern, the ambulatory ECG showed that preexcitation is intermittent in 65 percent of cases.[49] When the routine ECG is suggestive but not diagnostic of the WPW pattern, demonstration of more typical signs of preexcitation intermittently confirms the presence of this anomaly.

CARDIOMYOPATHIES

Hypertrophic obstructive cardiomyopathy is frequently associated with atrial and ventricular arrhythmias and occasionally with sudden death.[48,50,51] In a prospective study by Maron and associates,[51] 99 patients with hypertrophic cardiomyopathy had 24-hour ambulatory ECGs and were followed for 3 years. There was a significantly increased risk of sudden death for patients with asymptomatic ventricular tachycardia; the annual mortality rate among these patients was 8.6 percent.

Patients with dilated cardiomyopathy are known to have frequent complex ventricular arrhythmias. Patients with complex ventricular arrhythmias or nonsustained ventricular tachycardia and dilated cardiomyopathy were found to be at high risk of sudden death.[52,53]

CHRONIC OBSTRUCTIVE LUNG DISEASE

In patients with chronic obstructive lung disease, ambulatory ECG recording documented a 72 percent incidence of arrhythmia, most commonly multiform PVCs.[54] The incidence of atrial arrhythmia in this study was 52 percent. In hospitalized patients, however, supraventricular arrhythmias are more common.[55]

CHRONIC HEMODIALYSIS AND DIAGNOSTIC PROCEDURES

Morrison et al.[56] reported a 40 percent incidence of ventricular arrhythmias during and after dialysis, more prominently in patients receiving digitalis and exhibiting left ventricular hypertrophy. The arrhythmias were reduced as the potassium level in the dialysate was increased. Therefore ambulatory ECG monitoring may be of value in patients at risk of arrhythmia on dialysis.[55]

Ventricular and atrial ectopic complexes, tachyarrhythmias, and ST changes occurred in 38 percent of patients during gastroscopy.[57] A 40 percent incidence of new arrhythmia was reported during a barium enema.[58] Arrhythmias occur also in patients undergoing bronchoscopy.[55]

EVALUATING THE EFFICACY OF DRUG TREATMENT

The ambulatory ECG has gained widespread use for evaluating drug therapy for arrhythmias, especially ventricular arrhythmias. Readings are obtained before and after institution of antiarrhythmia therapy. Suppression of episodes of ventricular tachycardia or a significant reduction in ventricular ectopic complexes is considered to indicate the efficacy of the drug. In the electrocardiographic monitoring (ESVEM) trial, Holter monitoring compared favorably with intracardiac electrophysiologic studies for selecting effective antiarrhythmic drugs to treat ventricular tachyarrhythmias.[59]

The frequency of ventricular ectopic activity varies widely from hour to hour and from day to day. The spontaneous variation is even greater when the ambulatory ECG is repeated at weekly or longer intervals.[60] Such fluctuations in frequency have led to difficulty in deciding whether an observed reduction in ectopic activity is due to a drug effect or to spontaneous variations. It has been proposed that if a 24-hour Holter monitoring ECG is obtained before and another 1 to 2 weeks after therapy begins, a reduction by more than 85 percent of the total number of PVCs is necessary before the changes can be attributed to a drug effect.[60,61] It is almost impossible to distinguish a drug effect from spontaneous variation of the arrhythmias if the interval is longer than 3 months.[62] The detection of nonsustained VT in survivors of MI during Holter monitoring was found to be of limited value when selecting patients for a primary implantable cardioverter/defibrillator prevention trial.[63]

SLEEP APNEA SYNDROME

Cardiac arrhythmias and conduction disturbances during sleep were reported in patients with sleep apnea syndrome.[64,65] Among 23 patients with this syndrome monitored with 24-hour ECG, Miller[65] found episodes of marked sinus arrhythmia, extreme sinus bradycardia with a heart rate less than 30 beats/min, sinus pauses, and first- and second-degree AV block in a few cases. In a series of 400 patients reported by Guilleminault and associates, 48 percent had cardiac arrhythmias during the night of the Holter recording.[64] Nonsustained ventricular tachycardia was seen in 8 patients, sinus arrest lasting 2.5 to 13.0 seconds in 43, and second-degree AV block in 31. Seventy-five patients had frequent (>2 beats/min) PVCs during sleep. In 50 patients with significant arrhythmias who underwent tracheostomy, no arrhythmia other than PVC was seen by Holter monitoring after surgery. In patients with stable heart failure, the presence of sleep apnea was associated with a high incidence of atrial fibrillation and ventricular arrhythmias.[66]

Ambulatory monitoring revealed that ST segment depression is relatively common in patients with obstructive apnea during sleep. Moreover, the duration of ST segment depression is reduced by nasal continuous positive air pressure.[67]

VICTIMS OF CARDIAC ARREST

Several investigators have reported patients who had cardiac arrest or sudden death during Holter monitoring.[68–71] The terminal event at the time of cardiac arrest was ventricular tachyarrhythmia in most cases (about 80 percent),[69] but bradyarrhythmias and asystole were more common in one reported series of patients without apparent heart disease.[72] The ventricular tachyarrhythmias include ventricular tachycardia or flutter, torsade de pointes, and ventricular fibrillation. Ventricular fibrillation was always preceded by ventricular tachycardia or ventricular flutter. In patients with cardiac arrest due to bradyarrhythmia, the mechanism is mostly sinus arrest (Figure 27–12) with some cases of complete AV block. In patients who sustained ventricular fibrillation, there is usually an increased frequency of PVCs during the hour before the event.[69] The PVCs initiating ventricular tachycardia that degenerates into ventricular fibrillation do not display the R-on-T phenomenon in most instances.

Heart Rate Variability

Beat-to-beat variability in RR intervals is referred to as *heart rate variability*. It is determined by the interplay of the sympathetic and parasympathetic input. In normal subjects, age and heart rate are the major determinants of heart rate variability.[73] The variability is reduced in patients with congestive heart failure, left ventricular dysfunction, coronary artery disease, and diabetic neuropathy.[73] In these patients the sympathovagal balance shifts toward sympathetic predominance. Therefore more blunted heart variability occurs concomitantly with an elevated heart rate.[74] Conversely, increased heart rate variability by exercise training is attributed to an increase in parasympathetic tone.[75]

In survivors of acute MI, the degree of heart rate variability has been found to be a useful predictor of long-term prognosis. In a multicenter postinfarction study, Kleiger and associates[76] reported their findings from 808 patients who underwent 24-hour Holter recording 11 ± 3 days after acute MI and who were followed for a mean period of 31 months. Patients with heart rate variability (standard deviation of RR intervals) of less than 50 ms had a relative risk of all-cause mortality 5.3 times higher than those with heart rate variability of more than 100 ms. Subsequently, these results were confirmed in a 4-year follow-up study by the same group of investigators who analyzed the data in more detail and made adjustments for five covariates.[77]

Algra and associates[78] examined the relation between heart rate variability from the 24-hour ambulatory ECG and the 2-year risk for sudden

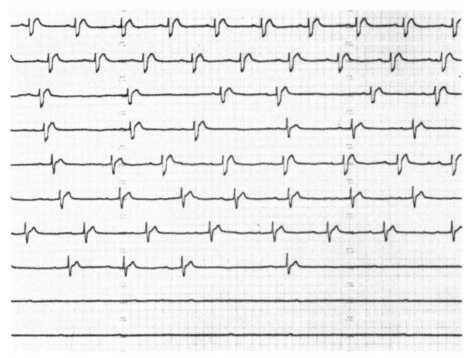

Figure 27–12 Ventricular asystole during Holter monitoring of a 74-year-old man with a history of recurrent dizziness. He had cardiac arrest while the ambulatory ECG was being recorded. The tracing shows sinus bradycardia, sinus pauses or sinoatrial block, first-degree and complete atrioventricular block, and ventricular asystole.

death. A total of 6693 consecutive patients were studied, 245 of whom died suddenly. Ten percent of the subjects studied were postinfarction patients. The others included those with symptoms suggestive of cardiac arrhythmia, such as palpitations, dizziness, and syncope (72 percent), and patients undergoing antiarrhythmia therapy (8 percent). They found that patients with a minimum mean per-minute heart rate of less than 65 beats/min had a double risk of sudden death compared with those with a minimum per-minute heart rate of more than 65 beats/min. The authors concluded that the findings support the theory that patients with low parasympathetic activity are at increased risk for sudden death independent of other risk factors. A more recent study of survivors of recent acute MI also confirmed a strong association between heart rate variability and mortality; but when other risk factors were considered, heart rate variability failed to add independent prognostic information.[79]

REFERENCES

1. Holter NJ: New method for heart studies: Continuous electrocardiography of active subjects over long periods is now practical. Science 134:1214, 1961.
2. Paustian RD: Holter monitoring: a review of current technology. Cardiology Special Edition: 31, 1999.
3. McClennen S, Zimetbaum PJ, Ho KKL, et al: Holter monitoring: are two days better than one?. Am J Cardiol 86:562, 2000.
4. Reiffel JA, Schwarzberg R, Murry M: Comparison of autotriggered memory loop recorders versus standard loop recorders versus 24-hour Holter monitors for arrhythmia detection. Am J Cardiol 95:1055, 2005.
5. Krahn AD, Klein GJ, Yee R, et al: The high cost of syncope. Cost implications of a new insertable loop recorder in the investigation of recurrent syncope. Am Heart J 137:870, 1999.
6. Salerno DM, Granrud G, Hodges M: Accuracy of commercial 24-hour electrocardiogram analyzers for quantitation of total and repetitive ventricular arrhythmias. Am J Cardiol 60:1299, 1987.
7. Knoebel SB, Crawford MH, Dunn MI, et al: Guidelines for ambulatory electrocardiography: a report of the American College of Cardiology/American Heart Association Task Force on Assessment of Diagnostic and Therapeutic Cardiovascular Procedures (Subcommittee on Ambulatory Electrocardiography). J Am Coll Cardiol 13:249, 1989.
8. Chou TC, Ceaser JH: Ambulatory electrocardiogram: clinical applications. In: Fowler NO (ed): Noninvasive Diagnostic Methods in Cardiology. Philadelphia, FA Davis, 1983, p 321.
9. DiMarco JP, Philbrick JT: Use of ambulatory electrocardiographic (Holter) monitoring. Ann Intern Med 113:53, 1990.
10. Kostis JB, Moreyra AE, Amendo MT, et al: The effect of age on heart rate in subjects free of heart disease: studies by ambulatory electrocardiography and maximal exercise stress test. Circulation 65:141, 1982.
11. Camm AJ, Evans KE, Ward DE, et al: The rhythm of the heart in active elderly subjects. Am Heart J 99:598, 1980.

12. Brodsky M, Wu D, Denes P, et al: Arrhythmias documented by 24 hour continuous electrocardiographic monitoring in 50 male medical students without apparent heart disease. Am J Cardiol 39:390, 1977.

13. Clarke JM, Shelton JR, Hamer J, et al: The rhythm of the normal human heart. Lancet 2:508, 1976.

14. Moss AJ, Wynar B: Tachycardia in house officers presenting cases at grand rounds. Ann Intern Med 72:255, 1970.

15. Talan DA, Bauernfeind RA, Washley WW, et al: Twenty-four continuous ECG recordings in long-distance runners. Chest 82:19, 1982.

16. Viitasalo MT, Kala R, Eisalo A: Ambulatory electrocardiographic recording in endurance athletes. Br Heart J 47:213, 1982.

17. Kantelip JP, Sage E, Duchene-Marullaz P: Findings on ambulatory electrocardiographic monitoring in subjects older than 80 years. Am J Cardiol 57:398, 1986.

18. Glasser SP, Clark PI, Appelbaum HJ: Occurrence of frequent complex arrhythmias detected by ambulatory monitoring: findings in an apparently healthy asymptomatic elderly population. Chest 75:565, 1979.

19. Southall DP, Johnston F, Shinebourne EA, et al: 24-Hour electrocardiographic study of heart rate and rhythm patterns in population of healthy children. Br Heart J 45:281, 1981.

20. Southall DP, Richards JM, Mitchell P, et al: Study of cardiac rhythm in healthy newborn infants. Br Heart J 43:14, 1980.

21. McHenry PL, Morris SN, Kavalier M, et al: Comparative study of exeircse-induced ventricular arrhythmias in normal subjects and patients with documented coronary artery disease. Am J Cardiol 37:609, 1976.

22. Taggart P, Carruthers M, Somerville W: Electrocardiogram, plasma catecholamines and lipids, and their modification by oxprenolol when speaking before an audience. Lancet 2:341, 1973.

23. Kim SG, Mercando AD, Fisher JD: Comparison of the characteristics of nonsustained ventricular tachycardia on Holter monitoring and sustained ventricular tachycardia observed spontaneously or induced by programmed stimulation. Am J Cardiol 60:288, 1987.

24. Schwab JO, Schmitt H, Coch M, et al: Results and significance of Holter monitoring after direct percutaneous transluminal coronary angioplasty for acute myocardial infarction. Am J Cardiol 87:466, 2001.

25. Kennedy HL, Caralis DG: Ambulatory electrocardiography: a clinical perspective. Ann Intern Med 87:729, 1977.

26. Surawicz B, Pinto RP: Symptoms in hospital patients and outpatients with ventricular arrhythmias during ambulatory ECG monitoring. J Ambulatory Monitor 4:83, 1991.

27. Rossen R, Kabat H, Anderson JP: Acute arrest of cerebral circulation in man. Arch Neurol Psychiatry 50:510, 1943.

28. Jonas S, Klein I, Dimant J: Importance of Holter monitoring in patients with periodic cerebral symptoms. Ann Neurol 1:470, 1977.

29. Fisher M: Holter monitoring in patients with transient focal cerebral ischemia. Stroke 9:514, 1978.

30. Kennedy HL, Wiens RD: Ambulatory (Holter) electrocardiography and myocardial ischemia. Am Heart J 117:164, 1989.

31. Stern S, Tzivoni D, Stern Z: Diagnostic accuracy of ambulatory ECG monitoring in ischemic heart disease. Circulation 52:1045, 1975.

32. Crawford MH, Mendoza CA, O'Rourke RA, et al: Limitations of continuous ambulatory electrocardiogram monitoring for detecting coronary artery disease. Ann Intern Med 89:1, 1978.

33. Armstrong WF, Jordan JW, Morris SN, et al: Prevalence and magnitude of S-T segment and T wave abnormalities in normal men during continuous ambulatory electrocardiography. Am J Cardiol 4:1638, 1982.

34. Figueras J, Singh BN, Ganz W, et al: Mechanism of rest and nocturnal angina: observations during continuous hemodynamic and electrocardiographic monitoring. Circulation 59:955, 1979.

35. Johnson SM, Mauritson DR, Winniford MD: Continuous electrocardiographic monitoring in patients with unstable angina pectoris: identification of high-risk subgroup with severe coronary disease, variant angina, and/or impaired early prognosis. Am Heart J 103:4, 1982.

36. Kerin NZ, Rubenfire M, Naini M, et al: Arrhythmias in variant angina pectoris: relationship of arrhythmias to ST-segment elevation and R-wave changes. Circulation 60:1343, 1979.

37. Miller DD, Waters DD, Szlachcic J, et al: Clinical characteristics associated with sudden death in patients with variant angina. Circulation 66:588, 1982.

38. Previtali M, Klersy C, Salerno JA, et al: Ventricular tachyarrhythmias in Prinzmetal's variant angina: clinical significance and relation to the degree and time course of S-T segment elevation. Am J Cardiol 52:19, 1983.

39. Plotnick GD, Fisher ML, Becker LC: Ventricular arrhythmias in patients with rest angina: correlation with ST segment changes and extent of coronary atherosclerosis. Am Heart J 105:32, 1983.

40. Balasubramanian V, Lahiri A, Green HL, et al: Ambulatory ST segment monitoring: problems, pitfalls, solutions and clinical application. Br Heart J 44:419, 1980.

41. Cecchi AC, Dovellini EV, Marchi F, et al: Silent myocardial ischemia during ambulatory electrocardiographic monitoring in patients with effort angina. J Am Coll Cardiol 1:934, 1983.

42. Cohn PF: Silent myocardial ischemia in patients with a defective anginal warning system. Am J Cardiol 45:697, 1980.

43. Mody FV, Nademanee K, Intarachot V, et al: Severity of silent myocardial ischemia on ambulatory electrocardiographic monitoring in patients with stable angina pectoris: relation to prognostic determinants during exercise stress testing and coronary angiography. J Am Coll Cardiol 12:1169, 1988.

44. Schang SJ, Pepine CJ: Transient asymptomatic S-T segment depression during daily activity. Am J Cardiol 39:396, 1977.

45. Lanza GA, Manzoli A, Pasceri V, et al: Ischemic-like ST-segment changes during Holter monitoring in patients with angina pectoris and normal coronary arteries but negative exercise testing. Am J Cardiol 79:1, 1997.

46. Bleifer SB, Bleifer DJ, Hansmann DR, et al: Diagnosis of occult arrhythmias by Holter electrocardiography. Prog Cardiovasc Dis 16:569, 1974.

47. Harrison DC, Fitzgerald JW, Winkle RA: Ambulatory electrocardiography for diagnosis and treatment of cardiac arrhythmias. N Engl J Med 294:373, 1976.

48. Winkle RA, Lopes MG, Fitzgerald JW, et al: Arrhythmias in patients with mitral valve prolapse. Circulation 52:73, 1975.

49. Hindman MC, Last JH, Rosen KM: Wolff-Parkinson-White observed by portable monitoring. Ann Intern Med 79:654, 1973.

50. McKenna WJ, Chetty S, Oakley CM, et al: Arrhythmia in hypertrophic cardiomyopathy: exercise and 48 hour ambulatory electrocardiographic assessment with and without beta adrenergic blocking therapy. Am J Cardiol 45:1, 1980.

51. Maron BJ, Savage DD, Wolfson JK, et al: Prognostic significance of 24 hour ambulatory electrocardiographic monitoring in patients with hypertrophic cardiomyopathy: a prospective study. Am J Cardiol 48:252, 1981.

52. Follansbee WP, Michelson EL, Morganroth J: Nonsustained ventricular tachycardia in ambulatory patients: characteristics and association with sudden cardiac death. Ann Intern Med 92:741, 1980.

53. Holmes J, Kubo SH, Cody RJ, et al: Arrhythmias in ischemic and nonischemic dilated cardiomyopathy: prediction of mortality by ambulatory electrocardiography. Am J Cardiol 55:146, 1985.

54. Kleiger RE, Senior RM: Long-term electrocardiographic monitoring of ambulatory patients with chronic airway obstruction. Chest 65:483, 1974.

55. Morganroth J, Kennedy HL: Ambulatory Holter electrocardiography: technology, clinical aplications, and limitations. In: Chatterjee K, Parmley WW (eds): Cardiology: An Illustrated Text/Reference. Philadelphia, JB Lippincott, 1991, 687–699.

56. Morrison G, Brown ST, Michelson EL, et al: Mechanism and prevention of cardiac arrhythmias during hemodialysis. Am J Cardiol 43:360, 1979.

57. Levy N, Abinader E: Continuous electrocardiographic monitoring with Holter electrocardiocorder throughout all stages of gastroscopy. Dig Dis 22:1901, 1977.

58. Higgins CB, Roeske WR, Karliner JS, et al: Predictive factors and mechanism of arrhythmias and myocardial ischemic changes in elderly patients during barium enema. Br J Cardiol 40:1023, 1976.

59. Mason JW: A comparison of electrophysiologic testing with Holter monitoring to predict antiarrhythmic-drug efficacy for ventricular tachyarrhythmias. N Engl J Med 329:445, 1993.

60. Anastasiou-Nana MI, Menlove RL, Nanas JN, et al: Changes in spontaneous variability of ventricular activity as a function of time in patients with chronic arrhythmias. Circulation 78:286, 1988.

61. Morganroth J, Michelson EL, Horowitz LN, et al: Limitations of routine long-term electrocardiographic monitoring to assess ventricular ectopic frequency. Circulation 58:408, 1978.

62. Schmidt G, Ulm K, Goedel-Meinen L, et al: Spontaneous variability of simple and complex ventricular premature contractions during long time intervals in patients with severe organic heart disease. Circulation 78:296, 1988.

63. Hohnloser SH, Klingenheben T, Zabel M, et al: Prevalence, characteristics and prognostic value during long-term follow-up of nonsustained ventricular tachycardia after myocardial infarction in the thrombolytic era. J Am Coll Cardiol 33:1895, 1999.

64. Guilleminault C, Connolly SJ, Winkle RA: Cardiac arrhythmia and conduction disturbances during sleep in 400 patients with sleep apnea syndrome. Am J Cardiol 52:490, 1983.

65. Miller WP: Cardiac arrhythmias and conduction disturbances in the sleep apnea syndrome. Am J Med 73:317, 1982.

66. Javaheri S, Parker TJ, Liming JD, et al: Sleep apnea in 81 ambulatory male patients with stable heart failure. Circulation 97:2154, 1998.

67. Hanly P, Sasaon Z, Zuberi N, et al: ST-segment depression during sleep apnea. Am J Cardiol 71:1341, 1993.

68. Nikolic G, Biship RL, Singh JB: Sudden death recorded during Holter monitoring. Circulation 66:218, 1982.

69. Panidis IP, Morganroth J: Sudden death in hospitalized patients: cardiac rhythm disturbances detected by ambulatory electrocardiographic monitoring. J Am Coll Cardiol 2:798, 1983.

70. Pratt CM, Francis MJ, Luck JC, et al: Analysis of ambulatory electrocardiograms in 15 patients during spontaneous ventricular fibrillation with special reference to preceding arrhythmic events. J Am Coll Cardiol 2:789, 1983.

71. Winkle RA: Current status of ambulatory electrocardiography. Am Heart J 102:757, 1981.

72. Weaver WD, Cobb LA, Hallstrom AP: Ambulatory arrhythmias in resuscitated victims of cardiac arrest. Circulation 66:212, 1982.

73. Tsuji H, Venditti FJ, Manders ES, et al: Determinants of heart rate variability. J Am Coll Cardiol 28:1538, 1996.

74. Hedman AE, Poloniecki JD, Camm AJ, et al: Relation of mean heart rate and heart variability in patients with left ventricular dysfunction. Am J Cardiol 84:225,1999.

75. Levy WC, Cerqueiro MD, Harp GD, et al: Effect of endurance exercise training on heart rate variability at rest in healthy young and older men. Am J Cardiol 82:1236, 1998.

76. Kleiger RE, Miller JP, Bigger JT, et al: Decreased heart rate variability and its association with increased mortality after acute myocardial infarction. Am J Cardiol 59:256, 1987.

77. Bigger JT, Fleiss JL, Steinman RC, et al: Frequency domain measures of heart period variability and mortality after myocardial infarction. Circulation 85:164, 1992.

78. Algra A, Tijssen JGP, Roelandt JR, et al: Heart rate variability from 24-hour electrocardiography and the 2-year risk for sudden death. Circulation 88:180, 1993.

79. Lanza GA, Guido V, Galeazzi MM, et al: Prognostic role of heart rate variability in patients with a recent acute myocardial infarction. Am J Cardiol 82:1323, 1998.

28 Normal Electrocardiograms in the Fetus, Infants, and Children

Heart Rate	S Waves
P Waves	ST Segment
PR Interval	T Waves
QRS Complex: Morphology, Duration, and Axis	QT Interval
Q Waves	Indications for Performance of ECGs in Pediatrics
R Waves	

In adults, an electrocardiogram (ECG) can be interpreted with the assumption of a common normal standard. Evaluation of the ECG in pediatric patients must consider dramatic variation of the normal standard with age. In the growing infant and child these variables change most rapidly in the first year of life. Davignon and colleagues published in 1979 the most extensive collection of age-dependent normal ECG parameters,[1] which are summarized in Table 28–1. This compilation of normal ECG parameters in pediatrics is limited by the preponderance of white (Caucasian) infants and children in this study population. The differences in ethnicity, racial background, and body mass index, as recognized in the ECG patterns in adults,[2] have been also recognized in children.[3–5] The most significant differences are in QRS voltage examined in the scalar ECGs and vectorcardiograms.[6] A large study in a more ethnically diverse population of children from birth to 6 years of age with normal left ventricular mass by echocardiogram has reported normal ranges for Q wave amplitude in leads III and V_6 and QRS voltage in precordial leads.[7] The voltages in most cases exceeded those in Davignon's study group and probably represent a better standard for current

patients. Extensive race-specific data are still lacking in the literature.

In recognition of improved technology in fetal electrocardiography and an anticipated transition of intervention for congenital heart disease from the newborn to the fetus, normal values for fetal ECGs are being developed[8,9] and are shown in Table 28–1.

Heart Rate

One of the most striking changes in the normal pediatric ECG is that affecting the resting heart rate with increasing age. The average resting heart rate increases from birth to 1 month of age and subsequently decreases.[1,10] The increase in heart rate in the first month of life is likely related to autonomic factors, but subsequent slowing of sinus node activity appears to be primarily related to the age-dependent changes in the "intrinsic" sinus node activity isolated from autonomic control[11]—a finding implying that changes in the autonomic control of heart rate in this age group are less important. Relative maturational changes in heart rate in the human have been shown to be similar to those seen in

TABLE 28–1   Normal Values for Pediatric ECG

Age/Gestation	Heart Rate (beats/min)	QRS Axis (degrees)	PR Interval (ms)	QRS Duration (ms)	Q (III) (mV)	R (V$_1$) (mV)	S (V$_1$) (mV)	R (V$_4$) (mV)	S (V$_4$) (mV)	R (V$_6$) (mV)	S (V$_6$) (mV)
20 weeks gestation	147	—	75.1–112.0	30.6–54.3	—	—	—	—	—	—	—
30 weeks gestation	143	—	80.7–129.2	35.4–62.9	—	—	—	—	—	—	—
40 weeks gestation	138	—	80.2–137.8	41.0–72.8	—	—	—	—	—	—	—
Days 0–1	122 (93–155)	59–193	79–161	21–76	0.01–0.51	0.5–2.6	0.1–2.3	0.3–3.0	0.3–2.8	0–1.2	0–1.0
1–3	122 (91–158)	64–196	81–139	22–67	0.01–0.51	0.5–2.7	0.1–2.1	0.6–3.0	0.2–2.7	0–1.2	0–1.0
3–7	128 (90–166)	77–193	73–136	21–68	0.01–0.48	0.3–2.4	0.1–1.7	0.6–2.9	0.3–2.6	0–1.2	0–1.0
7–30	149 (106–182)	65–161	72–138	22–79	0.01–0.56	0.3–2.1	0.1–1.1	0.8–2.9	0.3–2.3	0.2–1.7	0–1.0
Months 1–3	149 (120–179)	31–113	72–130	23–75	0.01–0.54	0.3–1.8	0.1–1.3	1.3–3.8	0.5–2.2	0.5–2.2	0–0.7
3–6	141 (106–186)	7–104	73–146	22–79	0–0.66	0.3–2.0	0.1–1.7	1.1–4.3	0.3–2.3	0.6–2.2	0–1.0
6–12	131 (108–169)	6–99	72–157	23–76	0–0.63	0.2–2.0	0.1–1.8	1.2–3.6	0.2–2.3	0.6–2.3	0–0.7
Years 1–3	119 (90–151)	7–101	81–148	27–75	0–0.53	0.3–1.8	0.1–2.1	1.1–3.5	0.3–2.0	0.6–2.3	0–0.7
3–5	109 (72–138)	6–104	83–161	30–72	0–0.42	0.2–1.8	0.2–2.2	1.3–4.5	0.2–1.8	0.8–2.4	0–0.5
5–8	100 (64–132)	11–143	90–163	32–79	0–0.32	0.1–1.4	0.3–2.3	1.2–4.4	0.2–1.9	0.8–2.7	0–0.4
8–12	91 (62–130)	9–114	88–171	32–85	0–0.27	0.1–1.2	0.3–2.5	1.1–4.2	0.2–1.9	0.9–2.6	0–0.4
12–16	80 (61–120)	11–130	92–176	34–88	0–0.30	0.1–1.0	0.3–2.2	0.7–3.9	0.1–1.8	0.7–2.3	0–0.4

Adapted from Davignon A, Rautuharju P, Boisselle E, et al: Normal ECG standards for infants and children. Ped Cardiol 1:123, 1979; and Taylor MJ, Smith MJ, Thomas M, et al: Non-invasive fetal electrocardiography in singleton and multiple pregnancies. BJOG 110:668, 2003.

smaller primates, although the absolute heart rates were markedly different.[12]

The interaction between heart rate, ventricular size, and cardiac output during development is of interest when considered from a teleologic viewpoint. Davignon's data[1] for heart rate and the body surface area of subjects make it apparent that the relationship of heart rate to body surface area is inverse and logarithmic. Akiba et al.[13] have shown an age-dependent increase in left ventricular volume and stroke volume that is logarithmic when indexed for body surface area. This increase is mirrored by a logarithmic decrease in heart rate, which creates a relatively constant product of heart rate and stroke volume, resulting in a stable cardiac output when indexed for body surface area.

P Waves

As in adults, the P wave axis in the frontal plane in sinus rhythm is normally directed to the left and inferiorly. Unlike the large variation in other ECG parameters with age, the P wave amplitude changes less in children. Thus the P wave in lead II for pediatric patients of all ages at the 50th percentile is approximately 1.5 mm and 2.5 mm for the 98th percentile.[1] Normal P wave duration and dispersion (range of P wave durations on a 12-lead ECG) are age dependent in the fetus[9] and in children,[14] probably due to an increase in atrial size with advancing age.

PR Interval

The mean PR interval increases from 102 to 110 ms from 18 to 22 weeks of gestational age to term in the normal fetus.[9] After birth, changes in atrioventricular (AV) nodal conduction, primarily influenced by autonomic factors, result in a decrease in the average PR interval from 107 ms at birth to 98 ms at 1 month of age.[1] From that age on, the duration of the PR interval increases due to slowing of AV nodal conduction related to intrinsic changes in the AV node, and in part to an increase in atrial size. The lower limit of normal for the PR interval of most children is 90 ms, which is considerably shorter than the accepted adult standard of 120 ms. The short PR interval may cause difficulties in the recognition of ventricular preexcitation. Perry et al. have suggested that the absence of Q waves in the left lateral precordial leads and presence of left axis deviation of the QRS complex in the frontal plane may suggest ventricular

preexcitation in children when the PR interval is less than 100 ms.[15] Ventricular preexcitation in children is usually due to conduction over an accessory AV connection but may also be due to conduction over a fasciculoventricular pathway.[16]

The upper limit of normal for the PR interval is 140 ms in the young infant and increases to 180 ms in the adolescent. When first-degree AV block is present, conduction slowing may be present either in the atrium, AV node, or His-Purkinje system.[17] In children with heart disease, this slowing usually occurs at only one of these sites.[18]

QRS Complex: Morphology, Duration, and Axis

The sequence of ventricular depolarization in children is the same as in adults. The amplitude of the QRS complex is dependent upon the relative mass of the right and left ventricles, cardiac position, body mass and habitus, and the impedance of the tissues. In contrast to the dominance of the left ventricle in the adult, the right ventricle of a term infant at birth is larger than the left.[19] At 1 month of age in a term infant the left ventricle is larger than the right, and the adult ratio of left-to-right ventricular size is usually reached by 6 months of age.[20] Thus term newborn infants usually demonstrate right ventricular preponderance with prominent R waves in the right precordium and deep S waves in the left lateral precordium. Notched R waves, which are recognized as a sign of right ventricular conduction delay in adults, are rarely seen in neonates, but notching of the R wave in lead V_1 is seen very frequently in normal infants after the age of 2 months. Regression of right ventricular dominance begins with a notch in the upstroke of the R wave in young infants and progresses to a notch in the downstroke of the R wave and ultimately in the S wave in older infants.[10]

Despite an equal ratio of left-to-right ventricular mass, the ECG of a 6-month-old infant differs from an adult-like pattern,[10] possibly due to a more vertical orientation of the heart in the infant. This results in more prominent midprecordial voltage and less voltage in the left lateral precordium.

During fetal life the left ventricular size exceeds the right ventricular size prior to 31 weeks of gestation.[19] Thus the right ventricular preponderance is frequently less pronounced in the preterm infant than in the term infant.[21] Right ventricular hypertrophy, however, may develop in these preterm infants due to lung disease of prematurity, and the ECG may be a useful tool in the follow-up of chronic residual lung disease in these infants.[22]

The QRS duration in the fetus and preterm infant is usually very short (Figure 28–1). Throughout childhood, the QRS complex demonstrates higher-frequency signals than in adult electrocardiograms, and higher bandwidth recording (250 Hz) may be required to accurately measure the QRS duration.[23]

The mean QRS duration increases from 47 ms at 18 to 22 weeks of gestation to 53 ms at term.[9] There is a subsequent continued increase in the QRS duration from birth to adolescence, with an increase from 50 ms at birth to 70 ms in the adolescent.[1,24] This increase parallels the increase in ventricular mass, which is probably responsible for it rather than a slower conduction.

As would be expected from the right ventricular preponderance of the term infant, the frontal plane QRS axis is usually directed rightward and inferiorly (Figure 28–2). Healthy preterm infants may have a more leftward and posteriorly directed vector.[21] In term infants, the rightward QRS axis changes to a more adult pattern, usually within the first year of life (Figure 28–3).

Q Waves

Q waves are normally seen in the inferior and left lateral precordial leads in pediatric patients. The duration of these Q waves is almost always less than 20 ms. The amplitude can be rather large (up to 14 mm)[7], especially in infants. Q waves are usually absent in leads I and aV_L in infants, and their presence is often suggestive of cardiac pathology. A deep ($\geq$3 mm) and broad ($\geq$30 ms) Q wave in leads I and aV_L, especially when accompanied by absence of Q waves in the inferior leads, may suggest the diagnosis of anomalous origin of the left coronary artery from the pulmonary artery.[25,26] Q waves in the right precordium are always pathologic and are commonly associated with right ventricular hypertrophy. Deep Q waves in the left lateral precordial leads are often seen with left ventricular hypertrophy of many etiologies. In the assessment of children and adolescents for familial hypertrophic cardiomyopathy, Q waves $\geq$3 mm in depth or $\geq$40 ms in duration in $\geq$2 leads other than lead V_1, V_2, or III have low sensitivity, but high specificity in the affected genetically tested children.[27]

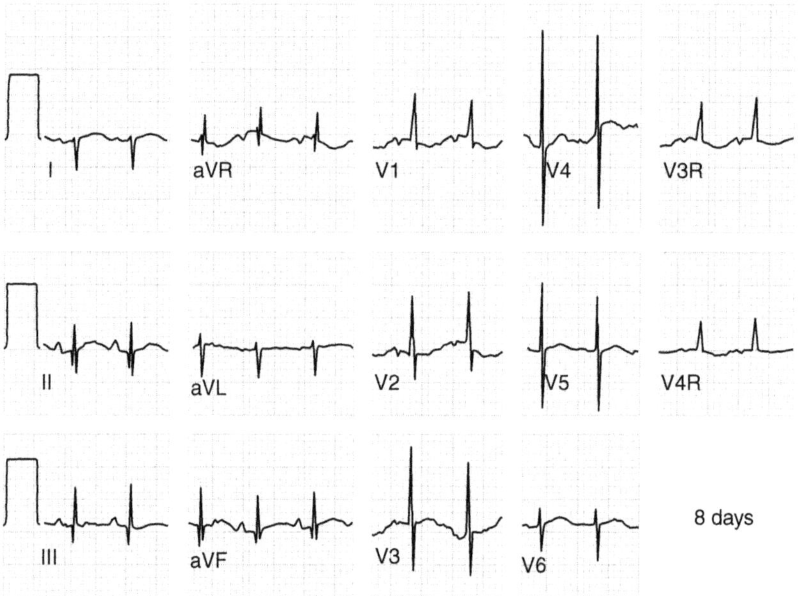

Figure 28–1 Normal ECG from an 8-day-old, 28-week-gestation premature infant. The frontal plane QRS axis is 150 degrees, there is a monophasic R wave in lead V_1, and the R/S ratio is less than 1 in lead V_6. This illustrates relative right ventricular preponderance without right ventricular hypertrophy. The QRS duration is less than 40 ms.

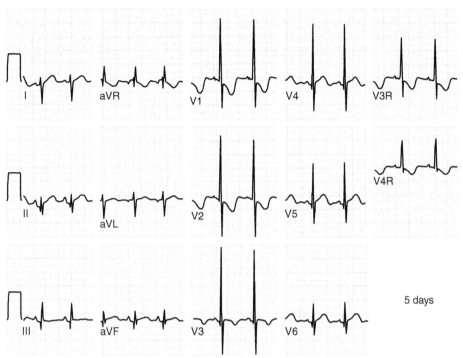

Figure 28–2   Normal ECG from a 5-day-old, term-gestation infant. The frontal plane QRS axis is 150 degrees. There is prominent voltage in the precordial leads and a suggestion of right ventricular preponderance but not right ventricular hypertrophy. The QRS duration is 60 ms.

R Waves

R waves are usually prominent in the right precordial leads in infants. An R wave in lead V_1 of up to 26 mm may be normal in a term newborn.[1] Right precordial R wave amplitude rapidly decreases in the first week of life[28] and undergoes further reduction later in life. Conversely the R wave in lead V_6 may be nearly absent in a term newborn but increases gradually from birth to adolescence (Figures 28–4 to 28–6). Substantial differences have been seen between black and white adolescents with higher voltage in the left lateral precordial leads in blacks.[4]

S Waves

Despite right ventricular preponderance in the term newborn, S waves are prominent in the right precordium and may be as large as 22 mm. The amplitude decreases to a minimum at 1 week to 1 month of age and then gradually increases with age and increasing left ventricular mass. The S waves in the left lateral precordium are frequently quite prominent at birth and may be up to 10 mm in lead V_6. Their amplitude then gradually decreases with age.[1]

ST Segment

Frequently in pediatric ECGs the true isoelectric line cannot be determined, because with faster heart rates the P wave falls on the preceding T wave. The PR segment may not be isoelectric due to the occurrence of atrial repolarization at that time. Despite such inherent drawbacks the PR segment is frequently used to assess the level of the ST segment. The elevation or depression of the ST segment >1 mm is rare in normal pediatric patients. When seen in normal children, ST elevation is most common in the precordial leads, especially those leads where the T wave is in transition. ST segment elevation related to "early repolarization" pattern has been shown to be gender specific,[29] with a high prevalence among adolescent males showing the "male pattern" with J point elevation exceeding 1 mm and ST angle greater than 20 degrees.[30]

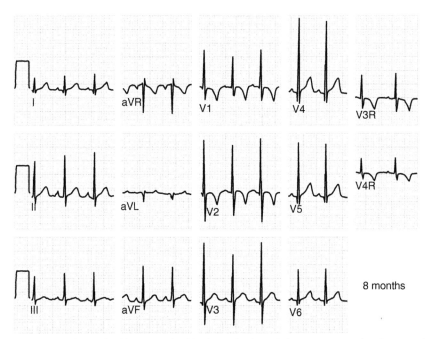

Figure 28–3   Normal ECG from a healthy 8-month-old infant. The frontal plane QRS axis is 60 degrees. There is less evidence of right ventricular preponderance than in the newborn tracing, with a smaller R wave in lead V_1 and smaller S wave in lead V_6.

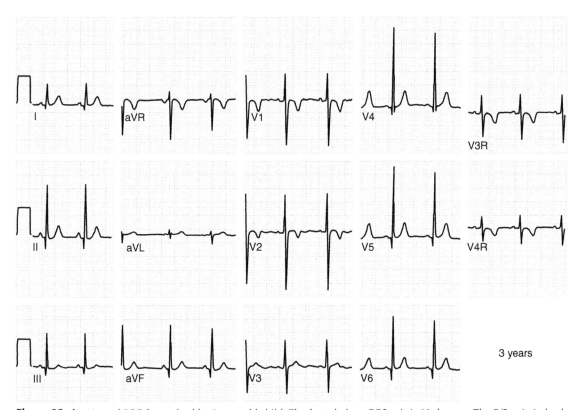

Figure 28–4   Normal ECG from a healthy 3-year-old child. The frontal plane QRS axis is 60 degrees. The R/S ratio in lead V_1 is less than 1, and there is no appreciable S wave in lead V_6. The R wave in lead V_6 is more prominent than that of the infant, suggesting more left ventricular preponderance but not left ventricular hypertrophy.

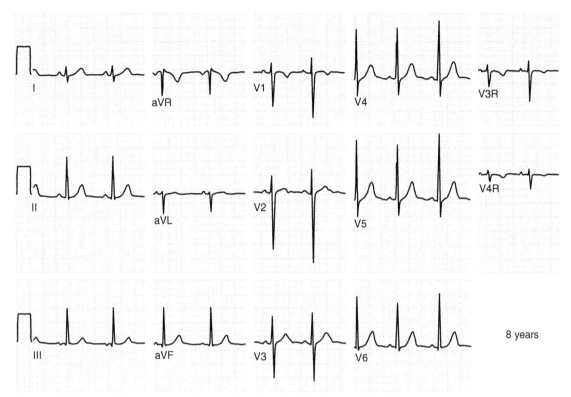

Figure 28–5   Normal ECG from a healthy 8-year-old child. The heart rate is 80 beats/min. The T wave transition is seen in lead V_2, farther to the right than in the younger child.

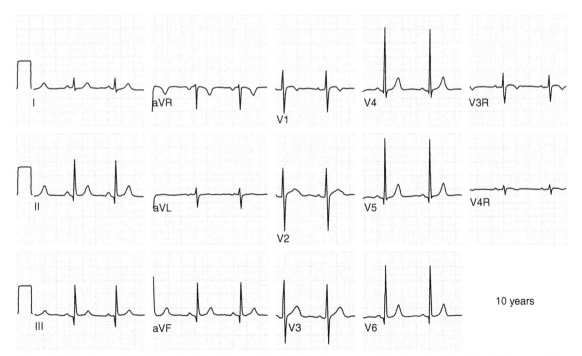

Figure 28–6   Normal ECG from a healthy 10-year-old child. The T wave transition is at lead V_1. It should be noted that although positive T waves in lead V_1 are normal, many individuals have negative T waves in the right precordium well into adulthood.

T Waves

The T waves of infants differ from those of adults in the right precordial leads. The T wave in lead V_1 is frequently upright in term newborn infants but becomes inverted by day 7 of life. These negative T waves generally persist until 7 years of life but frequently may remain inverted into adulthood, causing the so-called persistent juvenile T wave pattern. Upright T waves in the right precordium prior to age 7 years most commonly indicates right ventricular hypertrophy.

QT Interval

Exact measurement of the QT interval may be difficult for a number of reasons. The first is selection of the lead for measurement. In the era of single-channel ECG recording, lead II was the most commonly used.[31] With the ready availability of simultaneous multichannel ECG recordings, the QT interval can be measured from the earliest onset of the QRS complex in any lead to the end of the T wave where its terminal limb joins the baseline in any lead, excluding the measurement of distinct U waves.[32] When there is variation in the QT interval from lead to lead, the longest QT interval should be utilized.

A second problem in measuring the QT interval in young children is that the P wave may be superimposed on the preceding T wave. Extrapolation of the downslope of the T wave to the baseline is recommended in this case.

A third common problem in pediatric patients is the wide variation in RR intervals due to sinus arrhythmia and the slow adjustment of the QT interval to change with abrupt changes in heart rate.[33] Thus the determination of the RR interval to use for "correction" of the QT interval is difficult. It has been suggested that using the shortest RR interval with a diagnostic "cut-point" of 0.46 would place 3.8 percent of control patients in a "long QT" category, while 98.4 percent of patients with long QT syndrome would be included.[34] It may be more appropriate to use an RR interval that is averaged over several beats.[32] Sinus arrhythmia in children also affects the dispersion of the QT interval when corrected for heart rate, and as such it has been recommended that QT dispersion values not be corrected for heart rate in these patients.[35] There are no apparent differences in normal values for QT dispersion between adults and adolescents,[36] but data for younger children are lacking.

The formula used most commonly for "rate-correction" of the QT interval is the method of Bazett[37] (dividing the QT interval in seconds by the square root of the RR interval in seconds). More complex cube-root formulas (Fridericia) or tabular normal values for different heart rates (Framingham)[38] may be preferable but have not been widely applied, probably due to difficulty of use. However, as the "overcorrection" of the Bazett square-root formula in children results in a "corrected" QT interval that varies inversely with age and directly with heart rate,[39,40] whereas the "shorthand" rule that the rate-corrected QT interval will be normal if it is less than half of the RR interval has been validated, manual measurement and correction are preferred.[41]

It has been recognized that adult women have significantly longer corrected QT intervals than men. This gender difference has been confirmed in adolescents aged 14 to 18 years, but not in children from 10 to 13 years of age.[39] Also, infants do not have demonstrable gender differences in "rate-corrected" QT intervals.[42]

Exact measurement of the QT interval in pediatrics is critical in two situations. The first is in the diagnosis of the congenital long QT syndrome. For this application, the measurement of the QT interval with multi-lead recording and correction for heart rate with an RR interval averaged over a number of beats, using Bazett's formula with a normal range of <0.44, borderline range of 0.44 to 0.46, and abnormal range of >0.46, is reasonable.[31] Computer measurement of the QT interval has been shown to be unreliable in this situation.[43] The addition of clinical parameters and genetic studies improve diagnostic specificity.[44] Screening of large pediatric populations remains problematic given the overlap in normal and abnormal populations.[45] Assessment of QT interval response to exercise and measurement of the QT interval 1 minute into recovery from exercise has been proposed to discriminate prolonged QT syndrome from normal.[46,47] Epinephrine infusion has been proposed to unmask prolonged QT syndrome (especially LQT2) by development of a protuberance above the apex of the T wave in these individuals[48] and by substantially increasing the rate-corrected QT interval in LQT1 patients.[49] Beta-adrenergic blockers commonly used for treatment of children with the congenital long QT syndrome do not appear to affect the rate-corrected QT interval or QT dispersion.[50]

The second situation in which the assessment of QT interval is critical relates to changes in the QT interval in drug-treated patients in whom measurement of the QT interval at comparable heart rates is more reliable.[51] Assessment of a QT_{60} has also been proposed. This technique involves measurement of QT intervals at numerous heart rates from exercise testing or ambulatory ECG. The best mathematical relationship of the QT interval to heart rate is determined and the QT interval extrapolated to a heart rate of 60 beats/min.[52]

Indications for Performance of ECGs in Pediatrics

As the normal standards for pediatric ECGs differ from those of adults, indications for testing also vary. Many pediatric ECGs are performed to screen children for congenital heart disease, especially when a heart murmur is present. This practice is widespread, but one study found[53] that in a series of asymptomatic children presenting for evaluation of a heart murmur, the ECG did not affect the diagnosis assigned by a pediatric cardiologist, questioning its utility in this setting. Two other studies[54,55] agreed that the ECG was unlikely to disclose any unsuspected heart disease, but suggested that it may assist in reaching a lesion-specific diagnosis in the patient with underlying pathology. Yet another study[56] suggested that the ECG and chest x-ray were helpful in diagnosing heart disease in patients thought to have no disease by examination and in ruling out lesions in patients with possible heart disease in a population of pediatric patients referred for evaluation of heart murmurs or chest pain.

In diagnosed congenital heart disease, serial ECGs may be helpful in following the progression of disease and determining the need for intervention.

Another common use of the pediatric ECG is in the screening of clinically suspected arrhythmias. In this regard, the ECG may be helpful, both in demonstrating the arrhythmia or showing associated findings such as ventricular preexcitation or QT interval prolongation. Use of the ECG in screening pediatric patients with syncope has been shown to be reasonably cost effective when compared with other tests.[57] Routine ECG prior to noncardiac surgery has long been known to be unnecessary in adults unless cardiac signs or symptoms are present or the patient has high risk for occult heart disease.[58] A study in pediatrics[59] confirms that ECGs are unnecessary as a routine test in children before noncardiac surgery unless heart disease is suspected clinically.

The ECG is also indicated in the pediatric patient treated with drugs that may alter cardiac conduction or refractoriness, such as prokinetic agents, antidepressants, atypical antipsychotic drugs, stimulant medications used for attention deficit-hyperactivity disorder, and antiarrhythmic drugs.

ECGs are commonly performed in pediatric emergency departments. One study[60] showed that the indication for a majority of these studies was the evaluation of chest pain. Nearly half of the ECGs performed for the evaluation of chest pain in this study were performed on patients with chest pain reproducible by chest palpation. As expected all of these ECGs were normal. Of the patients with nonreproducible chest pain, approximately a third had abnormal findings on ECG including ventricular ectopy, QT interval prolongation, and ventricular hypertrophy. Another study showed no utility of the ECG in the emergency department when performed to evaluate acute chest pain.[61]

Other indications for ECG in the pediatric emergency department in this study included suspected arrhythmia (confirmed by ECG in nearly all patients tested) and seizure and syncope (demonstrating ventricular ectopy or QT interval prolongation in one fourth of patients tested). Less frequently identified indications included exposure to street drugs and patients with ingestion of drugs. In these patients, half had heart rate, conduction, and/or repolarization abnormalities.

Interpretation of ECGs by pediatric residents and emergency physicians has been shown to be relatively inaccurate,[62–64] suggesting that either further education, overreading by pediatric cardiologists,[65] or both may be advisable.

REFERENCES

1. Davignon A, Rautaharju P, Boisselle E, et al: Normal ECG standards for infants and children. Ped Cardiol 1:123, 1979.
2. Rautaharju PM, Zhou SH, Calhoun HP: Ethnic differences in ECG amplitudes in North American white, black, and Hispanic men and women. Effect of obesity and age. J Electrocardiol 27(Suppl):20, 1994.
3. Rao PS, Thapar MK, Harp RJ: Racial variations in electrocardiograms and vectorcardiograms between black and white children and their genesis. J Electrocardiol 17:239, 1984.
4. Rao PS: Racial differences in electrocardiograms and vectorcardiograms between black and white adolescents. J Electrocardiol 18:309, 1985.
5. Ito S, Okuni M, Hosaki J, et al: Effects of fatness on the electrocardiogram in children aged 12–15 years. Pediatr Cardiol 6:249, 1986.
6. Perry LW, Pipberger HV, Pipberger HA, et al: Scalar, planar, and spatial measurements of the Frank vectorcardiogram in normal infants and children. Am Heart J 111:721, 1986.
7. Rivenes SM, Colan SD, Easley KA, et al: Usefulness of the pediatric electrocardiogram in detecting left ventricular hypertrophy: results from the Prospective Pediatric

Pulmonary and Cardiovascular Complications of Vertically Transmitted HIV Infection (P2C2 HIV) multicenter study. Am Heart J 145:716, 2003.

8. Taylor MJ, Smith MJ, Thomas M, et al: Non-invasive fetal electrocardiography in singleton and multiple pregnancies. BJOG 110:668, 2003.

9. Chia EL, Ho TF, Rauff M, et al: Cardiac time intervals of normal fetuses using noninvasive fetal electrocardiography. Prenat Diagn 25:546, 2005.

10. Onat T, Ahunbay G: Regression of right ventricular dominance in the electrocardiogram after birth: a longitudinal follow-up of a healthy cohort from birth to 3 years. Pediatr Cardiol 19:197, 1998.

11. Marcus B, Gillette PC, Garson A Jr: Intrinsic heart rate in children and young adults: an index of sinus node function isolated from autonomic control. Am Heart J 119:911, 1990.

12. Brady AG, Johnson WH Jr, Botchin MB, et al: Developmental changes in ECG associated with heart rate are similar in squirrel monkey and human infants [published erratum appears in Lab Anim Sci 42:214, 1992]. Lab Anim Sci 41:596, 1991.

13. Akiba T, Nakasato M, Sato S, et al: Angiographic determination of left and right ventricular volumes and left ventricular mass in normal infants and children. Tohoku J Exp Med 177:153, 1995.

14. Kose S, Kilic A, Iyisoy A, et al: P wave duration and P dispersion in healthy children. Turk J Pediatr 45:133, 2003.

15. Perry JC, Giuffre RM, Garson A Jr: Clues to the electrocardiographic diagnosis of subtle Wolff-Parkinson-White syndrome in children. J Pediatr 117:871, 1990.

16. Sallee D III, Van Hare GF: Preexcitation secondary to fasciculoventricular pathways in children: a report of three cases. J Cardiovasc Electrophysiol 10:36, 1999.

17. Sarubbi B, Mercurio B, Ducceschi V, et al: A "multisite" atrioventricular block. Ital Heart J 5:64, 2004.

18. Sherron P, Torres-Arraut E, Tamer D, et al: Site of conduction delay and electrophysiologic significance of first-degree atrioventricular block in children with heart disease. Am J Cardiol 55:1323, 1985.

19. Emery JL, MacDonald MS: The weight of the ventricles in the later weeks of intra-uterine life. Br Heart J 22:563, 1960.

20. Emery JL, Mithal A: Weights of cardiac ventricles at and after birth. Br Heart J 23:313, 1961.

21. Sreenivasan VV, Fisher BJ, Liebman J, et al: Longitudinal study of the standard electrocardiogram in the healthy premature infant during the first year of life. Am J Cardiol 31:57, 1973.

22. Walsh EP, Lang P, Ellison RC, et al: Electrocardiogram of the premature infant at 1 year of age. Pediatrics 77:353, 1986.

23. Rijnbeek PR, Kors JA, Witsenburg M: Minimum bandwidth requirements for recording of pediatric electrocardiograms. Circulation 104:3087, 2001.

24. Macfarlane PW, McLaughlin SC, Devine B, et al: Effects of age, sex, and race on ECG interval measurements. J Electrocardiol 27(Suppl):14, 1994.

25. Johnsrude CL, Perry JC, Cecchin F, et al: Differentiating anomalous left main coronary artery originating from the pulmonary artery in infants from myocarditis and dilated cardiomyopathy by electrocardiogram. Am J Cardiol 75:71, 1995.

26. Chang RR, Allada V: Electrocardiographic and echocardiographic features that distinguish anomalous origin of the left coronary artery from pulmonary artery from idiopathic dilated cardiomyopathy. Pediatr Cardiol 22:3, 2001.

27. Charron P, Dubourg O, Desnos M, et al: Diagnostic value of electrocardiography and echocardiography for familial hypertrophic cardiomyopathy in genotyped children. Eur Heart J 19:1377, 1998.

28. Walsh SZ: The electrocardiogram during the first week of life. Br Heart J 25:784, 1963.

29. Bidoggia H, Maciel JP, Capalozza N, et al: Sex-dependent electrocardiographic pattern of cardiac repolarization. Am Heart J 140:430, 2000.

30. Surawicz B, Parikh SR: Prevalence of male and female patterns of early ventricular repolarization in the normal ECG of males and females from childhood to old age. J Am Coll Cardiol 40:1870, 2002.

31. Moss AJ: Measurement of the QT interval and the risk associated with QTc interval prolongation: a review. Am J Cardiol 72:23B, 1993.

32. Surawicz B, Knoebel SB: Long QT: good, bad or indifferent? J Am Coll Cardiol 4:398, 1984.

33. Brockmeier K, Khalil M, Sreeram N, et al: Repolarization analysis in children with the long QT syndrome. J Electrocardiol 36(Suppl):209, 2003.

34. Garson A Jr: How to measure the QT interval—what is normal? Am J Cardiol 72:14B, 1993.

35. Tutar HE, Ocal B, Imamoglu A, et al: Dispersion of QT and QTc interval in healthy children, and effects of sinus arrhythmia on QT dispersion. Heart 80:77, 1998.

36. Vialle E, Albalkhi R, Zimmerman M, et al: Normal values of signal-averaged electrocardiographic parameters and QT dispersion in infants and children. Cardiol Young 9:556, 1999.

37. Bazett HC: An analysis of the time relations of electrocardiograms. Heart 7:353, 1920.

38. Sagie A, Larson MG, Goldberg RJ, et al: An improved method for adjusting the QT interval for heart rate (the Framingham Heart Study). Am J Cardiol 70:797, 1992.

39. Pearl W: Effects of gender, age, and heart rate on QT intervals in children. Pediatr Cardiol 17:135, 1996.

40. Benatar A, Ramet J, Decraene T, et al: QT interval in normal infants during sleep with concurrent evaluation of QT correction formulae. Med Sci Monit 8:CR351, 2002.

41. Phoon CK: Mathematic validation of a shorthand rule for calculating QTc. Am J Cardiol 82:400, 1998.

42. Stramba-Badiale M, Spagnolo D, Bosi G, et al: Are gender differences in QTc present at birth? MISNES Investigators. Multicenter Italian Study on Neonatal Electrocardiography and Sudden Infant Death Syndrome. Am J Cardiol 75:1277, 1995.

43. Miller MD, Porter C, Ackerman MJ: Diagnostic accuracy of screening electrocardiograms in long QT syndrome I. Pediatrics 108:8, 2001.

44. Schwartz PJ, Moss AJ, Vincent GM, et al: Diagnostic criteria for the long QT syndrome. An update. Circulation 88:782, 1993.

45. Shannon DC: Method of analyzing QT interval can't support conclusions. Pediatrics 103(4 Pt 1):819, 1999.

46. Weintraub RG, Gow RM, Wilkinson JL: The congenital long QT syndromes in childhood. J Am Coll Cardiol 16:674, 1990.

47. Benatar A, Decraene T: Comparison of formulae for heart rate correction of QT interval in exercise ECGs from healthy children. Heart 86:199, 2001.

48. Khositseth A, Hejlik J, Shen WK, et al: Epinephrine-induced T-wave notching in congenital long QT syndrome. Heart Rhythm 2:141, 2005.

49. Vyas H, Hejlik J, Ackerman MJ: Epinephrine QT stress testing in the evaluation of congenital long-QT syndrome: diagnostic accuracy of the paradoxical QT response. Circulation 113:1385, 2006.

50. Kaltman JR, Ro PS, Stephens P, et al: Effects of beta-adrenergic antagonists on the QT measurements from exercise stress tests in pediatric patients with long QT syndrome. Pediatr Cardiol 24:553, 2003.

51. Funck-Brentano C, Jaillon P: Rate-corrected QT interval: techniques and limitations. Am J Cardiol 72:17B, 1993.

52. Davey P: How to correct the QT interval for the effects of heart rate in clinical studies. J Pharmacol Toxicol Methods 48:3, 2002.

53. Birkebaek NH, Hansen LK, Oxhoj H: Diagnostic value of chest radiography and electrocardiography in the evaluation of asymptomatic children with a cardiac murmur. Acta Paediatr 84:1379, 1995.

54. Newburger JW, Rosenthal A, Williams RG, et al: Noninvasive tests in the initial evaluation of heart murmurs in children. N Engl J Med 308:61, 1983.

55. Smythe JF, Teixeira OH, Vlad P, et al: Initial evaluation of heart murmurs: are laboratory tests necessary? [see comments]. Pediatrics 86:497, 1990.

56. Swenson JM, Fischer DR, Miller SA, et al: Are chest radiographs and electrocardiograms still valuable in evaluating new pediatric patients with heart murmurs or chest pain? Pediatrics 99:1, 1997.

57. Steinberg LA, Knilans TK: Syncope in children: diagnostic tests have a high cost and low yield. J Pediatr 146:355, 2005.

58. Goldberger AL, O'Konski M: Utility of the routine electrocardiogram before surgery and on general hospital admission. Critical review and new guidelines. Ann Intern Med 105:552, 1986.

59. von Walter J, Kroiss K, Hopner P, et al: Preoperative ECG in routine preoperative assessment of children. Anaesthesist 47:373, 1998.

60. Horton LA, Mosee S, Brenner J: Use of the electrocardiogram in a pediatric emergency department. Arch Pediatr Adolesc Med 148:184, 1994.

61. Massin MM, Bourguignont A, Coremans C, et al: Chest pain in pediatric patients presenting to an emergency department or to a cardiac clinic. Clin Pediatr (Phila) 43:231, 2004.

62. Snyder CS, Fenrich AL, Friedman RA, et al: The emergency department versus the computer: which is the better electrocardiographer? Pediatr Cardiol 24:364, 2003.

63. Snyder CS, Bricker JT, Fenrich AL, et al: Can pediatric residents interpret electrocardiograms? Pediatr Cardiol 26:396, 2005.

64. Giuffre RM, Nutting A, Cohen J, et al: Electrocardiogram interpretation and management in a pediatric emergency department. Pediatr Emerg Care 21:143, 2005.

65. Wathen JE, Rewers AB, Yetman AT, et al: Accuracy of ECG interpretation in the pediatric emergency department. Ann Emerg Med 46:507, 2005.

29 Abnormal Electrocardiograms in the Fetus, Infants, and Children

Atrial Abnormalities
Right Atrial Enlargement
Left Atrial Enlargement
Biatrial Enlargement

Ventricular Hypertrophy
Right Ventricular Hypertrophy
Left Ventricular Hypertrophy
Biventricular Hypertrophy

Ventricular Conduction Abnormalities

QT Interval Prolongation

Axis Deviation

Abnormal Q Waves

ST and T Abnormalities

The electrocardiographic (ECG) criteria for atrial end ventricular enlargement in children vary in some cases from those in adults, but in some cases are similar. Most abnormalities of the scalar ECG in pediatric patients must be determined based upon differences from the normal criteria for the patient's age, a factor infrequently considered in the ECG interpretation in adults. Changes in ventricular mass (absolute and relative [i.e., right versus left ventricle]) obtained from autopsy studies[1,2] and echocardiographic measurements[3,4] have been correlated with ECG abnormalities, but the correlations with the anatomic findings are less extensive in children than in adults.

Interpretation of the pediatric ECG is based on the combined knowledge from ECG and pathologic correlates in adults and the electrocardiographic measurement standards established for infants, children, and adolescents without cardiac pathology. Correlation of pediatric ECG findings with the echocardiographic findings in children with cardiac pathology also has been obtained.

The ECG criteria for atrial enlargement and ventricular hypertrophy assume the presence of sinus rhythm and normal ventricular conduction pattern, respectively.

Atrial Abnormalities

Data on P wave amplitudes in lead II in pediatric patients at various ages shows remarkable lack of age-related variation. In Liebman's study,[5] P wave amplitudes from birth to 16 years of age vary only from 1.5 to 1.8 mm at the 50th percentile and from 2.0 to 2.9 mm at the 95th percentile. In the study of Davignon et al.[6] in the same age groups P wave amplitudes at the 50th percentile varied only from 1.4 to 1.9 mm and at the 98th percentile from 2.4 to 2.9 mm. These values for the 98th percentile are similar to the 2.5 mm amplitude that is accepted as normal maximum for adults. P wave amplitudes in the right precordial leads in pediatrics have not been scrutinized to the same extent as those in lead II. In my experience it is rare for pediatric patients with normal hearts to have a positive deflection of the P wave in lead V_1 exceeding the adult normal amplitude of 1.5 mm.

The P wave duration, on the other hand, shows a progressive increase from early fetal gestation to adolescence.[5,7,8] Liebman's data[5] show a P wave duration of 51 ms at birth and 81 ms at 12 to 16 years at the 50th percentile. The 95th percentile increases from 65 to 95 ms in the same age groups.

RIGHT ATRIAL ENLARGEMENT

In the absence of appreciable age-related differences for P wave amplitude defining right atrial enlargement in the pediatric age range, the available diagnostic criteria for right atrial enlargement in adults may be applied to all age groups. In general, if the P wave exceeds 2.5 mm in lead II or the positive deflection of the P wave is greater than 1.5 mm in leads V_1 or V_2 in any age group, right atrial enlargement is suggested (Figure 29–1).

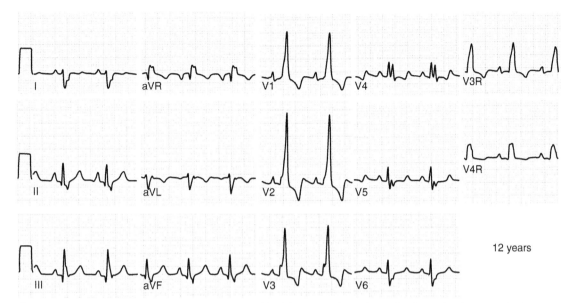

Figure 29–1   Right atrial enlargement in a 12-year-old adolescent with tetralogy of Fallot and right ventricular hypertension. The P waves are peaked in leads II, V_1, and V_2; they are 3 mm in amplitude in lead II and 2 mm in leads V_1 and V_2. Note also the presence of right axis deviation and right bundle branch block.

LEFT ATRIAL ENLARGEMENT

For reasons mentioned previously, the adult criteria for left atrial enlargement are applicable to children, notwithstanding the fact that the P wave duration in children gradually increases with age. It has been generally accepted that the product of the depth (in millimeters) and duration (in seconds) of the negative portion of the P wave in lead V_1 exceeding -0.04 mm × seconds suggests left atrial enlargement in all ages (Figure 29–2).

Notched P waves in lead II with a duration >95th percentile for age also suggest left atrial enlargement. The sensitivity of these criteria has been shown to be limited (44 percent), but the positive predictive value is acceptable (85 percent).[9]

The Macruz Index (the ratio of the duration of the P wave to the PR segment) is of little value in pediatrics. The normal index in children is higher than in adults,[5] probably due to more rapid conduction through the AV node in children. The variation of normal is so great that the index is not useful even if a higher cut-off point were to be established.

BIATRIAL ENLARGEMENT

As the right and left atria depolarize sequentially rather than simultaneously, ECG effects of enlargement of one atrium on the other is minimal. As in adults, the coexistence of ECG diagnostic criteria for both the left and right atrial enlargement suggest biatrial enlargement (Figure 29–3).

Ventricular Hypertrophy

Unlike P wave amplitudes, the amplitudes of Q, R, and S waves vary substantially in the age spectrum of normal pediatric patients. This is due to changes in ventricular mass, both absolute and relative to the patient's size, and the relation between the size of the right versus the left ventricle. Because of this marked variability, patient age must be considered in the assessment of ventricular hypertrophy.

RIGHT VENTRICULAR HYPERTROPHY

Right ventricular preponderance is the rule in the term newborn and young infants. Therefore when an ECG is interpreted as showing right ventricular hypertrophy (RVH) in this age group, the message to be conveyed is that the hypertrophy pattern is abnormal in comparison to that in normal patients of the same age, emphasizing to the referring physician that this diagnosis applies only to ECGs considered to be pathologic.

Traditional ECG criteria for RVH in pediatrics have included voltage, conduction abnormality, and Q wave and T wave criteria. Voltage criteria (R wave amplitude in lead V_1 or S wave amplitude in lead V_6 greater than the 98th percentile

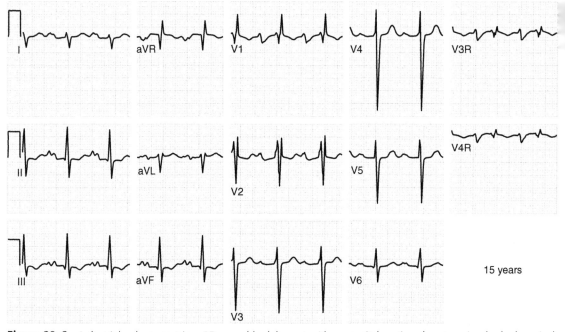

Figure 29–2   Left atrial enlargement in a 15-year-old adolescent with congenital aortic valve stenosis who had surgical intervention during infancy. Resultant left ventricular diastolic dysfunction caused elevation of the left ventricular end-diastolic and left atrial pressures. The P waves are notched in lead II and broad (P wave duration 160 ms). In lead V₁, the negative component is 2 mm deep and 100 ms in duration (−0.2 mm × seconds). Marked first-degree atrioventricular block is the result of antiarrhythmic drug therapy for atrial fibrillation that was seen in relation to the marked left atrial enlargement.

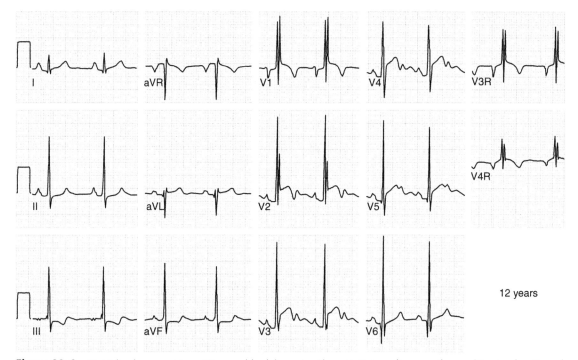

Figure 29–3   Biatrial enlargement in a 12-year-old adolescent with restrictive cardiomyopathy resulting in elevation of both right and left ventricular end-diastolic and right and left atrial pressures. The early portion of the P wave is peaked and 2.5 mm in amplitude in lead II, meeting criteria for right atrial enlargement. The P waves in lead V₁ are deeply negative and broad (3 mm × 50 ms = −0.15 mm × seconds), meeting criteria for left atrial enlargement.

for age and ratio of the R wave to the S wave in lead V_1 greater than the 98th percentile for age or in lead V_6 less than the 2nd percentile for age) have been sensitive for detection of RVH but seem to lack specificity (Figure 29–4). Right ventricular conduction delay secondary to hypertrophy, manifested as an rSR′ pattern in lead V_1 with normal QRS duration (Figure 29–5), is also suggestive of RVH, especially if the R′ wave is greater than the 98th percentile for age. The latter finding is also reasonably sensitive but less specific for the presence of RVH.

Enlargement of the right ventricle may occur with an increase in the thickness of the right ventricular wall, an increase in the ventricular cavity size, or both. Classically, increases in right ventricular wall thickness are related to an increase in right ventricular pressure, as seen in pulmonic stenosis or pulmonary hypertension. This type of hypertrophy is associated more commonly with increased voltage. An increase in the right ventricular cavity size is usually caused by higher than normal right ventricular volume load and is associated with an atrial

septal defect, anomalous pulmonary venous return, or tricuspid valve insufficiency. In these conditions there is typically right ventricular conduction delay. Despite the difference between the two different "classic" ECG patterns, either or both can be seen with both pathologic conditions (i.e., pressure and volume overload).

A qR complex in lead V_1 is abnormal in individuals of all ages and frequently suggests RVH. The Q wave is usually of low amplitude and is commonly associated with R wave amplitude of greater than the 98th percentile for age. Deeper Q waves and smaller R waves may suggest reversal of the normal depolarization of the ventricular septum and thus ventricular inversion. Although the finding of a qR complex in lead V_1 is highly specific for RVH, it is relatively insensitive and is usually only seen with severe RVH.

The T wave vector in the right precordial leads may also be helpful in assessment of RVH in pediatrics.[10] In normal children in the study of Davignon[6] the T waves were positive in lead V_1 in approximately half of all infants less than

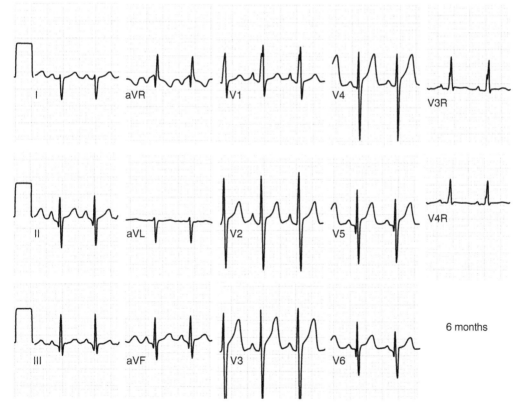

Figure 29–4 Right ventricular hypertrophy in a 6-month-old infant with valvar and supravalvar pulmonic stenosis. The pressure gradient across the stenosis measured at catheterization was 52 mmHg. This correlates well with reported formulas for right ventricular pressure (three times the amplitude of the R wave in lead V_1 + 47 mmHg). The T waves are positive in leads V_1 and V_{3R}. The S wave in lead V_6 is deeply negative, and the R/S ratio is less than 1.

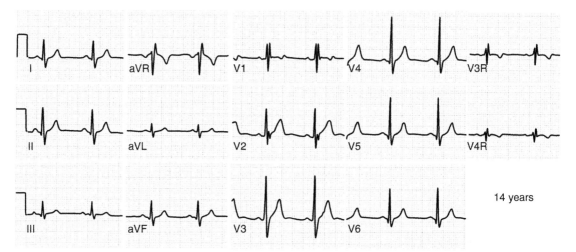

Figure 29–5 Right ventricular hypertrophy in a 14-year-old adolescent with a secundum-type atrial septal defect. The QRS duration is at the upper limits of normal, and the rSR' pattern in lead V_1 suggests right ventricular conduction delay. An echocardiogram showed significant enlargement of the right ventricular cavity with no increase in right ventricular wall thickness.

1 week of age. Between 1 week and 5 years of age the T wave amplitude in lead V_1 is distinctly negative even at the 98th percentile. Between 5 and 16 years of age the T wave amplitude in lead V_1 for the 50th percentile of the normal population becomes isoelectric and afterwards becomes positive in adults. For purposes of remembering the criteria, a T wave that is positive in lead V_1 between the ages of 7 days and 7 years should arouse suspicion of RVH. In my experience this is occasionally the only ECG manifestation of RVH. In older children, T wave inversion in the right precordial leads may signify right ventricular dilation, as in the setting of acute cor pulmonale.

The frontal plane QRS axis in pediatric patients is normally directed more rightward than in adults. This must be taken into consideration when assessing axis deviation from normal. Right axis deviation in the pediatric ECG is defined as a frontal plane QRS axis that is more rightward than the 98th percentile for age. The presence of a greater rightward axis for age should be considered as supportive evidence for RVH but is rarely the only criterion. Abreu-Lima and colleagues,[11] utilizing a Frank lead system, reported that determination of the frontal plane QRS axis was of little practical value in the diagnosis of RVH when used alone in adults but was useful for the prediction of RVH in pediatric patients. However, the proposed method of determining the area of QRS deflections on the vectorcardiogram is tedious, time consuming, and less accurate for the diagnosis than the more simple measurement of the amplitude of rightward forces. An evaluation of

the S wave amplitude alone, or determination of the R wave to S wave amplitude ratio in lead I compared with normal, may be as helpful or more helpful than calculation of the frontal plane axis. As in adults, right axis deviation with concomitant criteria for right atrial enlargement is highly suspicious for RVH.

Fretz and Rosenberg[12] reviewed the diagnostic value of ECG criteria RVH in 1000 pediatric patients. Of these, 434 had ECG criteria for RVH and a diagnosis based on clinical, echocardiographic, or angiographic criteria. Two thirds had a diagnosis consistent with RVH, but diagnoses were not separated by pressure or volume load. Upright T waves and the presence of Q waves in lead V_1 were found to be highly specific for RVH with specificities of 99 percent and 96 percent, respectively, and a sensitivity of approximately 13 percent for each criterion. Voltage criteria and presence of an rsR' pattern in lead V_1 were more sensitive (sensitivities of 63 percent and 74 percent, respectively) but were much less specific (specificities of 66 percent and 52 percent, respectively). This study confirmed the relatively poor predictive value of individual ECG criteria for RVH in most pediatric patients.

Puchalski et al. examined the value of the ECG in a pediatric population referred with suspicion of pulmonary hypertension.[13] Although there was a significant relationship between ECG and echocardiographic evidence for RVH, voltage, T wave, and Q wave criteria had a sensitivity of only 69 percent and a specificity of 82 percent for prediction of increased right ventricular wall thickness. The positive and negative predictive values were 67 percent and 84 percent, respectively. There was no relationship between estimated right ventricular pressure by tricuspid valve Doppler assessment and evidence for RVH by ECG. There was a statistically significant relationship between estimated RV pressure and echocardiographic assessment of right ventricular wall thickness.

LEFT VENTRICULAR HYPERTROPHY

ECG criteria for left ventricular hypertrophy (LVH) in pediatric patients have traditionally considered the QRS amplitude, the amplitude or absence of Q waves in the left precordial leads, and the morphology and polarity of T waves. Higher ECG voltage is seen in children and young adults than in older individuals, commonly resulting in "over-reading" of LVH when these criteria alone are used.[14] Increased posteriorly directed forces (the amplitude of S waves in lead V_1) and increased left lateral forces (the amplitude of R waves in lead V_6) or a sum of these amplitudes greater than the 98th percentile of normal have been considered as criteria for LVH.[15] These "voltage criteria" have been questioned for their lack of specificity.[16–18] The presence of Q waves in the left lateral precordial leads or the inferior leads greater than the 98th percentile of normal amplitude suggest hypertrophy of the interventricular septum, which usually accompanies hypertrophy of the left ventricle.[19] Absence of

Q waves in lead V_6 has been also considered as a criterion for LVH because it accompanies the incomplete left bundle branch block.[15] The absence of Q waves may also be related to displacement of the heart position related to the hypertrophy. These "Q wave criteria" are rather insensitive and also suffer from low specificity. The ST segment depression with upward convexity and T wave inversion in the left lateral precordial leads that is frequently accompanied by reciprocal changes in the right precordial leads manifested by ST segment elevation and a tall T wave[20] (Figure 29–6) represents a more specific but a less sensitive indicator of LVH.

As in the right ventricle, enlargement of the left ventricle may result from the increased thickness of the interventricular septum and left ventricular free wall, an increase in intracavitary volume, or both. Increased wall thickness occurs classically in situations of increased ventricular pressure such as aortic stenosis, coarctation of the aorta, or systemic hypertension. Increased wall thickness manifested by increased precordial lead voltage is also seen in storage disease such as Pompe's disease.[21] Increased intracavitary volume occurs in lesions such as ventricular septal defect, patent ductus arteriosus, aortic insufficiency, or mitral insufficiency.

Fogel and colleagues[22] compared the sensitivity and specificity of ECG criteria in pediatric populations with three conditions: aortic stenosis (increased pressure), ventricular septal defect

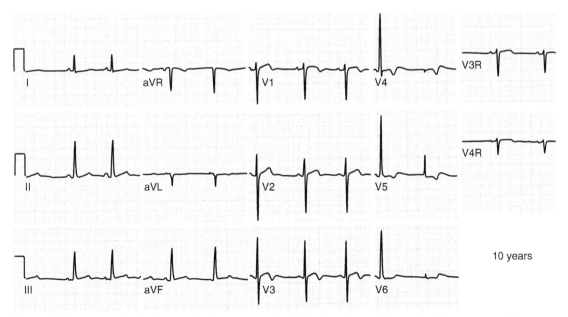

Figure 29–6 Left ventricular hypertrophy in a 10-year-old child with valvar aortic stenosis. The pressure gradient across the valve at catheterization was 40 mmHg. Prominent inferior, posterior, and left lateral precordial voltage is demonstrated for age. The ST segment and early portion of the T wave is depressed, suggesting a left ventricular "strain" pattern.

(increased volume), and normal patients. The findings with the highest sensitivity in the first two groups were voltage criteria (amplitude of S wave in lead V_1 plus R wave in lead V_6) with a sensitivity of 67 percent and 40 percent in the "pressure" and "volume" loaded groups, respectively. "Q wave criteria" (either an amplitude greater than the 98th percentile for age or absence in lead V_6) also showed similar sensitivity of 67 percent and 60 percent, respectively, in these groups. The specificity of "voltage criteria" in the normal patients was 95 percent, but for "Q wave criteria" it was only 71 percent. T wave criteria had a sensitivity of 50 percent in the pressure-loaded group, but only 10 percent in the volume-loaded group. The specificity of "T wave criteria" was 100 percent. When voltage and Q wave criteria were combined, the sensitivity increased to 89 percent in the pressure-loaded group and was unimproved over the individual criteria in the volume-loaded group. The specificity of the combined criteria was 71 percent. Fogel et al.[22] concluded that the sensitivity of ECG criteria for left ventricular enlargement in both pressure- and volume-loaded ventricles is at best modest and inferior to the serial assessment of left ventricular mass by echocardiography.

Another large study of children exposed to the human immunodeficiency virus (some with evidence for infection and others without) showed that in this population, ECG criteria were poor predictors of echocardiographic increase of left ventricular mass. When new age-adjusted predicted values were developed from the noninfected subjects, the sensitivity of voltage, Q wave, and T wave criteria was 17 percent and the specificity was 94 percent.[23] A study of a pediatric population with rheumatic heart disease has shown a somewhat higher sensitivity for height indexed left ventricular mass (71 percent) but lower specificity (74 percent).[24]

Obesity has been shown to affect precordial voltage in children,[25] and with the current epidemic of pediatric obesity, updated criteria for ECG voltage with consideration of the child's weight in different age groups may become necessary.

BIVENTRICULAR HYPERTROPHY

As evident from the previous sections on RVH and LVH, ECG criteria for each individual chamber must be applied with caution. Even among experienced cardiologists there is significant inter- and intraobserver variability in the interpretation of both RVH and LVH.[26] Computer analysis of pediatric ECGs for the diagnosis of RVH and LVH shows poor sensitivity but reasonable specificity when compared with cardiologist's interpretation.[27] Because right and left ventricular depolarization occur simultaneously rather than sequentially, the ECG effects from hypertrophy of one ventricle may substantially affect the recording from the other ventricle, making diagnosis of biventricular hypertrophy more difficult.

The ECG has a relatively low sensitivity for diagnosis of biventricular hypertrophy but has an acceptable specificity and positive predictive value.[28] A pattern of prominent mid-precordial voltage with biventricular hypertrophy secondary to large ventricular septal defects, known as the *Katz-Wachtel pattern*, was described in 1937.[29] If the R wave amplitude plus the S wave amplitude in the mid-precordial leads exceeds the 98th percentile for age, biventricular hypertrophy is suspected (Figure 29–7). Also, if the R and S wave amplitude in a relatively equiphasic mid precordial QRS complex is >6 mV or if there are several leads with R + S >5 mV, biventricular hypertrophy is likely.

Ventricular Conduction Abnormalities

Diagnostic criteria for bundle branch block, fascicular block, and conduction delay in pediatric patients are similar to those for adults. However, the duration of the QRS required for diagnosis is dependent upon the age of the patient. If the QRS duration is greater than 20 percent longer than the 98th percentile for age and other criteria for diagnosis are met, the terms *complete right bundle branch block* or *complete left bundle branch block* can be employed (Figures 29–8 and 29–9). Right bundle branch block is seen frequently in children with congenital heart disease, often as the result of surgical intervention, and may be seen in response to intrauterine events.[30] Left bundle branch block is less common in children. If the QRS duration is shorter but greater than the 98th percentile for age, the term *incomplete bundle branch block* may be used. If the QRS duration is greater than the 98th percentile for age and the criteria for right or left bundle branch block are not met, a nonspecific intraventricular conduction delay is diagnosed (Figure 29–10).

QT Interval Prolongation

The QT interval in pediatric patients may be prolonged in the presence of the congenital long QT syndrome, as in adults (see Chapter 24).

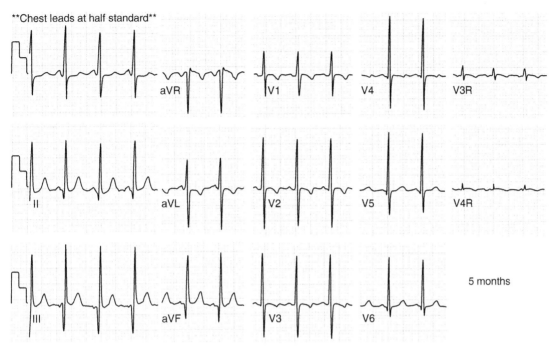

Chest leads at half standard

5 months

Figure 29–7 Biventricular hypertrophy in a 5-month-old infant with a large patent ductus arteriosus prior to intervention. Note that the precordial leads are recorded at a standard of 5 mm/mV. Prominent precordial voltage is seen in leads V_2–V_5 with R + S >5 mV in all of these leads. Deep and narrow Q waves are seen in the inferior leads, suggesting hypertrophy of the interventricular septum.

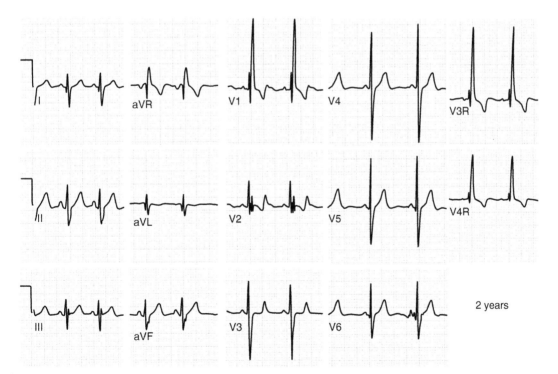

2 years

Figure 29–8 Right bundle branch block in a 2-year-old child following patch closure of a large infracristal ventricular septal defect. Note that the QRS duration of 100 ms exceeds the 98th percentile of normal by more than 20 percent. An rSR′ pattern in the right precordial leads is seen with a broad R′. A broad S wave is seen in the lateral leads.

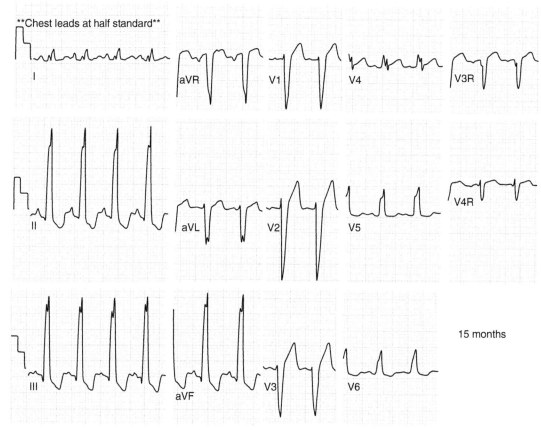

Figure 29–9 Left bundle branch block in a 15-month-old child with d-transposition of the great vessels with subaortic stenosis. It follows an arterial switch procedure and resection of the subaortic stenosis. The QRS duration of 120 ms is long enough to meet the criteria for bundle branch block in an adult and is far in excess of the 98th percentile of normal for age plus 20 percent. A broad, notched R wave is seen in the lateral leads, and Q waves are absent in these leads. The ST segments and T waves are displaced opposite the major QRS deflection.

Specific situations involving QT interval prolongation that are more commonly encountered in children than in adults include individuals on the ketogenic diet,[31] those with acute weight loss,[32] metabolic dilated cardiomyopathy,[33] and treatment with psychotropic drugs.[34–38] Children with Ullrich-Turner syndrome and those with sensory neural hearing loss have been shown to have QT interval prolongation.[39,40] Details on measurement and rate correction of the QT interval are discussed in Chapter 28.

Axis Deviation

In pediatrics, right axis deviation is most commonly seen in combination with other criteria for RVH (Figure 29–11). Left axis deviation is seen in ostium primum type atrial septal defect (Figure 29–12), AV canal, and inlet ventricular septal defects due to posterior and inferior displacement of the AV node and left bundle branch.[41,42] Left axis deviation is also commonly seen in tricuspid atresia.[43]

Abnormal Q Waves

Physiologic Q waves are common, especially in the inferior leads. They are usually less than 30 ms in duration. Q wave duration greater than 30 ms and amplitude greater than 0.4 mV may suggest myocardial infarction, especially in the context of Kawasaki syndrome[44] or anomalous left coronary artery arising from the pulmonary artery.[45] As previously discussed, Q waves in lead V_1 suggest RVH, and deep but narrow Q waves in the inferior and left lateral precordial leads may suggest LVH, especially that associated with hypertrophic cardiomyopathy.

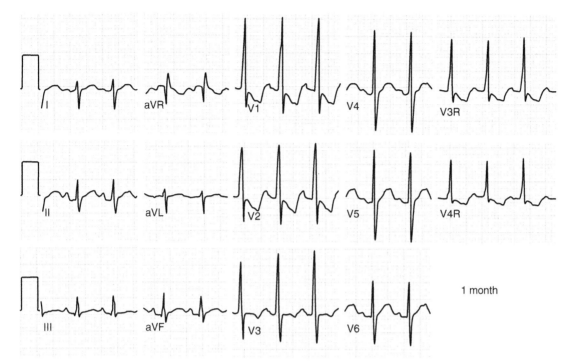

Figure 29–10   Nonspecific intraventricular conduction delay in a 1-month-old infant treated with flecainide. The QRS duration is 90 ms. The serum flecainide level was 0.89 μg/mL at the time of this ECG. Slowing of ventricular conduction by the drug resulted in the ECG finding.

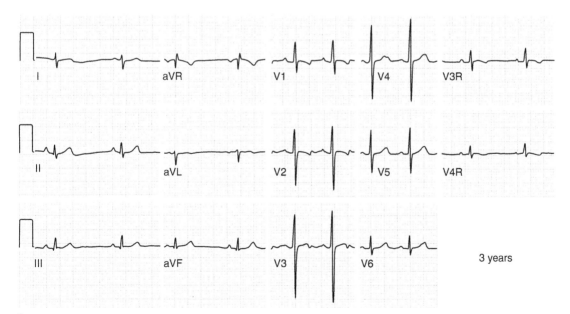

Figure 29–11   Right axis deviation in a 3-year-old child with mild valvar pulmonic stenosis. Doppler echocardiography estimated a gradient of 20 mmHg across the pulmonary valve. Right axis deviation may be the only ECG finding in pediatric patients with mild right ventricular hypertrophy.

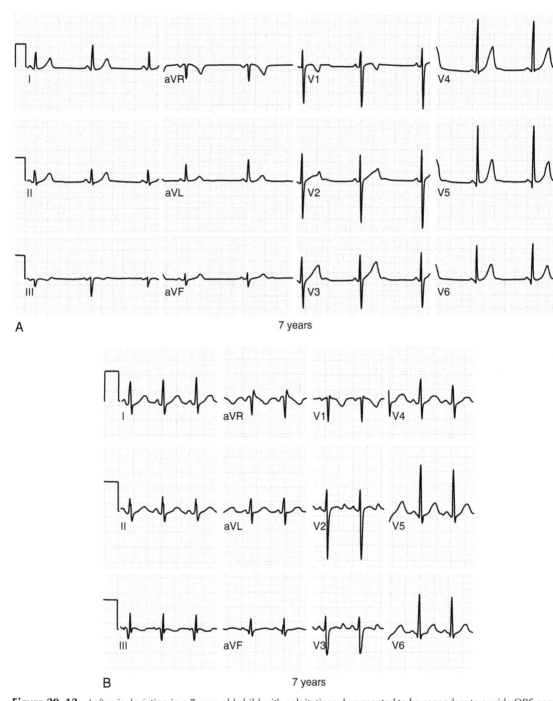

Figure 29–12 Left axis deviation in a 7-year-old child with palpitations documented to be secondary to a wide QRS complex tachycardia. **A,** Note that in the first ECG there is mild left axis deviation. The degree of left axis deviation appears to be somewhat variable (especially in lead III). Electrophysiologic study demonstrated that the patient had a right free wall accessory atrioventricular (AV) connection with decremental conduction properties that participated in an antidromic AV reentrant tachycardia (Mahaim fiber). **B,** The second ECG was recorded after radiofrequency catheter ablation of the accessory connection. The previously seen left axis deviation caused by subtle ventricular preexcitation has resolved.

ST and T Abnormalities

ST segment elevation of greater than 0.2 mV in several leads may be seen in myocarditis[46] and pericarditis.[47] Myocardial infarction is rare in pediatric patients but, if present, produces the same ST segment changes as in adults. Wide Q waves (longer than 35 ms) and prolonged QT interval corrected for heart rate (>440 ms) are reported to be highly specific for myocardial infarction when combined with ST segment elevation >2 mm.[46] ST segment depression has been reported in children with severe head injury.[48]

A "coved type" ST segment elevation has been reported in Brugada syndrome[49] (see Chapter 7). Presentation with arrhythmic syncope and cardiac arrest is rare in the pediatric age group,[50,51] and ECG changes are absent in most individuals with this sodium channel mutation before the age of 5 years.[52]

T wave inversion combined with ST segment depression in the left lateral precordial leads suggests LVH and is described as a "strain pattern" (see Figure 29–6). As previously mentioned, upright T waves in the right precordial leads between the ages of 7 days and 7 years suggest RVH.

REFERENCES

1. Emery JL, MacDonald MS: The weight of the ventricles in the later weeks of intra-uterine life. Br Heart J 22:563, 1960.
2. Emery JL, Mithal A: Weights of cardiac ventricles at and after birth. Br Heart J 23:313, 1961.
3. Devereux RB, Reichek N: Echocardiographic determination of left ventricular mass in man. Anatomic validation of the method. Circulation 55:613, 1977.
4. Reichek N, Devereux RB: Left ventricular hypertrophy: relationship of anatomic, echocardiographic and electrocardiographic findings. Circulation 63:1391, 1981.
5. Liebman J: Atrial hypertrophy. *In:* Liebman J, Plonsey R, Gillette P (eds): Pediatric Electrocardiography. Baltimore, Williams & Wilkins, 1982, p 140.
6. Davignon A, Rautuharju P, Boisselle E, et al: Normal ECG standards for infants and children. Ped Cardiol 1:123, 1979.
7. Chia EL, Ho TF, Rauff M, et al: Cardiac time intervals of normal fetuses using noninvasive fetal electrocardiography. Prenat Diagn 25:546, 2005.
8. Kose S, Kilic A, Iyisoy A, et al: P wave duration and P dispersion in healthy children. Turk J Pediatr 45:133, 2003.
9. Maok J, Krongrad E: Assessment of electrocardiographic criteria for left atrial enlargement in childhood. Am J Cardiol 53:215, 1984.
10. Cayler GG, Ongley P, Nadas AS: Relation of systolic pressure in the right ventricle to the electrocardiogram: a study of patients with pulmonary stenosis and intact ventricular septum. New Engl J Med 258:979, 1958.
11. Abreu-Lima C, Marques de Sa JP, Coelho G, et al: Frontal-plane QRS axis revisited: accuracy of current approximations and reappraisal of their merit in the diagnosis of right ventricular hypertrophy. J Electrocardiol 21:369, 1988.
12. Fretz EB, Rosenberg HC: Diagnostic value of ECG patterns of right ventricular hypertrophy in children. Can J Cardiol 9:829, 1993.
13. Puchalski MD, Lozier JS, Bradley DJ, et al: Electrocardiography in the diagnosis of right ventricular hypertrophy in children. Pediatrics 118:1052, 2006.
14. Walker CHM, Rose RL: Importance of age, sex and body habitus in the diagnosis of left ventricular hypertrophy from the precordial electrocardiogram in childhood and adolescence. Pediatrics 28:705, 1961.
15. Garson A Jr: The Electrocardiogram in Infants and Children: A Systematic Approach, 1st ed. Philadelphia, Lea and Febiger, 1983.
16. Aristimuno GG, Foster TA, Berenson GS, et al: Subtle electrocardiographic changes in children with high levels of blood pressure. Am J Cardiol 54:1272, 1984.
17. Hashida E, Nishi T: Constitutional and echocardiographic variability of the normal electrocardiogram in children. J Electrocardiol 21:231, 1988.
18. Morganroth J, Maron BJ, Krovetz LJ, et al: Electrocardiographic evidence of left ventricular hypertrophy in otherwise normal children. Clarification by echocardiography. Am J Cardiol 35:278, 1975.
19. Cabrera CE, Munroy JR: Systolic and diastolic loading of the heart. II: Electrocardiographic data. Am Heart J 43:669, 1952.
20. Wagner HR, Weidman WH, Ellison RC, et al: Indirect assessment of severity in aortic stenosis. Circulation 56 (1 Suppl):I20, 1977.
21. Ansong AK, Li JS, Nozik-Grayck E, et al: Electrocardiographic response to enzyme replacement therapy for Pompe disease. Genet Med 8:297, 2006.
22. Fogel MA, Lieb DR, Seliem MA: Validity of electrocardiographic criteria for left ventricular hypertrophy in children with pressure- or volume-loaded ventricles: comparison with echocardiographic left ventricular muscle mass. Pediatr Cardiol 16:261, 1995.
23. Rivenes SM, Colan SD, Easley KA, et al: Usefulness of the pediatric electrocardiogram in detecting left ventricular hypertrophy: results from the Prospective Pediatric Pulmonary and Cardiovascular Complications of Vertically Transmitted HIV Infection (P2C2 HIV) multicenter study. Am Heart J 145:716, 2003.
24. Sastroasmoro S, Madiyono B, Oesman IN: Sensitivity and specificity of electrocardiographic criteria for left ventricular hypertrophy in children with rheumatic heart disease. Paediatr Indones 31:233, 1991.
25. Ito S, Okuni M, Hosaki J, et al: Effects of fatness on the electrocardiogram in children aged 12–15 years. Pediatr Cardiol 6:249, 1986.
26. Hamilton RM, McLeod K, Houston AB, et al: Inter- and intraobserver variability in LVH and RVH reporting in pediatric ECGs. Ann Noninvasive Electrocardiol 10:330, 2005.
27. Hamilton RM, Houston AB, McLeod K, et al: Evaluation of pediatric electrocardiogram diagnosis of ventricular hypertrophy by computer program compared with cardiologists. Pediatr Cardiol 26:373, 2005.
28. Jain A, Chandna H, Silber EN, et al: Electrocardiographic patterns of patients with echocardiographically determined biventricular hypertrophy. J Electrocardiol 32:269, 1999.
29. Katz LN, Wachtel H: The diphasic QRS type of electrocardiogram in congenital heart disease. Am Heart J 13:202, 1937.

30. Benettoni A, Rustico MA: Pulmonary hypertension due to spontaneous premature ductal constriction in fetal life: association with right bundle branch block. Cardiol Young 12:581, 2002.

31. Best TH, Franz DN, Gilbert DL, et al: Cardiac complications in pediatric patients on the ketogenic diet. Neurology 54:2328, 2000.

32. Koch JJ, Porter CJ, Ackerman MJ: Acquired QT prolongation associated with esophagitis and acute weight loss: how to evaluate a prolonged QT interval. Pediatr Cardiol 26:646, 2005.

33. Ryerson LM, Giuffre RM: QT intervals in metabolic dilated cardiomyopathy. Can J Cardiol 22:217, 2006.

34. Blair J, Taggart B, Martin A: Electrocardiographic safety profile and monitoring guidelines in pediatric psychopharmacology. J Neural Transm 111:791, 2004.

35. Biswas AK, Zabrocki LA, Mayes KL, et al: Cardiotoxicity associated with intentional ziprasidone and bupropion overdose. J Toxicol Clin Toxicol 41:79, 2003.

36. Blair J, Scahill L, State M, et al: Electrocardiographic changes in children and adolescents treated with ziprasidone: a prospective study. J Am Acad Child Adolesc Psychiatry 44:73, 2005.

37. Francis PD: Effects of psychotropic medications on the pediatric electrocardiogram and recommendations for monitoring. Curr Opin Pediatr 14:224, 2002.

38. Rosenbaum TG, Kou M: Are one or two dangerous? Tricyclic antidepressant exposure in toddlers. J Emerg Med 28:169, 2005.

39. Dalla Pozza R, Bechtold S, Kaab S, et al: QTc interval prolongation in children with Ulrich-Turner syndrome. Eur J Pediatr 165:831, 2006.

40. El Habbal MH, Mahoney CO: QT interval in children with sensory neural hearing loss. Pacing Clin Electrophysiol 25(4 Pt 1):435, 2002.

41. Boineau JP, Moore EN, Patterson DF: Relationship between the ECG, ventricular activation, and the ventricular conduction system in ostium primum ASD. Circulation 48:556, 1973.

42. Feldt RH, DuShane JW, Titus JL: The atrioventricular conduction system in persistent common atrioventricular canal defect: correlations with electrocardiogram. Circulation 42:437, 1970.

43. Dick M, Fyler DC, Nadas AS: Tricuspid atresia: clinical course in 101 patients. Am J Cardiol 36:327, 1975.

44. Nakanishi T, Takao A, Kondoh C, et al: ECG findings after myocardial infarction in children after Kawasaki disease. Am Heart J 116:1028, 1988.

45. Johnsrude CL, Perry JC, Cecchin F, et al: Differentiating anomalous left main coronary artery originating from the pulmonary artery in infants from myocarditis and dilated cardiomyopathy by electrocardiogram. Am J Cardiol 75:71, 1995.

46. Towbin JA, Bricker JT, Garson AJr: Electrocardiographic criteria for diagnosis of acute myocardial infarction in childhood. Am J Cardiol 69:1545, 1992.

47. Spodick DH: Electrocardiogram in acute pericarditis. Distributions of morphologic and axial changes by stages. Am J Cardiol 33:470, 1974.

48. Dash M, Bithal PK, Prabhakar H, et al: ECG changes in pediatric patients with severe head injury. J Neurosurg Anesthesiol 15:270, 2003.

49. Antzelevitch C, Brugada P, Borggrefe M, et al: Brugada syndrome: report of the second consensus conference. Heart Rhythm 2:429, 2005.

50. Suzuki H, Torigoe K, Numata O, et al: Infant case with a malignant form of Brugada syndrome. J Cardiovasc Electrophysiol 11:1277, 2000.

51. Mivelaz Y, Di Bernardo S, Pruvot E, et al: Brugada syndrome in childhood: a potential fatal arrhythmia not always recognised by paediatricians. A case report and review of the literature. Eur J Pediatr 165:507, 2006.

52. Beaufort-Krol GC, van den Berg MP, Wilde AA, et al: Developmental aspects of long QT syndrome type 3 and Brugada syndrome on the basis of a single SCN5A mutation in childhood. J Am Coll Cardiol 46:331, 2005.

30 | The Electrocardiogram in Congenital Heart Disease

Acyanotic Lesions	Cyanotic Lesions
Atrial Septal Defect and AV Septal Defect	d-Transposition of the Great Vessels
Ventricular Septal Defect	Tetralogy of Fallot
Patent Ductus Arteriosus and Aortopulmonary Window	Truncus Arteriosus
Pulmonic Stenosis	Pulmonary Atresia with Intact Ventricular Septum
Aortic Stenosis	Ebstein's Anomaly of the Tricuspid Valve
L-Transposition of the Great Vessels	Tricuspid Atresia
Anomalous Origin of the Left Coronary Artery	Hypoplastic Left Heart Syndrome
Left Ventricular Noncompaction	Single Ventricle
	Fontan Palliation

Prior to the development of cardiac ultrasound, the electrocardiogram (ECG) was a vital component in the initial evaluation and follow-up of patients with congenital heart disease. Even now with widespread availability of echocardiography and other imaging technologies, the ECG remains a useful screening tool adjunct to the physical examination in the diagnosis of congenital heart disease and acquired heart disease in children. Evidence for atrial enlargement or ventricular hypertrophy on the ECG may help to confirm clinical suspicion of congenital heart lesion. Abnormalities of atrioventricular (AV) conduction might suggest ventricular inversion, whereas ventricular preexcitation suggests the possible association of Ebstein's anomaly of the tricuspid valve in the appropriate clinical circumstance. A leftward frontal plane QRS axis in an infant might suggest the presence of an ostium primum atrial septal defect, AV canal, or tricuspid atresia, depending upon the clinical correlates. A normal ECG, on the other hand, in the presence of a normal physical examination may be reassuring as to the absence of structural heart disease.

In addition to serving as a readily available screening tool for the diagnosis of congenital heart disease, in some forms of congenital heart disease the ECG may be used to monitor the severity and progression of the disease. This is the case in isolated valvar pulmonic stenosis, for which several formulas have been proposed to calculate right ventricular pressure based on ECG parameters.[1,2] In other diseases, the ECG has less utility in following the progression of disease. For example, in valvar aortic stenosis the ECG may be normal in the face of extreme stenosis and increased left ventricular pressure.[3]

Recent advances in technology have resulted in miniaturization of cardiac ultrasound and development of new imaging devices. The currently available "handheld" instruments[4] may replace the ECG for screening or establishing the presence of structural heart disease.

This chapter will review ECG abnormalities in congenital heart lesions and the reliability of the ECG in the diagnosis and assessment of disease severity. The lesions are grouped as either acyanotic or cyanotic at the time of initial clinical presentation.

Acyanotic Lesions

ATRIAL SEPTAL DEFECT AND AV SEPTAL DEFECT

The ECG in a child with a secundum-type atrial septal defect usually shows normal sinus rhythm. The preoperative abnormalities of sinus node function in children with this defect[5–8] are less common than in adults. Adults with unrepaired secundum-type atrial septal defect have an increased incidence of atrial flutter, atrial fibrillation, and sinus bradycardia with junctional escape rhythm.[9] Surgical closure of the atrial septal defect in adults has been shown to reduce the incidence of atrial flutter, but not atrial fibrillation.[10]

The child with a secundum-type atrial septal defect may have peaked P waves in lead II suggesting right atrial enlargement, but in the majority of patients the P wave amplitude and duration are normal. The PR interval[11] and (surprisingly) the HV interval of children with secundum-type atrial septal defects have been shown to be significantly longer than in normal children. These abnormalities are age related.[12] When the left-to-right shunt is significant, there is almost always right ventricular conduction delay[13] and right ventricular hypertrophy (RVH) with an rsR' pattern in lead V_1 (Figure 30–1). Zufelt and colleagues[14] examined the ECGs of pediatric patients with secundum-type atrial septal defects and defined criteria for RVH as a qR pattern or upright T wave in the right precordial leads, increased amplitude of R wave in lead V_1, S wave in lead V_6 greater than the 95th percentile, or abnormal R/S ratio in lead V_1 or V_6. They found that rsR' pattern in lead V_1, with or without other evidence of RVH, or other evidence for RVH without rsR' pattern in lead V_1 were 87 percent sensitive and 96 percent specific for this diagnosis when applied to a group with normal hearts. Cohen et al. found a high specificity of a notch near the apex of the R wave (crochetage pattern) in the inferior leads in children with secundum-type atrial septal defects,[15] confirming previous findings by Heller et al.[16] The sensitivity of this finding was only 32 percent, but the

specificity was 86 percent when the pattern was found in one inferior lead and 92 percent when found in all three inferior leads. Christensen and Vincent performed a review of patients with secundum atrial septal defects and found that 18 percent had normal ECGs and 7 percent had normal ECGs and normal physical examination.[17]

Surgical closure of secundum-type atrial septal defects has resulted in some studies[18] in decreased P wave duration and dispersion that were increased in children[19] and adults[20] prior to intervention, but did not restore them to normal levels. Other studies have not confirmed such improvement.[21] This may relate to a persistent risk of atrial fibrillation. Treatment with transcatheter devices resulted in partial or complete regression of ECG abnormalities in the majority of pediatric patients.[22–24] QT dispersion decreased significantly within 1 month after closure by the device, but other ECG intervals were not acutely changed.[24] Postprocedural AV block has been reported, but is typically transient.[25] Arrhythmias after device closure of secundum-type atrial septal defects are rare and benign, but long-term follow-up data are lacking.[26–28]

The distinctive feature of the ECG in an infant or child with an ostium primum atrial septal defect or AV septal defect (AV canal) is left axis deviation in the frontal plane. The QRS vector loop is inscribed in a counterclockwise fashion (Figures 30–2 and 30–3) due to the posterior and inferior

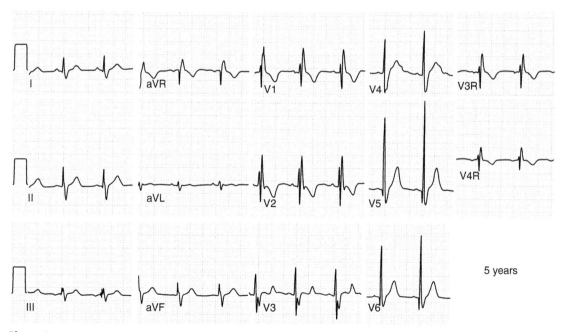

Figure 30–1 ECG of a 5-year-old child with an unrepaired secundum-type atrial septal defect. The rsR' pattern in the right precordial leads and incomplete right bundle branch block suggest right ventricular enlargement from a volume load. Echocardiography confirmed a large right ventricular chamber without an increase in wall thickness.

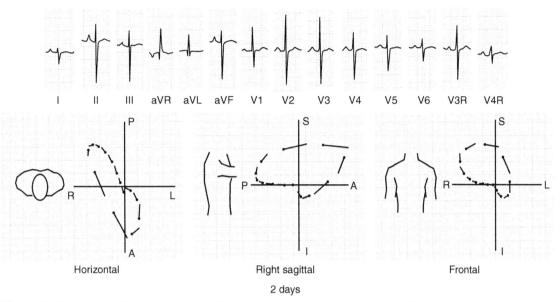

Figure 30–2 Vectorcardiogram of a 2-day-old infant with complete atrioventricular canal. The frontal plane QRS loop is inscribed in a counterclockwise direction, and the QRS loop is superior in the frontal and right sagittal planes. The grid represents a scale of 10 mm/mV, and each mark represents 4 ms.

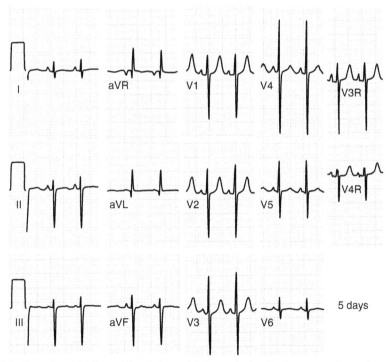

Figure 30–3 ECG of a 5-day-old infant with unbalanced, left ventricular dominant complete atrioventricular canal and coarctation of the aorta. The frontal plane QRS axis is −75 degrees. The precordial leads show more posteriorly directed voltage, consistent with a large left ventricle.

displacement of the AV node and left bundle branch. There is also a relative hypoplasia of the anterior left bundle branch.[29,30] P wave changes consistent with left or right atrial enlargement occur infrequently, but PR interval is prolonged in a majority of patients with AV septal defects secondary to prolonged intraatrial conduction.[31] Sinus node and AV node function are usually normal.[31,32] The conduction system is exposed to the risk of surgical repair, but modern surgical methods minimize the risk of postoperative AV block.[33] As in the children with secundum-type atrial septal defect, right ventricular conduction delay and hypertrophy are frequently seen in the presence of significant mitral valve insufficiency associated with cleft mitral valve. Evidence of left ventricular hypertrophy (LVH) may also be present in this setting.

In the less common sinus venosus type of atrial septal defect, the P wave axis in frontal plane in patients with sinus rhythm is either left and superior[34] or normal. Follow-up of patients after surgical repair of sinus venosus–type defects shows relatively high rates of sinus node dysfunction (6 percent) and age-related atrial fibrillation (14 percent).[35] Alternative operative techniques may reduce the frequency of sinus node dysfunction and arrhythmia.[36,37]

VENTRICULAR SEPTAL DEFECT

Changes in the ECG in children with ventricular septal defects reflect the degree of hemodynamic abnormality. A small isolated ventricular septal defect, with a small left-to-right shunt, will almost always be accompanied by a normal ECG

(Figure 30–4).[38–41] Moderate or large defects may result in RVH, especially if there is elevation of right ventricular pressure, but because the most predominant hemodynamic feature of the ventricular septal defect with large left-to-right shunt is left-sided volume overload from pulmonary overcirculation, left atrial enlargement and LVH are more frequently seen (Figure 30–5). The presence of associated RVH should suggest associated double-chamber right ventricle with obstruction between the inflow and outflow portions of the right ventricle.[42] Left atrial enlargement is usually suggested by a prominent wide terminal negative deflection in the P wave in lead V_1 and LVH by the presence of deep but narrow Q waves and prominent R waves in the inferior and left lateral precordial leads. Superior frontal plane QRS axis is commonly associated with AV septal defect and defects in the inlet portion of the ventricular septum. Shaw and colleagues[43] found superior frontal plane QRS axis in 6.2 percent of 1031 patients with a ventricular septal defect. In 59 percent of these patients, defects were in the inlet portion of the ventricular septum, but not in a ventricular septal defect of the AV canal type. Thus 41 percent of these

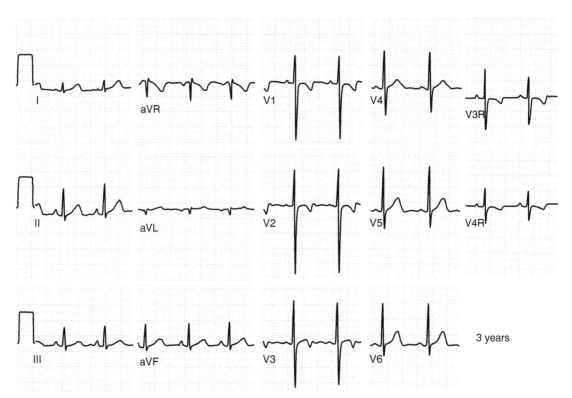

Figure 30–4 ECG of a 3-year-old child with a small ventricular septal defect. The ECG is essentially within normal limits for age. The frontal plane QRS axis is 60 degrees, and the precordial voltage pattern is normal. Echocardiography demonstrated a single small ventricular septal defect with an estimated pressure gradient across the defect by Doppler echocardiography of 70 mmHg (normal right ventricular pressure).

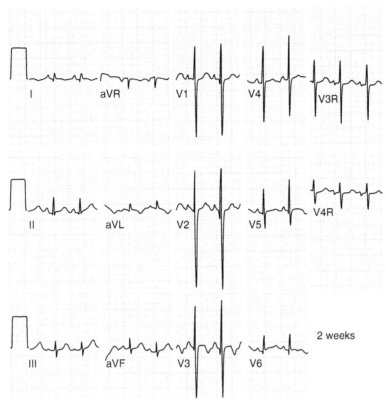

Figure 30–5   ECG of a 2-week-old infant with a moderate-size ventricular septal defect. Q waves in leads V_1 and V_2 and upright T wave in the right precordial leads suggest right ventricular hypertrophy. Prominent precordial voltage suggests possible biventricular hypertrophy.

patients had ventricular septal defects elsewhere, and the mechanism for a superior axis is uncertain. It is possible that defects in the inlet portion of the septum were present in fetal life and spontaneously closed or that the axis deviation is the remnant embryologic effect of faulty endocardial cushion development.[44] Aneurysm of the membranous septum has also been shown to be associated with left axis deviation in patients with perimembranous ventricular septal defects.[45,46]

The child with a large ventricular septal defect usually has ECG evidence of biventricular hypertrophy with large equiphasic QRS complexes in the mid-precordial leads, known as the *Katz-Wachtel pattern* (Figure 30–6).[40] One study of the natural history of ventricular septal defects demonstrated a higher than normal incidence of serious arrhythmia and sudden death. This risk was seen even in patients with small ventricular septal defects.[47] In a more recent study of patients with defects deemed small enough not to require intervention, follow-up was benign with no deaths, but incomplete or complete right bundle branch block (RBBB) was present in approximately 10 percent of all

patients.[48] No first-degree or higher AV block was seen, and LVH was seen in approximately 1 percent, with most of these patients having systemic arterial hypertension. Sinus node dysfunction requiring pacemaker placement was present in 4 percent of patients.[49]

Closure of ventricular septal defects with devices placed during cardiac catheterization has been performed with increasing frequency. Closure of perimembranous defects with devices resulted in RBBB and left anterior fascicular block in a minority of patients, and complete AV block occurred in 1 percent of interventions.[50]

PATENT DUCTUS ARTERIOSUS AND AORTOPULMONARY WINDOW

In patients with a small patent ductus arteriosus, the ECG is usually normal.[38] A larger patent ductus arteriosus with significant left-to-right shunt is usually associated with ECG evidence of left atrial enlargement and LVH (Figure 30–7). In low-birth-weight infants with patent ductus arteriosus determined to be hemodynamically significant by echocardiography, 22 percent of

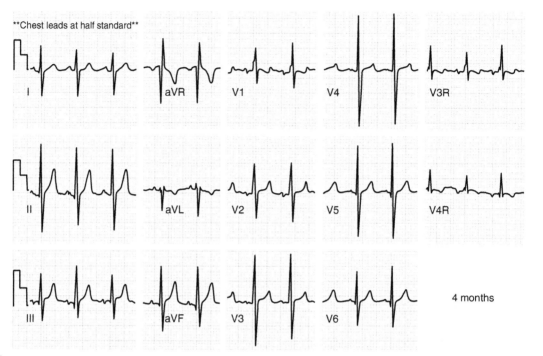

Figure 30–6   ECG of a 4-month-old infant with a large ventricular septal defect. Note that precordial leads are recorded at a standard of 5 mm/mV. Prominent precordial voltage suggests biventricular hypertrophy and meets "Katz-Wachtel" criteria. Cardiac catheterization demonstrated identical right and left ventricular pressure curves.

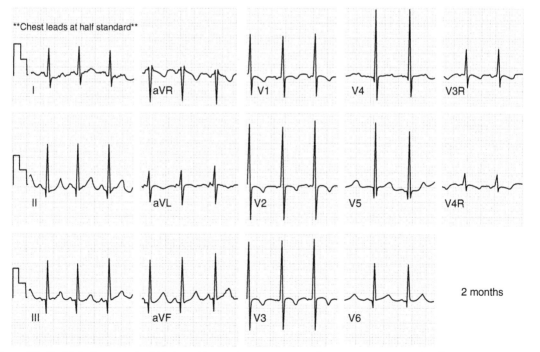

Figure 30–7   ECG of a 2-month-old infant with a moderate-size patent ductus arteriosus. Note that the precordial leads are recorded at a standard of 5 mm/mV. The precordial voltage is prominent with R+S >5mV in leads V_2–V_5.

patients had evidence of left atrial enlargement or LVH and 78 percent had normal ECGs, thus revealing very low sensitivity of the ECG in this diagnosis.[51]

An aortopulmonary window is usually associated with a larger left-to-right shunt and may show ECG evidence of biventricular hypertrophy similar to that in a large patent ductus arteriosus (Figure 30–8).

PULMONIC STENOSIS

The ECG is an excellent tool for evaluating the severity of valvar pulmonic stenosis.[1,2,52,53] In mild pulmonic stenosis the ECG may be normal or show mild right axis deviation in the frontal plane. In moderate pulmonic stenosis the R wave amplitude in lead V_1 exceeds the normal limits, and occasionally an rsR' pattern may be present (Figure 30–9).

In severe pulmonic stenosis, right axis deviation is usually marked and associated with a monophasic R wave in lead V_1, usually of >20 mm amplitude. Right atrial enlargement evidenced by peaked and tall P waves in leads

II and V_1 is also commonly seen in infants with critical valvar pulmonic stenosis. With very severe obstruction, Q waves are present in the right precordial leads.

In children and adolescents with isolated valvar pulmonic stenosis, there is good correlation between the height of the R wave in lead V_1 and the right ventricular systolic pressure.[54] The height of the R wave multiplied by 5 estimates the right ventricular systolic pressure in mmHg.[53]

AORTIC STENOSIS

Unlike in valvar pulmonic stenosis, the ECG may be a poor predictor of severity in valvar aortic stenosis. A completely normal or nearly normal ECG does not exclude severe stenosis.[3,55,56] The ECG is probably a better predictor of severity in valvar aortic stenosis in children younger than age 10 years than in older individuals,[55] but an overreliance on the ECG is hazardous at any age.[57] When present, abnormalities usually consist of increased R wave amplitude in lead V_6, increased S wave amplitude in lead V_1, and ST

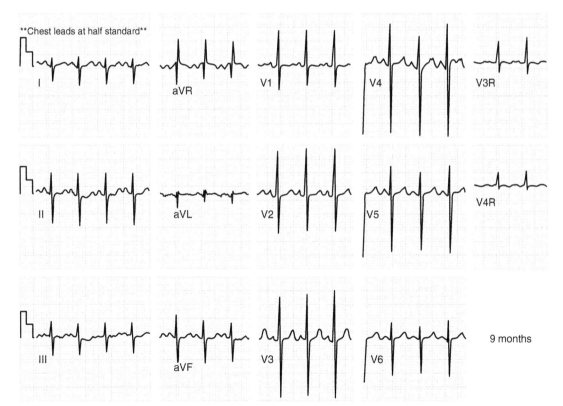

Figure 30–8 ECG of a 9-month-old infant with a large patent ductus arteriosus and pulmonary arterial hypertension with systemic pulmonary artery pressure. Note that precordial leads are recorded at a standard of 5 mm/mV. In comparison with the patient with a moderate-size patent ductus arteriosus, there is more marked right ventricular hypertrophy with an R/S ratio of <1 in lead V_6.

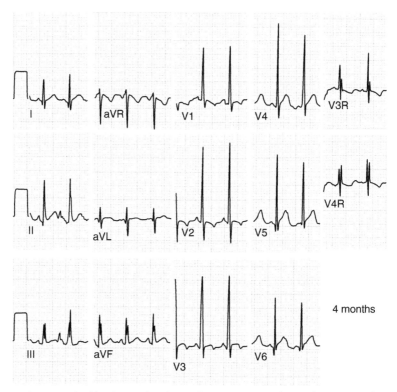

Figure 30–9 ECG of a 4-month-old infant with valvar pulmonic stenosis. The gradient across the pulmonary valve at catheterization was 46 mmHg. The R waves in leads V_1–V_3 are prominent.

segment depression and T wave inversion in the lateral precordial leads (i.e., the so-called left ventricular strain pattern) (Figure 30–10). Assessment of ECG parameters of LVH following aortic valve replacement for severe stenosis showed that no single ECG parameter performed well when measured against magnetic resonance imaging.[58]

P wave dispersion was greater in patients with aortic stenosis than in normal individuals, suggesting increased risk for atrial fibrillation.[59] QT interval dispersion has also been shown to be increased in individuals with aortic stenosis[60,61] and may be associated with sudden death in a small percentage of patients with this lesion. Balloon valvuloplasty and relief of severe aortic stenosis has been shown to reduce QT interval dispersion.

L-TRANSPOSITION OF THE GREAT VESSELS

Patients with ventricular inversion and *l*-transposition of the great vessels may have no symptoms. Their most characteristic ECG abnormality is the reversal of normal septal activation (Figure 30–11). Normally the intraventricular septum

is activated from left-to-right, producing Q waves in the left precordial leads. The inversion of the bundle branches associated with ventricular inversion results in Q waves in the right precordial leads.

Ventricular septal defect is present in as many as 80 percent of cases associated with the ventricular inversion.[62] Due to the inversion of the conduction system, closure of ventricular septal defects in this situation are most safely performed through the aorta to minimize the risk of conduction system damage.

Approximately 10 to 25 percent of patients with ventricular inversion have complete AV block with an equal incidence of first- or second-degree AV block.[63,64] Complete AV block may occur in these patients despite the absence of previous first- or second-degree AV block, sometimes spontaneously and unpredictably. Ebstein-like malformation of the systemic AV valve is also associated with ventricular inversion, with a common occurrence of accessory AV connections on the same side as the abnormal valve. Manifest ventricular preexcitation with Wolff-Parkinson-White syndrome, as well as concealed accessory AV connections,[65] may be present.

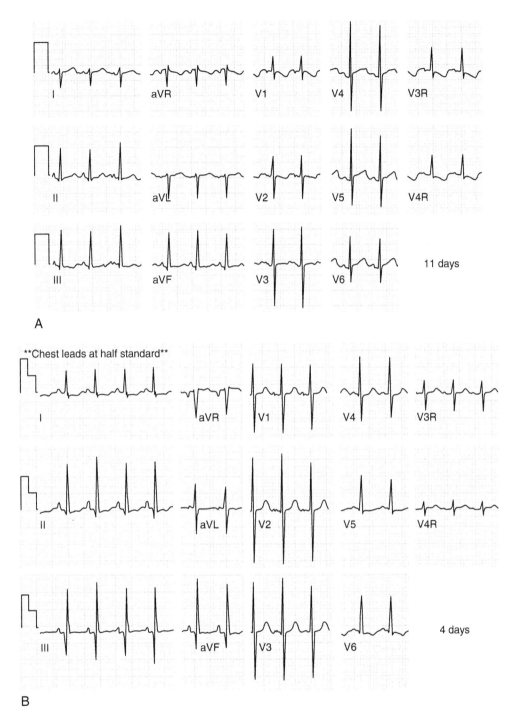

Figure 30–10   ECGs in two young infants with critical valvar aortic stenosis. **A,** This 11-day-old infant had a 112 mmHg gradient at catheterization prior to balloon valvuloplasty. The ECG is essentially within normal limits for age. The T waves in the inferior leads are slightly flat. **B,** This 4-day-old infant had a 60 mmHg gradient across a dysplastic aortic valve. The gradient was probably depressed by poor left ventricular function. Note that precordial leads are recorded at a standard of 5 mm/mV. Prominent precordial voltage suggests ventricular hypertrophy. ST segment depression and T wave inversion are seen in the inferior and left lateral precordial leads, consistent with left ventricular strain.

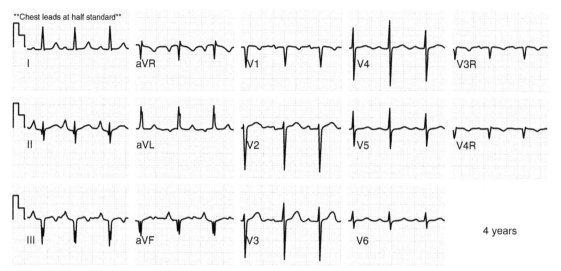

Figure 30–11   ECG of a 4-year-old child with *l*-transposition of the great vessels. Note the absence of Q waves in the left lateral precordial leads. Deep Q waves are seen in the inferior leads.

ANOMALOUS ORIGIN OF THE LEFT CORONARY ARTERY

Anomalous origin of the left coronary artery from the pulmonary artery results in coronary insufficiency due to inadequate perfusion pressure. Anterolateral infarction, manifested by deep and broad Q waves in leads I, aV$_L$, and left lateral precordial leads (Figure 30–12), is usually present at the time of diagnosis. This pattern may also be seen in pediatric patients with nonischemic cardiomyopathy and may make it difficult to establish the diagnosis by ECG alone.[66,67] Chang and Allada[68] proposed a scoring system using ECG and echocardiographic parameters to differentiate these diagnoses. They found that q waves wider than 30 ms in lead I and deeper than 3 mm in lead av$_L$ were more common in patients with anomalous origin of the left coronary artery. A QR pattern in lead aV$_L$ was the only ECG parameter considered in their scoring system derived by logistic regression,[68] but the typical pattern may be absent, especially in very young patients.[69]

The left coronary artery may also arise from the right sinus of Valsalva, and less commonly the right coronary artery arises from the left sinus of Valsalva. These abnormalities are associated with sudden death, usually during physical exertion. Unfortunately, prior to the occurrence of sudden death, the ECGs are usually normal[70] or show only minor abnormalities, such as ventricular ectopy and nonspecific T wave changes.[71]

LEFT VENTRICULAR NONCOMPACTION

Left ventricular noncompaction is an uncommon disorder of endocardial development demonstrating prominent ventricular trabeculations and deep intertrabecular recesses. It is seen in isolated form and also in combination with other forms of congenital heart disease. The diagnosis is typically made by echocardiography. The ventricular function is usually depressed. The ECG is often abnormal, most commonly with evidence for biventricular hypertrophy.[72] Abnormalities of sinus node and AV node function and ventricular arrhythmias are common in these patients.[73]

Cyanotic Lesions

d-TRANSPOSITION OF THE GREAT VESSELS

The ECG of the newborn infant with *d*-transposition of the great vessels is generally normal for age (Figure 30–13). Within the first weeks of life the ECG of an unoperated patient shows absence of expected regression of right ventricular predominance.[74] Biventricular hypertrophy is commonly seen when *d*-transposition of the great vessels is associated with a large ventricular septal defect. Isolated LVH is rare and should suggest associated right ventricular hypoplasia.

Without surgical intervention or with palliation, in cases in which atrial baffling retains the morphologic right ventricle as the systemic ventricle (Senning or Mustard procedure), the ECG continues to show RVH and frequently right axis deviation (Figure 30–14). Right atrial enlargement is also seen following this type of surgical palliation dependent upon the hemodynamic results. Sinus node dysfunction and atrial tachyarrhythmias are also common after

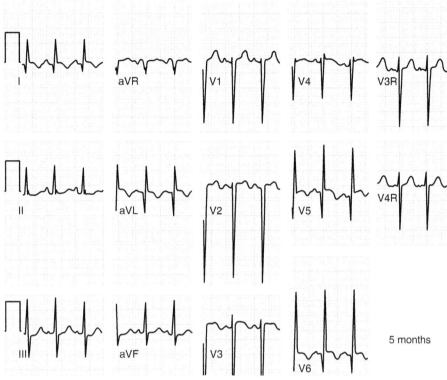

Figure 30–12 ECG of a 5-month-old infant with anomalous origin of the left coronary artery from the pulmonary artery. Note that precordial leads are recorded at a standard of 5 mm/mV. Deep and broad Q waves are seen in leads I, aV$_L$, V$_5$, and V$_6$. The usually prominent R waves in the right precordial leads are diminished, and there is prominent posteriorly directed voltage. This pattern is consistent with anterior and lateral myocardial damage secondary to poor coronary perfusion. The anomalous origin of the left coronary artery from the pulmonary artery and multiple anterior and lateral sites of myocardial infarction were confirmed at autopsy.

extensive atrial surgery. Sudden death is reported with disturbing frequency, but ECG findings do not appear to be predictive of sudden death.[75]

After arterial switch procedure, patients with *d*-transposition of the great vessels show resolution of right ventricular predominance. Midterm follow-up has shown normal ECGs at rest and with exercise, with normal sinus node function in some series[76,77] and chronotropic incompetence not affecting working capacity in as many as one third of patients in other series.[78] Right or left ventricular preponderance after this type of repair may suggest stenosis at the anastomotic sites in the great vessels.

TETRALOGY OF FALLOT

RVH is the hallmark ECG finding in the patient with tetralogy of Fallot and is of value in the differential diagnosis from ventricular septal defect. In the newborn, the ECG may be normal but over the first weeks of life normal regression of right ventricular preponderance is not seen.[79]

In those patients with tetralogy of Fallot who may remain acyanotic in infancy, the ECG (Figure 30–15) may offer a valuable diagnostic clue. Right axis deviation may accompany RVH, but left axis deviation suggests an associated complete AV canal.[79] Absence of left axis deviation does not exclude the associated defect of AV canal and is reportedly not seen in one third of patients.[80]

RBBB is common after surgical repair of tetralogy of Fallot, even when the repair is performed from a transatrial approach.[81,82] This is probably due to delayed activation of the right ventricular outflow tract caused by disruption of the right ventricular conduction system during resection of infundibular stenosis. Left anterior fascicular block is reported in 8 to 22 percent of patients after the repair of tetralogy of Fallot.[83,84]

Duration of the QRS complex greater than 150 ms and/or the presence of a right superior frontal plane QRS axis in pediatric patients with repaired tetralogy of Fallot has been associated with larger right ventricular volume and, when seen with pulmonary valve insufficiency, may

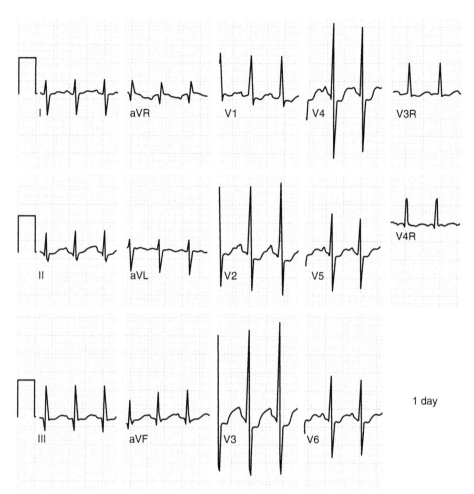

Figure 30–13 ECG of a 1-day-old infant with *d*-transposition of the great vessels. The prominent R waves in the right precordial leads and the deep S wave in lead V_6 suggest right ventricular preponderance.

suggest the need for pulmonary valve replacement.[85] QRST time integral values in the precordial leads have also been shown to correlate with right ventricular volume and pressure overload.[86]

QRS duration has been directly correlated with right ventricular volume and mass.[87] Residual right ventricular outflow tract obstruction[88] and pulmonary valve insufficiency[89] have also been associated with QRS prolongation. Pulmonary valve replacement postoperative following transannular patch repair has been shown to slow the progression of QRS widening.[90,91]

Sudden death is a late postoperative complication that is probably due to ventricular tachyarrhythmia.[92–94] Gatzoulis and colleagues[95] reported an association between QRS duration and ventricular tachycardia or sudden death in patients with repaired tetralogy of Fallot. They showed that in 178 adult survivors of repaired tetralogy of Fallot, 9 patients had sustained ventricular tachycardia (8 with near-miss sudden death). They also

reviewed the reports of four patients with sudden postoperative death. All patients with ventricular tachycardia or sudden death had QRS duration ≥180 ms. This finding was confirmed by Balaji and associates,[96] showing a 100 percent sensitivity and 96 percent specificity for QRS duration ≥180 ms in detecting clinical ventricular tachycardia late after tetralogy of Fallot repair. Other studies of patients following repair of tetralogy of Fallot suggested that narrow QRS complex on the resting ECG is associated with lower risk for sudden death.[97,98] More recent studies suggest that signal-averaged filtered QRS duration may be a better predictor of ventricular arrhythmia in this population than the standard ECG.[99,100]

Abnormal QT and JT dispersion have been noted in patients with ventricular tachycardia.[101,102] The increased QT and JT dispersion appears to be present in patients with tetralogy of Fallot preoperatively and increases further after surgical intervention, whereas ventricular

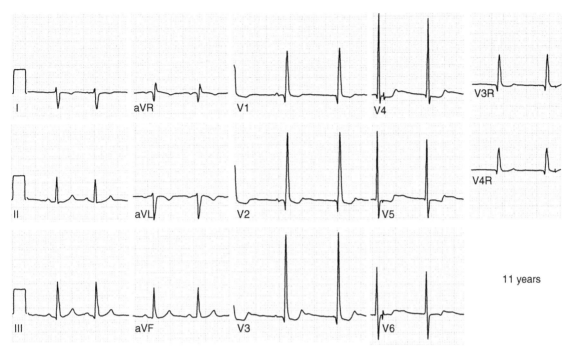

Figure 30–14   ECG of an 11-year-old child with *d*-transposition of the great vessels who underwent a Senning atrial baffle repair during infancy. A qR pattern is seen in the right precordial leads and a deep S wave in lead V_6, suggestive of extreme right ventricular hypertrophy. The T waves are diffusely flat in the precordial leads. Note that the rhythm is sinus in the first and second lead group recordings but becomes junctional escape rhythm at the end of the recording.

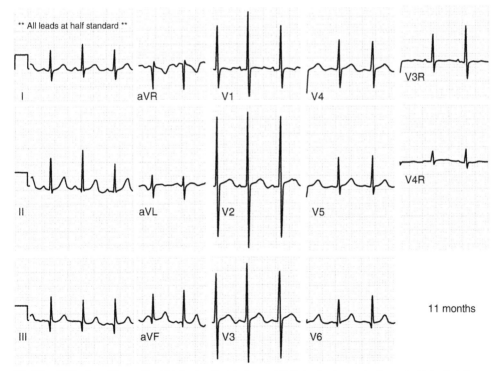

Figure 30–15   ECG of an 11-month-old infant with tetralogy of Fallot prior to surgical repair. Note that the precordial leads are recorded at a standard of 5 mm/mV. Prominent R waves are seen in leads V_1–V_3, and the T waves are upright in lead V_2 and isoelectric in the right precordial leads, suggesting right ventricular hypertrophy.

late potentials are not present prior to surgery but develop progressively following surgery, which suggests that they are the result of scarring.[103] Although these abnormalities have been used for risk stratification for ventricular arrhythmia,[104] their utility for predicting sudden death without consideration of other clinical factors has been questioned.[105]

Heart rate variability may also be a predictor of ventricular arrhythmia in those patients without other ECG risk factors.[106,107] Left ventricular size and dysfunction have also been suggested as an additional risk factor in these patients,[94,108,109] and microvolt T wave alternans is being investigated.[110]

Although not associated with life-threatening arrhythmia, atrial tachycardia and sinus node dysfunction are seen commonly following tetralogy of Fallot repair, and dispersion of the P wave duration has been shown to be a marker for these atrial rhythm abnormalities.[111]

TRUNCUS ARTERIOSUS

The ECG in infants with persistent truncus arteriosus is highly variable and depends in large part on the degree of pulmonary overcirculation. In the newborn period the ECG may show evidence of RVH (Figure 30–16). If pulmonary overcirculation is substantial, LVH and left atrial enlargement may also be seen. In the first days of life the ECG may be normal.[112]

Postsurgical anatomy and physiology of truncus arteriosus are similar to those of tetralogy of Fallot. It is unclear as to whether ventricular arrhythmia and late sudden death will afflict this population to the same extent, or whether risk stratification as proposed for tetralogy patients will be applicable to this smaller population.[113]

PULMONARY ATRESIA WITH INTACT VENTRICULAR SEPTUM

The ECG in patients with pulmonary atresia may show peaked and tall P waves in lead II suggestive of right atrial enlargement but at a much lower incidence than in tricuspid atresia (Figure 30–17).[114] The height of the P waves appears to correlate with the degree of tricuspid valve insufficiency (Figure 30–18). The frontal plane axis is usually leftward and inferior but may be rightward and inferior in the uncommon patient with pulmonary atresia and a normal or enlarged right ventricular cavity.[114] Most frequently posterior forces predominate, but prominent anterior forces may also be present, more commonly in the patient with a normal or enlarged right ventricular cavity.

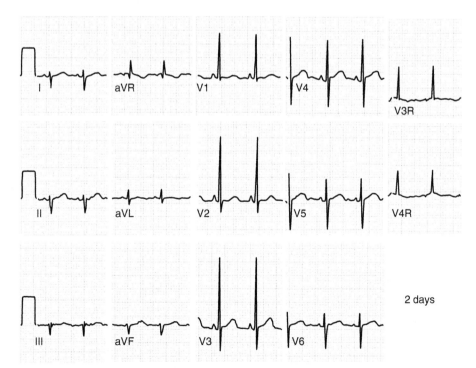

Figure 30–16 ECG of a 2-day-old infant with truncus arteriosus. A right superior axis is seen in the frontal plane. Prominent R waves in leads V_1–V_3 and an R/S ratio of <1 in leads V_5 and V_6 suggest right ventricular hypertrophy.

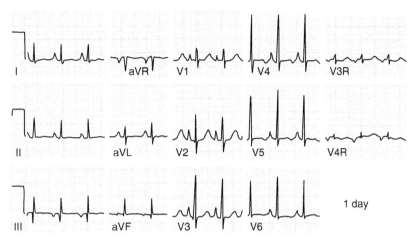

Figure 30–17　ECG of a 1-day-old infant with pulmonary atresia and intact ventricular septum. The tricuspid valve annulus was also small (Z score −3.5). The P waves are tall and peaked in leads V_1–V_4, suggesting right atrial enlargement. The combination of high right ventricular pressure and small right ventricular cavity dimension results in the absence of ECG evidence of right ventricular preponderance. The T waves are flat in the inferior and lateral leads, possibly secondary to myocardial ischemia from coronary cameral fistulas to the right ventricle.

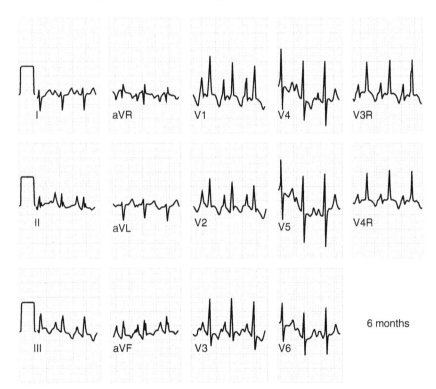

Figure 30–18　ECG of a 6-month-old infant with pulmonary atresia and intact ventricular septum. This is the same patient as in Figure 30–17 at an older age. A modified left Blalock-Taussig shunt was placed, but the patient did not have pulmonary valvotomy. The P waves are larger and more peaked than those seen at a younger age, and there is more evidence of right ventricular prominence.

EBSTEIN'S ANOMALY OF THE TRICUSPID VALVE

ECG evidence for right atrial enlargement is almost always seen in patients with Ebstein's anomaly of the tricuspid valve (Figure 30–19).[115]

Wolff-Parkinson-White syndrome is seen in 20 percent of patients, with the accessory AV connection being located on the right side. In those without ventricular preexcitation there is usually a right ventricular conduction delay, with

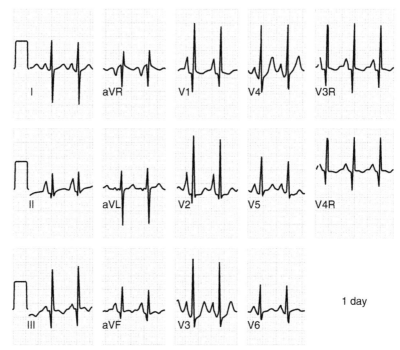

Figure 30–19 ECG of a 1-day-old infant with Ebstein's anomaly of the tricuspid valve and severe tricuspid valve insufficiency. The P waves are extremely tall and peaked in leads V_1–V_4, suggesting substantial right atrial enlargement. Deep Q waves are seen in the right precordial leads, suggesting right ventricular hypertrophy.

a characteristic low-amplitude, wide R′ wave.[116] Anterograde accessory pathway conduction may be associated with a longer than typical PR interval due to atrial conduction delay and, when fused with right ventricular conduction delay,[117] may not be readily identified as delta wave in ventricular preexcitation.[118] Tachyarrhythmia is common in this population.[119] Atrial arrhythmias (atrial reentrant tachycardia, atrial flutter, atrial fibrillation), AV reentrant tachycardia (orthodromic, antidromic, and "two-pathway"), and ventricular tachycardia[120] are seen frequently in patients with Ebstein's anomaly, both before and after surgical intervention.[121,122] "Mahaim type" accessory AV connections are also seen frequently.[123–125]

TRICUSPID ATRESIA

The ECG abnormalities in tricuspid atresia include atrial enlargement, QRS axis deviation, and ventricular hypertrophy. Tall P waves in lead II, V_{4R}, and V_1 are seen in 61 to 82 percent of patients with tricuspid atresia and are suggestive of right atrial enlargement.[126–129] Tricuspid atresia requires the presence of an intraatrial communication, which on rare occasion may be restrictive to blood flow. The detection of the latter is not facilitated by the ECG because of poor

correlation between P wave amplitude and the size of the intraatrial communication or right atrial pressure.[126,127] Prolongation of the PR interval is reported in 12 to 14 percent of cases and a short PR interval in 24 percent of cases. The latter may cause "pseudo-preexcitation," suggested by a delta-like wave without actual presence of an accessory pathway.[130] True ventricular preexcitation in the patient with tricuspid atresia is less common but has been reported.[131] It has been associated with right septal accessory pathways and also with connections from the right atrial appendage to the right ventricular outflow tract occurring as a complication of surgical intervention.[132,133]

A leftward and superior frontal plane QRS axis in a child with cyanotic heart disease suggests the presence of tricuspid atresia (Figure 30–20). In one large series, 87 percent of patients with tricuspid atresia and normally related great vessels had a leftward and superior frontal plane QRS axis.[126] This has been confirmed in other series.[134] Inferior frontal plane QRS axis was found in nearly 50 percent of patients with tricuspid atresia associated with d-transposition of the great vessels (Figure 30–21).[135] Inferior rightward QRS axes were rare but occurred in half of patients with the relatively uncommon association of tricuspid atresia with l-transposition of the great vessels.[126]

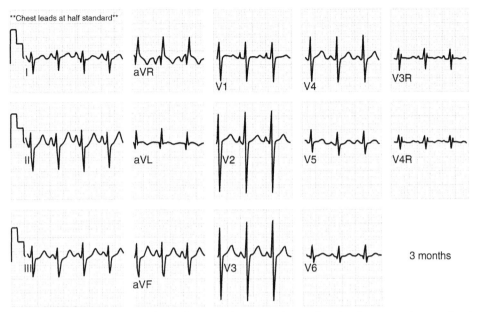

Figure 30–20   ECG of a 3-month-old infant with tricuspid atresia and normally related great vessels. Note that the precordial leads are recorded at a standard of 5 mm/mV. The tall P waves in lead II and tall and peaked P waves in leads V_1 and V_2 suggest right atrial enlargement. A right superior frontal plane QRS axis is seen.

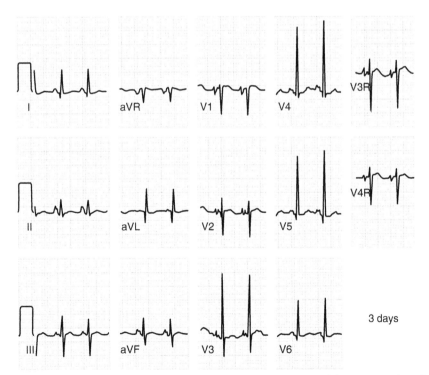

Figure 30–21   ECG of a 3-day-old infant with tricuspid atresia and *d*-transposition of the great vessels with coarctation of the aorta. The P waves are notched in lead II and biphasic in lead V_1 with a broad and deeply negative component, suggesting left atrial enlargement. In contrast to Figure 30–20 with tricuspid atresia with normally related great vessels, the frontal plane QRS axis here is normal.

The occurrence of a leftward and superior frontal plane QRS axis may be due to the early origin of the left bundle branch from the common bundle of His, possibly related to the absent diminution of the membranous septum.[127]

The precordial QRS pattern most frequently demonstrates left ventricular predominance with prominent S waves in the right precordial leads and tall R waves in the left precordial leads.[136] More prominent anteriorly directed forces are rarely seen but may correlate with more developed right ventricular size. One study demonstrated a poor correlation between the amplitude of the QRS and the size of the ventricular septal defect or thickness of the ventricular wall.[137]

Arrhythmias in patients with tricuspid atresia are common, especially atrial arrhythmias following Fontan palliation,[138] but AV reentrant and AV nodal reentrant tachycardia are also seen.[133,139] Accelerated ventricular rhythm has been reported in a fetus with tricuspid atresia.[140]

HYPOPLASTIC LEFT HEART SYNDROME

The newborn infant with hypoplastic left heart syndrome may present with few obvious identifying clinical features. The ECG almost always demonstrates RVH, commonly with a qR pattern in the right precordial leads (Figure 30–22). Left precordial R waves are diminutive, and deep S waves are usually seen in lead V_6.[141,142] Right atrial enlargement and right axis deviation are reported but less frequently. ST segment abnormalities may be observed and may reflect inadequate coronary perfusion from restriction of retrograde flow through a hypoplastic ascending aortic arch.

SINGLE VENTRICLE

Many types of single ventricle are seen with variation in the number of AV valves and the morphology of the ventricular chamber. The

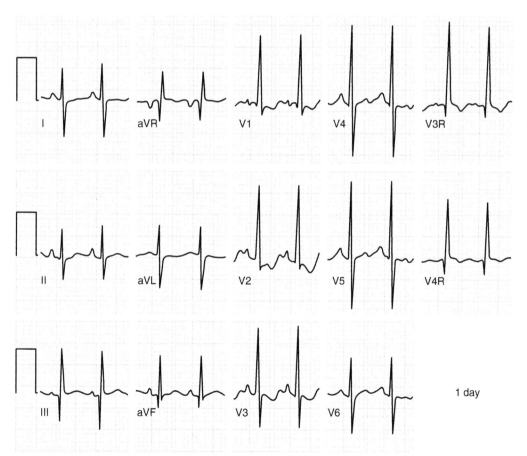

Figure 30–22   ECG of a 1-day-old infant with hypoplastic left heart syndrome with mitral and aortic valve atresia. Q waves in lead V_1 and V_{3R}, V_{4R} suggest right ventricular hypertrophy. Despite the near absence of left ventricular mass, well-developed R waves are seen from lead V_4 through lead V_6.

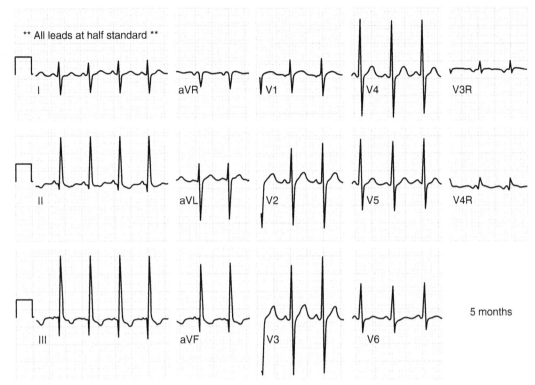

Figure 30–23 ECG of a 5-month-old infant with a double-inlet single ventricle. Note that all leads are recorded at a standard of 5 mm/mV. There is striking inferior and mid-precordial voltage. The T waves are inverted in the inferior leads, suggesting a ventricular strain pattern.

arrangement of the great vessels is also important to the physiologic and ECG appearance. Biventricular hypertrophy pattern is common, but depending on the chamber morphology and orientation, LVH or RVH may predominate (Figure 30–23). Atrial enlargement, when seen, usually reflects AV valve stenosis or insufficiency or the degree of ventricular dysfunction.

FONTAN PALLIATION

Modifications of the Fontan procedure (various connections of systemic venous return to the pulmonary arteries) have become common for palliation of patients with one functional ventricle (tricuspid atresia, hypoplastic left heart, and other, more complex forms of single ventricle anatomy). As described previously, the ECG appearance is highly variable depending on the specific physiology. Although the postoperative incidence of sudden death is low, many successfully operated patients show significant ST segment depression on ambulatory ECGs and during exercise testing.[143,144] These changes are likely to be secondary to ventricular hypertrophy with "ventricular strain" pattern, but ischemia can be difficult to exclude. Sinus node dysfunction

was common after earlier-performed total cavo-pulmonary connections[145] but appears to be less frequent with newer operative techniques. Atrial tachyarrhythmias occur frequently in association with increased duration of the P wave on signal-averaged recording[146] and increased P wave dispersion.[138]

REFERENCES

1. Cayler GG, Ongley P, Nadas AS: Relation of systolic pressure in the right ventricle to the electrocardiogram: a study of patients with pulmonary stenosis and intact ventricular septum. New Engl J Med 258:979, 1958.
2. Fowler RS, Newnham L, Jones M, et al: A simple method for ECG and VCG assessment of the severity of pulmonary valve stenosis. Eur J Cardiol 5:453, 1977.
3. Reynolds JL, Nadas AS, Rudolph AM, et al: Critical congenital aortic stenosis with minimal electrocardiographic changes. New Engl J Med 262:276, 1960.
4. Pandian NG, Ramasamy S, Martin P, et al: Ultrasound stethoscopy as an extension of clinical examination during hospital patient rounds: preliminary experience with a hand-held miniaturized echocardiography instrument (Abstract). J Am Soc Echocardiog 13:486, 2000.
5. Clark EB, Kugler JD: Preoperative secundum atrial septal defect with coexisting sinus node and atrioventricular node dysfunction. Circulation 65:976, 1982.
6. Ruschhaupt DG, Khoury L, Thilenius OG, et al: Electrophysiologic abnormalities of children with ostium secundum atrial septal defect. Am J Cardiol 53:1643, 1984.

7. Karpawich PP, Antillon JR, Cappola PR, et al: Pre- and postoperative electrophysiologic assessment of children with secundum atrial septal defect. Am J Cardiol 55:519, 1985.

8. Finley JP, Nugent ST, Hellenbrand W, et al: Sinus arrhythmia in children with atrial septal defect: an analysis of heart rate variability before and after surgical repair. Br Heart J 61:280, 1989.

9. Garson A Jr , Bink-Boelkens M, Hesslein PS, et al: Atrial flutter in the young: a collaborative study of 380 cases. J Am Coll Cardiol 6:871, 1985.

10. Berger F, Vogel M, Kramer A, et al: Incidence of atrial flutter/fibrillation in adults with atrial septal defect before and after surgery [see comments]. Ann Thorac Surg 68:75, 1999.

11. Bink-Boelkens MT, Bergstra A, Landsman ML: Functional abnormalities of the conduction system in children with an atrial septal defect. Int J Cardiol 20:263, 1988.

12. Shiku DJ, Stijns M, Lintermans JP, et al: Influence of age on atrioventricular conduction intervals in children with and without atrial septal defect. J Electrocardiol 15:9, 1982.

13. Azhari N, Shihata MS, Al-Fatani A: Spontaneous closure of atrial septal defects within the oval fossa. Cardiol Young 14:148, 2004.

14. Zufelt K, Rosenberg HC, Li MD, et al: The electrocardiogram and the secundum atrial septal defect: a reexamination in the era of echocardiography. Can J Cardiol 14:227, 1998.

15. Cohen JS, Patton DJ, Giuffre RM: The crochetage pattern in electrocardiograms of pediatric atrial septal defect patients. Can J Cardiol 16:1241, 2000.

16. Heller J, Hagege AA, Besse B, et al: "Crochetage" (notch) on R wave in inferior limb leads: a new independent electrocardiographic sign of atrial septal defect. J Am Coll Cardiol 27:877, 1996.

17. Christensen DD, Vincent RN, Campbell RM: Presentation of atrial septal defect in the pediatric population. Pediatr Cardiol 26:812, 2005.

18. Guray U, Guray Y, Mecit B, et al: Maximum p wave duration and p wave dispersion in adult patients with secundum atrial septal defect: the impact of surgical repair. Ann Noninvasive Electrocardiol 9:136, 2004.

19. Ho TF, Chia EL, Yip WC, et al: Analysis of P wave and P dispersion in children with secundum atrial septal defect. Ann Noninvasive Electrocardiol 6:305, 2001.

20. Guray U, Guray Y, Yylmaz MB, et al: Evaluation of P wave duration and P wave dispersion in adult patients with secundum atrial septal defect during normal sinus rhythm. Int J Cardiol 91:75, 2003.

21. Cua CL, Sparks EE, Chan DP, et al: Persistent electrical and morphological atrial abnormalities after early closure of atrial septal defect. Cardiol Young 14:481, 2004.

22. Schenck MH, Sterba R, Foreman CK, et al: Improvement in noninvasive electrophysiologic findings in children after transcatheter atrial septal defect closure. Am J Cardiol 76:695, 1995.

23. Di Bernardo S, Berger F, Fasnacht M, et al: Impact of right ventricular size on ECG after percutaneous closure of atrial septal defect with Amplatzer Septal Occluder. Swiss Med Wkly 135:647, 2005.

24. Santoro G, Pascotto M, Sarubbi B, et al: Early electrical and geometric changes after percutaneous closure of large atrial septal defect. Am J Cardiol 93:876, 2004.

25. Suda K, Raboisson MJ, Piette E, et al: Reversible atrioventricular block associated with closure of atrial septal defects using the Amplatzer device. J Am Coll Cardiol 43:1677, 2004.

26. Hessling G, Hyca S, Brockmeier K, et al: Cardiac dysrhythmias in pediatric patients before and 1 year after transcatheter closure of atrial septal defects using the amplatzer septal occluder. Pediatr Cardiol 24:259, 2003.

27. Chessa M, Carminati M, Butera G, et al: Early and late complications associated with transcatheter occlusion of secundum atrial septal defect. J Am Coll Cardiol 39:1061, 2002.

28. Celiker A, Ozkutlu S, Karakurt C, et al: Cardiac dysrhythmias after transcatheter closure of ASD with Amplatzer device. Turk J Pediatr 47:323, 2005.

29. Boineau JP, Moore EN, Patterson DF: Relationship between the ECG, ventricular activation, and the ventricular conduction system in ostium primum ASD. Circulation 48:556, 1973.

30. Feldt RH, DuShane JW, Titus JL: The atrioventricular conduction system in persistent common atrioventricular canal defect: correlations with electrocardiogram. Circulation 42:437, 1970.

31. Jacobsen JR, Gillette PC, Corbett BN, et al: Intracardiac electrography in endocardial cushion defects. Circulation 54:599, 1976.

32. Fournier A, Young ML, Garcia OL, et al: Electrophysiologic cardiac function before and after surgery in children with atrioventricular canal. Am J Cardiol 57:1137, 1986.

33. Baslaim G, Basioni A. Repair of complete atrioventricular septal defects: results with maintenance of the coronary sinus on the right atrial side. J Card Surg 21:545, 2006.

34. Davia JE, Cheitlin MD, Bedynek JL: Sinus venosus atrial septal defect: analysis of fifty cases. Am Heart J 85:177, 1973.

35. Attenhofer Jost CH, Connolly HM, Danielson GK, et al: Sinus venosus atrial septal defect: long-term postoperative outcome for 115 patients. Circulation 112:1953, 2005.

36. Pathi V, Guererro R, MacArthur KJ, et al: Sinus venosus defect: single-patch repair with caval enlargement. Ann Thorac Surg 59:1588, 1995.

37. Nicholson IA, Chard RB, Nunn GR, et al: Transcaval repair of the sinus venosus syndrome. J Thorac Cardiovasc Surg 119:741, 2000.

38. Driscoll DJ. Left-to-right shunt lesions. Ped Clin N Am 46:355, 1999.

39. DuShane JW, Weidman WH, Brandenburg RO, et al: The electrocardiogram in children with ventricular septal defect and severe pulmonary hypertension: correlation with response of pulmonary arterial pressure to surgical repair. Circulation 22:49, 1960.

40. Katz LN, Wachtel H: The diphasic QRS type of electrocardiogram in congenital heart disease. Am Heart J 13:202, 1937.

41. Atalay S, Imamoglu A, Dilek L, et al: Congenital isolated apical ventricular septal defects. Angiology 49:355, 1998.

42. Cil E, Saraclar M, Ozkutlu S, et al: Double-chambered right ventricle: experience with 52 cases. Int J Cardiol 50:19, 1995.

43. Shaw NJ, Godman MJ, Hayes A, et al: Superior QRS axis in ventricular septal defect. Br Heart J 62:281, 1989.

44. Swensson RE: QRS axis in isolated perimembranous ventricular septal defect. J Electrocardiol 34:205, 2001.

45. Farru-Albohaire O, Arcil G, Hernandez I: An association between left axis deviation and an aneurysmal defect in children with a perimembranous ventricular septal defect. Br Heart J 64:146, 1990.

46. Tutar HE, Atalay S, Turkay S, et al: QRS axis in isolated perimembranous ventricular septal defect and influences of morphological factors on QRS axis. J Electrocardiol 34:197, 2001.

47. Kidd L, Driscoll DJ, Gersony WM, et al: Second natural history study of congenital heart defects. Results of treatment of patients with ventricular septal defects. Circulation 87:I318, 1993.
48. Gabriel HM, Heger M, Innerhofer P, et al: Long-term outcome of patients with ventricular septal defect considered not to require surgical closure during childhood. J Am Coll Cardiol 39:1066, 2002.
49. Roos-Hesselink JW, Meijboom FJ, Spitaels SE, et al: Outcome of patients after surgical closure of ventricular septal defect at young age: longitudinal follow-up of 22–34 years. Eur Heart J 25:1057, 2004.
50. Masura J, Gao W, Gavora P, Sun K, et al: Percutaneous closure of perimembranous ventricular septal defects with the eccentric Amplatzer device: multicenter follow-up study. Pediatr Cardiol 26:216, 2005.
51. Shipton SE, van der Merwe PL, Nel ED: Diagnosis of haemodynamically significant patent ductus arteriosus in neonates—is the ECG of diagnostic help? Cardiovasc J S Afr 12:264, 2001.
52. Bassingthwaighte JB, Parkin TW, DuShane JW, et al: The electrocardiographic amd hemodynamic findings in pulmonary stenosis with intact ventricular septum. Circulation 28:893, 1963.
53. Mehran-Pour M, Whitney A, Liebman J, et al: Quantification of the Frank and McFee-Parungao orthogonal electrocardiogram in valvular pulmonic stenosis. Correlations with hemodynamic measurement. J Electrocardiol 12:69, 1979.
54. Ardura J, Gonzalez C, Andres J: Does mild pulmonary stenosis progress during childhood? A study of its natural course. Clin Cardiol 27:519, 2004.
55. Braunwald E, Goldblatt A, Aygen MM, et al: Congenital aortic stenosis: I. Clinical and hemodynamic findings in 100 patients. Circulation 27:426, 1963.
56. Reeve R, Kawamata K, Selzer A: Reliability of vectorcardiography in assessing the severity of congenital aortic stenosis. Circulation 34:92, 1966.
57. Ardura J, Gonzalez C, Andres J: Does mild valvular aortic stenosis progress during childhood? J Heart Valve Dis 15:1, 2006.
58. Beyerbacht HP, Bax JJ, Lamb HJ, et al: Evaluation of ECG criteria for left ventricular hypertrophy before and after aortic valve replacement using magnetic resonance imaging. J Cardiovasc Magn Reson 5:465, 2003.
59. Turhan H, Yetkin E, Atak R, et al: Increased p wave duration and p wave dispersion in patients with aortic stenosis. Ann Noninvasive Electrocardiol 8:18, 2003.
60. Orlowska-Baranowska E, Baranowski R, Zakrzewski D, et al: QT interval dispersion analysis in patients with aortic valve stenosis: a prospective study. J Heart Valve Dis 12:319, 2003.
61. Sarubbi B, Calvanese R, Cappelli Bigazzi M, et al: Electrophysiological changes following balloon valvuloplasty and angioplasty for aortic stenosis and coarctation of aorta: clinical evidence for mechano-electrical feedback in humans. Int J Cardiol 93:7, 2004.
62. Allwork SP, Bentall HH, Becker AE, et al: Congenitally corrected transposition of the great arteries: morphologic study of 32 cases. Am J Cardiol 38:910, 1976.
63. Bharati S, McCue CM, Tingelstad JB, et al: Lack of connection between the atria and the peripheral conduction system in a case of corrected transposition with congenital atrioventricular block. Am J Cardiol 42:147, 1978.
64. Gillette PC, Busch U, Mullins CE, et al: Electrophysiologic studies in patients with ventricular inversion and "corrected transposition." Circulation 60:939, 1979.
65. Bharati S, Rosen K, Steinfield L, et al: The anatomic substrate for preexcitation in corrected transposition. Circulation 62:831, 1980.
66. Johnsrude CL, Perry JC, Cecchin F, et al: Differentiating anomalous left main coronary artery originating from the pulmonary artery in infants from myocarditis and dilated cardiomyopathy by electrocardiogram. Am J Cardiol 75:71, 1995.
67. Towbin JA, Bricker JT, Garson A Jr : Electrocardiographic criteria for diagnosis of acute myocardial infarction in childhood. Am J Cardiol 69:1545, 1992.
68. Chang RR, Allada V. Electrocardiographic and echocardiographic features that distinguish anomalous origin of the left coronary artery from pulmonary artery from idiopathic dilated cardiomyopathy. Pediatr Cardiol 22:3, 2001.
69. Nakagawa M, Kimura K, Watanabe Y: Atypical electrocardiogram and echocardiogram in a patient with Bland-White-Garland syndrome in association with atrial septal defect. Cardiology 87:358, 1996.
70. Basso C, Maron BJ, Corrado D, et al: Clinical profile of congenital coronary artery anomalies with origin from the wrong aortic sinus leading to sudden death in young competitive athletes. J Am Coll Cardiol 35:1493, 2000.
71. Davis JA, Cecchin F, Jones TK, et al: Major coronary artery anomalies in a pediatric population: incidence and clinical importance. J Am Coll Cardiol 37:593, 2001.
72. Pignatelli RH, McMahon CJ, Dreyer WJ, et al: Clinical characterization of left ventricular noncompaction in children: a relatively common form of cardiomyopathy. Circulation 108:2672, 2003.
73. Celiker A, Ozkutlu S, Dilber E, et al: Rhythm abnormalities in children with isolated ventricular noncompaction. Pacing Clin Electrophysiol 28:1198, 2005.
74. Calleja HB, Hosier DM, Grajo MZ: The electrocardiogram in complete transposition of the great vessels. Am Heart J 69:31, 1965.
75. Kammeraad JA, van Deurzen CH, Sreeram N, et al: Predictors of sudden cardiac death after Mustard or Senning repair for transposition of the great arteries. J Am Coll Cardiol 44:1095, 2004.
76. Hovels-Gurich HH, Kunz D, Seghaye M, et al: Results of exercise testing at a mean age of 10 years after neonatal arterial switch operation. Acta Paediatr 92:190, 2003.
77. Hovels-Gurich HH, Seghaye MC, Ma Q, et al: Long-term results of cardiac and general health status in children after neonatal arterial switch operation. Ann Thorac Surg 75:935, 2003.
78. Mahle WT, McBride MG, Paridon SM: Exercise performance after the arterial switch operation for D-transposition of the great arteries. Am J Cardiol 87:753, 2001.
79. Feldt RH, DuShane JW, Titus JL: The anatomy of the atrioventricular conduction system in ventricular septal defect and tetralogy of Fallot: correlations with the electrocardiogram and vectorcardiogram. Circulation 34:774, 1966.
80. DiSciascio G, Bargeron LM Jr: The electrocardiogram in tetralogy of Fallot with complete atrioventricular canal. Tex Heart Inst J 9:163, 1982.
81. Goor DA, Lavee J, Smolinsky A, et al: Correction of tetrad of Fallot with reduced incidence of right bundle branch block. Am J Cardiol 48:892, 1981.
82. Horowitz LN, Simson MB, Spear JF, et al: The mechanism of apparent right bundle branch block after transatrial repair of tetralogy of Fallot. Circulation 59:1241, 1979.
83. Steeg CN, Krongrad E, Davachi F, et al: Postoperative left anterior hemiblock and right bundle branch block

following repair of tetralogy of Fallot. Clinical and etiologic considerations. Circulation 51:1026, 1975.

84. Kuzevska-Maneva K, Kacarska R, Gurkova B: Arrhythmias and conduction abnormalities in children after repair of tetralogy of Fallot. Vojnosanit Pregl 62:97, 2005.

85. Book WM, Parks WJ, Hopkins KL, et al: Electrocardiographic predictors of right ventricular volume measured by magnetic resonance imaging late after total repair of tetralogy of Fallot. Clin Cardiol 22:740, 1999.

86. Izumida N, Asano Y, Kiyohara K, et al: Precordial leads QRST time integrals for evaluation of right ventricular overload in children with congenital heart diseases. J Electrocardiol 30:257, 1997.

87. Neffke JG, Tulevski, II, van der Wall EE, et al: ECG determinants in adult patients with chronic right ventricular pressure overload caused by congenital heart disease: relation with plasma neurohormones and MRI parameters. Heart 88:266, 2002.

88. Galea N, Aquilina O, Grech V: Risk factors for QRS prolongation after repaired tetralogy of Fallot. Hellenic J Cardiol 47:66, 2006.

89. Abd El Rahman MY, Abdul-Khaliq H, Vogel M, et al: Relation between right ventricular enlargement, QRS duration, and right ventricular function in patients with tetralogy of Fallot and pulmonary regurgitation after surgical repair. Heart 84:416, 2000.

90. van Huysduynen BH, van Straten A, Swenne CA, et al: Reduction of QRS duration after pulmonary valve replacement in adult Fallot patients is related to reduction of right ventricular volume. Eur Heart J 26:928, 2005.

91. Kleinveld G, Joyner RW, Sallee D III, et al: Hemodynamic and electrocardiographic effects of early pulmonary valve replacement in pediatric patients after transannular complete repair of tetralogy of Fallot. Pediatr Cardiol 27:329, 2006.

92. Gillette PC, Yeoman MA, Mullins CE, et al: Sudden death after repair of tetralogy of Fallot. Electrocardiographic and electrophysiologic abnormalities. Circulation 56:566, 1977.

93. James FW, Kaplan S, Chou TC: Unexpected cardiac arrest in patients after surgical correction of tetralogy of Fallot. Circulation 52:691, 1975.

94. Gatzoulis MA, Elliott JT, Guru V, et al: Right and left ventricular systolic function late after repair of tetralogy of Fallot. Am J Cardiol 86:1352, 2000.

95. Gatzoulis MA, Till JA, Somerville J, et al: Mechanoelectrical interaction in tetralogy of Fallot. QRS prolongation relates to right ventricular size and predicts malignant ventricular arrhythmias and sudden death [see comments]. Circulation 92:231, 1995.

96. Balaji S, Lau YR, Case CL, et al: QRS prolongation is associated with inducible ventricular tachycardia after repair of tetralogy of Fallot. Am J Cardiol 80:160, 1997.

97. Nakazawa M, Shinohara T, Sasaki A, et al: Arrhythmias late after repair of tetralogy of fallot: a Japanese Multicenter Study. Circ J 68:126, 2004.

98. Gatzoulis MA, Balaji S, Webber SA, et al: Risk factors for arrhythmia and sudden cardiac death late after repair of tetralogy of Fallot: a multicentre study. Lancet 356:975, 2000.

99. Brili S, Aggeli C, Gatzoulis K, et al: Echocardiographic and signal averaged ECG indices associated with non-sustained ventricular tachycardia after repair of tetralogy of Fallot. Heart 85:57, 2001.

100. Russo G, Folino AF, Mazzotti E, et al: Comparison between QRS duration at standard ECG and signal-averaging ECG for arrhythmic risk stratification after surgical repair of tetralogy of fallot. J Cardiovasc Electrophysiol 16:288, 2005.

101. Berul CI, Hill SL, Geggel RL, et al: Electrocardiographic markers of late sudden death risk in postoperative tetralogy of Fallot children [published erratum appears in J Cardiovasc Electrophysiol 11:ix, 2000]. J Cardiovasc Electrophysiol 8:1349, 1997.

102. Gatzoulis MA, Till JA, Redington AN: Depolarization-repolarization inhomogeneity after repair of tetralogy of Fallot. The substrate for malignant ventricular tachycardia? Circulation 95:401, 1997.

103. Balkhi RA, Beghetti M, Friedli B: Time course of appearance of markers of arrhythmia in patients with tetralogy of Fallot before and after surgery. Cardiol Young 14:360, 2004.

104. Daliento L, Rizzoli G, Menti L, et al: Accuracy of electrocardiographic and echocardiographic indices in predicting life threatening ventricular arrhythmias in patients operated for tetralogy of Fallot. Heart 81:650, 1999.

105. Kugler JD: Predicting sudden death in patients who have undergone tetralogy of Fallot repair: is it really as simple as measuring ECG intervals? J Cardiovasc Electrophysiol 9:103, 1998.

106. Butera G, Bonnet D, Sidi D, et al: Patients operated for tetralogy of Fallot and with non-sustained ventricular tachycardia have reduced heart rate variability. Herz 29:304, 2004.

107. Folino AF, Russo G, Bauce B, et al: Autonomic profile and arrhythmic risk stratification after surgical repair of tetralogy of Fallot. Am Heart J 148:985, 2004.

108. Helbing WA, Roest AA, Niezen RA, et al: ECG predictors of ventricular arrhythmias and biventricular size and wall mass in tetralogy of Fallot with pulmonary regurgitation. Heart 88:515, 2002.

109. Chabrak S, Ammar S, Ammar N, et al: Cardiac involvement in emery Dreifuss muscular dystrophy: a case report. Tunis Med 84:361, 2006.

110. Cheung MM, Weintraub RG, Cohen RJ, et al: T wave alternans threshold late after repair of tetralogy of Fallot. J Cardiovasc Electrophysiol 13:657, 2002.

111. Hallioglu O, Aytemir K, Celiker A: The significance of P wave duration and P wave dispersion for risk assessment of atrial tachyarrhythmias in patients with corrected tetralogy of Fallot. Ann Noninvasive Electrocardiol 9:339, 2004.

112. Calder L, Van Praagh R, Van Praagh S, et al: Truncus arteriosus communis. Clinical, angiocardiographic, and pathologic findings in 100 patients. Am Heart J 92:23, 1976.

113. Huh J, Noh CI, Choi JY, et al: Sustained ventricular tachycardia in children after repair of congenital heart disease. J Korean Med Sci 16:25, 2001.

114. Gamboa R, Gersony WM, Nadas AS: The electrocardiogram in tricuspid atresia and pulmonary atresia with intact ventricular septum. Circulation 34:24, 1966.

115. Schiebler GL, Adams P, Anderson RC, et al: Clinical study of twenty-three cases of Ebstein's anomaly of the tricuspid valve. Circulation 19:165, 1959.

116. Van Lingen B, Bauersfeld SR: The electrocardiogram in Ebstein's anomaly of the tricuspid valve. Am Heart J 50:13, 1955.

117. Galvan O, Iturralde P, Basagoitia AM, et al: Ebstein's anomaly with the Wolff-Parkinson-White syndrome. Arch Inst Cardiol Mex 61:309, 1991.

118. Vora AM, Lokhandwala YY: Preexcited tachycardia in a patient with Ebstein's anomaly: is the preexcitation manifest during sinus rhythm? J Cardiovasc Electrophysiol 9:1012, 1998.

119. Jaiswal PK, Balakrishnan KG, Saha A, et al: Clinical profile and natural history of Ebstein's anomaly of tricuspid valve. Int J Cardiol 46:113, 1994.

120. Andress JD, Vander Salm TJ, Huang SK: Bidirectional bundle branch reentry tachycardia associated with Ebstein's anomaly: cured by extensive cryoablation of the right bundle branch. Pacing Clin Electrophysiol 14:1639, 1991.

121. Hebe J: Ebstein's anomaly in adults. Arrhythmias: diagnosis and therapeutic approach. Thorac Cardiovasc Surg 48:214, 2000.

122. Chauvaud SM, Brancaccio G, Carpentier AF: Cardiac arrhythmia in patients undergoing surgical repair of Ebstein's anomaly. Ann Thorac Surg 71:1547, 2001.

123. Aliot E, de Chillou C, Revault d'Allones G, et al: Mahaim tachycardias. Eur Heart J 19(Suppl E):E25, E52, 1998.

124. Berntsen RF, Gjesdal KT, Aass H, et al: Radiofrequency catheter ablation of two right Mahaim-like accessory pathways in a patient with Ebstein's anomaly. J Interv Card Electrophysiol 2:293, 1998.

125. Hluchy J: Mahaim fibers: electrophysiologic characteristics and radiofrequency ablation. Z Kardiol 89 (Suppl 3):136, 2000.

126. Dick M, Fyler DC, Nadas AS: Tricuspid atresia: clinical course in 101 patients. Am J Cardiol 36:327, 1975.

127. Guller B, Titus JL, DuShane JW: Electrocardiographic diagnosis of malformations associated with tricuspid atresia: correlation with morphologic features. Am Heart J 78:180, 1969.

128. O'Neill CA, Brink AJ: Left axis deviation in tricuspid atresia and single ventricle. Circulation 12:612, 1955.

129. Reddy SC, Zuberbuhler JR: Images in cardiovascular medicine. Himalayan P waves in a patient with tricuspid atresia. Circulation 107:498, 2003.

130. Zellers T, Porter CJ, Driscoll DJ: Pseudopreexcitation in tricuspid atresia. Texas Heart Inst J 18:124, 1991.

131. Dick MD, Behrendt DM, Byrum CJ, et al: Tricuspid atresia and the Wolff-Parkinson-White syndrome: evaluation methodology and successful surgical treatment of the combined disorders. Am Heart J 101:496, 1981.

132. Razzouk AJ, Gow R, Finley J, et al: Surgically created Wolff-Parkinson-White syndrome after Fontan operation. Ann Thorac Surg 54:974, 1992.

133. Hager A, Zrenner B, Brodherr-Heberlein S, et al: Congenital and surgically acquired Wolff-Parkinson-White syndrome in patients with tricuspid atresia. J Thorac Cardiovasc Surg 130:48, 2005.

134. Keating P, Van der Meulen H, Shipper JG: Tricuspid atresia—profile and outcome. Cardiovasc J S Afr 12:202, 2001.

135. Gyepes MT, Marcano BA, Desilets DT: Tricuspid atresia, transposition, and coatation of the aorta. Radiology 97:633, 1970.

136. Somlyo AP, Halloran KH: Tricuspid atresia: an electrocardiographic study. Am Heart J 63:171, 1962.

137. Davachi F, Lucas RV Jr , Moller JH: The electrocardiogram and vectorcardiogram in tricuspid atresia. Correlation with pathologic anatomy. Am J Cardiol 25:18, 1970.

138. Wong T, Davlouros PA, Li W, et al: Mechano-electrical interaction late after Fontan operation: relation between P wave duration and dispersion, right atrial size, and atrial arrhythmias. Circulation 109:2319, 2004.

139. Khairy P, Seslar SP, Triedman JK, et al: Ablation of atrioventricular nodal reentrant tachycardia in tricuspid atresia. J Cardiovasc Electrophysiol 15:719, 2004.

140. Yumoto Y, Satoh S, Koga T, et al: Prenatal diagnosis of slow-rate ventricular tachycardia using fetal electrocardiography. Prenat Diagn 24:463, 2004.

141. Strong WB, Liebman J, Perrin E: Hypoplastic left ventricle syndrome. Electrocardiographic evidence of left ventricular hypertrophy. Am J Dis Child 120:511, 1970.

142. Von Rueden TJ, Moller JH: The electrocardiogram in aortic valvular atresia. Chest 73:66, 1978.

143. Rydberg A, Teien DE, Rask P, et al: Electrocardiographic ST-segment depression in children with fontan circulation. Clin Physiol 20:69, 2000.

144. Rydberg A, Rask P, Teien DE, et al: Electrocardiographic ST segment depression and clinical function in children with Fontan circulation. Pediatr Cardiol 24:468, 2003.

145. Kavey RE, Gaum WE, Byrum CJ, et al: Loss of sinus rhythm after total cavopulmonary connection. Circulation 92(9 Suppl):II304, 1995.

146. Tuzcu V, Ozkan B, Sullivan N, et al: P wave signal-averaged electrocardiogram as a new marker for atrial tachyarrhythmias in postoperative Fontan patients. J Am Coll Cardiol 36:602, 2000.

31

Cardiac Arrhythmias in the Fetus, Infants, Children, and Adolescents with Congenital Heart Disease

Definitions

The normal range of heart rates is highly variable throughout fetal development, infancy, and childhood. On pediatric electrocardiograms (ECGs), *bradycardia* is defined as a heart rate less than the second percentile of normal for age, and *tachycardia* as a heart rate greater than the 98th percentile for age each when awake, and at rest. Typically there will be a substantial difference in heart rate from rest to an ambulatory situation or exercise state. Heart rates may be considerably slower or faster on ambulatory recordings due to changes in physiologic state.[1,2] Heart rates that may be "normal" for the physiologic state are nevertheless referred to as bradycardia or tachycardia if they are out of the normal heart rate range for awake resting conditions.[3]

An accelerated rhythm is a rhythm that is faster than anticipated for a given mechanism at a given age, but slower than the rate that is the 98th percentile for age. An escape rhythm is a rhythm that is slower than the normal mechanism but not necessarily slower than the second percentile for age.

Sinus Rhythms

The ECG appearance of sinus rhythm in infants and children is similar to that in adults. The P wave axis in the frontal plane is leftward and inferior, and the P wave is usually upright or diphasic in all precordial leads. Depending on the origin and exit of the impulse from the sinus node, there may be variation in the P wave morphology and axis (but always remaining leftward and inferior). This phenomenon is referred to as a *wandering atrial pacemaker.*

If sinus arrhythmia is defined as any variation in the sinus rate, it is nearly universal in patients of all ages[4] and is usually related to the respiratory pattern. Indeed, lack of rate variability is pathologic, and heart rate variability has been extensively evaluated for its ability to predict prognosis in a number of different conditions.[5] For purposes of assigning the diagnosis of sinus arrhythmia to an ECG, stricter criteria are usually applied. In adults, sinus arrhythmia is commonly defined as a difference in the PP interval of >0.16 second. Because the normal heart rate in infants and children is faster than in adults, a variation to this extent is less common, and we define sinus arrhythmia as a change in the PP interval of greater than 25 percent of the shortest PP interval. "Marked" sinus arrhythmia has been defined as a change in sinus cycle length of greater than 100 percent on adjacent beats.[6] Sinus arrhythmia to this extent is relatively rare in newborns but is not uncommon in older infants and children and may result in referral of children for ECG recording or pediatric cardiology consultation. Sinus arrhythmia independent of respiratory activity and dependent on ventricular activity is commonly seen in pediatric patients with atrioventricular (AV) dissociation due to AV block. The term "ventriculophasic" sinus arrhythmia is used in the presence of sinus cycle variability when the PP interval containing the ventricular complex is shorter than the PP interval without ventricular complex.

Sinus bradycardia in transient form commonly occurs in the fetus, infants, and children, especially the distressed fetus or the infant or child with systemic illness. Bradycardia may be secondary to hypoxia, acidosis, and intracranial events. Chronic sinus bradycardia is seen in patients with congenital heart disease as a manifestation of surgical trauma, but may also be due to congenital abnormality of the sinus node or cardiac ion channel abnormality.

Sinus node dysfunction from surgical trauma includes the sequelae of the atrial baffling procedures for *d*-transposition of the great vessels (Senning and Mustard) or the Fontan procedure.[7-10] Arterial switch procedure for *d*-transposition has been shown to result in less sinus node dysfunction than atrial baffling procedures,[11] whereas the early results of the modified Fontan procedure to minimize atrial involvement and reduce the incidence of bradycardia has produced conflicting results requiring a longer follow-up.[12-15]

Sinus node dysfunction from congenital abnormality is common in patients with left atrial isomerism[16] and may be also related to the destructive effects of maternal anti-SSA/Ro antibodies.[17] Sinus bradycardia or even atrial standstill has been associated with cardiac sodium ion channel abnormalities in children.[18,19] Ion channel abnormalities in patients with the congenital long QT syndrome have been associated with sinus bradycardia, especially in the fetus and newborn.[20-23] Antiarrhythmic drug therapy in pediatric patients, especially with β-adrenergic blockers,[24] frequently causes sinus bradycardia.[25] Fosphenytoin, a drug used as first-line therapy for status epilepticus in children, has been shown to cause sinus arrest.[26]

Mimickers of sinus bradycardia in children include non-conducted premature atrial contractions occurring in a pattern of bigeminy (Figure 31-1), 2:1 AV block with P waves concealed in the preceding T wave (Figure 31-2), and 2:1 AV block associated with a prolonged QT interval (Figure 31-3). Bigeminal atrial and ventricular ectopy may mimic bradycardia in the fetus. When fetal electrocardiography is not available in the obstetric clinic or delivery room, these arrhythmias, when assessed by fetal heart tones, may be mistaken for fetal distress and lead to premature cesarean section.

Sinus tachycardia is commonly seen in response to stress and in the setting of systemic illness, fever, and anemia. In the fetus and young infants, reactive sinus tachycardia may occur at rates as fast as 240 beats/min (a heart rate that would suggest another rhythm mechanism in adults). Drugs, especially some inotropic agents and β-adrenergic agonist bronchodilators, may also cause sinus tachycardia.

Automatic atrial tachycardia with a focus in the right atrium may mimic sinus tachycardia. When the ectopic atrial tachycardia causes cardiomyopathy, it may be difficult to discern this condition from sinus tachycardia in patients with

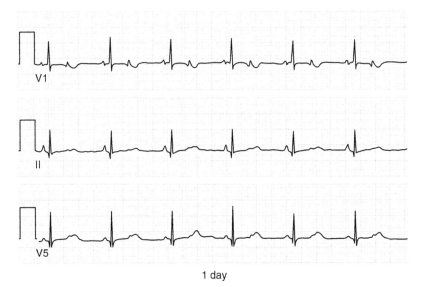

1 day

Figure 31–1 ECG of a 1-day-old infant with a structurally normal heart and frequent premature atrial contractions in a pattern of bigeminy that are nonconducted. This results in a slow ventricular rate for age and may mimic sinus bradycardia.

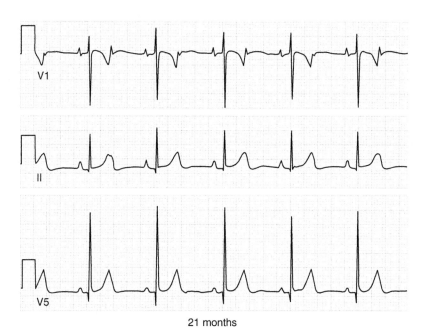

21 months

Figure 31–2   ECG of a 21-month-old child with sinus rhythm and 2:1 atrioventricular block. There is ventriculophasic sinus arrhythmia, and the sinus P wave interval containing the QRS complex is shorter than that without a QRS complex. This appears similar to Figure 31–1, but the morphology of conducted and nonconducted P waves are identical. Again, this pattern may mimic sinus bradycardia, especially in leads II and V_5, where the nonconducted P waves are not well seen.

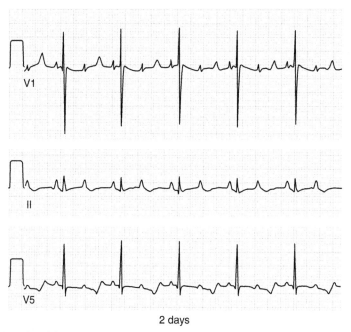

2 days

Figure 31–3   ECG of a 2-day-old infant with congenital prolonged QT interval. Sinus rhythm is seen with 2:1 atrioventricular block. Following the nonconducted P wave, a prominent T wave is seen, especially in lead V_1. The conduction block probably occurs with refractoriness at the level of the ventricular myocardium.

primary cardiomyopathy. Gelb and Garson[27] showed that in a comparison of patients with cardiomyopathy induced by right atrial automatic tachycardia and primary cardiomyopathy with sinus tachycardia, the P wave axis in the horizontal plane was more commonly less than 0 degrees (negative in lead V_2) and second-degree AV block was more common than in patients with primary cardiomyopathy and sinus tachycardia. The heart rates of patients with atrial tachycardia also tended to be higher than in those with primary cardiomyopathy, but there was significant overlap.

Sinus node reentrant tachycardia (Figure 31–4) is relatively uncommon and indistinguishable from sinus tachycardia on a standard ECG.[28,29] Abrupt initiation, frequently after a premature atrial contraction with P wave of different morphology and sudden termination, can establish the diagnosis. Ludomirsky and Garson[30] reported on 12 pediatric patients with sinus node reentrant tachycardia who were older than 2 years. The absence of younger patients in this study may be due to difficulty of diagnosing this arrhythmia at a young age rather than absence of this rhythm mechanism in a younger age group. Five of the 12 patients had no associated cardiac abnormality. One patient had unoperated and four had operated congenital heart disease, and two patients had congestive heart failure. The tachycardia-induced cardiomyopathy is well recognized with this arrhythmia.[31] Sinus node reentrant tachycardia has been reported in neonates, and isolated case reports suggest a favorable pattern of spontaneous resolution.[32]

Atrial Arrhythmias

Isolated premature atrial contractions are common in the fetus and in infants and children.[33] These ectopic beats, even when frequent, are usually benign. In one study approximately one in four term infants had more than five premature atrial contractions in 24 hours. The same infants, when monitored at 1 month of age, had no premature atrial contractions.[34] Atrial ectopy in the fetus and child may have two different relationships with supraventricular tachycardia. The first is that atrial ectopy not associated with the tachycardia mechanism may initiate reentrant tachycardia.[35] Several studies have confirmed that patients presenting with reentrant mechanisms of supraventricular tachycardia in

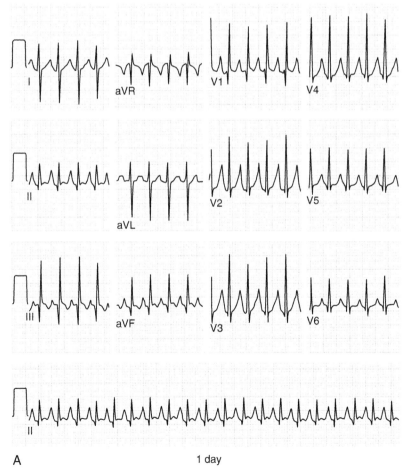

A   1 day

Figure 31–4   ECGs of a 1-day-old infant with Ebstein's anomaly of the tricuspid valve. **A,** The heart rate is 210 beats/min.

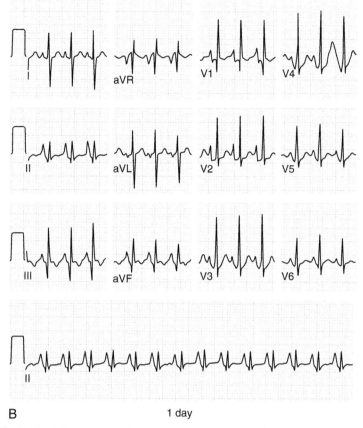

Figure 31–4 cont'd   B, The infant was noted to have abrupt changes in heart rate from this rate to a slower rate, 165 beats/min. Note that the P waves in both recordings appear identical, and the P wave axis and morphology are consistent with a sinus origin and marked right atrial enlargement. The abrupt change from a normal rate **(B)** to tachycardia **(A)** with no change in P wave morphology strongly suggests sinoatrial nodal reentrant tachycardia.

early infancy have a high likelihood of resolution of episodes of clinical tachycardia at 1 year of age, despite the persistent ability to induce the tachycardia with provocative testing. This is likely due to a decreased frequency of premature atrial contractions that can initiate these arrhythmias.[36,37] The second association with supraventricular tachycardia is present when the atrial ectopy is a manifestation of nonconducted accessory pathway echo beats.[38] This pattern will have a fixed interval from the preceding ventricular beat to the atrial ectopy and may be a harbinger for as yet unidentified supraventricular tachycardia.

Primary atrial arrhythmias are a relatively uncommon cause of narrow QRS complex tachycardia in the fetus and in infants and children. They represent 10 to 15 percent of all narrow QRS complex tachycardias in children.[39] The common mechanisms include enhanced or abnormal automaticity and reentry.

Automatic atrial tachycardia will typically resume immediately after atrial pacing or electrical cardioversion. Rate variability with "warm-up" at the initiation of tachycardia and "cool-down" just prior to termination are common. As the tachycardia is often not accompanied by an increase in sympathetic tone to enhance AV nodal conduction, there is frequently first-degree AV block and occasionally second-degree AV block.[27] The P wave morphology on the surface ECG may be helpful in localizing the focus of the atrial tachycardia in children and adults.[40] Kistler et al.[40] showed that a P wave in lead V_1 that was either negative or biphasic positive-negative was 100 percent specific for a right atrial focus, and P waves that were biphasic negative-positive, isoelectric, or positive were 100 percent specific for left atrial foci. Amiodarone is the most effective drug in treating automatic atrial tachycardia.[41] Propafenone, flecainide, and occasionally β-adrenergic blockade may also be successful.[42,43] Automatic atrial tachycardia in infancy is usually relatively persistent rather than paroxysmal. Children with ectopic atrial tachycardia may present with a tachycardia-induced cardiomyopathy, but this rhythm frequently undergoes spontaneous resolution over the course of years, both in pediatric and adult patients.[44] Spontaneous resolution in children diagnosed at less than 3 years of age is more common (78 percent) than that in children diagnosed after 3 years of age (16 percent).[45] The tachycardia can be cured with catheter ablation.[45–47]

Reentrant atrial tachycardia as a mechanism for primary atrial tachycardia in children is more common in patients with diseased or surgically damaged atria (see Figures 31–4 and 31–5).[48] This mechanism can be terminated with pacing or cardioversion. Electrocardiographically, other than by its initiation and termination patterns, it is indistinguishable from atrial automatic tachycardia. This type of atrial tachycardia is also amenable to catheter ablation[49] but may require placement of linear lesions, which result in conduction block in the reentrant circuit.[50,51] Antitachycardia pacemakers have also been shown to be effective.[52] Nonautomatic focal atrial tachycardia (likely micro-reentry) is seen in the pediatric and especially the adult congenital heart disease patient, commonly after repair of congenital heart disease.[53] It is indistinguishable from other forms of atrial reentrant tachycardia clinically and on the ECG and is commonly mistaken for atrial flutter prior to electrophysiology study. It is often amenable to focal catheter ablation.[53]

Atrial flutter is a form of reentrant atrial tachycardia with rapid, regular undulations on the ECG, giving rise to a sawtooth appearance in some leads. The atrial rate during atrial flutter in the fetus and in infants and children is faster than the 250 to 350 beats/min seen in adults. Atrial flutter occurs in the pediatric population in two relatively distinct patterns. The first type occurs in the fetus and newborn infant (Figure 31–6).

In the fetus, atrial flutter accounts for approximately one quarter of all documented tachyarrhythmias and has a median atrial rate of 450 beats/min (range 370 to 500 beats/min).[54] It is rarely seen before 27 weeks of gestation,[55] probably because the atrial size required to maintain the tachycardia cycle length is not reached until that gestational age. There is typically 2:1 AV conduction.

Hydrops fetalis occurs in about 40 percent of all fetuses with atrial flutter, and the overall mortality for affected gestations is 8 percent, an incidence that is not significantly different from that of supraventricular tachycardia.[54] Hydropic fetuses with atrial flutter have higher ventricular rates, but atrial rates are not significantly different than in fetuses with atrial flutter without hydrops.[54]

Texter et al. described a series of 50 infants with atrial flutter[56] not associated with structural heart disease. Most were diagnosed within the first 2 days of life. The average atrial and ventricular rates were 424 beats/min (range 340 to 580 beats/min) and 208 beats/min (range 125 to 280 beats/min), respectively. Twenty percent of the infants had also either a supraventricular tachycardia or an automatic atrial tachycardia. An association with the Wolff-Parkinson-White (WPW) syndrome and concealed accessory AV connections has been described.[57,58] In the study of Texter et al.,[56] atrial flutter recurred after conversion in only 12 percent of infants, in all cases within 5 days, and in most cases within 24 hours after initial conversion. All infants with recurrence had an associated supraventricular arrhythmia mechanism. The majority of patients in this series (88 percent) received antiarrhythmic medication following conversion (most commonly digoxin) as in other series,[59–61] although the reported risk for recurrence without drug therapy has been low.[62,63] Conversion to sinus rhythm can either

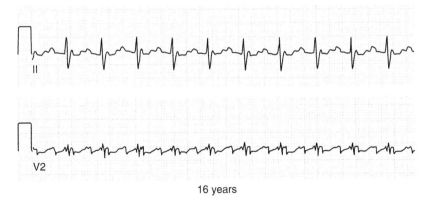

16 years

Figure 31–5 ECG of a 16-year-old adolescent with a double-inlet single ventricle. The patient presented with symptomatic palpitations. Atrial reentrant tachycardia is seen with 2:1 atrioventricular (AV) conduction. The recording in lead II mimics sinus rhythm with first-degree AV block, but the nonconducted P waves are easily seen in lead V₂.

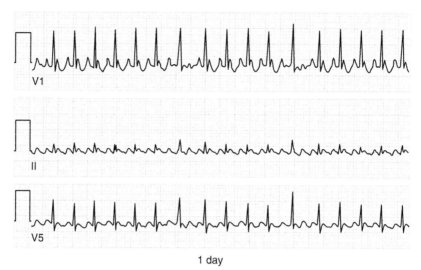

1 day

Figure 31–6 ECG of a 1-day-old infant (30 weeks' gestational age) with a structurally normal heart and atrial flutter. Note the presence of a "sawtooth" pattern at baseline. The atrial rate is approximately 400 beats/min, and there is variable but predominantly 2:1 atrioventricular (AV) conduction. The infant underwent synchronized cardioversion for treatment of this rhythm and developed orthodromic AV reentrant tachycardia (see Figures 31–10 and 31–11).

be accomplished with esophageal pacing[64] or more reliably with synchronized cardioversion.[56] Biphasic waveform cardioversion has been shown to be more effective at lower-delivered energy than monophasic waveform for the conversion of atrial flutter in infants.[65]

The second group of pediatric patients with atrial flutter includes the older infants, children, or adolescents. In a review by Garson, only 8 percent of these patients had structurally normal hearts.[66] The vast majority had congenital heart disease,[67] and some had cardiomyopathy.[68] The ECG appearance and atrial rates during atrial flutter in these patients were similar to those in adults. In contrast to patients with atrial flutter in the newborn period or early infancy, recurrence of atrial flutter is common and as a rule requires catheter or surgical ablation or long-term drug therapy.

Chaotic atrial tachycardia is rarely seen in children. Unlike adults, in whom chaotic atrial tachycardia is usually seen with chronic obstructive pulmonary disease, most infants with this arrhythmia have structurally normal hearts,[69] although frequently there are contributing noncardiac conditions.[70] Coexisting respiratory infections were reported in one third of infants with this rhythm in one series and structural heart disease in a similar number in the same series.[71] The ECG diagnosis requires three or more ectopic P wave morphologies, irregular PP intervals, an isoelectric baseline between p waves, and a rapid atrial rate.[71] Chaotic atrial tachycardia is usually a well-tolerated and self-

limited rhythm in most pediatric patients[72] but has been reported to result in a tachycardia-induced cardiomyopathy in as many as one fourth of affected infants.[71] This rhythm in infants frequently has an excellent outcome with spontaneous resolution by 1 year of age.[71] If the ventricular rate can not be adequately controlled with digoxin, beta-blockade, or calcium channel blocker, conversion to sinus rhythm can usually be accomplished with amiodarone, flecainide, or propafenone. Electrical cardioversion is not effective.

Atrial fibrillation is seen more commonly in the adolescent or adult patient with congenital heart disease or cardiomyopathy.[73] It often coexists with atrial reentrant tachycardia. Kirsh et al.[74] reviewed a series of 149 patients with congenital heart disease undergoing cardioversion for reentrant atrial tachycardia or atrial fibrillation. They found that as many as one third of patients in this population had atrial fibrillation in addition to the more common reentrant atrial tachycardia. They did not find a tendency of progression of atrial tachycardia to atrial fibrillation, but they did find that both arrhythmias required intervention with increasing frequency over time. Patients with unoperated congenital heart disease or those with residual left ventricular valvular lesions appeared to be more prone to atrial fibrillation than those after a more adequate surgical repair or palliation. Rheumatic fever with severe mitral regurgitation was a more common cause of atrial fibrillation in the distant past but is now rarely seen.

Atrial fibrillation in the infant or child with a structurally normal heart is extremely rare.[73] It has been reported with abuse of alcohol, inhalants, and other illicit drugs in children and adolescents[75,76] and rarely in a familial form.[77] In the adolescent with a structurally normal heart, atrial fibrillation is most commonly associated with WPW syndrome but can also be seen in patients with concealed accessory pathways (Figure 31–7). Atrial fibrillation in patients with accessory pathways with short refractory periods for anterograde conduction may cause hemodynamic collapse and cardiac arrest (see later discussion). In our experience, adolescents with WPW syndrome and frequent episodes of atrial fibrillation usually cease to have atrial fibrillation after successful radiofrequency catheter ablation of the accessory pathway.

Atrial fibrillation has been reported to result from administration of adenosine for treatment of supraventricular tachycardia.[78,79] Adenosine is used when resuscitative facilities are available to abort hemodynamic collapse from rapid anterograde conduction over an accessory pathway during atrial fibrillation.[80]

AV Junctional Arrhythmias

Junctional escape beats and **junctional escape rhythm** are seen commonly in normal children, especially on ambulatory recordings during sleep,[1,2,81] but are less common on routine ECG

in pediatric patients who are awake and at rest. It is usually seen in two clinical situations in pediatrics. The first is in the fetus, newborn infant, or child with congenital complete AV block. In this setting, there is usually sinus rhythm and AV dissociation is present. The junctional escape rate at rest is usually between 45 and 60 beats/min but may exceed 100 beats/min with exercise. The QRS morphology is the same as in atrial rhythm mechanisms.

The second group of pediatric patients with junctional escape rhythm includes those with sinus node dysfunction, especially following atrial baffle procedures for *d*-transposition of the great vessels (Figure 31–8), and after Fontan palliation for single ventricle physiologies, as well as patients with heterotaxy syndromes with congenital absence of the sinus node.[16] There is frequently retrograde conduction from the junction to the atrium and simultaneous contraction of the atrium and the ventricle. Depending upon the junctional escape rate, ventricular function, and clinical symptoms, these patients may benefit from permanent pacing. Junctional escape rhythm is also seen in individuals with atrial standstill (Figure 31–9). Atrial activity on the surface ECG may be difficult to discern when retrograde P waves are concealed within the QRS complex. The uncommon atrial standstill has been associated with muscular dystrophy,[82] ventricular noncompaction,[83] and inherited conditions with cardiac sodium channel mutations.[18,19]

Accelerated junctional rhythm or **automatic junctional tachycardia** is most often seen in the

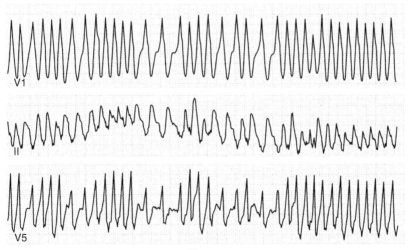

15 years

Figure 31–7 ECG of a 15-year-old adolescent with Wolff-Parkinson-White syndrome. Atrial fibrillation with rapid ventricular response over an accessory atrioventricular connection is seen. The shortest preexcited RR interval was 160 ms. The patient presented with syncope related to this rhythm and underwent radiofrequency catheter ablation of the accessory pathway.

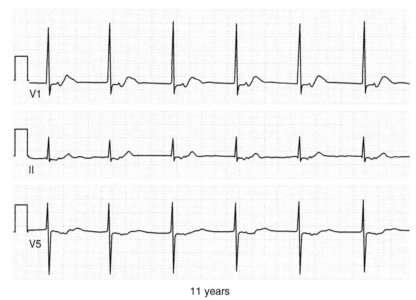

11 years

Figure 31–8   ECG of an 11-year-old child with *d*-transposition of the great vessels following Senning baffle palliation. A junctional escape rhythm with retrograde conduction to the atrium is seen. This rhythm is common in older patients following both Senning and Mustard-type atrial baffle palliations owing to sinus node damage from the surgical intervention.

pediatric population following cardiac surgery.[84] It is more common after procedures that involve manipulation of the AV junction, such as ventricular septal defect repair, but it can be caused by other procedures. When it occurs following surgical manipulations remote from the bundle of His, pressure on the area from cardiopulmonary bypass cannulae or coronary sinus cannulation for retrograde cardioplegia usually can be implicated. The mechanism is thought to be abnormal automaticity, and the arrrhythmia in this setting is usually transient but can be potentially life threatening if not adequately controlled. Reducing dose of inotropic agents if possible, atrial

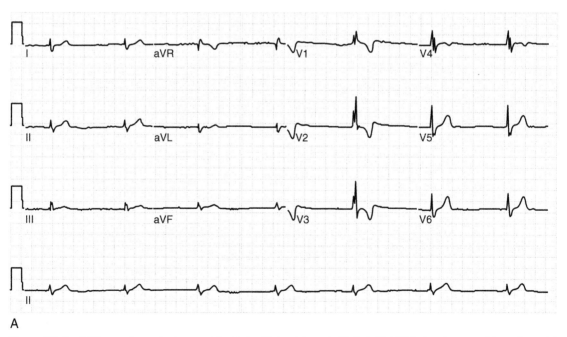

A

Figure 31–9   ECG recordings of a 6-year-old with familial atrial standstill. **A,** Initial ECG showing no evidence for atrial activity and a wide QRS complex escape rhythm at a rate of 40 beats/min.

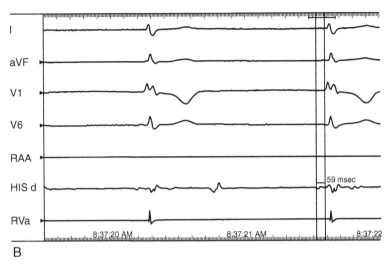

B

Figure 31–9 cont'd   B, Intracardiac recordings showing no evidence of atrial activity, even at high recording gain, and a His bundle deflection preceding each QRS complex with a somewhat prolonged HV interval of 59 ms.

pacing at a slightly faster rate to maintain AV synchrony, sedation, systemic cooling,[85] and many antiarrhythmic drugs including intravenously administered amioadorone have been reported to be effective.[86–88] Intravenous flecainide has also been shown to be effective[89] but is not currently available in the United States. Rarely, aggressive support with extracorporeal circulation[90] or ventricular assist may be required.

Transient accelerated junctional rhythm is also seen during radiofrequency catheter ablation of the slow AV nodal pathway for treatment of AV nodal reentrant tachycardia and can be a helpful marker, indicating appropriate catheter position for successful ablation.[91]

Congenital automatic junctional tachycardia (Figure 31–10) in infancy is rare and frequently familial.[92,93] AV dissociation is most commonly seen in these patients, but retrograde conduction to the atrium can also be seen. Sudden death is reported in infants and children with this arrhythmia. This may be due to sudden complete AV block as the result of degeneration of the conduction system,[94] extremely rapid ventricular rates and hemodynamic instability, or proarrhythmic effects of antiarrhythmic drugs.[93,95] Amiodarone appears to be the most effective antiarrhythmic drug in treating this rhythm[92] but can be associated with proarrhythmia.[93] Propafenone[96] and flecainide[93] have also been shown to be effective in controlling the ventricular rate and preventing tachycardia-induced cardiomyopathy. Frequent ECG monitoring for AV block, proarrhythmia, and extreme junctional acceleration and echocardiographic monitoring for ventricular dysfunction are critical for prevention of

undesirable outcomes in these infants. Catheter ablation of the automatic junctional focus has been reported to preserve normal AV conduction, even in neonates.[97,98]

AV nodal reentrant tachycardia has been previously considered to be rare in infants and was thought to be more common later in childhood and in adolescence.[39,99] This perception of prevalence has been based on esophageal electrophysiology studies in infants, aimed at differentiating orthodromic AV reentrant tachycardia from AV nodal reentrant tachycardia and primarily relying on the VA interval >70 ms for the diagnosis of orthodromic AV reentry. This perception has been further supported by diagnostic concordance between esophageal and subsequent invasive electrophysiology studies in children.[100] We have seen numerous infants following cardiac surgery with an unusual form of AV nodal reentrant tachycardia and VA interval greater than 70 ms, and the diagnosis was proven by electrophysiology study using postoperative epicardial atrial and ventricular pacing wires. The tachycardia is often initiated with atrial pacing with extrastimuli with or without an abrupt increase in the AV interval, and is not due to AV reentry even though the VA interval is greater than 70 ms. The atrial activity is not "preexcited" even with placement of very early ventricular extrastimuli in small hearts, inconsistent with orthodromic AV reentry (Figure 31–11). The tachycardia can be terminated with very early ventricular extrastimuli that do not conduct to the atrium, ruling out atrial tachycardia. It is unclear whether this tachycardia is more frequent in infants with congenital heart disease or immediately following cardiac surgery. This tachycardia

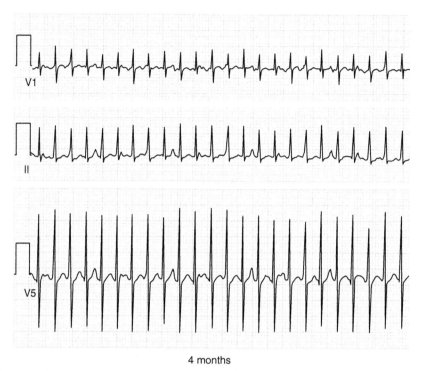

4 months

Figure 31–10   ECG of a 4-month-old child with a structurally normal heart and automatic junctional tachycardia. The tachycardia is regular with a ventricular rate of 285 beats/min. There is atrioventricular dissociation with a slower atrial rate of 170 beats/min. P waves are easily seen in leads II and V₅.

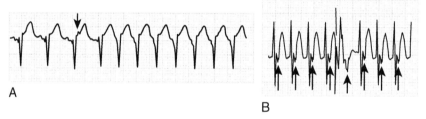

A

B

Figure 31–11   ECGs from an 11-day-old infant with double outlet right ventricle and atrioventricular (AV) nodal reentrant tachycardia 6 days after arterial switch procedure. **A,** Initiation of the tachycardia with a premature atrial contraction (arrow) conducted with a long PR interval (320 ms), probably indicating conduction over a slow AV nodal pathway. **B,** A premature ventricular contraction, introduced using postoperative epicardial pacing wires preceding the next expected QRS complex (preexcitation index) by 120 ms, results in a slight delay in atrial activity. Atrial activity is augmented by epicardial atrial wires (electrograms marked with arrows).

may be similar to "slow/slow" AV nodal reentrant tachycardia, which has been described in adults and is frequently confused with orthodromic AV reentry.[101] In the usual clinical setting, ventricular stimulation, which is required for diagnosis, is not readily available in infants with supraventricular tachycardia, and because this rhythm tends to resolve spontaneously after infancy, the affected infants would not be included in comparative studies performed in later childhood at the time of invasive electrophysiology study for purposes of catheter ablation.

As in adults, AV nodal reentrant tachycardia in older children occurs in typical and atypical forms. The ECG appearance is similar to that in adults with sudden onset (usually from a premature atrial contraction) and P waves that are often concealed within the QRS complex in the typical form (anterograde conduction using the slow AV nodal pathway and retrograde conduction using the fast AV nodal pathway) or P waves that occur midway between ventricular contractions in the atypical form (anterograde conduction using the fast or a second slow AV nodal pathway and retrograde conduction using the slow AV nodal pathway). The presence of dual AV nodal physiology in children using previously defined adult criteria of a 50-ms increase in H_1H_2 interval is seen in only half of pediatric patients,[102] and decreasing the interval that defines a "jump" in AV nodal conduction did not reliably demonstrate the dual AV nodal pathways.[103] This is probably due to overlapping refractory period durations of the slow and fast pathways in young patients. Kannankeril and Fish noted in pediatric patients with AV nodal reentrant tachycardia that "sustained slow pathway conduction" (PR interval exceeding RR interval during incremental atrial pacing) is seen more commonly (75 percent) than dual AV nodal physiology (52 percent).[104] Sustained slow pathway conduction was more frequently abolished by catheter ablation of the slow AV nodal pathway (persistent in 13 percent) than traditional markers of dual AV nodal physiology (persistent in 31 percent).

The rate of AV nodal reentrant tachycardia in children is somewhat faster than in adults, ranging from 180 to 260 beats/min. Digoxin, β-adrenergic blockers, and calcium channel blockers are effective in treatment of this rhythm. Radiofrequency catheter modification of the slow AV nodal pathway has been effective in treatment of this rhythm with a relatively low risk of AV block.[105] Cryothermal catheter ablation of the slow AV nodal pathway has also been effective, with a lower risk of AV block but a higher recurrence rate.[106–109] Occasionally, suspected AV nodal reentrant tachycardia is not inducible at electrophysiology study. Catheter modification of the slow AV nodal pathway may be helpful in this situation to eliminate recurrence of tachycardia.[110] The low risk of AV block from cryothermal AV node modification allows for this approach with minimal risk of complication.

A special form of reentrant tachycardia utilizing two distinctly separate AV nodes and His bundles, termed "twin" AV nodes, has been observed in patients with congenital heart disease.[111] This anatomic conduction system arrangement has been seen most commonly in patients with AV discordance and malaligned complete AV canal. These patients often have two distinct non-preexcited QRS morphologies during sinus rhythm. (Figure 31–12). Catheter ablation of one of the AV nodes prevented recurrence of tachycardia.[111]

AV Reentrant Arrhythmias

AV reentrant rhythms use accessory AV connections. Next to the AV nodal reentrant tachycardia, **orthodromic atrioventricular reentrant tachycardia** is the most common narrow QRS complex tachycardia in childhood.[39] This may be seen in subjects with both manifest (ventricular preexcitation) and unidirectional (concealed)

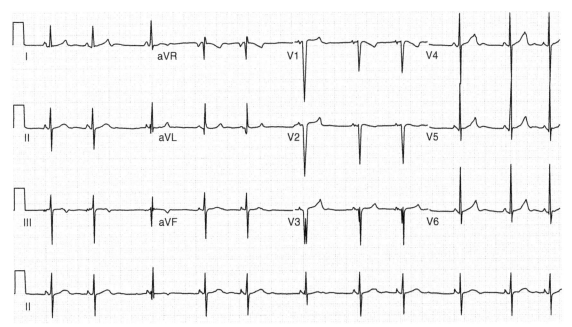

Figure 31–12 ECG of a 3-year-old with double inlet left ventricle and d-transposition of the great vessels. Sinus rhythm with two distinct QRS morphologies. The third and sixth beats in lead II at the bottom are conducted with a normal QRS axis over one atriventricular (AV) node and conduction system, and the other beats are conducted with left axis deviation over a second AV node and conduction system.

AV conduction. As in adults, the onset of tachycardia is of sudden onset, usually with a premature ventricular or premature atrial contraction. The P waves are usually inscribed within the ST segment with an RP interval of >70 ms (see Figure 31–12). Jaeggi et al.[112] have proposed an algorithm for differentiation of AV reentrant tachycardia from AV nodal reentrant tachycardia based on the 12-lead ECG in children. If a pseudo r′ pattern in lead V_1 or a pseudo S pattern are present in the inferior leads, AV nodal reentry is suggested. If the RP interval is greater than 100 ms, AV reentry is suggested. When the RP interval is less than 100 ms, or P waves are not visible and ST segment depression is greater than 2 mm, the algorithm suggests AV reentry, but if the ST depression is less than 2 mm, then AV nodal reentry is favored. Functional bundle branch block on the same side as the accessory pathway increases the VA interval and frequently slows the rate of tachycardia (Figure 31–13). This response confirms the participation of an ipsilateral accessory pathway in the tachycardia. Although most accessory AV connections are congenital, surgically created accessory pathways have been reported with connection of the right atrial appendage to the right ventricular outflow tract.[113]

Antidromic AV reentrant tachycardia (Figure 31–14) is less common in children. It uses the accessory pathway in anterograde direction from the atrium to the ventricle and the AV node to conduct retrogradely from the ventricle to the atrium. This results in a wide QRS complex tachycardia with the early part of the QRS being similar to the delta wave during sinus rhythm. This rhythm or other preexcited tachycardias, including atrial tachycardia conducted over an accessory pathway or automaticity from an accessory pathway, may easily be mistaken for ventricular tachycardia (VT) on a surface ECG.[114]

Similar to adults, pediatric patients with WPW syndrome are prone to developing rapid rates during atrial tachyarrhythmias with anterograde conduction over an accessory pathway. This may be especially dangerous during atrial fibrillation, which may result in the development of ventricular fibrillation. In the pediatric population this occurs most commonly in adolescents, frequently during vigorous physical activity. A prospective study in children and adults with asymptomatic ventricular preexcitation showed that cardiac arrest occurred in 3 of 212 patients during 5 years of follow-up.[115] Each of these 3 patients had multiple accessory pathways and the shortest preexcited RR interval during atrial fibrillation <230 ms. Assessment of anterograde conduction over an accessory pathway during intermittent ventricular preexcittion may be performed noninvasively with an exercise or an ambulatory ECG. There should be careful inspection for the cause of accessory pathway block, as "phase 4 block" may not

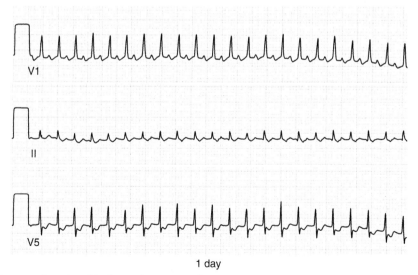

V1

II

V5

1 day

Figure 31–13   ECG of a 1-day-old infant with a structurally normal heart (see Figure 31–6). After synchronized cardioversion for atrial flutter the infant developed this rhythm, a narrow QRS complex tachycardia at a rate of 250 beats/min with a 1:1 atrioventricular (AV) relation, and an RP interval of 100 ms. Atrial activity is seen best in lead V_1 with positive P waves. This rhythm was shown to be orthodromic AV reentrant tachycardia with the development of left bundle branch block (see Figure 31–11); it was confirmed at invasive electrophysiology study and catheter ablation due to drug refractory tachycardia.

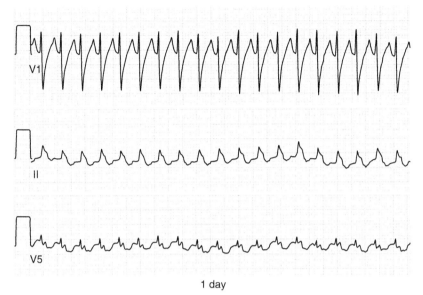

1 day

Figure 31–14   ECG of a 1-day-old infant with a structurally normal heart (see Figure 31–10). A wide QRS complex tachycardia is seen with a left bundle branch block (LBBB) pattern. A 1:1 atrioventricular (AV) relation is seen with an RP interval of 140 ms. An increase in the ventriculoatrial (VA) interval suggests that this is orthodromic AV reentrant tachycardia with LBBB aberrant conduction in a patient with a left-sided accessory AV connection. Note that the ventricular rate is slower than in Figure 31–10.

predict slow pathway conduction during atrial fibrillation.[116] When cycle length–dependent accessory pathway block can not be demonstrated by noninvasive means, minimally invasive esophageal electrophysiology studies on asymptomatic children with ventricular preexcitation can be performed to select appropriate patients for catheter ablation.[117–119]

The **permanent form of junctional reciprocating tachycardia** (Figures 31–15 and 31–16) is the most common type of incessant tachycardia in children.[120] The term is somewhat misleading, as the mechanism of the incessant tachycardia is usually an AV reentry over the AV node in the anterograde direction and a slowly and usually decrementally conducting unidirectional accessory AV connection in the retrograde direction. The accessory pathways associated with this rhythm have been localized at multiple sites.[121] The incessant nature of tachycardia frequently results in a tachycardia-induced cardiomyopathy. The tachycardia may be erroneously diagnosed as atrial because of long RP interval. For drug treatment for this condition, the reader is referred to the study of Lindinger et al.,[122] who found propafenon and flecainide to be most effective, but catheter ablation is the preferred treatment for older patients.[123] Both radiofrequency and cryothermal catheter ablation have been effective.[124,125] Due to the possibility of spontaneous resolution of tachycardia and higher

procedural risk in infants, Lindinger and others[126] recommended initial therapy with antiarrhythmic agents in this young population, reserving catheter ablation for infants who failed drug therapy or have left ventricular dysfunction.

Ventricular Arrhythmias

Ventricular escape beats or **ventricular escape rhythm** may be seen in patients with sinus node dysfunction or AV block with inadequate junctional escape rhythm. Pediatric patients with AV block and ventricular escape rhythm (Figure 31–17) are at higher risk for sudden death, and permanent pacing is recommended.[127]

Premature ventricular contractions are seen commonly in pediatric patients. One study showed an incidence of 18 percent in term infants on the first day of life.[34] Similar to premature atrial contractions, they occur less frequently in older infants, and as previously mentioned, this may account for a decreased occurrence of supraventricular arrhythmia due to an absence of initiating factors.[37,128] A cricadian pattern to the frequency of the premature ventricular contractions has been shown in children, similar to that in adults.[129] Premature ventricular contractions may occur with disturbing frequency in some infants and children. Frequent premature ventricular contractions,

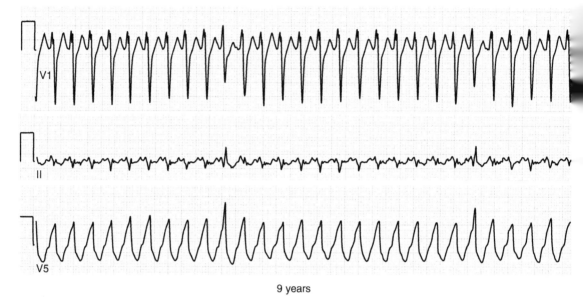

9 years

Figure 31–15   ECG of a 9-year-old child with Wolff-Parkinson-White syndrome. There is a wide QRS complex tachycardia, and the morphology mimicked the patient's delta wave morphology. Initially antidromic tachycardia was suspected, but narrower "fused" complexes seen on the 10th and 23rd beats of the recording suggested that the atrioventricular (AV) node was conducting anterogradely intermittently during the tachycardia. Either preexcited atrial tachycardia or "two-pathway" AV reentrant tachycardia was suspected. Electrophysiologic study confirmed the tachycardia to be "two-pathway" AV reentrant tachycardia with anterograde conduction occurring over a right free-wall accessory AV connection and retrograde conduction over a posterior septal accessory AV connection. Both were successfully ablated with radiofrequency energy.

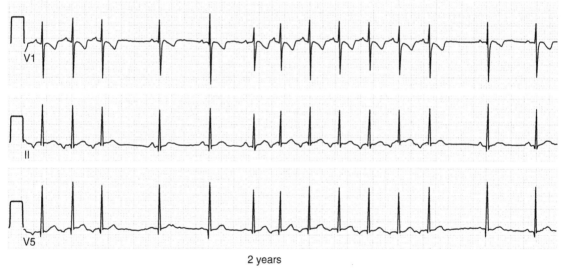

2 years

Figure 31–16   ECG of a 2-year-old child with paroxysms of a relatively slow, narrow QRS complex tachycardia. This rhythm was nearly incessant and shows P waves that are negative in the inferior leads preceding the QRS complexes. This is consistent with the permanent form of junctional reciprocating tachycardia.

especially ventricular couplets or nonsustained VT in children, may be of concern but are usually benign when they occur in a structurally normal heart.[130,131] Suppression of premature ventricular contractions with physical activity and increasing sinus rate usually supports the

benign nature,[132–134] although this has not been proven. Several studies found that isolated premature ventricular contractions and even ventricular couplets in young patients with structurally normal hearts were benign.[131,135–137] Iwamoto et al. reported that even the presence of up to 5 beats of nonsustained monomorphic ventricular tachycardia in children with structurally normal hearts does not require treatment and has good long-term prognosis.[138]

Accelerated ventricular rhythm (ventricular rhythm faster than sinus rhythm but slower than the 98th percentile of normal) is not associated with hemodynamic instability and, when seen in association with a structurally normal heart, is considered to be benign.[139–141]

Ventricular tachycardia (VT) is rare in the pediatric population. The QRS duration may be narrow when compared with VT in adults but is usually longer than normal for the patient's age. As in adults, the onset and termination of VT are usually abrupt. Less frequently than in adults there is AV dissociation, and not uncommonly there is retrograde conduction to the atrium. AV dissociation, if seen, is clearly helpful in the diagnosis. Capture and fusion beats are rarely seen in pediatric patients but are helpful diagnostically when present. Supraventricular tachycardia with preexisting or rate-dependent aberrant conduction or conduction over an accessory AV connection can mimic VT on the electrocardiogram.[114]

Monomorphic VT is most commonly seen in pediatric patients with repaired congenital heart disease, especially tetralogy of Fallot (Figure 31–18), ventricular septal defect, and double-outlet right ventricle. This tachycardia usually originates from the right ventricular outflow tract or the intraventricular septum.[142] Most commonly it presents with a left bundle branch block (LBBB) pattern, but it may have a right bundle branch block (RBBB) pattern if it exits to the left side of the septum.

Monomorphic VT may be seen in patients with structurally normal hearts. Two clinical forms are common. The first is idiopathic left VT. This is frequently misdiagnosed as supraventricular tachycardia due to the relatively narrow QRS complexes that can be seen during tachycardia (Figure 31–18). The QRS morphology is an RBBB pattern with a superior frontal plane QRS axis. It is frequently responsive to verapamil and can be cured with radiofrequency catheter ablation. Ablation can be complicated by inability to induce the tachycardia, and in such cases a linear ablation lesion strategy has been shown to be effective.[143] The second common form of monomorphic VT in children with structurally normal hearts is right ventricular outflow tract tachycardia. It has a QRS morphology of LBBB pattern with an inferior frontal plane axis (Figure 31–19). It is frequently responsive to adenosine. Cure of this tachycardia has been reported with radiofrequency catheter ablation.[144] Origin of the tachycardia from the left aortic sinus cusp has also been reported.[145] Monomorphic VT may also be related to ventricular hamartoma, rhabdomyoma, cardiac fibroma,[146] focal myocarditis, or arrhythmogenic right ventricular dysplasia.[147] Treatment requires consideration of the rate of tachycardia, resultant symptoms, patient age, and concomitant heart disease.[131] In some

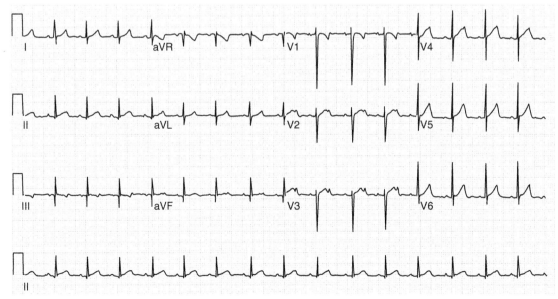

Figure 31–17 ECGs of a 7-month-old child with presumed myocarditis. **A,** Presenting ECG with sinus rhythm at a rate of 132 beats/min with complete atrioventricular (AV) block and a wide QRS complex ventricular escape rhythm.

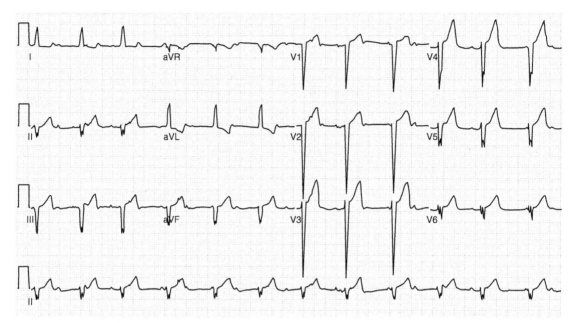

Figure 31–17 cont'd   B, ECG recorded the next day with sinus rhythm at a rate of 90 beats/min with normal AV conduction.

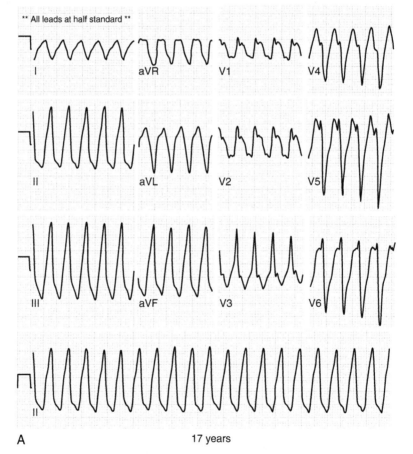

A   17 years

Figure 31–18   ECGs of a 17-year-old adolescent with tetralogy of Fallot. The patient sustained resuscitated sudden cardiac death. **A,** This ECG was recorded after induction of ventricular tachycardia with ventricular extrastimuli. The tachycardia was mapped to the right ventricular outflow tract and ablated.

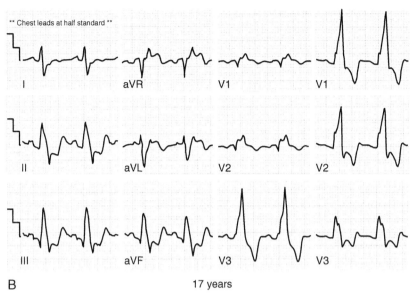

Figure 31–18   B, The ECG in sinus rhythm demonstrates a wide QRS complex due to right bundle branch block, with morphology different from that during the tachycardia.

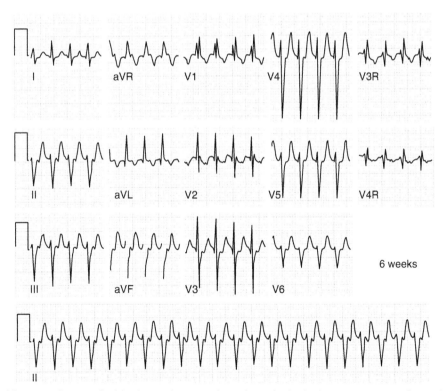

Figure 31–19   ECG of a 6-week-old infant with ventricular tachycardia (VT). There is 1:1 retrograde conduction to the atrium with an RP interval of 120 ms. The QRS complexes are somewhat narrow, and the tachycardia was thought to be supraventricular in origin prior to cardiac electrophysiology consultation. The morphology is consistent with idiopathic left VT.

cases no therapy is required; in others, antiarrhythmic drug therapy, catheter or surgical ablation, or antitachycardia pacing and implanted defibrillators are options for treatment.

Polymorphic VT is seen in pediatric patients in several different clinical situations. The **congenital long QT syndrome** is associated with "torsades de pointes" VT, in which the axis of the QRS complex changes as though to twist around the baseline. The pathophysiology is possibly related to triggered early afterdepolarizations. The congenital long QT syndrome has been shown to result from a number of abnormalities of sodium and potassium cardiac ion channels related to genetic defects.[148–150] Therapy of pediatric patients with the congenital long QT syndrome includes β blockade, left cervical sympathectomy, permanent pacing, and more rarely antiarrhythmic drugs such as mexiletine, flecainide, and α-adrenergic blockade. Implantable defibrillators are another option for treatment in patients with arrhythmia recalcitrant to medical therapy or those presenting with resuscitated cardiac arrest.

Polymorphic VT may also be seen in an entity described as **catecholaminergic polymorphic VT**. Leenhardt and colleagues[151] reported a group of children with stress- or emotion-induced syncope secondary to polymorphic VT. They frequently demonstrated multiform premature ventricular contractions at rest and development of polymorphic VT with a high catecholamine state. Thirty percent of their patients had a family history of syncope or sudden death. β-adrenergic blockade reduced the frequency of tachycardia, but 2 of 21 patients died suddenly in a follow-up period of 7 years. Other reports have confirmed the benefits of β-blockade in this disorder.[152] Estimated mortality of untreated cases ranges from 30 to 50 percent by the third decade of life.[153] Diagnosis can be difficult, and implanted loop recorders may be helpful in documenting the arrhythmia.[154] Recently genes on chromosome 1, with mutations in the ryanodine receptor gene and calsequestrin gene, have been identified in families that exhibit catecholaminergic polymorphic VT.[153,155,156] It is hoped that this discovery will result in improved therapies for this serious disorder.

Another genetic syndrome associated with polymorphic VT is the **Andersen-Tawil syndrome**. Mutations in the KCNJ2 gene, which encodes a potassium channel subunit, are seen in more than half of all affected inidividuals and result in a decrease in IK1 current.[33,157,158] Affected individuals have periodic paralysis and frequent multiform premature ventricular contractions, ventricular couplets, and nonsustained polymorphic VT (Figure 31–21). The QT intervals in these individuals are normal or borderline prolonged.[33] Despite extremely frequent ventricular ectopy, these patients are often asymptomatic but are at

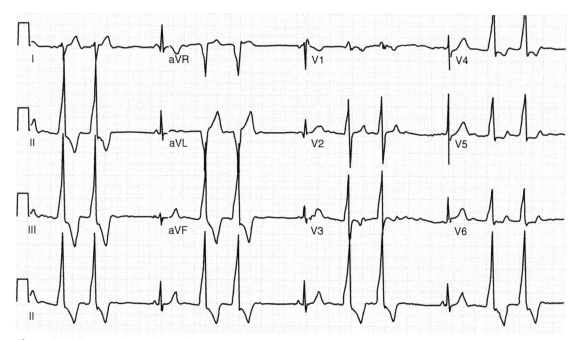

Figure 31–20   ECG of an 18-year-old with monomorphic ventricular tachycardia originating from the right ventricular outflow tract as proven by intracardiac mapping and radiofrequency catheter ablation (not shown). Sinus beats with ventricular couplets of the same morphology as the tachycardia are seen.

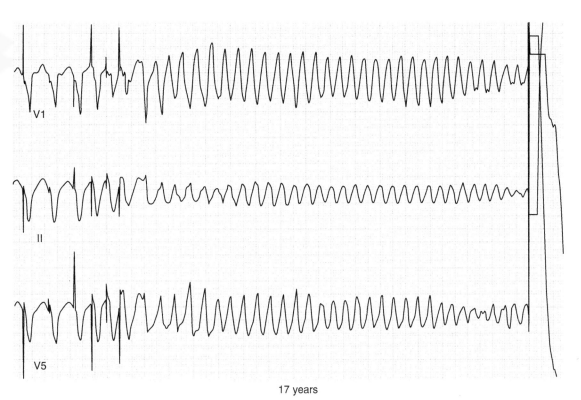

Figure 31–21 ECG of a 17-year-old adolescent with a structurally normal heart who sustained resuscitated sudden cardiac death at age 14. This recording was obtained during a test of an implanted cardioverter defibrillator. Polymorphic ventricular tachycardia is initiated with ventricular pacing from the defibrillator at a cycle length of 400 ms with three ventricular extrastimuli. The device appropriately detects the tachycardia and converts it to sinus rhythm with a 5-joule endocardial shock at the end of the recording.

risk for degeneration to ventricular fibrillation and sudden death. Therapy or risk stratification for these individuals has not been well defined. Anecdotally, we have found elevation of serum potassium with supplemental potassium and potassium-sparing diuretics to reduce the frequency of ventricular ectopy and syncopal events in symptomatic patients. The place of implanted defibrillators has not been defined in this syndrome.

Brugada syndrome, first described in 1992, is now thought to account for as many as 20 percent of all sudden deaths in adults with structurally normal hearts.[159] The disease is inherited in an autosomal dominant fashion related to a sodium channel mutation. The resting ECG demonstrates a "coved type" ST segment elevation in the right precordial leads. The ECG pattern is dynamic and often concealed. The ECG findings can be unmasked with administration of sodium channel–blocking drugs and also by febrile state or vagotonic agents. The average age of presentation is 40 years,[160] and occurrence of symptomatic arrhythmia in children or

adolescents is rare but has been reported even in infants.[161,162]

Ventricular fibrillation is a rare presenting rhythm in cardiac arrest in young children and becomes more common in older children.[163] Samson et al.[164] showed a better outcome from resuscitation of children with in-hospital cardiac arrest when ventricular fibrillation was the presenting arrhythmia as opposed to those patients who presented with other rhythms and developed ventricular fibrillation in the course of resuscitation. Conversion of pediatric ventricular fibrillation often fails,[165] and although spontaneous circulation returns in one third of children, the chances for long-term survival in patients resuscitated with ventricular fibrillation are small.[166]

AV Block

AV block in children may be of first, second, or third degree. First-degree AV block in pediatrics is defined as a PR interval >98th percentile for age. This definition is necessary due to the natural increase in the PR interval with age and development (see Chapter 28). Second-degree AV block may be either Mobitz type I (Wenckebach pattern) or Mobitz type II. Mobitz type I second-degree AV block is usually associated with AV nodal conduction block and Mobitz type II AV block with His-Purkinje block. Mobitz type I AV block is rarely responsible for symptoms, but pediatric patients with Mobitz type II AV block may have syncope and are often candidates for permanent pacing.

AV block is present in a mitochondrial disorder known as *Kearns-Sayre syndrome*, with external opthalmoplegia and pigmentary retinopathy.

Progressive infranodal block with RBBB and left anterior fascicular block may require that prophylactic permanent pacing be performed prior to the development of complete AV block.[167,168]

In rare cases, paroxysmal AV block is seen in pediatric patients, often resulting in syncope and requiring cardiac pacing.[169]

Acquired AV block in pediatric patients can occur in Lyme disease[170] and rheumatic heart disease.[171] In both conditions AV block frequently resolves spontaneously and does not require permanent pacing.

Complete AV block in pediatric patients (Figure 31–23) is usually congenital and most frequently associated with maternal collagen vascular disease or congenital structural heart disease. It can be also secondary to surgical disruption of the AV conduction system. In each of the above conditions, the escape rhythm is most commonly junctional.

The diagnosis of complete AV block in the fetus with a structurally normal heart identifies a high-risk pregnancy. Treatment with maternal dexamethasone in cases of autoantibody mediated AV block has been beneficial in case reports[172] and small uncontrolled series. Sympathomimetic agents administered to the mother may increase the ventricular rate and forestall the development of fetal hydrops.[173] AV block in the fetus with structural heart disease has poor prognosis,[174] and hydrops fetalis in affected fetuses should prompt delivery as soon as the biophysical profile is favorable.[175]

Michaelsson et al.[176] prospectively analyzed a large group of adults with congenital AV block and recommended prophylactic pacemaker treatment in asymptomatic adults because of the high incidence of Stokes-Adams attacks associated with considerable mortality, but asymptomatic children with congenital complete AV block and an adequate junctional escape rhythm may not require permanent pacing. The junctional escape rhythm is considered to be inadequate with ventricular rates of <55/min, <45/min, and <40/min for infants, children, and adolescents, respectively, and is an indication for pacing in asymptomatic subjects with structurally normal hearts. These heart rates

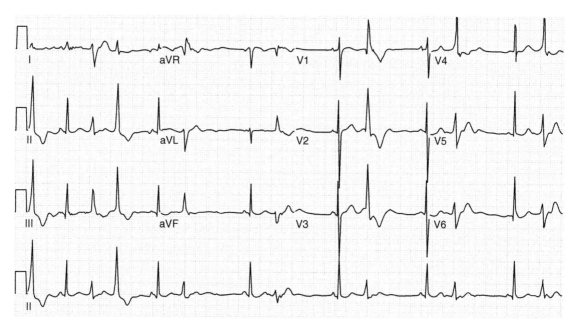

Figure 31–22 ECG of an asymptomatic 12-year-old female with Andersen-Tawil syndrome. Occasional normally conducted sinus beats are seen with frequent multiform ventricular ectopy.

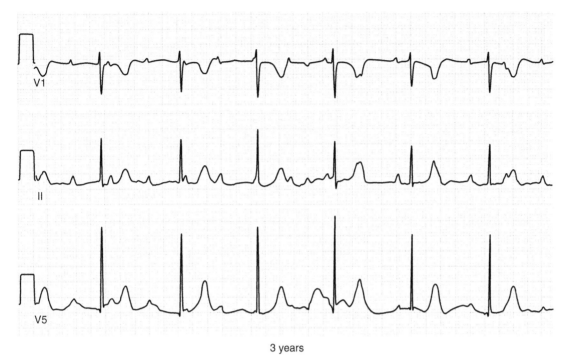

3 years

Figure 31–23   ECG of a 3-year-old child who presented with a history of a seizure disorder. The ECG demonstrates the atrial mechanism to be sinus and the ventricular mechanism to be a junctional escape rhythm secondary to complete atrioventricular block. The patient was asymptomatic with no further "seizures" after placement of a permanent pacemaker.

were selected to prevent congestive heart failure and sudden death,[127,177] but the benefit of the suggested approach requires confirmation in studies of patients with implanted pacemakers.[178] The presence of QT prolongation and significant structural heart disease are factors supporting early pacing. Presence of wide QRS escape rhythm is currently considered to indicate permanent pacing, but this approach is not supported by data from Michaelsson's study.[176] It is not known whether pacing can prevent ventricular dysfunction and mitral valve insufficiency in adults with congenital complete AV block, but permanent pacing in asymptomatic older children and adolescents with this disorder is advisable.

Postoperative complete AV block carries a much higher risk of mortality, and in all cases where AV block persists more than 10 to 14 days after surgery, permanent pacing is indicated. In as many as one third of patients with postoperative AV block receiving pacemakers, AV conduction is restored during long-term follow-up.

REFERENCES

1. Southall DP, Richards J, Mitchell P, et al: Study of cardiac rhythm in healthy newborn infants. Br Heart J 43:14, 1980.

2. Southall DP, Johnston F, Shinebourne EA, et al: 24-hour electrocardiographic study of heart rate and rhythm patterns in population of healthy children. Br Heart J 45:281, 1981.

3. Davignon A, Rautuharju P, Boisselle E, et al: Normal ECG standards for infants and children. Ped Cardiol 1:123, 1979.

4. Massin MM, Bourguignont A, Gerard P: Study of cardiac rate and rhythm patterns in ambulatory and hospitalized children. Cardiology 103:174, 2005.

5. Massin M, von Bernuth G: Clinical and haemodynamic correlates of heart rate variability in children with congenital heart disease. Eur J Pediatr 157:967, 1998.

6. Garson A Jr , Gillette PC, McNamara DG: A Guide to Cardiac Dysrhythmias in Children. New York, Grune & Stratton, 1980.

7. Deanfield J, Camm J, Macartney F, et al: Arrhythmia and late mortality after Mustard and Senning operation for transposition of the great arteries. An eight-year prospective study. J Thorac Cardiovasc Surg 96:569, 1988.

8. Manning PB, Mayer JE Jr , Wernovsky G, et al: Staged operation to Fontan increases the incidence of sinoatrial node dysfunction. J Thorac Cardiovasc Surg 111:833, 1996; discussion 839.

9. Vetter VL, Tanner CS, Horowitz LN: Electrophysiologic consequences of the Mustard repair of d-transposition of the great arteries. J Am Coll Cardiol 10:1265, 1987.

10. Cohen MI, Rhodes LA. Sinus node dysfunction and atrial tachycardia after the Fontan procedure: the scope of the problem. Semin Thorac Cardiovasc Surg Pediatr Card Surg Annu 1:41, 1998.

11. Rhodes LA, Wernovsky G, Keane JF, et al: Arrhythmias and intracardiac conduction after the arterial switch operation. J Thorac Cardiovasc Surg 109:303, 1995.

12. Nurnberg JH, Ovroutski S, Alexi-Meskishvili V, et al: New onset arrhythmias after the extracardiac conduit Fontan operation compared with the intraatrial lateral tunnel procedure: early and midterm results. Ann Thorac Surg 78:1979, 2004; discussion 1988.

13. Kumar SP, Rubinstein CS, Simsic JM, et al: Lateral tunnel versus extracardiac conduit Fontan procedure: a concurrent comparison. Ann Thorac Surg 76:1389, 2003; discussion 1396.

14. Bae EJ, Lee JY, Noh CI, et al: Sinus node dysfunction after Fontan modifications—influence of surgical method. Int J Cardiol 88:285, 2003.

15. Dilawar M, Bradley SM, Saul JP, et al: Sinus node dysfunction after intraatrial lateral tunnel and extracardiac conduit fontan procedures. Pediatr Cardiol 24:284, 2003.

16. Wu MH, Wang JK, Lin JL, et al: Cardiac rhythm disturbances in patients with left atrial isomerism. Pacing Clin Electrophysiol 24:1631, 2001.

17. Costedoat-Chalumeau N, Amoura Z, Villain E, et al: Anti-SSA/Ro antibodies and the heart: more than complete congenital heart block? A review of electrocardiographic and myocardial abnormalities and of treatment options. Arthritis Res Ther 7:69, 2005.

18. Benson DW, Wang DW, Dyment M, et al: Congenital sick sinus syndrome caused by recessive mutations in the cardiac sodium channel gene (SCN5A). J Clin Invest 112:1019, 2003.

19. Makita N, Sasaki K, Groenewegen WA, et al: Congenital atrial standstill associated with coinheritance of a novel SCN5A mutation and connexin 40 polymorphisms. Heart Rhythm 2:1128, 2005.

20. Hofbeck M, Ulmer H, Beinder E, et al: Prenatal findings in patients with prolonged QT interval in the neonatal period. Heart 77:198, 1997.

21. Donofrio MT, Gullquist SD, O'Connell NG, et al: Fetal presentation of congenital long QT syndrome. Pediatr Cardiol 20:441, 1999.

22. Beinder E, Grancay T, Menendez T, et al: Fetal sinus bradycardia and the long QT syndrome. Am J Obstet Gynecol 185:743, 2001.

23. Chang IK, Shyu MK, Lee CN, et al: Prenatal diagnosis and treatment of fetal long QT syndrome: a case report. Prenat Diagn 22:1209, 2002.

24. Celiker A, Ayabakan C, Ozer S, et al: Sotalol in treatment of pediatric cardiac arrhythmias. Pediatr Int 43:624, 2001.

25. Burri S, Hug MI, Bauersfeld U: Efficacy and safety of intravenous amiodarone for incessant tachycardias in infants. Eur J Pediatr 162:880, 2003.

26. Adams BD, Buckley NH, Kim JY, et al: Fosphenytoin may cause hemodynamically unstable bradydysrhythmias. J Emerg Med 30:75, 2006.

27. Gelb BD, Garson A Jr: Noninvasive discrimination of right atrial ectopic tachycardia from sinus tachycardia in "dilated cardiomyopathy." Am Heart J 120:886, 1990.

28. Gomes JA, Hariman RJ, Kang PS, et al: Sustained symptomatic sinus node reentrant tachycardia: incidence, clinical significance, electrophysiologic observations and the effects of antiarrhythmic agents. J Am Coll Cardiol 5:45, 1985.

29. Gomes JA, Mehta D, Langan MN: Sinus node reentrant tachycardia. Pacing Clin Electrophysiol 18:1045, 1995.

30. Ludomirsky A, Garson A Jr: Supraventricular tachycardia in children. In: Gillette PC, Garson A Jr (eds): Pediatric Arrhythmias: Electrophysiology and Pacing. Philadelphia, Saunders, 1990, pp 380–426.

31. Streanga V, Dimitriu AG, Iordache C, et al: Arrhythmic cardiomyopathy. Case report. Rev Med Chir Soc Med Nat Iasi 108:592, 2004.

32. Ozer S, Schaffer M: Sinus node reentrant tachycardia in a neonate. Pacing Clin Electrophysiol 24:1038, 2001.

33. Zhao BW, Pan M, Zhang SY, et al: Application of fetal echocardiography in detection of fetal arrhythmia and its clinical significance. Zhonghua Fu Chan Ke Za Zhi 39:365, 2004.

34. Nagashima M, Matsushima M, Ogawa A, et al: Cardiac arrhythmias in healthy children revealed by 24-hour ambulatory ECG monitoring. Pediatr Cardiol 8:103, 1987.

35. Respondek M, Wloch A, Kaczmarek P, et al: Diagnostic and perinatal management of fetal extrasystole. Pediatr Cardiol 18:361, 1997.

36. Etheridge SP, Judd VE, Yowell RL: Spontaneous resolution of ventricular arrhythmias with left bundle branch block morphology and abnormal endomyocardial biopsy. Pediatr Cardiol 20:364, 1999.

37. Lemler MS, Schaffer MS: Neonatal supraventricular tachycardia: predictors of successful treatment withdrawal. Am Heart J 133:130, 1997.

38. Wakai RT, Strasburger JF, Li Z, et al: Magnetocardiographic rhythm patterns at initiation and termination of fetal supraventricular tachycardia. Circulation 107:307, 2003.

39. Ko JK, Deal BJ, Strasburger JF, et al: Supraventricular tachycardia mechanisms and their age distribution in pediatric patients. Am J Cardiol 69:1028, 1992.

40. Kistler PM, Roberts-Thomson KC, Haqqani HM, et al: P wave morphology in focal atrial tachycardia: development of an algorithm to predict the anatomic site of origin. J Am Coll Cardiol 48:1010, 2006.

41. Paul T, Guccione P: New antiarrhythmic drugs in pediatric use: amiodarone. Pediatr Cardiol 15:132, 1994.

42. Mehta AV, Sanchez GR, Sacks EJ, et al: Ectopic automatic atrial tachycardia in children: clinical characteristics, management and follow-up. J Am Coll Cardiol 11:379, 1988.

43. von Bernuth G, Engelhardt W, Kramer HH, et al: Atrial automatic tachycardia in infancy and childhood. Eur Heart J 13:1410, 1992.

44. Klersy C, Chimienti M, Marangoni E, et al: Factors that predict spontaneous remission of ectopic atrial tachycardia. Eur Heart J 14:1654, 1993.

45. Salerno JC, Kertesz NJ, Friedman RA, et al: Clinical course of atrial ectopic tachycardia is age-dependent: results and treatment in children <3 or >or =3 years of age. J Am Coll Cardiol 43:438, 2004.

46. Walsh EP, Saul JP, Hulse JE, et al: Transcatheter ablation of ectopic atrial tachycardia in young patients using radiofrequency current [see comments]. Circulation 86:1138, 1992.

47. Kistler PM, Sanders P, Fynn SP, et al: Electrophysiological and electrocardiographic characteristics of focal atrial tachycardia originating from the pulmonary veins: acute and long-term outcomes of radiofrequency ablation. Circulation 108:1968, 2003.

48. Muller GI, Deal BJ, Strasburger JF, et al: Electrocardiographic features of atrial tachycardias after operation for congenital heart disease [published erratum appears in Am J Cardiol 71:375, 1993]. Am J Cardiol 71:122, 1993.

49. Triedman JK, Saul JP, Weindling SN, et al: Radiofrequency ablation of intra-atrial reentrant tachycardia after surgical palliation of congenital heart disease. Circulation 91:707, 1995.

50. Paul T, Windhagen-Mahnert B, Kriebel T, et al: Atrial reentrant tachycardia after surgery for congenital heart disease: endocardial mapping and radiofrequency catheter ablation using a novel, noncontact mapping system. Circulation 103:2266, 2001.

51. Kriebel T, Tebbenjohanns J, Janousek J, et al: Intraatrial reentrant tachycardias in patients after atrial switch procedures for d-transposition of the great arteries. Endocardial mapping and radiofrequency catheter ablation primarily targeting protected areas of atrial tissue within the systemic venous atrium. Z Kardiol 91:806, 2002.

52. Drago F, Silvetti MS, Grutter G, et al: Long term management of atrial arrhythmias in young patients with sick sinus syndrome undergoing early operation to correct congenital heart disease. Europace 8:488, 2006.

53. Seslar SP, Alexander ME, Berul CI, et al: Ablation of non-automatic focal atrial tachycardia in children and adults with congenital heart disease. J Cardiovasc Electrophysiol 17:359, 2006.

54. Krapp M, Kohl T, Simpson JM, et al: Review of diagnosis, treatment, and outcome of fetal atrial flutter compared with supraventricular tachycardia. Heart 89:913, 2003.

55. Jaeggi E, Fouron JC, Drblik SP: Fetal atrial flutter: diagnosis, clinical features, treatment, and outcome. J Pediatr 132:335, 1998.

56. Texter KM, Kertesz NJ, Friedman RA, et al: Atrial flutter in infants. J Am Coll Cardiol 48:1040, 2006.

57. Lubbers WJ, Losekoot TG, Anderson RH, et al: Paroxysmal supraventricular tachycardia in infancy and childhood. Eur J Cardiol 2:91, 1974.

58. Till J, Wren C: Atrial flutter in the fetus and young infant: an association with accessory connections. Br Heart J 67:80, 1992.

59. Martin TC, Hernandez A: Atrial flutter in infancy. J Pediatr 100:239, 1982.

60. Rowland TW, Mathew R, Chameides L, et al: Idiopathic atrial flutter in infancy: a review of eight cases. Pediatrics 61:52, 1978.

61. Chotivittayatarakorn P, Uerpairojkit B, Khonphatthanayothin A, et al: Atrial flutter in fetuses and early childhood: a report of eight cases. J Med Assoc Thai 84 (Suppl 1):S39, 2001.

62. Mendelsohn A, Dick MD, Serwer GA: Natural history of isolated atrial flutter in infancy. J Pediatr 119:386, 1991.

63. Lisowski LA, Verheijen PM, Benatar AA, et al: Atrial flutter in the perinatal age group: diagnosis, management and outcome. J Am Coll Cardiol 35:771, 2001.

64. Brockmeier K, Ulmer HE, Hessling G: Termination of atrial reentrant tachycardias by using transesophageal atrial pacing. J Electrocardiol 35(Suppl):159, 2002.

65. Batra AS, Hasan BS, Hurwitz RA: Efficacy of biphasic waveform compared to monophasic waveform for cardioversion of atrial flutter in pediatric patients. Pediatr Cardiol 27:230, 2006.

66. Garson A Jr , Bink-Boelkens M, Hesslein PS, et al: Atrial flutter in the young: a collaborative study of 380 cases. J Am Coll Cardiol 6:871, 1985.

67. Satomi K, Shimizu W, Suyama K, et al: Macroreentrant atrial flutter around a common atrioventricular canal in an infant with complicated congenital heart anomaly. Pacing Clin Electrophysiol 25:1530, 2002.

68. Suda K, Matsumura M, Hayashi Y: Myotonic dystrophy presenting as atrial flutter in childhood. Cardiol Young 14:89, 2004.

69. Liberthson RR, Colan SD: Multifocal or chaotic atrial rhythm: report of nine infants, delineation of clinical course and management, and review of the literature. Pediatr Cardiol 2:179, 1982.

70. Yeager SB, Hougen TJ, Levy AM: Sudden death in infants with chaotic atrial rhythm. Am J Dis Child 138:689, 1984.

71. Bradley DJ, Fischbach PS, Law IH, et al: The clinical course of multifocal atrial tachycardia in infants and children. J Am Coll Cardiol 38:401, 2001.

72. Bisset GSd, Seigel SF, Gaum WE, et al: Chaotic atrial tachycardia in childhood. Am Heart J 101:268, 1981.

73. Radford DJ, Izukawa T: Atrial fibrillation in children. Pediatrics 59:250, 1977.

74. Kirsh JA, Walsh EP, Triedman JK: Prevalence of and risk factors for atrial fibrillation and intra-atrial reentrant tachycardia among patients with congenital heart disease. Am J Cardiol 90:338, 2002.

75. Koul PB, Sussmane JB, Cunill-De Sautu B, et al: Atrial fibrillation associated with alcohol ingestion in adolescence: holiday heart in pediatrics. Pediatr Emerg Care 21:38, 2005.

76. Madhok A, Boxer R, Chowdhury D: Atrial fibrillation in an adolescent—the agony of ecstasy. Pediatr Emerg Care 19:348, 2003.

77. Bertram H, Paul T, Beyer F, et al: Familial idiopathic atrial fibrillation with bradyarrhythmia. Eur J Pediatr 155:7, 1996.

78. Crosson JE, Etheridge SP, Milstein S, et al: Therapeutic and diagnostic utility of adenosine during tachycardia evaluation in children. Am J Cardiol 74:155, 1994.

79. Paul T, Pfammatter JP: Adenosine: an effective and safe antiarrhythmic drug in pediatrics. Pediatr Cardiol 18:118, 1997.

80. Kaltman JR, Tanel RE, Shah MJ, et al: Induction of atrial fibrillation after the routine use of adenosine. Pediatr Emerg Care 22:113, 2006.

81. Scott O, Williams GJ, Fiddler GI: Results of 24 hour ambulatory monitoring of electrocardiogram in 131 healthy boys aged 10 to 13 years. Br Heart J 44:304, 1980.

82. Chabrak S, Ammar S, Ammar N, et al: Cardiac involvement in emery Dreifuss muscular dystrophy: a case report. Tunis Med 84:361, 2006.

83. El Menyar AA, Gendi SM: Persistent atrial standstill in noncompaction cardiomyopathy. Pediatr Cardiol 27:364, 2006.

84. Grant JW, Serwer GA, Armstrong BE, et al: Junctional tachycardia in infants and children after open heart surgery for congenital heart disease. Am J Cardiol 59:1216, 1987.

85. Walsh EP, Saul JP, Sholler GF, et al: Evaluation of a staged treatment protocol for rapid automatic junctional tachycardia after operation for congenital heart disease. J Am Coll Cardiol 29:1046, 1997.

86. Bash SE, Shah JJ, Albers WH, et al: Hypothermia for the treatment of postsurgical greatly accelerated junctional ectopic tachycardia. J Am Coll Cardiol 10:1095, 1987.

87. Perry JC, Knilans TK, Marlow D, et al: Intravenous amiodarone for life-threatening tachyarrhythmias in children and young adults. J Am Coll Cardiol 22:95, 1993.

88. Laird WP, Snyder CS, Kertesz NJ, et al: Use of intravenous amiodarone for postoperative junctional ectopic tachycardia in children. Pediatr Cardiol 24:133, 2003.

89. Bronzetti G, Formigari R, Giardini A, et al: Intravenous flecainide for the treatment of junctional ectopic tachycardia after surgery for congenital heart disease. Ann Thorac Surg 76:148, 2003; discussion 151.

90. Walker GM, McLeod K, Brown KL, et al: Extracorporeal life support as a treatment of supraventricular tachycardia in infants. Pediatr Crit Care Med 4:52, 2003.

91. Epstein MR, Saul JP, Fishberger SB, et al: Spontaneous accelerated junctional rhythm: an unusual but useful observation prior to radiofrequency catheter ablation for atrioventricular node reentrant tachycardia in young patients. Pacing Clin Electrophysiol 20:1654, 1997.

92. Villain E, Vetter VL, Garcia JM, et al: Evolving concepts in the management of congenital junctional ectopic tachycardia. A multicenter study [see comments]. Circulation 81:1544, 1990.

93. Sarubbi B, Musto B, Ducceschi V, et al: Congenital junctional ectopic tachycardia in children and adolescents: a 20 year experience based study. Heart 88:188, 2002.

94. Henneveld H, Hutter P, Bink-Boelkens M, et al: Junctional ectopic tachycardia evolving into complete heart block. Heart 80:627, 1998.

95. Yap SC, Hoomtje T, Sreeram N: Polymorphic ventricular tachycardia after use of intravenous amiodarone for postoperative junctional ectopic tachycardia. Int J Cardiol 76:245, 2000.

96. Paul T, Reimer A, Janousek J, et al: Efficacy and safety of propafenone in congenital junctional ectopic tachycardia. J Am Coll Cardiol 20:911, 1992.

97. Fukuhara H, Nakamura Y, Ohnishi T: Atrial pacing during radiofrequency ablation of junctional ectopic tachycardia—a useful technique for avoiding atrioventricular bloc. Jpn Circ J 65:242, 2001.

98. Bae EJ, Kang SJ, Noh CI, et al: A case of congenital junctional ectopic tachycardia: diagnosis and successful radiofrequency catheter ablation in infancy. Pacing Clin Electrophysiol 28:254, 2005.

99. Blaufox AD, Rhodes JF, Fishberger SB: Age related changes in dual AV nodal physiology. Pacing Clin Electrophysiol 23:477, 2000.

100. Samson RA, Deal BJ, Strasburger JF, et al: Comparison of transesophageal and intracardiac electrophysiologic studies in characterization of supraventricular tachycardia in pediatric patients. J Am Coll Cardiol 26:159, 1995.

101. Oh S, Choi YS, Sohn DW, et al: Differential diagnosis of slow/slow atrioventricular nodal reentrant tachycardia from atrioventricular reentrant tachycardia using concealed posteroseptal accessory pathway by 12-lead electrocardiography. Pacing Clin Electrophysiol 26:2296, 2003.

102. Lee PC, Chen SA, Chiang CE, et al: Clinical and electrophysiological characteristics in children with atrioventricular nodal reentrant tachycardia. Pediatr Cardiol 24:6, 2003.

103. Blurton DJ, Dubin AM, Chiesa NA, et al: Characterizing dual atrioventricular nodal physiology in pediatric patients with atrioventricular nodal reentrant tachycardia. J Cardiovasc Electrophysiol 17:638, 2006.

104. Kannankeril PJ, Fish FA: Sustained slow pathway conduction: superior to dual atrioventricular node physiology in young patients with atrioventricular nodal reentry tachycardia? Pacing Clin Electrophysiol 29:159, 2006.

105. Van Hare GF, Javitz H, Carmelli D, et al: Prospective assessment after pediatric cardiac ablation: demographics, medical profiles, and initial outcomes. J Cardiovasc Electrophysiol 15:759, 2004.

106. Collins KK, Dubin AM, Chiesa NA, et al: Cryoablation in pediatric atrioventricular nodal reentry: electrophysiologic effects on atrioventricular nodal conduction. Heart Rhythm 3:557, 2006.

107. Kirsh JA, Gross GJ, O'Connor S, et al: Transcatheter cryoablation of tachyarrhythmias in children: initial experience from an international registry. J Am Coll Cardiol 45:133, 2005.

108. Papez AL, Al-Ahdab M, Dick M II, et al: Transcatheter cryotherapy for the treatment of supraventricular tachyarrhythmias in children: a single center experience. J Interv Card Electrophysiol 15:191, 2006.

109. Kriebel T, Broistedt C, Kroll M, et al: Efficacy and safety of cryoenergy in the ablation of atrioventricular reentrant tachycardia substrates in children and adolescents. J Cardiovasc Electrophysiol 16:960, 2005.

110. Fishberger SB: Radiofrequency ablation of probable atrioventricular nodal reentrant tachycardia in children with documented supraventricular tachycardia without inducible tachycardia. Pacing Clin Electrophysiol 26:1679, 2003.

111. Epstein MR, Saul JP, Weindling SN, et al: Atrioventricular reciprocating tachycardia involving twin atrioventricular nodes in patients with complex congenital heart disease. J Cardiovasc Electrophysiol 12:671, 2001.

112. Jaeggi ET, Gilljam T, Bauersfeld U, et al: Electrocardiographic differentiation of typical atrioventricular node reentrant tachycardia from atrioventricular reciprocating tachycardia mediated by concealed accessory pathway in children. Am J Cardiol 91:1084, 2003.

113. Hager A, Zrenner B, Brodherr-Heberlein S, et al: Congenital and surgically acquired Wolff-Parkinson-White syndrome in patients with tricuspid atresia. J Thorac Cardiovasc Surg 130:48, 2005.

114. Moak JP, Moore HJ, Lee SW: Case report: spontaneous atriofascicular pathway automaticity simulating ventricular tachycardia. J Interv Card Electrophysiol 5:455, 2001.

115. Pappone C, Santinelli V, Rosanio S, et al: Usefulness of invasive electrophysiologic testing to stratify the risk of arrhythmic events in asymptomatic patients with Wolff-Parkinson-White pattern: results from a large prospective long-term follow-up study. J Am Coll Cardiol 41:239, 2003.

116. Cnota JF, Ross JE, Knilans TK, et al: Does intermittent accessory pathway block during slow sinus rhythm always imply a low risk for rapid AV conduction of preexcited atrial fibrillation? Cardiology 98:106, 2002.

117. Campbell RM, Strieper MJ, Frias PA, et al: Survey of current practice of pediatric electrophysiologists for asymptomatic Wolff-Parkinson-White syndrome. Pediatrics 111:e245, 2003.

118. Niksch AL, Dubin AM: Risk stratification in the asymptomatic child with Wolff-Parkinson-White syndrome. Curr Opin Cardiol 21:205, 2006.

119. Sarubbi B: The Wolff-Parkinson-White electrocardiogram pattern in athletes: how and when to evaluate the risk for dangerous arrhythmias. The opinion of the paediatric cardiologist. J Cardiovasc Med (Hagerstown) 7:271, 2006.

120. Trigo C, Paixao A, da Silva MN, et al: Permanent junctional reciprocating tachycardia: an incessant tachycardia in children. Rev Port Cardiol 22:767, 2003.

121. Ticho BS, Saul JP, Hulse JE, et al: Variable location of accessory pathways associated with the permanent form of junctional reciprocating tachycardia and confirmation with radiofrequency ablation. Am J Cardiol 70:1559, 1992.

122. Lindinger A, Heisel A, von Bernuth G, et al: Permanent junctional re-entry tachycardia. A multicentre long-term follow-up study in infants, children and young adults. Eur Heart J 19:936, 1998.

123. Semizel E, Ayabakan C, Ceviz N, et al: Permanent form of junctional reciprocating tachycardia and tachycardia-induced cardiomyopathy treated by catheter ablation: a case report. Turk J Pediatr 45:338, 2003.

124. Kriebel T, Kroll M, Paul T: Radiofrequency catheter ablation therapy in the young: current status. Expert Rev Cardiovasc Ther 1:421, 2003.

125. Gaita F, Montefusco A, Riccardi R, et al: Cryoenergy catheter ablation: a new technique for treatment of permanent junctional reciprocating tachycardia in children. J Cardiovasc Electrophysiol 15:263, 2004.

126. Drago F, Silvetti MS, Mazza A, et al: Permanent junctional reciprocating tachycardia in infants and children:

effectiveness of medical and non-medical treatment. Ital Heart J 2:456, 2001.

127. Karpawich PP, Gillette PC, Garson A Jr, et al: Congenital complete atrioventricular block: clinical and electrophysiologic predictors of need for pacemaker insertion. Am J Cardiol 48:1098, 1981.

128. Etheridge SP, Judd VE: Supraventricular tachycardia in infancy: evaluation, management, and follow-up. Arch Pediatr Adolesc Med 153:267, 1999.

129. Massin MM, Maeyns K, Withofs N, et al: Dependency of premature ventricular contractions on heart rate and circadian rhythms during childhood. Cardiology 93:70, 2000.

130. Scagliotti D, Deal BJ: Benign cardiac arrhythmias in the newborn. *In:* Riemenschneider TA, Allen HD, Gutgesell HP (eds): Heart Disease in Infants, Children, and Adolescents, 5th ed. Baltimore, Williams & Wilkins, 1995, p 628.

131. De Rosa G, Butera G, Chessa M, et al: Outcome of newborns with asymptomatic monomorphic ventricular arrhythmia. Arch Dis Child Fetal Neonatal Ed 91:F419, 2006.

132. Bricker JT, Traweek MS, Smith RT, et al: Exercise-related ventricular tachycardia in children. Am Heart J 112:186, 1986.

133. Jacobsen JR, Garson A Jr, Gillette PC, et al: Premature ventricular contractions in normal children. J Pediatr 92:36, 1978.

134. Rozanski JJ, Dimich I, Steinfeld L, et al: Maximal exercise stress testing in evaluation of arrhythmias in children: results and reproducibility. Am J Cardiol 43:951, 1979.

135. Attina DA, Mori F, Falorni PL, et al: Long-term follow-up in children without heart disease with ventricular premature beats. Eur Heart J 8(Suppl D):21, 1987.

136. Montague TJ, McPherson DD, MacKenzie BR, et al: Frequent ventricular ectopic activity without underlying cardiac disease: analysis of 45 subjects. Am J Cardiol 52:980, 1983.

137. Paul T, Marchal C, Garson A Jr: Ventricular couplets in the young: prognosis related to underlying substrate. Am Heart J 119:577, 1990.

138. Iwamoto M, Niimura I, Shibata T, et al: Long-term course and clinical characteristics of ventricular tachycardia detected in children by school-based heart disease screening. Circ J 69:273, 2005.

139. Gaum WE, Biancaniello T, Kaplan S: Accelerated ventricular rhythm in childhood. Am J Cardiol 43:162, 1979.

140. MacLellan-Tobert SG, Porter CJ: Accelerated idioventricular rhythm: a benign arrhythmia in childhood. Pediatrics 96:122, 1995.

141. Van Hare GF, Stanger P: Ventricular tachycardia and accelerated ventricular rhythm presenting in the first month of life [see comments]. Am J Cardiol 67:42, 1991.

142. Stevenson WG, Delacretaz E, Friedman PL, et al: Identification and ablation of macroreentrant ventricular tachycardia with the CARTO electroanatomical mapping system. Pacing Clin Electrophysiol 21:1448, 1998.

143. Lin D, Hsia HH, Gerstenfeld EP, et al: Idiopathic fascicular left ventricular tachycardia: linear ablation lesion strategy for noninducible or nonsustained tachycardia. Heart Rhythm 2:934, 2005.

144. O'Connor BK, Case CL, Sokoloski MC, et al: Radiofrequency catheter ablation of right ventricular outflow tachycardia in children and adolescents. J Am Coll Cardiol 27:869, 1996.

145. Gonzalez y Gonzalez MB, Will JC, Tuzcu V, et al: Idiopathic monomorphic ventricular tachycardia originating from the left aortic sinus cusp in children: endocardial mapping and radiofrequency catheter ablation. Z Kardiol 92:155, 2003.

146. Wong JA, Fishbein MC: Cardiac fibroma resulting in fatal ventricular arrhythmia. Circulation 101:E168, 2000.

147. Zeigler VL, Gillette PC, Crawford FA Jr, et al: New approaches to treatment of incessant ventricular tachycardia in the very young. J Am Coll Cardiol 16:681, 1990.

148. Towbin JA, Vatta M: The genetics of cardiac arrhythmias. Pacing Clin Electrophysiol 23:106, 2000.

149. Ching CK, Tan EC: Congenital long QT syndromes: clinical features, molecular genetics and genetic testing. Expert Rev Mol Diagn 6:365, 2006.

150. Roden DM, Viswanathan PC: Genetics of acquired long QT syndrome. J Clin Invest 115:2025, 2005.

151. Leenhardt A, Lucet V, Denjoy I, et al: Catecholaminergic polymorphic ventricular tachycardia in children. A 7-year follow-up of 21 patients. Circulation 91:1512, 1995.

152. De Rosa G, Delogu AB, Piastra M, et al: Catecholaminergic polymorphic ventricular tachycardia: successful emergency treatment with intravenous propranolol. Pediatr Emerg Care 20:175, 2004.

153. Francis J, Sankar V, Nair VK, et al: Catecholaminergic polymorphic ventricular tachycardia. Heart Rhythm 2:550, 2005.

154. Ormaetxe JM, Saez R, Arkotxa MF, et al: Catecholaminergic polymorphic ventricular tachycardia detected by an insertable loop recorder in a pediatric patient with exercise syncopal episodes. Pediatr Cardiol 25:693, 2004.

155. Priori SG, Napolitano C, Memmi M, et al: Clinical and molecular characterization of patients with catecholaminergic polymorphic ventricular tachycardia. Circulation 106:69, 2002.

156. Thomas NL, George CH, Lai FA: Role of ryanodine receptor mutations in cardiac pathology: more questions than answers? Biochem Soc Trans 34:913, 2006.

157. Smith AH, Fish FA, Kannankeril PJ: Andersen-Tawil syndrome. Indian Pacing Electrophysiol J 6:32, 2006.

158. Tsuboi M, Antzelevitch C: Cellular basis for electrocardiographic and arrhythmic manifestations of Andersen-Tawil syndrome (LQT7). Heart Rhythm 3:328, 2006.

159. Antzelevitch C, Brugada P, Borggrefe M, et al: Brugada syndrome: report of the second consensus conference. Heart Rhythm 2:429, 2005.

160. Juang JM, Huang SK: Brugada syndrome—an under-recognized electrical disease in patients with sudden cardiac death. Cardiology 101:157, 2004.

161. Suzuki H, Torigoe K, Numata O, et al: Infant case with a malignant form of Brugada syndrome. J Cardiovasc Electrophysiol 11:1277, 2000.

162. Mivelaz Y, Di Bernardo S, Pruvot E, et al: Brugada syndrome in childhood: a potential fatal arrhythmia not always recognised by paediatricians. A case report and review of the literature. Eur J Pediatr 165:507, 2006.

163. Smith BT, Rea TD, Eisenberg MS: Ventricular fibrillation in pediatric cardiac arrest. Acad Emerg Med 13:525, 2006.

164. Samson RA, Nadkarni VM, Meaney PA, et al: Outcomes of in-hospital ventricular fibrillation in children. N Engl J Med 354:2328, 2006.

165. Berg MD, Samson RA, Meyer RJ, et al: Pediatric defibrillation doses often fail to terminate prolonged

out-of-hospital ventricular fibrillation in children. Resuscitation 67:63, 2005.

166. Rodriguez-Nunez A, Lopez-Herce J, Garcia C, et al: Pediatric defibrillation after cardiac arrest: initial response and outcome. Crit Care 10:R113, 2006.

167. Roberts NK, Perloff JK, Kark RA: Cardiac conduction in the Kearns-Sayre syndrome (a neuromuscular disorder associated with progressive external ophthalmoplegia and pigmentary retinopathy). Report of 2 cases and review of 17 published cases. Am J Cardiol 44:1396, 1979.

168. Charles R, Holt S, Kay JM, et al: Myocardial ultrastructure and the development of atrioventricular block in Kearns-Sayre syndrome. Circulation 63:214, 1981.

169. Silvetti MS, Grutter G, Di Ciommo V, et al: Paroxysmal atrioventricular block in young patients. Pediatr Cardiol 25:506, 2004.

170. Lo R, Menzies DJ, Archer H, et al: Complete heart block due to lyme carditis. J Invasive Cardiol 15:367, 2003.

171. Zalzstein E, Maor R, Zucker N, et al: Advanced atrioventricular conduction block in acute rheumatic fever. Cardiol Young 13:506, 2003.

172. Jaeggi ET, Silverman ED, Yoo SJ, et al: Is immune-mediated complete fetal atrioventricular block reversible by transplacental dexamethasone therapy? Ultrasound Obstet Gynecol 23:602, 2004.

173. Jaeggi ET, Fouron JC, Silverman ED, et al: Transplacental fetal treatment improves the outcome of prenatally diagnosed complete atrioventricular block without structural heart disease. Circulation 110:1542, 2004.

174. Berg C, Geipel A, Kohl T, et al: Atrioventricular block detected in fetal life: associated anomalies and potential prognostic markers. Ultrasound Obstet Gynecol 26:4, 2005.

175. Jaeggi ET, Hamilton RM, Silverman ED, et al: Outcome of children with fetal, neonatal or childhood diagnosis of isolated congenital atrioventricular block. A single institution's experience of 30 years. J Am Coll Cardiol 39:130, 2002.

176. Michaelsson M, Jonzon A, Riesenfeld T: Isolated congenital complete atrioventricular block in adult life. A prospective study [see comments]. Circulation 92:442, 1995.

177. Smith RT. Pacemakers for bradycardia. In:Garson A Jr, Bricker JT, McNamara DG (eds): The Science and Practice of Pediatric Cardiology. Philadelphia, Lea and Febiger, 1990, p 2135.

178. Breur JM, Cate FE, Kapusta L, et al: Potential additional indicators for pacemaker requirement in isolated congenital atrioventricular block. Pediatr Cardiol 27:564, 2006.

INDEX

A

Aberrant intraventricular conduction, 413, 414*f*

Aberrant ventricular conduction perpetuation of, 473, 476

Ablation, 367

Accelerated atrial rhythm, 349, 634, 635*f*

Accelerated atrioventricular conduction, 499–500

Accelerated atrioventricular junctional rhythm, 390–391
AV dissociation caused by, 388*f*

Accelerated junctional rhythm, 694, 701–703

Accelerated ventricular rhythm, 184, 420, 428*f*, 429*f*, 709

Accessory pathways
electrophysiologic properties of, 494–495
radiofrequency ablation of, 504–505

Acquired immune deficiency syndrome, 294–296

Acyanotic lesions
anomolous origin of the left coronary artery, 680
aortic stenosis, 677–678
aortopulmonary window, 675–677
atrial septal defect, 671–674
AV defect, 671–674
l-transposition of the great vessels, 678–680
left ventricular noncompaction, 680
patent ductus arteriosus, 675–677
pulmonic stenosis, 677
ventricular septal defect, 674–675

Adam-Stokes disease, 116

Adenosine, 510
and ATP, 520
on AV reentrant tachycardia, 520*f*
and dipyridamole, administration of, 242
vagal stimulation and, 446–447

Adenosine triphosphate (ATP), 510

Adipose tissue, accumulation of, 55

Adrenal insufficiency, 290

Age
in ECG diagnosis of LVH, 54
heart disease with, 113
sinus rate decreases with, 328

Alternans
of conduction, 579–580
diagnosis of, 580
of T wave, U wave, and QT interval, 579

Alternans (*Continued*)
total, 580
type of, 582

Ambulatory electrocardiogram, 631
continuous record, 370*f*
to evaluate chest pain, 637
monitoring, 631
in normal subjects, 635
in patients with pacemakers, 627–628
with premature ventricular complexes, 632*f*
strips recorded during, 467*f*

Amiodarone, 515–518
accumulation and dissipation, 516
antiarrhythmia drug, 516
in treating automatic atrial tachycardia, 698–699

Amyloidosis, 292–293

Andersen-Tawil syndrome, 571, 712–713, 714*f*

Aneurysm, 145
results of aneurysmectomy, 146–147

Angina, 205, 232
stable, 210
variant, 144*f*, 217, 233–234, 640
arrhythmias and, 640
ECG monitoring with, 639–640
exercise-induced ST elevation and, 233–234
with recurrent angina, 155*f*

Angina pectoris, 232
during exercise test, 222, 232
pulmonale in, 35
torsade de pointes in, 443, 443*f*
unstable, 205, 211–213, 574
variant, 217
U wave in, 575

Antiarrhythmia drugs, 513–522
administration, 512
class I, 511
class II, 511
class III, 512
class IV, 512
class V, 512
classification, 512
clinical application, 512
depress normal automaticity, 512
evaluating efficacy of, 641–642
individual drugs, 520–522
proarrhythmic effects of, 512–513

Aorta, coarctation of, 51*f*

Aorticopulmonary septal defect, 313

Aortic stenosis, 677–678
with bifascicular block, 118
calcific, 470
congenital, 56
false-positive exercise in, 239*f*

Aortic valve disease, 118, 273
with left ventricular hypertrophy, 50*f*

Aortic valvular stenosis, sclerotic or calcific, 273

Arborization block, 172

Arm cables
with leg cables, reversal of, 590–592
reversal of left and right, 586

Arm leads, reversal of, 586

Arrhythmias
atrial, 245–246, 284–285, 697–701
and AV conduction, 281
primary, 698
refractory period, shortening, 526
and cardiogenic syncope, 637
common, 268–270
etiology of, 338–339
with hypocalcemia, 542
incidence of, 424–425
during ischemic episode, 217
occlusion, 155
during reperfusion, 184
after secundum-type atrial septal defects, 672
with tricuspid atresia, 688
ventricular. *See* Ventricular arrhythmias.

Arrhythmogenic right ventricular dysplasia (ARVD), 145–146, 279–280

Arsenic intoxication, chronic, 528–529

Artifacts, on ECG, 594–596
affects lead III, 595*f*
affects leads II and aVR, 595*f*

ARVD. *See* Arrhythmogenic right ventricular dysplasia (ARVD).

Ashman phenomenon, 379, 413

Asynchronous ventricular pacing, 606*f*

Atria, 580
and conduction fibers, sequence of activation of, 9*f*
and ectopic atrial pacemaker, abnormalities in, 40

Atrial abnormalities, 659
analysis of, 29
atrial depolarization, 31–32
correlation with precordial P wave mapping, 30
P wave abnormalities, 30
unicentric and multicentric pacemaker, 29–30
atrial enlargement, 41–42
atrial repolarization, 42–43
biatrial enlargement, 659
diagnostic criteria, 40
left atrial abnormality, 36, 40
clinical and anatomic correlation, 38
echocardiographic correlations, 40
leftward shift of P wave axis, 40
wide and notched P waves, 38–40
left atrial enlargement, 659, 660*f*
right atrial abnormalities, 35–36

Printed in the United States
By Bookmasters